ɔital – ɔ

Plea

PSYCHO-ONCOLOGY

Psycho-Oncology

SECOND EDITION

EDITED BY

Jimmie C. Holland, M.D.

Wayne E. Chapman Chair in Psychiatric Oncology, Department of Psychiatry and Behavioral Sciences, Memorial Sloan-Kettering Cancer Center

Professor, Department of Psychiatry, Weill Medical College of Cornell University, New York, New York

William S. Breitbart, M.D.

Chief, Psychiatry Service, and Vice-Chairman, Department of Psychiatry and Behavioral Sciences, Memorial Sloan-Kettering Cancer Center

Professor of Clinical Psychiatry, Weill Medical College of Cornell University, New York, New York

Paul B. Jacobsen, Ph.D.

Chair, Department of Health Outcomes and Behavior, Moffitt Cancer Center

Professor, Department of Psychology, University of South Florida, Tampa, Florida

Marguerite S. Lederberg, M.D.

Attending Psychiatrist, Department of Psychiatry and Behavioral Sciences, Memorial Sloan-Kettering Cancer Center

Professor of Clinical Psychiatry, Weill Medical College of Cornell University, New York, New York

Matthew J. Loscalzo, M.S.W.

Liliane Elkins Professor in Supportive Care Programs

Administrative Director, Sheri & Les Biller Patient and Family Resource Center

Executive Director, Department of Supportive Care Medicine

Professor, Department of Population Sciences, City of Hope, Duarte

Ruth McCorkle, Ph.D., R.N., F.A.A.N.

Florence Schorske Wald Professor, Yale School of Nursing

Professor, Department of Epidemiology and Public Health, School of Medicine

Program Leader, Population Sciences and Cancer Control, Yale Cancer Center

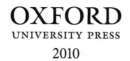

OXFORD
UNIVERSITY PRESS
2010

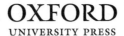

OXFORD
UNIVERSITY PRESS

Oxford University Press, Inc., publishes works that further
Oxford University's objective of excellence
in research, scholarship, and education.

Oxford New York
Auckland Cape Town Dar es Salaam Hong Kong Karachi
Kuala Lumpur Madrid Melbourne Mexico City Nairobi
New Delhi Shanghai Taipei Toronto

With offices in
Argentina Austria Brazil Chile Czech Republic France Greece
Guatemala Hungary Italy Japan Poland Portugal Singapore
South Korea Switzerland Thailand Turkey Ukraine Vietnam

Published by Oxford University Press, Inc.
198 Madison Avenue, New York, New York 10016
www.oup.com

Library of Congress Cataloging-in-Publication Data

Psycho-oncology / edited by Jimmie C. Holland ... [et al.]. — 2nd ed.
p. ; cm.
Includes bibliographical references and index.
ISBN 978-0-19-536743-0
1. Cancer—Psychological aspects.   2. Cancer—Patients—Mental health.
I. Holland, Jimmie C.
[DNLM: 1. Neoplasms—psychology.   2. Neoplasms—complications.
3. Neoplasms—therapy.   QZ 200 P9743 2010]
RC262.P7825 2010
616.99′40019—dc22
2009015792

3 5 7 9 8 6 4 2
Printed in the United States of America
on acid-free paper

PREFACE

It has been my honor and privilege to write the preface for the two prior Oxford Psycho-Oncology texts—the *Handbook of Psychooncology*, in 1989, which I edited with Julia Rowland, and the textbook, *Psycho-Oncology*, in 1998, with William Breitbart, Paul Jacobsen, Marguerite Lederberg, Matthew Loscalzo, Mary Jane Massie and Ruth McCorkle. This Second Edition of *Psycho-Oncology*, for publication in 2010, looks at the field over its 35 year development, since its beginning in the mid 1970s when cancer came "out of the closet" and the stigma diminished so that patients knew their diagnosis and could talk with us about their illness. Through the 1980s, research of necessity addressed the absence of reliable and valid instruments to measure cancer patient's subjective symptoms (e.g., pain, anxiety, depression, delirium), previously considered unreliable. Armed with reliable and valid instruments, research in the 1990s focused on randomized controlled trials of interventions from which changes in outcomes, particularly quality of life, were accurately measured.

The first 20 years of research has opened new horizons for clinical care: the recognition that there now exist a sufficiently strong evidence base to mandate that the psychosocial domain must be integrated into routine cancer care. In fact, the report of the US Institute of Medicine, National Academies of Science states that "quality cancer care today has a new standard that demands cancer care for the whole patient." (See Chapter 97).

Parallel to this research and scientific stream of work has been increasing attention to an equally important arena: impacting health policy to assure that evidence-based findings are converted to clinical interventions to help patients and their families cope with cancer. Psycho-Oncology in the present decade is seeking to address these crucial issues across the globe. The International Psycho-Oncology Society (IPOS) has a key international role, in relationship with the UICC and soon, the WHO, to bring global attention to the need for attention to the "human" side of cancer care. The Federation of National Psycho-Oncology Societies, established by IPOS, now includes over 30 countries which address the unique cultural issues in each country. The IPOS core curriculum is available free online (www.ipos-society.org) in nine languages with outreach efforts to address health disparities, especially in emerging and developing countries. Pocket handbooks for oncology clinicians are now available for quick reference in the clinic. The development of standards and clinical practice guidelines for psychosocial care are providing a new standard of quality care in several countries. The first guidelines in the United States for psychosocial care, through the National Cancer Centers Network, addressed the attitudinal barrier of stigma related to psychosocial care by suggesting use of the word "distress" as an encompassing word that avoided labeling as "psychiatric or psychological," which is a barrier to both oncology staff and patients. The fact that oncologists can now self-audit their practices, using valid quality indicators of psychosocial care is a major advance that will allow "report cards" to be given for quality of psychosocial care, even in community practices where most cancer care is given.

The guidelines have supported the routine screening of all new patients for distress level and psychosocial needs. This innovation begins to remove the barrier of psychosocial care being seen as something separate and apart from medical care. While there is a downside to more electronic communication (at the expense of face to face), there is a new opportunity for providing support for patients through new media, such as touch screens and chat rooms, which clearly can make free psychosocial information and interaction available.

Our work in cancer over the 35 years in cancer parallels the centuries-old efforts within medical education to make care more "patient-centered" (the name for this has changed over time, but not the core issues). And the "human" needs of people who are ill have not changed—they have remained identical through the centuries. Unfortunately, the barriers to delivery of truly patient-centered care have also changed very little. Harris reviewed classics from the *JAMA* archives that have contributed to "the science of care" (*JAMA*, 2009;301:1710–12). Adolf Meyer noted early in the twentieth century the need for a framework for medical care that would consider the patient as a "whole person" (*JAMA*, 1915;65:861–863). Peabody in 1927 wrote about the importance of knowing the patient as a person, noting: "One of the essential qualities of the clinician is interest in humanity, for the secret of the care of the patient is in caring for the patient" (*JAMA*, 1927;88:877–882). Engel continued the tradition by defining the biopsychosocial model (*NEJM*, 1977;140:1514–1518). Lewis Thomas brought this crucial issue to cancer care, lamenting in the foreword of the first *Handbook* in 1989, that "cancer treatment is extremely technical…given by professionals working at a rather impersonal distance from the patient as an individual—who have for too long overlooked or ignored psychological factors. He saw psycho-Oncology as "an emerging respectable field…improving the lot of cancer patients as to make these new (psycho-oncology) professionals indispensable."

This Second Edition of *Psycho-Oncology* continues in the tradition of these pioneers—presenting the many ways in which patients' experience of illness can be understood and improved: the core of all psychosocial interventions, noted by Peabody noted 1927: the need of patients to feel that those providing their care are interested in them as a person. One recent patient of mine, 80 years later, said it well: "I need to know that someone taking care of me *cares* about me."

I wish to thank the co-editors of the Second Edition, Drs. Breitbart, Jacobsen, Lederberg, Loscalzo, and McCorkle for their superb work. We thank Dr. Sonia Ancoli-Israel for the figure "Actigraph of breast cancer patient before and after treatment." I thank Marilla Owens at the American Psychosocial Oncology Society (APOS) for coordinating editors and authors. The privilege of seeing the development of psycho-oncology from its beginning and to have been a loving historian of the field has been quite unique. I am grateful for having had that role. The groundwork is laid for exponential progress in coming years in research and in the policy arena. We are closer to our goal of assuring that patients around the world experience their cancer care as directed toward them as a "whole person"; that their psychosocial needs are viewed as an integral part of their cancer care. There is much that remains to be done, however, by the next generation of psycho-oncologists. The Second Edition provides a strong base from which to move with confidence into the second decade of the twenty-first century.

Jimmie C. Holland, M.D.
June 26, 2009
New York, NY

PREFACE TO THE FIRST EDITION

Nearly a decade ago, Julia Rowland, psychologist, and I edited the *Handbook of psychooncology*. Written in the late eighties, its seven hundred forty-nine pages easily covered the available information about the psychological issues in the care of patients with cancer. The rationale for the edited volume was to provide a single resource in which the widely scattered information could be found; the corollary was that the book be written in nonjargon language that would make it readable and useful to all disciplines working in oncology, from the classical clinical disciplines to the mental health professionals who were increasingly being invited to join cancer centers and participate in multidisciplinary research teams. At that time, it was feasible to develop the *Handbook* by asking only individuals from our own cancer center to participate. They based their reviews on the sparse but growing empirical research and their experiences with patients. The Preface noted that the authors had learned from the "true experts" our patients with cancer and their families, whose courage in the face of illness taught us many lessons about living and dying. While we proudly touted the presence of a new subspecialty on the scene, psycho-oncology, it was in fact in its infancy. Almost 10 years later, it is reassuring to look back and see that the field did continue to grow and that it has made and continues to make significant contributions to both patient care and research.

Lewis Thomas, in the Foreword to that handbook, observed that the time was right for such a volume. He noted:

The clinical oncologists of all stripes have, for too long, overlooked or ignored the psychological factors that may, for all we know at present, play a surprisingly large role in individual susceptibility to neoplasia. They are certainly influential in affecting the course of treatment, the adaptation to the illness, and hence, in some ways, not all of which are yet understood, affect the outcome of treatment.

He felt that intensive cancer treatment had

come to be an extremely technical undertaking,…involving the strenuous efforts of highly specialized professionals, each taking his or her responsibility for a share of the patient's problem, but sometimes working at a rather impersonal distance from the patient as an individual. To many patients, stunned by the diagnosis, suffering numerous losses and discomforts, moved from place to place for one procedure after another, the experience is bewildering and frightening; at worst, it is like being trapped in the workings of a huge piece of complicated machinery.…

Within less than a decade, the term psycho-oncology, viewed at first with deep suspicion by most oncologists, has at last emerged as a respectable field for both application and research. In my own view, having passed through both stages as a skeptical clinician and administrator, the appearance on the scene of psychiatrists and experimental psychologists has so vastly improved the lot of cancer patients as to make these new professionals indispensable.

This present volume describes the many ways in which mental health professionals have indeed contributed to improving the lot of the cancer patient. The parts of the book reveal the whole new areas that have come under psycho-oncology's purview. First, there is a large section of the book devoted to the present understanding of psychological, social, and behavioral factors that contribute to cancer risk and survival. Changing habits and behaviors to reduce the toll of preventable cancer deaths has come very much into the domain of behavioral psycho-oncology. Smoking cessation is reviewed by Gritz and colleagues; sun exposure by Berwick. Research showing the impact of social class and socioeconomic factors in altering risk is also reviewed, by Balfour and Kaplan. Social ties, coping, treatment adherence, are all critiqued by experts as to their role in risk and survival. Fox provides a critical review of such research, fulfilling his long-respected role of monitor of the quality of the science in this area. Two chapters explore the brain-endocrine-immune connections and how they may contribute to risk and survival.

Advances in cancer treatment bring new psychological issues. Several parts of the book are devoted to the vastly extended "worried well" population emerging from the cancer information today—people who are physically healthy but who bear the knowledge of a positive tumor marker (without clinical signs of disease) or those who have a strong family history of a particular cancer and who must deal with whether to pursue gene testing or not. These individuals vary in their responses—from denial leading to refusal to follow surveillance guidelines to anxiety levels causing almost constant self-monitoring and almost immobilizing anxiety. The psychological issues raised are clinically very important to assure appropriate screening behaviors. Counseling with genetic testing, and attention to its psychological, social, and ethical consequences, is a critical part of the national agenda for dealing with this new issue.

Ten years has led to a widely expanded discussion of interventions. Many controlled trials have shown efficacy for psychosocial interventions which represent a far wider array of ways to improve patient's quality of life, using psychological, psychoeducational, and behavioral methods. The management of psychiatric disorders complicating cancer is greatly enhanced by the array of psychopharmacological agents available to relieve distressing psychological symptoms, and many of these agents have been found useful in the control of the pain, nausea and vomiting, and fatigue that often accompany cancer. Group therapies have become familiar in most settings. Nontraditional therapies, such as art, meditation, and alternative and complementary therapies, have come into greater use in traditional medical settings. Greater appreciation of spiritual and religious beliefs and the importance of including spiritual care in total patient care has occurred, with greater collaboration and dialogue with members of the clergy.

The ethical issues of cancer care have received far more attention. First, this related to clinical trials and the ethics of informed consent, as outlined by Dubler and Post. The more recent agenda, coming out of the public debate about physician-assisted suicide, has been devoted to end-of-life and palliative care; Emanuel provides a critique of this area. Psycho-oncology is particularly attuned to the complexity of issues that are intertwined with psychology and ethics, as outlined by Lederberg. Special issues in care of the family of the cancer patient, the psychological care of children with cancer, and patients with special needs, such as the elderly and underserved populations, are presented and discussed.

Last, the research agenda for psycho-oncology has become more central to oncology in general as the outcome measures for treatments have come to include not only length of survival but quality of life as well. The valid measurement of quality of life, a multidimensional construct that involves subjective evaluation of the domains of living that are important to people, has become a major research endeavor. Methods are being developed and refined to relate scores to clinical situations and treatment decisions. Cella provides a useful overview of the status of this research area. Ingham and Portenoy outline research methods in evaluation of pain and symptoms common in palliative care, providing a basis for clinical trials of interventions.

In 1997, it is encouraging that far greater attention is being given to patient's own reports of their symptoms and their quality of life. Dr. Thomas, who died in 1995, would be pleased that psycho-oncology has indeed achieved a "respectable place in application and research" in cancer. Care is more patient-centered, less fragmented, and the treatment teams more commonly include a mental health professional. Almost all cancer centers have an identified psycho-oncology unit, although often small, with a staff responsible for identifying and treating patients having trouble coping with illness and treatment. The larger units are engaged in training and in conducting psychosocial and behavioral research as well. In the late nineties, an exciting new agenda for psycho-oncology is being developed, based on advances in oncology that have themselves led to new forms of psychological and social problems. Fortunately, the field itself has generated a body of solid research that has defined clinical problems more clearly, has provided empirical data on interventions and their efficacy, and has devised research methods that include quality of life as a bona fide treatment goal.

I thank the co-editors who have joined me in this endeavor, Drs. Breitbart, Jacobsen, Lederberg, Loscalzo, Massie, and McCorkle. Each has done excellent editorial work. They represent the major disciplines working in psycho-oncology today. The authors of the chapters have been outstanding in their willingness to write, and sometimes revise, their contributions to fit them into the whole. Jeff House at Oxford University Press has provided the guidance to assure that the effort came to fruition And last, and most important, my co-editors join me in giving much thanks to Ivelisse Belardo and Wanda Cintron, who truly made it possible to compile the chapters and collate the large amount of information. We are saddened by the untimely death of Ms. Cintron in November 1996. It is a source of great sadness that she is not here to share in the pleasure of the publication of the book. This Preface is dedicated to her memory, with great appreciation for her contributions to this volume and to our lives and our work.

J.C.H.
April, 1997
New York, NY.

CONTENTS

III SCREENING FOR CANCER IN NORMAL AND AT-RISK POPULATIONS

PAUL B. JACOBSEN, ED

IV SCREENING AND TESTING FOR GENETIC SUSCEPTIBILITY TO CANCER

PAUL B. JACOBSEN, ED

V PSYCHOLOGICAL ISSUES RELATED TO SITE OF CANCER

RUTH McCORKLE, ED

VI MANAGEMENT OF SPECIFIC SYMPTOMS

WILLIAM S. BREITBART, ED

IX INTERVENTIONS

MATTHEW J. LOSCALZO, ED

XIV ETHICAL ISSUES

MARGUERITE S. LEDERBERG, ED

XV THE FUTURE OF PSYCHO-ONCOLOGY RESEARCH

PAUL B. JACOBSEN, ED

XVI INTERNATIONAL PSYCHO-ONCOLOGY

JIMMIE C. HOLLAND, ED

XVII POLICY ISSUES

JIMMIE C. HOLLAND, ED

CONTRIBUTORS

Tim A. Ahles, Ph.D.   Member, Department of Psychiatry and Behavioral Sciences, and Director, Neurocognitive Research Laboratory, New York, NY

Yesne Alici, M.D.   Attending Psychiatrist, Geriatrics Services Unit, Central Regional Hospital, New Butner, NC

Lia Amakawa, M.A.   Research Associate, Department of Psychiatry and Behavioral Sciences, Memorial Sloan-Kettering Cancer Center, New York, NY

Barbara L. Andersen, Ph.D.   Professor, Department of Psychology and Comprehensive Cancer Center and Solove Research Institute, The Ohio State University, Columbus, OH

Michael A. Andrykowski, Ph.D.   University of Kentucky Provost's Distinguished Service Professor, Department of Behavioral Science, University of Kentucky College of Medicine, Lexington, KY

Terry A. Badger, Ph.D., PMHCNS-BC, F.A.A.N.   Professor and Division Director, Systems College of Nursing, The University of Arizona, Tucson, AZ

Neil J. Berman, D.Phil.   Former Executive Director, Canadian Strategy for Cancer Control, Vancouver, British Columbia, Canada

Marianne Berwick, Ph.D.   Professor and Chief, Division of Epidemiology, and Associate Director-CRTC, and Co-Leader – Population Health Sciences, Cancer Health Disparities and Cancer Control Program, University of New Mexico, Albuquerque, NM

Kelly A. Biegler, Ph.D.   Postdoctoral Fellow, Department of Medicine, University of California–Irvine, Irvine, CA

Joan R. Bloom, Ph.D.   Professor, Department of Health Policy and Management, School of Public Health, University of California, Berkeley, CA

Thomas H. Brandon, Ph.D.   Professor, Department of Psychology and Department of Interdisciplinary Oncology, University of South Florida and Director, Tobacco Research and Intervention Program, H. Lee Moffitt Cancer Center and Research Institute, Tampa, FL

Ilana M. Braun, M.D.   Director, Cancer-Related Fatigue Clinic, Massachusetts General Hospital, Boston, MA

William S. Breitbart, M.D.   Chief, Psychiatry Service, Vice-Chairman, Department of Psychiatry and Behavioral Sciences, Memorial Sloan-Kettering Cancer Center, and Professor of Clinical Psychiatry, Weill Medical College of Cornell University, New York, NY

Brittany M. Brothers, Ph.D.   Program Director, The Ohio State University LIVESTRONG Survivorship Center of Excellence, Comprehensive Cancer Center and Solove Research Institute, The Ohio State University, Columbus, OH

Richard F. Brown, Ph.D.   Assistant Professor, Social and Behavioral Health, Virginia Commonwealth University School of Medicine, Richmond, VA

Julia A. Bucher, Ph.D., R.N. Associate Professor, Department of Nursing, York College of PA, York, PA

Barry D. Bultz, Ph.D. Director, Department of Psychosocial Resources, Tom Baker Cancer Centre, and Adjunct Professor and Chief, Division of Psychosocial Oncology, Department of Oncology, Faculty of Medicine, University of Calgary, Calgary, Alberta, Canada

Phyllis Butow, Ph.D., M.P.H. Professor, Centre for Medical Psychology and Evidence-based Medicine (CeMPED), School of Psychology, University of Sydney, Sydney, NSW, Australia

Carma L. Bylund, Ph.D. Assistant Attending Psychologist, Psychiatry and Behavioral Sciences, Memorial Sloan-Kettering Cancer Center, New York, NY

Andrea L. Canada, Ph.D. Assistant Professor, Department of Behavioral Sciences, Rush University Medical Center, Chicago, IL

Linda E. Carlson, Ph.D. Associate Professor, Department of Oncology, University of Calgary, Calgary, Alberta, Canada

Jeanne Carter, Ph.D. Assistant Attending Psychologist, Department of Psychiatry and Behavioral Sciences, Memorial Sloan-Kettering Cancer Center, New York, NY

Danielle R. Casden, Ph.D. Licensed Clinical Psychologist, Education and Psychosocial Program Development Manager, Moores University of California San Diego Cancer Center, La Jolla, CA

Juskaran S. Chadha, Undergraduate Student College of Arts and Sciences, New York University, New York, NY

Karen L. Clark, M.S. Program Manager, Sheri & Les Biller Patient and Family Resource Center, Department of Supportive Care Medicine, City of Hope, Duarte, CA

Lorenzo Cohen, Ph.D. Professor, Departments of Behavioral Science and General Oncology, and Director, Integrative Medicine Program, The University of Texas M. D. Anderson Cancer Center, Houston, TX

Yvette Colón, Ph.D., A.C.S.W., B.C.D. Director of Education and Support, American Pain Foundation, Baltimore, MD

Stephen R. Connor, Ph.D. Senior Executive, Worldwide Palliative Care Alliance, London, UK; Senior Research and International Consultant, National Hospice and Palliative Care Organization (US), Alexandria, VA; and Palliative Care Consultant, Open Society Institute and Soros Foundations Network, New York, NY

Mary E. Cooley, Ph.D., R.N. Nurse Scientist, Phyllis F. Cantor Center; Research in Nursing and Patient Care, Dana Farber Cancer Center; and Assistant Professor, University of Massachusetts-Boston, College of Nursing and Health Sciences, Boston, MA

Denise D. Correa, Ph.D., ABPP-CN Assistant Attending, Board Certified in Clinical Neuropsychology, Department of Neurology, Memorial Sloan-Kettering Cancer Center, New York, NY

Kerry S. Courneya, Ph.D. Professor and Canada Research Chair in Physical Activity and Cancer, and Faculty of Physical Education and Recreation, University of Alberta, Edmonton, Alberta

Liliana De Lima, M.S., M.H.A. Executive Director, International Association for Hospice and Palliative Care (IAHPC), Houston, TX

Wendy Demark-Wahnefried, Ph.D., R.D. Professor of Behavioral Science, The University of Texas M. D. Anderson Cancer Center, Houston, TX

Gerald M. Devins, Ph.D. Head, Psychosocial Oncology and Palliative Care Research, Princess Margaret Hospital; Senior Scientist, Division of Psychosocial Oncology and Palliative Care, Ontario Cancer Institute; and Professor of Psychiatry, Department of Psychosocial Oncology and Palliative Care, University of Toronto, Toronto, Ontario, Canada

Joel E. Dimsdale, M.D. Distinguished Professor of Psychiatry, Department of Psychiatry, University of California, San Diego School of Medicine, La Jolla, CA

Joanna S. Dognin, Psy.D.   Assistant Professor/Behavioral Science Faculty, Department of Family and Social Medicine, Montefiore Medical Center, Albert Einstein College of Medicine, Bronx, NY

Lucy A. Epstein, M.D.   Attending Psychiatrist, Psychiatric Consultation-Liaison Service, New York Presbyterian Hospital, and Assistant Professor of Clinical Psychiatry, Columbia University, New York, NY

Andrea Farkas Patenaude, Ph.D.   Director of Psycho-Oncology Research, Division of Pediatric Oncology, Dana-Farber Cancer Institute, and Associate Professor, Department of Psychology, Harvard Medical School, Boston, MA

Christopher A. Fausel, Pharm.D., B.C.P.S., B.C.O.P.   Clinical Director, Oncology Pharmacy Services, Indiana University Simon Cancer Center, Indianapolis, IN

Sara Fernandes-Taylor, Doctoral Candidate   Department of Health Services and Policy Analysis, University of California, Berkeley, CA

Betty Ferrell, Ph.D., M.A., F.A.A.N., F.H.P.N.   Research Scientist, Division of Nursing Research and Education, Department of Population Sciences, City of Hope National Medical Center, Duarte, CA

Richard Fielding, Ph.D., F.F.P.H.   Professor of Medical Psychology and Public Health, and Head, Behavioural Sciences Unit and Centre for Psychochooncology Research and Training, School of Public Health, The University of Hong Kong, Hong Kong, HKSAR, China

Betsy L. Fife, Ph.D., R.N.   Senior Research Scientist, Indiana University School of Nursing, Indiana University Simon Cancer Center, Indianapolis, IN

Margaret I. Fitch, Ph.D., R.N.   Head, Oncology Nursing/Co-Director, Patient and Family Support Program, Odette Cancer Centre, Sunnybrook Health Sciences Centre, Toronto, Ontario, Canada

George Fitchett, Ph.D.   Associate Professor, Department of Religion, Health and Human Values, Rush University Medical Center, Chicago, IL

Marian L. Fitzgibbon, Ph.D.   Professor and Chief, Section of Health Promotion Research, Department of Medicine, University of Illinois at Chicago, and Associate Director, Center for Management of Complex Chronic Care (CMC³), Jesse Brown Veterans Affairs Medical Center, Chicago, IL

Stewart B. Fleishman, M.D.   Director, Cancer Supportive Services, Continuum Cancer Centers of New York: Beth Israel and St. Luke's-Roosevelt, and Associate Chief Medical Officer, Continuum Hospice Care, New York, NY

Kilah Fox, Research Intern   Phyllis F. Cantor Center, Research in Nursing and Patient Care, Dana Farber Cancer Center, Boston, MA

Moshe Frenkel, M.D.   Medical Director, Department of General Oncology, The University of Texas M. D. Anderson Cancer Center, Houston, TX

Patricia A. Ganz, M.D.   Professor, UCLA Schools of Medicine and Public Health, Division of Cancer Prevention and Control Research, Jonsson Comprehensive Cancer Center, Los Angeles, CA

Linda Ganzini, M.D., M.P.H.   Director of Health Services Research and Development, Portland Veterans Affairs Medical Center, Portland, OR

M. Kay Garcia, Dr.P.H., M.S.N., R.N., L.Ac.   Clinical Nurse Specialist/Acupuncturist, Integrative Medicine Program, The University of Texas M. D. Anderson Cancer Center, Houston, TX

Barbara A. Given, Ph.D., R.N., F.A.A.N.   University Distinguished Professor, Associate Dean for Research and Doctoral Program, College of Nursing, Michigan State University, East Lansing, MI

Charles W. Given, Ph.D.   Professor, Department of Family Medicine/College of Human Medicine, Michigan State University, East Lansing, MI

Mitch Golant, Ph.D.   Senior Vice President Research and Training, Department of Research and Training, The Wellness Community, Washington, DC

Alejandro González-Restrepo, M.D.   Staff Psychiatrist, Department of Psychiatry, Saint Francis Hospital and Medical Center, Hartford, CT

Carolyn C. Gotay, Ph.D.   Professor, Canadian Cancer Society Chair in Cancer Primary Prevention, School of Population and Public Health, and Faculty of Medicine, University of British Columbia, Vancouver, Canada

Luigi Grassi, M.D.   Professor and Chair of Psychiatry, Department of Medical Disciplines of Communication and Behavior, Section of Psychiatry, University of Ferrara, Ferrara, Italy

Erin E. Hahn, M.P.H.   Program Coordinator, UCLA-LIVESTRONG Survivorship Center of Excellence, Division of Cancer Prevention and Control Research, Jonsson Comprehensive Cancer Center at UCLA, Los Angeles, CA

Sarah Hales, M.D.   Staff Psychiatrist, Psychosocial Oncology and Palliative Care, Princess Margaret Hospital, and Lecturer, University of Toronto, Toronto, Ontario, Canada

Sheri J. Hartman, Ph.D.   Postdoctoral Fellow, Department of Psychiatry and Human Behavior, Centers for Behavioral and Preventive Medicine, The Miriam Hospital and W. Alpert Medical School of Brown University, Providence, RI

Jennifer Hay, Ph.D.   Assistant Attending Psychologist, Department of Psychiatry and Behavioral Sciences, Memorial Sloan-Kettering Cancer Center, New York, NY

Vicki S. Helgeson, Ph.D.   Professor, Psychology Department, Carnegie Mellon University, Pittsburgh, PA

Barb Henry, APRN-BC, M.S.N.   Psychiatric Nurse Practitioner, University of Cincinnati Central Clinic and Psycho-Oncology Associates, LLC, Cincinnati, OH

Michael A. Hoge, Ph.D.   Professor of Psychology (in Psychiatry), Department of Psychiatry, Yale School of Medicine, New Haven, CT

Jimmie C. Holland, M.D.   Wayne E. Chapman Chair in Psychiatric Oncology, Department of Psychiatry and Behavioral Sciences, Memorial Sloan-Kettering Cancer Center, and Professor, Department of Psychiatry, Weill Medical College of Cornell University, New York, NY

Penelope Hopwood, M.D. F.R.C.Psych.   Visiting Professor of Psycho-Oncology, ICR Clinical Trials and Statistics Unit (Section of Clinical Trials), The Institute of Cancer Research, Sutton, Surrey, UK, and Honorary Professor of Pscyho-Oncology, School of Health, Sport and Rehabilitation Sciences, University of Salford, Salford, UK

Jonathan C. Irish, M.D., M.Sc., F.R.C.S.C., F.A.C.S.   Chief, Department of Surgical Oncology; Professor, Otolaryngology-Head and Neck Surgery, Department of Otolaryngology/Surgical Oncology, Princess Margaret Hospital, University of Toronto, Toronto, Ontario, Canada

Scott A. Irwin, M.D., Ph.D.   Director, Palliative Care Psychiatry Programs, The Institute for Palliative Medicine at San Diego Hospice, and Clinical Professor of Psychiatry, University of California, San Diego, CA

Paul B. Jacobsen, Ph.D.   Chair, Department of Health Outcomes and Behavior, Moffitt Cancer Center, and Professor, Department of Psychology, University of South Florida, Tampa, FL

Christoffer Johansen, M.D., Ph.D., D.MSc   Head, Department of Psychosocial Cancer Research, Institute of Cancer Epidemiology, The Danish Cancer Society, Copenhagen, Denmark, and Professor, The National Centre for Cancer Rehabilitation Research, Institute of Public Health, Southern Danish University, Odense, Denmark

Maria Kangas, Ph.D.   Senior Lecturer, Centre for Emotional Health, Department of Psychology, Macquarie University, Sydney, NSW, Australia

Aviva M. Katz, B.A.   Research Assistant, Department of Psychiatry and Behavioral Sciences, Memorial Sloan-Kettering Cancer Center, New York, NY

Anne E. Kazak, Ph.D., A.B.P.P.   Professor and Director, Psychology Research Department of Pediatrics, University of Pennsylvania School of Medicine; Deputy Director, Behavioral Health Center; and Director, Department of Psychology, The Children's Hospital of Philadelphia, Philadelphia, PA

Victoria Kennedy, M.S.W., L.C.S.W.   Vice President, Program Development and Quality Assurance, The Wellness Community, Washington, DC

Youngmee Kim, Ph.D.   Associate Professor, Department of Psychology, University of Miami, Coral Gables, FL

Stephen D. W. King, Ph.D.   Manager, Chaplaincy, Seattle Cancer Care Alliance, Seattle, Washington, DC

David W. Kissane, M.B.B.S., M.P.M., M.D., F.R.A.N.Z.C.P., F.A.Ch.P.M.   Attending Psychiatrist, Jimmie C. Holland Chair and Chairman, Department of Psychiatry and Behavioral Sciences, Memorial Sloan-Kettering Cancer Center, and Professor of Psychiatry, Weill Medical College of Cornell University, New York, NY

James L. Klosky, Ph.D.   Assistant Member, Department of Behavioral Medicine, St. Jude Children's Research Hospital, Memphis, TN

Robert S. Krouse, M.D., F.A.C.S.   Staff General and Oncologic Surgeon, and Director of Surgical Research, Southern Arizona Veterans Affairs Health Care System, and Professor of Surgery, Department of Surgery, University of Arizona College of Medicine, Tucson, AZ

Marguerite S. Lederberg, M.D.   Attending Psychiatrist, Department of Psychiatry and Behavioral Sciences, Memorial Sloan-Kettering Cancer Center, and Professor of Clinical Psychiatry, Weill Medical College of Cornell University, New York, NY

Tomer T. Levin, M.B., B.S., F.A.P.M., A.C.T.   Assisting Attending Psychiatrist, Department of Psychiatry and Behavioral Sciences, Memorial Sloan-Kettering Cancer Center, New York, NY

Frances Marcus Lewis, Ph.D., M.N., R.N.   The Virginia and Prentice Bloedel Professor, School of Nursing, University of Washington, and Affiliate Fellow, Public Health Division, The Fred Hutchinson Cancer Research Center, Seattle, Washington, DC

Madeline Li, M.D., Ph.D.   Staff Psychiatrist, Psychosocial Oncology and Palliative Care, Princess Margaret Hospital, and Assistant Professor, University of Toronto, Toronto, Ontario, Canada

Wendy G. Lichtenthal, Ph.D.   Instructor, Department of Psychiatry and Behavioral Sciences, Memorial Sloan-Kettering Cancer Center, New York, NY

Matthew J. Loscalzo, M.S.W., L.C.S.W.   Liliane Elkins Professor in Supportive Care Programs; Administrative Director, Sheri & Les Biller Patient and Family Resource Center; Executive Director, Department of Supportive Care Medicine; and Professor, Department of Population Sciences, City of Hope, Duarte, CA

Paola M. Luzzatto, Ph.D., ATR-BC (Art Therapist Registered and Board Certified).   Teacher and Supervisor, Art Therapy Italiana, Bologna, Italy

Julie Lynch, B.S.N., M.B.A.   Doctoral Student, University of Massachusetts-Boston, College of Nursing and Health Sciences, Boston, MA

Lucanne Magill, D.A., MT-BC   Assistant Professor and Coordinator, Music Therapy Program, School of Music, University of Windsor, Ontario, Canada

Mary Jane Massie, M.D.   Attending Psychiatrist, Department of Psychiatry and Behavioral Sciences, Memorial Sloan-Kettering Cancer Center, and Professor of Clinical Psychiatry, Department of Psychiatry, Weill Medical College of Cornell University, New York, NY

Ruth McCorkle, Ph.D., R.N., F.A.A.N.   Florence Schorske Wald Professor, Yale School of Nursing; Professor, Department of Epidemiology and Public Health, School of Medicine; and Program Leader, Population Sciences and Cancer Control, Yale Cancer Center, New Haven, CT

John M. McLaughlin, M.S. Graduate Research Associate, Comprehensive Cancer Center, and Ph.D. Candidate, Division of Epidemiology, College of Public Health, The Ohio State University, Columbus, OH

Amy McQueen, Ph.D. Assistant Professor, Division of Health Behavior Research, Washington University School of Medicine, St. Louis, MO

Abigail L. McUmber, B.S. Kinship/Adoption Caseworker, Family Services of Northwestern Pennsylvania, Meadville, PA

Franklin G. Miller, Ph.D. Bioethicist, Department of Bioethics, Clinical Center, National Institutes of Health, Bethesda, MD

Kimberley Miller, M.D., F.R.C.P.C. Attending Psychiatrist, Lecturer, Psychosocial Oncology and Palliative Care, Princess Margaret Hospital, University of Toronto, Toronto, Ontario, Canada

Suzanne M. Miller, Ph.D. Professor and Director, Psychosocial and Biobehavioral Medicine Program, Fox Chase Cancer Center, Philadelphia, PA

Alex J. Mitchell, M.B.B.S.. M.R.C.Psych Consultant and Honorary Senior Lecturer in Psycho-Oncology, Department of Cancer and Molecular Medicine, University of Leicester, Leicester, Leicestershire, UK

Cynthia W. Moore, Ph.D. Parenting At a Challenging Time (PACT) Program, Department of Psychiatry, Massachusetts General Hospital Cancer Center, and Clinical Instructor in Psychiatry, Harvard Medical School, Boston, MA

Stirling Moorey, M.D. Trust Head of Psychotherapy, South London and Maudsley NHS Foundation Trust, Maudsley Psychotherapy Service, Maudsley Hospital, Denmark Hill, London, UK

Catherine E. Mosher, Ph.D. Postdoctoral Research Fellow, Department of Psychiatry and Behavioral Sciences, Memorial Sloan-Kettering Cancer Center, New York, NY

Diwani B. Msemo, M.D. Consultant in Clinical Oncology, Department of Radiotherapy and Oncology, Ocean Road Cancer Institute, Dar Es Salaam, Tanzania

Ronald E. Myers, Ph.D. Professor and Director, Division of Population Science, Department of Medical Oncology, Thomas Jefferson University, Philadelphia, PA

Christian J. Nelson, Ph.D. Assistant Attending Psychologist, Department of Psychiatry, Memorial Sloan-Kettering Cancer Center, New York, NY

Twalib A. Ngoma, M.D. Executive Director, Ocean Road Cancer Institute, Dar Es Salaam, Tanzania

Laurel L. Northouse, Ph.D., R.N., F.A.A.N. Mary Lou Willard French Professor of Nursing, School of Nursing, University of Michigan, Ann Arbor, MI

Shirley Otis-Green, M.S.W., L.C.S.W., A.C.S.W., OSW-C Senior Research Specialist, Division of Nursing Research and Education, Department of Population Sciences, City of Hope National Medical Center, Duarte, CA

Kristen J. Otto, M.D., Assistant Professor, Department of Otolaryngology and Communicative Sciences, University of Mississippi Medical Center, Jackson, MS

Jessica Park, B.S. Research Associate, Department of Psychiatry and Behavioral Sciences, Memorial Sloan-Kettering Cancer Center, New York, NY

Electra D. Paskett, Ph.D. Marion N. Rowley Professor of Cancer Research, Division of Epidemiology, College of Public Health; Associate Director of Population Sciences, Comprehensive Cancer Center; Program Co-Leader, Cancer Control Program, Comprehensive Cancer Center; and Program Director, Diversity Enhancement Program, The Arthur G. James Cancer Hospital and Richard J. Solove Research Institute, The Ohio State University, Columbus, OH

Steven D. Passik, Ph.D. Associate Attending Psychologist, Memorial Sloan-Kettering Cancer Center and Associate Professor of Psychiatry, Weill College of Medicine, Cornell University Medical Center, New York, NY

Haley Pessin, Ph.D.   Research Associate, Department of Psychiatry and Behavioral Sciences, Memorial Sloan-Kettering Cancer Center, New York, NY

Susan K. Peterson, Ph.D., M.P.H.   Associate Professor, Department of Behavioral Science, The University of Texas M. D. Anderson Cancer Center, Houston, TX

Bernardine M. Pinto, Ph.D.   Professor (Research), Department of Psychiatry and Human Behavior, Centers for Behavioral and Preventive Medicine, The Miriam Hospital and W. Alpert Medical School of Brown University, Providence, RI

William F. Pirl, M.D., M.P.H.   Director, Center for Psychiatric Oncology and Behavioral Sciences, Massachusetts General Hospital, Boston, MA

Holly G. Prigerson, Ph.D.   Associate Professor of Psychiatry, Brigham and Women's Hospital, Harvard Medical School, and Director, Center for Psychosocial Oncology and Palliative Care Research, Dana-Farber Cancer Institute, Boston, MA

Kavitha Ramchandran, M.D.   Clinical Fellow, Department of Medicine, Division of Hematology/Oncology, Feinberg School of Medicine and the Robert H. Lurie Comprehensive Cancer Center, Northwestern University, Chicago, IL

Paula K. Rauch, M.D.   Director, Parenting At a Challenging Time (PACT) Program, Department of Psychiatry, Massachusetts General Hospital Cancer Center, and Associate Professor, Harvard Medical School, Boston, MA

Gary M. Rodin, M.D., F.R.C.P.C.   Professor, Department of Psychiatry, University of Toronto, and Head, Department of Psychosocial Oncology and Palliative Care, Princess Margaret Hospital, University of Toronto, University Health Network, Toronto, Ontario, Canada

Lauren J. Rogak, M.A.   Health Outcomes Research Coordinator, Department of Epidemiology and Biostatistics, Memorial Sloan-Kettering Cancer Center, New York, NY

Donald L. Rosenstein, M.D.   Professor, Department of Psychiatry, and Director, Comprehensive Cancer Support Program, University of North Carolina, Chapel Hill, NC

Andrew J. Roth, M.D.   Attending Psychiatrist, Department of Psychiatry and Behavioral Sciences, Memorial Sloan-Kettering Cancer Center, New York, NY

Pagona Roussi, Ph.D.   Assistant Professor, Department of Psychology, Aristotle University of Thessaloniki, Thessaloniki, Greece

Julia H. Rowland, Ph.D.   Director, Office of Cancer Survivorship, Division of Cancer Control and Population Sciences, National Cancer Institute, NIH/DHHS, Bethesda, MD

Lisa M. Ruppert, M.D.   Chief Resident, Department of Rehabilitation Medicine, New York Presbyterian Hospital-University Hospitals of Columbia and Cornell, New York, NY

Nancy Russell, Ph.D.   Houston, TX

Leonard B. Saltz, M.D.   Attending Oncologist, Division of Solid Tumor Oncology, Department of Medicine, Memorial Sloan-Kettering Cancer Center, New York, NY

Sheila J. Santacroce, Ph.D., A.P.R.N., C.P.N.P.   Associate Professor and Beerstecher-Blackwell Distinguished Scholar, The University of North Carolina at Chapel Hill School of Nursing, Chapel Hill, NC

Linda Sarna, D.N.Sc, R.N., F.A.A.N.   Professor, University of California-Los Angeles, School of Nursing, Los Angeles, CA

Lisa A. Schwartz, Ph.D.   Psychologist, Division of Oncology, The Children's Hospital of Philadelphia, Philadelphia, PA

Peter A. Selwyn, M.D., M.P.H.   Professor and Chairman, Department of Family and Social Medicine, Montefiore Medical Center, Albert Einstein College of Medicine, Bronx, NY

Felicia A. Smith, M.D. Chief, Acute Psychiatry Service, Massachusetts General Hospital, and Instructor in Psychiatry, Harvard Medical School, Boston, MA

Kathryn M. Smolinski, M.S.W., L.M.S.W. Oncology Social Work Consultant, Ypsilanti, MI

Robert Socherman, Ph.D. Psychologist, Mental Health Division, Portland Veterans Affairs Medical Center, Portland, OR

Barbara M. Sourkes, Ph.D. Associate Professor of Pediatrics, Stanford University School of Medicine, and Kriewall-Haehl Director, Pediatric Palliative Care Program, Lucile Packard Children's Hospital at Stanford, Palo Alto, CA

James L. Spira, Ph.D., M.P.H., ABPP. Senior Psychologist; Health, Social, and Economic Research Division, RTI International, San Diego, CA

Sheri L. Spunt, M.D. Associate Member, Department of Oncology, and Associate Professor, Department of Pediatrics, University of Tennessee School of Medicine, Memphis, TN

Annette L. Stanton, Ph.D. Professor, Departments of Psychology and Psychiatry/Biobehavioral Sciences, University of California, Los Angeles, CA

Tatiana D. Starr, M.A. Clinical Research Coordinator, Department of Psychiatry and Behavioral Sciences, Memorial Sloan-Kettering Cancer Center, New York, NY

Michael Stefanek, Ph.D. Vice President, Behavioral Research, American Cancer Society, Atlanta, GA

Theodore A. Stern, M.D. Chief, Psychiatric Consultation Service, Massachusetts General Hospital, and Professor of Psychiatry, Harvard Medical School, Boston, MA

Jessica Stiles, B.A. Graduate Student, Columbia School of Nursing, New York, NY

Melinda R. Stolley, Ph.D. Assistant Professor, Section of Health Promotion Research, Department of Medicine, University of Illinois at Chicago, and Research Health Scientist, Center for Management of Complex Chronic Care (CMC³), Jesse Brown Veterans Affairs Medical Center, Chicago, IL

E. Alessandra Strada, Ph.D. Attending Psychologist, Department of Pain Medicine and Palliative Care, Beth Israel Medical Center, New York, NY; Assistant Professor of Neurology and Psychiatry, Albert Einstein School of Medicine, New York, NY; and Assistant Professor of East-West Psychology, California Institute of Integral Studies, San Francisco, CA

Michael D. Stubblefield, M.D. Assistant Attending Physiatrist, Rehabilitation Medicine Service, Department of Neurology, Memorial Sloan-Kettering Cancer Center, and Assistant Professor of Rehabilitation Medicine, Weill Medical College of Cornell University, New York, NY

Antonella Surbone, M.D., Ph.D., F.A.C.P. Professor of Medicine, Department of Medicine, New York University Medical School, New York, NY

Kim Thiboldeaux President and CEO, The Wellness Community, Washington, DC

Lisa M. Thornton, Ph.D. Postdoctoral Fellow, Department of Psychology, The Ohio State University, Columbus, OH

Peter C. Trask, Ph.D., M.P.H. Senior Director-Oncology, Global Outcomes Research, Pfizer Inc., New London, CT

Marina Unrod, Ph.D. Applied Research Scientist, Tobacco Research and Intervention Program, H. Lee Moffitt Cancer Center and Research Institute, Tampa, FL

Mary L. S. Vachon, Ph.D., R.N. Professor, Department of Psychiatry and Behavioral Science, University of Toronto, Ontario, Canada

Alan D. Valentine, M.D. Professor, Department of Psychiatry, The University of Texas M. D. Anderson Cancer Center, Houston, TX

Anne Vandenhoeck, Ph.D. Researcher and supervisor, Academic Center for Practical Theology, Faculty of Theology, Catholic University of Louvain, Louvain, Belgium

Sally W. Vernon, M.A., Ph.D. Director, Division of Health Promotion and Behavioral Sciences and Blair Justice, Ph.D. Professorship in Mind-Body Medicine and Public Health, Division of Health Promotion and Behavioral Sciences, University of Texas Houston School of Public Health, Houston, TX

Charles F. von Gunten, M.D., Ph.D. Provost, The Institute for Palliative Medicine at San Diego Hospice, and Clinical Professor of Medicine, University of California, San Diego, CA

Jamie H. Von Roenn, M.D. Professor of Medicine, Department of Medicine, Division of Hematology/Oncology, Feinberg School of Medicine and the Robert H. Lurie Comprehensive Cancer Center, Northwestern University, Chicago, IL

Edward H. Wagner, M.D., M.P.H. Director, MacColl Institute for Healthcare Innovation, Group Health Research Institute, Seattle, WA

Maggie Watson, Ph.D. Head of Service, Psychological Medicine, Royal Marsden Hospital NHS Trust; Honorary Senior Lecturer, Institute of Cancer Research, Sutton, Surrey, UK; and Honorary Professor, University College London, London, UK

Talia R. Weiss, B.A. Doctoral Student, Department of Psychiatry, Ferkauf Graduate School, Memorial Sloan-Kettering Cancer Center, New York, NY

Branlyn E. Werba, Ph.D. Psychologist, Division of Oncology, The Children's Hospital of Philadelphia, Philadelphia, PA

John David Wynn, M.D. Clinical Professor, Department of Psychiatry and Behavioral Science, University of Washington School of Medicine, and Medical Director, Division of PsychoOncology, Swedish Cancer Institute, Seattle, Washington, DC

Herbert J. Yue, M.D. Pulmonary Fellow, Department of Medicine, Division of Pulmonary/Critical Care, University of California, San Diego School of Medicine, La Jolla, CA

James R. Zabora, D.S.W. Dean, School of Social Work, Catholic University, Washington, DC

Talia Irit Zaider, Ph.D. Psychologist/Instructor, Department of Psychiatry and Behavioral Sciences, Memorial Sloan-Kettering Cancer Center, New York, NY

Brad J. Zebrack, Ph.D., M.S.W., M.P.H. Associate Professor, University of Michigan School of Social Work, University of Michigan Comprehensive Cancer Center, Socio-Behavioral Program, Ann Arbor, MI

PART I

Introduction

CHAPTER 1

History of Psycho-Oncology

Jimmie C. Holland and Talia R. Weiss

We are not ourselves when nature, being oppressed, commands the mind to suffer with the body. -King Lear, Act II, Sc. IV.

INTRODUCTION

The formal beginnings of psycho-oncology date to the mid-1970s, when the stigma making the word "cancer" unspeakable was diminished to the point that the diagnosis could be revealed and the feelings of patients about their illness could be explored for the first time. However, a second stigma has contributed to the late development of interest in the psychological dimensions of cancer: negative attitudes attached to mental illness and psychological problems, even in the context of medical illness. It is important to understand these historical underpinnings because they continue to color contemporary attitudes and beliefs about cancer and its psychiatric comorbidity and psychosocial problems. Over the last quarter of the past century, psycho-oncology became a subspecialty of oncology with its own body of knowledge contributing to cancer care. In the new millennium, a significant base of literature, training programs, and a broad research agenda have evolved with applications at all points on the cancer continuum: behavioral research in changing lifestyle and habits to reduce cancer risk; behaviors and attitudes to ensure early detection; psychological issues related to genetic risk and testing; symptom control (anxiety, depression, delirium, pain, and fatigue) during active treatment; management of psychological sequelae in cancer survivors; and management of the psychological aspects of palliative and end-of-life care. Links between psychological and physiological domains of relevance to cancer risk, quality of life, and survival are being actively explored through translational research relating to cytokines and genetic patterns. At the start of the third millennium, psycho-oncology has come of age as one of the youngest subspecialties of oncology, and as one of the most clearly defined subspecialties of consultation-liaison psychiatry and psychosomatic medicine. It is an example of the value of a broad multidisciplinary application of the behavioral and social sciences to a particular disease.

The brief history of psycho-oncology is interesting for contemporary review because it has, over 30 years, produced a model in which the psychological domain has been integrated, as a subspecialty, into the disease-specific specialty of oncology. As such, the field today contributes to the clinical care of patients and families, to the training of staff in psychological management, and to collaborative research.[1] Given the centrality of psychological issues in cancer, it is surprising that the formal history of psycho-oncology began only in the mid-1970s. It becomes understandable, however, when one realizes that it was only then that the stigma attached to cancer diminished to the point that most patients in western countries were told their diagnosis, which made it possible to openly explore and study their psychological responses.

Although the development of psycho-oncology occurred primarily over the last quarter of the twentieth century, it is crucial to understand the attitudes of society toward cancer and toward mental illness (including psychiatric comorbidity and psychological issues in medical illness) because they still impact on contemporary attitudes, albeit in an attenuated form today. Internationally, they continue to present barriers to optimal psychosocial care and research.

This chapter explores the history of psycho-oncology with attention to the barriers arising from longstanding beliefs about cancer and mental illness that produced difficulties in the development of the psychosocial and psychiatric care of the medically ill.

HISTORICAL BARRIERS RELATED TO CANCER

In the 1800s, like the preceding centuries, a cancer diagnosis was viewed as the equivalent of death. There was no known cause or cure. Revealing the diagnosis to a patient was considered cruel and inhumane because the patient would lose all hope and could cope better by not knowing. This was viewed as an acceptable "white lie," although the patient's family was always told. Tolstoy's story *The death of Ivan Ilyich*[2] graphically describes the consequences which Ilyich felt in nineteenth-century Russia when his family and doctor pretended that his intense stomach pain (likely cancer) was nothing serious. He struggled alone with his pain and awareness that he was mortally ill while his family and physician maintained a conspiracy of silence.

Fear of cancer was so great that the family would not reveal the diagnosis to others because of the stigma that became attached to the family. Shame and guilt were dominant emotions, combined with the fear that it was contagious. Care of the indigent dying from cancer was done by religious groups. The hospice in Beaune, France, which still stands, dates back several centuries. Early in the twentieth century, as surgery improved and anesthesia was developed, it became possible (though uncommon) to cure a cancer if the tumor was found early and could be removed before it had spread. For the first time, educating the public about cancer became important. Educational programs began encouraging people in Europe to seek consultation for symptoms suspicious of cancer. The American Cancer Society, formed in 1913, was the first attempt in the United States to alter the public's fatalistic attitudes toward cancer. The Society's mandate was to "disseminate knowledge concerning the symptoms, treatment and prevention of cancer."[3] These efforts were undertaken to counter the ignorance, fatalism, and fears. Such slogans as "Fight cancer with knowledge" were used to combat the fears. Despite the greater public information, however, many people neglected the danger signals, largely because of these attitudes, and they sought consultation only after delaying too long for surgery to be effective.

Radiation joined surgery as a treatment for cancer early in the first quarter of the twentieth century, thanks to the pioneering work of Marie Curie in Paris. However, it was offered mainly as palliation, often after surgical failure, and people feared it as they did surgery.[4] The radiation dose was often poorly calibrated and burns were common. In 1937, the National Cancer Institute was created in the United States as the first of the National Institutes of Health. In 1948, the first temporary remissions of childhood acute leukemia occurred with aminopterin, followed by the early responses of Hodgkin's disease to nitrogen mustard.[4] This began an active search for new chemotherapeutic drugs; thus, chemotherapy was added as the third treatment modality for cancer, combined with increasingly more effective surgery and radiation.

The first *chemotherapy cure* of a cancer, choriocarcinoma, a tumor common in Asian women, by the single agent methotrexate, was achieved in the early 1950s. The introduction of chemotherapy to the treatment armamentarium dramatically altered the prognosis for several, previously fatal, tumors of children and young adults, notably childhood acute lymphocytic leukemia, testicular cancer, and Hodgkin's disease. These cures in the 1960s, of previously fatal cancers, did much to reduce the fear, stigma, and pessimism about cancer and stimulated a new optimism.

This period coincided with the awakening of concerns about the importance of patients' right to give informed consent for treatment, which could occur only in the context of an open dialogue with the doctor about the diagnosis and treatment options. Patients' rights became more important as revelations of the post-World War II Nuremberg trials disclosed experimentation on humans without consent. The repercussions, plus evidence of several clinical trials on patients in the United States without their consent, led to the promulgation of federal guidelines for research on human subjects. The era of social upheaval in America (1960s–1970s) contributed to movements for the rights of women, consumers, and finally patients, who began to recognize their right to know their diagnosis, prognosis, and treatment options.

During the post-World War II years, the only formal psychological support for cancer patients was through the American Cancer Society's "visitor" programs.[3] Patients who had had a laryngectomy or colostomy were asked to speak with patients who feared undergoing these frightening and disabling—yet often curative—procedures. Self-help groups were formed by patients as laryngectomy and ostomy clubs. These were followed by "Reach to Recovery," started in the 1950s by the American Cancer Society as a program in which women who had had a mastectomy (usually radical in those days) visited women in the postoperative period.

Despite widespread endorsement by patients, these organizations had an uphill battle to gain acceptance in the medical community. Except in special situations, physicians were slow to acknowledge that there was a unique and useful role for patients who were survivors to support and encourage others with the same diagnosis and treatment, even though few adverse effects were reported. The strong bias against encouraging patients to talk with one another continued into the last quarter of the twentieth century, when experience began to show that the benefits of the social support far outweighed the risks.

Table 1–1 outlines the major advances by decade in cancer medicine since 1800; the changes in societal attitudes toward cancer and death in each period; and the progress made in the psychological and psychiatric care of the medically ill, including cancer patients. Readers who are interested in the historical details of cancer medicine and the social attitudes associated with it are referred to Shimkin,[4] Patterson,[5] and Holland.[6]

HISTORICAL BARRIERS RELATED TO PSYCHOLOGICAL ISSUES

The centuries-old stigma attached to mental illness and its treatment had a profound impact on developing psychological care for medically ill patients. Mental illness, like cancer, had no known cause or cure. It was as feared as cancer. Demonic possession was a common attribution; the person was blamed and ostracized and often brutalized in some societies.[7,8]

In the United States, the nineteenth and early twentieth centuries saw mental patients and their physicians (called "alienists" because they removed the mentally ill person from society) isolated in mental hospitals in pastoral settings, which were located at a distance from general hospitals. By the latter 1800s, however, interest was developing to bring the treatment of mental illness into general medicine by placing psychiatric units in general hospitals and by teaching physicians and medical students to recognize and treat psychiatric comorbidity in medical patients.[9] Adolph Meyer did much to bring the unifying concept of "psychobiology" to the awareness of academic physicians. From his position as Professor at Johns Hopkins, he and his students had a major impact on medicine, by encouraging treatment of the "whole person." In 1902, the first psychiatric ward was opened in a general hospital in Albany, New York. Psychiatric consultations to medical patients began to develop in the 1930s, fostered in part by the Rockefeller Foundation, which supported several centers of excellence whose prominence in academic medicine did much to expand the concepts of psychosomatic medicine and psychiatric care of the medically ill.

However, the early attitudes toward the participation of a psychiatrist on the medical wards of the general hospital varied from hostile to indifferent. In 1929, George Henry,[10] a psychiatrist, documented his experience:

For several years, it has been my privilege to be engaged in making practical applications of psychiatry in general hospitals and after having dealt with the problems of more than two thousand cases, I am attempting to formulate my experiences. Very few exceptions can be taken to the statement that when psychiatry is first introduced into a general hospital there is likely to be indifference or even resistance on the part of the hospital staff.…In one hospital, the superintendent received the proposal of psychiatric aid with the remark that in his experience, "insanity" was a hopeless disease and furthermore there were no "insane" patients in the hospital.

Henry proposed that every general hospital should have a psychiatrist available.

The principles enunciated by Henry in 1929 are still applicable. He suggested the importance of a psychiatrist as a part of medical services to bring the attention of teaching doctors and medical students to comorbid psychiatric problems and common psychological factors contributing to medical illness or symptoms.

Such were the beginnings of what became known in the United States as consultation-liaison psychiatry. In Europe the field has been called Psychological Medicine. These initial endeavors came out of the experiences in psychiatric units that cared for patients with medical illness and psychiatric comorbidity and also from the psychiatric consultations done on patients on the floors of the general hospitals.[9] Patients with cancer were treated in the general wards of the hospital by general physicians. The disease did not attract much academic interest or study since it was viewed as having little "science" attached to it. Patients sensed that they were regarded as largely untreatable as doctors spent less time at their bedside, following the custom of not discussing the diagnosis and prognosis and avoiding questions that would lead to such a discussion.

The 1930s saw the arrival of many psychoanalysts from Europe to the United States. The impact of psychoanalysis on American psychiatry and society was immense. Flanders Dunbar and Franz Alexander were well-known figures whose research focused on a possible psychoanalytic base for several medical diseases. The psychosomatic movement sought psychodynamic formulations or traumatic events that were antecedents to a range of physical illnesses whose etiologies were unknown, particularly rheumatoid arthritis, ulcer, asthma, hypertension, and cancer. In cancer, the research focused on patients with a specific malignancy, who were then studied psychiatrically by a retrospective life review to identify the problems that were assumed to have had a possible physiological impact and contributed to the development of cancer.

Several studies published in *Psychosomatic Medicine* reflect research methods and direction at the time. In 1954, Blumberg and colleagues[11] described "A possible relationship between psychological factors and human cancer." The same issue contained an article by Stephenson and Grace[12] on "Life stress and cancer of the cervix." In 1955, Reznikoff[13] reported "Psychological factors in breast cancer: a preliminary study of some personality trends in patients with cancer of the breast." In 1956, Fisher and Cleveland[14] described the "Relationship of body image to site of cancer." Greene and Miller[15] described psychological factors and family dynamics in children who developed leukemia. These studies were of theoretical interest to mental health professionals and were reported in psychiatric and psychoanalytic journals, but they were not of interest to the developing field of oncology. Unfortunately, the studies were usually not done in collaboration with cancer physicians and surgeons, who had little or no interest in these speculative approaches to etiology. The "disconnect" between these early investigators and physicians working in cancer led to a delay in the development of prospective studies of patients that explored both medical and psychological perspectives and ensured an integrated approach to their care.

Hackett[16] offered a critique of this period:

the message [from psychosomatic studies] came across quite distinctly that the pay dirt was embedded in psychology. Placing such weight on the importance of emotional issues in the etiology of an illness disengaged the attention of internist and surgeon alike. The psychosomatic

Table 1–1. Advances in cancer treatment and changes affecting psychological care

Decade	Advances in cancer treatment	Societal attitudes		Psychological/psychiatric care
		Cancer	Death/supportive services	
1800s	Mortality high from infectious diseases; tuberculosis common	Cancer = death; diagnosis not revealed	Patient is in "God's hands"; physician's role is to comfort; "death is a part of life"; person died at home	Major mental illness treated in asylums isolated from general hospitals
	Effective cancer treatment unknown	Stigma, shame, guilt associated with having cancer; fears of transmission	Fatalism about cancer diagnosis; death is inevitable	By 1850s efforts made to bring psychiatry into medicine but largely unsuccessful
	Introduction of anesthesia (1847) and antisepsis; opened way for surgical excision of cancer	Fatalism about cancer diagnosis		
1900s–1920s	Successful surgical removal of some early cancers	In 1890s, efforts in Europe and United States to inform public of warning signs of cancer		First psychiatric unit in a general hospital, Albany, NY (1902)
	Radiation used for palliation	Era of home remedies and quack cures for cancer		Psychobiological approach of Adolf Meyer had strong impact on U.S. psychiatry
	American Cancer Society (ACS) started in 1913			
1930s	National Cancer Institute and International Union Against Cancer formed in 1937	ACS began visitor–volunteer programs for patients with functional deficits (colostomy, laryngectomy)	Deaths in hospitals; embalming, elaborate funerals; person "only sleeping" as euphemism for death	Beginning psychiatric consultation and psychiatric units in general hospitals through grants from Rockefeller Foundation
	Beginning of research in cancer treatment			Psychosomatic movement with psychoanalytic orientation
1940s	Nitrogen mustards, developed in W W II, found to have an antitumor action in lymphomas	Pervasive pessimism of public and doctors about outcome of cancer treatment	Expression of grief encouraged; concern for handling of death	Search for a cancer personality and life events as cause of cancer; efforts not related to cancer care
	First remission of acute leukemia by use of drug, aminopterin, folic acid antagonist		Funeral "industry"	First scientific study of acute grief by Lindemann
1950s	Beginning of cancer chemotherapy; first cure of choriocarcinoma by drugs alone (1951)	Debates about the practice of not revealing cancer diagnosis; public is better informed	Post-WWII concerns about informed consent and patient autonomy	First papers on psychological reactions to cancer (1951–1952)
	Improvement of radiation therapy techniques			Psychiatrists favor revealing cancer diagnosis
				Biopsychosocial approach of Engel and his group in Rochester, NY
				First psychiatric unit established at MSKCC under Sutherland in 1951 and at Massachusetts General Hospital
				Feinberg at Karolinska uses psychoanalytical approach with dying
1960s	Combined modalities lead to first survivors of childhood leukemia and Hodgkin's disease	More optimism about cancer; survivors' concerns heard	U.S. federal guidelines for patient participation in research	Kubler-Ross challenged taboo of not talking to dying patients about their imminent death
	Hospice movement started	Public concern grows for prevention research in cancer		Dame Cecily Saunders, London, advocates training in palliative care
	Tobacco related to lung cancer			U.S. Surgeon General's report on smoking and lung cancer (1964); behavioral studies of smoking

(Continued)

Table 1–1. Continued

Decade	Advances in cancer treatment	Cancer	Death/supportive services	Psychological/psychiatric care
1970s	National Cancer Plan (1972) with rehabilitation and cancer control; psychosocial included Informed consent for treatment protocols; increased patient autonomy Two cooperative groups, CALGB and EORTC, established committees to study quality of life (QOL) and psychosocial issues	Diagnosis usually revealed in U.S. and several other countries Guidelines for protection of patients' rights Women's, consumers and patients' rights movements	Prognosis more likely not revealed First hospice in U.S. (1974) Guidelines for care of hopelessly ill (DNR) (1976) Pain service, MSKCC, Kathy Foley Palliative Care Unit, McGill, Montreal, Dr. Balfour Mount	First federal support for psychosocial studies First psychiatric comorbidity studies in cancer First National Conference on Psychosocial Research (1975) Psychiatry committee Cancer and Leukemia Group B (1976) QOL Committee for training and research in cancer European Organization Psychosocial Collaborative Oncology Group (1976–1981) and Project Omega at Massachusetts General Hospital (1977–1984) Faith Courtland Psychosocial Unit, Kings College Medical School, London (Pettingale, Green Tee, Brinkley) (1971–1986) Full Time Psychiatry Service at MSKCC established (1977)
1980s	ACS assisted development of psycho-oncology, sponsoring four conferences on research methods ACS Peer Review Committee established for psychosocial research (1989) Better analgesics and antiemetics developed	Eight million cancer survivors in U.S. "out of the closet" National cancer survivors organizations Concern for QOL and symptom control increases	Ethical issues explored; impact of U.S. President's Commission for Study of Ethical Problems in Medicine Health proxy assignment encouraged in United States	British Psychosocial Oncology Society (1982) International Psycho-Oncology Society (1984) Royal Marsden Unit/Greer and Watson (1986) American Psycho-Oncology Society (1986) Health psychologists contribute to clinical care and research in cancer Development of psychoneuroimmunology Handbook of psychooncology published (1989)
1990–2000	U.S. Federal Drug Administration designates QOL change as basis for approval of new anticancer agents (1985) Identification of genetic basis of several cancer and gene therapy Immunological therapies (monoclonal antibody, allogeneic transplants)	Pain initiatives for public and professional education on pain Increased public interest in cancer prevention, lifestyle changes, decreased smoking Improved symptom control and palliative care; public debate over physician-assisted suicide	U.S. physicians required to discuss wishes about resuscitation (DNR) Greater interest in end-of-life care; first Chair of Palliative Medicine in United States Improved treatment of pain, fatigue, nausea and vomiting, anxiety, depression, delirium	Research in psychological issues associated with genetic risk and testing Greater range of psychosocial and behavioral interventions, especially groups Psycho-Oncology journal published (1992) Standards of care and clinical practice guidelines for psychosocial distress (1998) National Cancer Centers Network

	Combined chemotherapy agents Improved radiotherapy (brachytherapy, conformal) Laparoscopic surgery First decrease in cancer mortality	Public fear of cancer diminished, but strong beliefs in psychological causes of cancer and as factors in survival Increased use of alternative/complementary therapies	More formal study of grief Research in teaching doctor–patient communication	International Psycho-Oncology World Congresses (France 1992, Japan 1994, Germany 1996, Australia 2000) Psychiatric complications of immunologic therapies (interferon, stem-cell transplant) Quality-of-life assessment with innovative therapies First Department of Psychiatry and Behavioral Sciences established in a cancer center (MSKCC, 1996)
2001–2008	Oral-targeted chemotherapy agents developed (2007) Stem-cell transplants Better diagnostic tools (PET, CT scans)	Clinical Practice Guidelines for Psychosocial care: Canada, Australia, United Kingdom, United States Institute of Medicine Report: "Cancer Care for the Whole Patient: Meeting Psychosocial Health Needs" (2007) evidence base for psychosocial care integrated in routine cancer care	Palliative care expanded worldwide National Psycho-Oncology Societies join Federation of International Psycho-Oncology Society (2008)	APOS—20 lectures in English free on website (www.apos-society.org) IPOS and European School of oncology—website core curriculum in psycho-oncology in six languages (http://www.ipos-society.org/) IPOS seeks WHO nongovernmental organization member status

movement, with some exceptions, loosened even more the moorings of psychiatry to medical pragmatism.

By the 1960s and 1970s, clinical and experimental psychologists began to study patients with more quantitative measures and finally with methods that permitted exploration of interactions between the physiological and the psychological, as exemplified by the work of Mason[17] and colleagues.

The psychosomatic medicine movement later branched into two areas relevant to cancer: psychoneuroimmunology and consultation-liaison psychiatry (presently the certified subspecialty of psychiatry) now renamed Psychosomatic Medicine. The work of Ader and Cohen[18] established the beginnings of psychoneuroimmunology in 1975, when they reported a conditioned taste aversion, using saccharin as the stimulus, that resulted in a conditioned immune response in rats. The work in this area was important in fostering research in cancer because it contributed to the understanding of conditioned nausea and vomiting as a learned response in patients undergoing chemotherapy. Studies have shown that patients, years after chemotherapy is finished, are sensitive to visual and olfactory stimuli that are reminders of chemotherapy and that such sights and smells still produce transient nausea and anxiety. For example, the sight of the nurse or doctor, the smell of an antiseptic, or the perfume worn by the nurse will elicit these symptoms.[19]

Psychoneuroimmunology used newer techniques that tracked biological events and measured psychological phenomena in a far more precise way, truly embodying the biopsychosocial concept of Engel.[20] Researchers also explored the impact of stress and coping on immune function during the course of cancer treatment.[21,22] The significance of psychoimmune mechanisms as factors in cancer risk and survival remains unclear, and investigators have been modest in their interpretation of the findings in cancer.[23] But psychoneuroimmunology clearly has become an independent field. Its future appears bright as our field begins to explore translational research opportunities which examines the impact of genetic, immune, endocrine, and the social environment on physical status, psychological symptoms, quality of life, and survival.[24,25]

The second identifiable field that grew out of psychosomatic medicine was consultation-liaison psychiatry, which, in terms of cancer, focused on understanding the psychological burden of patients with cancer. Eissler in 1955[26] and Norton in 1963[27] made detailed and sensitive observations of their patients who, during psychoanalysis, developed cancer. These fortuitous studies provided rich material for those beginning to work in the field in the 1960s as to how patients coped with progressive stages of illness and approaching death.

In the early 1950s, several prospective studies began to examine the psychological response of hospitalized patients to cancer, providing the first opportunity for collaborative research with the physicians treating cancer. The shared research effort led to more trust between psychiatry and medicine and to closer collaboration. The first reports of psychological adaptation to cancer and its treatment were made by the psychiatric group at the Massachusetts General Hospital, under the direction of Finesinger, and the psychiatric research group at Memorial Sloan-Kettering Cancer Center, under Sutherland, also a psychiatrist. By 1955, these two centers had published the initial papers documenting the psychological reactions to cancer and its treatment.[28–31] Guilt and shame were described by Abrams and Finesinger[28] related to the stigma of cancer. Shands and colleagues,[29] also at Massachusetts General Hospital, observed how patients' communication patterns changed over the stages of illness, noting that communication became more limited as the disease progressed, likely as they responded to the expectation that progressing illness was not to be discussed. It is important to note the early contributions of social work to the psychological care of cancer patients. Ruth Abrams, a social worker at the Massachusetts General Hospital, contributed to these early observations of patients, as did other social workers, by providing the first psychosocial services to patients with cancer. Much credit goes to these pioneers. Also the early contributions of nurses at the bedside must be recognized. They intuitively provided psychological support and later were increasingly trained in psychosocial care and guided by early nursing researchers, such as

Jeanne Quint Benoliel, who trained a second generation of psychosocial nurse researchers represented by Ruth McCorkle.

The group at Memorial Sloan-Kettering Cancer Center focused on the patients' responses to the radical surgical procedures of the day for gynecological, breast, and colon cancer. Major physical and functional deficits were the cost of possible cure. The group described, in two seminal papers that are still highly relevant, the responses to colostomy and radical mastectomy.[30,31] The psychiatric groups at these two hospitals (comprising psychiatrists, psychologists, and social workers) began to forge clinical and research ties with treating surgeons, radiotherapists, and oncologists; thus, collaborative work began to establish the first building blocks of what later became psycho-oncology.

Another early area of psychological intervention occurred in the 1960s, when the first debate began in this country about the wisdom of never revealing the diagnosis of cancer to the patient. Psychiatrists were active as participants (on the "do tell" side) of these lively debates with oncologists, who were often on the "never tell" side. In a survey by Oken in 1961,[32] more than 90% of physicians in this country did not reveal the diagnosis to the patient. The argument that many people preferred to know the truth and more harm was done by telling a lie began to be persuasive. The same questions asked in a survey in 1978 showed that 97% of the doctors in the same geographic area were then telling patients their cancer diagnosis.[33] Over the course of those intervening 17 years, the public's knowledge about cancer increased, and we saw patients, consumers, and women mount their respective rights movements, encouraging a more equitable and less paternalistic dialogue about diagnosis and treatment. Also, as more types of cancer were cured, optimism about outcome made it easier to discuss these matters.[34]

Another factor in the 1960s was new attention beginning in the United Kingdom, given to palliative and end-of-life care started by Dame Cecily Saunders in London. In the United States, heightened interest in psychological issues in cancer resulted from the work of psychiatrist Elizabeth Kubler-Ross. She challenged the taboo against talking to cancer patients about their impending death and challenged doctors and nurses to stop avoiding these patients and to listen to their concerns. Kubler-Ross[35] galvanized both public and medical attention to recognize the isolation of dying patients and their need for dialogue about their situation. Her contributions were crucial to the beginning of the thanatology movement in this country, to fostering the concept of hospice care, and to humanizing end-of-life care.

FORMAL BEGINNING OF PSYCHO-ONCOLOGY: 1975

The subspecialty of psycho-oncology began formally around the mid-1970s, when the barrier to revealing the diagnosis fell and it became possible to talk with patients about their cancer diagnoses and their reactions. This coincided with several social changes. First, the public felt a greater sense of optimism about cancer, due principally to the presence of increasing numbers of cancer survivors who were vocal about their successful outcomes, in contrast to prior times, when they remained silent because of the illness' stigma and the fear of repercussions at their job. Second, celebrities began to permit the media to report their illness revealing both the diagnosis and treatment. Most notable examples were Betty Ford and Happy Rockefeller in 1975, as major national figures, as well as Betty Rollin who wrote *First, you cry*,[36] an account of her breast cancer. Last, this period saw a surge of powerful social movements championing human rights that were the legacy of the Vietnam era, directing the nation's attention to previously underserved individuals: women, consumers, and patients. As a result of all these factors, cancer "came out of the closet," and the door opened for exploration of the psychological dimension of cancer.

In England, a group of psychosocial investigators at the Faith Courtauld Unit of the King's College Medical School established a research unit in 1971 headed by a rotating directorship of Pettingale, Greer, Tee, and Brinkley. Morris and Watson were Research Fellows whose work began there. Their early work examined women with breast cancer in which they explored factors in survival and developed one of the first quantitative scales to measure psychological aspects of coping. Greer and Watson moved to the Royal Marsden Hospital in 1986 where they continued their psychological research. They also established the British Psychosocial Oncology Society in 1982.

Early during this same period, Feigenberg at the Karolinska Institute, in Stockholm, made significant contributions to patient care, using a psychoanalytic approach. Christina Bolund continued this pioneering work.

In the Netherlands, Fritz Van Dam developed the first psychosocial research unit in Amsterdam. His pioneering work led to measurement of quality of life and psychological variables in the European Organization for Research and Training in Cancer (EORTC) (the European multicenter cooperative clinical trials group) in 1976. He, with Aaronson, developed a multilanguage quality-of-life scale which was of great importance to research in the field.

Simultaneously, in 1976 in the United States, the National Cancer Institute (NCI)-supported national clinical trials group, the Cancer and Leukemia Group B, was mandated to become multidisciplinary. A Psychiatry Committee was formed by Holland which undertook quality of life in patients undergoing treatment protocol. The first studies of early survivors who were treated by protocol came from this group.[37] The group also introduced the use of a centralized interviewer to collect psychosocial data by telephone which improved quality and improved data points.[38]

Razavi in Belgium provided early studies of doctor–patient communication and interventions to reduce patient's distress. Marget van Kerekjarto in Hamburg and Kawano in Japan were early contributors to our international collaborations.

In Australia, the impetus for the growth of psycho-oncology came from three forces. First, cancer prevention and population control was organized through State Cancer Councils, which drove behavioral science research in achieving success with tobacco control, sun screen protection, and screening for early detection of cancer. Second, patient advocacy groups pushed government for the creation of a National Breast Cancer Center, which became a platform through which psychosocial research was able to be coordinated. Third, social forces around end-of-life care lobbied for the development of palliative care as a national agenda, which in turn spurred the creation of academic training and research units funded by government. The partnership between psycho-oncology and palliative care was strong. The Clinical Oncology Society of Australia operated a Psycho-Oncology group, while the Australian and New Zealand Society of Palliative Care helped promote collaborative research. Activities directed at developing national guidelines for psychosocial care brought academics together. The creation of government funding for PhD and postdoctoral scholarships helped train a future workforce. The Section of Consultation-Liaison Psychiatry within the Australian and New Zealand College of Psychiatrists and University Departments of Psychology supported the growth of scholars in each state, leading to the development of steadily stronger clinical and research programs that have advanced the field.

A similar pattern developed in Canada with a strong alliance between palliative care under Balfour Mount at McGill, and psychosocial research, particularly Vachon and later the group headed by Chochinov in Winnipeg, Bultz in Calgary, and Rodin in Toronto. The Canadian Association for Psychosocial Oncology produced one of the earliest standards for psychosocial care, and Bultz has been instrumental in obtaining federal support for making "distress" the sixth vital sign (see Chapter 96 by Bultz).

In the United States the door was further opened for psychosocial and psychiatric cancer research in 1975, when the small group of clinical investigators gathered in San Antonio, TX, for the first national research conference on psycho-oncology,[39] organized by Bernard Fox, early proponent of the highest quality of psychosocial research. The 25 colleagues addressed the barrier posed by the lack of quantitative instruments to measure subjective symptoms such as pain, anxiety, and depression. Instruments designed for the study of physically healthy patients with psychiatric disorders were not calibrated to measure these types of distress in the medically ill. The American Cancer Society supported several research conferences which fostered instrument development to quantitatively measure subjective symptoms of pain, anxiety, nausea, depression, and delirium and health-related quality of life.

The American Cancer Society also acknowledged Psycho-Oncology as a legitimate area of cancer research and established the first peer-review mechanism for psychosocial and behavioral research. The psychiatric group at Memorial Sloan-Kettering *Cancer Center*, which began in 1951 and dispersed in 1961, was reestablished in 1977 as a full-time academic program which began to develop clinical services, a postgraduate clinical and research training program, and research.[40] As a critical mass developed, the group (collaborating with the American Cancer Society and the NCI) has served as a major force for national and international development of psycho-oncology. Today, over 300 professionals have been trained there. Many of them constitute major contributors to the research and clinical work in the field.

By the mid-1970s, the consultation-liaison psychiatrists working on inpatient cancer floors or in psycho-oncology units were the first wave of investigators; as such, they explored the epidemiology of comorbid psychiatric disorders that most often complicated cancer care: depression, anxiety, and delirium.[41] The Psychosocial Collaborative Oncology Group under Schmale led to the multicenter, cross-sectional study by Derogatis and colleagues[42] of the frequency and type of DSM-III diagnoses in cancer patients, which showed a 47% prevalence of psychiatric disorder, most often adjustment disorder. Studies began to document the frequency of depression by site and stage of cancer, acknowledging the difficulties in separating physical from psychological symptoms; the causes and course of delirium; the causes, both functional and treatment-related, of anxiety; the relationship of all to the presence of pain and impaired cognitive functioning. The seminal studies of Weisman and Worden through Project Omega at Massachusetts General Hospital provided much information about responses to cancer diagnosis, which they called "existential plight." Clinical trials began of psychosocial and psychopharmacologic interventions. An account of this research literature and clinical experience appeared in the first handbook of psycho-oncology published in 1989.[40] The opportunity for teaching oncology staff about these issues increased as a curriculum and research studies became available for use in teaching rounds, in-service workshops, and national conferences. Group sessions for doctors and nurses explore counter-transference, staff-patient communication, and the impact of stress on oncology staff.[43] The research in and training of doctors and nurses in communication skills has grown exponentially with major contributions in the United Kingdom, Australia, and Canada.

The behavioral medicine movement in the United States began around the late 1970s and brought a second wave of researchers to the psychosocial and behavioral aspects of cancer. Health psychologists brought a new and valuable dimension to this research. They began to study theoretical models of effective coping. They brought cognitive-behavioral models of psychological interventions that have proved widely acceptable and efficacious. The development of theoretical models on which to build psychosocial and behavioral interventions has been critically important. Behavioral psychologists have given cancer prevention its strongest boost by their studies of how to change lifestyle to reduce cancer incidence. Their work in smoking cessation research is seminal and provides insight into promoting lifestyle changes in sun exposure, diet, and exercise to reduce cancer risk.

Several quality-of-life scales were developed in the early 1980s to provide outcome measures in cancer clinical trials.[44–46] Aaronson[45] in Europe (European Organization for Research and Training in Cancer) and Cella and colleagues[46] in the United States have developed extensively used scales comprising a core set of questions with modules to apply to specific tumor sites. Evaluation of a new drug or cancer treatment today assesses not only impact on length of survival and disease-free interval but also quality of life as a quantifiable outcome measure. Combining quality-of-life data with survival data now permits statistical approaches to determine "quality-adjusted life years." Many other instruments have been developed by others for symptom assessment, patients' unmet needs, and screening for psychosocial distress. All add to the range of instruments that are available to the psychosocial or behavioral researcher in cancer.

Other important contributions, in recent years, to psycho-oncology have come from nursing researchers. This cadre of contributors often combine their astute insights gleaned from a nursing background with psychological research methodology to make unique contributions to symptom measurement and control,[47] palliative care,[48] pain management,[49] and psychosocial support[50] and relief of caregiver burden.

As mentioned earlier, social workers were the first, alongside nurses, to attend to the psychological and social problems of cancer patients and their families. They have continued as the "front line" in clinical care and as important researchers in psycho-oncology. Studies of children's and parent's reactions, distress management, caregivers' burden, and especially palliative care, have been contributions.[50-53] *The Journal of Psychosocial Oncology*, established in 1983, was the first journal dedicated to informing the field about current research.

Only in recent years have the contributions to psycho-oncology by clergy and pastoral counselors been acknowledged and has recognition been given to the fact that the psychosocial aspects of dealing with the existential crisis of life-threatening illness and death includes the spiritual and religious domains, reflecting the patients' need to find a tolerable meaning in the situation. In fact, serious illness has been called a "psychospiritual" crisis by some.[54] This newest area of psycho-oncology has received major contributions to methodology by Pargament,[55] a psychologist, and others. Scales to measure patients' spiritual beliefs and reliance on them in coping with cancer have been developed, as have spiritual assessment tools for clinicians. A special issue of *Psycho-Oncology* in 1999[56] reviewed spiritual and religious belief studies in psycho-oncology.

One of the accomplishments in the past decade within psycho-oncology has been the careful investigation of personality, stress and grief, and cancer. Johansson and his group in Denmark explored some of the myths about psychological causes of cancer. Using the Denmark Cancer and Demographic Registry, the group has shown that neither personality, stress, nor grief lead to greater cancer incidence. This work has laid to rest some of the assumptions from the early psychosocial papers in the field (see Chapter 7 by Johansen).

The discrete areas of psycho-oncology, and the remarkably expanded range of interventions, were described in the multiauthored *Handbook of psychooncology* and the first edition textbook *Psycho-oncology*, published in 1989 and 1998, respectively.[1,40] The monthly journal *Psycho-Oncology*, begun in 1992 to cover the psychological, social, and behavioral dimensions of cancer, makes new research findings available from each area and thereby serves as an integrating force as the official journal of the International Psycho-Oncology Society (http://www.ipos-society.org/), the British Psychosocial Oncology Society, and the American Psychosocial Oncology Society (APOS) (http://www.apos-society.org/). The IPOS website has a core curriculum in six languages available free online. A free core curriculum on the APOS website in English provides 20 basic lectures with certification following taking an examination on the lecture.

Psycho-oncology is defined as the subspecialty of oncology dealing with two psychological dimensions: (1) the psychological reactions of patients with cancer and their families at all stages of disease and the stresses on staff; and (2) the psychological, social, and behavioral factors that contribute to cancer cause and survival. This definition has broadened to include concern for survivors and their psychosocial issues.[57-62] The fact that most cancer care has moved to outpatient clinics has increased the family caregiver burden.[63]

Psychiatric complications of palliative care have received more attention as end-of-life care has received a greater focus, especially the study of depression.[64,65] Research has also addressed the clinical evaluation and measurement of the severity of the delirium and its pharmacologic management[66] which remains a major issue with palliative care.[66]

Research model. We developed an integrative research model in the 1990s (Fig. 1–1). It has guided our work since the 1990s. Cancer (and its treatment) is the independent variable; quality of life (in all its dimensions, including psychological) and survival are the outcome variables. The mediating variables (and interventions to affect them) are the core of psycho-oncologic research. Studies explore (1) the personal variables of sociodemography, personality and coping style, beliefs, and prior adjustment; (2) the variables associated with stage of illness, rehabilitation options, illness-related behaviors, and the relationship to the treatment team; (3) the availability of social supports (family, friends, community, and sociocultural influences); and (4) concurrent stresses related to illness that add to the psychological burden, such as loss of a spouse (Fig. 1–2).

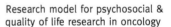

Research model for psychosocial & quality of life research in oncology

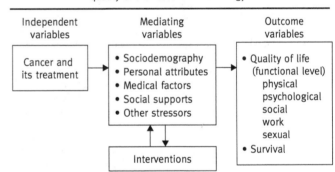

Fig. 1–1. Model of research in psycho-oncology.

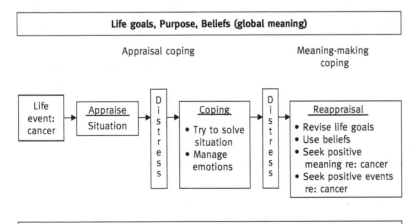

Fig. 1–2. Revised model of Folkman's original Lazarus and Folkman stress and coping paradigm. *Source:* Copyright © [1997] by the American Psychological Association. Adapted with permission. Park CL. Folkman S. Meaning in the context of stress and coping. *Rev Gen Psychol.* 1997;12:115–144. The use of APA information does not imply endorsement by APA.

Standards for psychosocial care and clinical practice guidelines. These changes are occurring at the time when the range of psychosocial, psychotherapeutic, and behavioral interventions is broader than it has ever been.[67] As efficacy has been shown for psychosocial interventions, it has become possible to develop standards and guidelines.[68,69]

NCCN standard and guidelines. In 1997, the National Comprehensive Cancer Network (NCCN), an organization of 18 comprehensive cancer centers, established a multidisciplinary panel which developed the first standard for psychosocial care in cancer and clinical practice guidelines for the disciplines providing supportive services.[70] The standard, similar to that developed for pain, requires that all patients be evaluated initially and monitored for the level and nature of their psychosocial "distress" (a word chosen to be least stigmatizing). A rapid screening tool is recommended for use in the waiting room given verbally or by pen and paper or computer based, called the Distress Thermometer (0–10 scale in a thermometer form). Tested against the Hospital Anxiety and Depression Scale (HADS), it was acceptable to patients and staff and identifies a score of 4 or greater as equivalent to "caseness" using the HADS scale. The decision-tree guideline provides that a score of 4 or more is the algorithm that triggers the oncology staff to refer the patient to mental health, social work, or pastoral counseling for further evaluation, depending on the nature of the problem. A multicenter trial for validity and feasibility conducted by Jacobsen and colleagues, confirmed their validity.[71] Mitchell has reported a meta-analysis "ultra short screening tools," confirming that they work as well as a first broad screen, best followed by a second assessment to determine the cause and intervention needed.[72]

The American College of Surgeons' Commission on Standards and the Association of Community Cancer Centers adapted their standards to incorporate these concepts.

In Australia, Canada, and the United Kingdom, evidence-based clinical practice guidelines have been developed. In Canada, Bultz has worked with the Cancer Advocacy Council to make "distress" the sixth vital sign after pain—assuring that it will be a part of routine care. The Institute of Medicine (IOM) Report on Care for the Whole Patient adds weight to these policy changes and suggested that a new quality of care dimension has been added.[69] On the basis of the review of evidence, psychosocial interventions are efficacious and screening of all cancer patients for distress/psychosocial needs is necessary to meet the new standards.

Institute of Medicine: standard and guidelines. In 2007, the IOM presented the report from a 16-member committee charged with exploring the barriers to psychosocial care in cancer and other chronic diseases. The report of the IOM "Cancer Care for the Whole Patient: Meeting Psychosocial Health Needs" in 2007 is a landmark study which confirms the evidence base for psychological, psychiatric, psychosocial, and psychopharmacologic interventions.[69] The standard mandated by the IOM is that quality cancer care today demands that the psychosocial needs of patients be integrated into routine cancer care. The credibility given to psycho-oncology by the report will have an impact on training, clinical care, and policy. An alliance of 9 professional organizations and 25 have joined to ensure that there is dissemination and implementation of the guidelines. A simple model is recommended: screening for psychosocial needs, developing a treatment plan, and referral to a program resource for help (see Chapter 97).

CONCLUSION

As we approach the second decade of the new millennium, the good news is that a psycho-oncology unit exists in virtually all cancer centers and community hospitals; these units, ideally, are composed of a multidisciplinary group that offers psychosocial services and maintains attention to these issues in patient care. However, there remains a dearth of these resources in the busy outpatient oncology offices and clinics where *most* cancer care is given.

The training of psycho-oncologists and the encouragement of young clinicians and investigators into the field remains critically important to address clinical and research needs worldwide. Die-Trill in Madrid and Alarcon in Columbia have written textbooks in Spanish and Die-Trill has a graduate program in psycho-oncology for psychologists.[73] Other countries have similar programs. Trainees from psychiatry are needed in psycho-oncology, particularly in palliative care and symptom control. Health psychologists form the central cadre of investigators, especially in cancer prevention, early detection, genetic testing, and the emerging field of psychoneuroimmunology, where the possible links to cancer risk and survival are being explored. This pool of investigators is small and funding limits jeopardize it.

Psycho-oncology is almost 35 years old, and much progress has been made in that short period. The discipline has an accepted place at the table within the oncology community, both in clinical care and in research. The traditional domain of inpatient consultation has expanded greatly along the continuum of cancer care. Our present body of information rests on a strong literature database which was recognized in the recent IOM Reports.[69,74] Implementation of what we know *now* could greatly improve the psychological well-being and quality of life of patients. As noted by Greer,[75] "The most immediately important task of psycho-oncology is to close the yawning gap between current knowledge and actual clinical care of patients."

REFERENCES

1. Holland JC, ed. *Psycho-oncology.* New York, NY: Oxford University Press; 1998.
2. Tolstoy L. The death of Ivan Ilyich. In: Maude L, Maude A, trans. *Great short works of Leo Tolstoy.* New York, NY: Harper & Row; 1967. Original work published in 1886.
3. American Cancer Society. *Fact book for the medical and related professional.* New York, NY: American Cancer Society; 1980.
4. Shimkin M. *Contrary to nature.* Washington, DC: US Department of Health and Human Services, Public Health Service; 1977.
5. Patterson J. *The dread disease: cancer and modern American culture.* Cambridge, MA: Harvard University Press; 1987.
6. Holland JC. History of psycho-oncology: overcoming attitudinal and conceptual barriers. *Psychosom Med.* 2002;64:206–221.
7. Fabrega H Jr. Psychiatric stigma in the classical and medieval period: a review of the literature. *Compr Psychiatry.* 1990;31:289–306.
8. Fabrega H Jr. The culture and history of psychiatric stigma in early modern and modern western societies: a review of recent literature. *Compr Psychiatry.* 1991;32:97–119.
9. Lipowski ZJ. Consultation-liaison psychiatry at century's end. *Psychosomatics.* 1992;33:128–133.
10. Henry GW. Some modern aspects of psychiatry in general hospital practice. *Am J Psychiatry.* 1929;86:481–499.
11. Blumberg EM, West PM, Ellis FW. A possible relationship between psychological factors and human cancer. *Psychosom Med.* 1954;16:277–286.
12. Stephenson JH, Grace WJ. Life stress and cancer of the cervix. *Psychosom Med.* 1954;16:287–294.
13. Reznikoff M. Psychological factors in breast cancer: a preliminary study of some personality trends in patients with cancer of the breast. *Psychosom Med.* 1955;17:96–108.
14. Fisher S, Cleveland SE. Relationship of body image to site of cancer. *Psychosom Med.* 1956;18:304–309.
15. Greene W, Miller G. Psychological factors and reticuloendothelial disease: IV. Observations on a group of children and adolescents with leukemia: an interpretation of disease development in terms of the mother child unit. *Psychosom Med.* 1958;20:124–144.
16. Hackett TP. The psychiatrist: in the mainstream or on the banks of medicine? *Am J Psychiatry.* 1977;134:432–434.
17. Mason JW. The scope of psychoendocrine research. *Psychosom Med.* 1968;30:565–575.
18. Ader R, Cohen N. Behaviorally conditioned immunosuppression. *Psychosom Med.* 1975;37:333–340.
19. Kornblith AB, Herndon JE II, Zuckerman E, et al. Comparison of psychosocial adaptation of advanced stage Hodgkin's disease and acute leukemia survivors: cancer and *Leukemia* Group B. *Ann Oncol.* 1998;9:297–306.
20. Engel G. The biopsychosocial model and medical education: who are to be the teachers? *N Engl J Med.* 1982;306:802–805.
21. Spiegel D, Kraemer H, Bloom JR, Gottheil D. Effect of psychosocial treatment on survival of patients with metastatic breast cancer. *Lancet.* 1989;2:888–891.
22. Kiecolt-Glaser J, Glaser R. Psychological influences on immunity. *Psychosomatics.* 1986;27:621–624.

23. Bovbjerg DH, Valdimarsdottir HB. Psychoneuroimmunology: implications for psycho-oncology. In: Holland JC, ed. *Psycho-oncology*. New York: Oxford University Press; 1998:125–134.

24. Brown TM. The rise and fall of psychosomatic medicine [lecture]. *New York Acad Med*. November 29, 2000.

25. Weiner H. Praise be to psychosomatic medicine. *Psychosom Med*. 1999;61:259–262.

26. Eissler KR. *The psychiatrist and the dying patient*. New York, NY: International Universities Press; 1955.

27. Norton J. Treatment of a dying patient. *Psychoanal Study Child*. 1963;18:541–560.

28. Abrams RD, Finesinger JE. Guilt reactions in patients with cancer. *Cancer*. 1953;6:474–482.

29. Shands HC, Finesinger JE, Cobb S, Abrams RD. Psychological mechanisms in patients with cancer. *Cancer*. 1951;4:1159–1170.

30. Sutherland AM, Orbach CE, Dyk RB, Bard M. The psychological impact of cancer and cancer surgery. I. Adaptation to the dry colostomy: preliminary report and summary of findings. *Cancer*. 1952;5:857–872.

31. Bard M, Sutherland AM. The psychological impact of cancer and its treatment. IV. Adaptation to radical mastectomy. *Cancer*. 1955;8:656–672.

32. Oken D. What to tell cancer patients: a study of medical attitudes. *JAMA*. 1961;175:1120–1128.

33. Novack DH, Plumer R, Smith RL, Ochitill H, Morrow GR, Bennett JM. Changes in physicians' attitudes toward telling the cancer patient. *JAMA*. 1979;241:897–900.

34. Holland JC, Geary N, Marchini A, Tross S. An international survey of physician attitudes and practice in regard to revealing the diagnosis of cancer. *Cancer Invest*. 1987;5:151–154.

35. Kubler-Ross E. *On death and dying*. New York, NY: Macmillan; 1969.

36. Rollin B. *First, you cry*. New York, NY: Harper-Perennial Library; 2000.

37. Rowland JH, Glidwell OJ, Sibley RF, et al. Effects of different forms of central nervous system prophylaxis on neuropsychologic function in childhood leukemia. *J Clin Oncol*. 1984;2:1327–1336.

38. Kornblith AB, Holland JC. Model for quality of life research from the Cancer and Leukemia Group B: the telephone interview, conceptual approach to measurement, and theoretical framework. *J Natl Cancer Inst*. 1996;88:661–667.

39. Cullen JW, Fox BH, Isom RN, eds. *Cancer: the behavioral dimensions*. Washington, DC: National Cancer Institute; 1976.

40. Holland JC, Rowland JH, eds. *Handbook of psychooncology: psychological care of the patient with cancer*. New York, NY: Oxford University Press; 1989.

41. Massie MJ, Holland JC. Overview of normal reactions and prevalence of psychiatric disorders. In: Holland JC, Rowland JH, eds. *Handbook of psychooncology: psychological care of the patient with cancer*. New York, NY: Oxford University Press; 1989:273–282.

42. Derogatis LR, Morrow GR, Fetting J, et al. The prevalence of psychiatric disorders among cancer patients. *JAMA*. 1983;249:751–757.

43. Artiss LK, Levine AS. Doctor-patient relation in severe illness: a seminar for oncology fellows. *N Engl J Med*. 1973;288:1210–1214.

44. Schipper H, Clinch J, McMurray A, Levitt M. Measuring the quality of life of cancer patients: the Functional Living Index-Cancer: development and validation. *J Clin Oncol*. 1984;2:472–483.

45. Aaronson NK. Methodologic issues in assessing the quality of life of cancer patients. *Cancer*. 1991;67:844–850.

46. Cella DF, Tulsky DS, Gray G, et al. The Functional Assessment of Cancer Therapy (FACT) scale: development and validation of the general measure. *J Clin Oncol*. 1993;11:570–579.

47. Coyle N, Layman-Goldstein M, Passik S, Fishman B, Portenoy R. Development and validation of a patient needs assessment tool (PNAT) for oncology physicians. *Cancer Nurs*. 1996;19:81–92.

48. Schacter S, Coyle N. Palliative home care—impact on families. In: Holland JC, ed. *Psycho-oncology*. New York, NY: Oxford University Press; 1998.

49. Ferrell BR, Dean GE, Grant M, Coluzzi P. An institutional commitment to pain management. *J Clin Oncol*. 1995;13:2158–2165.

50. Fawzy FI, Fawzy NW, Hyun CS, et al. Malignant melanoma. Effects of an early structured psychiatric intervention, coping, and affective state on recurrence and survival 6 years later. *Arch Gen Psychiatry*. 1993;50:681–689.

51. Zabora JR. Screening procedures for psychosocial distress. In: Holland JC, ed. *Psycho-oncology*. New York, NY: Oxford University Press; 1998:653–661.

52. Jacobs J, Ostroff J, Steinglass P. Family therapy: a systems approach to cancer care. In: Holland JC, ed. *Psycho-oncology*. New York, NY: Oxford University Press; 1998:994–1003.

53. Zabora JR, Fetting JH, Shanley VB, Seddon CF, Enterline JP. Predicting conflict with staff among families of cancer patients during prolonged hospitalizations. *J Psychosoc Oncol*. 1989;7:103–111.

54. Kass JD, Friedman R, Leserman J, Zuttermeister PC, Benson H. Health outcomes and a new index of spiritual experience. *J Sc Stud Rel*. 1991;30: 203–211.

55. Pargament KI. *The psychology of religion and coping: theory, research, practice*. New York, NY: Guilford Press; 1997.

56. Lederberg M, Fitchett G, Russak SM. Spirituality and coping with cancer. *Psycho-Oncology*. 1999;8:375–466.

57. Folkman S. Positive psychological states and coping with severe stress. *Soc Sci Med*. 1997;45:1207–1221.

58. Koocher GP, O'Malley JE. *Damocles' syndrome: psychological consequences of surviving childhood cancer*. New York, NY: McGraw-Hill; 1981.

59. Andrykowski MA, Cordova MJ. Factors associated with PTSD symptoms following treatment for breast cancer: test of the Andersen model. *J Trauma Stress*. 1998;11:189–203.

60. Jacobsen PB, Bovbjerg DH, Schwartz M, Hudis CA, Gilewski TA, Norton L. Conditioned emotional distress in women receiving chemotherapy for breast cancer. *J Consult Clin Psychol*. 1995;63:108–114.

61. Jacobsen PB, Widows MR, Hann DM, Andrykowski MA, Kronish LE, Fields KK. Posttraumatic stress disorder symptoms after bone marrow transplantation for breast cancer. *Psychosom Med*. 1998;60:366–371.

62. Auchincloss S. Sexual dysfunction in cancer patients: issues in evaluation and treatment. In: Holland JC, ed. *Handbook of psychooncology: psychological care of the patient with cancer*. New York, NY: Oxford University Press; 1989:383–413.

63. Baider L, Cooper C, Kaplan De-Nour A. *Cancer and the family*. Chichester, England: John Wiley & Sons; 2000.

64. Chochinov HM, Wilson KG, Enns M, Lander S. Depression, hopelessness, and suicidal ideation in the terminally ill. *Psychosomatics*. 1998;39:366–370.

65. Chochinov HM, Wilson KG, Enns M, et al. Desire for death in the terminally ill. *Am J Psychiatry*. 1995;152:1185–1191.

66. Breitbart W, Cohen KR. Delirium. In: Holland JC, ed. *Psycho-oncology*. New York, NY: Oxford University Press; 1998:564–575.

67. Jacobsen PB, Jim HS. Psychosocial interventions for anxiety and depression in adult cancer patients: achievements and challenges. *CA Cancer J Clin*. 2008;58:214–230.

68. Meyer T, Mark M. Effects of psychosocial interventions with adult cancer patients: a meta-analysis of randomized experiments. *Health Psychol*. 1995;14:101–108.

69. IOM. *Cancer care for the whole patient*. Washington, DC: The National Academies Press; 2007.

70. Holland JC. Update. NCCN practice guidelines for the management of psychosocial distress. *Oncology*. 1999;(Suppl 13):459–507.

71. Jacobsen P, Donovan K, Trask M, et al. Screening for psychological distress in ambulatory cancer patients: a multicenter evaluation of the distress thermometer. *Cancer*. 2005;103:1494–1502.

72. Mitchell AJ, Coyne JC. Do ultra-short screening instruments accurately detect depression in primary care? *Br J Gen Pract*. 2007;57 144–151.

73. Maria Die-Trill JH. A model curriculum for training in psycho-oncology. *Psycho-Oncology*. 1995;4:169–182.

74. IOM. *From cancer patient to cancer survivor: lost in transition*. Washington, DC: The National Academies Press; 2005.

75. Greer S. Psycho-oncology: its aims, achievements and future tasks. *Psycho-Oncology*. 1994;3:87–101.

PART II

Behavioral and Psychological Factors in Cancer Risk

Paul B. Jacobsen, ED

CHAPTER 2

Tobacco Use and Cessation

Thomas H. Brandon and Marina Unrod

TOBACCO AND CANCER

Each year over 185,000 Americans die of cancer caused by tobacco smoking.[1] Smoking is responsible for approximately 40% of all cancer deaths among men, and 26% of cancer deaths among women. Lung cancer alone now causes approximately 140,000 smoking-attributable deaths annually in the United States. Cigarette smoking accounts for 89% of all lung cancer mortalities, and also contributes significantly to mortality rates for oral cancer, and cancers of the esophagus, larynx, bladder, stomach, pancreas, kidney, and cervix. In addition to cancer, smoking contributes significantly to coronary heart disease, chronic obstructive pulmonary disease, cardiovascular disease, stroke, and ulcer disease. Indeed, 21% of all U.S. deaths can be attributed to smoking.[1] From the individual perspective, a given smoker has about a 50% chance of dying from smoking, with the average smoker living 10 years less than a non-smoker.[2] Use of smokeless tobacco (chew, snuff) is also associated with increased risk of oral cancer and premature death. But because tobacco smoking has much higher prevalence as well as relative risk, this chapter will focus on smoking.[3] Nevertheless, patients should be advised to cease all forms of tobacco use.

Smoking cessation is associated with decreased mortality and morbidity from cancer and other diseases. Stopping smoking at age 30 restores 9 years of life expectancy, whereas stopping at age 60 still restores an expected 3 years of life, compared to continuing to smoke.[2] Although quitting smoking does not appear to reduce the absolute risk of lung cancer, it significantly retards the steeply increasing risk associated with continued smoking.[4] Fig. 2–1 illustrates the reduced lung cancer mortality among men associated with quitting smoking at various ages, compared to continuing to smoke. Thus, great potential for cancer prevention lies with efforts toward long-term cessation of smoking. In this chapter, we begin by reviewing the evidence-based treatments for tobacco use and dependence, emphasizing primarily qualitative and meta-analytic reviews. In particular, we draw upon the 2008 update of the U.S. Public Health Service's Clinical Practice Guideline, Treating Tobacco Use and Dependence.[5] This update, the first since 2000, was released in May 2008, and is based on a review of 8700 research articles, with treatment recommendations derived from meta-analyses of most treatment modalities. We then discuss special issues of relevance for treating cancer patients. And finally, we address the accelerating trend of medical centers enacting tobacco-free campus policies.

TREATMENT OF TOBACCO USE AND DEPENDENCE

Tobacco dependence has multiple motivational influences within and across individual smokers.[6] Among these are physical dependence on nicotine (abstinence produces craving and aversive withdrawal symptoms), tolerance to the toxic effects of cigarette smoke, operant and classical conditioning processes, environmental and social factors, cognitive expectancies about the benefits of smoking, perceived mood regulation from smoking, possible cognitive benefits of nicotine (i.e., to attention and concentration), and desire for weight control. Given the complexity of the factors influencing smoking, it is not surprising that single treatment approaches have limited success, with the best long-term outcomes obtained from multimodal treatments. In this section, we will review pharmacological interventions, followed by social/behavioral interventions, broadly defined, and finally discuss combination treatments.

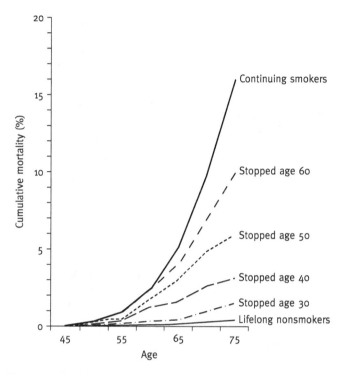

Fig. 2–1. Effect of stopping smoking at various ages on the cumulative risk of death from lung cancer up to age 75, at death rates for men in the United Kingdom in 1990. Reproduced from Richard Peto, Sarah Darby, Harz Deo, et al. Smoking, smoking cessation, and lung cancer in the UK since 1950: combination of national statistics with two case-control studies. *BMJ.* 2000;321:323–329. With permission from BMJ Publishing Group Ltd.

Pharmacotherapy. There are currently seven FDA-approved pharmacotherapies for smoking cessation, and two second-line medications that are not FDA-approved for treating tobacco dependence. All nine of these medications have been found to approximately double the odds of long-term abstinence (with one, varenicline, tripling the odds), and the Clinical Practice Guidelines recommends that pharmacotherapy be routinely offered to smokers to quit.[5] The seven first-line pharmacotherapies are summarized in Table 2–1.

Nicotine replacement therapies. Nicotine replacement therapy (NRT) aids smoking cessation by partially replacing nicotine in circulation, thereby reducing nicotine cravings and symptoms of nicotine withdrawal (e.g., depression, anxiety, irritability and other negative effect, sleep disturbance, difficulty concentrating, hunger, and weight gain) and possibly reducing the reinforcement derived from any cigarettes smoked. Five types of NRT have FDA approval: chewing gum, transdermal patches, intranasal spray, inhaler devices, and lozenges. In general, NRT is used during the first 8–12 weeks of abstinence, when

Table 2-1. FDA-approved pharmacotherapies

Medication	Availability	Dosage	Duration	Side effects	Contraindications
Nicotine gum	OTC	<25 cpd: 2 mg gum ≥25 cigarettes / day: 4 mg gum Use up to 24 pieces/day	Up to 12 weeks	Mouth soreness; dyspepsia	
Nicotine patch	OTC	21 mg patch for 4 weeks; 14 mg/patch for 2 weeks; 7 mg patch for 2 weeks	8 weeks total	Skin irritation; insomnia	Caution in unstable cardiac disease
Nicotine nasal spray	Prescription	1–2 sprays/hour, up to 40 doses daily	3–6 months	Nasal irritation	Caution with asthma, rhinitis, sinusitis, and nasal polyps
Nicotine inhaler	Prescription	6–16 cartridges/ day	Up to 6 months	Oral cavity irritation	
Nicotine lozenge	OTC	2 mg and 4 mg available Use up to 20 pieces/day	Up to 12 weeks	Nausea, hiccups, heartburn, insomnia, mouth irritation	
Bupropion SR	Prescription	150 mg daily for 3 days, then 150 mg twice daily Begin at least 1 week before quitting smoking	Up to 12 weeks (mainte-nance up to 6 months)	Insomnia, dry mouth	Caution with history of seizures, eating disorders, alco-holism, significant head trauma
Varenicline	Prescription	0.5 mg daily for 3 days; 0.5 mg twice daily for 4 days; 1 mg twice daily thereafter Begin at least 1 week before quitting smoking	Up to 12 weeks (mainte-nance up to 3 months)	Nausea, sleep disturbance Anecdotal reports of agitation, depression, suicidality Use caution while driving	Monitor for agitation, depressed mood, behavior change, suicidal ideation

ABBREVIATIONS: FDA, Food and Drug Administration; OTC, Over-the-counter
Adapted from Fiore et al. (2008).[5]

nicotine withdrawal symptoms are greatest, and they deliver approximately 1/3–1/2 of the plasma nicotine levels achieved by smoking.[7] Of the five NRT delivery methods, the nicotine nasal spray reaches its peak concentration most rapidly, whereas the transdermal patch provides the slowest, but most consistent serum nicotine levels over the course of a day. The gum, patch, and lozenge are available over the counter in the United States, whereas the nasal spray and inhaler remain available only by prescription.

Meta-analyses reported in the Clinical Practice Guideline indicate roughly equivalent efficacies for the five NRT products, with odds ratios ranging from 1.5 (for nicotine gum) to 2.3 (for nasal spray) compared to placebo.[5] Estimated 6-month abstinence rates are approximately 20%–25%. Although patients are usually instructed to begin NRT use when they cease smoking, some recent research suggests that abstinence rates may be further increased by beginning use before making a quit attempt.[8,9] However, this approach is not yet recommended by the guideline.

Because NRT delivers nicotine without the harmful by-products of smoked tobacco, it is considered a far safer alternative to smoking. Each product is associated with specific contraindications and cautions primarily related to its particular mode of drug delivery. Most notable, however, is that none of these products have been approved for use in pregnant women.

Bupropion SR (Zyban®). Bupropion was the first non-nicotine medication to be approved by the Food and Drug Administration (FDA) for treating tobacco dependence. Also marketed as an atypical antidepressant (Wellbutrin'), bupropion approximately doubles tobacco abstinence rates compared to placebo. It attenuates nicotine withdrawal and cigarette cravings, and can reduce postcessation weight gain. The practice guideline reports an average odds ratio of 2.0, and an abstinence rate of approximately 24%.[5]

Bupropion's mechanism of action in not fully understood, but it appears to inhibit the neuronal reuptake of dopamine and norepinephrine—key neurotransmitters in the maintenance of nicotine dependence.[10] It may also have antagonistic effects on nicotinic receptors, attenuating perceived satisfaction from smoking. Despite its antidepressant properties, it is not differentially effective for smokers with a history of depression.[11]

To reach steady-state blood levels before quitting smoking, the smoker should begin using bupropion SR 1 week before the target quit date. Contraindications include a history of seizure disorders or factors known to increase the risk of seizures (e.g., bulimia or anorexia nervosa, serious head trauma, alcoholism). The safety of bupropion during pregnancy has not been established.

Varenicline (Chantix™). Varenicline is the most recently approved pharmacotherapy for treating nicotine dependence. It is an orally administered partial agonist of α4β2 nicotinic acetylcholine receptors (nAChRs). Varenicline appears to reduce nicotine cravings and withdrawal symptoms, and its agonistic properties may attenuate the reinforcing effects of smoking, including perceived satisfaction. Similar to bupropion, varenicline use should be initiated 1 week before the target quit date. Current evidence suggests that it is the most effective of the smoking cessation medications, with the practice guideline reporting an average odds ratio of 3.1, producing 33% abstinence.[5] It has outperformed bupropion in head-to-head studies.[12,13]

The main adverse effect of varenicline is mild to moderate nausea. However, because of anecdotal postmarketing reports of changes in behavior, agitation, depressed mood, suicidal ideation, and actual suicidal behavior, the FDA issued an advisory in early 2008, and product labeling was revised to advise patients and caregivers that the patient should stop taking CHANTIX and contact their healthcare provider immediately if agitation, depressed mood, or changes in behavior that are not typical for them are observed, or if the patient develops suicidal ideation or suicidal thoughts. Varenicline is not approved for use with pregnant women.

Second-Line agents. The Clinical Practice Guideline lists two pharmacotherapies that have demonstrated efficacy levels in the same range as the seven FDA-approved medications.[5] These include clonidine (FDA-approved as an antihypertensive) and nortriptyline (an antidepressant). Their respective estimated odds ratios are 2.1 and 1.8, with associated abstinence rates of 23%–25%. However, because these medications are not FDA-approved for smoking cessation, and because of prominent side effects (e.g., sedation and dizziness for clonidine, and risk of arrhythmias and postural hypotension for nortriptyline), the guideline classifies them as second-line agents to be tried only if the seven FDA-approved medications are either contraindicated or found ineffective for a given patient.

Combination pharmacotherapies. Recent research has tested the efficacy of combining different forms of pharmacotherapy. The general model has been to combine a long-acting, relatively stable medication, such as the nicotine patch, with a shorter acting medication that can be used ad lib. In this manner, both tonic and phasic nicotine cravings and withdrawal symptoms can be addressed. The most recent Clinical Practice Guideline concluded that the combination of nicotine patch with gum, nasal spray, or inhaler had evidence of significant efficacy, as did the combination of the patch and bupropion SR.[5]

Social/behavioral treatments. The nonpharmacological therapies described in this section span a wide range of intensity and duration, from minimal self-help interventions to intensive individual counseling. Clinicians should be aware of the availability of these options and be willing to refer patients for what they are unable to provide themselves.

Self-help. Self-help refers to materials that can be provided to smokers, such as pamphlets, booklets, or audio–visual media. Their primary advantages are low cost and ease of distribution. Unfortunately, the efficacy of self-help materials appears to be quite limited. Meta-analyses for both the Clinical Practice Guideline[5] and a Cochrane Review[14] indicated that self-help materials improve cessation rates by about 1% compared to no-treatment controls. Self-help materials can also be "tailored" to the characteristics of individual smokers. The Cochrane meta-analysis found that tailored materials produced slightly superior outcomes over standard, nontailored materials. However, many of the original studies suffered methodological and design limitations, and there is also recent evidence that the benefits of tailoring may be due to the superficial personalization of the materials rather than to the theory-based tailored content.[15,16]

In contrast to the very modest efficacy of self-help materials designed to aid initial smoking cessation, two controlled studies indicate that print materials may have greater efficacy for preventing smoking relapse when provided to smokers shortly after they quit smoking.[17,18] These *Forever Free* booklets produced significant reduction in relapse through 2 years of follow-up, and appear to be highly cost-effective.

Telephone quitlines. The growth of smoking cessation quitlines over the past two decades has been exponential. They exist in all U.S. states, the District of Columbia, and five territories. One number (1–800-QUIT-NOW) serves as a central access point that automatically routes calls to the appropriate state or federal quitline service. In addition, all Canadian provinces now have smoking quitlines, and they have expanded to Mexico, South America, Europe, South Africa, Australia, New Zealand, and some Asian countries. A 2004–2005 analysis of state quitlines found an average utilization rate of about 1%.[19] In other words, approximately 400,000 smokers called state quitlines during that 12-month period, and the Centers for Disease Control (CDC) advised funding quitlines with the goal of reaching up to 10% of smokers annually.[20]

Quitline services differ in the amount and frequency of counseling offered, the provision of ancillary materials, referrals to local smoking cessation agencies, the provision of free or subsidized pharmacotherapies, and whether calls are proactive (call-out), reactive (call-in), or both. Quitlines have the advantage of providing more personal and intensive help than self-help materials, while also having greater potential reach than face-to-face counseling. All quitlines report providing some degree of standard cognitive-behavioral counseling.[19]

Two recent meta-analyses concluded that quitlines were efficacious, with overall odds ratios of 1.2–1.6 compared to control conditions, which translates into differential long-term abstinence rates of at least 3%–5%.[5,21]

Brief interventions. Healthcare providers have the opportunity to deliver relatively brief face-to-face interventions, although studies indicate that no more than 50% of physicians give their patients advice about quitting smoking, and psychologists are similarly negligent.[22,23] Meta-analyses have indicated that physician advice increases abstinence rates by approximately 2.3%–2.5%.[5,14] Because 70% of smokers visit their physician each year, the potential cumulative effect of even this small effect is sizable. Moreover, there is a dose–response relationship between contact time and abstinence outcomes, with minimal counseling (<3 minutes) yielding 13.4% abstinence, low intensity counseling (3–10 minutes) yielding 16.0%, and higher intensity counseling (>10 minutes) yielding 22.1% abstinence. Abstinence rates also increase with the number of counseling meetings and/or the number of clinician types delivering the cessation messages.[5] The basic content of brief interventions (e.g., the "Five A's") will be covered in a later section of this chapter.

Intensive interventions. The most intensive interventions tend to be multisession treatments typically offered through smoking cessation clinics, in either group or individual formats. Of the empirically supported intensive interventions, the most common approach is cognitive-behavioral counseling. Key elements of this approach include patient education regarding the nature of tobacco dependence and withdrawal, advice for surviving the withdrawal syndrome without smoking, identifying high-risk situations ("triggers") that produce urges to smoke, teaching and practicing cognitive and behavioral responses for coping with urges, discussion of long-term risk factors such as depression and weight gain, and discussion of how to respond in the event of an initial "slip" or "lapse." The most recent Clinical Practice Guideline classifies this general approach as "Practical Counseling," but it has also been labeled Coping Skills Training, General Problem Solving, Multicomponent Behavior Therapy, and Relapse Prevention Training. It usually involves multiple sessions over multiple weeks, and may begin before the target quit date. It is offered in both groups or individual formats, and therapy manuals exist.[24] The Clinical Practice Guideline analysis found Practical Counseling to be effective, with an odds ratio of 1.5 compared to no counseling and an average abstinence rate of 16.2% compared to 11.2%.[5] Other analyses and reviews have also supported this general approach.[25–27]

In addition to Practical Counseling, the guideline also finds evidence for Intratreatment Social Support, and it therefore recommends providing support and encouragement as part of treatment. Although analyzed as a separate treatment approach, in fact support and encouragement would normally be incorporated into any respectable form of cognitive-behavioral counseling. Although the guideline meta-analysis of behavioral therapies (which was not updated from the earlier, 2000, edition of the guideline) also found empirical support for two other treatment approaches—aversive smoking, and garnering extra-treatment social support—it did not recommend these approaches due to more recent literature that cast doubt on their effectiveness, and in the case of aversive smoking, the side effects of the treatment.

Another behavioral approach, which is not included in the guideline but has garnered empirical support, is scheduled reduced smoking, in which the therapist (using a computer algorithm) determines when a patient can have a cigarette, gradually reducing the number smoked per day. The notion is that this process dissociates smoking from personally relevant cues and periods of potentially high reinforcement from tobacco use. This treatment was found to produce 44% abstinence at 1 year, which was superior to multiple control conditions.[28] In a review of health-related interventions, scheduled reduced smoking was listed as a "possibly efficacious" treatment that warranted additional research.[27]

Combining counseling and pharmacotherapy. A key conclusion of the most recent guideline is that the combination of counseling and medication is more effective than either alone in producing long-term tobacco abstinence. Moreover, as noted earlier, higher abstinence rates tend to be produced with more intensive counseling. Thus, the guideline meta-analysis produced an estimated abstinence rate of approximately 33%, when medication was combined with nine or more sessions of counseling, compared to 22% when no more than one counseling session was provided. Conversely, the guideline reported an odds ratio of 1.7 for the combination of medication and counseling, compared to counseling alone.[5] Earlier reviews have reached similar conclusions.[29] Counseling and medication appear to provide complimentary benefits. Whereas medication reduces withdrawal symptoms and craving, counseling can teach cognitive and behavioral coping strategies and provide valuable social support. Therefore, whenever medication is recommended or provided to patients, they should also be offered counseling or given a referral for counseling.

How clinicians can intervene. The Clinical Practice Guideline is highly relevant to clinicians who provide cancer prevention and treatment services. The office visit presents a critical teachable moment for delivery of smoking cessation interventions within the context of educating patients about the link between tobacco use and cancer. Because motivation to quit smoking increases following cancer diagnosis, clinicians can seize this unique window of opportunity to intervene and assist in the cessation process.[30–32] The five essential steps to screening, assessing, and treating tobacco dependence are referred to as the "5 A's" (*Ask, Advise, Assess, Assist,* and *Arrange*), which the Guideline recommends implementing with every patient who uses tobacco.[5] Special cancer-related treatment issues will be discussed in the next section.

Effective identification and assessment of tobacco use status is the first step in treating tobacco dependence. To that end, the guideline recommends that clinicians systematically identify and document tobacco use status for every patient at every visit (*Ask*); urge every tobacco user to quit in a clear, strong, and personalized manner (*Advise*); and determine the willingness of all tobacco users to make a quit attempt at this time

Table 2–2. Key elements of assisting patients with quitting smoking

Key elements	Specific strategies
Assisting patients willing to quit	
Help with a quit plan	Set a quit date, ideally within 2 weeks
	Advise to tell family, friends, co-workers, and gather support
	Help anticipate challenges
	Advise to remove all tobacco products from patient's environment
	Discuss medication options
Provide practical counseling and support	Strive for total abstinence and build on past quit attempts
	Develop coping skills: anticipate, avoid, or prepare for triggers, reduce stress, exercise, take deep breaths, substitute, and keep mouth busy
	Avoid or limit alcohol consumption
	Encourage other smokers in the household to quit or not smoke in patient's presence
	Offer a supportive clinical environment and encouragement
Provide basic information	Provide information about withdrawal symptoms and effects of smoking cessation medications
	Provide supplementary materials, including information on quitlines
	Offer referral to comprehensive program for patients in need of more intensive treatment
Assisting patients unwilling to quit	
Enhance motivation to quit by discussing the "5 R's"	**Relevance**—Why may quitting be particularly helpful to this patient?
	Risks—What are the negative consequences of smoking?
	Rewards—What are the benefits of quitting?
	Roadblocks—What are the barriers to quitting? How can the barriers be addressed?
	Repetition—Repeat the motivational intervention at every office visit

Adapted from Fiore et al. (2008).[5]

(*Assess*). With respect to *Assisting* tobacco users, the Guideline offers specific strategies to guide clinicians in the provision of brief interventions. For patients willing to quit, clinicians should assist in developing a quit plan, provide practical counseling and support, offer pharmacotherapy, and provide supplementary materials. Finally, they should *Arrange* for follow-up contact, preferably within the first week after the quit date. Patients interested in more intensive treatment, particularly those with a history of multiple unsuccessful quit attempts, should be referred to a comprehensive smoking cessation program or a telephone quitline. For patients unwilling to make a quit attempt, clinicians should provide a brief motivational intervention designed to increase future quit attempts. This intervention is captured by the "5 R's": *Relevance, Risks, Rewards, Roadblocks,* and *Repetition.* See Table 2–2 for key aspects of assisting patients.

SPECIAL ISSUES WITH CANCER PATIENTS

With advances in cancer treatments, the number of cancer survivors is significantly increasing, emphasizing the importance of improving health outcomes and quality of life within this high-risk population.[33] Cigarette smoking places individuals with a cancer history at risk for multiple health problems. There is a growing body of evidence that smoking following cancer diagnosis has a negative impact on cancer treatment efficacy, treatment-related complications and side effects, cancer recurrence and second malignancies, and overall survival.[33] In this section, we will describe the benefits of smoking cessation in cancer patients, review factors associated with cessation and relapse, and summarize the current knowledge regarding cessation interventions targeted to cancer patients.

Benefits of quitting smoking. Continued smoking following cancer diagnosis has been found to diminish treatment effects of radiation therapy, chemotherapy, and surgery.[34-36] In addition, smoking contributes to increased occurrence of treatment complications such as infection, poor wound healing, and exacerbated side effects, such as oral mucositis.[37,38] Cancer and treatment-related suppression of immune function and weight loss may be exacerbated in smokers due to nicotine's suppressive effects on natural killer cell activity and appetite.[39,40]

Smoking after cancer diagnosis has a negative impact on overall survival in patients with lung, head and neck, prostate, breast, and cervical cancer.[34,41-44] Studies have also shown that failure to quit smoking upon initial diagnosis of lung or head and neck cancer is associated with higher risk of second malignant or primary tumors.[45,46]

Smoking cessation results in several health benefits among cancer patients. Medical complications can be diminished when patients stop smoking at least 4 weeks before surgery.[47] Other key benefits include decreased risk of subsequent malignancies and increased survival rate.[48,49] Finally, some research indicates that patients who remain smoke-free following cancer treatment report lower levels of depression and anxiety relative to patients who continue to smoke.[50] In summary, there is significant evidence that smoking cessation after a cancer diagnosis improves quality of life, increases survival, and decreases cancer recurrence and psychological distress.

Smoking cessation and relapse among cancer patients. Despite the benefits of quitting, smoking prevalence at the time of cancer diagnosis falls within a reported range of 46%–75%, with 14%–58% of cancer patients continuing to smoke posttreatment.[51] However, studies with this population also indicate that many cancer patients who smoke at the time of diagnosis make an attempt to quit, consistent with the notion that a cancer diagnosis motivates tobacco cessation. For example, one study of head and neck cancer patients found that 84% made at least one quit attempt and 69% made multiple quit attempts.[32] Of note is that most quit attempts appear to occur at the time of diagnosis and treatment, suggesting that the period between cancer diagnosis and end of treatment may represent the optimal window of opportunity for provision of smoking cessation interventions.[52]

There is less research on long-term abstinence rates among cancer patients. Estimates of smoking relapse range from 13% to 44%.[53,54]

Studies of patients with early-stage non-small-cell lung cancer reveal that approximately half of the patients returned to smoking after cancer diagnosis or treatment.[55,56] Unlike the general population of smokers for whom relapse most often occurs within a week after cessation, the majority of relapse among cancer patients occurs 1 month following a quit attempt, again reflecting the initial motivational impact of a cancer diagnosis.[57]

Among cancer patients, predictors of cessation and maintained tobacco abstinence include being female, older age, higher education level, later stage cancer diagnosis, and more extensive disease.[58,59] Psychosocial factors associated with continued smoking include lower levels of both perceived health risk and quitting self-efficacy, fatalistic beliefs, and alcohol use.[60,61]

Interventions for cancer patients. Very few studies have empirically tested smoking cessation interventions with cancer patients, although interest in this area is growing. A review of eight cessation studies for cancer patients included nurse-delivered inpatient counseling, distribution of educational materials, and follow-up phone calls. Although the overall findings were mixed, larger abstinence rates were observed with a greater number of sessions, underscoring the benefits of more intensive interventions.[58] A more recent nurse-based tailored intervention for head and neck cancer patients resulted in higher 6-month quit rates among the intervention group relative to the usual care group, 47% and 31%, respectively.[62] This study highlighted the importance of simultaneously treating comorbid depression and problem drinking, both factors known to be associated with lower smoking cessation rates. Finally, there is suggestive evidence that even brief physician-delivered advice to abstain from smoking can have potent effects at producing long-term tobacco abstinence among cancer patients.[31]

When implementing smoking cessation interventions with cancer patients, clinicians should be mindful of several unique cancer-related issues. For instance, the delay in relapse among cancer patients described earlier may suggest a waning of motivation as patients physically recover and return to their prediagnosis lifestyles. Thus, smoking relapse prevention interventions may be particularly important as patients recover. Another issue to consider is related to potential medical contraindications with the use of smoking cessation pharmacotherapy. With respect to NRT, for example, although nicotine is not itself carcinogenic, preclinical research suggests that it can accelerate tumor growth, and that it can suppress cancer cell death caused by several chemotherapy agents.[36,63] In addition, NRTs such as nicotine gum, spray, inhaler, or lozenge may not be appropriate for individuals with oral cancers, whereas bupropion is contraindicated for patients with a history of central nervous system (CNS) tumors due to an increased risk of seizures. Hence, clinicians must take extra care in selecting appropriate cessation medications that address cancer patients' unique needs.

Lastly, several studies offer guidance with regard to tailoring cessation interventions to cancer patients. For instance, given that cessation rates have been reported to be higher for patients with tobacco-related cancers,[30,31] raising awareness of the link between cancer diagnosis and smoking status is likely to facilitate cessation. Findings from a study with newly diagnosed cancer patients who were followed for 12 months indicate that targeting perceived risk of cancer recurrence may be useful in motivating smoking cessation after the acute cancer treatment is over.[64]

In summary, the importance of quitting smoking for all cancer patients is clear. Clinicians who treat cancer patients must capitalize on the window of opportunity during cancer diagnosis and treatment to identify smokers and make cessation interventions readily available to these high-risk patients. Cancer patients who stop smoking and remain abstinent after treatment are likely to reap significant benefits, including improved quality of life and prolonged survival.

SMOKE-FREE MEDICAL FACILITIES

To this point we have focused on individually targeted smoking cessation interventions. We now wish to mention a relevant institutional-level tobacco control intervention: smoke-free campus policies. It has been well established that environmental tobacco smoke (ETS) is a significant cause of illness including the development of cancers, and that there is no safe level of exposure to ETS.[65] Therefore, in 1992, the Joint Commission introduced a standard prohibiting smoking inside all U.S. hospitals, resulting in the nation's first industry-wide ban on smoking in the workplace.[66] The adoption of indoor smoke-free hospital policy has led to a decline in cigarette use and increase in cessation among employees.[67,68] In addition, healthcare providers became better prepared to promote smoking cessation with patients, seizing the "teachable moment" presented by inpatient hospitalizations.[69]

However, patients and employees continue to be exposed to tobacco smoke from smoking that occurs in designated outdoor areas on hospital campuses. Furthermore, research has revealed that complete smoking bans are more effective than such restrictions in reducing exposure to ETS.[68,70] Consequently, many hospitals and healthcare centers nationwide have been expanding their tobacco-free policies, prohibiting smoking on the entire hospital campus, including at entranceways, on grounds, and in parking areas.[71] Although little is known about how many hospitals to date have adopted 100% smoke-free campus policies, it is quickly becoming a national trend.

The rationale for these policies is based largely on the belief that 100% smoke-free facilities project a healthy image, protect patients and staff, and encourage smoking cessation. This rationale is particularly relevant to cancer centers, where permitting smoking on campus stands in stark contrast to cancer centers' mission of treating and preventing cancer. Conversely, a comprehensive smoke-free policy encourages abstinence, helps to reduce the risk of relapse among former smokers, diminishes the level of smoking among current users, and makes messages to patients about the health risks of tobacco use more credible.[68]

Despite the significant benefits, administrators are often reluctant to implement comprehensive smoke-free policies, mainly due to unfounded fears related to negative employee morale and lack of acceptance by patients. Research has shown, however, that campus-wide smoke-free policy has no detrimental effect on employee or patient attitudes or behaviors.[72] On the contrary, a few formal evaluations of hospital outdoor smoke-free policies revealed large cessation rates among employees, the majority of whom found the effect of the policy to be positive.[73] A national survey of hospitals found very few barriers to policy implementation and insignificant levels of negative employee morale or patient nonacceptance.[69]

Several key points regarding successful implementation of tobacco-free campus policies have been identified.[71] First, administrative support and a clear plan for enforcement are critical for successful implementation. Second, patient and employee support is enhanced by eliciting the opinions and assessing the needs of affected individuals. Perhaps the most important component of a successful policy is to provide easy access to pharmacotherapy and other smoking cessation interventions to employees and patients who are either motivated to make a quit attempt or unable to tolerate involuntary abstinence.

CONCLUSION

Tobacco use by cancer patients appears to be influenced by the same range of biopsychosocial factors as it is in the general population. However, cancer diagnosis and treatment offers a unique and potentially powerful opportunity for healthcare providers to intervene by offering cessation advice and assistance. To date, there is little research to recommend specialized smoking cessation interventions for cancer patients above and beyond the general recommendations of the Clinical Practice Guidelines.[5] However, it is likely that targeted treatments that capitalize on the teachable moment could be highly effective, and research has been increasing in this area. Meanwhile, the greatest progress in both cancer prevention and recovery depends on consistent action by all aspects of the healthcare system to promote tobacco cessation. This includes coverage of smoking cessation interventions by third-party payers, establishment of smoke-free campuses by hospital administrators, and strong cessation advice and assistance by every healthcare provider.

ACKNOWLEDGMENTS

Preparation of this chapter was supported by National Cancer Institute grants R01 CA94256 and R03 CA134203. We thank Vani Nath Simmons, Ph.D., for her assistance on the manuscript.

Disclosure: Dr. Brandon receives research funding from Pfizer, Inc., and has served on a scientific advisory board for Pfizer, Inc.

REFERENCES

1. Peto R, Lopez AD, Boreham J, Thun M, Heath C Jr. *Mortality from smoking in developed countries 1950–2000*. Oxford: Oxford University Press; 1994 (revised 2006).
2. IARC. *Reversal of risk after quitting smoking*. Lyon, France: IARC Handbooks of Cancer Prevention, Tobacco Control; 2007:11.
3. Levy DT, Mumford EA, Cummings KM, et al. The relative risks of a low-nitrosamine smokeless tobacco product compared with smoking cigarettes: estimates of a panel of experts. *Cancer Epidemiol Biom Prev.* 2004;13:2035–2042.
4. Peto R, Darby S, Deo H, Silcocks P, Whitley E, Doll R. Smoking, smoking cessation, and lung cancer in the UK since 1950: combination of national statistics with two case-control studies. *BMJ.* 2000;321:323–329.
5. Fiore MC, Jaén CR, Baker TB, et al. *Treating tobacco use and dependence: 2008 update. Clinical Practice Guideline*. Rockville, MD: U.S. Department of Health and Human Services, Public Health Service; May 2008.
6. Baker TB, Brandon TH, Chassin L. Motivational influences on cigarette smoking. *Annu Rev Psychol.* 2004;55:463–491.
7. Balfour DJ, Fagerstrom KO. Pharmacology of nicotine and its therapeutic use in smoking cessation and neurodegenerative disorders. *Pharmacol Ther.* 1996;72:51–81.
8. Schuurmans MM, Diacon AH, van Biljon X, et al. Effect of pre-treatment with nicotine patch on withdrawal symptoms and abstinence rates in smokers subsequently quitting with the nicotine patch: a randomized controlled trial. *Addiction.* 2004;99:634–640.
9. Rose JE, Behm FM, Westman EC, Kukvich, P. Precessation treatment with nicotine skin patch facilitates smoking cessation. *Nicotine Tob Res.* 2006;8:89–101.
10. Dwoskin LP, Rauhut AS, King-Pospisil KA, Bardo MT. Review of the pharmacology and clinical profile of bupropion, an antidepressant and tobacco use cessation agent. *CNS Drug Rev.* 2006;12:178–207.
11. Hayford KE, Patten CA, Rummans TA, et al. Efficacy of bupropion for smoking cessation in smokers with a former history of major depression or alcoholism. *Br J Psychiatry.* 1999;174:173–178.
12. Jorenby DE, Hays JT, Rigotti NA, et al. Efficacy of varenicline, an alpha4-beta2 nicotinic acetylcholine receptor partial agonist, vs placebo or sustained-release bupropion for smoking cessation: a randomized controlled trial. *JAMA.* 2006;296:56–63.
13. Gonzales D, Rennard SI, Nides M, et al. Varenicline, an alpha4beta2 nicotinic acetylcholine receptor partial agonist, vs sustained-release bupropion and placebo for smoking cessation: a randomized controlled trial. *JAMA.* 2006;296(1):47–55.
14. Lancaster T, Stead LF. Self-help interventions for smoking cessation. *Cochrane Database Syst Rev.* 2005;3.
15. Webb MS, Simmons VN, Brandon TH. Tailored interventions for motivating smoking cessation: using placebo-tailoring to examine the influence of personalization and expectancies. *Health Psychol.* 2005;24:179–188.
16. Webb MS, Hendricks PS, Brandon TH. Expectancy priming of smoking cessation messages enhances the placebo effect of tailored interventions. *Health Psychol.* 2007;26:598–609.
17. Brandon TH, Collins BN, Juliano LM, Lazev AB. Preventing relapse among former smokers: a comparison of minimal interventions via telephone and mail. *J Consult Clin Psychol.* 2000;68:103–113.
18. Brandon TH, Meade CD, Herzog TA, Chirikos TN, Webb MS, Cantor AB. Efficacy and cost-effectiveness of a minimal intervention to prevent smoking relapse: dismantling the effects of content versus contact. *J Consult Clin Psychol.* 2004;72:797–808.
19. Cummins SE, Bailey L, Campbell S, Koon-Kirby C, Zhu Shu-Hong. Tobacco cessation quitlines in North America: a descriptive study. *Tob Control.* 2007;16:9–15.
20. Centers for Disease Control and Prevention. *Best Practices for Comprehensive Tobacco Control Programs—2007*. Atlanta, GA: U.S. Department of Health and Human Services, Centers for Disease Control and Prevention, National Center for Chronic Disease Prevention and Health Promotion, Office on Smoking and Health; 2007.
21. Stead LF, Perera R, Lancaster T. Telephone counseling for smoking cessation. *Cochrane Database Syst Rev.* 2006;3.

22. Ellerbeck EF, Ahluwalia JS, Jolicoeur DG, Gladden J, Mosier MC. Direct observation of smoking cessation activities in primary care practice. *J Fam Pract.* 2001;50:688–693.

23. Phillips KM, Brandon TH. Do psychologists adhere to the clinical practice guidelines for tobacco cessation? A survey of practitioners. *Prof Psychol Res Pr.* 2004;35:281–285.

24. Perkins KA, Conklin CA, Levine MD. *Cognitive-behavioral therapy for smoking cessation: a practical guidebook to the most effective treatments.* New York: Routledge; 2007.

25. Stead LF, Lancaster T. Group behaviour therapy programs for smoking cessation. *Cochrane Database Syst Rev.* 2005;2.

26. Irvin JE, Bowers CA, Dunn ME, Wang MC. Efficacy of relapse prevention: a meta-analytic review. *J Consult Clin Psychol.* 1999;67:563–570.

27. Compas BE, Haaga DAF, Keefe FJ, Leitenberg H, Williams DA. Sampling of empirically supported psychological treatments from health psychology: smoking, chronic pain, cancer, and bulimia nervosa. *J Consult Clin Psychol.* 1998;66:89–112.

28. Cinciripini PM, Lapitsky LG, Seay S, Wallfisch A, Kitchens K, Van Vunakis H. The effects of smoking schedules on cessation outcome: can we improve on common methods of gradual and abrupt nicotine withdrawal. *J Consult Clin Psychol.* 1995;63:388–399.

29. Hughes JR. Combining behavioral therapy and pharmacotherapy for smoking cessation: an update. In: Onken LS, Blaine JD, Boren JJ, eds. *Integrating behavior therapies with medication in the treatment of drug dependence: NIDA research monograph.* Monograph no. 150. Washington, DC: U.S. Government Printing Office; 1995:92–109.

30. Gritz ER, Nisenbaum R, Elashoff RE, Holmes EC. Smoking behavior following diagnosis in patients with stage I non-small cell lung cancer. *Cancer Causes Control.* 1991;2:105–112.

31. Gritz ER, Carr CR, Rapkin D, et al. Predictors of long-term smoking cessation in head and neck cancer patients. *Cancer Epidemiol Biomarkers Prev.* 1993;2:261–270.

32. Ostroff JS, Jacobsen PB, Moadel AB, et al. Prevalence and predictors of continued tobacco use after treatment of patients with head and neck cancer. *Cancer.* 1995;75:569–576.

33. Klosky JL, Tyc VL, Garces-Webb DM, Buscemi J, Klesges RC, Hudson MM. Emerging issues in smoking among adolescent and adult cancer survivors. *Cancer.* 2007;110(11):2408–2417.

34. Browman GP, Wong G, Hodson I, et al. Influence of cigarette smoking on the efficacy of radiation therapy in head and neck cancer. *N Engl J Med.* 1993;328(3):159–163.

35. Cinciripini PM, Gritz ER, Tsoh JY, Skaar KL. Smoking cessation and cancer prevention. In: Holland JC, ed. *Psycho-oncology.* New York: Oxford University Press; 1998.

36. Dasgupta P, Kinkade R, Bharat J, Decook C, Haura E, Chellappan S. Nicotine inhibits apoptosis induced by chemotherapeutic drugs by up-regulating XIAP and surviving. *Proc Natl Acad Sci USA.* 2006;103:6332–6337.

37. Arcavi L, Benowitz NL. Cigarette smoking and infection. *Arch Intern Med.* 2004;164(20):2206–2216.

38. Goodwin SJ, McCarthy CM, Pusic AL, et al. Complication in smokers after postmastectomy tissue expander/implant breast reconstruction. *Ann Plast Surg.* 2005;55:16–19.

39. Tollerud DJ, Clark JW, Brown LM. The effects of cigarette smoking on T cell subsets: a population-based survey of healthy Caucasians. *Am Rev Respir Dis.* 1989 Jun;139(6):1446–1451.

40. Gritz ER, Vidrine DJ, Lazev AB. Smoking cessation in cancer patients: never too late to quit. In: Green CW, Given B, Champion VL, Kozachik S, Devoss DN, eds. *Evidence-based cancer care and prevention: behavioral interventions.* New York: Springer Publishing Co.; 2003:107–140.

41. Lippman SM, Lee JJ, Karp DD, et al. Randomized phase III intergroup trial of isotretinoin to prevent second primary tumors in stage I non-small-cell lung cancer. *J Natl Cancer Inst.* 2001;93:605–618.

42. Bako G, Dewar R, Hanson J, Hill G. Factors influencing the survival of patients with cancer of the prostate. *Can Med Assoc J.* 1982;127:727–729.

43. Calle EE, Miracle-McMahill HL, Thun MJ, Heath CW Jr. Cigarette smoking and risk of fatal breast cancer. *Am J Epidemiol.* 1994 May 15;139(10):1001–1007.

44. Kucera H, Enzelsberger H, Eppel W, Weghaupt K. The influence of nicotine abuse and diabetes mellitus on the results of primary irradiation in the treatment of carcinoma of the cervix. *Cancer.* 1987;60(1):1–4.

45. Do KA, Johnson MM, Lee JJ, et al. Longitudinal study of smoking patterns in relation to the development of smoking-related secondary primary tumors in patients with upper aerodigestive tract malignancies. *Cancer.* 2004;101(12):2837–2842.

46. Silverman S Jr, Gorsky M, Greenspan D. Tobacco usage in patients with head and neck carcinomas: a follow-up study on habit changes and second primary oral/oropharyngeal cancers. *J Am Dent Assoc.* 1983;106(1):33–35.

47. Dresler CM, Gritz ER. Smoking, smoking cessation and the oncologist. *Lung Cancer.* 2001;34:315–323.

48. Kawahara M, Ushijima S, Kamimori T, et al. Second primary tumors in more than 2-year disease-free survivors of small-cell lung cancer in Japan: the role of smoking cessation. *Br J Cancer.* 1998;78(3):409–412.

49. Ebbert JO, Williams BA, Sun Z, et al. Duration of smoking abstinence as a predictor for non small lung cancer survival in women. *Lung Cancer.* 2005;47:165–172.

50. Humphris GM, Rogers SN. The association of cigarette smoking and anxiety, depression and fears of recurrence in patients following treatment of oral and oropharyngeal malignancy. *Eur J Cancer Care.* 2004;13:328–335.

51. Cox LS, Africano NL, Tercyak KP, Taylor KL. Nicotine dependence treatment for patients with cancer. *Cancer.* 2003;98(3):632–644.

52. Vander Ark W, DiNardo LJ, Oliver DS. Factors affecting smoking cessation in patients with head and neck cancer. *Laryngoscope.* 1997;107(7):888–892.

53. Dresler CM, Bailey M, Roper CR, Patterson GA, Cooper JD. Smoking cessation and lung cancer resection. *Chest.* 1996;110(5):1199–1202.

54. Davison G, Duffy M. Smoking habits of long-term survivors of surgery for lung cancer. *Thorax.* 1982;37:331–333.

55. Walker MS, Vidrine DJ, Gritz ER, et al. Smoking relapse during the first year after treatment for early-stage non-small-cell lung cancer. *Cancer Epidemiol Biomarkers Prev.* 2006;15(12):2370–2377.

56. Baser S, Shannon VR, Eapen GA, et al. Smoking cessation after diagnosis of lung cancer is associated with a beneficial effect on performance status. *Chest.* 2006;130(6):1784–1790.

57. Gritz ER, Schacherer C, Koehly L, Nielsen IR, Abemayor E. Smoking withdrawal and relapse in head and neck patients. *Head & Neck.* 1999;21(5):420–427.

58. Cox L Sanderson, Patten CA, Ebbert JO, et al. Tobacco use outcomes among patients with lung cancer treated for nicotine dependence. *J Clin Oncol.* 2002;20:3461–3469.

59. Chan Y, Irish JC, Wood SF, et al. Smoking cessation in patient diagnosed with head and neck cancer. *J Otolaryngol.* 2004;33:75–81.

60. Schnoll RA, Zhang B, Rue M, et al. Brief physician-initiated quit-smoking strategies for clinical oncology settings: a trial coordinated by the Eastern Cooperative Oncology Group. *J Clin Oncol.* 2003;15(2):355–365.

61. Lambert MT, Terrell JE, Copeland LA, Ronis DL, Duffy SA. Cigarettes, alcohol, and depression: characterizing head and neck cancer survivors in 2 systems of care. *Nicotine Tob Res.* 2005;7:233–241.

62. Duffy SA, Ronis DL, Valenstein M, et al. A tailored smoking, alcohol, and depression intervention for head and neck cancer patients. *Cancer Epidemiol Biomarkers Prev.* 2006;15(11):2203–2208.

63. Heeschen C, Jang JJ, Weis M, et al. Nicotine stimulates angiogenesis and promotes tumor growth and atherosclerosis. *Nat Med.* 2001;7:833–839.

64. Hay JL, Ostroff J, Burkhalter J, Li Y, Quiles Z, Moadel A. Changes in cancer-related risk perception and smoking across time in newly-diagnosed cancer patients. *J Behav Med.* 2007;30(2):131–142.

65. U.S. Department of Health and Human Services. *The health consequences of involuntary exposure to tobacco smoke: a report of the Surgeon General.* Atlanta, GA: Office on Smoking and Health; 2006.

66. U.S. Joint Commission on Accreditation of Healthcare Organizations. *Accreditation manual for hospitals.* Oakbrook Terrace, IL: Joint Commission on Accreditation of Healthcare Organizations; 1992.

67. Longo DR, Feldman MA, Kruse RL, Brownson RC, Petroski GF, Hewett JE. Implementing smoking bans in American hospitals: results of a national survey. *Tobacco Control.* 1998;7:47–55.

68. Fichtenberg CM, Glantz SA. Effect of smoke-free workplaces on smoking behaviour: systematic review. *BMJ.* 2002;325:188–195.

69. Orleans TC, Kristeller JL, Gritz ER. Helping hospitalized smokers quit: new directions for treatment and research. *J Consult Clin Psychol.* 1993;61(5):778–779.

70. Hopkins DP, Briss PA, Ricard CJ, et al. Reviews of evidence regarding interventions to reduce tobacco use and exposure to environmental tobacco smoke. *Am J Prev Med.* 2001;20(2S):16–66.

71. Kunyk D, Els C, Predy G, Haase M. Development and introduction of a comprehensive tobacco control policy in a Canadian regional health authority. *Prev Chron Dis.* 2007;4(2):1–8.

72. Wheeler JG, Pulley L, Felix HC, et al. Impact of a smoke-free hospital campus policy on employee and consumer behavior. *Public Health Rep.* 2007;122(6):744–752.

73. Bloch M, Shopland DR. Outdoor smoking bans: more than meets the eye. *Tobacco Control.* 2000;9:97–99.

CHAPTER 3

Diet and Cancer

Marian L. Fitzgibbon and Melinda R. Stolley

THE SCOPE OF THE PROBLEM

The relationship between diet and cancer has been a topic of significant interest in both the scientific and the popular press for decades.[1] Overall, it is estimated that dietary factors account for approximately 30% of cancers in developed countries and 20% of cancers in developing countries.[1] Only tobacco is considered a stronger, modifiable cause of cancer.[2]

The role of diet, however, in the development of cancer is complex.[3] In recent years, it has become increasingly clear that cancer is not a single disease, but an expression of multiple alterations in the normal process of cell growth and death.[1] Therefore, it is important to analyze which foods affect cancer risk and how they interact with the chain of cellular events that lead to carcinogenesis and cancer.[4] Most foods contain a variety of components, making it difficult to identify which components, individually or in combination, affect cell function.

Because of the complexity of both carcinogenesis and dietary intake, the true relationship between diet and cancer is difficult to determine. For example, the results of some recent epidemiological studies,[5] and randomized trials [6] do not support the hypothesis that fruits and vegetables play a protective role.[7] That said, some null findings may be a function of faulty methodology, and the relationship between diet and cancer may become clearer as methodological factors are refined. Limitations from past studies include measurement errors in the timing and length of exposures, intervention length, insufficient follow-up periods, and a lack of appreciation for genomic variations in the population studied.[8]

Part of the complexity in how diet affects cancer risk lies in the fact that there can be both a direct and indirect effect. For example, diet can affect cancer development directly, through long-term exposure to certain nutrients,[9] but also indirectly through the effect of diet on energy balance, body fat, and obesity.[10] A negative balance through physical activity has been shown to reduce cancer risk in a number of epidemiological reviews,[11] but excess body weight that develops from an imbalance between energy intake over energy expenditure may increase risk.[12] Positive energy balance is highly prevalent in both developed and developing countries.[13] The estimated total number of overweight (body mass index [BMI] ≥25 kg/m^2) and obese (BMI ≥30 kg/m^2) adults worldwide in 2005 was 937 million and 396 million, respectively.[14] In 2002, the International Agency for Research on Cancer concluded that there was convincing evidence that being overweight or obese is associated with an increased risk of cancer in both men and women.[15]

The purpose of this chapter is fivefold: to summarize established associations of diet-related factors with increased and decreased cancer risk; to summarize the results of recent dietary clinical trials; to highlight nutritional recommendations for cancer risk reduction; to identify barriers to healthy eating; and to discuss preventive dietary behaviors in the era of genomics.

DIET-RELATED FACTORS AND CANCER RISK

This section presents an overview of the best-established associations between diet and the top 10 causes of cancer deaths worldwide.[16,17] For many of these factors, the specific mechanism that causes or prevents carcinogenesis is unknown, but instead a number of plausible mechanisms have been suggested. Hence, only those mechanisms that have been clearly established in the scientific literature are presented. The diet-related factors described represent only a fraction of those being studied; the data on those not presented are either too limited or too inconsistent to consider. Most of the associations discussed below are based on observational data; only a few have been tested in randomized, controlled trials.

Lung cancer. Lung cancer is both the most common cause of cancer death and the most commonly occurring cancer worldwide.[18] The highest incidence is seen in high-income countries, and the primary risk factor is smoking, accounting for an estimated 80% of lung cancers in developed countries.[19]

Increases risk. The most established dietary risk factor for lung cancer is arsenic in drinking water.[16] The World Health Organization (WHO) reports that Bangladesh, India (West Bengal), China, and parts of the United States (western states) have levels of arsenic in the drinking water that are above the recommended limit.[20]

β-Carotene supplements are also associated with increased risk for lung cancer, particularly among smokers.[21] This association was largely unexpected, since several epidemiological studies had shown a relationship between a diet rich in β-carotene and a decreased incidence of lung cancer.[22] On the basis of the results of these observational studies, two large randomized trials were conducted to test whether β-carotene supplements could reduce the incidence of lung cancer in high-risk individuals. The Beta-carotene and Retinol Efficacy Trial (CARET) was conducted in the United States and enrolled male and female smokers and former smokers, along with men with occupational exposure to asbestos. The Alpha-Tocopherol, Beta-Carotene (ATBC) Cancer Prevention Study was conducted in Finland and enrolled male smokers. Both studies found an increase in risk for lung cancer in the group assigned to take β-carotene supplements. Risk decreased once participants stopped taking the supplements.[21]

Decreases risk. To date, only fruits and foods containing carotenoids show sufficient evidence to suggest a protective effect against lung cancer.[16]

Stomach (gastric) cancer. Stomach cancer is the second most common cause of cancer death. It is the fourth most common cancer worldwide with highest incidence noted among men and in certain regions of Asia and Latin America.[18] Infection with *Helicobacter pylori*, a bacteria found in the stomach, is the main risk factor for stomach cancer, accounting for 80% or more of stomach cancers, particularly in developing countries.[19] The incidence of stomach cancer has been steadily declining in many developed countries. This is likely due to improved methods for preserving and storing foods (e.g., refrigeration), leading to reduced intake of salted foods and increased consumption of fresh fruits and vegetables.[18]

Increases risk. Salt and salt-preserved foods have the strongest association with increased risk for stomach cancer.[16] This association may help to explain the high rates of stomach cancer observed in parts of Asia and Latin America where salt-preserved foods are frequently consumed.[23]

Decreases risk. The protective effects of fruits for stomach cancer have been consistently supported in case-control and cohort studies.[16] Data for nonstarchy and allium vegetables are also consistent, but limited to case-control studies.[16] There is some limited evidence that foods containing selenium may also reduce risk by providing protection against *H pylori*.[16]

Liver cancer. Liver cancer is the third most common cause of cancer death and the sixth most common type of cancer worldwide. It is more prevalent in developing countries, with China having the highest prevalence.[18] Liver cancer is also more prevalent in men. Hepatitis B (HBV) and C (HCV) viruses are the primary risk factors, accounting for 75% of cases worldwide.[18]

Increases risk. The most significant dietary-related risk factor is exposure to aflatoxins.[16,24] Aflatoxins are produced by mold, which develops when foods are stored in hot, wet conditions.[16,24] Foods most commonly affected include grains and nuts. Exposure to aflatoxins in combination with HBV further increases risk for hepatocellular cancer, the most common form of liver cancer.[18] While aflatoxin exposure is the primary dietary risk factor in developing countries, it is much less common in developed countries, where alcohol consumption is the main dietary risk factor.[16,19] There is consistent evidence from both case-control and cohort studies to suggest that alcohol intake increases risk for liver cancer through the development of cirrhosis and alcoholic hepatitis.[16]

Decreases risk. To date, little is known about the protective effects of diet against liver cancer. Data suggest that fruits may decrease risk, but this association is not yet firmly established.[16]

Colorectal cancer. Colorectal cancer is the fourth most common cause of cancer death and the third most common form of cancer.[16,18] Incidence is somewhat higher in men than in women. It is also higher in North America and Europe than in Africa or Asia.[16,18] A number of lifestyle-related factors influence risk, including physical activity, obesity, alcohol consumption, and diet.[25]

Increases risk. Multiple studies have shown convincing evidence that red meat (e.g., beef, veal, pork, and lamb) and processed meats increase risk for colorectal cancer.[26] Processed meats are meats preserved by methods other than freezing, such as smoking, salting, air drying, or heating. Ham, bacon, sausages, and canned meats are all examples of processed meats. Alcohol intake also increases risk, particularly in men and in people with low folate levels.[16]

Decreases risk. For many years, there has been ongoing debate about the relationship between fiber and colorectal cancer. Despite conflicting reports, American Institute for Cancer Research (AICR) and other investigators agree that fiber likely decreases colon cancer risk, with the greatest reduction noted for higher fiber intakes.[16] There is also probable evidence that calcium and milk reduce colorectal cancer risk; however, the effect for milk is, in part, mediated by calcium.[27] Finally, in the past 10 years there has been growing evidence that garlic protects against colorectal cancer.[16]

Breast cancer. Breast cancer is the most commonly occurring cancer and the most common cause of cancer death among women worldwide.[16,18] Overall, it is the fifth most common cause of cancer death.[16] Incidence is more common in high-income countries, but in recent years it has increased in less-developed regions such as Africa, Asia, and Latin America.[18] Because it is a hormone-related cancer, risk is most affected by factors that influence exposure to estrogen, including menopausal status.

Increases risk. There is significant evidence that consuming high levels of alcohol is a risk factor for both pre- and postmenopausal breast cancer.[28] For many years, dietary fat was also considered a risk factor

based on data from international correlation studies, animal studies, and case-control studies.[29] However, pooled analyses of cohort studies do not support these findings.[30]

Decreases risk. To date, there is insufficient evidence to support the protective effects of any diet-related factors against breast cancer. However, recent data from the Women's Health Initiative (WHI) suggest a small protective effect for a low-fat diet.[31] Results from the 10-year follow-up should help to clarify this relationship.

Esophageal cancer. Cancer of the esophagus is the sixth most common cause of cancer death and the eighth most commonly occurring cancer worldwide.[16,18] Esophageal cancer is strongly related to lifestyle behaviors, including tobacco use, alcohol consumption, and diet.[16]

Increases risk. Consistent evidence from cohort and case-control studies suggests that alcohol contributes to the development of esophageal cancer.[16] Maté (a tea-like beverage, served very hot and consumed through a metal straw) is also associated with increased risk.[16] The traditional practice of drinking maté is related to higher rates of esophageal cancer in Uruguay, southern Brazil, and northern Argentina.[18]

Decreases risk. A number of studies have found that nonstarchy vegetables, foods containing β-carotene, foods containing vitamin C, and fruits decrease risk for esophageal cancer.[16]

Cancers of the mouth, pharynx, and larynx. These cancers have the seventh highest incidence worldwide and are the seventh most common cause of cancer death.[16,18] These cancers are more common in men than in women. Alcohol and tobacco use are the primary risk factors, particularly in higher income, developed countries.[16] Other risk factors may be more important in developing countries. For example, in the Indian subcontinent it is common to chew gutka (betel leaf with tobacco), a carcinogen associated with oral and esophageal cancers.

Increases risk. Dietary items that may increase risk are alcohol and maté.[16] IARC considers alcohol to be a Class I carcinogen for cancers of the mouth, pharynx, and larynx.[19]

Decreases risk. Sufficient evidence exists to suggest that nonstarchy vegetables, fruits, and foods containing carotenoids decrease risk for cancers of the mouth, pharynx, and larynx and that there is a dose-response relationship.[16]

Cervical cancer. Cervical cancer is the second most common cancer among women worldwide and the third most common cause of cancer death in women.[16] It is most common in Africa, Latin America, and parts of Asia. The primary risk factor is infection with the human papilloma viruses.

Increases/decreases risk. On the basis of the literature to date, there are no identified dietary factors that play a significant role in either increasing or decreasing cervical cancer risk.[16]

Pancreatic cancer. Pancreatic cancer is the thirteenth most common cancer worldwide and the ninth most common cause of cancer deaths.[16,18] Incidence is higher in men than in women and higher in high-income countries. Particularly low rates are found in Africa and Asia.[16,18] Established risk factors are smoking and body fatness.[16]

Increases risk. Data from case-control studies suggest that red meat consumption increases risk; however, results from cohort studies are less consistent. At one time, coffee consumption was considered a possible risk factor,[32] but this is currently not supported.[16]

Decreases risk. A limited number of cohort studies suggest a possible dose-response relationship between foods containing folate and

Table 3–1. Dietary factors showing convincing or probable evidence of association with the top 10 causes of cancer death worldwide

Cancer	Increases risk	Decreases risk
Lung	Arsenic in water β-Carotene supplements	Fruits Foods containing carotenoids
Stomach	Salt and salt-preserved foods Deficient fruits and vegetables	Fruits Foods containing selenium
Liver	Exposure to aflatoxins Alcohol	None
Colorectal	Red meat Processed meats Alcohol	Fiber Calcium Garlic
Breast	Alcohol	None
Esophageal	Alcohol Maté	Nonstarchy vegetables Foods containing β-carotene Foods containing vitamin C Fruits
Mouth, pharynx, larynx	Alcohol Maté	Nonstarchy vegetables Fruits Foods containing carotenoids
Cervical	None	None
Pancreatic	Red meat	Foods containing folate
Prostate	Animal fat Calcium	Selenium Lycopene

decreased risk for pancreatic cancer.[16] Folate-rich foods include green leafy vegetables, cruciferous vegetables, oranges, legumes, and whole grains. Folic acid supplements, however, have not shown a protective effect.[16] There is also some evidence that fruits may decrease risk.[16]

Prostate cancer. Prostate cancer is the second most common cancer in men, the sixth most common cause of cancer deaths in men, and the tenth most common cause of cancer death worldwide. Incidence is much higher in developed countries.

Increases risk. Ecological studies, animal studies, and some case-control studies support a positive relationship between dietary fat, particularly animal fat, and prostate cancer risk.[33] A number of studies also suggest that high calcium intake increases risk for prostate cancer.[16] These studies, however, did not adjust for dietary fat, and it is possible that results were confounded by this factor. One study did report reduced risk for users of calcium channel blockers.[34]

Decreases risk. Dietary factors that may protect against prostate cancer include selenium, lycopene, and α-tocopherol (vitamin E).[16] Evidence is strongest and most consistent for selenium and lycopene. For example, the Nutritional Prevention of Cancer Trial in the United States found a 65% reduction in prostate cancer incidence among those receiving selenium supplementation compared with those receiving a placebo.[35] A meta-analysis of studies of lycopene found a 10%–25% reduction in risk for men with the highest lycopene intake and for men consuming the highest number of cooked tomato products.[36] Table 3–1 shows the dietary factors showing convincing or probable evidence of association with the top 10 causes of cancer death worldwide.

DIETARY CLINICAL TRIALS

This section analyzes the results of U.S.-based large randomized trials that have examined the effects of dietary factors on cancer prevention or control and includes a description of ongoing dietary large randomized trials.

Women's Healthy Eating and Living (WHEL) study. This randomized trial (1995–2006) assessed whether a significant increase in vegetable,

fruit and fiber intake, and a decrease in dietary fat intake could reduce the risk of recurrent and new primary breast cancer and "all cause" mortality among 3088 survivors of early-stage breast cancer.[37] Women randomized to the intervention group received telephone counseling, along with cooking classes and newsletters that promoted daily intake of five vegetable servings plus 16 oz of vegetable juice, three fruit servings, 30 g of fiber, and 15%–20% of energy intake from fat. Women randomized to the comparison group received written materials consistent with the "5-a-Day" dietary guidelines. Although the intervention group did adhere to the prescribed diet, there was no effect on breast cancer events or mortality among early-stage breast cancer survivors.

Women's Intervention Nutrition Study (WINS). This Phase III clinical trial (1994–2001) examined the relationship between dietary fat intake and breast cancer among 2437 women with resected, early-stage breast cancer.[38] Women randomized to the intervention group were counseled to reduce their dietary fat intake to 15% of calories during a 4-month intervention period followed by monthly group sessions. The comparison group received no dietary counseling. Interim results at 60 months showed that dietary fat intake and body weight were significantly lower in the intervention group compared to the control group. In addition, women in the intervention group, particularly those with estrogen receptor negative tumors, were less likely to experience a recurrence. Longer-term follow-up will be conducted in the coming years.

Women's Health Initiative (WHI). The WHI was a large, complex study of over 45,000 postmenopausal women (1993–2004) that included a clinical trial of three intervention arms, two of which were diet and cancer related.[39] The first of these tested a low-fat eating pattern (less than 20% of total calories; five servings a day of fruits and vegetables, six servings a day of whole grains) on breast cancer and colorectal cancer. Women in the intervention group attended a number of intensive behavioral modification sessions delivered by study nutritionists, while control group participants received the Department of Agriculture (USDA) Dietary Guidelines for Americans. Follow-up at 8.1 years showed no significant reduction in the incidence of breast cancer or colon cancer among women in the intervention group.[31] However, breast cancer incidence was 9% lower among women in the intervention group. Further follow-up is expected. The second trial examined the effects of calcium

Table 3-2. Recommendations for good health and cancer prevention

2005 Dietary Guidelines for Americans[50]	American Cancer Society[53]	American Institute for Cancer Research[52]
Maintain body weight in a healthy range	Consume at least five servings of fruits and vegetables daily as well as grain products such as cereals, bread, and pasta plus beans daily	Choose a diet high in a variety of plant-based foods
Engage in regular physical activity		Eat plenty of vegetables and fruits
Consume a variety of fruits, vegetables, whole grains, and low-fat dairy products each day	Limit intake of high-fat food, particularly from animal sources	Maintain a healthy weight and be physically active
Consume less fat, keeping trans fatty acid consumption as low as possible	Be physically active and achieve and maintain a healthy weight	Drink alcohol in moderation, if at all
Choose fiber-rich fruits, vegetables, and whole grains often	Limit consumption of alcoholic beverages, if you drink at all	Select foods low in fat and salt
Consume and prepare foods with little salt and choose potassium-rich foods		Prepare and store foods safely
Those who choose to drink alcoholic beverages should do so sensibly and in moderation		Do not use tobacco in any form
Keep food safety in mind during preparation, storing, and serving		

and vitamin D supplementation on colorectal cancer. Over an average of 7 years, there was no significant difference in colorectal cancer incidence between the intervention and control groups.[40] The extended period of time over which colorectal cancer develops may have led to these null findings; further follow-up is expected.

Polyp Prevention Trial (PPT). The PPT was a randomized controlled study of the effects of a low-fat (20% of total energy intake), high-fiber (18 g/1000 kcal), high fruit and vegetable (5–8 daily servings) diet on the recurrence of colorectal adenomas among individuals who had had a polyp removed in the previous 6 months.[41] Participants ($N = 2079$) were randomized to the intervention group in which they received intensive nutritional counseling, or the control group in which they received a brochure on healthy eating. At the 4-year follow-up, results suggested that adopting a low-fat, high-fiber diet, and increasing fruit and vegetable consumption did not affect the risk of recurrence for colorectal adenomas.[6] These results are similar to those reported by the Toronto Polyp Prevention Trial and the Australian Polyp Prevention Trial.[42] Further follow-up at 8 years supported the initial findings.[43]

Calcium Polyp Prevention Study. This randomized trial (1998–1992) examined the effects of calcium supplements on the recurrence of colorectal polyps.[44] Individuals with a history of colorectal polyps were randomized to receive either calcium supplements (1200 mg) or placebo daily for 4 years. Initial results showed that calcium supplements were associated with a decreased risk of recurrent colorectal adenomas. At the 5-year follow-up, results showed a prolonged effect of calcium supplementation on risk of recurrent colorectal adenomas.[45]

Selenium and Vitamin E Cancer Prevention Trial (SELECT). The SELECT trial is currently investigating the individual and additive effects of selenium and vitamin E on prostate cancer incidence.[46] The rationale for the study is based on results from secondary analyses of data from previous intervention trials for other cancers that found a significant effect of selenium and vitamin E on prostate cancer risk. Secondary outcomes include the incidence of lung, colorectal, and all cancers combined. The study began in 2001 and has enrolled over 35,000 men. Results are expected in 2013.

NUTRITIONAL STRATEGIES FOR CANCER RISK REDUCTION

The role of diet in an overall healthy lifestyle is not a new concept. More than 2500 years ago, Hippocrates is quoted as saying "Leave your drugs in the chemist's pot if you can heal the patient with good food." Advice on food choices and food preparation has a long history, and as our understanding of the role of food and nutrition has evolved, so have

dietary recommendations.[47] Currently, both public and private organizations publish nutrition guidelines.[48] However, the complexity of the human diet makes simple recommendations a challenge. Over time, recommendations have progressed from a rather narrow focus on nutrient adequacy to a broader focus that incorporates chronic disease risk reduction and health promotion.[49]

Overall, both national and international dietary recommendations highlight the importance of increased fruit, vegetable, and whole grain intake; decreased red meat consumption; and limited or no alcohol consumption as strategies for cancer risk reduction.[16,48] In the United States, *Dietary Guidelines for Americans* has been published jointly every 5 years beginning in 1980 by the Department of Health and Human Services (DHHS) and the USDA.[50] These guidelines, which are used in conjunction with the Food Guide Pyramid (MyPyramid), provide advice on how healthy dietary patterns can promote health and reduce risk for a number of chronic diseases.[51] MyPyramid presents various food groups including grains, vegetables, fruits, dairy, and meat and nonmeat protein, each shown with the number of servings needed to provide for adequate daily nutrition.[51]

The AICR and the American Cancer Society (ACS), two nongovernmental organizations dedicated to cancer control, have developed similar guidelines,[52,53] which are generally more qualitative and less quantitative than the recommendations in MyPyramid. Overall, these dietary recommendations encourage eating a plant-based diet that includes a variety of fruits, vegetables, and whole grains, and limiting the consumption of red meats and excessive alcohol.[52,53] Table 3–2 shows an overview of current dietary and lifestyle recommendations.

BARRIERS TO HEALTHFUL EATING

A limitation of the dietary recommendations discussed in the preceding section is that they are seldom published in conjunction with a well-funded marketing campaign to explain the material to the consumer.[54] However, the Nutrition Labeling and Education Act (NLEA) has ensured that important information about the nutrient content of foods and their associated health implications is available. The act, which was passed by Congress in 1990, introduced a new regulatory system for food labeling and health claims, and packaged foods were required to meet the new standards beginning in 1994.[55]

Despite nutritional recommendations, foods labels, and health claims, individuals often continue to make food choices based on taste, cost, and convenience, rather than health.[56] In general, people do not eat recommended foods on a regular basis.[56] For example, estimated fruit and vegetable intake in the United States is 3.4 total servings of fruits and vegetables per day, while the 2005 Dietary Guidelines recommends 5–13 servings each day. Especially worrisome is the fact that only 2% of children (aged 2–19 years) eat a diet consistent with the USDA guidelines.[57] There may be several reasons why guidelines are not followed.

First, foods that are energy-dense often are more satisfying than foods that are not.[58] Clinical studies show that foods that are high in fat, sugar, or both are usually the targets of cravings, and the intrinsic reward associated with these foods may perpetuate their consumption.[59] Second, there is a disturbing trend toward an increased reliance on pre-packaged and fast food, requiring little or no preparation.[60] Consumer spending at fast food restaurants in the United States has increased more than 15-fold over the past two decades.[3] Equally unhealthful is the prevalence of high-temperature cooking, high-fat content in red meat and fried potatoes, and sugar sweetened drinks offered at fast food restaurants. This runs counter to a number of guidelines of the World Cancer Research Fund and the AICR.[61] Unfortunately, healthful foods such as fish, whole grains, and fresh fruits and vegetables tend to be more expensive, less accessible, and require more preparation.[62] Data from the Bureau of Labor Statistics indicate that income disparities do affect dietary choices.[63] Limited economic resources may shift dietary choices toward an energy-dense, highly palatable diet that provides more calories for less cost.[64]

Third, the relationship between the neighborhood food environment and eating behavior has recently come under increased scrutiny.[65] A positive relationship between the consumption of fruits and the availability of healthy options in nearby grocery stores has been noted.[66] Better access to grocery stores has been found in higher versus lower socioeconomic areas.[66] Overall, some communities have less access than others to the food necessary to meet current dietary recommendations to reduce cancer risk.

Fourth, the role culture plays in influencing food choices and how nutrition recommendations are received needs increased exploration.[67] Cultural influences affect adult eating behaviors and parental feeding practices.[68] It may be that certain foods, such as meat and other high-fat foods, are more highly valued in certain cultures because they are associated with past unavailability, even though they are now plentiful and relatively inexpensive.[67] Given that dietary guidelines change with advances in the field, information can be confusing and even appear contradictory. Therefore, some individuals may be skeptical about changing their diet based on the latest research.[69] This may be a particularly salient concern in communities that feel marginalized or are linguistically isolated,[70] highlighting the importance of recognizing and responding to culturally based beliefs and attitudes.

PREVENTION, DIET, AND CANCER IN THE ERA OF GENOMICS

The completion of the sequencing of the human genome in 2001 marked the onset of a basic shift in biomedical research that will expand our knowledge of the complex relationships between genotype, diet, lifestyle, and the environment.[71] Research in the area of nutritional genomics has the potential to identify which components in foods influence changes in cancer risk.[1] However, even though genes may, in time, be able to provide important information about the increased risk of a disease, in many cases genes will not determine the actual cause of the disease.[72] Behavior will still play a critical role in the translation and adoption of biomedical advances, particularly associations between molecular markers of disease and environmental factors.[73] Thus, turning to the human genome to provide the ultimate solution to most chronic illnesses may be unrealistic. For example, observational studies suggest that as individuals migrate from one country to another (e.g., from Japan to the United States) the chance of being diagnosed with a chronic illness is determined by the country migrated to, not the country of origin.[19] For the most part, our environment and lifestyle determine the risk of most chronic illnesses, including cancer.[72]

CONCLUSIONS

Providing definitive evidence for the effects of specific dietary factors on cancer risk is a challenge and for some relationships may not be possible.[74] Nonetheless, taken cumulatively, there are data to support diet and

energy balance (combined diet and physical activity) as determinants of cancer risk.[9,72] Therefore, establishing a healthy and cancer-preventing lifestyle should be a public health priority. A number of recommendations reflect current research findings: maintaining a BMI between 18.5 and 25 kg/m^2, avoiding preserved or red meat, salt-preserved foods, and extremely hot beverages as well as limiting alcohol intake and dietary exposure to aflatoxin, and increasing physical activity and fruit and vegetable intake. These are factors consistent with the available evidence and should be part of public health policy.

REFERENCES

1. Milner JA. Diet and cancer: facts and controversies. *Nutr Cancer.* 2006;56(2): 216–224.
2. McGinnis JM, Foege WH. The immediate vs the important. *JAMA.* 2004;291(10):1263–1264.
3. Uauy R, Solomons N. Diet, nutrition, and the life-course approach to cancer prevention. *J Nutr.* 2005;135(suppl 12):2934S-2945S.
4. Davis CD, Uthus EO. DNA methylation, cancer susceptibility, and nutrient interactions. *Exp Biol Med (Maywood).* 2004;229(10):988–995.
5. Michels KB, Edward G, Joshipura KJ, et al. Prospective study of fruit and vegetable consumption and incidence of colon and rectal cancers [erratum appears in J Natl Cancer Inst. 2001 Jun 6;93(11):879]. *J Natl Cancer Inst.* 2000;92(21):1740–1752.
6. Schatzkin A, Lanza E, Corle D, et al. Lack of effect of a low-fat, high-fiber diet on the recurrence of colorectal adenomas. Polyp Prevention Trial Study Group. *N Engl J Med.* 2000;342(16):1149–1155.
7. Riboli E, Norat T. Epidemiologic evidence of the protective effect of fruit and vegetables on cancer risk. *Am J Clin Nutr.* 2003;78(suppl 3):559S-569S.
8. Robbins RJ, Keck A-S, Banuelos G, Finley JW. Cultivation conditions and selenium fertilization alter the phenolic profile, glucosinolate, and sulforaphane content of broccoli. *J Med Food.* 2005;8(2):204–214.
9. Key TJ, Schatzkin A, Willett WC, Allen NE, Spencer EA, Travis RC. Diet, nutrition and the prevention of cancer. *Public Health Nutr.* 2004;7(1A):187–200.
10. Rolls BJ, Ello-Martin JA, Tohill BC. What can intervention studies tell us about the relationship between fruit and vegetable consumption and weight management? *Nutr Rev.* 2004;62(1):1–17.
11. Willett WC. Diet and cancer: an evolving picture. *JAMA.* 2005; 293(2): 233–234.
12. Calle EE, Rodriguez C, Walker-Thurmond K, Thun MJ. Overweight, obesity, and mortality from cancer in a prospectively studied cohort of U.S. adults. *N Engl J Med.* 2003;348(17):1625–1638.
13. Bleich S, Cutler D, Murray C, Adams A. Why is the developed world obese? *Annu Rev Public Health.* 2008;29:273–295.
14. Kelly T, Yang W, Chen CS, Reynolds K, He J. Global burden of obesity in 2005 and projections to 2030. *Int J Obes.* 2008;1–7. http://www.nature.com/ijo/journal/vaop/ncurrent/pdf/ijo2008102a.pdf. Accessed October 8, 2009.
15. International Agency for Research on Cancer (IARC). Weight control and physical activity. In: Vainio H, Biachini F, eds. *IARC handbooks of cancer prevention: cancer preventive effects.* Lyons, France: IARC Press; 2002.
16. World Cancer Research Fund/American Institute for Cancer Research. *Food, nutrition and physical activity, and the prevention of cancer: a global perspective.* Washington, DC: American Institute for Cancer Research (AICR); 2007.
17. Cancer Research U.K. Commonly diagnosed cancers worldwide. http://info.cancerresearchuk.org/cancerstats/geographic/world/commoncancers/. Accessed August 21, 2008.
18. Parkin DM, Bray F, Ferlay J, Pisani P. Global cancer statistics, 2002. *CA Cancer J Clin.* 2005;55(2):74–108.
19. International Agency for Research on Cancer (IARC). Cancer: causes, occurrence and control. *IARC Sci Publ.* 1990;(100):1–352.
20. World Health Organization. *Arsenic in drinking water.* Fact sheet No. 210. 2001. http://www.who.int/mediacentre/factsheets/fs210/en/. Accessed August 21, 2008.
21. Goodman GE, Thornquist MD, Balmes J, et al. The beta-carotene and retinol efficacy trial: incidence of lung cancer and cardiovascular disease mortality during 6-year follow-up after stopping beta-carotene and retinol supplements. *J Natl Cancer Inst.* 2004;96(23):1743–1750.
22. National Research Council. *Diet, nutrition, and cancer.* Washington, DC: National Academy Press; 1982.
23. Tsugane S, Sasazuki S, Kobayashi M, Sasaki S. Salt and salted food intake and subsequent risk of gastric cancer among middle-aged Japanese men and women. *Br J Cancer.* 2004;90(1):128–134.
24. National Institute of Environmental Health Services (NIEHS). *Aflatoxin & Liver Cancer.* http://www.niehs.nih.gov/health/impacts/aflatoxin.cfm. Accessed August 21, 2008.

25. Howard RA, Freedman DM, Park Y, Hollenbeck A, Schatzkin A, and Leitzmann MF. Physical activity, sedentary behavior, and the risk of colon and rectal cancer in the NIH-AARP Diet and Health Study. *Cancer Causes Control.* 2008. http://www.springerlink.com/content/f51208p34745684u/fulltext.pdf. Accessed August 27, 2008.

26. Larsson SC, Wolk A. Meat consumption and risk of colorectal cancer: a meta-analysis of prospective studies. *Int J Cancer.* 2006;119(11):2657–2664.

27. Cho E, Smith-Warner SA, Spiegelman D, et al. Dairy foods, calcium, and colorectal cancer: a pooled analysis of 10 cohort studies [erratum appears in *J Natl Cancer Inst.* 2004 Nov 17;96(22):1724]. *J Natl Cancer Inst.* 2004;96(13):1015–1022.

28. Smith-Warner SA, Spiegelman D, Yaun SS, et al. Alcohol and breast cancer in women: a pooled analysis of cohort studies. *JAMA.* 1998;279(7):535–540.

29. Smith-Warner SA, Spiegelman D, Adami HO, et al. Types of dietary fat and breast cancer: a pooled analysis of cohort studies. *Int J Cancer.* 2001;92(5):767–774.

30. Boyd NF, Stone J, Vogt KN, Connelly BS, Martin LJ, Minkin S. Dietary fat and breast cancer risk revisited: a meta-analysis of the published literature. *Br J Cancer.* 2003;89(9):1672–1685.

31. Prentice RL, Caan B, Chlebowski RT, et al. Low-fat dietary pattern and risk of invasive breast cancer: the Women's Health Initiative Randomized Controlled Dietary Modification Trial. *JAMA.* 2006;295(6):629–642.

32. Binstock M, Krakow D, Stamler J, et al. Coffee and pancreatic cancer: an analysis of international mortality data. *Am J Epidemiol.* 1983;118(5):630–640.

33. Connolly JM, Coleman M, Rose DP. Effects of dietary fatty acids on DU145 human prostate cancer cell growth in athymic nude mice. *Nutr Cancer.* 1997;29(2):114–119.

34. Debes JD, Roberts RO, Jacobson DJ, et al. Inverse association between prostate cancer and the use of calcium channel blockers. *Cancer Epidemiol Biomarkers Prev.* 2004;13(2):255–259.

35. Li H, Stampfer MJ, Giovannucci EL, et al. A prospective study of plasma selenium levels and prostate cancer risk. *J Natl Cancer Inst.* 2004;96(9):696–703.

36. Etminan M, FitzGerald JM, Gleave M, Chambers K. Intake of selenium in the prevention of prostate cancer: a systematic review and meta-analysis. *Cancer Causes Control.* 2005;16(9):1125–1131.

37. Pierce JP, Natarajan L, Caan BJ, et al. Influence of a diet very high in vegetables, fruit, and fiber and low in fat on prognosis following treatment for breast cancer: the Women's Healthy Eating and Living (WHEL) randomized trial. *JAMA.* 2007;298(3):289–298.

38. Chlebowski RT, Blackburn GL, Thomson CA, et al. Dietary fat reduction and breast cancer outcome: interim efficacy results from the Women's Intervention Nutrition Study. *J Natl Cancer Inst.* 2006;98(24):1767–1776.

39. Anonymous. Design of the Women's Health Initiative clinical trial and observational study. The Women's Health Initiative Study Group. *Control Clin Trials.* 1998;19(1):61–109.

40. Wactawski-Wende J, Kotchen JM, Anderson GL, et al. Calcium plus vitamin D supplementation and the risk of colorectal cancer [erratum appears in *N Engl J Med.* 2006 Mar 9;354(10):1102]. *N Engl J Med.* 2006;354(7):684–696.

41. Schatzkin A, Lanza E, Freedman LS, et al. The Polyp Prevention Trial I: rationale, design, recruitment, and baseline participant characteristics. *Cancer Epidemiol Biomarkers Prev.* 1996;5(5):375–383.

42. MacLennan R, Macrae F, Bain C, et al. Randomized trial of intake of fat, fiber, and beta carotene to prevent colorectal adenomas. The Australian Polyp Prevention Project. *J Natl Cancer Inst.* 1995;87(23):1760–1766.

43. Lanza E, Yu B, Murphy G, et al. The polyp prevention trial continued follow-up study: no effect of a low-fat, high-fiber, high-fruit, and -vegetable diet on adenoma recurrence eight years after randomization. *Cancer Epidemiol Biomarkers Prev.* 2007;16(9):1745–1752.

44. Baron JA, Beach M, Mandel JS, et al. Calcium supplements for the prevention of colorectal adenomas. Calcium Polyp Prevention Study Group. *N Engl J Med.* 1999;340(2):101–107.

45. Grau MV, Baron JA, Sandler RS, et al. Prolonged effect of calcium supplementation on risk of colorectal adenomas in a randomized trial. *J Natl Cancer Inst.* 2007;99(2):129–136.

46. Klein EA, Lippman SM, Thompson IM, et al. The Selenium and Vitamin E Cancer Prevention Trial. *World J Urol.* 2003;21(1):21–27.

47. Centers for Disease Control and Prevention. Safer and healthier foods. *MMWR Morbid Mortal Wkly Rep.* 1999;48(40):905–913.

48. U.S. Department of Health and Human Services (USDHHS). *Healthy People 2010: understanding and improving health.* 2nd ed. Washington, DC: U.S. Government Printing Office; 2000.

49. Fitzgibbon M, Gans KM, Evans WD, et al. Communicating healthy eating: lessons learned and future directions. *J Nutr Educ Behav.* 2007;39(suppl 2): S63–S71.

50. U.S. Department of Health and Human Services and U.S. Department of Agriculture. *Dietary guidelines for Americans, 2005.* 6th ed. Washington, DC: U.S. Government Printing Office; 2005.

51. United States Department of Agriculture (USDA). *My Pyramid.gov steps to a healthier you.* http://www.mypyramid.gov/. Accessed August 19, 2008.

52. American Institute for Cancer Research. http://www.aicr.org/site/PageServer. Accessed August 19, 2008.

53. American Cancer Society (ACS). http://www.cancer.org/docroot/PED/ped_3_1x_ACS_Guidelines.asp?sitearea=PED. Accessed August 19, 2008.

54. Kuehn BM. Experts charge new US dietary guidelines pose daunting challenge for the public. *JAMA.* 2005;293(8):918–920.

55. Nutrition Labeling and Education Act of 1990. Pub L No. 101–535, 104 Stat 2353.

56. Glanz K, Basil M, Maibach E, Goldberg J, Snyder D. Why Americans eat what they do: taste, nutrition, cost, convenience, and weight control concerns as influences on food consumption. *J Am Diet Assoc.* 1998;98(10):1118–1126.

57. Munoz KA, Krebs-Smith SM, Ballard-Barbash R, Cleveland LE. Food intakes of US children and adolescents compared with recommendations [erratum appears in *Pediatrics.* 1998 May;101(5):952–953]. *Pediatrics.* 1997;100(3, pt 1): 323–329.

58. Drewnowski A, Henderson SA, Barratt-Fornell A. Genetic taste markers and food preferences. *Drug Metab Dispos.* 2001;29(4, pt 2):535–538.

59. Yanovski S. Sugar and fat: cravings and aversions. *J Nutr.* 2003;133(3):835S–837S.

60. Chou S, Grossman M, Saffer H. An economic analysis of adult obesity: results from the Behavioral Risk Factor Surveillance System. *J Health Econ.* 2004;23(3):565–587.

61. World Cancer Research Fund. *Food, nutrition and the prevention of cancer: a global perspective.* Washington, DC: American Institute for Cancer Research; 1997.

62. Drewnowski A, Darmon N. Food choices and diet costs: an economic analysis. *J Nutr.* 2005;135(4):900–904.

63. Kaufman PR, MacDonald JM, Lutz SM, Smallwood DM. *Do the poor pay more for food? Item selection and prices differences affect low-income household food costs.* Washington, DC: Economic Research Service, U.S. Department of Agriculture; 1997.

64. Drewnowski A. Obesity and the food environment: dietary energy density and diet costs. *Am J Prev Med.* 2004;27(suppl 3):154–162.

65. Story M, French S. Food advertising and marketing directed at children and adolescents in the US. *Int J Behav Nutr Phys Act.* 2004;1(1):3.

66. Morland K, Wing S, Diez Roux A, Poole C. Neighborhood characteristics associated with the location of food stores and food service places. *Am J Prev Med.* 2002;22(1):23–29.

67. Kumanyika SK. Environmental influences on childhood obesity: ethnic and cultural influences in context. *Physiol Behav.* 2008;94(1):61–70.

68. Mintz LB, O'Halloran SM, Mulholland AM, Schneider PA. Questionnaire for eating disorder diagnoses: reliability and validity of operationalizing DSM-IV criteria into a self-report format. *J Counsel Psychol.* 1997;44:63–79.

69. Wasserman J, Flannery MA, Clair JM. Rasing the ivory tower: the production of knowledge and distrust of medicine among African Americans. *J Med Ethics.* 2007;33(3):177–180.

70. Corbie-Smith G, Thomas SB, St George DMM. Distrust, race, and research. *Arch Intern Med.* 2002;162(21):2458–2463.

71. Guttmacher AE, Collins FS. Welcome to the genomic era [comment]. *N Engl J Med.* 2003;349(10):996–998.

72. Anand P, Kunnumakara AB, Sundaram C, et al. Cancer is a preventable disease that requires major lifestyle changes. *Pharm Res.* 2008;25(9):2097–2116.

73. McBride CM, Lipkus IM, Jolly D, Lyna P. Interest in testing for genetic susceptibility to lung cancer among Black college students "at risk" of becoming cigarette smokers. *Cancer Epidemiol Biomarkers Prev.* 2005;14(12):2978–2981.

74. Willett W. *Nutritional epidemiology.* 2nd ed. New York, NY: Oxford University Press; 1998.

CHAPTER 4

Exercise and Cancer

Bernardine M. Pinto and Sheri J. Hartman

INTRODUCTION

Cancer is the second leading cause of death in developed countries and the third leading cause of death in developing countries. It is estimated that there will be more than 12 million new cancer cases in 2007 worldwide, and by 2050, the global burden is expected to grow to 27 million new cancer cases.[1] Although there have been considerable improvements in early detection and treatment of cancer; preventing the disease by targeting modifiable factors such as tobacco use, diet, and inactivity has received considerable attention. The role of physical activity (PA; defined as any bodily movement produced by skeletal muscles that results in energy expenditure) or exercise (defined as PA that is planned, structured, repetitive, and directed to the improvement or maintenance of physical fitness)[2] (We used the term physical activity to encompass both exercise and physical activity.) in preventing cancer has been examined in numerous epidemiological studies and several reviews of the literature (e.g., see references 3–8). This chapter reviews more recent publications (2002–2008) on the effects of PA on risk for the most prevalent cancers in the developed countries[1]: breast (women), colorectal, lung, and prostate (men).

METHODS

Literature review. To provide a review of the recent research on PA and cancer, we included studies published (or published online) in the past 5 years (5/15/2002–5/15/2008) and written in English. Articles to be included were identified through a systematic review of literature available on PubMed. A combination of the following terms was used to search the database: PA, exercise, prevention, risk, cancer, breast, colorectal, colon, prostate, and lung. Reference lists from identified studies and recent reviews on this topic were scanned to identify additional studies.

To obtain a comprehensive view of PA, there are various types of PA that should be considered: for example, occupational, leisure, transportation, and household activities. We limited this review to studies that, at a minimum, assessed occupational and leisure activity. When the type of PA assessed could not be determined, we chose to keep it in the review.[9] Companion papers that assessed leisure activity in one article and occupational activity in another article were also included.[10,11]

Breast cancer. In 2002, the International Agency for Research on Cancer (IARC) in their review concluded that the evidence of an inverse association between PA and breast cancer risk was convincing.[5] Our review included six cohort studies[12–17] and 10 case-control studies[9,18–26] that assessed both occupational and leisure activity. (Note: the study by Tehard and colleagues[17] did not directly assess occupational activity, but was retained because a majority of women in the sample were teachers, and, hence, occupational activity was likely to be similar among the participants.) The studies have been conducted chiefly among middle-aged and older women in Japan, several European countries, and the United States. A majority of studies presented data for women irrespective of menopausal status, although in a few studies, data were presented separately for pre- and postmenopausal women (Table 4–1).[12,19,20,23]

Twelve studies found that PA conferred protective benefits (case-control studies;[9,17–24,26] cohort studies[12,14]) and four studies did not find such evidence (three cohort studies[13,15,16] and one case-control study[25]).

Previous reviews have found that breast cancer risk reduction associated with PA is about 20%.[8,27] The more recent research shows considerable variation in risk estimates. For example, in a case-control study, Kruk[21] found that lifetime total PA among women was associated with 72% reduced risk for total PA of at least 55 hours/week/year (>150 Metabolic equivalent or MET hours/week/year, odds ratio [OR] = 0.43). Tehard and colleagues[17] found a 38% reduction in risk among women who reported more than 5 hours/week of vigorous leisure activity. Among the studies that did not find evidence for protective benefits, one utilized two questions to assess PA,[16] in another, lifetime activity was not assessed,[15] and in the third, the sample consisted largely of premenopausal women.[13] The one case-control study that did not find any benefits was conducted among premenopausal women only.[25]

As noted in previous reviews (e.g., see reference 8), case-control studies have found protective benefits of PA among younger women but cohort studies tend not to find these benefits. The same trend was found in the current review with only two of the six cohort studies finding such benefits[12,14] (Lahmann and colleagues[12] found that household PA but not total PA was associated with reduced risk in premenopausal women). It is worthwhile to summarize the findings from four studies that analyzed data separately for pre- and postmenopausal women. In a large cohort study of 218,169 pre- and postmenopausal women (participants in the European Prospective Investigation into Cancer and Nutrition [EPIC] study), household activity was associated with reduced risk in premenopausal (hazard ratio [HR] = 0.71) and postmenopausal women (HR = 0.81).[12] Among the case-control studies, Slattery and colleagues[23] found reduced risk (OR = 0.62) among premenopausal non-Hispanic white women who exercised at least 30 MET hours/week or more in the referent year. Among postmenopausal women, PA had greatest benefit among women not recently exposed to hormones. In the third study, John and colleagues[20] found that lifetime PA reduced risk in both pre- (OR = 0.74) and postmenopausal women (OR = 0.81). Finally, Dorn and colleagues[19] found that strenuous PA was associated with reduced breast cancer risk in both pre- and postmenopausal women.

How much activity provides benefits? In general, greater activity (intensity/duration/energy expenditure as reflected in MET hours) has been associated with greater protection. Peplonska and colleagues[22] found that women in the highest quartiles of moderate/vigorous leisure PA, outdoor activities, and heavy physical work (as measured in MET hours/week/lifetime) had lower risk. Tehard and colleagues[17] found a linear decrease in risk with increasing amounts of moderate (at least 14 hours/week, relative risk [RR] = 0.89) and vigorous activity (5 or more hours/week, RR = 0.62). In a case-control study among Asian American women, Yang and colleagues[26] found reduced risk with increasing lifetime energy expenditure in leisure PA (OR = 0.65 with >3–6 MET hours/week, OR = 0.53 with >6–12 MET hours/week, and OR = 0.47 with >12 MET hours/week). In the Nurses' Health Study II cohort, Maruti and colleagues[14] found that women who engaged in 39 or more MET hours/week of total activity on average during their lifetime (equivalent to 13 hours/week of walking or 3.25 hours/week of running) had a 23% lower risk of premenopausal breast cancer.

Interaction effects: Some studies found that benefits of PA toward risk reduction were not affected by age,[20] weight,[17] parity,[14,17,20] family history,[17,20] hormone use,[17,20] menopausal status,[17,26] and body mass index (BMI).[14,20,26] Yet others have found benefits to be found only among those

Table 4–1. Summaries of studies on breast cancer

Breast cancer case-control studies

Authors	Sample	Activity measure	Factors adjusted	Results
Carpenter et al., 2003	N = 1883 post-menopausal cases N = 1628 post-menopausal controls United States	Lifetime history of exercise activity where duration of activity was at least 2 hrs/wk for 1 year Constructed several PA variables including average MET-hrs/wk from menarche to referent year, number of years exercised more than 4 hrs/wk, and average MET-hrs/wk in the 10-year period before referent year	Age at first term pregnancy Age at menopause Interviewer BMI at reference date	Decreased risk among women who maintained on average 17.6 MET-hrs of activity per week from menarche onward (OR = 0.66, CI = 0.48–0.90) Risk reduction associated with exercise activity adjusting for BMI was limited to women without a family history (hx) of breast cancer (BC)
Dorn et al., 2002	N = 301 pre-menopausal cases N = 316 pre-menopausal controls N = 439 post-menopausal cases N = 494 post-menopausal controls United States	Leisure activity assessed with two questions of the frequency of engaging in strenuous activity at age 16 and 2, 10, and 20 years before the interview Computed summary of lifetime PA by summing the totals for 2, 10, and 20 years before interview Occupational PA—all jobs held for 1 year or longer and used the NCI's Job Exposure Matrix to determine the number of years worked at sedentary, moderate, or vigorous jobs	Age Education Age at menarche Relative with BC Benign BC BMI Age at first pregnancy	Strenuous PA generally associated with reduced BC risk Among women active at all four periods strong significant protective effect observed for postmenopausal (OR = 0.5, CI = 0.28–0.90) but not for premenopausal women (OR = 1.06, CI = 0.54–2.08) Strong protective effect observed for activity performed 20 years prior in both groups Walking was generally unrelated to risk Some indication of increased risk for the upper category on occupational PA for postmenopausal women
Hirose et al., 2003	N = 2376 cases N = 18,977 controls Japan	No details provided	Age Visit year Age at menarche Menopausal status Family hx Parity Age at first full-term pregnancy Drinking Intake of fruit Dietary restriction Hx of stomach cancer screening BMI Occupation	Decreased risk for women who regularly exercised twice a week or more (OR = 0.81, CI = 0.69–0.94) irrespective of menopausal status Greater risk reduction for some subgroups including women who were parous, no family hx, or nondrinkers Among premenopausal women, strong protective effect of PA was observed for women with BMI ≥25 (OR = 0.57, CI = 0.28–1.15) Risk reduction found for postmeno-pausal women who's BMI was 22–25 (OR = 0.71, CI = 0.5–1.01)
John et al., 2003	N = 403 premeno-pausal cases N = 483 premeno-pausal controls N = 847 post-menopausal cases N = 1065 post-menopausal controls United States	In-person structured interview assessed frequency, duration, and type of recreational activity engaged in for at least 1 hr/wk for 4 months throughout lifetime Assessed daily living activities: walk-ing/biking to school or work at least 20 min/day for 4 months and stren-uous household and outdoor chores at least 2 hrs/wk for 4 months Occupational activity—all jobs held for at least 1 year self-assessed level of activity	Age Race/ethnicity Country of birth Education Family hx of BC Prior biopsy for benign BC Age of menarche Parity Age at first full-term pregnancy Breast-feeding BMI Other components of total activity Age at menopause	Reduced risk in both pre- and postmeno-pausal women with the highest vs. lowest tertile of average lifetime activity (premenopausal OR = 0.74, CI = 0.52–1.05; postmenopausal OR = 0.81, CI = 0.64–1.02) Similar risk reduction in three assessed racial/ethnic groups For premenopausal women, risk reductions were similar for different types of activities For postmenopausal women, risk reduction only for occupational activity Risk reduction similar for moderate and vigorous activities

(Continued)

Table 4–1. Continued

Breast cancer case-control studies

Authors	Sample	Activity measure	Factors adjusted	Results
Kruk, 2007	N = 250 cases N = 301 controls Poland	Details about recreational, occupational, and household activities were recorded in a table format using a modified version on the Friedenreich et al and Kriska et al questionnaires Recreational activity was assessed at ages 14–20, 21–34, 35–50, and >50 For occupational activity, asked to identify jobs held for at least 2 years outside of home out of list of the 20 most popular occupations Assessed frequency and duration of household activities Also indicated the intensity of each activity from 1 to 3	Age BMI Material conditions Parity Breast-feeding Active cigarette smoking	Lifetime total PA was associated with reduced risk (OR = 0.28, CI = 0.16–0.50) Analyses by type of lifetime activity for household (OR = 0.32, CI = 0.18–0.58) and recreational activities (OR = 0.37, CI = 0.20–0.67) showed significant risk reduction For lifetime occupational activity a modest association could not be ruled out (OR = 0.58, CI = 0.33–1.00) Women who started recreational activity after age 20 had much higher BC risk than either those who were active between 14 and 20 and were inactive after age 20 or those who continued their activity throughout adulthood
Peplonska et al., 2008	N = 2176 cases N = 2326 controls Poland	Assessed total number of hours spent in five categories of recreational activities in five age ranges (age 20–24, 24–29, 30–34, 35–39, 40–50) Subjects over 50 were asked if they had changed their level of PA since their 40s Occupational PA assessed level of activity in all jobs held for longer than 6 months	Age Study site Education BMI Age at menarche Menopausal status Age at menopause Number of full-term births Age at first full-term birth Breast-feeding Family hx of BC Previous mammography screening	Total adult lifetime activity reduced risk of BC in highest compared to lowest quartiles (OR = 0.8, CI = 0.67–.096) Reduced risks were most consistent for the highest quartile of moderate to vigorous recreational activity, outdoor activities, heavy physical work, and combined high-intensity activities Reductions in risk with moderate/vigorous recreational activities were stronger for larger tumors and those with nodal involvement Women who increased their recreational activity in their 50s had significantly reduced risk with those in the highest tertile of change being at a 27% lower risk
Slattery et al., 2007	N = 1527 Non-Hispanic whites (NHW) cases N = 1601 NHW controls N = 798 Hispanic/American Indian (HAI) cases N = 924 HAI controls United States	PA questionnaire adapted from the Cross-Cultural Activity Participation Study Asked to report the amount, intensity, and duration of activities they performed during referent year and at ages 15, 30, and 50 Lifetime activity score Total MET values assigned to each activity based on the Compendium of Physical Activities	Age Center Parity BMI Energy intake	Among premenopausal women only, high total MET during referent year was associated with reduced risk in NHW (OR = 0.62, CI = 0.43–0.91) Among postmenopausal women, PA had the greatest influence on women not recently exposed to hormones—among these women high total lifetime activity reduced risk for both NHW (OR = 0.60, CI = 0.36–1.02) and HAI (OR = 0.52, 0.23–1.16) High total MET at age 30 (OR = 0.56, CI = 0.37–0.85) and age 15 (OR = 0.57, CI = 0.38–0.88) associated with reduced risk among postmenopausal NHW not recently exposed to hormones Among HAI women, more recent activity performed during the referent year at age 50 appeared to have the greatest influence on BC risk
Sprague et al., 2007	N = 7630 controls N = 1689 in situ BC cases N = 6391 invasive BC cases United States	Lifetime history of multiple recreational activities assessed by reporting their age when the activity was started and stopped, the number of months per year, and the number of hours per week	Age State Menopausal status Family hx of BC Parity Age at first birth Age at menarche Age at menopause	Neither lifetime recreational nor strenuous occupational PA associated with risk of BC in situ Women averaging >6 hrs/wk of strenuous recreational activity over their lifetime had a 23% reduction in risk of invasive BC compared to women reported no recreational activity (OR = 0.77, CI = 0.65–0.92)

Authors	Sample	Activity measure	Factors adjusted	Results
		Lifetime average hours of exercise per week assessed from age 14 to 1 year before reference date Occupational activity—any job held at least 1 year, job titles coded and classified into one of five intensity ratings Total PA combined recreational and occupational activity	HRT used Education Alcohol BMI Weight change since 18	Inverse association observed for PA age 14–22 (OR = 0.87, CI = 0.74–1.01), age 22 to menopause (OR = 0.70, CI = 0.53–0.91) in postmenopausal years (OR = 0.80, CI = 0.64–1.00), and in recent past (0.86, CI = 0.75–0.98), but only for women with no family hx of BC Lifetime strenuous occupational activity not associated with invasive BC risk
Steindorf et al., 2003	N = 360 cases N = 886 controls Germany	PA assessed during adolescence (12–19) and young adulthood (20–30) with questionnaire assessing frequency and intensity (light, moderate, heavy, or variable) of walking, cycling, household tasks, and 41 sports Lifetime occupational activity assessed for all jobs held more than 1 year and intensity classified as sedentary, standing/walking, or strenuous	First-degree family hx of BC Number of full-term pregnancies Height Change in BMI between ages 20 and 30 Total months breast-feeding Mean daily alcohol consumption	No association between total PA and premenopausal BC found in either age periods Decreased risk when active in both age periods (OR = 0.83, CI = 0.60–1.14) When both age periods were combined only moderately high PA showed a significant decrease in risk when compared to the lowest quartile of PA (OR = 0.68, CI = 0.46–0.99) Analysis by type of activity showed a protective effects for women who reported the highest level of cycling (OR = 0.66, CI = 0.45–0.97)
Yang et al., 2003	N = 501 cases N = 594 controls Asian Americans	Assessed amount of recreational PA participated in for at least 1 hr/wk from age 10 to referent year Summary recreational PA variables included total years, average hours per week, average MET-hrs/wk of PA Occupational PA assessed by identifying three jobs of longest duration held outside of the home as an adult. Categorized into 1 of 4 job-related PA categories: sedentary, mixed, active white collar jobs only, active blue collar jobs	Age Ethnic group Parity Family hx of BC Menopausal status Years with active jobs Job activity category Soy intake during adolescence and adult life	Increasing years and levels of lifetime recreational activity were associated with significant reduced risk of BC Compared with women who had no lifetime recreational PA, reduced risk was associated with increased levels of lifetime PA (<3 MET-hrs/wk: OR = 0.91, CI = 0.55–1.49; 3–6 MET-hrs/wk: OR = 0.65, CI = 0.39–1.1; 6–12 MET-hrs/wk: OR = 0.53, CI = 0.31–0.90; >12 MET-hrs/wk: OR = 0.47, CI = 0.28–0.80) Women who reported some recreational PA during adolescence and adulthood had decreased risk compared to women with no activity (OR = 0.57, CI = 0.36–0.91) Risk inversely associated with occupational PA, but results not significant

BC prospective cohort studies

Authors	Sample	Activity measure	Factors adjusted	Results
Lahmann et al., 2007	N = 218,169 Europe	Assessed occupational, household activity, recreational activity for past year Total activity calculated by combining household and recreational activity in MET-hrs/wk and divided into quartiles	Age Study center Age at menarche Age at first pregnancy Parity Current oral contraceptive use HRT use	Increasing total PA was associated with a reduction in risk among postmenopausal women Household activity associated with risk reduction for postmenopausal (HR = 0.81, CI = 0.70–0.93) and premenopausal women (HR = 0.71, CI = 0.55–0.90) Occupational and recreational activity were not significantly related to risk in either pre- or postmenopausal women
Margolis et al., 2005	N = 99,504 Norway and Sweden	Rated level of PA at three time points: age 14, 30, at enrollment of study on a scale of 1 very low to 10 very high in Norway and 1 very low to 5 very high in Sweden (collapsed 10-point scale to make comparable to 5-point scale)	Age at enrollment Education BMI Height Smoking status Alcohol intake Age at menarche Parity	Compared to inactive women, women with high levels of PA at enrollment had similar risk of BC (RR = 1.24, CI = 0.85–1.82) PA at age 30 or 14 did not decrease risk of BC

(Continued)

Table 4–1. Continued

		Breast cancer case-control studies		
Authors	Sample	Activity measure	Factors adjusted	Results
		Categorized based on changes of PA over time dichotomizing as active or inactive at each time point	Age at first birth Number of months breast-feeding Oral contraceptive use Family hx of BC Menopausal status Country of origin	Consistently high level of PA from younger age to enrollment did not decrease risk of BC
Maruti et al., 2008	N = 64,777 United States	Assessed three categories of leisure activity in five age periods and in the year before assessment Occupational activity assessed in 1997—asked to describe work activity during two age periods	Age Average childhood body shape Duration and recency of oral contraceptive use History of benign breast disease Mother or sister with BC Parity Age at first birth Current alcohol consumption Height	Strongest associations were for total leisure-time activity during participants' lifetime rather than for any one intensity or age period Active women engaging in ≥39 MET per week of total activity during their lifetime has a 23% lower risk of premenopausal BC than women reporting less activity High levels of PA during ages 12–22 contributed most strongly to the association
Mertens et al., 2006	N = 7994 United States	Modified version of the Baecke PA questionnaire to assess sport, leisure, and work activity	Age Race Center Age at first live birth Age at menopause Family hx of BC	No statistically significant associations of BC incidence with baseline PA for leisure, sport, or work Highest compared with lowest quartile: Leisure HR = 1.0, CI = 0.64–1.54 Sport HR = 1.31, CI = 0.87–1.96 Work HR = 0.87, CI = 0.61–1.24
Moradi et al., 2002	N = 9539 Sweden	Leisure activity assessed with one question: "How much physical exercise have you had from age 25 to 50?" Assigned to intensity level based on answers: hardly any activity, light exercise, regular exercise involving sports, hard physical training Occupational activity was assessed with one question: "Has your work been mainly (1) sedentary, (2) active, (3) physically strenuous?"	Age BMI	No association between PA and BC risk Women aged 51–70 at baseline who reported regular leisure-time activity had a borderline significant lower risk compared to those with no activity (RR = 0.6, CI = 0.4–1.0). Decreased risk was confined to women with a low BMI after the age of 50 and to women with a high BMI during premenopausal period No evidence that work activity reduced risk of BC
Tehard et al., 2006	N = 90,509 France	PA assessed with six questions concerning daily distance walked, daily number of flights of stairs climbed, weekly time spent doing light household activity, heavy household activity, and vigorous recreational activity		Linear decrease in risk with increasing amounts of moderate (at least 14 hrs/wk, RR = 0.89) and vigorous (≥5 hrs/wk, RR = 0.62) recreational activity Decreased risk for more than 5 hrs/wk of vigorous recreational activity compared to no recreational activity (RR = 0.62, CI = 0.49–0.78)

ABBREVIATIONS: BC, breast cancer; BMI, body mass index; CI, confidence interval; HR, hazard ratio (the effect of an explanatory variable on the hazard or risk of an event); HRT, hormone replacement therapy; hx, history; MET, metabolic equivalent; OR, odds ratio (the ratio of the odds of an event occurring in one group to the odds of it occurring in another group); N, number of people; PA, physical activity; RR, relative risk or incidence rate in a particular category of exposure divided by the corresponding rate in the comparison category.

who were parous[9] or had no family history of breast cancer.[9,18] Slattery and colleagues[23] found that increased PA among postmenopausal women not recently on hormones was found to be protective, but such benefits were not found among women who had recently been on hormone treatment. Ethnicity did not seem to produce differential effects (e.g., John and colleagues[20] found similar risk reductions associated with lifetime PA among Latinas, African American, and white women) but this variable has not been extensively studied.

When is activity most beneficial? In the case-control studies where lifetime exposure to PA was examined, attention was paid to determining when activity might be most beneficial. Kruk[21] found that women who had been engaged in leisure activity at ages 14–20 had lowered risk.

Maruti and colleagues[14] reported that women with high levels of PA during ages 12–22 years derived the most benefits (RR = 0.75). Yang and colleagues[26] found reduced breast cancer risk (OR = 0.57) with leisure PA reported during both adolescence and adulthood. Long-term maintenance of activity also seems to be protective: for example, Dorn and colleagues[19] found that postmenopausal women who were consistently active over time had lowered risk (OR = 0.50).

Assessment of PA. There continues to be considerable variability in the methods used to assess PA. In some studies, validated questionnaires were administered,[14,15] or modified versions of validated questionnaires that were tested for reliability were used.[21] On the other hand, Hirose and colleagues[9] had only one question about exercise and it was not clear what types of activities were included; Moradi and colleagues[16] in their cohort study had two questions on exercise. Variations occur in the duration of activities that are included for analyses; for example, Carpenter and colleagues[18] used in-person interviews and cognitive interviewing techniques to assess lifetime exercise and included activities that were at least 2 hours/week for a year. Such criteria were not used consistently across the studies, making it difficult to make cross study comparisons. In case-control studies that examined lifetime activity, the specific ages at which PA was recalled varied; for example, Slattery and colleagues[23] assessed household, exercise, work, and activity at age 15, 30, 50 years as well as the referent year; yet other case-control studies (e.g., see reference 19) required women to recall activity at other ages. While recall bias may influence the results in case-control studies, on the other hand, lifetime PA was not assessed in cohort studies.[12,15,17] On a positive note, household activity has been assessed in more recent studies (e.g., see references 12 and 23) and is appropriate because such activities may contribute to a sizable proportion of women's PA. Again, more recent studies have used a comprehensive approach to assessment, examining the frequency, duration, and intensity of activity within the broader categories of recreational, household, and occupational activity across the lifetime.[21] The strengths of many of the studies lies in the attention to assessment and statistical controlling for confounder variables such as age, age at first live birth, age at menopause, family history of breast cancer in a first degree relative, BMI, hormone use, contraceptive use, smoking, and alcohol intake.[12,14,15,17,21,23]

Mechanisms. The relationship of PA and breast cancer risk has been linked to various biological mechanisms that have been reviewed previously.[6,8,27] Heavy exercise is associated with delayed menarche, irregular and anovulatory menstrual cycle, and a shortened luteal phase. If exercise contributes to a delay in menarche and in the onset of regular cycles, young women may gain protective effects for hormone-sensitive cancers. Another mechanism is that regular exercise may help to reduce women's risk for breast cancer by reducing body fat. Obesity is associated with increased conversion of androgen to estrogen and the metabolism of estrogen to more potent forms. Postmenopausal women who are active had been shown to have lower levels of androgens.[28] Other mechanisms include positive effects of PA on the immune and antioxidant systems and regulation of insulin sensitivity. Much work is needed to further explore these mechanisms.

Colon and rectal cancers. In 2002, on the basis of their review, the IARC concluded there is sufficient evidence for preventive effect of PA for colon cancer and inadequate evidence for rectal cancer.[5] Our review of more recently published papers (seven cohort and six case-control studies) suggests that these conclusions continue to hold. Four studies examined only colon cancer and excluded cases of rectal cancer,[29–32] and one study combined the two cancers.[33] Of the seven cohort studies, four included both men and women,[30,34–36] one was restricted to men,[37] and two were restricted to women[29,33]; the seven case-control studies included both men and women. The studies were conducted in several European countries, Japan, and the United States. The study populations were middle-aged and older.

Of the seven cohort studies and six case-control studies that examined the relationship between PA and colon cancer: five cohort studies[33–37]

and five case-control studies[31,32,38–40] suggested protective benefits of PA for colon cancer; two cohort studies did not find such associations.[29,30] The remaining study examined the interaction between gene polymorphisms with energy balance and did not examine the independent effects of PA.[41] Of the two studies that did not find protective benefits, one may have been limited by a small number of cancer cases[30] and the other by possible misclassification of activities (women's only sample) (Table 4–2).[29]

Colon cancer. Previous reviews have concluded that PA helps to reduce risk of colon cancer by about 30%[8] or more (e.g., 40%–50%[27]). In a large European cohort study of over 400,000 individuals, PA was associated with reduced colon cancer risk among both men and women (OR = 0.80).[34] In a case-control study, Steindorf and colleagues[40] found that those with the highest quartile of PA (occupational combined with leisure activity) had lower risk (OR = 0.37) compared those in the lowest quartile. Similarly, Slattery and Potter[31] in a case-control study found that long-term vigorous activity (more than 1000 kCal/week) reduced risk by 40% (OR = 0.60). There has been continued interest in examining whether the protective benefits of PA apply for both men and women: one cohort study found reduced risk for colon cancer with increased PA among both men and women[35] and another identified reduced risk only among men.[36] It appears that there may be gender differences by anatomic subsite: for example, among men, dose–response relationships have been found, with increased PA offering protection against proximal[35,36] and for distal colon cancers.[35] In a cohort study of women, Calton and colleagues[29] did not find a significant association of PA and colon cancer risk by subsite or intensity of PA. Hence, the evidence for protective benefits of increased PA among women is less consistent.

There has been increasing interest in determining whether the relationship of PA and colon/rectal cancer risk varies across gender and by the type of activity. A case-control study[38] found that among men and women, increased occupational PA was associated with reduced risk for distal colon cancer (men, OR = 0.60; women, OR = 0.40). Steindorf and colleagues[40] found protective effects for colon cancer only for occupational PA and not for leisure PA. The differential benefits of occupational versus leisure activity may be traced to the varying patterns of each class of activity that can influence the etiology of colon cancer. Occupational PA may be less intensive but systematic and performed over long periods whereas leisure activity such as sports can be intensive but of shorter duration and irregular. Finally, in a study that examined the combined effects of occupational and leisure activity, risk for colon cancer was lowest for those with the greatest activity in both categories.[32]

Next arises the question of how much PA is needed to lower the risk of colon cancer? Larsson and colleagues[37] found reduced risk for colon and rectal cancer among men who participated in 60 minutes or more/day of leisure activity (walking, biking, and exercising) compared to those who exercised less than 10 minutes/day. In another study, men who participated in exercise/sports five or more times per week for at least 20 minutes each time had lower risk of colon cancer (RR = 0.79) versus those who did not or rarely exercised.[35] At the lower end of the continuum of PA "dose," in their case-control study, Zhang and colleagues[32] found lowered risk (OR = 0.70) for colon cancer among men and women who reported moderate/strenuous leisure time activity two or more times/week (for at least 10 minutes each time). For occupational activity, the answer is obscured due to difficulties in determining the duration of moderate and hard activity.[38] Steindorf and colleagues[40] found that over 146.7 MET hours/week of lifetime occupational PA was associated with reduced risk (OR = 0.39) for colon cancer. In summary, consistent with a previous review[8] about 30–60 minutes/day of moderate to vigorous intensity PA appears to reduce risk for colon cancer.

Another question of interest to PA promotion efforts is when is PA the most beneficial? A cohort study found that among men more recent PA (at ages 35–39) was associated with reduced colon cancer than activity at earlier ages (15–18 and 19–29 years).[35] In a case-control study, Steindorf and colleagues[40] found that lifetime high exercisers (occupational and leisure PA) had substantially reduced risk compared to lifetime nonexercisers.

Table 4-2. Summary of studies on colorectal cancer

Colorectal cancer case-control studies				
Authors	*Sample*	*Activity measure*	*Factors adjusted*	*Results*
Isomura et al., 2006	N = 778 cases N = 767 controls Japan	Questions about type of job, activities in commuting, housework, shopping, and leisure-time activities 5 years before interview Intensity of nonjob PA was classified into three levels based on distribution of PA among controls Job-related PA categorized into sedentary, moderate, and hard	Smoking Alcohol consumption Age BMI	In males, greater job-related PA associated with decreased risk of cancer in the distal colon (OR = 0.6, CI = 0.4–1.0) and rectum (OR = 0.6, CI = 0.4–0.9) In males, total moderate and hard leisure activity associated with decreased cancer in rectum (OR = 0.5, CI = 0.3–0.8) In females, job-related PA and moderate and hard leisure PA associated with decreased risk of cancer in distal colon only (OR = = 0.04, CI = 0.2–0.8 and OR = 0.5, CI = 0.3–1.1, respectively)
Slattery et al., 2002	N = 1993 cases N = 2410 controls United States	Assessed moderate and vigorous home and leisure activities for at least 1 hr in any month of the referent year Asked to recall their activity patterns for the referent year, 10 years and 20 years ago People were ranked according to their overall amount of long-term activity	None	Differences in effects of diet and lifestyle factors were identified depending on the level of PA Statistically significant interactions between PA and high-risk dietary pattern and vegetable intake, in that the relative importance of diet was dependent on the level of PA
Slattery et al., 2003	N = 952 cases N = 1205 controls United States	Assessed moderate and vigorous home and leisure activities for at least 1 hr in any month of the referent year Reported up to three full- or part-time jobs during the referent year and to recall any moderate or vigorous level activities on those jobs Long-term PA—amount of time performed moderate and vigorous home, leisure, and work activities for 10 and 20 years before the interview date	Age BMI Energy intake	Vigorous PA associated with reduced risk of rectal cancer in both men and women (OR = 0.60, CI = 0.44–0.81 for men; OR = 0.59, CI = 0.40–0.86 for women) Among men, moderate levels of PA associated with reduced risk of rectal cancer (OR = 0.70, CI = 0.51–0.97) Participation in vigorous activity over the past 20 years had greatest protection for both men and women (OR = 0.55, CI = 0.39–0.78 for men; OR = 0.44, CI = 0.30–0.67 for women)
Slattery et al., 2005	N = 1956 cases N = 2174 controls United States	Questionnaire assessing frequency and intensity of PA during referent period and 10 and 20 years before referent date Long-term vigorous PA was calculated as the sum of all vigorous activities reported	Age BMI Calcium Energy intake Dietary fiber Cigarette smoke	Colon and rectal cancer patients engaged in significantly less exercise than controls ($p < 0.01$)
Steindorf et al., 2005	N = 239 cases N = 239 controls Poland	Occupational and recreational PA assessed at ages 20, 30, 40, 50, and 60 through interview Reported time spent on each activity per week was multiplied by its typical MET Total PA was estimated as the sum of all reported data	Age Gender BMI Total energy intake Alcohol intake Calcium intake Fiber intake Smoking packs per year	Lifetime mean PA decreased risk for the highest quartile of PA (OR = 0.37, CI = 0.17–0.84) Decreased risk for lifelong constantly high exercisers compared with lifelong nonexercisers (OR = 0.26, CI = 0.08–0.84) Decreased risk for the highest quartile of occupational activity (>146.7 MET-hrs/wk; OR = 0.31, CI = 0.15–0.71) but not for the highest quartile of recreational activity (>74.4 MET-hrs/wk; OR = 0.91, CI = 0.43–1.92) Decreased risk for lifetime exercisers in the highest quartile compared to lifetime nonexercisers (OR = 0.36, CI = 0.17–0.77)

		Colorectal cancer case-control studies		
Authors	Sample	Activity measure	Factors adjusted	Results
Zhang et al., 2006	N = 585 cases N = 2172 controls United States	Leisure activity—one question: "During most of your adult life, how often did you usually do strenuous or moderate exercise such as jogging, swimming laps, gardening, or walking briskly for 10 min?" with four response categories Occupational PA—reported all jobs held for ≥5 years since age 16 and classified into one of three activity levels based on the Standard Industry Classification and Standard Occupational Classification Manual codes	Age Gender Level of education Dietary intake of fat and fiber FDR with colon cancer	30% risk reduction of colon cancer for all sites and 40% risk reduction for cancer of the right colon for those who reported recreational activity more than twice per week Occupational PA associated with reduced risk Risk lowest for those with both high occupational and recreational PA (OR = 0.5, CI = 0.3–0.8)

Colorectal cancer prospective cohort studies

Authors	Sample	Activity measure	Factors adjusted	Results
Calton et al., 2006	N = 31,783 United States	Asked to estimate the number of hours they spent per day sleeping and engaging in light, moderate, and vigorous activities and to sum these four categories to equal 24 hours	BMI Education Family hx of colorectal cancer Smoking status HRT use Aspirin use Alcohol consumption Energy-adjusted intakes of total calcium and red meat	No association observed between PA and risk of colon cancer Relationship between PA and colon cancer risk did not vary by anatomic subsite or across subgroups defined by age, BMI, fiber intake, menopausal status, HRT use, or aspirin use
Friedenreich et al., 2006	N = 413,044 Europe	Questions derived from the more extensive modified Baecke questionnaire	Age Center Energy intake Education Smoking Height Weight Fiber intake	Decreased risk when most active compared with inactive: colon cancer HR = 0.78, CI = 0.59–1.03; right-sided colon tumors HR = 0.65, CI = 0.43–1.0 Decreased colon cancer risk when active and BMI <25 compared with inactive (HR = 0.63, CI = 0.21–0.68) Interaction between BMI and activity was seen for right-sided colon cancer; among moderately active and active participants with BMI <25 compared with inactive with BMI >30 No decreased risks observed for rectal cancer for any type of PA for any subgroup analyses or interaction
Howard et al., 2008	N = 448,720 United States	Baseline questionnaires asked number of times in past 12 months engaged in vigorous activity for at least 20 min with six forced choice options Asked to indicate which of five categories best described their routine throughout the day at home or work Second questionnaire asked about PA during four different age periods	Age Smoking Alcohol consumption Education Race Family hx of CC Total energy and energy-adjusted intake of red meat, calcium, whole grains, fruits, and vegetables HRT	Decreased risk of colon and rectal cancer comparing men who engaged in exercise/sports five or more times a week for at least 20 min each to men who never or rarely exercise (colon cancer RR = 0.79, CI = 0.68–0.91; rectal cancer RR = 0.76, CI = 0.61–0.94) In men, inverse relations of both low intensity (RR = 0.81, CI = 0.65–1.0) and moderate to vigorous intensity (RR = 0.82, CI = 0.67–0.99) for colon cancer In men, positive relationship between sedentary behavior and colon cancer (RR = 1.61, CI = 1.14–2.27) In men, decreased risk associated with PA at ages 35–39 (RR = 0.76, CI = 0.64–0.91) but no association with decreased risk at ages 15–18 and 19–29 Similar but less pronounced relations observed in women

(Continued)

Table 4-2. Continued

Colorectal cancer case-control studies

Authors	Sample	Activity measure	Factors adjusted	Results
Johnsen et al., 2006	N = 28,356 women N = 26,122 men Denmark	Leisure PA assessed with 12 questions covering the average number of hours per week spent in the past year on six types of PA Occupational PA assessed with one question about intensity of PA with four options	Occupational PA BMI Education NSAID Present use of HRT Smoking Intake of total energy, fat, dietary fiber, red meat, and alcohol	No associations between risk of colon cancer and occupational activity, MET-hrs/wk of total leisure-time activity Borderline significant association was found with the number of activities in which the participants were active—for each additional activity IRR = 0.87, CI = 0.76–1.0 for women and IRR = 0.88, CI = 0.78–1.0 for men
Larsson et al., 2006	N = 45,906 Sweden	Questionnaire to assess activity at work, home/housework, walking/bicycling, exercise, inactivity, sleeping, and sitting/lying down in the year before the study Reported time spent at each activity per day was multiplied by its typical METS and added together to create a MET-hrs/day score	Age at baseline Education Family hx of colorectal cancer Hx of diabetes Smoking Aspirin use BMI	Sixty minutes or more of leisure PA per day associated with decreased risk when compared with <10 min/day (colorectal cancer: HR = 0.57, CI = 0.41–0.79; colon cancer: HR =0.56, CI = 0.37–0.83; rectal cancer: HR = 0.59, CI = 0.34–1.02) Home/housework activity inversely associated with colon cancer risk (HR= 0.68, CI = 0.48–0.96) No association observed for work/occupational PA
Lee et al., 2007	N = 65,022 Japan	Reported average time per day spent for each of the following activities: heavy physical work or strenuous exercise, sedentary activity, and walking or standing with three choices of duration for each MET-hrs/day were estimated by multiplying reported time spent at each activity per day by its assigned MET intensity	Age Study area Family hx of colorectal cancer Smoking status Alcohol intake BMI Intake of red meat Dietary fiber and folate	Significant inverse association between PA and risk of developing colorectal cancer, particularly colon cancer, among men Relative to men in the lowest level of MET-hrs/day, those in the highest level had a RR = 0.69, CI = 0.49–0.97 Significant decrease in risk of colon cancer was associated with increasing MET-hrs/day among men, no significant decrease seen among women
Nazeri et al., 2006	N = 6908 Sweden	Leisure PA assessed by asking questions about duration of low intensity PA and more intensive PA Occupational PA based on working status and self-reported intensity of work Women divided into high, intermediate, and low PA regarding their work and leisure activity levels	Parity BMI Smoking	Positive association between low PA and risk of colorectal cancer (p = 0.04)

ABBREVIATIONS: BMI, body mass index; CC, colon cancer; CI, confidence interval; FDR, first-degree relative; HR, hazard ratio (the effect of an explanatory variable on the hazard or risk of an event); HRT, hormone replacement therapy; hx, history; IRR, incidence rate ratio; MET, metabolic equivalent; N, number of people; NSAID, nonsteroidal anti-inflammatory drugs; OR, odds ratio (the ratio of the odds of an event occurring in one group to the odds of it occurring in another group); PA, physical activity; RR, relative risk or incidence rate in a particular category of exposure divided by the corresponding rate in the comparison category.

However, the data are too sparse to reach conclusions about the most effective timing of interventions to promote PA for cancer prevention.

Assessment of PA. A majority of studies assessed PA via self-administered questionnaires, although a few used interviewers to collect data.[31,39–41] There is variation in the type of activity assessed: in some studies, occupational and recreational activities were assessed separately; in others, these two types of activity were combined into overall activity.[29,36] In general household activities were not assessed separately,

although household activities such as scrubbing floors were subsumed within vigorous activity in a women's cohort study.[29] Several studies used validated instruments[30,31,34,39,41] or reported reliability indices.[36,37] The case-control studies (and one cohort study[35]) required respondents to recall activity at various prior time periods. As with the breast cancer literature, careful attention was given to assessing and evaluating the effects of various confounding variables such as dietary intake, BMI, alcohol use, family history of colon cancer, smoking, aspirin use, and education (see Table 4–2).

Mechanisms. Several potential biological mechanisms have been hypothesized to underlie the benefits of increased PA against colon cancer (see reviews by Kruk and Aboul-Enein[6] and McTiernan[27]) such as increased PA is associated with lower levels of colonic mucosal prostaglandin, PA increases stool transit by stimulating peristalsis resulting in reduced exposure of the intestinal epithelium to potential carcinogens and mutagens, and PA may also increase colon blood flow so that potential carcinogens or mutagens may be carried away. Also, increased PA is associated with decreased insulin and insulin-like growth factors (IGFs) and enhanced immune functioning that confers protective benefits. The general agreement is that a combination of these and other factors may underlie the relationship of PA and colon cancer. However, there are few empirical studies to support any of the hypothesized biological mechanisms for these protective effects.

Rectal cancer. The IARC reviewed two cohort studies and 10 case-control studies and only four case-control studies suggested a protective association (2002).[5] In our review, four cohort studies[34–37] and three case-control studies[38–40] assessed the effects of PA on rectal cancer risk. Four studies found that PA protected against rectal cancer[35,37–39] and three did not.[34,36,40]

The EPIC cohort study did not show protective effects of PA for rectal cancer[34]; however, two other cohort studies showed reduced risk for rectal cancer among men who were physically active.[35,37] A case-control study[38] found that increased occupational PA (OR = 0.6), total activity, nonoccupational activity (OR = 0.50), as well as moderate intensity or hard intensity nonoccupational activity appeared to protect men from rectal cancer (OR = 0.50). Slattery and colleagues[39] with a large sample (952 cases) found that vigorous activity reduced risk of rectal cancer in men (OR = 0.60) and women (OR = 0.59). There was also a dose-response relationship with reductions in risk for rectal (and colon) cancer with increased PA of 30–45 minutes/day. There are little data[39] to address the question of when activity is most beneficial. However, at this time, across the studies reviewed, there is less convincing evidence supporting positive effects of PA on rectal cancer risk.

Lung cancer. Four prospective cohort studies were identified that examined the relationship between PA and lung cancer risk in the past 5 years.[42–45] One study was of males only,[44] while the others included both males and females. Two studies consisted of samples of smokers[42,44] and two had mixed samples of smokers and nonsmokers.[43,45] The studies were conducted in several European countries and the United States (Table 4–3).

In general, occupational, leisure, and total PA were not associated with decreased risk of lung cancer in men or women. However, two studies that examined the interaction between PA and age[42,44] found a decreased risk of lung cancer in younger smokers who exercised (OR = 0.84[42]; RR = 0.77[44]). When examining specific activities by gender, there was reduction of lung cancer risk in men engaged in the highest tertile of sports versus inactive (RR = 0.71), and for women in the highest tertile of cycling versus inactive (RR = 0.73).[45] Bak and colleagues[43] also found that when examining specific activities by gender there was reduction in lung cancer risk. Women showed reduced risk in four out of six activities, sport (incidence rate ratio [IRR] = 0.61), cycling (IRR = 0.56), walking (IRR = 0.60), and gardening (IRR = 0.73), whereas men had a decreased risk for only two activities, sports (IRR = 0.40) and gardening (IRR = 0.71), compared to nonactive men.

These findings are in contrast to a recent review[8] and meta-analysis[7] which found an inverse relationship between PA and lung cancer risk. However, this relationship was stronger for women than for men,[7] which is partially consistent with the findings for specific activities by Bak and colleagues.[43] Lee and Oguma[8] also noted that the association was stronger for case control than for cohort studies. This may explain the lack of relationship found in recent studies as they were all cohort studies.

Assessment of PA. Although all were prospective studies, PA was only assessed at one time point. All four studies used self-administered questionnaires to assess PA, but some participants were interviewed.[45] Assessment of PA varied with three of the four studies separately assessing

leisure and occupational activity in the past year.[43–45] Household activity was included within leisure activity for two of the three studies.[43,45] Alfano and colleagues[42] assessed overall PA, including leisure, household, sports, and occupational activity, in an average weekday and weekend over the past 5 years. All of the studies controlled for smoking status and diet.

Mechanisms. There are several biological mechanisms hypothesized for the association between PA and lung cancer risk. First, PA may impact growth factors, such as IGFs and their binding proteins (IGFBPs). Some research has found that high levels of IGF-I were associated with increased risk of lung cancer and high levels of IGFBP-3 were associated with decreased risk of lung cancer; however, other research has found no relationship with lung cancer risk.[7,45] Second, PA can lower insulin, glucose, and triglycerides, and raise high-density lipopolysaccharide (HDL) cholesterol, which may decrease cancer risk.[7] Third, PA can increase pulmonary ventilation and perfusion that can reduce the concentration of carcinogens in the airways.[7,45] Further, long-term PA may enhance immune functioning therefore decreasing cancer risk.[7,45]

Prostate cancer. Six studies[46–51] and one set of companion papers[10,11] were identified that examined the relationship between PA and prostate cancer risk in the past 5 years. Two were prospective cohort studies and the remaining were case-control studies. The studies were conducted in several European countries, the United States, Canada, and China (Table 4–4).

There were mixed findings for the relationship between occupational, leisure, and total PA with risk of prostate cancer. About half of the studies generally found no significant relationship with PA.[10,11,47,48,51] Three studies found that occupational activity, but not leisure activity, was associated with decreased risk (RR = 0.41,[46] OR = 0.75,[49] OR = 0.46[50]). In contrast, increased risk of prostate cancer was found in one study comparing the highest quartile of occupational activity to the lowest quartile (OR = 1.33).[11] The authors speculated that this inconsistent finding may be due to methodological differences between studies or due to potentially high levels of stress in physically strenuous work. Of the two studies that assessed leisure activity at specific ages throughout the lifespan, one found no relationship at any age;[49] the other only found a relationship for strenuous activity in early 50s, but not in mid-teens or early 30s.[10] One study assessed occupational activity at specific ages throughout the lifespan and found a significantly decreased risk of prostate cancer in the highest tertile compared to the lowest tertile of occupational activity for ages 30–39 (OR = 0.78) and 50–59 (OR = 0.75), but not for age 12 (OR = 0.84) and age 15–19 (OR = 0.94).[49] It should be noted that occupational activity among teenagers is likely to be limited as compared to later ages. Two studies examined the relationship between PA and risk of localized versus advanced prostate cancer. One found no relationship,[51] while the other found a decreased risk for localized but not for advanced prostate cancer.[50] Friedenreich and colleagues[47] examined the influence of family history and found that men with a family history of prostate cancer in the highest quartile of lifetime PA had a decreased risk of prostate cancer (OR = 0.48), while PA was not significantly related to risk in men without a family history of prostate cancer.

These findings are consistent with previous reviews that found inconsistent relationships between PA and prostate cancer risk.[3,5,8] However, Friedenreich[3] stated that although the findings are mixed, there is strong evidence that PA is associated with decreased risk of prostate cancer with the majority of studies observing about 10%–30% risk reduction. Lee and Oguma,[8] on the other hand, concluded that "the epidemiological data on the whole do not provide support for an inverse relationship between PA and the risk of [prostate] cancer," with a median 10% risk reduction in cohort studies and median 20% risk reduction in case-control studies. The IARC[5] interpreted the mixed results to suggest that PA may protect against prostate cancer, as a majority of the studies reviewed suggested a moderate protective effect, sometimes only observed in subgroup analyses.

Assessment of PA. PA was only assessed at one time point in all the studies reviewed. About half of the studies used self-administered questionnaires to assess PA,[10,11,46,47,51] while the others used in-person interviews.[48–50] Assessment of PA varied greatly across the studies. Two

Table 4–3. Summary of studies on lung cancer

		Lung cancer prospective cohort studies		
Authors	Sample	Activity measure	Factors adjusted	Main results
Alfano et al., 2004	N = 7045 United States	Self-administered section from the Paffenberger Physical Activity Questionnaire Total activity during past year: average weekday and weekend day hours of activity and five categories of intensity	Smoking (pack per year history) Age BMI Gender	Decreased risk of lung cancer only for younger participants (HRR = 0.84, CI = 0.69–1.03) and women (HRR = 0.68, CI = 0.53–0.89) Decreased risk of lung cancer mortality only for younger participants (HRR = 0.75, CI = 0.59–0.94) and women (HRR = 0.69, CI = 0.53–0.90)
Bak et al., 2005	N = 54,422 Denmark	Self-administered questionnaires Leisure activity during past year: average number of hours per week spent on six types of leisure activities during summer and winter Occupational activity during past year: five categories of intensity for occupational activity	Active/nonactive status Smoking (duration, intensity, time since cessation) Education Intake of fruit and vegetables Possible occupational exposure to lung carcinogen	No significant association between number of hours per week spent on six types of leisure activity and lung cancer risk For each type of leisure activity, decreased risk of lung cancer active compared to nonactive women, but for men, decreased risk observed for only two leisure activities Higher levels of occupational PA has no protective effect
Colbert et al., 2002	N = 27,087 Finland	Self-administered questionnaires Leisure activity during past year: one question with three categories of intensity Occupational activity during past year: one question with five categories of intensity	Age Supplement group BMI Cigarettes smoked per day Years of smoking Education Energy intake Vegetable intake	No significant association between occupational, leisure, or combined PA with lung cancer risk Some modest risk reduction associated with leisure activity among younger smokers—with increasing quartiles of age the RRs for men active in leisure activity compared to sedentary men were 0.77 (CI = 0.54–1.09), 0.74 (CI = 0.57–0.95), 1.09 (CI = 0.89–1.33), and 1.03 (CI = 0.88–1.21)
Steindorf et al., 2006	N = 416,227 10 European countries	In-person interviews or self-administered standardized questionnaire Typical week in past year Categorical frequencies and durations of occupational, recreational, and household activities	Age Center Smoking status, duration, intensity, time since cessation Weight Height Education Total energy intake without energy from alcohol Alcohol intake Fruit intake Vegetable intake Red and processed meat intake Occupational exposure to lung carcinogens	No inverse association between recent occupational, recreational, or household PA and lung cancer in either males or females Some reduction in lung cancer risk associated with sports in males (RR = 0.71, CI = 0.50–0.98; highest tertile vs. inactive group), cycling in women (RR = 0.73, CI = 0.54–0.99), and nonoccupational vigorous PA Lung cancer risk was increased for unemployed men (RR = 1.57, CI = 1.2–2.05) and men with standing occupations (RR = 1.35, CI = 1.02–1.79) compared to sitting occupations

ABBREVIATIONS: CI, confidence interval; HR, hazard ratio (the effect of an explanatory variable on the hazard or risk of an event); HRR = hazard rate ratio; N,number of people; PA, physical activity; RR, relative risk or incidence rate in a particular category of exposure divided by the corresponding rate in the comparison category.

studies assessed total PA that incorporated leisure and occupational activity[46,48] and the remaining studies assessed leisure and occupational activity separately. Household activity was also assessed in three of the studies: included within leisure activity,[48] included within occupational activity,[46] and assessed separately.[47] Zeegers and colleagues,[51] assessed transportation activity and history of sports participation along with leisure and occupational activity.

Mechanisms. There are several biological mechanisms hypothesized for the association between PA and prostate cancer risk. First, prostate cancer is hormonally mediated and PA may influence hormone levels.[3,48] Second, obesity may increase prostate cancer risk and PA may prevent weight gain.[48] Finally, long-term PA may enhance immune functioning therefore decreasing cancer risk.[48]

Table 4–4. Summary of studies on prostate cancer

Prostate cancer case-control studies

Authors	Sample	Activity measure	Factors adjusted	Main results
Darlington et al., 2007	N = 752 cases N = 1613 controls Canada Same sample as Sass-Kortsak et al., 2007	Questions about recreational PA were derived from the National Enhanced Cancer Surveillance Study in Canada Frequency and intensity of recreational PA for at least 20 min based on three periods of life (mid-teens, early 30s, and early 50s) Participants classified as participated in activities at less than three times per week or equal to or greater than three times per week	Age Family history (hx) of PC Quartiles of recent BMI SES Education Type of occupation of longest duration	Strenuous PA by men in their early 50s, but not mid-teens or early 30s, was associated with reduced risk (OR = 0.8, CI = 0.6–0.9)
Friedenreich et al., 2004	N = 988 cases N = 1063 controls	Lifetime Total Physical Activity Questionnaire—measured occupational, household, and recreational activity levels from childhood until diagnosis	Age Region Education BMI Waist/hip ratio Total caloric intake Average lifetime total alcohol intake First-degree family hx of PC Number of time had PSA test Number of digital rectal examinations	No association for total lifetime PA and prostate cancer risk (OR = 0.87, CI = 0.65–1.17) Risks were decreased for occupational (OR = 0.90, CI = 0.66–1.22) and recreational (OR = 0.80, CI = 0.61–1.05) activity, but were increased for household (OR = 1.36, CI = 1.05–1.76) activity when comparing the highest and lowest quartiles Activity done during the first 18 years of life (OR = 0.78, CI = 0.59–1.04) decreased risk Vigorous activity decreased PC risk (OR = 0.70, CI = 0.54–0.92) Decreased risk for men with a family hx of prostate cancer in the highest quartile of lifetime PA (OR = 0.48, CI = 0.21–1.11) but not for men with no family hx
Jian et al., 2005	N = 130 cases N = 274 controls China	Weekly average intensity and duration of occupational, leisure, and household activity Intensity categorized as moderate or vigorous Calculated MET/hr	Age Locality Education Family income Marital status Age at marriage Number of children Years in workforce Family hx of PC BMI Average daily caloric intake	Moderate PA was inversely related to prostate cancer risk (OR = 0.20, CI = 0.07–0.62 for upper vs. lower quartiles of weekly metabolic equivalent task-hours) Significant dose-response
Pierotti et al., 2005	N = 1294 cases N = 1451 controls Italy	Self-reported levels leisure and occupational activity Assessed four periods of their life: 12, 15–19, 30–39, and 50–59 PA during leisure time classified into four categories of hrs/week Occupational PA classified into five categories of intensity Scores of the two highest and two lowest groups were combined	Age Center Education Social class BMI Total energy intake Smoking Alcohol Family hx of PC	Lowest level compared to highest level of occupational PA: OR = 0.94 (CI = 0.75–1.17) at age 15–19, OR = 0.78 (CI = 0.63–0.97) at age 30–39, and 0.75 (CI = 0.61–0.93) at age 50–59 Significant inverse trend in risk was found for activity at work at ages 30–39 and 50–59

(Continued)

Table 4–4. Continued

Prostate cancer case-control studies

Authors	Sample	Activity measure	Factors adjusted	Main results
Sass-Kortsak et al., 2007	N = 760 cases N = 1632 controls Canada Same sample as Darlington et al., 2007	Rated each job for the usual level of workplace PA Response options included specific examples: sitting, light, moderate, or strenuous Composite workplace PA score computed	Age Family hx	Highest vs. lowest quartile of workplace PA showed a significant positive association (OR = 1.33, CI = 1.02–1.74) No statistically significant associations were found for any other occupational category or exposure
Strom et al., 2008	N = 176 cases N = 174 controls United States	Recreational PA dichotomized as less than once a week vs. greater than or equal to once a week Occupational PA coded using a validated job-exposure matrix Average level of PA for each person was calculated based on level of intensity and duration of each job held divided by total number of years worked	Age Education Screening history First- degree family hx of PC Agrichemical exposure	Compared to controls, cases were 54% less likely to work in jobs with moderate/high PA (OR = 0.46, CI = 0.28–0.77) Cases with organ-confined PC were 56% less likely to have moderate/high levels of occupational PA (OR = 0.44, CI = 0.26–0.76) Increased risk of being diagnosed with advanced PC not associated with occupational PA No significant difference between cases and controls on leisure-time PA

Prostate cancer prospective cohort studies

Authors	Sample	Activity measure	Factors adjusted	Main results
Calton et al., 2007	N = 328,316 United States	Intensity of daily activity routine at work or home Vigorous PA defined as times/week defined as PA that lasted at least 20 min and caused increased breathing or heart rate or working up a sweat	Age BMI Height Education Race Family hx of PC Smoking status Vigorous PA Supplemental vitamin E Supplemental zinc Alcohol intake Quintiles of energy-adjusted intakes of multiple foods	Inverse association between diabetes and PC was particularly strong among men in the highest category of routine PA at work or home (RR = 0.41, CI = 0.23–0.74)
Zeegers et al., 2005	N = 58,279 Netherlands	Baseline nonoccupational PA based on two questions to obtain overall measure in min/day Past sports activity was assessed by asking about the hrs/wk and the years spent playing each sport Occupational PA—asked about last five jobs—activity based on job title	Age Alcohol intake from wine BMI Energy intake Family history Education	No relationship with PC risk for nonoccupational PA (RR = 1.01, CI = 0.81–1.25, for >90 vs. <30 min/day), history of sports participation (RR = 1.04, CI = 0.90–1.22 for ever vs. never participated), occupational PA (RR = 0.91, CI = 0.70–1.18, for >12 vs. <8 kJ/min energy expenditure in the longest held job) Increased risk of PC for men who were physically active for >1 hr/day in obese men and men with a high baseline energy intake

ABBREVIATIONS: CI, confidence interval; HR, hazard ratio (the effect of an explanatory variable on the hazard or risk of an event); MET, metabolic equivalent; N, number of people; OR, odds ratio (the ratio of the odds of an event occurring in one group to the odds of it occurring in another group); PA, physical activity; PC prostate cancer; RR, relative risk or incidence rate in a particular category of exposure divided by the corresponding rate in the comparison category; SES, socio-economic status.

FUTURE DIRECTIONS

As seen in this review of the recent literature, there are more data to support the benefits of PA in reducing risk of breast cancer in women and colon cancer in men and women. A strength of the studies is that these relationships have been examined, after assessing and controlling for the effects of confounding variables (as described previously), and the relationships have been upheld. The effects of PA in reducing risk for lung, prostate, and rectal cancers are inconsistent among these more recent studies.

To help guide future research efforts, certain key areas merit further attention: (1) Cancer risk varies in population subgroups: for example, the protective benefits of increased PA are more consistently demonstrated among postmenopausal versus premenopausal women. Age, sex, race/ethnicity, and BMI may be some of the factors that can differentially affect the relationship of PA to cancer risk. The studies we reviewed have been largely conducted in developed countries and for the most part, among white non-Hispanic participants. (2) Improve PA assessments. To develop public health messages (e.g., what exercise dose offers the greatest protection against which type[s] of cancer) aimed at cancer prevention), it is important to identify the type of PA (such as occupational, leisure, household, transportation), intensity (e.g., metabolic equivalents or energy expended), duration (e.g., number of minutes or hours per day), and frequency (number of days/week) that offers the greatest benefit. Many studies have not assessed all these dimensions of PA. In addition, there are insufficient data to identify when such activity should be initiated and how long activity should be sustained for protective benefits. It is not clear whether energy expenditure in all activities is of importance, but it does appear to be a limitation when investigators assess only leisure activity, overlooking occupational and household activities that may be more prevalent in subgroups such as people of lower socioeconomic strata, women, and minorities. It is encouraging to note that there have been recent studies that have assessed household activities particularly when the samples include women.[12,23,29] The measurement of PA continues to show variability with some studies utilizing very brief assessments (1–2 questions) whose reliability and validity have not been established. Investigators are encouraged to use measures that have established reliability and validity for the populations that are to be studied, or at a minimum establish indices of reliability and validity before an observational study is launched. Assessing PA over long periods is challenging but is required if definitive answers are to be obtained to answer the question of when is it important to become and stay active to reduce cancer risk. Researchers are encouraged to use tested approaches to enhance accurate recall of lifetime activity. (3) Approximately 10 years ago, there was a call to go beyond observational epidemiological studies to clinical trials that examine the effects of exercise interventions on specific biological mechanisms (including differentiating the effects of PA from weight loss) to help obtain evidence on the mechanisms that underlie the effects of PA on cancer risk.[52] The type of studies that are needed require identifying high-risk populations, identifying intermediate end points/biomarkers, conducting pilot feasibility studies, replicating results in other populations and settings, and then initiating large-scale intervention trials. Studies examining the effects of exercise alone or in combination with a dietary intervention on biomarkers for breast cancer have already been launched (ALPHA trial, PI, C. Friedenreich, SHAPE, PI: E. Monninkof; NEW trial; PI: A. McTiernan, WISER trial, PI: M. Kurzer as cited in McTiernan[27]).

Currently, the PA guidelines for reducing cancer risk are a minimum of 30 minutes/day of moderate to vigorous intensity activity on 5 days/week or more (American Cancer Society, *United States Department of Health and Human Services* [USDHHS], International Union against Cancer, Canadian Cancer Society, and Health Canada). There has been progress in understanding the relationship between PA and cancer risk, but much more needs to be done by researchers and funding agencies before definitive public health recommendations can be offered. The challenge of the worldwide burden of cancer requires no less.

REFERENCES

1. American Cancer Society. *Global cancer facts and figures.* Atlanta, GA: American Cancer Society; 2007.

2. Caspersen CJ, Powell KE, Christenson GM. Physical activity, exercise, and physical fitness: definitions and distinctions for health-related research. *Public Health Rep.* 1985;100(2):126–131.

3. Friedenreich CM. Physical activity and cancer prevention: from observational to intervention research. *Cancer Epidemiol Biomarkers Prev.* 2001; 10(4):287–301.

4. Friedenreich CM, Orenstein MR. Physical activity and cancer prevention: etiologic evidence and biological mechanisms. *J Nutr.* 2002;132(suppl 11):3456S–3464S.

5. International Agency for Research on Cancer (IARC). *IARC handbooks of cancer prevention: weight control and physical activity.* Vol 6. Lyon, France: IARC Press; 2002.

6. Kruk J, Aboul-Enein HY. Physical activity in the prevention of cancer. *Asian Pac J Cancer Prev.* 2006;7(1):11–21.

7. Tardon A, Lee WJ, Delgado-Rodriguez M, et al. Leisure-time physical activity and lung cancer: a meta-analysis. *Cancer Causes Control.* 2005;16(4):389–397.

8. Lee I-M, Oguma Y. Physical activity. In: Schottenfeld DF, Joseph F, ed. *Cancer epidemiology and prevention.* Vol 3. New York, NY: Oxford University Press; 2006.

9. Hirose K, Hamajima N, Takezaki T, Miura S, Tajima K. Physical exercise reduces risk of breast cancer in Japanese women. *Cancer Sci.* 2003;94(2):193–199.

10. Darlington GA, Kreiger N, Lightfoot N, Purdham J, Sass-Kortsak A. Prostate cancer risk and diet, recreational physical activity and cigarette smoking. *Chronic Dis Can.* 2007;27(4):145–153.

11. Sass-Kortsak AM, Purdham JT, Kreiger N, Darlington G, Lightfoot NE. Occupational risk factors for prostate cancer. *Am J Ind Med.* 2007;50(8):568–576.

12. Lahmann PH, Friedenreich C, Schuit AJ, et al. Physical activity and breast cancer risk: the European Prospective Investigation into Cancer and Nutrition. *Cancer Epidemiol Biomarkers Prev.* 2007;16(1):36–42.

13. Margolis KL, Mucci L, Braaten T, et al. Physical activity in different periods of life and the risk of breast cancer: the Norwegian-Swedish Women's Lifestyle and Health cohort study. *Cancer Epidemiol Biomarkers Prev.* 2005; 14(1):27–32.

14. Maruti SS, Willett WC, Feskanich D, Rosner B, Colditz GA. A prospective study of age-specific physical activity and premenopausal breast cancer. *J Natl Cancer Inst.* 2008;100(10):728–737.

15. Mertens AJ, Sweeney C, Shahar E, Rosamond WD, Folsom AR. Physical activity and breast cancer incidence in middle-aged women: a prospective cohort study. *Breast Cancer Res Treat.* 2006;97(2):209–214.

16. Moradi T, Adami HO, Ekbom A, et al. Physical activity and risk for breast cancer a prospective cohort study among Swedish twins. *Int J Cancer.* 2002;100(1):76–81.

17. Tehard B, Friedenreich CM, Oppert JM, Clavel-Chapelon F. Effect of physical activity on women at increased risk of breast cancer: results from the E3N cohort study. *Cancer Epidemiol Biomarkers Prev.* 2006;15(1):57–64.

18. Carpenter CL, Ross RK, Paganini-Hill A, Bernstein L. Effect of family history, obesity and exercise on breast cancer risk among postmenopausal women. *Int J Cancer.* 2003;106(1):96–102.

19. Dorn J, Vena J, Brasure J, Freudenheim J, Graham S. Lifetime physical activity and breast cancer risk in pre- and postmenopausal women. *Med Sci Sports Exerc.* 2003;35(2):278–285.

20. John EM, Horn-Ross PL, Koo J. Lifetime physical activity and breast cancer risk in a multiethnic population: the San Francisco Bay area breast cancer study. *Cancer Epidemiol Biomarkers Prev.* 2003;12(11 pt 1):1143–1152.

21. Kruk J. Lifetime physical activity and the risk of breast cancer: a case-control study. *Cancer Detect Prev.* 2007;31(1):18–28.

22. Peplonska B, Lissowska J, Hartman TJ, et al. Adulthood lifetime physical activity and breast cancer. *Epidemiology.* 2008;19(2):226–236.

23. Slattery ML, Edwards S, Murtaugh MA, et al. Physical activity and breast cancer risk among women in the southwestern United States. *Ann Epidemiol.* 2007;17(5):342–353.

24. Sprague BL, Trentham-Dietz A, Newcomb PA, Titus-Ernstoff L, Hampton JM, Egan KM. Lifetime recreational and occupational physical activity and risk of in situ and invasive breast cancer. *Cancer Epidemiol Biomarkers Prev.* 2007;16(2):236–243.

25. Steindorf K, Schmidt M, Kropp S, Chang-Claude J. Case-control study of physical activity and breast cancer risk among premenopausal women in Germany. *Am J Epidemiol.* 2003;157(2):121–130.

26. Yang D, Bernstein L, Wu AH. Physical activity and breast cancer risk among Asian-American women in Los Angeles: a case-control study. *Cancer.* 2003;97(10):2565–2575.

27. McTiernan A. Mechanisms linking physical activity with cancer. *Nat Rev Cancer.* 2008;8(3):205–211.

28. McTiernan A, Tworoger SS, Rajan KB, et al. Effect of exercise on serum androgens in postmenopausal women: a 12-month randomized clinical trial. *Cancer Epidemiol Biomarkers Prev.* 2004;13(7):1099–1105.

29. Calton BA, Lacey JV Jr, Schatzkin A, et al. Physical activity and the risk of colon cancer among women: a prospective cohort study (United States). *Int J Cancer.* 2006;119(2):385–391.

30. Johnsen NF, Christensen J, Thomsen BL, et al. Physical activity and risk of colon cancer in a cohort of Danish middle-aged men and women. *Eur J Epidemiol.* 2006;21(12):877–884.

31. Slattery ML, Potter JD. Physical activity and colon cancer: confounding or interaction? *Med Sci Sports Exerc.* 2002;34(6):913–919.

32. Zhang Y, Cantor KP, Dosemeci M, Lynch CF, Zhu Y, Zheng T. Occupational and leisure-time physical activity and risk of colon cancer by subsite. *J Occup Environ Med.* 2006;48(3):236–243.

33. Nazeri K, Khatibi A, Nyberg P, Agardh CD, Lidfeldt J, Samsioe G. Colorectal cancer in middle-aged women in relation to hormonal status: a report from the Women's Health in the Lund Area (WHILA) study. *Gynecol Endocrinol.* 2006;22(8):416–422.

34. Friedenreich C, Norat T, Steindorf K, et al. Physical activity and risk of colon and rectal cancers: the European prospective investigation into cancer and nutrition. *Cancer Epidemiol Biomarkers Prev.* 2006;15(12):2398–2407.

35. Howard RA, Freedman DM, Park Y, Hollenbeck A, Schatzkin A, Leitzmann MF. Physical activity, sedentary behavior, and the risk of colon and rectal cancer in the NIH-AARP Diet and Health Study. *Cancer Causes Control.* 2008;19(9):939–953.

36. Lee KJ, Inoue M, Otani T, Iwasaki M, Sasazuki S, Tsugane S. Physical activity and risk of colorectal cancer in Japanese men and women: the Japan Public Health Center-based prospective study. *Cancer Sci.* 2006;97(10):1099–1104.

37. Larsson SC, Rutegard J, Bergkvist L, Wolk A. Physical activity, obesity, and risk of colon and rectal cancer in a cohort of Swedish men. *Eur J Cancer.* 2006;42(15):2590–2597.

38. Isomura K, Kono S, Moore MA, et al. Physical activity and colorectal cancer: the Fukuoka Colorectal Cancer Study. *Cancer Sci.* 2006;97(10):1099–1104.

39. Slattery ML, Edwards S, Curtin K, et al. Physical activity and colorectal cancer. *Am J Epidemiol.* 2003;158(3):214–224.

40. Steindorf K, Jedrychowski W, Schmidt M, et al. Case-control study of lifetime occupational and recreational physical activity and risks of colon and rectal cancer. *Eur J Cancer Prev.* 2005;14(4):363–371.

41. Slattery ML, Murtaugh M, Caan B, Ma KN, Neuhausen S, Samowitz W. Energy balance, insulin-related genes and risk of colon and rectal cancer. *Int J Cancer.* 2005;115(1):148–154.

42. Alfano CM, Klesges RC, Murray DM, et al. Physical activity in relation to all-site and lung cancer incidence and mortality in current and former smokers. *Cancer Epidemiol Biomarkers Prev.* 2004;13(12):2233–2241.

43. Bak H, Christensen J, Thomsen BL, et al. Physical activity and risk for lung cancer in a Danish cohort. *Int J Cancer.* 2005;116(3):439–444.

44. Colbert LH, Hartman TJ, Tangrea JA, et al. Physical activity and lung cancer risk in male smokers. *Int J Cancer.* 2002;98(5):770–773.

45. Steindorf K, Friedenreich C, Linseisen J, et al. Physical activity and lung cancer risk in the European Prospective Investigation into Cancer and Nutrition Cohort. *Int J Cancer.* 2006;119(10):2389–2397.

46. Calton BA, Chang SC, Wright ME, et al. History of diabetes mellitus and subsequent prostate cancer risk in the NIH-AARP Diet and Health Study. *Cancer Causes Control.* 2007;18(5):493–503.

47. Friedenreich CM, McGregor SE, Courneya KS, Angyalfi SJ, Elliott FG. Case-control study of lifetime total physical activity and prostate cancer risk. *Am J Epidemiol.* 2004;159(8):740–749.

48. Jian L, Shen ZJ, Lee AH, Binns CW. Moderate physical activity and prostate cancer risk: a case-control study in China. *Eur J Epidemiol.* 2005;20(2):155–160.

49. Pierotti B, Altieri A, Talamini R, et al. Lifetime physical activity and prostate cancer risk. *Int J Cancer.* 2005;114(4):639–642.

50. Strom SS, Yamamura Y, Flores-Sandoval FN, Pettaway CA, Lopez DS. Prostate cancer in Mexican-Americans: identification of risk factors. *Prostate.* 2008;68(5):563–570.

51. Zeegers MP, Dirx MJ, van den Brandt PA. Physical activity and the risk of prostate cancer in the Netherlands cohort study, results after 9.3 years of follow-up. *Cancer Epidemiol Biomarkers Prev.* 2005;14(6):1490–1495.

52. McTiernan A, Schwartz RS, Potter J, Bowen D. Exercise clinical trials in cancer prevention research: a call to action. *Cancer Epidemiol Biomarkers Prev.* 1999;8(3):201–207.

CHAPTER 5

Sun Exposure and Cancer Risk

Marianne Berwick and Jennifer Hay

All substances are poisons; there is none which is not a poison. The right dose differentiates a poison and a remedy[1]

Sunlight, critical to human health, provides light and warmth and aids the body in the formation of vitamin D. Yet too much may be lethal. Excessive exposure to the sun invites the most common cancer of all: skin cancer, melanoma, and nonmelanoma. This chapter will, first, summarize both aspects of sunlight exposure—its risk for cancer as well as its protective aspect—and so help provide an informed basis for evaluating sun exposure. Second, the chapter will review the literature examining psychosocial and behavioral approaches to minimizing sun exposure.

A critical evaluation of the role of sun exposure in cancer risk is particularly important today. There is a great deal of evidence that ultraviolet (UV) exposure has both positive and negative effects.[2] A systematic review of the literature identified risk from sun exposure for melanoma skin cancer, cancer of the lip, basal cell carcinoma (BCC) of the skin, and squamous cell carcinoma (SCC) of the skin but potential protection for other cancers such as prostate, non-Hodgkin's lymphoma, breast, and colon cancer. Although sun protection messages are important to prevent diseases associated with UV exposure, some sun exposure is probably essential to avoid diseases of vitamin D deficiency.[2]

MELANOMA

The association with melanoma, the most deadly form of skin cancer, is still not totally clear. Although "too much" sun exposure may cause melanoma, how much is "too much" is highly individual; the characteristics of susceptibility have not been as thoroughly defined as possible to make prevention effective.

Sun exposure plays a complex role in causing melanoma skin cancer and its precursor lesions. Lifetime sun exposure is difficult to measure; most people cannot recall episodes of sunburn or amount of sun exposure reliably.[3] Some studies have found that sunburn increases risk for cutaneous malignant melanoma (CMM), as noted by Whiteman and Green.[4] Our own work[5] shows no effect of one sunburn, but an increased risk as the number of burns increases. Westerdahl's data are somewhat similar[6]; this group found an increased risk of 1.9 for 3 or more sunburns per year when compared with subjects who had never had a sunburn.

Hersey and colleagues[7,8] found a reduced immune function in volunteers both immediately after and 2 weeks after exposure to commercial suntanning beds. Changes included reduced responses to carcinogens, slightly reduced blood lymphocyte numbers, changes in the proportion of lymphocyte subpopulations, changes in suppressor T-cell activity, and a depression of natural killer (NK) cell activity.

The use of sunscreens that block UVB but not UVA may be associated with an increase in melanoma rates. Also, most people do not apply sunscreen thickly enough (as directed) to afford the protection signified by the sun protection factor (SPF) on the label.[9] Garland and colleagues[10] first suggested that the use of sunscreens may encourage excessive exposure of the skin to UVA (where 90%–95% of the UV energy in the solar spectrum occurs). New biological evidence supports this hypothesis,[11] and an epidemiologic study in Sweden has reported an increased risk for melanoma with the use of sunscreens.[12] Therefore, traditional means of avoiding overexposure to the sun, such as wearing hats and long sleeves and limiting sunbathing, may be more appropriate than a heavy reliance on sunscreens.

NONMELANOMA SKIN CANCER

Sun exposure plays a relatively clear role in causing nonmelanoma skin cancer (BCC and SCC) and its precursor lesions, such as actinic keratoses.[13] Clinicians diagnose approximately 100,000 SCC and 200,000 BCC each year in the United States.[14] Approximately 2% of SCC will metastasize[15]; BCC rarely metastasizes.[16] Mortality from nonmelanoma skin cancers is low, but the associated morbidity (illness) places a burden on the healthcare system[17] and is expected to increase as the population ages.

Nonmelanoma skin cancers occur primarily at sunexposed body sites such as the head, neck, and arms, in people who are sensitive to the sun, and possibly among those who have a reduced capacity to repair DNA damage.[18] Individual pigmentary risk factors are critical determinants of skin cancer risk. Subjects with light skin, light hair color, light eye color, a tendency to freckle, a tendency to burn on first exposure to sunlight, and an inability to tan after repeated exposures have a greater risk of developing all forms of skin cancer. Conversely, light pigmentation and sun exposure may decrease risk of colon, breast, prostate, and ovarian cancer at higher latitudes if the hypothesized association between sun exposure and vitamin D_3 in relation to carcinogenesis is correct.

Each individual has a different "dangerous dose" of sun depending on their genetic predisposition and cutaneous phenotype, or coloring. This explanation may account for the conflicting results from epidemiologic studies. Several studies have found that the effects of sun exposure differ depending on individual susceptibility; for those who tan poorly, sun exposure increases risk (or shows no effect) compared with those who tan well, and sun exposure protects against melanoma for those who tan well. White and colleagues[19] reported that tanning ability can modify melanoma risk due to sun exposure in childhood. Poor tanners showed no effect of sun exposure at ages 2–10 or ages 11–20 years. In contrast, people who reported a deep or moderate tan in reaction to chronic sun exposure appeared to be protected from melanoma with increasing sun exposure at ages 2–10 and at ages 11–20 years.

NON-HODGKIN'S LYMPHOMA

Data for a relationship between sun exposure and cancers other than melanoma have been more limited. Several researchers have suggested that sun exposure plays a causal role in the incidence of non-Hodgkin's lymphoma.[20,21] This relationship may be due to the immunosuppressive role of sun exposure, or to the mutation of a tumor suppressor gene which may have a similar function in both non-Hodgkin's lymphoma and cutaneous melanoma.[22] Boffetta et al. (2008) recently demonstrated that this protective relationship is quite strong (odds ratio for highest vs. lowest quartile of exposure 0.6, 95% confidence interval [CI] 0.4–0.9).

CANCER OF THE COLON, BREAST, PROSTATE, OVARY, AND LEUKEMIA

Mortality rates for colorectal and other cancers decrease from North to South; this association has led to the hypothesis that sunlight exposure might be important in preventing some cancers by enhancing vitamin D_3 and calcium formation, which are inversely associated with colorectal cancer incidence.[23] In a cohort of 25,000 subjects, even moderately elevated concentrations of 25-hydroxyvitamin D were associated with large reductions in the incidence of colorectal cancer.[24]

Melanin, the pigment responsible for dark skin, has for long been thought to be photoprotective.[25]

However, racial pigmentation also determines the magnitude of increase in serum vitamin D_3 levels following whole-body exposure to UVB irradiation; serum levels of vitamin D_3 were highest in whites and lowest in blacks.[26] Some evidence shows that low levels of sun exposure may result in higher cancer incidence, particularly among subsets of individuals, such as older people who would benefit from exposure to sunlight because of problems with micronutrient absorption or darker-skinned people who may have moved to higher latitudes.[27] For example, Pakistani women living in Oslo, Norway, traditionally avoid the sun, have a low dietary intake of vitamin D, use few or no supplements, and have lower serum vitamin D levels.[28]

The relationship of vitamin D to colorectal cancer is the strongest of the protective associations, but even that is not terribly strong. One study[29] has compared black and white males in relationship to dietary, lifestyle, and medical risk factors that might act as proxies for vitamin D levels. Not surprisingly, black men were at higher risk of total cancer incidence (relative risk [RR] 1.3, 95% CI 1.1–1.6) and total cancer mortality (RR 1.9, 95% CI 1.4–2.6). The highest risk was found for digestive system cancer mortality (RR 2.2, 95% CI 1.4–3.7). Surprisingly, among white men with the same number of risk factors for vitamin D insufficiency, the cancer incidence was significantly increased not by very much and few other risk factors were considered (RR 1.1, 95% CI 1.0–1.1), while cancer mortality was similar to incidence for whites. It should be noted that the number of blacks in this study were quite small (n = 63).

Other cancers, such as breast cancer,[30,31] prostate cancer,[32–34] and ovarian cancer[35] may be inversely associated with sunlight exposure through a lack of vitamin D produced in the skin. However, the data available are still conflicting and difficult to interpret.[36]

SUN EXPOSURE BEHAVIOR

Sun exposure and protection is behaviorally controlled. Acute or intermittent sun exposure produces sunburn; chronic exposure, such as occupational exposure, where the skin has adapted to the sun, produces thickening of the stratum corneum and tanning, and may afford protection for many people. Epidemiologic studies[37,38] have shown that people such as farmers and construction workers who are outdoors constantly have a lower relative mortality from melanoma than people who work indoors, such as office workers. Intermittent sun exposure is probably more risky; indoor workers have a higher risk of melanoma incidence and mortality and thus may be a more important group to target for behavioral intervention than individuals who are chronically exposed. Fluorescent light exposure appears not to increase risk, notwithstanding an early suggestion of an association.[39]

Sun protection behaviors are recommended for both primary and secondary melanoma prevention.[40] The American Cancer Society[41] recommends sun protection strategies including sun avoidance between 10 a.m. and 4 p.m., and when sun cannot be avoided that umbrellas, protective hats and clothing, and sunscreen of SPF of 15 or more be used for protection. Total avoidance of artificial UV sources such as tanning beds is also recommended. Unfortunately, less than half (47%) of the U.S. population engages in any sun protection[42] and 59% report that they have sunbathed in the past year.[43] Recently, Coups and colleagues (2008) examined data from over 28,000 individuals in the 2005 National Health Interview Survey[44] and found that only approximately half (43%–51% across age groups) reported frequent (sometimes/most of the time/always) use of sunscreen, 65%–80% did not usually stay in the shade when outside on a sunny day, and 15%–51% used sun protection clothing; for each behavior younger age was related to higher levels of risk behavior. Recently, the Centers for Disease Control reported that about a third of U.S. adults reported at least one sunburn in the past year over the 1999, 2003, and 2004 Behavioral Risk Factor Surveillance System Surveys.[45]

Measurement of intermittent sun exposure or recreational sun exposure represents an important research challenge because measures of past sun exposure necessarily depend on subject recall of exposure, which is not always a reliable measure.[3] Epidemiologic studies have invariably shown weak associations between episodes of sunburn and melanoma incidence.[4,46] Estimates of the effect of intermittent exposure have ranged from a protective effect reported by MacKie and Aitchison[47] of 0.44 (0.21–0.91) to an adverse risk of 8.41 (3.63–19.6) estimated by Grob and colleagues.[48] In contrast to popular notions, estimates of the effects of sun exposure on melanoma incidence vary widely and are frequently not statistically significant.[46] It is likely that the imprecise measurement associated with self-reports is an important rate-limiting factor in determining the relationship between sun exposure and melanoma incidence.

Other methods of assessment of recent sun exposure have been developed, and may increase measurement reliability,[49] although they are not helpful in determining lifetime cumulative dose. For example, direct measures of UV exposure include redemption of a sunscreen coupon on the beach,[50] and biological measures as well as direct visual inspection of the skin.[49,51] In addition, daily diary methods, which involve self-reports made on a day-by-day basis are a useful strategy.[52] All of these alternatives to cumulative, retrospective self-report may circumvent poor participant recall of sun exposure, as well as underestimates of sun exposure due to social desirable responding, or the tendency to underestimate cancer risk behavior that is common in many self-reports.

PSYCHOSOCIAL AND BEHAVIORAL RESEARCH ON SUN PROTECTION

Given the fact that sun exposure represents the most modifiable risk factor for skin cancer, behavioral scientists and health communication experts have been active over the past two decades in identifying strategies to increase knowledge of skin cancer and skin cancer risks, and to encourage consistent sun protection and sun avoidance across diverse populations and different environmental contexts.

Rutten Finney and colleagues[53] have recently shown that individuals drawn from the general population have relatively accurate understandings concerning methods of skin cancer prevention. However, it has been clear for many years that high levels of knowledge about the risks of skin cancer do not necessarily ensure consistent sun protection.[54–57] Indeed, this is the case for knowledge concerning diet and exercise recommendations as well, where knowledge is necessary but not adequate to motivate behavior change.

The content of sun protection interventions has been shaped by multiple elements. Health behavior theories, such as Social Cognitive Theory,[58] the Health Belief Model,[59] and the Trans-theoretical Model,[60] have provided useful guidance in the development of interventions to modify sun protection behavior, because these theories advance our conceptual knowledge of the predisposing factors and psychological processes necessary to enhance individuals' motivation to change behaviors regarding their health. In addition, the empirical examination of psychosocial factors related to the adoption of various sun protection strategies has also proven useful in the development of interventions to promote the adoption of sun protection. For example, there are relatively consistent findings that those who have heightened perceptions of risk for developing skin cancer are most likely to adopt sun protection behaviors[56,61] and that those who value the appearance of being tan are less likely to adopt sun protection behaviors.[62]

General population approaches to improve the overall sun protection have been adopted most prominently in Australia. For example, the Australian state of Victoria adopted the SunSmart program integrating environmental change and mass media public education to address sun protection across the entire population, and this work documents that a mix of strategies is highly effective in improving sun protection behaviors.[63] However, in the United States, targeted approaches to specific higher-risk populations have been the predominant approach to intervention development. For example, interventions targeted at children are arguably quite important given the fact that children spend a greater proportion of their time outdoors, and because sun exposure and sunburns in particular before age 18 represent a large proportion of the lifetime environmental risk of skin cancer. Accordingly, Buller and Borland[64] reviewed the sun protection programs for children, which include interventions focused on parent behaviors, preschool children, and school-age children. Many of these interventions have been implemented in schools and hospitals, and in general, those multiunit programs that occur over several sessions with intensive instruction work best. However, widespread dissemination of these interventions may be limited by shrinking resources and competing demands in the school and other institutional environments. Another population that has been recently targeted for intervention has included those with a family history of melanoma, who face increased risks for skin cancer over and above the general population. For instance, Geller and colleagues[65] developed a novel telephone motivational interviewing and tailored education material approach, but the intervention did not show differential improvement in the treatment over the control group. Other targeted groups have included those with outdoor occupations such as postal employees[66] and farmers.[67]

Given the prevailing belief that a suntan is attractive, concerns for appearance is a barrier to sun protection campaigns.[68] Accordingly, another important approach to promoting sun protection involves the use of appearance appeals, which are designed to emphasize the harm to physical appearance associated with sun exposure, or to increase the perceived attractiveness of untanned skin. Not surprisingly, these appeals to physical appearance have been used most often with teenagers and young adults, and they integrate novel elements such as photoaging information and UV photography to accentuate the appearance of sun damage, as well as social norms information regarding their peers' opinion of sun protection.[69-76] Given that sunless tanning is quite prevalent,[77] it represents another important focus for intervention is amenable to appearance appeals.

A final distinct intervention approach includes those interventions that are specific to various higher-risk environments, and thus capitalize on the local situational cues in certain environments. For example, a program implemented at a zoo contained signage linking sun protection to animals' strategies of skin protection, tip sheets for parents, children's activities, and discounted sun protection was useful in increasing sales of sunscreen and hats compared to a control zoo.[78] Environmentally specific interventions have also been instituted at beaches,[79] ski resorts,[80] and swimming pools.[81] Glanz and colleagues have been quite successful in documenting that their intervention has been successfully implemented by pool staff at selected swimming pools in the United States.[82]

On the whole, these educational messages may, however, be based on an inaccurate assessment of the causes of skin cancer.[83] Although sunscreen use is important in reducing erythema (sunburn), clear evidence that it is associated with a reduction in melanoma or basal cell skin cancer is lacking, and the public may realize this. In the coming years, behavioral and psychosocial approaches will be important in addressing challenges on the horizon for skin cancer control. For example, the availability of genomic testing for melanoma may raise new questions on how to encourage sun protection in those who are tested to be genetically susceptible to melanoma or other skin cancers.[84] The value and strategies concerning sun protection in melanoma survivors has received some recent attention in the behavioral literature.[85,86] Finally, the value of sun protection versus screening in melanoma control[87] will have implications for the focus of behavioral intervention approaches, with both higher-risk and general population cohorts.

SUMMARY AND FUTURE DIRECTIONS

As epidemiologists, behavioral scientists and laboratory scientists become more accurate in ascertaining the role of sun exposure in the etiology of melanoma and other cancers, public health educators will be able to make use of the research on motivation for safe sun behavior. Perception of risk appears to be a major *sine qua non* for adopting appropriate sun protection. As the scientific community develops the ability to define risk more carefully and accurately, public health research into behavior change and the public health messages will become more appropriate.

The most important aid for the recognition of the healing power and avoidance of the destructive effects of natural and artificial UV radiation remains still the human intelligence.[88]

REFERENCES

1. Pagel W. *Paracelsus: an introduction to philosophical medicine in the era of the Renaissance.* New York, NY: S. Karger; 1958.
2. Lucas RM, McMichael A, Armstrong B, Smith W. Estimating the global disease burden due to ultraviolet radiation exposure. *Int J Epidemiol.* 2008;37(3):654–667.
3. Berwick M, Chen YT. Reliability of reported sunburn history in a case-control study of cutaneous malignant melanoma. *Am J Epidemiol.* 1995;141(11):1033–1037.
4. Whiteman D, Green A. Melanoma and sunburn. *Cancer Causes Control.* 1994;5(6):564–572.
5. Berwick M, Begg CB, Fine JA, Roush GC, Barnhill RL. Screening for cutaneous melanoma by skin self-examination. *J Natl Cancer Inst.* 1996;88(1):17–23.
6. Westerdahl J, Olsson H, Ingvar C. At what age do sunburn episodes play a crucial role for the development of malignant melanoma. *Eur J Cancer.* 1994;30A(11):1647–1654.
7. Hersey P, Bradley M, Hasic E, Haran G, Edwards A, McCarthy, WH. Immunological effects of solarium exposure. *Lancet.* 1983;1(8324):545–548.
8. Hersey P, MacDonald M, Henderson C, et al. Suppression of natural killer cell activity in humans by radiation from solarium lamps depleted of UVB. *J Invest Dermatol.* 1988;90(3):305–310.
9. Bech-Thomsen N, Wulf HC. Sunbathers' application of sunscreen is probably inadequate to obtain the sun protection factor assigned to the preparation. *Photodermatol Photoimmunol Photomed.* 1992;9(6):242–244.
10. Garland CF, Garland FC, Gorham ED. Rising trends in melanoma. An hypothesis concerning sunscreen effectiveness. *Ann Epidemiol.* 1993;3(1):103–110.
11. Setlow RB, Grist E, Thompson K, Woodhead AD. Wavelengths effective in induction of malignant melanoma. *Proc Natl Acad Sci USA,* 1993;90(14):6666–6670.
12. Westerdahl J, Olsson H, Másbäck A, Ingvar C, Jonsson N. Is the use of sunscreens a risk factor for malignant melanoma? *Melanoma Res.* 1995;5(1):59–65.
13. Ananthaswamy HN, Pierceall WE. Molecular mechanisms of ultraviolet radiation carcinogenesis. *Photochem Photobiol.* 1990;52(6):1119–1136.
14. Preston DS, Stern RS. Nonmelanoma cancers of the skin. *N Engl J Med.* 1992;327(23):1649–1662.
15. Nixon RL, Dorevitch AP, Marks R. Squamous cell carcinoma of the skin. Accuracy of clinical diagnosis and outcome of follow-up in Australia. *Med J Aust.* 1986;144(5):235–239.
16. Miller SJ. Biology of basal cell carcinoma (Part I). *J Am Acad Dermatol.* 1991;24(1):1–13.
17. Johnson ML, Johnson KG, Engel A. Prevalence, morbidity, and cost of dermatologic diseases. *J Am Acad Dermatol.* 1984;11(5 pt 2):930–936.
18. Wei Q, Matanoski GM, Farmer ER, Hedayati MA, Grossman L. DNA repair and aging in basal cell carcinoma: a molecular epidemiology study. *Proc Natl Acad Sci USA.* 1993;90(4):1614–1618.
19. White E, Kirkpatrick CS, Lee JA. Case-control study of malignant melanoma in Washington State. I. Constitutional factors and sun exposure. *Am J Epidemiol.* 1994;139(9):857–868.
20. Adami J, Frisch M, Yuen J, Glimelius B, Melbye M. Evidence of an association between non-Hodgkin's lymphoma and skin cancer. *BMJ.* 1995;310(6993):1491–1495.
21. Zheng T, Mayne ST, Boyle P, Holford TR, Liu WL, Flannery J. Epidemiology of non-Hodgkin lymphoma in Connecticut. 1935–1988. *Cancer.* 1992;70(4):840–849.
22. Boffetta P, van der Hel O, Kricker A, et al. Exposure to ultraviolet radiation and risk of malignant lymphoma and multiple myeloma—a multicentre European case-control study. *Int J Epidemiol.* 2008;37(5):1080–1094.
23. Garland CF, Garland FC. Do sunlight and vitamin D reduce the likelihood of colon cancer? *Int J Epidemiol.* 1980;9(3):227–231.
24. Bostick RM, Potter JD, Sellers TA, McKenzie DR, Kushi LH, Folsom AR. Relation of calcium, vitamin D, and dairy food intake to incidence of colon cancer among older women. The Iowa Women's Health Study. *Am J Epidemiol.* 1993;137(12):1302–1317.
25. Barker D, Dixon K, Medrano E, et al. Comparison of the responses of human melanocytes with different melanin contents to ultraviolet B irradiation. *Cancer Res.* 1995;55(18):4041–4046.
26. Matsuoka LY, Wortsman J, Haddad JG, Kolm P, Hollis BW. Racial pigmentation and the cutaneous synthesis of vitamin D. *Arch Dermatol.* 1991;127(4):536–538.
27. Studzinski GP, Moore DC. Sunlight—can it prevent as well as cause cancer? *Cancer Res.* 1995;55(18):4014–4022.
28. Henriksen C, Brunvand L, Stoltenberg C, Trygg K, Haug E, Pedersen JI. Diet and vitamin D status among pregnant Pakistani women in Oslo. *Eur J Clin Nutr.* 1995;49(3):211–218.

29. Giovannucci E, Liu Y, Willett WC. Cancer incidence and mortality and vitamin D in black and white male health professionals. *Cancer Epidemiol Biomarkers Prev.* 2006;15(12):2467–2472.

30. Furst CJ, et al. DNA pattern and dietary habits in patients with breast cancer. *Eur J Cancer.* 1993;29A(9):1285–1288.

31. Gorham ED, Garland FC, Garland CF. Sunlight and breast cancer incidence in the USSR. *Int J Epidemiol.* 1990;19(4):820–824.

32. Hanchette CL, Schwartz GG. Geographic patterns of prostate cancer mortality. Evidence for a protective effect of ultraviolet radiation. *Cancer.* 1992;70(12):2861–2869.

33. Schwartz GG, Hulka BS. Is vitamin D deficiency a risk factor for prostate cancer? [Hypothesis]. *Anticancer Res.* 1990;10(5A):1307–1311.

34. Schwartz GG, Hulka BS, Morris D, Mohler JL. Prostate cancer and vitamin (hormone) D: a case control study. *J Urol.* 1992;147(Suppl):294A.

35. Lefkowitz ES, Garland CF. Sunlight, vitamin D, and ovarian cancer mortality rates in US women. *Int J Epidemiol.* 1994;23(6):1133–1136.

36. Soerjomataram I, Louwman WJ, Lemmens VEPP, Coebergh JWW, de Vries, E. Are patients with skin cancer at lower risk of developing colorectal or breast cancer? *Am J Epidemiol.* 2008;167(12):1421–1429.

37. Holman CD, Armstrong BK. Cutaneous malignant melanoma and indicators of total accumulated exposure to the sun: an analysis separating histogenetic types. *J Natl Cancer Inst.* 1984;73(1):75–82.

38. Lee JA, Strickland D. Malignant melanoma: social status and outdoor work. *Br J Cancer.* 1980;41(5):757–763.

39. Beral V, Shaw H, Evans S, Milton G. Malignant melanoma and exposure to fluorescent lighting at work. *Lancet.* 1982;2(8293):290–293.

40. Rogers RS III. Malignant melanoma in the 21st century. *Int J Dermatol.* 2000;39(3):178–179.

41. American Cancer Society. *Facts and figures, 2007.* 2007. http://www.cancer.org/downloads/STT/CAFF2007PWSecured.pdf. Accessed 2008.

42. Hall HI, May DS, Lew RA, Koh HK, Nadel M. Sun protection behaviors of the U.S. white population. *Prev Med.* 1997;26(4):401–407.

43. Koh HK, Bak SM, Geller AC, et al. Sunbathing habits and sunscreen use among white adults: results of a national survey. *Am J Public Health.* 1997;87(7):1214–1217.

44. Coups EJ, Manne SL, Heckman CJ. Multiple skin cancer risk behaviors in the U.S. population. *Am J Prev Med.* 2008;34(2):87–93.

45. Centers for Disease Control and Prevention. Sunburn prevalence among adults—United States, 1999, 2003, and 2004. *MMWR Morb Mortal Wkly Rep.* 2007;56(21):524–528.

46. Armstrong BK. Epidemiology of malignant melanoma: intermittent or total accumulated exposure to the sun? *J Dermatol Surg Oncol.* 1988;14(8):835–849.

47. MacKie RM, Aitchison T. Severe sunburn and subsequent risk of primary cutaneous malignant melanoma in Scotland. *Br J Cancer.* 1982;46(6):955–960.

48. Grob JJ, Gouvernet J, Aymar D, et al. Count of benign melanocytic nevi as a major indicator of risk for nonfamilial nodular and superficial spreading melanoma. *Cancer.* 1990;66(2):387–395.

49. Glanz K, Mayer JA. Reducing ultraviolet radiation exposure to prevent skin cancer methodology and measurement. *Am J Prev Med.* 2005;29(2):131–142.

50. Detweiler JB, Bedell BT, Salovey P, Pronin E, Rothman AJ. Message framing and sunscreen use: gain-framed messages motivate beach-goers. *Health Psychol.* 1999;18(2):189–196.

51. Creech LL, Mayer JA. Ultraviolet radiation exposure in children: a review of measurement strategies. *Ann Behav Med.* 1997;19(4):399–407.

52. O'Riordan DL, Glanz K, Gies P, Elliott T. A pilot study of the validity of self-reported ultraviolet radiation exposure and sun protection practices among lifeguards, parents and children. *Photochem Photobiol.* 2008;84(3):774–748.

53. Rutten Finney L, et al. Public understanding of cancer prevention, screening, and survival: comparison with state-of-science evidence for colon, skin, and lung cancer. *J Cancer Educ.* 2008. In press.

54. Arthey S, Clarke VA. Suntanning and sun protection: a review of the psychological literature. *Soc Sci Med.* 1995;40(2):265–274.

55. Berwick M, Fine JA, Bologna JL. Sun exposure and sunscreen use following a community skin cancer screening. *Prev Med.* 1992;21(3):302–310.

56. Grob JJ, Guglielmina C, Gouvernet J, Zarour H, Noe C, Bonerandi JJ. Study of sunbathing habits in children and adolescents: application to the prevention of melanoma. *Dermatology.* 1993;186(2):94–98.

57. Rossi JS, et al. Preventing skin cancer through behavior change. Implications for interventions. *Dermatol Clin.* 1995;13(3):613–622.

58. Bandura A. Social foundations of thought and action: a social cognitive theory. Englewood Cliff, NJ: Prentice-Hall; 1986.

59. Rosenstock IM. Historical origins of the health belief model. *Health Educ Monogr.* 1974;2(4):328–335.

60. Prochaska JO, DiClemente CC, Norcross JC. In search of how people change. Applications to addictive behaviors. *Am Psychol.* 1992;47(9):1102–1114.

61. von Schirnding Y, Strauss N, Mathee A, Robertson P, Blignaut R. Sunscreen use and environmental awareness among beach-goers in Cape Town, South Africa. *Public Health Rev.* 1991;19(1–4):209–217.

62. Jackson KM, Aiken LS. A psychosocial model of sun protection and sunbathing in young women: the impact of health beliefs, attitudes, norms, and self-efficacy for sun protection. *Health Psychol.* 2000;19(5):469–478.

63. Dobbinson SJ, Wakefield MA, Jamsen KM, et al. Weekend sun protection and sunburn in Australia trends (1987–2002) and association with SunSmart television advertising. *Am J Prev Med.* 2008;34(2):94–101.

64. Buller DB, Borland R. Skin cancer prevention for children: a critical review. *Health Educ Behav.* 1999;26(3):317–343.

65. Geller AC, Emmons KM, Brooks DR, et al. A randomized trial to improve early detection and prevention practices among siblings of melanoma patients. *Cancer.* 2006;107(4):806–814.

66. Mayer JA, Slymen DJ, Clapp EJ, et al. Promoting sun safety among US Postal Service letter carriers: impact of a 2-year intervention. *Am J Public Health.* 2007;97(3):559–565.

67. Silk KJ, Parrott RL. All or nothing… or just a hat? Farmers' sun protection behaviors. *Health Promot Pract.* 2006;7(2):180–185.

68. Leary MR, Jones JL. The social psychology of tanning and sunscreen use: self-presentational motives as a predictor of health risk. *J Appl Soc Psychol.* 1993:1390–1406.

69. Broadstock M, Borland R, Gason R. Effects of suntan on judgements of healthiness and attractiveness by adolescents. *J Appl Soc Psychol.* 1992;22:157–172.

70. Gibbons FX, Gerrard M, Lane DJ, Mahler HI, Kulik JA. Using UV photography to reduce use of tanning booths: a test of cognitive mediation. *Health Psychol.* 2005;24(4):358–363.

71. Jones JL, Leary MR. Effects of appearance-based admonitions against sun exposure on tanning intentions in young adults. *Health Psychol.* 1994;13(1):86–90.

72. Mahler HI, Kulik JA, Butler HA, Gerrard M, Gibbons FX. Social norms information enhances the efficacy of an appearance-based sun protection intervention. *Soc Sci Med.* 2008;67(2):321–329.

73. Mahler HI, Kulik JA, Gerrard M, Gibbons FX. Long-term effects of appearance-based interventions on sun protection behaviors. *Health Psychol.* 2007;26(3):350–360.

74. Mahler HI, Kulik JA, Gibbons FX, Gerrard M, Harrell J. Effects of appearance-based interventions on sun protection intentions and self-reported behaviors. *Health Psychol.* 2003;22(2):199–209.

75. Mahler HI, Kulik JA, Harrell J, Correa A, Gibbons FX, Gerrard M. Effects of UV photographs, photoaging information, and use of sunless tanning lotion on sun protection behaviors. *Arch Dermatol.* 2005;141(3):373–380.

76. Vail-Smith K, Felts WM. Sunbathing: college students' knowledge, attitudes, and perceptions of risks. *J Am Coll Health.* 1993;42(1):21–26.

77. Hoerster KD, Mayer J, Woodruff S, Malcarne V, Roesch S, Clapp, E. The influence of parents and peers on adolescent indoor tanning behavior: findings from a multi-city sample. *J Am Acad Dermatol.* 2007;57(6):990–997.

78. Mayer JA, Slymen DJ, Clapp EJ, et al. Promoting sun safety among zoo visitors. *Prev Med.* 2001;33(3):162–169.

79. Weinstock MA, et al. Randomized controlled community trial of the efficacy of a multicomponent stage-matched intervention to increase sun protection among beach goers. *Prev Med.* 2002;35(6):584–592.

80. Buller DB, Andersen PA, Walkosz BJ, et al. Randomized trial testing a worksite sun protection program in an outdoor recreation industry. *Health Educ Behav.* 2005;32(4):514–535.

81. Glanz K, et al. A randomized trial of skin cancer prevention in aquatics settings: the Pool Cool program. *Health Psychol.* 2002;21(6):579–587.

82. Glanz K, Mayer JA. Diffusion of an effective skin cancer prevention program: design, theoretical foundations, and first-year implementation. *Health Psychol.* 2005;24(5):477–487.

83. Young AR, et al. Photoprotection and 5-MOP photochemoprotection from UVR-induced DNA damage in humans: the role of skin type. *J Invest Dermatol.* 1991;97(5):942–948.

84. Hay JL, Meischke HW, Bowen DJ, et al. Anticipating dissemination of cancer genomics in public health: a theoretical approach to psychosocial and behavioral challenges. *Ann Behav Med.* 2007;34(3):275–286.

85. Manne S, Lessin S. Prevalence and correlates of sun protection and skin self-examination practices among cutaneous malignant melanoma survivors. *J Behav Med.* 2006;29(5):419–434.

86. Mujumdar U, Hay JL, Monroe-Hinds YC, et al. Sun protection and skin self-examination in melanoma survivors. *Psycho-Oncology.* 2008;. 9999(9999): In press.

87. Wartman D, Weinstock M. Are we overemphasizing sun avoidance in protection from melanoma? *Cancer Epidemiol Biomarkers Prev.* 2008;17(3):469–470.

88. Breit R. *Roting und Braunnung durch UVA.* Munich: W. Zucherschwert Verlag; 1987.

Socioeconomic Status and Psycho-Oncology

Sara Fernandes-Taylor and Joan R. Bloom

The challenge in overcoming cancer is not only to find therapies that will prevent or arrest the disease quickly, but also to map the middle ground of survivorship and minimize its medical and social hazards.

These words of physician and cancer survivor Hugh Mullan[1] epitomize the focus of this chapter: How to understand the "social hazards" affecting the development of cancer. A better understanding of these hazards may lead to measures that minimize the risk. The social hazards referenced are the resource-based and prestige-based characteristics of individuals and the places they live, which comprise "socioeconomic status" (SES). These "social hazards" can be found at all points along the cancer care continuum beginning with the etiology of cancer, screening and early detection, diagnosis and treatment, survivorship, and mortality. Even though cancer outcomes have improved in the past two decades, those individuals with lower SES have not improved as quickly as those with higher SES.[2] Moreover, the impact of SES on health is much broader than cancer. SES affects the chances of contracting both acute and chronic illnesses. In general, poorer people have a higher risk of getting most acute and chronic health conditions.

In the chapter that follows, the definition of SES is explicated along with both the resource-based (income, wealth, education) and prestige-based (indices, occupation) measures. The methodological implications are discussed. Cancer incidence, mortality, and survival rates as they are associated with SES are also presented. Finally, the implications for SES across the cancer care continuum, prevention (or primary prevention), screening and early diagnosis (secondary prevention), and survival (tertiary prevention) are considered.

SOCIOECONOMIC STATUS IN HEALTH RESEARCH: MEASUREMENT AND PATHWAYS

Although the links between SES and health are well established, SES itself is a dynamic and multifactorial construct that is measured in a number of different ways. Generally, SES is defined as "a broad concept that refers to the placement of persons, families, households, and census tracts or other aggregates with respect to the capacity to create or consume goods that are valued in our society."[3] Taking into account the complexities and multiple components of the construct, Krieger, Williams, and Moss[4] define SES as follows:

An aggregate concept that includes both resource-based and prestige-based measures, as linked to both childhood and adult social class position. Resource-based measures refer to material and social resources and assets, including income, wealth, educational credentials; terms used to describe inadequate resources include "poverty" and "deprivation." Prestige-based measures refer to [an] individual's rank or status in a social hierarchy, typically evaluated with reference to people's access to and consumption of goods, services, and knowledge, as linked to their occupational prestige, income, and educational level.

This definition of SES underscores (1) the various elements of SES—education, wealth, income, education, occupation; (2) the dynamic nature of SES over the lifespan; and (3) the levels of analysis at which SES can be measured—individual, family, household, neighborhood, and so on. Each element likely affects health via distinct pathways. As Shavers[5] notes, a significant lack of precision and reliability underlies SES measures in health research. Therefore, this section will provide a brief overview of the ways in which SES is measured and the ways in which SES can affect health.

Education. Owing to the relative ease of data collection, education is probably the most widely used measure of SES in health research.[5] Education is often represented as the number of years of education or as credentials, such as having high school or college degree.[5,6] Better-educated individuals are likely to have better information processing and literacy skills, greater health-related knowledge, increased ability to navigate bureaucracies, social prestige, and better interactions with health professionals.[5,6] In addition, education is indicative of behaviors that contribute to good health (e.g., gym membership, a good diet, insurance, etc.).[4,7] However, education does not serve as an adequate proxy for income and wealth.[6]

Measuring SES using education has significant advantages and disadvantages. Whereas measuring SES via occupation and individual income excludes or misclassifies people who are not in the labor force (e.g., retirees and homemakers), education excludes and misclassifies fewer individuals.[4,5] In addition, education remains relatively stable beyond early adulthood and likely reflects certain lifestyle choices and health behaviors. Therefore, cross-sectional measurement of education may be indicative of the effect of education on health over the lifespan whereas the cross-sectional measurement of income may not be a valid measure when examining the effect of income on health.[5] However, the same level of education has different social implications in different time periods and cultural settings. For example, economic returns to education differ depending on race and gender.[8] Also, education (being relatively stable) does not represent variations in income and wealth over the lifespan that may affect health and does not serve as a good proxy measure for other SES indicators.[5,9]

Income. Ostensibly, income is a simple measure of SES represented by, for example, annual household income. However, it represents a multitude of revenue sources, such as wages, dividends, accrued interest, alimony, child support, and pensions.[4] Income may also be measured using a normative poverty construct in which individuals are classified as being above or below an income level defined relative to a certain subsistence level or to the national median income.[4,6] Economic resources, commonly income and wealth, lead to better health via access to material goods and services, such as nutrition, recreational facilities, housing, and healthcare.[5,7] In addition, low-income individuals may experience chronic stress related to job insecurity and financial strain, greater environmental exposures to toxins both at work and at home, and less social support, which in turn adversely affect health.[7] An increased prevalence of behavioral risk factors for poor health, such as smoking, alcohol consumption, and a sedentary lifestyle, is also found among lower-income populations.[10–12] The relationship between income and health has often been modeled as linear, but evidence indicates that small increases in income may lead to greater health benefits among lower-income groups.[13,14]

Income also has significant shortcomings as a measure of SES. Income is age dependent and fluctuates considerably over short periods of time.[5,15] Therefore, cross-sectional measures of income may inadequately represent the relationship between SES and health, particularly given the demonstrated persistence of the relationship between childhood SES and adult health.[16,17] In addition, income as a measure of SES does not account for accumulated assets (wealth) or benefits and may not adequately capture purchasing power, given that the quality of goods and services in poorer neighborhoods is worse and prices are higher.[5,18,19] Nonresponse for income measures also tends to be systematically higher among individuals with higher income.[20]

Wealth. As previously mentioned, wealth is also used as an economic measure of SES and is not interchangeable with income.[6] Wealth is represented using accumulated assets, such as investments, savings, and home and car ownership, and serves as a proxy for fiscal security and social prestige.[4,5] It is valuable as a measure of SES because it represents the ability to absorb emergencies and financial upsets and is more strongly linked to social class than income.[5,6] Wealth may also serve as a better indicator for SES than income among retirees, whose income may not accurately reflect their accumulated resources.[4] Wealth among whites is also significantly greater than wealth among blacks of the same income level in the United States.[21] Therefore, it may shed some light on racial health disparities that persist after controlling for income and education. However, it is difficult to calculate and is susceptible to high error rates.[5]

Occupation. Occupation is a particularly common measure of SES in western European health research, but has also been used in the United States and other areas.[4,6] It can be measured using employment status (employed, unemployed, student, retired, etc.) or using an aggregated occupational group (professional, intermediate, skilled nonmanual, skilled manual, partly skilled, unskilled).[4,5,22] Examining occupation's link to health has several benefits. Occupation provides a link between education and income and positions individuals in a social structure, serving as a proxy for both prestige and skill.[4] It is also a more stable measure of SES than income.[5] Furthermore, occupation accounts for salient environmental conditions, such as an individual's control over his or her work, exposure to toxins, and the psychological demands of a given job.[7,23]

However, classifications of occupation have been developed chiefly on the basis of men and may misclassify unemployed individuals, such as retirees and homemakers.[5,6] Moreover, occupational classifications may be heterogeneous with wide variation in education, income, and prestige within each category.[5] Occupation measures also fail to account for gender and race inequities within occupation; women and minorities systematically receive lower pay for the same job.[24] Finally, using occupation as a measure of SES may create circularity problems; does employment lead to better health or vice versa?[25]

Index measures. Some research utilizes indices that compile multiple measures of SES. Index SES measures are most common in the United Kingdom and in sociological research, but are also used in health research.[4] Socioeconomic indices fall into two general categories: (1) material and social deprivation measures and (2) social standing and prestige-based measures.[5] These indices can include income, occupation, and education within a single variable. Although indices have the advantage of including multiple measures of SES, index measures have not been validated and likely conflate the various pathways by which SES affects health.[4,5]

Area level. Geographically aggregated measures of SES are increasingly common in health disparities research. Areas may be represented by neighborhoods, census tracts, census blocks, census block groups, zip/postal codes, states, or general regions of a country.[4] In general, smaller, more homogenous areas are best for estimating area-level effects; zip/postal codes (developed for mail delivery and not for population research) are less ideal.[4] Area-level SES measures are as numerous as the geographic areas they represent. Researchers have used average house value, median rental value, percent unemployment, per capita income, among other area-level SES measures.[4]

Although most studies do not include both individual and area SES measures, area-level measures do not serve as a proxy for individual SES, and area-level measures generally correlate poorly with individual-level measures.[5] Rather, they represent the architectural, social, and service environments that affect individuals' health via multiple pathways, such as recreation areas, tobacco and alcohol advertisements, noise and crowding, and access to grocers carrying fresh produce.[7] These measures also represent geographic access to medical care and pharmacies. Area-level SES measures are more stable than many individual measures, can be used to estimate population-level prevalence, and can be applied similarly to homemakers, retirees, and working individuals in the same area.[4]

However, there are significant shortcomings to using area-level SES without controlling for individual SES. Area SES measures are susceptible to the ecological fallacy, which involves drawing incorrect inference about individuals from aggregated data.[4] The possibility of reverse causality is also an issue; do environmental conditions affect health, or do people with certain health-related proclivities cluster in certain areas?[26]

Overall, socioeconomic is a term that encompasses multiple individual and area-level social characteristics. These characteristics, in turn, produce health disparities that are (1) systematic, (2) social produced, and (3) unfair.[27] Moreover, growing income inequalities in the United States and worldwide will likely lead to greater socioeconomic health disparities.[27] Therefore, better understanding of the links between SES and health is essential to both research and policy.

INCIDENCE AND ETIOLOGY

Cancer incidence refers to the number of newly diagnosed cases and is often expressed as the absolute number of new cases in a given year. Incidence may also be expressed as the rate of new cases per 100,000 people, allowing for comparison between different populations as well as the identification of trends within populations over time.[28] Cancer incidence is related to SES both directly and inversely.[29] The incidence of some types of cancer, such as lung and stomach, increases with decreasing SES. The incidence of other types of cancer, such as breast and prostate, generally increases with increasing SES. In addition, socioeconomic gradients for cancer incidence differ between nations,[28] and the availability and quality of data are variable. Therefore, global estimates of cancer incidence involve extrapolation and "best guesses," but represent the best available knowledge.[28]

At a global level, the incidence of some cancers is more prevalent among low-resource, or developing, countries while high-resource, or developed/industrialized, nations have higher rates of other cancers. Discrepancies in cancer incidence between nations are often explained by differences in access to preventive healthcare services and differential patterns of behavioral risk, such as smoking. Although differences in cancer incidence between low- and high-resource countries are not true socioeconomic disparities, they reflect systematic differences between those areas of the world with high income and those with relatively low income. As the quality and availability of global cancer incidence data increase, between-nation disparities and internationally pooled data will likely become central in understanding SES-related cancer incidence patterns. Therefore, these disparities are summarized by cancer type. The cancer types discussed encompass some of the most common cancers in the world with notable SES gradients among men and women in both low- and high-resource countries.[28] In addition, within-nation, SES-related patterns of cancer incidence and etiology are discussed.

Prostate cancer. According to global estimates for 2002, prostate cancer is the most common type of cancer diagnosed among men in high-resource nations.[28] The prevalence of prostate cancer in high-resource nations may be partially explained by the higher rates of screening and prostate-specific antigen (PSA) testing in those nations, which leads to the detection of cancers that would not otherwise be discovered.[30] Within countries, prostate cancer tends to be more prevalent among high SES individuals than among people of low SES. This has historically been true both in countries without universal healthcare[31,32] and in countries with universal coverage, such as England and Canada.[33,34] This observed trend may be due to lower utilization of preventive care among low SES individuals,[35,36] although observed associations between occupation and prostate cancer incidence are less readily explained.[30,37]

However, recent data from population-based registries suggest that this trend is changing in the United States. Although prostate cancer incidence was higher among low-poverty counties and for all racial/ethnic groups from 1988 to 1992, data from the 1990s show that incidence rates in high-poverty counties now surpass those in low-poverty counties.[32] Additional research examining data from the United Kingdom from 1986 through 2000 indicates that prostate cancer incidence rates have decreased in high SES areas.[38] However, the inverse association between prostate cancer incidence and SES has persisted in other countries, such as Denmark[39] and Norway.[37]

Lung cancer. Lung cancer is the second most common cancer diagnosed among men and third among women in high-resource nations. Among low-resource nations, however, lung cancer is the most common type of cancer among men (fourth among women) due largely to high rates of tobacco smoking.[28] Lung cancer is also more prevalent among low SES populations within countries. High rates of smoking, exposure to air pollution, and occupational hazards (e.g., asbestos exposure) explain lung cancer incidence among low SES individuals.[40,41] In the United States, incidence rates are 12% higher among men and 11% higher among women in areas of high poverty compared to areas of low poverty.[32] Similar results have been obtained in France,[42] Canada, and Denmark.[33,39,43] In the United Kingdom, incidence rates in deprived areas are more than double those in the least deprived areas, and the deprivation gap is widening due to decreased incidence rates in the least deprived areas.[34]

Colorectal cancers. Among men in high-resource countries, incidence rates of lung cancer are followed by cancers of the bowel. Colon cancer is also the second most commonly diagnosed cancer among women in high-resource nations (after breast cancer).[28] The high incidence of colorectal cancer in developed nations is explained by high rates of meat and animal fat consumption, low fiber intake, and physical inactivity.[28] Nonetheless, the relationship between SES and colon cancer incidence within nations is relatively unclear. Recent data from both the United Kingdom and Denmark demonstrate no clear association between colon cancer incidence and SES.[34,39] However, research in Italy has documented a higher prevalence of colon cancer among high SES individuals.[44] In the United States, there has been a recent reversal of the relationship between colon cancer incidence and SES; whereas colon cancer was more prevalent in high SES areas in 1975, incidence rates in low SES areas are now higher.[32,45] In a similar vein, data from Finland for the years 1971–1995 show that increasing incidence rates among low SES men have narrowed the gap between high and low SES men, with the former having historically high colon cancer incidence; no trend was observed for women.[46]

Major risk factors for colon cancer were once more prevalent among high SES populations, but have recently become more common among low SES communities.[11,12] Because colon cancer develops over a long time, the reversal of risk factor prevalence in high versus low SES populations may explain the current lack of a definitive association between SES and colon cancer.[29] However, controlling for known risk factors did not eliminate the association between low education and increased colon cancer incidence in a Canadian study, which suggests that current knowledge of causal pathways is incomplete.[47]

Breast cancer. In women, breast cancer is the most common type of cancer in both high- and low-resource countries, although breast cancer rates in high-resource nations are higher. Porter[48] suggests that recent increases in breast cancer incidence rates in low-resource nations are due partly to the "westernization" of the developing world including the widespread adoption of behavioral risk factors for breast cancer that have historically been more prevalent in developed countries—certain dietary patterns, decreased physical activity, delayed and decreased childbearing, increased exposure to hormones (via birth control and hormone replacement therapy), and lower rates of breast-feeding. However, higher rates of breast cancer in high-resource countries have also been attributed to widespread screening, which, like prostate cancer, may result in the detection of cancers that would not otherwise be found.[49]

Within countries, breast cancer incidence is higher among high SES women due to the aforementioned risk factors as well as relatively early menarche and later menopause.[33,50–52] Although data from the United States show that incidence rates are increasing in high SES areas more than in low SES areas,[32] the incidence gap between low and high SES areas does not appear to be changing in the United Kingdom.[34]

SCREENING AND DIAGNOSIS

Screening for asymptomatic disease. Screening for asymptomatic cancer is the major way that cancer can be prevented in some types of cancers (e.g., cervical, skin, and colorectal cancer). Screening can detect precancerous growths and prevent cancer from occurring or detect cancers at early stages when there are usually more options for treatment and better outcomes. In the United States, the gold standard for cancer screening tests is that screening reduces mortality. Currently, the only cancers for which this standard has been demonstrated are for cancers of the breast, cervix, and colon/rectum. There are both national and international studies indicating that socioeconomic factors, regardless of how they are measured, are related to screening. For example, Ross and colleagues[36] used pooled data from the 1996, 1998, and 2000 surveys of a nationally representative sample of older community-dwelling adults in the United States to assess variations in the use of preventive behaviors. They found that the working poor were significantly less likely to receive breast cancer, prostate cancer, and cholesterol screening but not cervical cancer screening or influenza vaccine. Moreover, a study in Ontario, Canada, found that being in the highest quintile for income was related to receiving any screening and higher odds of receiving a colonoscopy.[53] A large, cross-sectional study of French women also found that mammography screening was related to income and education.[54] Similar findings have been obtained in the United States and Geneva, Switzerland.[55,56] Perhaps due to a lack of universal health care in the United States, the focus on screening and SES is greater than in countries with universal coverage. For example, there are several studies that focus on the underserved and have tried to separate the effects of race/ethnicity from SES. In general, they find that by controlling for SES, the effects of race are mitigated. Also, later stages of breast and cervical cancer are associated with lack of screening.[56,57]

In general, screening programs are more likely to be found in high-resource countries (Western Europe, Canada, the United States, Australia, New Zealand, and Japan) than in middle and low-resource countries. Measures of screening program effectiveness include the success of initial efforts to enroll the target population, high rescreening rates, and timely diagnosis and treatment of cancers. An example of such a screening program is the National Breast and Cervical Cancer Early Detection Program (NBCCEDP) created in 1991 by the U.S. Centers for Disease Control and Prevention.[58] For the reasons described above, it focuses on low-income women who are uninsured or underinsured. The program provides screening support in all 50 states, the District of Columbia, five U.S. territories, and twelve American Indian/ Alaska Native tribes or tribal organizations and helps low-income, uninsured, and underinsured women gain access to breast and cervical cancer screening and diagnostic services.

Since 1991, the NBCCEDP has served more than 3.1 million women, provided more than 7.5 million screening examinations, and diagnosed 32,996 breast cancers, 2035 invasive cervical cancers, and 106,904 precursor cervical lesions, of which 43% were high grade. The program has been successful in enrolling its target population (minority women),[59] somewhat successful in rescreening efforts,[60] and timely in provision of diagnosis and treatment relative to comparisons.[61,62] Therefore, one can conclude that there is little disparity in follow-up treatment for underserved, poor women participating in interventions such as the BCCEDP National Program.[59,62] National screening programs exist in other countries that have been evaluated in a manner similar to the BCCEDP program. A program to ensure an equal standard of care for women with breast cancer was established in the 1970s in Stockholm. In this program, albeit within a single payer system, socioeconomic gradients in both clinical stage at presentation and survival were found.[63] High income, skilled work, and more education were all associated with less advanced tumors, and hence better survival. The authors concluded that "the results indicate social inequalities regarding awareness of the disease and/or access to early detection."

Symptom recognition and timely diagnosis. Symptom recognition by the patient and confirmation by the physician have been considered as explanations of socioeconomic differences in stage of disease at diagnosis, a major predictor of cancer survival. Two literature reviews on this topic have been conducted in the past decade,[64,65] and the following conclusion was made by the authors of the more recent study:

Overall, the idea that socio-economic differences in the stage of disease at diagnosis are the result of differential delays in diagnosis, whether by the patient or by the provider, is not supported by strong research evidence.[65]

Primary access to care versus socioeconomic status. Primary access to care refers to having health insurance and a physician or access to another source of preventive care.[66] For most high-resource countries that have single payer systems, lack of health insurance is a nonissue. In the United States, 46.5 million people do not have health insurance, and 80% of these are citizens. Most of the uninsured in the United States work either full- (71%) or part-time (11%) and are at 100% of poverty level. Many policy advocates believe that providing a national health insurance program will eliminate socioeconomic disparities. However, U.S. systems such as the Department of Veterans Affairs (VA) and Military Health System provide access, yet lower utilization persists among those of low socioeconomic position.[67] In addition, studies from France, Switzerland, Canada, and elsewhere provide evidence that, even when there is universal primary access, the problem of SES disparities in the provision of primary and secondary prevention through cancer screening continues.[53–55] Several explanations of this phenomenon exist. The working poor may have limited opportunity to receive preventive care.[35] An additional explanation is that physicians who provide care to low SES communities (have greater practice revenue from Medicaid) are less likely to provide recommended primary care.[68] Underutilization of primary care may also reflect widespread preferences and beliefs in low SES communities.[35]

CANCER TREATMENT

Concerns have been raised that diagnostic delays and receipt of standard treatment are related to SES. One source of diagnostic delay is the time that occurs between screening for cancer and entering the healthcare system as well as the system's slow responsiveness to people already in the medical care system. These delays are often a result of lack of coordination between systems (i.e., the screening program and the treatment system) or bureaucratic barriers within one system. For example, using patient reported data from the National Health System in the United Kingdom, Neal and Allgar[69] found systematic diagnostic delays for six cancers among lower social classes. In Italy, researchers found that being admitted with a more advanced or urgent diseases as well as having longer intervals between onset of symptoms, surgical referral, and hospital admission were more common among less educated individuals.[70] Receiving state-of-the-art treatment is another potential source of inequality due to socioeconomic factors. Studies of treatment outcomes where patients have equal access to comprehensive cancer treatment (including supportive care) demonstrate that similar treatment yields similar outcomes.[71,72] Therefore, the aforementioned U.S. studies that find unequal treatment among groups provides evidence of disparities. There may be patient-level factors, such as education or literacy, or physician level factors, such as subtle prejudice, that affect the treatment that patients are offered and/or select. For example, by linking data from Medicaid with U.S. national cancer registry data, low SES was found to be associated with nonreceipt of surgical treatment and the likelihood of receiving breast-conserving treatment among those receiving surgery, controlling for race/ethnicity, Medicaid enrollment, and clinical factors.[73] In another U.S. study using ecological measures of SES, women with early-stage breast cancer were less likely to be treated with breast-conserving surgery and radiation if they resided in poorer, compared

with more affluent, census tracts.[32] Socioeconomic disparities in palliative care, "active total care of patients whose disease is not responsive to curative treatment,"[74] are generally due to the lack of hospice care and pain management. For example, Morrison et al.[75] found that pharmacies in low-income neighborhoods failed to stock opioid analgesics whereas pharmacies in higher-income neighborhood had plentiful stocks.

High-resource countries are more able to provide state-of-the-art treatment. However, across the globe, there are differences in the availability of state-of-the-art treatment. This is true even when the provision of such treatment would be cost-effective, as in the provision of radiotherapy in low- and middle-resource countries[76] where the proportion of cancer cases will increase from 60% to 70% by the year 2020. Most countries in this group have limited access to radiotherapy, while 22 countries in Asia and African have no service capability at all. This concern is growing in importance as novel-targeted therapies are becoming a reality in oncology. Compelling new technologies such as gene profiling, circulating tumor cells, and proteomix are becoming major tools for prognostic assessment and prediction of response to certain treatments.[77] Since these technologies are expensive, lack of access among low SES individuals and in low-income countries may result in unprecedented inequalities in cancer care.

MORTALITY

According to Parkin and colleagues,[28] "mortality is the number of deaths occurring, and the mortality rate is the number of deaths per 100,000 persons per year. Mortality is the product of the incidence and the fatality for a given cancer." Although SES-incidence gradients for cancer vary by cancer site, the burden of cancer mortality disproportionately falls on people of lower SES regardless of the site[29] due to disparities in psychosocial factors, health behaviors, access to care, screening, treatment, and other areas of care outlined in the previous sections. In addition, low-resource countries largely bear the burden of cancer mortality.

International patterns of cancer mortality. In 2002, Parkin and others[28] report an estimated 6.7 million cancer deaths worldwide. In general, survival rates are higher in high-resource regions with the exception of Eastern Europe, which has particularly high cancer fatalities.[28,78] Recent data from the global, population-based CONCORD study indicate that 5-year relative survival estimates are highest in North America, Australia, Japan, and Europe (northern, western, and southern) and appear lower in Algeria, Eastern Europe, and Brazil.[79] Although cancer incidence rates are highest in North America, fatalities are greatest in Eastern Europe and East Africa for men and women, respectively. For men, cumulative cancer mortality is slightly greater in high-resource than in low-resource nations, while female cumulative cancer mortality rates are higher in low-resource countries. In addition, men are far more likely to die of cancer than women due to the higher prevalence of cancers with relatively low survival rates among men.[28] Although the incidence of some cancers is higher in high-resource countries, a lack of access to appropriate screening and care in low-resource countries contributes to inequalities in mortality rates.

The disproportionate burden of cancer mortality on low-resource countries is illustrated by Fig. 6–1,[80] which depicts the 2002 global estimates for prostate and breast cancer incidence and mortality. As previously noted, prostate cancer is the most common cancer among men in high-resource nations, and breast cancer is the most common cancer among women worldwide, although incidence rates are higher in high-resource nations. However, low-resource countries have disproportionately high mortality rates from these cancers despite higher incidence rates in high-resource countries. Whereas prostate cancer incidence rates are highest in North America, Western and Northern Europe, and Australia, mortality is disproportionately high in the Caribbean and parts of Africa. Similarly, breast cancer mortality in West Africa and regions of the South Pacific are similar to mortality rates in North America, despite significantly greater incidence in North America.[28] These disparities are most often attributed to the differential provision of screening and appropriate treatment in low- versus high-income countries.

Within-country SES patterns of cancer mortality. Within countries, people of lower SES have higher cancer mortality rates than those of high SES. This is true both in countries with universal access to care[39,41,55,81–91] and countries without universal access, such as the United States and Eastern Europe.[32,78,86,92–96] Some research still notes higher colorectal and breast cancer mortality among high SES individuals, although these trends appear to be reversing.[32,97] Although differential stage at diagnosis and treatment factors are the most widely cited reasons for the SES mortality gradient,[98] a number of studies have found independent associations between cancer mortality and SES after controlling for stage of disease and treatment/surgery factors.[55,73]

In addition to disease stage and treatment factors, some of the socioeconomic disparities in cancer mortality are explained by SES disparities in all-cause mortality.[99] Additional factors that may contribute to SES-cancer (and all-cause) mortality gradients are differences in the psychosocial characteristics of low versus high SES individuals and the higher prevalence of comorbid conditions in low SES populations. Widespread differences in coping styles and social support are hypothesized to contribute to SES-cancer mortality patterns, but evidence is scant.[29,100] Moreover, psychosocial factors, such as coping and social support, are known to contribute to health in general via immunosuppressive endocrine pathways, and fewer coping skills and low social support are likely more prevalent among low SES communities.[7,29] In addition, chronic stress from, for example, financial insecurity may contribute to poorer health and subsequent cancer fatalities among low SES individuals.[7] Dalton and others[82] provide additional evidence demonstrating that a

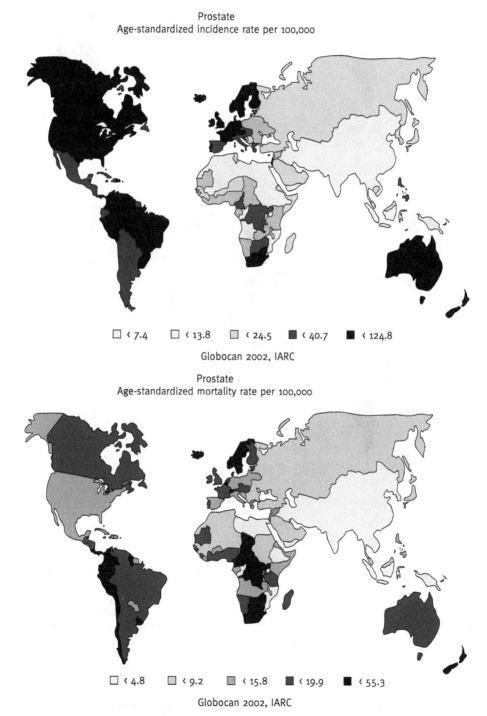

Fig. 6–1. Age-standardized incidence and mortality rates for prostate and breast cancer. Reprinted with permission from CancerMondial. International Agency for Research on Cancer Globocan 2002 Cancer Maps. http://www-dep.iarc.fr/.

Breast
Age-standardized incidence rate per 100,000

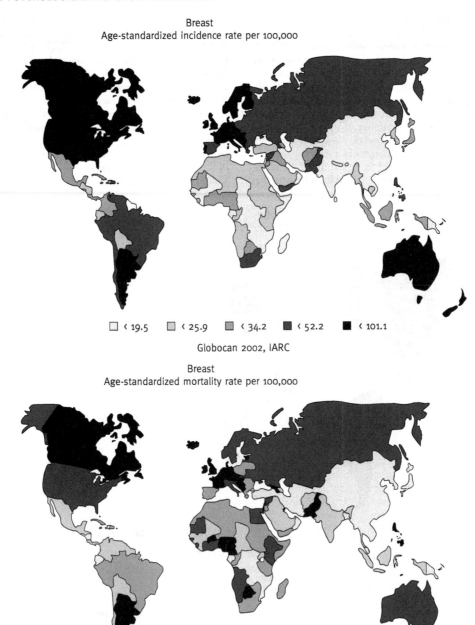

☐ ‹ 19.5   ▨ ‹ 25.9   ▨ ‹ 34.2   ▨ ‹ 52.2   ■ ‹ 101.1

Globocan 2002, IARC

Breast
Age-standardized mortality rate per 100,000

☐ ‹ 10.3   ▨ ‹ 13.9   ▨ ‹ 17.0   ▨ ‹ 20.0   ■ ‹ 29.6

Globocan 2002, IARC

Fig. 6–1. Continued.

failure to manage comorbid conditions partially explains SES-related cancer mortality disparities. Overall, the psychosocial and behavioral factors that contribute to SES disparities in cancer mortality warrant further research.

Between-country differences and time trends in SES-cancer mortality. Despite an overall negative SES-cancer mortality gradient, patterns vary between countries and by site. Menvielle and her colleagues (2005)[88] studied cancer mortality in France from 1975 to 1990 and noted large differences in SES-gradients by cancer type, with high inequalities for aerodigestive cancers in men, no inequalities in mortality rates for colon or liver cancers in men, and lessened inequalities for cancers in women. Strand et al.[101] examined breast cancer mortality in Europe and found higher mortality among high SES women, except

in Finland, France, and Barcelona. Also, cancer mortality appears to be declining by approximately 7.3% per year in the European Union, Switzerland, and Scandinavian countries, but is rising by 2.4% in Central and Eastern Europe.[102] These international trends are related to gross national product, national health expenditures, unemployment, smoking, alcohol consumption, and air quality, among other factors. Mackenbach and colleagues[87] similarly found widening SES inequalities in cancer mortality in some countries, but not others. As data are increasingly pooled internationally, between-country differences in SES-related cancer mortality patterns will likely become integral to understanding the behavioral, psychosocial, and biological factors that underlie SES-cancer mortality disparities. In France, England/Wales, Scotland, and the United States, overall cancer mortality is declining while SES gaps in cancer mortality are widening.[81,89,90] In addition, cancer has overtaken cardiovascular disease as the principal driver of SES mortality inequalities in New Zealand, despite universal healthcare coverage.[83,103] In the United States, socioeconomic inequalities in cancer mortality are frequently discussed in parallel with racial disparities, which are pervasive in the United States. For example, black men bear a significant mortality burden from prostate cancer[30] and have significantly higher cancer mortality than other demographic groups in the United States.[79] However, within each race/ethnic group, socioeconomic disparities in cancer mortality have persisted despite stabilized or decreasing overall cancer mortality.[32] Although race has historically been used as a proxy for SES in U.S. research, race has been shown to be an inappropriate measure of SES, and that practice has largely ceased.

FROM CANCER PATIENT TO CANCER SURVIVOR

Owing to earlier diagnosis and improved treatment, especially in developed, high-resource countries, more people are becoming cancer survivors, denoting people who have completed cancer therapy regardless of whether their cancer is in remission. Because there may be social and psychological differences between those who are undergoing treatment and those who are disease- or recurrence-free, most research separates survivors on the basis of whether they are symptomatic or disease free. Excitement about progress in treating cancer has been accompanied by a myriad of questions about who long-term survivors are, what the late effects of treatment are, and how well survivors have reintegrated into society.

Late effects of treatment. There is some evidence that indicators of one's SES influence the late effects of treatment. This is evident in a large Canadian study of pediatric cancer survivors 17 years of age or younger. When compared to matched controls, survivors were more likely to have problems at school, such as repeating a grade or being in special programs, to have fewer friends, and to be less likely to have a friend as a confidant. These educational and social problems were greater if the cancer survivor had cranial irradiation, but were less likely if the child had higher self-esteem and if their parents had postsecondary education.[104] In this case, increased educational level of the family appears to have mitigated the late effects of the treatment. Although there is limited direct evidence of the relationship between SES and late effects of cancer and its treatment, some indirect evidence exists that people of lower SES report poorer quality of life after cancer.[105,106]

Reintegrating into society: work and income. Regardless of the type of cancer or the country in which the study takes place, most research reports that cancer survivors compared to cancer-free controls of the same age and gender are less likely to be working and are more likely to retire early. And for those survivors who lose their job, reemployment may take more time. Accordingly, of 47% of survivors who lost their jobs, only 30% of participants in a Korean study were reemployed over a period of 69–72 months of follow-up. When mediating factors are considered, researchers inevitably find that survivors of lower SES, whether measured by income, education, or place of residence, are more likely to be out of the workforce either by their own choice (retirement), their health, or involuntary separation and slower reemployment.[107–109] Chirikos and colleagues[110] studied the long-term economic consequences for breast cancer survivors in a U.S. sample. Most of the income loss was due to survivors' reduced work effort when compared to women of the same age without a cancer history. A Canadian team also found wage losses among breast cancer survivors,[111,112] which were predicted by lower level of education, self-employment, shorter job tenure, and part-time work. These income reductions have consequences for survivors' access to resources to maintain their health.[109]

Access to resources to maintain health. There are few studies of the relationship between secondary access factors and SES among cancer survivors. Secondary access factors focus on the way care is provided once a person has entered the system.[66] These can include the difficulties in navigating complex bureaucratic systems in seeking care and the characteristics of the systems themselves that are not welcoming. Historically, cancer care services have been fragmented and poorly coordinated from the perspective of the survivor. This makes access particularly problematic for people with limited health literacy, who are poor, and who have less education. Accordingly, the impact of cancer is found to be greater for individuals with poorer living conditions, which serves as evidence of lower SES.[113] Also, Macleod et al.[114] found evidence that relatively affluent women with breast cancer in the United Kingdom were more likely to receive information from their physicians and nurses. In addition, affluent patients were more likely to report using health information sources external to the clinical encounter, such as the Internet.

CONCLUSIONS AND IMPLICATIONS

The association between SES and cancer is established for all points along the cancer care continuum: prevention (primary, secondary, tertiary), incidence, etiology, screening, diagnosis, access to care (including clinical trials), treatment, survival, morbidity, and mortality.[115] The sources of these inequalities vary and are attributed to a combination of environmental, biological, behavioral, psychosocial, and healthcare factors. The interplay of these factors accounts for much of the observed inequalities in the burden of cancer, but it also makes the association between SES and cancer particularly complex. Accordingly, SES is measured in a multitude of different ways, and the pathways through which SES affects cancer initiation, promotion, and progression are not completely understood.[29] Furthermore, the multiple sources of inequality are rarely accounted for in a single research study. Often times, population-based datasets measure SES inadequately and rarely do they account for the various psychological and behavioral variables that may generate SES inequalities in cancer incidence, treatment, and outcomes.

Another fundamental feature of cancer disparities is their dynamic nature. The associations between SES and cancer change radically by place and time period. By and large, SES disparities in cancer mortality appear to be widening. Moreover, cancer incidence patterns have altered significantly in the past 30 years. For example, breast and colorectal cancers, which have historically been more prevalent among high SES populations in the United States, are now more prevalent in low SES regions.[32] These longitudinal patterns have been attributed in part to widespread changes in behavior that are systematic by SES. This phenomenon begs the questions: "Why do social groups adopt certain patterns that may increase or decrease risk of health and mortality? Why are risk factors clustered and graded by socioeconomic group?"[29]

A number of approaches are essential to understanding and mitigating SES disparities in cancer. From a research perspective, the utilization of population-based, longitudinal public health data systems to monitor, understand, and alleviate SES-related cancer inequalities is essential.[116] In addition to research efforts in SES disparities, policy interventions are needed to mitigate persistent and sometimes widening SES health disparities. Adler and her colleagues[117] outline policies that fall under two general goals: (1) policy interventions to lessen income, educational, and occupation inequalities; and (2) policy interventions to decrease the health-related impact of being low SES. Policies that fall under the former goal include equalizing access to quality primary and secondary education, eliminating financial barriers to higher education, minimum wage increases, tax credits, fiscal policies that encourage financial security, and opportunities for job skills training. Policies that fall under the latter goal include providing affordable housing, restricting noise and pollution, reducing crime, decreasing stress and exposure to toxins in the workplace, and promoting health behaviors. This bilateral approach to reducing health disparities would work both to abolish inequalities in health that are systematic by SES and to change the underlying social structure that creates disparities.

Overall, socioeconomic inequalities in cancer remain pervasive both globally and within individual countries. The pathways by which SES affects cancer incidence, care, and survival are numerous and complicated, and advances in research are needed to fully understand and document the extent of these disparities. However, a significant evidence base exists for cancer disparities, and policy interventions are currently needed to begin to address these disparities.

REFERENCES

1. Mullan F. Seasons of survival: reflections of a physician with cancer. *NEJM.* 1985;313(4):270–273.

2. Ries LAG, Melbert D, Krapcho M, et al. *SEER Cancer Statistics Review, 1975–2005.* Bethesda, MD: National Cancer Institute; 2008.

3. Miech RA, Hauser RM. Socioeconomic status (SES) and health at midlife: a comparison of educational attainment with occupation-based indicators. *Ann Epidemiol.* 2001;11:75–84.

4. Krieger N, Williams DR, Moss NE. Measuring social class in U.S. public health research: concepts, methodologies, and guidelines. *Annu Rev Public Health.* 1997;18:341–378.

5. Shavers VL. Measurement of socioeconomic status in health disparities research. *J Natl Med Assoc.* 2007;99(9):1013–1023.

6. Braveman PA, Cubbin C, Egerter S, et al. Socioeconomic status in health research: one size does not fit all. *JAMA.* 2005;294(22):2879–2888.

7. Adler NE, Newman K. Socioeconomic disparities in health: pathways and policies. *Health Aff.* 2002;21(2):60–76.

8. *US Bureau of the Census current population reports, Series P-60, No. 174 money income of households, families, and persons in the United States.* Washington, DC: US GPO; 1991.

9. Smith GD, Hart C, Hole D, et al. Education and occupational social class: which is the more important indicator of mortality risk? *J Epidemiol Community Health.* 1994;52:153–160.

10. Pamuk E, Makuc D, Heck K, Reuben C, Lochner K. *Socioeconomic status and health chartbook.* Hyattsville, MD: National Center for Health Statistics; 1998.

11. Hjartaker A, Lund E. Relationship between dietary habits, age, lifestyle, and socio-economic status among adult Norwegian women. The Norwegian Women and Cancer Study. *Eur J Clin Nutr.* 1998;52(8):565–572.

12. Wardle J, Jarvis MJ, Steggles N, et al. Socioeconomic disparities in cancer-risk behaviors in adolescence: baseline results from the Health and Behaviour in Teenagers Study (HABITS). *Prev Med.* 2003;36(6):721–730.

13. Stewart J. Economic status. John D. and Catherine T. MacArthur Research Network on socioeconomic status and health. http://www.macses.ucsf.edu/Research/Social%20Environment/notebook/economic.html. Accessed July 24, 2008.

14. Backlund E, Sorlie PD, Johnson NJ. The shape of the relationship between income and mortality in the United States—evidence from the National Longitudinal Mortality Study. *Ann Epidemiol.* 1996;24:12–20.

15. Duncan GJ. Income dynamics and health. *Int J Health Serv.* 1996;26:419–444.

16. Galobardes B, Lynch JW, Smith GD. Childhood socioeconomic circumstances and cause-specific mortality in adulthood: systematic review and interpretation. *Epidemiol Rev.* 2004;26:7–21.

17. Smith GD, Hart C, Blane D, Hole D. Adverse socioeconomic conditions in childhood and cause specific adult mortality: prospective observational study. *BMJ.* 1998;316:1631–1635.

18. Sooman A, Macintyre S, Anderson A. Scotland's health—a more difficult challenge for some? The price and availability of healthy foods in socially contrasting localities in the West of Scotland. *Health Bull.* 1993;51:276–284.

19. Kaplan G. People and places: contrasting perspectives on the association between social class and health. *Int J Health Serv.* 1996;26:507–519.

20. Hauser RM, Carr D. *Measuring poverty and socioeconomic status in studies of health and well-being.* Madison, WI: Center for Demography and Ecology, University of Wisconsin; 1995.

21. Orzechowski S, Sepielli P.*Net worth and asset ownership of households: 1998 and 2000.* Washington, DC: U.S. Census Bureau; May 2003.

22. Szreter SRS. The genesis of the Registrar General's social classification of occupations. *Br J Sociol.* 1984;35:522–546.

23. Marmot MG, Bosma H, Hemingway H, Brunner E, Stansfeld S. Contribution of job control and other risk factors to social variations in coronary heart disease incidence. *Lancet.* 1997;350:235–239.

24. Altonji JG, Blank RM. Race and gender in the labor market. In: Ashenfelter O, Card D, eds. *Handbook of labor economics.* Vol 3c. Amsterdam: North-Holland; 1999:3143–3259.

25. Ross CE, Mirowsky J. Does unemployment affect health? *J Health Soc Behav.* 1995;36:230–243.

26. Duncan C, Jones K, Moon G. Context, composition and heterogeneity: using multilevel models in health research. *Soc Sci Med.* 1998;46:97–117.

27. Whitehead M, Dahlgren G. *Concepts and principles for tackling social inequities in health: levelling up Part 1.* Copenhagen, Denmark: World Health Organization; 2006.

28. Parkin M, Bray F, Ferlay J, Pisani P. Global Cancer Statistics, 2002. *CA Cancer J Clin.* 2005;55(2):74–108.

29. Balfour J, Kaplan G. Social class/socioeconomic factors. In: Holland J, ed. *Psycho-oncology.* New York: Oxford University Press; 1998:78–90.

30. Gilligan T. Social disparities and prostate cancer: mapping the gaps in our knowledge. *Cancer Causes Control.* 2005;16(1):45–53.

31. Liu L, Cozen W, Bernstein L, Ross RK, Deapen D. Changing relationship between socioeconomic status and prostate cancer incidence. *J Natl Cancer Inst.* 2001;93(9):705–709.

32. Singh GK, Miller BA, Hankey BE, Edwards BK. *Area socioeconomic variations in U.S. cancer incidence, mortality, stage, treatment, and survival, 1975–1999.* Bethesda, MD: National Cancer Institute; 2003.

33. Mackillop WJ, Zhang-Salomons J, Boyd CJ, Groome PA. Associations between community income and cancer incidence in Canada and the United States. *Cancer.* 2000;89(4):901–912.

34. Rowan S. Trends in cancer incidence by deprivation, England and Wales, 1990–2002. *Health Stat Q.* 2007;Winter(36):24–35.

35. Ross JS, Bernheim SM, Bradley EH, Teng HM, Gallo WT. Use of preventive care by the working poor in the United States. *Prev Med.* 2007;44(3):254–259.

36. Ross JS, Bradley EH, Busch SH. Use of health care services by lower-income and higher-income uninsured adults. *JAMA.* 2006;295(17):2027–2036.

37. Lund Nilsen TI, Johnsen R, Vatten LJ. Socio-economic and lifestyle factors associated with the risk of prostate cancer. *Br J Cancer.* 2000;82(7):1358–1363.

38. Dutta Roy S, Philip J, Javle P. Trends in prostate cancer incidence and survival in various socioeconomic classes: a population-based study. *Int J Urol.* 2005;12(7):644–653.

39. Dalton SO, Schuz J, Engholm G, et al. Social inequality in incidence of and survival from cancer in a population-based study in Denmark, 1994–2003: summary of findings. *Eur J Cancer.* 2008.: 44(14):2074–2085.

40. Ward E, Jemal A, Cokkinides V, et al. Cancer disparities by race/ethnicity and socioeconomic status. *CA Cancer J Clin.* 2004;54:78–93.

41. Rosengren A, Wilhelmsen L. Cancer incidence, mortality from cancer and survival in men of different occupational classes. *Eur J Epidemiol.* 2004;19(6):533–540.

42. Melchior M, Goldberg M, Krieger N, et al. Occupational class, occupational mobility and cancer incidence among middle-aged men and women: a prospective study of the French GAZEL cohort*. *Cancer Causes Control.* 2005;16(5):515–524.

43. Mao Y, Hu J, Ugnat AM, Semenciw R, Fincham S. Socioeconomic status and lung cancer risk in Canada. *Int J Epidemiol.* 2001;30(4):809–817.

44. Tavani A, Fioretti F, Franceschi S, et al. Education, socioeconomic status and risk of cancer of the colon and rectum. *Int J Epidemiol.* 1999;28(3):380–385.

45. Palmer RC, Schneider EC. Social disparities across the continuum of colorectal cancer: a systematic review. *Cancer Causes Control.* 2005;16(1):55–61.

46. Weiderpass E, Pukkala E. Time trends in socioeconomic differences in incidence rates of cancers of gastro-intestinal tract in Finland. *BMC Gastroenterol.* 2006;6:41.

47. Goy J, Rosenberg MW, King WD. Health risk behaviors: examining social inequalities in bladder and colorectal cancers. *Ann Epidemiol.* 2008;18(2):156–162.

48. Porter P. "Westernizing" women's risks? Breast cancer in lower-income countries. *NEJM.* 2008;358(3):213–216.

49. International Agency for Research on Cancer (IARC). *IARC Handbook on Cancer Prevention No. 7.* Lyon, France: IARC; 2002.

50. Bigby J, Holmes MD. Disparities across the breast cancer continuum. *Cancer Causes Control.* 2005;16(1):35–44.

51. Hussain SK, Altieri A, Sundquist J, Hemminki K. Influence of education level on breast cancer risk and survival in Sweden between 1990 and 2004. *Int J Cancer.* 2008;122(1):165–169.

52. Robert SA, Strombom I, Trentham-Dietz A, et al. Socioeconomic risk factors for breast cancer: distinguishing individual- and community-level effects. *Epidemiology.* 2004;15(4):442–450.

53. Singh SM, Paszat LF, Li C, He J, Vinden C, Rabeneck L. Association of socioeconomic status and receipt of colorectal cancer investigations: a population-based retrospective cohort study. *CMAJ.* 2004;171(5):461–465.

54. Duport N, Ancelle-Park R. Do socio-demographic factors influence mammography use of French women? Analysis of a French cross-sectional survey. *Eur J Cancer.* 2006;15(3):219–224.

55. Bouchardy C, Verkooijen HM, Fioretta G. Social class is an important and independent prognostic factor of breast cancer mortality. *Int J Cancer.* 2006;119(5):1145–1151.

56. Williams BA, Lindquist K, Sudore RL, Covinsky KE, Walter LC. Screening mammography in older women. Effect of wealth and prognosis. *Arch Intern Med.* 2008;168(5):514–520.

57. MacKinnon JA, Duncan RC, Huang Y, et al. Detecting an association between socioeconomic status and late stage breast cancer using spatial analysis and area-based measures. *Cancer Epidemiol Biomarkers Prev.* 2007;16(4):756–762.

58. Centers for Disease Control and Prevention. National Breast and Cervical Cancer Early Detection Program. http://www.cdc.gov/cancer/NBCCEDP/. Accessed : July 15, 2008.

59. Schootman M, Fuortes LJ. Early indicators of the effect of a breast cancer screening program for low-income women. *Cancer Detect Prev.* 2001;25(2):138–146.

60. Song L, Fletcher R. Breast cancer rescreening in low-income women. *Am J Prev Med.* 1998;15(2):128–133.

61. Liu MJ, Hawk H, Gershman ST, et al. The effects of a National Breast and Cervical Cancer Early Detection Program on social disparities in breast cancer diagnosis and treatment in Massachusetts. *Cancer Causes Control.* 2005;16(1):27–33.

62. Richardson LC, Schulman J, Sever LE, Lee NC, Coate RJ. Early-stage breast cancer treatment among medically underserved women diagnosed in a national screening program, 1992–1995. *Breast Cancer Res Treat.* 2001;69(2):133–142.

63. Rutqvist LE, Bern A. Socioeconomic gradients in clinical stage at presentation and survival among breast cancer patients in the Stockholm area 1977–1997. *Int J Cancer.* 2006;119(6):1433–1439.

64. Kogevinas M, Porta M. Socioeconomic differences in cancer survival: a review of the evidence. In: Kogevinas M, Pearce M, Susser M, Boffetta M, eds. *Social inequalities and cancer, IARC scientific publications no. 138.* Lyon, France: IARC; 1997:177–206.

65. Woods LM, Rachet B, Coleman MP. Choice of geographic unit influences socioeconomic inequalities in breast cancer survival. *Br J Cancer.* 2005;92(7):1279–1282.

66. Lurie N. Studying access to care in managed care environments. *HSR.* 1997;32(5):691–701.

67. Tarman GJ, Kane CJ, Moul JW, et al. Impact of socioeconomic status and race on clinical parameters of patients undergoing radical prostatectomy in an equal access health care system. *Urology.* 2000;56(6):1016–1020.

68. Pham HH, Schrag D, Hargraves JL, Bach PB. Delivery of preventive services to older adults by primary care physicians. *JAMA.* 2005;294:473–481.

69. Neal RD, Allgar VL. Sociodemographic factors and delays in the diagnosis of six cancers: analysis of data from the "National Survey of NHS Patients: Cancer". *Br J Cancer.* 2005;92(11):1971–1975.

70. Ciccone G, Prastaro C, Ivaldi C, Giacometti R, Vineis P. Access to hospital care, clinical stage and survival from colorectal cancer according to socioeconomic status. *Ann Oncol.* 2000;11(9):1201–1204.

71. McCollum AD, Catalano PJ, Haller DG, et al. Outcomes and toxicity in African-American and Caucasian patients in a randomized adjuvant chemotherapy trial for colon cancer. *J Natl Cancer Inst.* 2002;94:1160–1167.

72. Dignam JJ. Differences in breast cancer prognosis among African-American and Caucasian women. *CA Cancer J Clin.* 2000;50:50–64.

73. Bradley CJ, Given CW, Roberts C. Race, socioeconomic status, and breast cancer treatment and survival. *J Natl Cancer Inst.* 2002;94(7):490–496.

74. Institute of Medicine. *Improving palliative care for cancer.* Foley KM, Gelband H, (Eds). Washington, DC: National Academy Press; 2001.

75. Morrison RS, Wallenstein S, Natale DK, Senzel RS, Huang LL. "We don't carry that"—failure of pharmacies in predominantly nonwhite neighborhoods to stock opioid analgesics. *NEJM.* 2000;342:1023–1026.

76. Barton MB, Frommer M, Shafiq J. Role of radiotherapy in cancer control in low-income and middle-income countries. *Lancet Oncol.* 2006;7(7):584–595.

77. Mano M. The burden of scientific progress: growing inequalities in the delivery of cancer care. *Acta Oncol.* 2006;45(1):84–86.

78. Plavinski SL, Plavinskaya SI, Klimov AN. Social factors and increase in mortality in Russia in the 1990s: prospective cohort study. *BMJ.* 2003;326(7401):1240–1242.

79. Coleman MP, Quaresma M, Berrino F, et al. Cancer survival in five continents: a worldwide population-based study (CONCORD). *Lancet Oncol.* 2008;9:730–756.

80. Cancer*Mondial.* International Agency for Research on Cancer Globocan 2002 Cancer Maps. http://www-dep.iarc.fr/. Accessed July 25, 2008.

81. Coleman MP, Rachet B, Woods LM, et al. Trends and socioeconomic inequalities in cancer survival in England and Wales up to 2001. *Br J Cancer.* 2004;90(7):1367–1373.

82. Dalton SO, Ross L, During M, et al. Influence of socioeconomic factors on survival after breast cancer—a nationwide cohort study of women diagnosed with breast cancer in Denmark 1983–1999. *Int J Cancer.* 2007;121(11):2524–2531.

83. Fawcett J, Blakely T. Cancer is overtaking cardiovascular disease as the main driver of socioeconomic inequalities in mortality: New Zealand (1981–99). *J Epidemiol Community Health.* 2007;61(1):59–66.

84. Gentil-Brevet J, Colonna M, Danzon A, t al. The influence of socio-economic and surveillance characteristics on breast cancer survival: a French population-based study. *Br J Cancer.* 2008;98(1):217–224.

85. Hussain SK, Lenner P, Sundquist J, Hemminki K. Influence of education level on cancer survival in Sweden. *Ann Oncol.* 2008;19(1):156–162.

86. Jha P, Peto R, Zatonski W, Boreham J, Jarvis MJ, Lopez AD. Social inequalities in male mortality, and in male mortality from smoking: indirect estimation from national death rates in England and Wales, Poland, and North America. *Lancet.* 2006;368(9533):367–370.

87. Mackenbach JP, Bos V, Andersen O, et al. Widening socioeconomic inequalities in mortality in six Western European countries. *Int J Epidemiol.* 2003;32(5):830–837.

88. Menvielle G, Leclerc A, Chastang JF, Luce D. Social inequalities in breast cancer mortality among French women: disappearing educational disparities from 1968 to 1996. *Br J Cancer.* 2006;94(1):152–155.

89. Menvielle G, Leclerc A, Chastang JF, Melchior M, Luce D. Changes in socioeconomic inequalities in cancer mortality rates among French men between 1968 and 1996. *Am J Public Health.* 2007;97(11):2082–2087.

90. Shack LG, Rachet B, Brewster DH, Coleman MP. Socioeconomic inequalities in cancer survival in Scotland 1986–2000. *Br J Cancer.* 2007;97(7):999–1004.

91. Shaw C, Blakely T, Crampton P, Atkinson J. The contribution of causes of death to socioeconomic inequalities in child mortality: New Zealand 1981–1999. *N Z Med J.* 2005;118(1227):U1779.

92. Albano JD, Ward E, Jemal A, et al. Cancer mortality in the United States by education level and race. *J Natl Cancer Inst.* 2007;99(18):1384–1394.

93. Du XL, Fang S, Vernon SW, et al. Racial disparities and socioeconomic status in association with survival in a large population-based cohort of elderly patients with colon cancer. *Cancer.* 2007;110(3):660–669.

94. Grann V, Troxel AB, Zojwalla N, Hershman D, Glied SA, Jacobson JS. Regional and racial disparities in breast cancer-specific mortality. *Soc Sci Med.* 2006;62(2):337–347.

95. Lee DJ, Fleming LE, Leblanc WG, et al. Occupation and lung cancer mortality in a nationally representative U.S. Cohort: The National Health Interview Survey (NHIS). *J Occup Environ Med.* 2006;48(8):823–832.

96. Singh GK, Miller BA, Hankey BF, Edwards BK. Persistent area socioeconomic disparities in U.S. incidence of cervical cancer, mortality, stage, and survival, 1975–2000. *Cancer.* 2004;101(5):1051–1057.

97. Steenland K, Hu S, Walker J. All-cause and cause-specific mortality by socioeconomic status among employed persons in 27 US states, 1984–1997. *Am J Public Health.* 2004;94(6):1037–1042.

98. Woods LM, Rachet B, Coleman MP. Origins of socio-economic inequalities in cancer survival: a review. *Ann Oncol.* 2006;17(1):5–19.

99. Dickman PW, Auvinen A, Voutilainen ET, Hakulinen T. Measuring social class differences in cancer patient survival: is it necessary to control for social class differences in general population mortality? A Finnish population-based study. *J Epidemiol Community Health.* 1998;52(11):727–734.

100. Lehto US, Ojanen M, Dyba T, Aromaa A, Kellokumpu-Lehtinen P. Baseline psychosocial predictors of survival in localised breast cancer. *Br J Cancer.* 2006;94(9):1245–1252.

101. Strand BH, Kunst A, Huisman M, et al. The reversed social gradient: higher breast cancer mortality in the higher educated compared to lower educated. A comparison of 11 European populations during the 1990s. *Eur J Cancer.* 2007;43(7):1200–1207.

102. Antunes JL, Toporcov TN, de Andrade FP. Trends and patterns of cancer mortality in European countries. *Eur J Cancer Prev.* 2003;12(5):367–372.

103. Shaw C, Blakely T, Sarfati D, Fawcett J, Peace J. Trends in colorectal cancer mortality by ethnicity and socio-economic position in New Zealand, 1981–99: one country, many stories. *Aust N Z J Public Health.* 2006;30(1):64–70.

104. Barrera M, Shaw AK, Speechley KN, Maunsell E, Pogany L. Educational and social late effects of childhood cancer and related clinical, personal, and familial characteristics. *Cancer.* 2005;104(8):1751–1760.

105. Penson DF, Stoddard ML, Pasta DJ, Lubeck DP, Flanders SC, Litwin MS. The association between socioeconomic status, health insurance coverage, and quality of life in men with prostate cancer. *J Clin Epidemiol.* 2001;54(4):350–358.

106. Short PF, Mallonee EL. Income disparities in the quality of life of cancer survivors. *Med Care.* 2006;44(1):16–23.

107. Park JH, Park EC, Park JH, Kim SG, Lee SY. Job loss and re-employment of cancer patients in Korean employees: a nationwide retrospective cohort study. *J Clin Oncol.* 2008;26(8):1302–1309.

108. Lee MK, Lee KM, Bae JM, et al. Employment status and work-related difficulties in stomach cancer survivors compared with the general population. *Br J Cancer.* 2008;98(4):708–715.

109. Ell K, Xie B, Wells A, Nedjat-Haiem F, Lee PJ, Vourlekis B. Economic stress among low-income women with cancer: effects on quality of life. *Cancer.* 2008;112(3):616–625.

110. Chirikos TN, Russell-Jacobs A, Cantor AB. Indirect economic effects of long-term breast cancer survival. *Cancer Pract.* 2002;10(5):248–255.

111. Lauzier S, Maunsell E, Drolet M, et al. Wage losses in the year after breast cancer: extent and determinants among Canadian women. *J Natl Cancer Inst.* 2008;100(5):321–332.

112. Maunsell E, Drolet M, Brisson J, Brisson C, Masse B, Deschenes L. Work situation after breast cancer: results from a population-based study. *J Natl Cancer Inst.* 2004;96(24):1813–1822.

113. Gudbergsson SB, Fossa SD, Ganz PA, Zebrack BJ, Dahl AA. The associations between living conditions, demography, and the 'impact of cancer'

scale in tumor-free cancer survivors: a NOCWO study. *Support Care Cancer.* 2007;15(11):1309–1318.

114. Macleod U, Ross S, Fallowfield L, Watt GC. Anxiety and support in breast cancer: is this different for affluent and deprived women? A questionnaire study. *Br J Cancer.* 2004;91(5):879–883.

115. Krieger N. Defining and investigating social disparities in cancer: critical issues. *Cancer Causes Control.* 2005;16(1):5–14.

116. Koh HK, Judge CM, Ferrer B, Gershman ST. Using public health data systems to understand and eliminate cancer disparities. *Cancer Causes Control.* 2005;16(1):15–26.

117. Adler NE, Stewart J, Cohen S, et al. *Reaching for a Healthier Life: facts on socioeconomic status and health in the U.S.* San Francisco, CA: The John D. and Catherine T. MacArthur Foundation Research Network on Socioeconomic Status and Health; 2008.

CHAPTER 7

Psychosocial Factors

Christoffer Johansen

INTRODUCTION

This topic has many diverse and complimentary scientific disciplines involved ranging from epidemiology to biological mechanistic investigations. There are so many conflicting opinions about mind as a risk factor for cancer, created on different interpretations of the data available, that it is almost impossible to contain everything in one chapter. Nevertheless, in scientific studies published during the past 75 years and in reviews of the literature, little is said about cancer causation as such. It is important that this subject be raised, in order to emphasize that the criteria for causation originally stated by Austin Bradford Hill[1] in the early 1960s also apply to psychosocial risk factors. It is therefore of interest to evaluate the extent to which the risk factors in epidemiological studies cause cancer. Hill (1965) listed nine criteria for progressing from observation of an association to a verdict of causation. He suggested that the following issues be considered to distinguish association from causation: strength, temporality, coherence, consistency, specificity, biological gradient, strength of the association, analogy, and biological plausibility. Hill stated, "None of these nine standards can bring indisputable evidence for or against the cause-and-effect hypothesis and none can be required as a sine qua non." This cannot be considered a final list of factors that establish causality, but they must be taken into account in determining the weight of evidence. Hill (1965) also warned against overemphasis on statistical significance testing, writing: "The glitter of the *t* table diverts attention from the inadequacies of the fare." The theory of causality has developed since Hill's time, increasing the complexity of establishing causality and requiring new levels of sophistication in epidemiology.[2]

Few studies in psychosocial cancer research discuss how psychosocial factors fit into the context of cancer causation in terms of initiation or promotion, latency, duration and timing, and pattern of exposure. None of the studies published so far has taken into account the fact that several standards must be included in discussions of the mind as a risk factor for cancer, and various factors and phenomena have been used to represent the mind factor as the exposure under study, including bereavement, loss of a close relative, depression, personality traits, and exposure to well-defined major life events. The overwhelming body of the scientific literature on psychosocial risk ignores fundamental methodological issues. Only recently has it become mandatory to discuss whether bias, confounding, or chance might be an alternative explanation for a result, and only recently has there been discussion of how study design influences important methodological factors. The many studies in this area with a case-control design are therefore probably not adequate to answer the basic scientific question. Taking this statement further, one can say that psychosocial risk factors can be addressed only in studies designed for that purpose. Recall bias, lack of adjustment for disease-specific factors or comorbidity, use of unbiased data sources, exclusion of interviewer bias, and so on have been ignored by researchers working in this area. Today, however, more studies in this area fully acknowledge the need for such considerations in the search for possible psychosocial risk factors in cancer.

WHAT IS A RISK FACTOR FOR CANCER?

Researchers on psychosocial risk factors for cancer should refer to the guidelines for cancer causation published by the International Agency for Research in Cancer (IARC) in Lyon, France, in the worldwide effort to identify cancer-causing agents. Since 1969, working groups convened by IARC have assessed the degree of evidence for the carcinogenicity to humans of some 800 biological, physical, chemical, and occupational factors and have ranked risk factors for cancer according to the degree of evidence for causality. Psychological factors have not been reviewed in this context, but a brief review of psychological factors associated with cancer was included in another IARC publication on cancer prevention and control in 1990.[3] No conclusion was reached about the degree of evidence, but it was stated that future epidemiological studies should include standardized instruments and data on potential confounders in order to be credible.

The evaluation of psychosocial factors in the causation of cancer must be addressed in the context of certain methodological problems, which are summarized briefly below on the basis of the preamble to the IARC Monographs.[3] It is essential to take into account the possibilities of bias, confounding, and chance in interpreting any study. "Bias" is the effect of factors in study design or execution that lead erroneously to a stronger or weaker association than in fact exists between an agent—in this case the mind factor—and disease. "Confounding" is a form of bias that occurs when the relation with disease is made to appear stronger or weaker than it truly is as a result of an association between the apparent causal factor and another factor that is associated with either an increase or decrease in the incidence of the disease. The role of chance is related to variation in the broadest aspect of the word and the influence of sample size on the precision of estimates of effect.

In evaluating the extent to which these factors have been minimized in a study, consideration must be given to aspects of the design and analysis. For example, when suspicion of carcinogenicity arises largely from a single small study, care must be taken in interpreting subsequent studies that include the same data in a larger population. Most such considerations apply equally to case-control, cohort, and correlation studies. Lack of clarity in any of the aspects of reporting of a study can decrease its credibility and the weight given to it in a final evaluation of exposure.

First, the study population, disease, and exposure should have been well defined by the authors. Cases of disease in the study population should have been identified in a way that was independent of the exposure of interest—in this case, the mind factor. The exposure should have been assessed in a way that was not related to disease status.

Second, the authors should have taken into account the study design and analysis of other variables that can influence the risk for disease and might have been related to the exposure of interest. Potential confounding by such variables should have been dealt with either in the design of the study, such as by matching, or in the analysis, by statistical adjustment. In cohort studies, comparisons with local rates of disease may or may not be more appropriate than those with national rates. Internal comparisons of frequency of disease among individuals at different levels of exposure are also desirable in cohort studies, as they minimize the potential for confounding related to the difference in risk factors between an external reference group and the study population.

Third, the authors should have reported the basic data on which the conclusions are founded, even if sophisticated statistical analyses were employed. At the very least, they should have given the numbers of exposed and unexposed cases and controls in a case-control study and the numbers of cases observed and expected in a cohort study. Further tabulations by time since exposure began and other temporal factors are also important. In a cohort study, data on all cancer sites and all causes of death should have been given, to reveal the possibility of reporting bias. In a case-control study, the effects of investigated factors other than the exposure of interest should have been reported.

Finally, the statistical methods used to obtain estimates of relative risk, absolute rates of cancer, confidence intervals and significance, and to adjust for confounding should have been clearly stated by the authors.

When an agent is discussed by the independent working groups convened by IARC, evidence from studies in humans and experimental animals is evaluated together, and the strength of the mechanistic evidence is also characterized. The groups then decide on the strength of the association between the exposure under review and carcinogenicity. An agent is assigned to one of five groups[3]:

Group 1: The agent is *carcinogenic to humans.*
Group 2A: The agent is *probably carcinogenic to humans.*
Group 2B: The agent is *possibly carcinogenic to humans.*
Group 3: The agent is *not classifiable as to its carcinogenicity to humans.*
Group 4: The agent is *probably not carcinogenic to humans.*

These considerations should be of interest to clinicians and researchers working in the field of psychosocial risk factors for cancer. They stimulate attention to the design and interpretation of scientific studies and form part of the discussion of the current state of the art in this intriguing area of research.

RESEARCH ON PSYCHOSOCIAL RISK FACTORS IN CANCER

In the 1930s, several psychoanalytically inspired psychologists went to the United States and introduced a psychoanalytical formulation of disease, including cancer, which became an immense, deeply rooted interpretation of illness. The lay public and numerous oncologists are convinced that this is an explanation for the random occurrence of cancer. Despite many years of research that revealed the major causes of cancer, including tobacco smoking, alcohol consumption, diet, ultraviolet radiation, and asbestos, the idea that psychological factors are the cause of at least some cases of cancer has been almost impossible to prove. In the middle of the 1950s, the first publications that claimed that psychological factors such as stress, personality trends, and body image were important risks for cancer were published.[4] The research effort was not guided by collaboration among disciplines, and the psychodynamic movement placed so much weight on emotional aspects in cancer causation that health providers who actually worked with cancer patients lost interest in the idea. The psychosomatic approach is of interest for a number of reasons related to the biopsychosocial concept as defined by Engel (1982)[5] and the treatment of cancer patients; but this aspect is out of the scope of this chapter. In the subsequent decades, access to modern statistical software packages and continuous interest in the association between mind and cancer resulted in numerous publications in the scientific literature, implicating one or more psychological factors as risk factors for cancer.

The three psychosocial factors that have been most rigorously studied in investigations of psychosocial cancer risks are major life events or stress, depression or depressive mood, and personality or personality traits. The commentary in this chapter does not represent a systematic review; it covers only studies conducted as prospective or retrospective cohort studies and case-control studies in which the information on psychosocial variables was collected independently of the outcome, thereby reducing the possibility of selection and recall bias. The findings of some of the best-designed studies published since 2000 are summarized briefly later.

Major life events and stress. Numerous studies have investigated the association between major life events, stress in daily life or work-related stress, and the risk for cancer. Breast cancer has been a focus in this research tradition.

With regard to work-related stress, a large Finnish prospective cohort study of 10,519 women aged 18 years or more investigated the relation between stress in daily activities and breast cancer. Daily stress was assessed twice, in 1975 and 1981, by a self-administered questionnaire, and study subjects were divided into three groups: no stress (23% of women), some stress (68%), and severe stress (9%). The authors identified 205 incident cases of breast cancer by linkage to the nationwide, population-based cancer registry, and observed that the hazard ratio for breast cancer in women with "some stress" was 1.11 (95% confidence interval [CI], 0.78–1.57) when compared with women with "no stress." For women with "severe stress," the hazard ratio for breast cancer was 0.96 (95% CI, 0.53–1.73) when compared with those with "no stress." The analysis included detailed information on reproductive factors, anthropometrics, and lifestyle. Neither shifting the cut-off point for stress nor restricting the analysis to women who reported the same level of stress at the two measurements altered the results.[6]

The same group investigated the same hypothesis in a cohort of 10,808 women sampled in the Finnish Twins Registry and obtained information on exposure to life events by using a standardized life event inventory. They examined the effect of accumulation of life events, placing emphasis on events experienced 5 years before completion of the questionnaire. They observed that experience of divorce or the death of a husband was followed by a significant twofold increase in the hazard ratio for breast cancer; the death of a close relative or friend also significantly increased the risk by almost 40%. The analysis included some information on reproductive factors, anthropometrics, and lifestyle. It is notable that the authors investigated the effect of cumulative exposure to life events.[7]

In the Nurses' Health Study of 69,886 women aged 46–71 at baseline in the United States, the women answered questions on informal caregiving. The authors hypothesized that hours and self-reported levels of stress from informal caregiving would be associated with breast cancer incidence. A total of 1700 incident cases of breast cancer were identified between 1992 and 2000, in which period the women reported caregiving twice, in 1992 and 1996. The analysis included information on reproductive factors; family history of breast cancer; psychosocial factors such as depressive symptoms, social network, and self-reported level of stress; anthropometrics; and lifestyle factors. The authors did not find that stress due to caregiving increased the risk for breast cancer.[8]

Two reports based on the Nurses' Health Study in the United States and the Danish Nurse Cohort study of job stress and risk for breast cancer found no increase in the risk of women who reported high levels of strain in their daily working lives. Both studies were conducted as cohort studies, with morbidity from breast cancer as the outcome and adjustment for a number of factors of relevance for breast cancer risk.[9,10] The Danish study also investigated the association between stress and the stage of disease at diagnosis but did not find that stress affected the prognostic characteristics of disease.

In summary, almost none of the large population-based studies with information from administrative registers, in which information on exposure is collected independently of scientific hypotheses, found evidence that work-related stress or major life events are associated with an increased risk for cancer. Although a few well-designed studies have shown an increased risk,[7,11] the strong consistency among the presumably unbiased studies indicates that explanations for the elevated risk may include selection bias, residual confounding, or chance. This conclusion comes close to the overall conclusion in previous reviews.[12]

Depression and depressive mood. In a nationwide Danish cohort study of the cancer risk of patients hospitalized for depression, all 89,491 adults who had been admitted to a hospital with depression, as defined in the International Classification of Diseases, Eighth Revision, between 1969 and 1993 were identified. A total of 9922 cases of cancer were diagnosed in the cohort, with 9434.6 expected, yielding a standardized incidence ratio of 1.05 (95% CI, 1.03–1.07). The risk for cancer increased during the first year after hospital admission, brain cancer in particular, occurring more frequently than expected. When the first year of follow-up was excluded, the increase was attributable mainly to an increased risk for tobacco-related cancers, with standardized incidence ratios for non–tobacco-related cancers of 1.00 (95% CI, 0.97–1.03) after 1–9 years of follow-up and 0.99 (95% CI, 0.95–1.02) after 10 or more years of follow-up. These findings provide no support for the hypothesis that depression independently increases the risk for cancer, but they emphasize the deleterious effect that depression can have on lifestyle.[13]

In a Dutch prospective follow-up study of 5191 women living in Eindhoven and born in the Netherlands between 1941 and 1947, all the participants answered a questionnaire about the presence of depressive symptoms measured on the Edinburgh Depression Scale. The outcome was morbidity from cancer recorded in the regional cancer registry, which reported incident breast cancer cases up to 5 years after the questionnaire screening. The analyses were adjusted for information on 15 demographic, medical, and lifestyle factors known to be associated with the risk for breast cancer. Breast cancer was diagnosed in 58 women during the follow-up period, yielding an odds ratio of 0.29 (95% CI, 0.09–0.92), which suggested that depressive symptoms may be protective against breast cancer.[14]

The same design was used in a study in Finland in which 10,892 women aged 48–50 years at the time of inclusion were followed-up for breast cancer 6–9 years later. The questionnaire includes items on depression, personality traits, attitudes to illness, life events, and health history. The incident cancer cases were obtained from the nationwide Finnish cancer registry, which has almost complete population-based coverage. The multivariate analysis was controlled for socioeconomic factors, family history of cancer, parity and health behavior, and identified a nonsignificantly increased risk of 1.15 (95% CI, 1.0–1.28) for breast cancer among women aged 50–59 when compared with the general population. There was no evidence that depression, anxiety, cynical distrust, or coping increased the risk for cancer.[15]

A large prospective study was conducted of the association between depressive symptoms as measured by the mental health index, which is a subscale of the short form of the 36 Health Status Survey, and risks for colorectal cancer and colorectal adenomas. The scores ranged from 0 to 100, and women (who were all part of the Nurses' Health Study) who scored between 0 and 52 were defined as having significant depressive symptomatology. A total of 33 of the 400 cases of colorectal cancer filled this definition, as did 45 out of 680 cases of distal adenoma. The authors created other categories across the range of mental health index scores and reported a nonsignificantly elevated risk of 1.43 (95% CI, 0.97–2.11) for colorectal cancer in women with the highest score on the index, with a stronger association in overweight women. Depressive symptoms did not increase the risk for adenomas. The analysis included several factors known to be associated with colorectal cancer.[16]

A large population-based record-linkage study in the Oxford National Health Service region in the United Kingdom addressed people who had been admitted to hospitals for depression or anxiety. A reference cohort of 525,436 people was constructed by selecting records for admission for various other medical and surgical conditions as "controls." The outcome was identified as either death from cancer or hospital care for any cancer. The authors excluded people who had the cancer at the first recorded admission for the psychiatric disorder or a comparison condition to avoid misclassification. The authors did not identify an increased risk for all cancers among the 27,818 people with depression or in the 24,292 people with anxiety. When the first year of follow-up was excluded, the relative risk for lung cancer was significantly increased in both cohorts (1.30; 95% CI, 1.14–1.48 in the depression cohort and 1.21; 1.03–1.36 in the anxiety cohort).[17]

In most of the studies in which total cancer risk was assessed, no statistically significant increase was seen, or increases were seen in only some strata. Increased risks were observed for smoking-associated cancers such as lung cancer. One researcher in this field stated that "the literature on depression as a predictor of cancer incidence is mixed, although chronic and severe depression may be associated with elevated cancer risk."[18] It is the lifestyle of depressed people that is probably the most straightforward explanation for the positive findings in some studies, although a depressive component cannot be excluded.

Personality traits. In a large Finnish study based on the above-mentioned Twins Cohort, 12,032 women answered questions about life satisfaction and neuroticism in 1975 and 1981. During the 21 years of follow-up, 238 cases of breast cancer were identified in the Finnish Cancer Registry. The authors reported no association between the measures of life satisfaction, neuroticism, and the risk for breast cancer. Subsequent nested case-cohort analyses and analyses that included changes in the levels of neuroticism and life satisfaction at the two times led the authors to conclude that there was no evidence that breast cancer is more likely to occur in unhappy, dissatisfied, anxious women.[19] These findings were confirmed in additional analyses that included Eysenck extroversion, Bortner type A behavior, and an author-constructed measure of hostility.[20]

A smaller prospective cohort study in Germany of 5114 women and men aged 40–65 measured mortality from and incidence of cancer. A number of personality scales were included in a questionnaire, and participants were followed-up for a median of 8.5 years. During this time, 240 people developed a cancer or died from the disease. The authors reported no association between the personality measures and cancer occurrence after adjustment for lifestyle, comorbidity, and family history of cancer.[21]

"Ikigai" is a Japanese concept believed to be an essential factor for maintaining health. Japanese dictionaries define "ikigai" as something to live for, the joy and goal of living or the happiness and benefit of being alive. In a cohort of 31,992 Japanese women aged 40–79 years, a total of 149 cases of breast cancer were identified from either mortality records or diagnostic information. The mean follow-up was 7.5 years. Women who expressed "ikigai" were at a significantly lower risk for breast cancer (relative risk, 0.66; 95% CI, 0.47–0.94), as were women who expressed decisiveness (0.56; 0.36–0.94). Two other factors investigated, ease of anger arousal and self-perceived stress of daily life, were not associated with breast cancer risk.[22]

In a cohort of 9705 women in Nijmegen, the Netherlands, the authors investigated the association between 10 personality traits as measured with the SAQ-N, a questionnaire developed by this group. The participation rate was 34%, which somewhat limits the conclusions. The medical risk factors included in the analysis were family history of breast cancer, parity, age at birth of first child, estrogen use, age at menarche, and body mass index. The authors reported no association between any of the personality traits and the risk for breast cancer.[23]

In summary, these studies do not point to an association between personality traits and the risk for cancer, in particular breast cancer. This statement is based on well-designed prospective studies that covered fairly large populations, clear definition of the "exposure," an acceptable length of follow-up, and adjustment for some factors that might be confounders. The outcome was based on either information on morbidity or close follow-up of mortality to exclude misclassification. Furthermore, the hypothesis was established independently of the cohort formation, and none of the data sources was biased by interviewers or information to cohort members. The use of administrative sources almost completely excludes selection bias.

Mechanism. A number of investigations have been conducted of the possible pathways between mind factors and the risk for cancer. These now form a complete research area, named psychoneuroimmunology, which is an important component, with human studies, of a new field that bridges biology, epidemiology, and cancer risk research.

It has been hypothesized that the mind factor (major life events or stress, depression or depressive mood, and personality or personality traits) acts like stress through the hypothalamic-pituitary-adrenal axis in a complex feedback system between the mind, the immune system, and actual cortisol levels, which adversely affect overall immune function. It has been further hypothesized that the immune system is involved in eliminating mutated cells, and it is possible that reduced immunity could lead to more rapid development of cancer. Furthermore, the mind factor may also act as a promoter of faulty DNA repair and an inhibitor of apoptosis and DNA repair. These systems and changes in function are suggested to be precursors of certain types of cancer, such as hormonal and hematological–lymphatic cancers.

Despite the plausibility of these mechanisms, little or no epidemiological evidence has arisen during the past 50 years of research on psychosocial risk factors in cancer. The association between diseases characterized by immune deficiency and breast cancer is weak, although several studies have demonstrated a reverse causation.[24,25] In a large Scandinavian case-control study, however, a personal or family history of certain autoimmune conditions was strongly associated with an increased risk for Hodgkin's lymphoma. The association between both personal and family histories of sarcoidosis and a statistically significantly increased risk for Hodgkin's lymphoma suggests a shared susceptibility for these conditions.[26] This points to the possibility that mechanisms linking the mind factor with cancer differ, depending on the cancer site.

Alternatively, the mechanism may be driven more by changes in behavior. It is well known that people under severe stress, in depression or expressing certain personality traits differ from others with regard to health behavior. This is true for smoking, alcohol consumption, diet, and physical activity. Some studies have confirmed this pattern, finding higher risks for cancers associated with these behaviors.[27-29] Thus, our understanding of psychosocial risk factors might have a larger public health impact if we focused on prevention and changes in the lifestyles of people exposed to stress or major life events who exhibit certain personality traits and experience depression or depressive mood.

DISCUSSION

This review covers studies of associations between cancer and psychological factors such as acute life events, work stress, coping style, personality, and depression.[29,30] Other reviews have been limited to one type of cancer, notably breast cancer,[31] a number of meta-analyses[32] have been conducted, and some reviews have mixed studies of risk and prognosis.[12] During the past 10 years, more than 15 reviews have been published, although they are of uneven quality. Some did not describe the design of the studies, others summarized the findings of all studies, despite methodological differences, while some reviews focused on breast cancer. The conclusions reached out in two directions: one group of reviewers found small or putative associations, while the other group found no or only a small etiological fraction reserved for psychosocial risk factors because of methodological limitations in the studies reviewed.

Any conclusion must take into account the quality of the studies, whether pro or con. From a methodological viewpoint, it is incorrect to use a case-control design, as such studies have serious problems that are exacerbated in this area of research. Researchers need information on psychological and social circumstances, which the exposed person must recall differently from the control. This design can be used only if information on exposure is obtained from administrative sources, in which information is collected for purposes that have nothing to do with the hypothesis of the study, as illustrated by Ewertz (1986).[33] She conducted a nationwide case-control study of 1792 cases of breast cancer diagnosed in Denmark in 1983-1984 and identified from the cancer register, with 1939 population-based controls, and found that divorce and widowhood did not increase the age-adjusted risk for breast cancer. Among the requirements for future research, therefore, are prospective data, clearer definitions of exposure, and repeated measures during follow-up; we also need longer follow-up to identify more cases and to investigate psychosocial factors with the same rigorous methods as used in other areas of research.

We must include information on other well-defined risk factors for the disease under study to find out how they confound or interact with each other in relation to the association investigated. This is being recognized in more and more studies. The socioeconomic aspects of the exposure under study, comorbidity, and health behavior are new aspects of our understanding of the association between mind and cancer risk. We must consider carefully whether health behavior is an intermediate rather than a confounding factor, as this will have profound implications for our understanding of the possible association between psychological factors and the risk for cancer. It has also been noted that this field of research would be more comprehensive if not just one but several psychosocial factors were included.[12]

We need to use the quality criteria defined by IARC (2006)[3] in this research area and reflect the findings of studies of psychosocial risk factors in the effects of other risk factors for cancer.

Psychosocial factors such as stress, depression, and personality traits do not appear to play a major role in cancer causation. All the studies published so far have limitations, making it difficult to reach a definitive decision about causality. On the basis of the data available, excluding studies with inadequate methods and applying sound epidemiological methodological principles, psychosocial factors would be placed in IARC Group 3 or even Group 4.

REFERENCES

1. Hill AB. The environment and disease: association or causation? *Proc R Soc Med*. 1965;58:295–300.

2. Greenland S, Pearl J, Robins JM. Causal diagrams for epidemiologic research. *Epidemiology*. 1999;10:37–48.

3. IARC. 2006. www.iarc.fr.

4. Holland JC. History of psycho-oncology: overcoming attitudinal and conceptual barriers. *Psychosom Med*. 2002;64:206–221.

5. Engel G. The biopsychosocial model and medical education: who are to be the teachers? *N Engl J Med*. 1982;306:802–805.

6. Lillberg K, Verkasalo PK, Kaprio J, Teppo L, Helenius H, Koskenvuo M. Stress of daily activities and risk of breast cancer: a prospective cohort study in Finland. *Int J Cancer*. 2001;91:888–893.

7. Lillberg K, Verkasalo PK, Kaprio J, Teppo L, Helenius H, Koskenvuo M. Stressful life events and risk of breast cancer in 10,808 women: a cohort study. *Am J Epidemiol*. 2003;157:415–423.

8. Kroenke CH, Hankinson SE, Schernhammer ES, Colditz GA, Kawachi I, Holmes MD. Caregiving stress, endogenous sex steroid hormone levels, and breast cancer incidence. *Am J Epidemiol*. 2004;159:1019–1027.

9. Schernhammer ES, Hankinsin SE, Rosner B, et al. Job stress and cancer risk. The Nurses' Health Study. *Am J Epidemiol*. 2004;160:1079–1086.

10. Nielsen NR, Stahlberg C, Strandberg-Larsen K, et al. Are work-related stressors associated with diagnosis of more advanced stages of incident breast cancer? *Cancer Causes Control*. 2008;19:297–303.

11. Levav I, Kohn R, Iscovich J, Abramson JH, Tsai WY, Vigdorovich D. Cancer incidence and survival following bereavement. *Am J Public Health*. 2000;90:1601–1607.

12. Garssen B. Psychological actors and cancer development: evidence after 30 years of research. *Clin Psychol Rev*. 2004;24:315–338.

13. Dalton SO, Mellemkjaer L, Olsen JH, Mortensen PB, Johansen C. Depression and cancer risk: a register-based study of patients hospitalized with affective disorders, Denmark, 1969–1993. *Am J Epidemiol*. 2002;155:1088–1095.

14. Nyklicek I, Louwman WJ, Van Nierop PW, Wijnands CJ, Coebergh JW, Pop VJ. Depression and the lower risk for breast cancer development in middle-aged women: a prospective study. *Psychol Med*. 2003;33:1111–1117.

15. Aro AR, De Koning HJ, Schreck M, Henriksson M, Anttila A, Pukkala E. Psychological risk factors of incidence of breast cancer: a prospective cohort study in Finland. *Psychol Med*. 2005;35:1515–1521.

16. Kroenke CH, Bennett GG, Fuchs C, et al. Depressive symptoms and prospective incidence of colorectal cancer in women. *Am J Epidemiol*. 2005;162:839–848.

17. Goldacre MJ, Wotton CJ, Yeates D, Seagroatt V, Flint J. Cancer in people with depression or anxiety: a record-linkage study. *Soc Psychiatry Psychiatr Epidemiol*. 2007;42:683–689.

18. Spiegel D, Giese-Davis J. Depression and cancer: mechanisms and disease progression. *Biol Psychiatry*. 2003;54:269–282.

19. Lillberg K, Verkasalo PK, Kaprio J, Teppo L, Helenius H, Koskenvuo M. A prospective study of life satisfaction, neuroticism and breast cancer risk (Finland). *Cancer Causes Control*. 2002;13:191–198.

20. Lillberg K, Verkasalo PK, Kaprio J, Teppo L, Helenius H, Koskenvuo M. Personality characteristics and the risk of breast cancer: a prospective cohort study. *Int J Cancer*. 2002;100:361–366.

21. Stürmer T, Hasselbach P, Amelang M. Personality, lifestyle, and risk of cardiovascular disease and cancer: follow-up of population based cohort. *BMJ*. 2006;332:1359–1365.

22. Wakai K, Kojima M, Nishio K, et al. Psychological attitudes and risk of breast cancer in Japan: a prospective study. *Cancer Causes Control*. 2007;18:259–267.

23. Bleiker EMA, Hendriks JHCL, Otten JDM, Verbreek ALM, van der Ploeg HM. Personality factors and breast cancer risk: a 13 year follow-up. *J Natl Cancer Inst*. 2008;100:213–218.

24. Stewart T, Tsai SC, Grayson H, Henderson R, Opelz G. Incidence of de-novo breast cancer in women chronically immune suppressed after organ transplantation. *Lancet*. 1995;346:796–798.

25. Frisch M, Biggar RJ, Engels EA, Goerdert JJ. Association of cancer with AIDS-related immune suppression in adults. *JAMA*. 2001;285:1736–1745.

26. Landgren O, Engels EA, Pfeiffer RM, et al. Autoimmunity and susceptibility to Hodgkin lymphoma: a population-based case–control study in Scandinavia. *J Natl Cancer Inst*. 2006;98:1321–1330.

27. Schapiro IR, Ross-Petersen L, Saelan H, Garde K, Olsen JH, Johansen C. Extroversion and neuroticism and the associated risk of cancer: a Danish cohort study. *Am J Epidemiol.* 2001;153:757–763.

28. Schapiro IR, Nielsen LF, Jørgensen T, Boesen EH, Johansen C. Psychic vulnerability and the associated risk for cancer. *Cancer.* 2002;94:3299–3306.

29. Dalton SO, Boesen EH, Ross L, Schapiro IR, Johansen C. Mind and cancer. Do psychological factors cause cancer? *Eur J Cancer.* 2002;38:1313–1323.

30. Chida Y, Hamer M, Wardle J, Steptoe A. Do stress-related psychosocial factors contribute to cancer incidence and survival? *Nat Clin Pract Oncol.* 2008;5:466–475.

31. Nielsen NR, Grønbaek M. Stress and breast cancer: a systematic update on the current knowledge. *Nat Clin Pract Oncol.* 2006;3:612–620.

32. Duijts SFA, Zeegers MPA, Borne BVD. The association between stressful events and breast cancer risk: a meta-analysis. *Int J Cancer.* 2003;107:1023–1029.

33. Ewertz M. Bereavement and breast cancer. *Cancer.* 1986;53:701–703.

Social Environment and Cancer

Vicki S. Helgeson and Abigail L. McUmber

There is a wealth of literature on the relation of the social environment to psychological adjustment to cancer leading to the clear conclusion that the social environment can have both helpful and deleterious effects on adjustment.[1-3] Although there is much less research on the role of the social environment in cancer risk and survival, this body of research is growing. About 10 years ago, we provided a theoretical model as to how the social environment might influence cancer risk and survival and reviewed the literature on this topic in this handbook. Because the number of articles on this topic has doubled in the past decade, we provide an update to that review.

We review studies that examine the impact of the social environment on cancer incidence and mortality among healthy people (Table 8-1), and the impact of the social environment on survival for people who have been diagnosed with cancer (Table 8-2).

There are fewer studies that examine cancer incidence and mortality compared to survival. Incidence and mortality studies require extremely large sample sizes, and often abstract data from medical records or large national databases. Many of the studies employ a case-control methodology in which a group of people with cancer are matched to a healthy comparison group and social environment differences between the two groups are examined. Survival studies typically measure an aspect of the social environment at cancer diagnosis and then follow those patients for some period to predict survival. We do not include studies in this review that manipulate the social environment or create new social environments (i.e., social support interventions), as that literature has proliferated over the past 10 years and been subject to its own review. Please see Zimmerman et al.,[33] Graves,[34] Sheard and Maguire[35] for reviews of support interventions and Chow et al.[36] and Coyne[37] for reviews that explicitly address survival.

The literature that we review includes studies of both structural and functional characteristics of the social environment. *Structural measures* of the social environment describe the existence of connections with network members. Three types of structural measures have been evaluated: marital status, network size, and social integration. Marital status variables range from a comparison of married to all other groups of individuals to more specific comparisons among married, widowed, divorced, and separated people. Network size is measured by a count of family and friends. Social integration typically includes a variety of structural measures such as marital status, group membership, and frequency of contact with network members. One frequently employed measure of social integration is the Social Network Index (SNI).[38] *Functional measures* of the social environment tap the receipt of support resources or the perception that support resources are available. The most common functions or kinds of support assessed are emotional support, instrumental support, and informational support. Before we review the studies that examine the relation of the social environment to cancer, we present a theoretical model that describes how the social environment could predict cancer outcomes.

PATHWAYS LINKING THE SOCIAL ENVIRONMENT TO CANCER

We present a theoretical model of how the social environment could be related to cancer that is similar to the one we presented 10 years ago (see Fig. 8-1).

Social structure represents the presence of social network members, such as marital status, network size, and social integration. One of the primary pathways by which social structure is expected to influence health is by the provision of support functions, such as emotional

Table 8-1. Studies linking the social environment to incidence of/mortality from cancer

Author	Cancer	N	Sex	Race/ethnicity	Marital	Structural	Functional Design
Bleiker et al.[4]	Breast	9705 healthy	100% women	Holland		0	Prospective, I
Hemminki and Li[5]	All cancers	2.42 million	50% women	Sweden	Mixed		Case–control, I
Kravdal[6]	All cancers	Entire population	-----	Norway	+		Mortality
Kvikstad et al.[7]	All cancers	17,235 cancer 34,460 healthy	100% women	Norway	Mixed		Case–control, I
Kvikstad et al.[8]	Breast	4491 cancer 44,910 healthy	100% women	Norway	0		Case–control, I
Randi et al.[9]	All cancers	17,976 cancer 15,343 controls	64% women 56% women	Italy	0		Case–control, I
Tomaka et al.[10]	All cancers	755 seniors	59% women	72% white	0	0	Case–control, I

NOTE: +, incidence/mortality benefit; –, incidence/mortality deficit; 0, no relation to incidence/mortality; ------, information not provided; I, incidence.

Table 8-2. Studies linking the social environment to survival from cancer

Author	Cancer	N	Sex	Race/ethnicity	Marital	Structural	Functional	Length of follow-up
Allard et al.[11]	Variety, terminal	1081	48% women	Quebec	−			*Md* 11 days
Butow et al.[12]	Melanoma, metastatic	125	38% women	Australia	+		0,0~	0–2 years
Butow et al.[13]	Breast, metastatic	99	100% women	Australia			0~	*Md* 29 months
Cousson-Gelie et al.[14]	Breast	75	100% women	France	+		0/−	10 years
Frick et al.[15]	Bone marrow transplant	99	42% women	Germany			0/+~	up to 1 year
Giraldi et al.[16]	Breast	95	100% women	Italy			0	6 yrs
Herndon et al.[17]	Lung, advanced	206	26% women	------ (U.S.)			0	until death
Kroenke et al.[18]	Breast cancer	2835	100% women	------ (U.S.)	0	+	0	0–12 years, *Md* 6
Krongrad et al.[19]	Prostate	146,979	100% men	86% white	+			0–27 years
Kvikstad et al.[20]	Variety	14,231	100% women	Norway	+			1–25 years, *Md* 4.5
Lai et al.[21]	Variety, metastatic	261,070	44% women	84% white	+			0–27 years
Lehto et al.[22]	Melanoma, nonmetastatic	59	100% men	Finland			0	7–10 years
Maunsell et al.[23]	Breast, nonmetastatic	224	100% women	Quebec			+	7 years
Neale[24]	Breast cancer	10,778	100% women	86% white 14% black	0			10 years
Reynolds et al.[25]	Breast, all stages	1011	100% women	52% black 48% white		0	+,0~	5–6 years
Reynolds et al.[26 a]	Breast	847	100% women	52% black 48% white			+~	7–8 years
Rodrigue et al.[27]	Bone marrow transplant	92	47% women	------- (U.S.)			+	--------
Saito-Nakaya et al.[28]	Lung, nonmetastatic	238	39% women	Japan	0		0,0~	0–8 years
Saito-Nakaya et al.[29]	Lung, all stages	1230	30% women	Japan	+ men only			0–5 years
Tammemagi et al.[30]	Lung	1154	41% women	60% white 40% black	+			5 years
Vigano et al.[31]	Variety, terminal	227	64% women	92% white			0	min 20 months
Weihs et al.[32]	Breast	90	100% women	51% white 41% black			+, +	8–9 years

NOTE: +, survival benefit; −, survival deficit; 0, no relation to survival; -----, information not available; ~. support measure was cancer-specific.
[a]This study used the same sample as Reynolds et al.[25]

and instrumental support. Both social structure and support functions may influence the incidence and mortality from cancer as well as cancer survival via cognitive, affective, and behavioral pathways. Cognitive pathways include access to information that comes directly from network members or indirectly via network members' social connections. Other cognitive benefits stem from simply being part of a social network or from the support functions that network members provide. These include positive feelings about the self (i.e., self-esteem), positive beliefs about the future (i.e., optimism), and beliefs in personal control. Affective benefits include the increase in positive emotions and the reduction in negative emotions that come from belonging to a network, being part of a family, or from the support provided by network members. Behavioral benefits include a decrease in risk behavior and an increase in preventive health care among healthy people and a timely response to symptoms and adherence to treatment among those with cancer. These effects can be indirect as people involved in social networks take better care of themselves because network members depend on them or direct as network members are more likely to urge one to reduce risk behavior (e.g., smoking), enhance health promotion behaviors (e.g., regular checkups), and seek treatment for symptoms. The cognitive, affective, and behavioral benefits (which are likely to be interconnected) of social ties and social support could impact cancer incidence, mortality, and survival by altering biological pathways. Biological pathways include cardiovascular, neuroendocrine, and immune function. Research has linked social support to better functioning in all three domains.[39] Health behaviors, such as smoking, exercise, diet, and treatment adherence also may directly affect cancer outcomes.

REVIEW OF THE LITERATURE: SOCIAL ENVIRONMENT PREDICTING CANCER INCIDENCE AND MORTALITY

Our previous review showed no clear relation of marital status to cancer incidence or mortality, and suggested that the effect of marriage may vary by gender and ethnicity. There were only a few studies of structural measures of support, none finding a relation to cancer incidence and only suggestive evidence for a protective relation in terms of cancer mortality. There were even fewer studies that examined the relation of support functions to cancer incidence and mortality. Since that time, six studies of cancer incidence and one study of cancer mortality have been published. These studies are shown in Table 8-1. Most focus on marital status.

Marital status. Two very large studies examined the relation of marital status to cancer incidence and found a complicated set of results. A study in Sweden compared 60,000 divorced and 47,000 widowed people to a comparison group of married individuals.[5] Marital status was assessed in 1960 and 1970. Only individuals whose marital status remained unchanged were included in the study. Individuals were followed for cancer incidence between 1971 and 1998. There was no effect of widowhood on cancer risk. The overall risk of cancer for divorced individuals was slightly *less* than that for married individuals. The risk among divorced individuals, however, really depended on the cancer site. Divorce was associated with an increased risk of lung cancer, pancreatic cancer, digestive tract cancers, cervical cancer, and anal cancer, whereas divorce was associated with a decreased risk of colon, kidney,

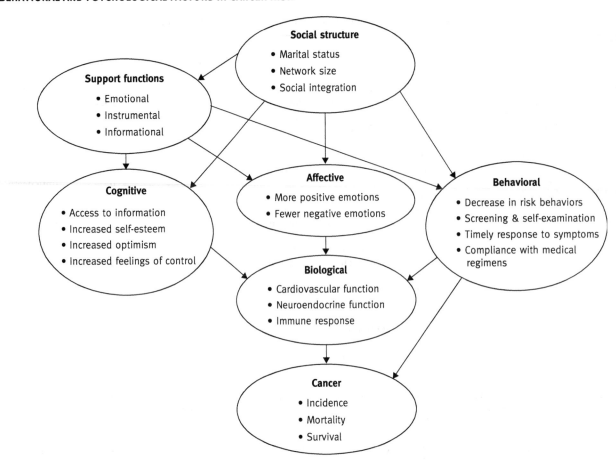

Fig. 8–1. Pathways by which the social environment might influence cancer outcomes.

breast, endometrial, ovarian, and prostate cancer. For some cancers, the increased risk was larger for males than females. The authors suggested that the increased risk was associated with cancers for which lifestyle factors such as tobacco, alcohol, and sexual behavior are more likely to play a role.

A study in Norway examined the relation of marital status to cancer in a group of 34,460 healthy women and 17,235 women with cancer.[7] There was no risk of cancer for widowed compared to married women. Like the previous study, the relation of divorce to cancer incidence depended on the cancer site. Divorce was associated with a reduced risk of breast, endometrial, thyroid, and colorectal cancers, but an elevated risk of lung and cervical cancer. Again, the authors suggested that lifestyle factors such as smoking and sexual behavior could explain the heightened risk. Unlike the previous study, however, not all of the marital status changes were taken into consideration. Never married people were excluded from this study.

Two cross-sectional studies showed no relation of marital status to cancer incidence. One case-control study in Italy compared 17,976 people with cancer to 15,343 controls admitted to the hospital for acute noncancer-related reasons.[9] Twenty different cancers were examined. Compared to married individuals, never married people had an increased risk of oral and pharynx cancer but a decreased risk of colon, liver, kidney, bladder, breast, and thyroid cancer. There was no excess risk of cancer for divorced or widowed people. Overall, the study authors concluded that marital status was not associated with cancer risk. A second case-control study in Norway compared 4491 women with breast cancer to 44,910 healthy women (all born between 1935 and 1954 and followed through 1990) and found no increased risk of breast cancer for either widowed women or divorced women.[8]

The one study of cancer mortality found evidence for a protective effect of marriage. The population of Norway was studied during 1960 through 1991 using the population and cancer registries.[6] The incidence of 11 different kinds of cancer for women and 8 different kinds of cancer for men were examined. Results showed that unmarried people had higher mortality rates than married people for 13 out of the 19 cancers; divorced and separated people had higher mortality rates than married people for 7 out of the 19 cancers; and widowed people had higher mortality rates than married people for 5 out of the 19 cancers. When data were pooled across cancer sites, there was a significantly higher mortality for unmarried, divorced/separated, and widowed compared to married people. The risk was higher for men than women. The highest risk was associated with being never married. These findings held even when stage of disease was controlled.

STRUCTURAL AND FUNCTIONAL MEASURES

Only two studies examined the relation of other kinds of support measures to cancer incidence. In one study, researchers sent questionnaires, which included a nonspecific measure of social support, to women ages 43 and older in a city in Holland.[4] Of the 9705 questionnaires returned (34% response rate), 131 women developed breast cancer during the 0–5 years of follow-up. In comparison to women who did not develop breast cancer, social support did not distinguish the two groups. In a second study, a survey was administered via random digit dialing to 755 seniors in New Mexico between the ages of 60 and 92.[10] None of the support measures (received support from family and friends, living alone, or feeling socially isolated) was associated with the presence of cancer. Both studies are limited by small sample sizes, especially the latter.

Summary. The relation of marital status to cancer incidence and cancer mortality appears to depend on the cancer site. This provides some support for the behavioral pathway linking social ties to cancer outcomes. Whereas cognitive and affective benefits of social ties would not seem to be uniquely tied to specific cancer sites, behavioral benefits of social ties may be linked to particular kinds of cancer. The literature also is becoming increasingly complex in recognizing that not all unmarried groups of individuals are equal. In the few studies reviewed here, the hazards of being unmarried appeared to be strongest for the divorced and weakest for the widowed.

There was little evidence for benefits of other structural or functional aspects of support to cancer incidence, but to be fair these were evaluated by only two studies with fairly small sample sizes.

REVIEW OF THE LITERATURE: SURVIVAL AMONG INDIVIDUALS WITH CANCER

Marital status. Our earlier review did not show a consistent association of marital status with cancer survival. The only studies that showed protective effects of marriage employed very large samples extracting data from medical records. Over the past decade, 11 new studies have examined the relation of marital status to cancer survival.

Two large-scale studies using Surveillance Epidemiology and End Results (SEER) data showed positive effects of being married. In one study, 146,979 men with prostate cancer were followed for up to 27 years.[19] Married men had longer survival times than single, divorced, or widowed men for all stages of cancer, when age, demographic variables, and treatment were statistically controlled. A study of 261,070 people with metastatic cancer showed that married people survived longer and were more likely to be alive at follow-up (up to 27 years later) than single, separated, divorced, or widowed people.[21] Single people had the poorest rate of survival. These findings held when demographic and treatment variables were statistically controlled. The relation of marital status to survival also was stronger in men than in women. The authors noted that this is the first study of people with advanced cancer to show a link of marriage to survival.

Another large-scale study of 14,231 people with a variety of cancers in Norway showed that divorced people had higher mortality rates than married people but this finding was limited to breast, lung, and cervical cancer.[20] There was no difference between married and widowed people, with the exception of colorectal cancer for which widowed people suffered a 2.5 times higher mortality rate.

Several smaller studies also have found benefits of marital status on cancer survival. A study of 1230 Japanese people with lung cancer showed that married men had higher survival rates compared to widowed men but there was no difference between the married and single, divorced, or separated individuals.[29] There were no effects of marital status for women. A study of 125 people from Australia with metastatic melanoma showed that married people were less likely to die within 2 years than single, widowed, or separated individuals.[12]

Some studies revealed more equivocal relations of marital status to survival. A small study of 75 women with breast cancer showed that widowed and divorced women had lower rates of 10-year survival compared to married people but this relation disappeared when disease characteristics were statistically controlled.[14] Similarly, a study of 1154 people with lung cancer showed that married people survived longer than unmarried people, but this finding disappeared when disease stage and adverse symptoms were statistically controlled.[30] The fact that disease stage mediates the finding of marital status to survival does not necessarily negate the significance of marital status; however, it may simply imply that married people are more likely to be diagnosed at an earlier stage of disease which then contributes to their prolonged survival.

Three studies found no significant relation of marital status to survival. One study found a weak but nonsignificant relation of marital status ($p = 0.09$) to survival from breast cancer among 10,778 women, in the direction of married people being more likely to survive 10 years later compared to unmarried people.[24] A study of 2835 women with breast cancer revealed no relation of marital status to survival.[18] A study of a smaller group of people with nonmetastatic lung cancer

($n = 238$) treated with surgery showed no association of marital status with survival.[28]

Only one study showed a disadvantage in terms of cancer survival for married individuals. In a study of terminally ill people with a variety of cancers, marital status predicted slightly shorter survival times following hospital admission for palliative care.[11] The authors suggested that married people may have arrived at the hospital with more advanced disease because they had a spouse at home to care for the patient during the earlier stages of physical decline.

Social integration. The previous review found substantial evidence that social integration was associated with increased cancer survival. The one limitation was that the majority of the studies focused on breast cancer, limiting the generalizability of the findings. To date, two new studies have appeared in the literature—both focusing on women with breast cancer.

Social integration as assessed with the SNI predicted lower cancer mortality as well as lower all-cause mortality in 2835 women with breast cancer from the Nurses' Health Study.[18] This study is noteworthy because it is the first study to have assessed the SNI before the cancer diagnosis. The authors also noted a threshold effect, such that those who were the least socially integrated had the highest mortality rates. Despite the fact that the least integrated women were more likely to smoke and less likely to exercise, findings held when these health behaviors were statistically controlled. However, the SNI did not predict survival in a study of 1011 women with breast cancer.[25]

Functional measures. There were only a handful of studies that examined the relation of support functions to cancer survival in the previous review. Findings were mixed, which made any kind of conclusion premature. To date, many more investigators are examining support functions, with 15 new studies in this review.

Three studies of women with breast cancer have found clear benefits of social support to cancer survival. A study of 224 women in Quebec with local and regional breast cancer showed that confiding in someone following surgery was associated with higher survival rates 7 years later.[23] In addition, survival rates increased with more than one confidant. A larger study of 1011 women with breast cancer showed that perceived emotional support with respect to cancer was associated with longer survival whereas perceived instrumental support was not.[25] These findings held when age, disease stage, and other demographic variables were statically controlled. A subsequent follow-up of this sample confirmed these findings and showed that cancer-specific emotional support interacted with emotional expression to predict survival.[26] Women who scored low on emotional support and low on emotional expression were at greater risk for poor survival compared to women who scored high on both. In addition, these findings were stronger for women who had an earlier stage of disease, such that early stage women who scored low on both were four times as likely to die as early stage women who scored high on both. Finally, a study of 90 women with breast cancer showed that perceived availability of support and amount of contact with these support providers predicted longer survival.[32]

Two studies of people with cancer who were treated with bone marrow transplants showed relations of support functions before the transplant to posttransplant survival. One study showed that social support stability, as assessed by strong interpersonal ties, was associated with being alive at follow-up controlling for demographic and disease variables.[27] A second study showed no relation of cancer-specific support to 1-year survival but a relation of negative illness support (i.e., negative interactions) to poorer survival, controlling for performance status, treatment, and depression.[15]

However, there are a large number of studies that do not show a relation between social support and cancer survival. Three studies of women with breast cancer conducted outside the United States showed no benefits of received support to survival. A study of 95 women from Italy showed that neither received support from close relations nor received support from more diffuse network members was associated with mortality or recurrence status 6 years later.[16] A study of 99 women with metastatic breast cancer from Australia showed no link between cancer-specific received support from a close other to survival.[13] A study of 75 women from France showed no relation of support satisfaction with survival and an inverse relation of perceived support with survival, such that those who perceived more support had an increased risk of death, when adjusting for medical variables.[14]

Other studies also have failed to find relations of functional support to cancer survival. A study of 59 men from Finland with nonmetastatic melanoma found no relation of perceived support to survival.[22] Neither cancer-specific received support nor satisfaction with received support was related to survival in a study of 125 people with melanoma.[12] Two studies measured the presence of a confidant (presumably a source of emotional support) and did not find a relation. In a group of people with nonmetastatic lung cancer, having someone with whom they could discuss the illness was not associated with cancer-specific or all-cause mortality.[28] Satisfaction with that relation also did not predict mortality. In a study of 2835 women with breast cancer, neither the presence of a confidant nor the extent of contact with a confidant predicted cancer or all-cause mortality.[18] Two studies of people with advanced cancer also failed to detect a relation between support functions and survival. First, there was no relation between either of the two indices of received emotional support and survival among 206 people with advanced lung cancer.[17] Second, social support (mix of perceived and received) was not related to survival in a study of people with terminal breast, lung, or gastrointestinal cancer.[31]

Summary. The strongest evidence for the relation of the social environment to cancer survival comes from studies that examine marital status. The majority of these studies find positive links between being married and longer cancer survival. The effects also seem to be stronger among men. It is not clear from this literature which unmarried status (never married, divorced, widowed) has the greatest survival disadvantage.

Recent research has not greatly expanded our knowledge of the relation of social integration to cancer survival. There were only two new studies, one finding a survival benefit for social integration and one finding no relation. Because the methodologically stronger study was the one that found a survival benefit, we believe that our conclusion from the past review holds—that social integration seems to be related to cancer survival. This area of research still suffers from the bias of being heavily weighted toward breast cancer.

Whereas we were not able to draw conclusions about the relation of support functions to cancer survival in the previous review because of the dearth of studies, this is not the case today. Many more researchers have examined the relation of support functions to cancer survival, with the majority finding no relation. There does not seem to be an easy way to distinguish studies that do and do not find a relation of support functions to survival. Whether support was received or perceived, whether support was specific to cancer (noted by "~" in Table 8-2) or not, and sample characteristics (e.g., gender, disease stage) did not distinguish between the two groups.

BIOLOGICAL PATHWAYS LINKING THE SOCIAL ENVIRONMENT TO CANCER

Researchers have long speculated that one of the pathways by which the social environment influences health is biological (see Fig. 8–1). As the field of health psychology has become increasingly sophisticated both conceptually and methodologically, researchers are now investigating this pathway. We present three relatively recent studies that have examined links between the social environment and biology. A study of 103 women with metastatic breast cancer found that network size was not associated with cortisol levels but that perceived support was associated with lower cortisol levels.[40] None of the support measures were associated with the cortisol slope. A study of 72 women with metastatic breast cancer showed that neither network size, positive support, or aversive social relationships were associated with immune response.[41] However, the authors found that network size interacted with stressful life events to predict immune response. A large social network was associated with a better immune response when there were a large number of stressful

life events but a worse immune response when there were few stressful life events. The authors suggested that social networks are beneficial under conditions of high stress. Finally, a third study showed that seeking instrumental support was associated with lower interleukin (IL)-6, a cytokine involved in tumor progression, among 21 women with gynecological cancer.[42] Seeking instrumental support also was associated with better functional and clinical status (i.e., more likely to be alive) 1 year later, but this effect was not mediated by IL-6. Thus, evidence for a biological link between the social environment and cancer is growing.

CONCLUSIONS

As in the previous review, we again found stronger relations between the social environment and disease progression or cancer survival than cancer incidence. How might the social environment contribute to cancer survival? First, people who have stronger social ties and more social support may engage in better health behavior and may be more adherent to treatment recommendations. Second, social ties and support may lead to earlier treatment-seeking in response to symptoms, which could result in earlier detection of the disease. One study showed that marital status was linked to an earlier stage of diagnosis for breast and prostate cancers.[43] Third, social ties and support may enable one to cope more effectively with the distress surrounding the diagnosis and treatment for cancer, potentially having an impact on biological pathways.

One reason that we found less evidence for an influence of the social environment on cancer incidence is that cancer takes years to develop and the social environment changes over time.[44] A major challenge for studies in this area is to track changes in the social environment over time. Most incidence and mortality studies focus on structural measures of the social environment, especially marital status. There may be changes in marital status over the period of follow-up. Case-control studies assess marital status and cancer incidence simultaneously, but often without regard to the person's marital history. There is some evidence from other research that marital transitions rather than marital statuses are associated with poor health outcomes. One study showed that the consistently married were less distressed than the consistently single and separated/divorced but similar to the consistently widowed.[45] In that study, transitions out of marriage were associated with short-term increases in distress whereas the transition into marriage was associated with a short-term decrease in distress.

Among the studies of the social environment and cancer survival, we found stronger evidence for the relation of marital status and social integration (structural measures of support) to survival than for the relation of functional support to survival. This is a bit perplexing as functional support is often considered to be one pathway by which structural measures influence health (see Fig. 8–1). There are a couple of possible explanations for these findings. The first explanation is methodological. Measures of functional support may be more susceptible to response biases and may be influenced by the demands of the illness in a way that marital status and other structural measures of support are not. Functional support is assessed after diagnosis. It is not clear if people are describing support functions in response to the illness or support functions that existed before the illness. The fact that some support measures are cancer-specific and others are not makes it even more difficult to synthesize across studies. The severity of the illness also might influence support functions. People who have a more severe disease or are having more problems coping with the side effects of treatment may need more support and thus receive more support. In that case, disease progression is leading to support receipt rather than support receipt leading to disease progression. Some studies measure received support, whereas others measure the perceived availability of support. The two are not the same. There is a great deal of literature documenting that relations of perceived support to good health outcomes are stronger and more consistent than relations of received support.[46] At any rate, marital status does not suffer from these difficulties. Marital status before cancer can be easily recalled after diagnosis and is not typically affected by the onset or severity of disease. Thus, it is still possible that marital status influences cancer survival via support functions but measurement difficulties make it difficult to discern this effect.

A second explanation for the stronger relation of marital status compared to support functions to cancer survival is that the positive effects of marriage on cancer survival are not due to the benefits of being married but due to the hazards associated with not being married. One study of health outside the cancer arena showed that marital status differences in health were due to the strain of marital dissolution rather than the benefits of being married.[47] In that study, self-ratings of health of the continually divorced and never married were similar to the continually married. Negative effects on self-rated health were tied to the transition to widowhood and divorce. A similar conclusion was reached by another set of investigators who tracked marital history and mortality over a 40-year period.[48] The consistently married lived longer than those who had experienced a breakup, but this was not due to the benefit of marriage per se. There was no difference in mortality between the consistently married and the consistently unmarried. In addition, those who had separated/divorced and remarried had a similar mortality to those who remained separated and divorced. Thus, it may be the strain of widowhood and divorce that have health costs rather than marriage having health benefits. It also may be that only supportive marriages are health beneficial, rather than marriage per se.

FUTURE DIRECTIONS

There are several differences between the studies that have been conducted more recently and the studies that were reviewed in our earlier article. One difference is that more studies are examining the specific cancer site. Interestingly, the two incidence studies that examined different cancer sites not only found that the results differed by site but also concurred on those differences.[5,7] In both cases, there was some evidence that the social environment played a role in cancers associated with behavioral risk factors. These findings suggest that the pathways by which the social environment might lead to cancer outcomes could differ by site. Future research should continue to investigate the differences between the kinds of cancers and determine whether there are some cancers for which the social environment plays a stronger role.

Another difference is that the studies presented in this chapter are from countries all over the world, with an emphasis on Western cultures. To the extent that the role of the social environment in people's lives differs across cultures, the effect of the social environment may differ and the pathways by which health effects occur could differ. For example, marriage may not have the same connections to support functions in countries where marriages are arranged. There are other ways in which the research in this area has not advanced as far as one would have liked. Researchers typically fail to investigate interactive effects between the social environment and demographic, disease variables, or stress—a point noted by Garssen.[49] There are a large number of studies of general health (not specific to cancer) that show the relation of the social environment to health differs for men and women, most notably that relations of marital status to good health are stronger for men than women.[38,50] Only a few studies in the area of cancer examined whether gender moderated the relations of the social environment to health, an incidence study finding relations stronger for males than females[5] and two survival studies finding relations stronger for males than females.[21,29] In fact, many of the null findings for marital status occurred in studies that consisted entirely of females. One reason that marital status might be more strongly related to cancer outcomes among males than females is that wives' have a stronger influence on husbands' health behavior than vice versa.[51,52] The authors of the study of people with lung cancer suggested that unmarried males may be more likely than unmarried females to continue to smoke after diagnosis.[29] Future research should routinely examine gender when examining the relation of marital status to cancer outcomes.

The extent to which the social environment interacts with stressful life events to predict cancer incidence or interacts with disease severity to predict cancer survival was rarely investigated. There are two models by which social support is said to influence health—the direct or main effects model and the interactive or stress-buffering model.[53] The direct effects model holds that social support is good for health, regardless of the level of stress in one's life. The stress-buffering hypothesis holds that social support is beneficial for one's health only under conditions of high stress. The pathways by which social support influences health differ for the two models. In the area of cancer, one might expect the direct effects model to hold for cancer incidence and mortality but the stress-buffering model to hold for cancer survival. The question is whether cancer in and of itself is a sufficient stressor so that support leads directly to survival or whether level of stress, distress, or stage of disease should be taken into consideration.

Despite the fact that research has shown that the negative aspects of relationships are more strongly related to health than the positive aspects of relationships,[54] only a few research studies reviewed here have taken this point into consideration. Only one study assessed both the positive and negative aspects of social relations and found no relations of positive support to survival but a hazardous relation of negative relations to survival.[15] More research needs to examine the negative side of the social environment.

ACKNOWLEDGMENT

Preparation of this chapter was partially supported by a grant from the National Cancer Institute (CA104078).

REFERENCES

1. Helgeson VS, Cohen S. Social support and adjustment to cancer: reconciling descriptive, correlational, and intervention research. *Health Psychol.* 1996;15:135–148.
2. Lepore SJ, Helgeson VS. Social constraints, intrusive thoughts, and mental health after prostate cancer. *J Soc Clin Psychol.* 1998;17:89–106.
3. Manne SL. Intrusive thoughts and psychological distress among cancer patients: the role of spouse avoidance and criticism. *J Consult Clin Psychol.* 1999;67:539–546.
4. Bleiker EM, ven der Ploeg HM, Hendriks JH, Ader HJ. Personality factors and breast cancer development: a prospective longitudinal study. *J Natl Cancer Inst.* 1996;88:1478–1482.
5. Hemminki K, Li X. Lifestyle and cancer: effects of widowhood and divorce. *Cancer Epidemiol Biomarkers.* 2003;12:899–904.
6. Kravdal O. The impact of marital status on cancer survival. *Soc Sci Med.* 2001;52:357–368.
7. Kvikstad A, Vatten LJ, Tretli S, Kvinnsland S. Widowhood and divorce related to cancer risk in middle-aged women. A nested case-control study among Norwegian women born between 1935 and 1954. *Int J Cancer.* 1994;58:512–516.
8. Kvikstad A, Vatten LJ, Tretli S, Kvinnsland S. Death of a husband or marital divorce related to risk of breast cancer in middle-aged women. A nested case-control study among Norwegian women born between 1935 and 1954. *Eur J Cancer.* 1994;30A:473–477.
9. Randi G, Altieri A, Gallus S, et al. Marital status and cancer risk in Italy. *Prev Med.* 2004;38:523–528.
10. Tomaka J, Thompson S, Palacios R. The relation of social isolation, loneliness, and social support to disease outcomes among the elderly. *J Aging Health.* 2006;18:359–384.
11. Allard P. Factors associated with length of survival among 1081 terminally ill cancer patients. *J Palliat Care.* 1995;11:20–24.
12. Butow PN, Coates AS, Dunn SM. Psychosocial predictors of survival in metastatic melanoma. *J Clin Oncol.* 1999;17:2256–2263.
13. Butow PN, Coates AS, Dunn SM. Psychosocial predictors of survival: metastatic breast cancer. *Ann Oncol.* 2000;11:469–474.
14. Cousson-Gelie F, Bruchon-Schweitzer M, Dilhuydy JM, Jutand M-A. Do anxiety, body image, social support, and coping strategies predict survival in breast cancer? A ten-year follow-up study. *Psychosom J Consult Liaison Psychiatry.* 2007;48:211–216.
15. Frick E, Motzke C, Fischer N, Busch R, Bumeder I. Is perceived social support a predictor of survival for patients undergoing autologous peripheral blood stem cell transplantation. *Psycho-Oncology.* 2005;14:759–770.
16. Giraldi T, Rodani MG, Cartei G, Grassi L. Psychosocial factors and breast cancer: a 6-year Italian follow-up study. *Psychother Psychosom.* 1997;66:229–236.
17. Herndon JE II, Fleishman S, Kornblith AB, Kosty M, Green MR, Holland J. Is quality of life predictive of the survival of patients with advanced nonsmall cell lung carcinoma? *Cancer.* 1999;85:333–340.
18. Kroenke CH, Kubzansky LD, Schernhammer ES, Holmes MD, Kawachi I. Social networks, social support, and survival after breast cancer diagnosis. *J Clin Oncol.* 2006;24:1105–1111.
19. Krongrad A, Lai H, Burke M, Goodkin K, Lai S. Marriage and mortality in prostate cancer. *J Urol.* 1996;156:1696–1700.

20. Kvikstad A, Vatten LJ, Tretli S. Widowhood and divorce in relation to overall survival among middle-aged Norwegian women with cancer. *Br J Cancer.* 1995;71:1343–1347.

21. Lai H, Lai S, Krongrad A, Trapido E, Page JB, McCoy CB. The effect of marital status on survival in late-stage cancer patients: an analysis based on surveillance, epidemiology and end results (SEER) data, in the United States. *Int J Behav Res.* 1999;6:150–176.

22. Lehto U-S, Ojanen M, Dyba T, Aromaa A, Kellokumpu-Lehtinen P. Baseline psychosocial predictors of survival in localized melanoma. *J Psychosom Res.* 2007;63:9–15.

23. Maunsell E, Brisson J, Deschenes L. Social support and survival among women with breast cancer. *Cancer.* 1995;76:631–637.

24. Neale AV. Racial and marital status influences on 10 year survival from breast cancer. *J Clin Epidemiol.* 1994;47:475–482.

25. Reynolds P, Boyd PT, Blacklow RS, et al. The relationship between social ties and survival among black and white breast cancer patients. National Cancer Institute Black/White Cancer Survival Study Group. *Cancer Epidemiol Biomarkers.* 1994;3:253–259.

26. Reynolds P, Hurley S, Torres M, Jackson J, Boyd P, Chen VW. Use of coping strategies and breast cancer survival: results from the Black/White Cancer Survival Study. *Am J Epidemiol.* 2000;152:940–949.

27. Rodrigue JR, Pearman TP, Moreb J. Morbidity and mortality following bone marrow transplant: predictive utility of pre-BMT affective functioning, compliance, and social support stability. *Int J Behav Med.* 1999;6:241–254.

28. Saito-Nakaya K, Nakaya N, Fujimori M, et al. Marital status, social support and survival after curative resection in non-small cell lung cancer. *Cancer Sci.* 2006;97:206–213.

29. Saito-Nakaya K, Nakaya N, Akechi T, et al. Marital status and non-small cell lung cancer survival: the Lung Cancer Database Project in Japan. *Psycho-Oncology.* 2008;17(9):869–876.

30. Tammemagi CM, Neslund-Dudas C, Simoff M, Kvale P. Lung carcinoma symptoms—an independent predictor of survival and an important mediator of African-American disparity in survival. *Cancer.* 2004;101:1655–1663.

31. Vigano A, Bruera E, Jhangri GS, Newman SC, Fields AL, Suarez-Almazor ME. Clinical survival predictors in patients with advanced cancer. *Arch Intern Med.* 2000;160:861–868.

32. Weihs KL, Simmens SJ, Mizrahi J, Enright TM, Hunt ME, Siegel RS. Dependable social relationships predict overall survival in stages II and III breast carcinoma patients. *J Psychosom Res.* 2005;59:299–306.

33. Zimmermann T, Heinrichs N, Baucom DH. "Does one size fit all?" Moderators in psychosocial interventions for breast cancer patients: a meta-analysis. *Ann Behav Med.* 2007;34:225–239.

34. Graves KD. Social cognitive theory and cancer patients' quality of life: a meta-analysis of psychosocial intervention components. *Health Psychol.* 2003;22:210–219.

35. Sheard T, Maguire P. The effect of psychological interventions on anxiety and depression in cancer patients: results of two meta-analyses. *Br J Cancer.* 1999;80:1770–1780.

36. Chow E, Tsao MN, Harth T. Does psychosocial intervention improve survival in cancer? A meta-analysis. *Palliat Med.* 2004;18:25–31.

37. Coyne JC. Psychotherapy and survival in cancer: the conflict between hope and evidence. *Psychol Bull.* 2007;133:367–394.

38. Berkman LF, Syme SL. Social networks, host resistance, and mortality: a nine-year follow-up study of Alameda County residents. *Am J Epidemiol.* 1979;109:186–204.

39. Uchino BN, Cacioppo JT, Kiecolt-Glaser JK. The relationship between social support and physiological processes: a review with emphasis on underlying mechanisms and implications for health. *Psychol Bull.* 1996;119:488–531.

40. Turner-Cobb JM, Sephton SE, Koopman C, Blake-Mortimer J, Spiegel D. Social support and salivary cortisol in women with metastatic breast cancer. *Psychosom Med.* 2000;62:337–345.

41. Turner-Cobb JM, Koopman C, Rabinowitz JD, Terr AI, Sephton SE, Spiegel D. The interaction of social network size and stressful life events predict delayed-type hypersensitivity among women with metastatic breast cancer. *Int J Psychophysiol.* 2004;54:241–249.

42. Lutgendorf SK, Anderson B, Sorosky JI, Buller RE, Lubaroff DM. Interleukin-6 and use of social support in gynecologic cancer patients. *Int J Behav Med.* 2000;7:127–142.

43. Nayeri K, Pitaro G, Feldman JG. Marital status and stage at diagnosis in cancer. *N Y State J Med.* 1992;92:8–11.

44. Spiegel D, Kato PM. Psychosocial influences on cancer incidence and progression. *Harv Rev Psychiatry.* 1996;4:10–26.

45. Strohschein L, McDonough P, Monette G, Shao Q. Marital transitions and mental health: are there gender differences in the short-term effects of marital status change? *Soc Sci Med.* 2005;61:2293–2303.

46. Wills TA, Shinar O. Measuring perceived and received social support. In: Cohen S, Underwood LG, Gottlieb BH, eds. *Social support measurement and intervention: a guide for health and social scientists.* New York, NY: Oxford University Press;2000:86–135.

47. Williams K, Umberson D. Marital status, marital transitions, and health: a gendered life course perspective. *J Health Soc Behav.* 2004;45:81–98.

48. Tucker JS, Wingard DL, Friedman HS, Schwartz JE. Marital history at midlife as a predictor of longevity: alternative explanations to the protective effect of marriage. *Health Psychol.* 1996;15:94–101.

49. Garssen B. Psychological factors and cancer development: evidence after 30 years of research. *Clin Psychol.* 2004;24:315–338.

50. Kaplan RM, Kronick RG. Marital status and longevity in the United States. *J Epidemiol Community Health.* 2006;60:760–765.

51. Schone BS, Weinick RM. Health-related behaviors and the benefits of marriage for elderly persons. *Gerontologist.* 1998;38:618–627.

52. Umberson D. Family status and health behaviors: social control as a dimension of social integration. *J Health Soc Behav.* 1987;28:306–319.

53. Cohen S, Wills TA. Stress, social support, and the buffering hypothesis. *Psychol Bull.* 1985;98:310–357.

54. Lincoln KD. Social support, negative social interactions, and psychological well-being. *Soc Serv Rev.* 2000;74:231–252.

PART III

Screening for Cancer in Normal and At-Risk Populations

Paul B. Jacobsen, ED

CHAPTER 9

Colorectal Cancer Screening

Sally W. Vernon and Amy McQueen

INTRODUCTION

The overall goal of colorectal cancer screening (CRCS) is to reduce morbidity and mortality from colorectal cancer (CRC). CRC is the second leading cause of cancer deaths in the United States, with estimates of 148,810 new cases and 49,960 deaths in 2008.[1] From 2000 to 2004, the average annual incidence rates of CRC were 60.4 and 44.0 per 100,000 in white men and women and 72.6 and 55.0 per 100,000 in black men and women.[2] During the same period, average annual mortality rates were 22.9 for white men and 15.9 for white women; they were 32.7 for black men and 22.9 for black women. Regular screening with the fecal occult blood test (FOBT) or sigmoidoscopy (SIG) facilitates earlier detection of CRC and lowers mortality.[3–7] Screening colonoscopy (COL) may decrease CRC incidence through early detection and removal of precancerous polyps.[8] Other than cervical cancer, CRC is the only cancer for which both incidence and mortality can be reduced through population-based screening.

Professional organizations agree that, for those at average risk, CRCS should begin at age 50.[9] The most recent guidelines distinguish between tests that detect cancer early (i.e., annual guaiac-based FOBT, annual fecal immunochemical test, or stool DNA testing) and tests that also can prevent cancer through the detection and removal of polyps (i.e., COL every 10 years or SIG, double-contrast barium enema, or computed tomographic colonography/virtual COL every 5 years).[10] Behavioral scientists interested in conducting research on cancer screening need to be aware of changes in the guidelines so that their research will be based on sound scientific evidence that links a target screening behavior to a reduction in incidence or mortality.[11]

Two national sources of prevalence data on CRC test use in the United States are the National Health Interview Survey (NHIS) and the Behavioral Risk Factor Surveillance System (BRFSS). Differences in the methods of data collection have resulted in slightly different estimates of CRCS prevalence; however, both sources show a gradual increase in overall test use. BRFSS data show an increase from 53.9% in 2002 to 60.8% in 2006 for FOBT in the past year or SIG or COL in the past 10 years.[12] NHIS data from 2000 to 2005 show that most of the increase was due to increased use of COL (Fig. 9–1). Despite this increase, the prevalence of CRCS in the United States is low compared with breast and cervical cancer screening.[13] Implementation of the screening guidelines is essential if we are to impact morbidity and mortality from CRC.

The primary purpose of this chapter is to review behavioral research on CRCS access and use in the United States and to identify directions for future research based on this evidence.

FACTORS ASSOCIATED WITH CRCS

Studies of factors associated with CRCS are used to inform the selection of target populations for intervention and to inform the content of interventions. The major categories of factors that have been studied in relation to CRCS behaviors include sociodemographic, healthcare access, health status, health behavior, cognitive, psychosocial, and more recently, environmental. Demographic variables are useful for identifying population subgroups for whom we can target interventions. They are less amenable to change and are therefore not as useful in interventions designed to motivate and enable screening test use. Most of this literature is based on cross-sectional study designs that can only establish

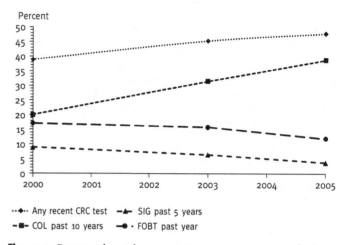

Percent

Fig. 9–1. Recent colorectal cancer test usage among respondents age 50 and older: National Health Interview Survey 2000, 2003, and 2005.[a] ABBREVIATIONS: COL, colonoscopy; CRC, colorectal cancer; FOBT, fecal occult blood test; SIG, sigmoidoscopy. [a]Percentages are standardized to the 2000 standard population by 5-year age groups.

associations, although a few studies have used prospective designs. More recent studies have begun to test hypotheses about causal pathways by examining mediators and moderators. Because CRCS is unique in that multiple test options are available, the role of test preferences and informed decision making (IDM) in CRCS test use have begun to be examined.

Although numerous studies have identified factors related to CRCS, there have been few attempts to systematically review this literature. Early reviews reported on correlates and predictors of FOBT[14–16] and SIG use.[15,17] Hiatt et al.[18] reviewed studies using cancer-screening data from the NHIS that were published from 1980 to 2001, but few studies addressed CRCS.

Sociodemographic, healthcare access, health status, and health behavior factors. Studies of sociodemographics, access to healthcare, health status, and health behavior have used data from national surveys. Meissner et al.[13] reviewed trends using NHIS data from 1987 to 2003 and reported several positive correlates of CRCS over time: age 65 years and older, male gender, non-Hispanic race/ethnicity, married, former smoker, higher education, health insurance, a usual source of healthcare, and more visits to a provider in the past year. More recent data from the 2005 NHIS were generally consistent with those findings; however, there were no differences in test use by gender for either FOBT or endoscopy. Blacks and Hispanics were less likely to report endoscopy use, but they reported similar rates of FOBT.[19] Engaging in other preventive health behaviors was positively associated with CRCS including reporting a recent mammogram or Pap test among women or a recent prostate-specific antigen (PSA) test among men,[13,19–23] cholesterol tests, dental visits,[24] seat belt use, fruit and vegetable consumption, and physical activity.[22] Some differences have been observed in the pattern of associations by test type, but few studies have made direct comparisons. Compared with FOBT, the likelihood of completing an endoscopic test is increased among people with a family history of CRC,[19,21,25] access to regular health care,[19,23] health insurance[19,21] fewer concerns about cost,[23] and higher perceived CRC risk.[23] Poorer health status was associated with less FOBT use but was not associated with endoscopic test use.[26]

Colorectal cancer screening is the only type of cancer screening that is recommended for both males and females, but few studies have examined whether correlates differ by gender. Cokkinides et al.[20] found some differences in analyses stratified by age group and gender suggesting that being single and unable to see a provider due to cost were important CRCS barriers for women but not for men. McQueen et al.[23] examined gender-specific correlates by CRCS test type using 2003 Health Information National Trends Survey data and found some consistent positive correlates of CRCS for both genders including age, recent physician visit, recent breast or PSA screening, and knowledge of test-specific screening intervals. Correlates that differed by gender included comparative perceived risk, belief that CRCS was too expensive, fear of finding CRC if tested, and attention to and trust in media sources of health information. Such differences may inform the use of gender-specific messages or intervention strategies to increase CRCS test use.

Survey data also have been used to examine reasons for not being screened among nonscreeners. The consistent and most common reasons for not having a CRC test include lack of awareness or no reason and no physician recommendation.[19,21,23,26,27] These reasons do not appear to differ by gender.[23] Cross-sectional studies report that a physician's recommendation for CRCS is important for patient adherence, but prospective studies suggest that a recommendation is not sufficient for increasing CRCS uptake to desired levels.[28,29]

Cognitive and psychosocial factors

Correlates. Health behavior theories are used to identify cognitive and psychosocial variables that may influence behavior. Many key constructs overlap across the most commonly used behavior change theories or models (e.g., benefits and barriers from the health belief model[30] and pros and cons from the trans-theoretical model[31]). Table 9–1 summarizes the most frequently studied correlates and predictors found to be associated with CRCS. It does not account for the numerous studies that reported nonsignificant associations between these variables and CRCS. Consistent correlates of CRCS include preventive health orientation, physician recommendation, knowledge of cancer risk factors, and perceived benefits (pros) and barriers (cons) to screening. Most, but not all, studies of perceived risk report a positive association with CRCS. Self-efficacy also is positively associated with CRCS, although there is less consensus about how to conceptualize and measure it. Existing measures include items specific to a particular test as well as to screening decisions in general.[32] Fear and worry about CRC or the screening test itself have small, if any, direct effects on CRCS behavior, possibly due to low levels of worry even among high-risk populations.[33] Specifying the source of worry has shown that cancer worries are positively associated with screening, whereas worries about the test may act as a barrier to screening.[34] Hypotheses of a curvilinear effect of worry or anxiety have not been supported.[33]

Few studies have examined affect and social influence in relation to CRCS (Table 9–1). McQueen et al.[35] found positive associations between family members' support and CRCS. Trait-level personality characteristics such as dispositional optimism[36–38] or conscientiousness have seldom been studied. Additional factors related to CRCS are suggested from qualitative studies and warrant further examination.[39–41] For example, low perceived need for CRCS, perceived importance of symptoms for necessitating CRCS,[39,41] perceived risk for competing health conditions,[41] and avoidant and self-exemption tendencies[40] should be explored as important barriers to CRCS in future studies.

Predictors. Relatively few psychosocial constructs have been examined in prospective studies, and fewer have been examined across

Table 9–1. Psychosocial correlates and predictors associated with FOBT, SIG, and COL use

Constructs	Correlates			Predictors		
	FOBT	SIG/COL	Any test	FOBT	SIG/COL	Any test
Preventive health orientation	+	++	++	-	+	
Knowledge of cancer risk factors	+	+	+			
Perceived benefits/pros/outcome expectations	+	+	+	+		+
Perceived barriers/cons[a]	--	--	--		-	
Self-efficacy/perceived behavioral control[b]	+	+		+		+
Perceived risk/susceptibility	+	+/-	+	+		+
Perceived severity	+/-	-		+		
Fear of screening test		-		-		
Fear or worry about CRC	-	-				-
Cancer fatalism	-					
Depression or hostility	-	-				
Dispositional optimism and optimistic beliefs	+	+	+			+
Social influence			+			+
Physician recommendation	++	++	++	+		
Locus of control	+					
Intention	+	+		+		+

ABBREVIATIONS: COL, colonoscopy; CRC, colorectal cancer; FOBT, fecal occult blood test; SIG, sigmoidoscopy.
NOTE: +, ≤ three studies and ++, > three studies report positive associations; -, ≤ three studies and --, > three studies report negative associations.
[a]Includes scales of multiple barriers or a single barrier item (e.g., busy or embarrassed).
[b]Includes general self-efficacy and self-efficacy specific to CRCS.

studies.[14] Even when the same constructs were used, they were often defined and operationalized differently, and few measures of psychosocial constructs have been validated.[17,32,42,43] Nevertheless, cumulative evidence based on prospective study designs and multivariable analyses suggest consistent independent associations between CRCS perceived benefits and barriers, self-efficacy, and intention (Table 9–1). Future research should confirm the predictive utility of cognitive and psychosocial variables, both those previously examined and those not yet examined, with CRCS and explore their interrelations in theory-based causal models.

Causal models. Very few studies have tested hypothesized causal pathways. Health behavior models that posit only direct effects between predictors and intention and behavior may underestimate the total effects of CRCS determinants through other mediating and moderating pathways. Three studies, informed by the health belief model,[30] examined different mediation models predicting CRCS interest,[38] intent,[44] or behavior[45] among U.K. citizens,[38] siblings of CRC patients,[44] and women adherent to mammography recommendations.[45] Wardle et al.[38] reported that attitudes toward medical tests, family history of CRC, and bowel symptoms had direct and indirect effects on interest in getting CRCS through perceived susceptibility, worry, barriers, and benefits. Manne et al.[44] found significant indirect effects of perceived severity of CRC, physician and family support, and sibling closeness on CRCS intention through perceived benefits and barriers. Hay et al.[45] found no support for benefits and barriers as significant mediators of the effects of comparative perceived risk, perceived severity, self-efficacy, and physician recommendation on CRCS. Studies are needed to extend previous research, all of which[38,44,45] used cross-sectional data to test hypothesized causal models. Similarly, future studies should examine hypothesized mediators of intervention effects on CRCS intention and behavior.

Intermediate outcomes. Basic causal models are formed when intermediate behavioral outcomes are examined as mediators. Variables that have been examined as intermediate outcomes of CRCS include intention, knowledge, risk perceptions, and, more recently, preferences and IDM, but their association with CRCS is not well established. Intention is a frequently studied intermediate outcome because it is a strong predictor of behavior. Different intervention strategies may be needed to increase CRCS, depending on individuals' behavioral intentions.[46,47] Understanding how to effectively tailor intervention messages or strategies is informed by process evaluation; however, few studies have reported thorough evaluations of participants' responses to CRCS informational materials[48,49] or examined an intervention's effect on behavioral intentions before a large-scale trial.[50–52]

Community-level interventions have attempted to raise public awareness of CRC and CRCS[53] and individual-level interventions have attempted to influence knowledge[51,52,54] and CRC risk perceptions[55–57] in order to increase CRCS behaviors, but the direct effects on behavior are largely unknown (awareness, knowledge) or small and often not statistically significant (perceived susceptibility). Treatment of these variables as effect modifiers, as well as or instead of intervention mediators, may provide new ways of thinking about the underlying mechanisms relating cognitions and behaviors.

Preferences for specific CRCS tests vary by screening goals and test characteristics (e.g., see references 58–61) and by patient-level variables,[61–63] but only one prospective study examined the effect of patient preferences on subsequent CRCS.[64] They found that only about half of the sample received the test they preferred. More longitudinal studies investigating patient and provider preferences for CRCS, and the effect of potential mismatches in test preferences on CRCS adherence are needed.

IDM also may be an intermediate outcome in CRCS. Braddock et al.[65] created a checklist of nine criteria to assess IDM. Two recent studies used this checklist to evaluate IDM in CRCS discussions between patients and physicians. Wackerbarth et al.[66] conducted physician interviews to elicit typical recommendations for CRCS, and Ling et al.[67] audiotaped patient-physician visits and reviewed medical records. Both studies found that CRCS discussions between patients and physicians included little evidence of IDM. Communication between patients and providers appears to be essential to patients' satisfaction and preventive care use,[68,69] but the nature of patient-provider discussions about cancer screening are poorly understood. Not all CRCS discussions lead to CRCS adherence; therefore, we need to better understand which components of these discussions or which IDM criteria are important for increasing CRCS uptake.[28,67] Future studies will need to examine whether these factors are indeed significant mediators of the effect of interventions on CRCS. Evidence of mediation, if demonstrated, may elucidate the different pathways of influence on CRCS behavior and suggest optimal intervention targets.

Environment. Studies using multilevel statistical analysis can examine the independent and interactive effects of individual- and area-level variables on CRCS and potentially identify screening disparities in specific geographic areas that could be targeted for interventions or CRCS programs. A systematic review of U.S. studies found small positive associations between area-level socioeconomic factors and CRCS after controlling for individual-level socioeconomic factors, although not all were statistically significant.[70] Independent of individual-level factors, health maintenance organization (HMO) market-level factors (e.g., penetration, competition, proportion of staff/group/network HMOs) have been shown to affect CRCS use among Asian American and Pacific islanders, but not among whites.[71] Studies of other health behaviors have examined the effects of geographic residence,[72] the "built" environment,[73] social-psychological norms,[74] and workplace conditions and policies,[75] which may help identify important area-level influences on CRCS that warrant investigation. Future research is needed to further elucidate the mechanisms of influence underlying observed associations between area-level factors and CRCS. Valid and reliable measures of socioeconomic status and other area-level variables also are needed.

INTERVENTIONS TO PROMOTE CRCS

Efforts to promote the uptake of CRCS began in the 1980s and accelerated in 1997 upon publication of consensus screening guidelines.[76] There have been relatively few systematic reviews or meta-analyses of the effectiveness of interventions on CRCS test use[14,15,77–81] and those reviews focused on FOBT. We summarize findings for FOBT using published systematic reviews. More recent studies have promoted the uptake of CRCS tests other than or in addition to FOBT, and these studies are reviewed in more detail.

Interventions to promote the uptake of FOBT. Snell and Buck[77] conducted a meta-analysis of multiple cancer-screening behavioral interventions directed at patients, providers, or both in studies that were published between 1989 and 1994. The strongest summary effect size for FOBT (measured as the difference between treatment groups in the proportion or frequency of patients who were screened) was found for patient and provider interventions combined (20.6%; 95% confidence interval [CI] = 19.0–22.2%). Stone et al.[78] conducted a meta-analysis of FOBT interventions published from 1966 through February 1999. Using the odds ratio as the summary effect size measure, they reported a range of effect sizes for different intervention types: 1.18 (95% CI = 0.98–1.43) for minimal interventions using provider feedback; 1.38 (95% CI = 0.84–2.25) for patient education; 1.46 (95% CI = 1.15–1.85) for provider reminders; 1.82 (95% CI = 1.35–2.46) for patient financial incentives; 2.75 (95% CI = 1.90–3.97) for patient reminders; 3.01 (95% CI = 1.98–4.56) for provider education; and 17.6 (95% CI = 12.3–25.2) for interventions that targeted organizational change. It is noteworthy that the summary effect size measure for systems-level interventions involving organizational change was much larger than for any of the patient- or provider-directed interventions.

The Task Force on Community Preventive Services systematic reviews included studies of FOBT published through 2004. Interventions were classified into three broad categories with subtypes. The three categories were as follows: client-directed interventions to increase community demand for screening,[79] client-directed interventions to increase community access to screening services,[80] and interventions to increase recommendation and delivery of screening by healthcare providers.[81] The measure of effect size for individual studies was the absolute percentage point change from a baseline or comparison value in completed FOBT screening attributable to the intervention; the summary effect size measure was the median percentage point increase postintervention and interquartile interval (IQI). Interventions to increase community demand for screening included client reminders, client incentives, mass media, small media, group education, and one-on-one education.[79] They found support for the effectiveness of client reminders (median = 11.5 percentage points; IQI = 8.9, 20.3) and small media (median = 12.7 percentage points; IQI = 0, 26.4) but not for other subtypes of interventions in this category. Interventions to reduce barriers to access included those that reduced structural barriers and those that reduced out-of-pocket costs to clients.[80] Only interventions designed to reduce barriers such as mailing FOBT kits were effective at increasing completion (median = 16.1 percentage points; IQI = 12.1, 22.9). Interventions to increase delivery of CRCS by healthcare providers included provider assessment and feedback and provider incentives.[81] There was sufficient evidence to recommend the use of provider assessment and feedback (median = 13 percentage points; IQI = 12, 23) but not incentives.[81]

Interventions conducted in the United States to promote CRCS with tests other than or in addition to FOBT.

Characteristics of intervention studies that promoted CRCS with tests other than or in addition to FOBT are summarized in Table 9–2. All but four studies[82–85] were conducted in healthcare settings. All but one[84] was of average-risk people; Rawl et al. studied first-degree relatives of CRC patients. Most of the study populations included both men and women and were predominantly white. Most studies offered multiple CRCS test options, although two promoted only COL.[86,87] Most measured the outcome with objective data sources such as medical records.

A description of the interventions including effect size estimates is shown in Table 9–3. If available, we report the postintervention difference between the intervention and control groups. We organize our discussion by whether the intervention was directed at patients or at providers and/or their practices. We classified patient-directed interventions based on the primary approach as tailored, education/motivation, or navigation. We chose to be inclusive and included a few recent pilot studies of innovative approaches.

Patient-directed interventions

Tailored interventions. Five studies used tailored print materials[82,84,95] or telephone counseling.[83,88] Tailoring is a process of creating individualized messages matched to a person's profile of measured constructs.[99] The rationale for tailoring a communication to a person's specific needs, concerns, emotions, and values is that it is more likely to reduce "noise" and consequently bring about intended behavior change than generic messages.[100]

Marcus et al.[82] evaluated tailored mailed print materials using constructs from the health belief[30] and trans-theoretical[31] models. Callers to the Cancer Information Service received one of four interventions, three of which were tailored and varied in the source of data used to tailor messages and in the frequency of delivery. At 6-month follow-up, there was no difference in self-reported CRCS across the four groups. At 14-months, only one of the three tailored conditions differed statistically from the single untailored condition. In a study of first-degree relatives of CRC patients, Rawl et al.[84] found that a mailed tailored print brochure based on the health belief and trans-theoretical models was no more effective than generic print materials. Myers et al.[95] used constructs from the preventive health model[101] and the decision stage construct from the precaution adoption process model[102] to develop tailored print messages. The three intervention groups differed from the usual care control group but not from each other, indicating that tailored and untailored intervention materials were equally effective and that the addition of a telephone call did not increase screening rates above that achieved with mailed materials. Costanza et al.[88] also found no difference in CRCS completion for patients receiving a mailed print brochure based on decision stage[102] followed by a computer-assisted tailored telephone counseling call compared with a survey-only control

group. Basch et al.[83] evaluated tailored telephone outreach compared with mailed generic print materials in a predominantly Black urban population and found participants in the telephone outreach group were more likely to complete CRCS.

Education/motivation interventions. Five studies evaluated educational interventions using constructs from behavior change theories or from models of health services utilization to motivate patients to be screened.[58,59,85,87,98] Pignone et al.[59] randomized patients to view a video on CRCS or automobile safety. After viewing the CRCS video, patients chose a brochure based on the trans-theoretical model stages of change construct that reflected their current readiness to be screened, and a card that identified the patient's stage was attached to the chart before the provider encounter. Patients who viewed the CRCS video were more likely to be screened than patients in the attention-control condition. Denberg et al.[87] evaluated the efficacy of an educational brochure in promoting scheduling and completing screening COL among patients who received a referral from a primary care provider. The brochure was personalized with the name of the patient's primary care provider and contained information about CRC and CRCS including risks of COL. Compared with usual care, patients receiving the brochure were more likely to complete COL. Zapka et al.[98] found that an educational video based on the precede/proceed model[103] and constructs from social cognitive theory[104] that encouraged patients to discuss CRCS, especially SIG, with their provider was no more effective than usual care in promoting CRCS uptake. Dolan[58] compared a patient decision aid based on multicriteria decision-making theory with an educational session. The decision aid was intended to help patients choose a CRCS test based on their judgment of factors such as the importance of avoiding CRC, avoiding side effects from screening tests, and avoiding false positive results. There was no difference between the study groups in CRCS completion. In a community-based study, Thompson et al.[85] developed an intervention targeting multiple cancer prevention behaviors, including CRCS, based on principles of community organization. There were no statistically significant differences in CRCS rates between the intervention and control communities.

Patient navigation. Recent studies have investigated navigation strategies to increase CRCS in healthcare settings. Although not explicitly based on behavioral science theory, navigation involves addressing patient and system barriers to accessing healthcare, such as scheduling and completing CRCS,[105] which likely increase behavioral capacity and self-efficacy. Dietrich et al.[89,90] evaluated interventions that involved navigation to promote breast, cervical, and colon cancer screening among women; they evaluated a single call compared with a series of calls to educate and assist women in scheduling and completing appointments.[89] Women who received a series of calls were more likely to complete CRCS. In another study, a mammography outreach program was modified to include information and recommendations for cervical and colon cancer screening and was compared with an enhanced version of that program.[90] The enhanced intervention showed a modest positive effect on CRCS completion.

Chen et al.[106] reported a case series in which patients referred for COL were navigated through the healthcare system. Of those who received some contact from the navigator, 66% completed COL. In a pilot study of 21 patients in the same setting, Christie et al.[86] found that 7 of 13 patients randomized to navigation completed COL compared with 1 of 8 patients in the nonnavigated group. In another small-scale study, Jandorf et al.[93] found that patients randomized to navigation were more likely than patients receiving usual care to complete endoscopy; there was a nonsignificant increase for FOBT. A pilot study by Myers and colleagues[107] used a pre/post-design to assess the feasibility of tailored navigation. On the basis of a patient's decision stage for FOBT and COL, ascertained during a single telephone call, a navigator guided patients through the process needed to complete the test. Eighteen of thirty-two patients who decided to do FOBT and 45 of 122 patients who decided to do COL completed the test by study's end. This pilot led to two randomized controlled trials that are currently in the field.

Table 9–2. Selected characteristics of U.S. randomized controlled trials of interventions to increase the uptake of colorectal cancer screening

Primary author	Data collection	Study setting	Age range	% Women	% White	Targeted CRCS test/primary outcome	Follow-up interval	Outcome measurement
Basch, C (2006)[83]	2000–2002	Membership lists of a health benefit fund	≥52	71	16	FOBT, SIG, COL, BE	6 months	SR, MR, AD
Christie, J (2008)[86]	2004	1 community health center	>50	75	8[a]	COL	6 months	MR
Costanza, ME (2007)[88]	2001–2004	37 community-based primary care practices	52–77	57	92	FOBT, SIG, COL	17–22 months	MR
Denberg, T (2006)[87]	2005	2 general internal medicine practices	≥50	62	57	COL	4 months	AD
Dietrich, A (2006)[89]	2001–2004	11 community and migrant health centers	50–69	100	NR	FOBT, SIG, COL, BE	18 months	MR
Dietrich, A (2007)[90]	2005	6 community health centers	50–69	100	NR	FOBT, SIG, COL, BE	11 months	AD
Dolan, JG (2002)[58]	NR	2 internal medicine practices	≥50	53	98	FOBT, SIG, COL, BE	2–3 months	MR
Ferreira, MR (2005)[91]	2001–2003	2 VA general medicine clinics	≥50	0	45	FOBT, SIG, COL	6–18 months	MR
Ganz, P (2006)[92]	2000–2002	36 provider organizations	52–83	52	64	FOBT, SIG, COL	24 months	MR
Jandorf, L (2005)[93]	2002	1 primary care practice	≥50	74	NR	FOBT, SIG, COL	6 months	MR
Lane, DS (2008)[94]	2004–2006	8 community health centers	≥50	63	22[a]	FOBT, SIG, COL	12 months	MR
Marcus, A (2005)[82]	NR	9 NCI Cancer Information Service call centers	≥50	83	85	FOBT, SIG, COL	6 and 14 months	SR
Myers, RE (2007)[95]	2002	1 primary care practice	50–74	67	42	FOBT, SIG, COL, BE[b]	24 months	SR, MR
Pignone, M (2000)[59]	1998	3 community primary care practices	50–75	61	87	FOBT, SIG	3–6 months	MR
Rawl, S (2008)[84]	NR	Relatives of CRC patients identified through cancer registries and oncology clinics	≥40	69	77	FOBT, SIG, COL	3 months	SR
Ruffin, M (2004)[96]	1994–1998	22 primary care practices	≥50	50	51	FOBT, SIG	Annually for 4 years	MR
Thompson, B (2006)[85]	2003–2005	20 farming communities	≥50	55	70	FOBT, SIG, COL	30 months	SR
Walsh, J (2005)[97]	2000–2001	Community and academic general internal medicine practices	50–79	57	NR	FOBT, SIG, COL	12 months	MR
Zapka, J (2004)[98]	1999–2000	5 clinics, most were internal medicine or family practice	50–74	57	NR	FOBT, SIG, COL, BE[b]	4–6 months	SR

ABBREVIATIONS: AD, administrative data; BE, barium enema; COL, colonoscopy; CRCS, colorectal cancer screening; FOBT, fecal occult blood test; MR, medical record; NCI, National Cancer Institute; NR, not reported; SIG, sigmoidoscopy; SR, self-report.

[a]Christie et al.: Of the 21 participants, 2 (8%) were classified as "other", the rest (n = 19) were Hispanic or African American. Lane et al.: 78% of the sample was classified as nonwhite; the race/ethnicity of the other 22% was not specified.

[b]Myers et al. promoted FOBT and SIG in the intervention materials, but measured completion of FOBT, SIG, COL, or BE. Zapka et al. promoted SIG, but measured completion of FOBT, SIG, COL, or BE.

Provider and practice-directed interventions. Three studies targeted providers[91,92,94] and two[91,97] targeted both patients and providers. Some approaches included changing the organization of healthcare delivery in addition to provider-directed interventions. Ferreira et al.[91] found that screening rates increased at a clinic where providers received a 2-hour workshop on CRCS and on improving communication with low-literacy patients in addition to periodic feedback on the clinic's and their own performance. The intervention was particularly effective among low-literacy patients. Lane et al.[94] found significant positive effects in clinics exposed to an intervention that combined continuing medical education with a team-building strategic planning exercise. In contrast, Ganz et al.[92] found no intervention effect in a large-scale effectiveness trial of a quality-improvement intervention that focused on system changes to increase offering and completion of CRCS.

Table 9–3. Characteristics of interventions to promote colorectal cancer screening

Primary author	Delivery channel(s)	Theoretical framework	Control group	Final sample	Intervention description	% CRCS[a]
Patient-directed interventions						
Tailored						
Basch, C(2006)[83]	Mail and telephone	"several behavioral sciences and educational theories" (p. 2247)	Active	446	G1: Generic printed materials consisting of a cover letter and a Centers for Disease Control brochure G2: Telephone education based on behavioral science theories. Goals of the intervention were to establish rapport with the participant; reinforce accurate knowledge and health beliefs, correct misconceptions, and bolster motivation to obtain CRCS based on the participant's readiness and cognitive factors; address barriers and skill deficits; provide social and emotional support to obtain CRCS; and elicit a verbal commitment to obtain CRCS	G1: 6 G2: 27[b]
Costanza, ME(2007)[88]	Mail and telephone	Precaution adoption process model	Survey-only	2448	G1: Survey-only G2: Mailed print brochure based on stages of adoption construct followed 3 months later by computer-assisted tailored telephone counseling call. The protocol included a motivational counseling segment for subjects who were not planning to get tested	G1: 24 G2: 25[c]
Marcus, A(2005)[82]	Mail	Health belief model; trans-theoretical model	Active	4014	G1: Single untailored print brochure (single untailored) G2: Single tailored booklet (single tailored) G3: 4 tailored booklets over a 12-month period using information obtained at baseline (multiple tailored) G4: 4 tailored booklets over a 12-month period using information obtained at baseline (first booklet) and at a 6-month telephone follow-up (second through fourth booklets) (multiple retailored) All participants received a brief educational message encouraging CRCS at the completion of the baseline interview	G1: 42 G2: 44 G3: 51 G4: 48[d]
Myers, RE(2007)[95]	Mail and telephone	Preventive health model	Survey-only	1546	G1: Survey-only G2: Standard intervention consisting of a personalized invitation letter, informational booklet, FOBT, and reminder letter G3: Standard intervention plus two tailored message pages addressing personal barriers to CRCS identified on the baseline survey G4: Standard intervention and message pages plus a phone call from a trained health educator who reviewed the mailed materials and encouraged CRCS	G1: 33 G2: 46 G3: 44 G4: 48[e]
Rawl, S(2008)[84]	Mail	Health belief model; trans-theoretical model	Active	140	G1: Generic print brochure from the American Cancer Society G2: Tailored print booklet	G1: 21 G2: 14[c]
Education/motivation						
Denberg, T(2006)[87]	Mail	None reported	No contact	781	G1: Usual care G2: Usual care plus an informational brochure with the name of the patient's primary care physician, information CRC and CRCS, and encouragement to call and schedule a procedure	G1: 59 G2: 71[b]

Primary author	Delivery channel(s)	Theoretical framework	Control group	Final sample	Intervention description	% CRCS[a]
Dolan, JG(2002)[58]	Telephone	Analytic hierarchy process	Active	96	G1: An interview consisting of a preliminary phase and an educational phase. The first phase described CRC, administered a survey to collect demographic and medical history data, and CRCS test preference. The second phase described CRCS tests and urged patients to discuss CRCS with their physician at their upcoming visit G2: Same as phase 1. Phase 2 consisted of a detailed analysis of the decision regarding the recommended CRCS options using the analytic hierarchy process. This process resulted in a choice of a CRCS test and patients were encouraged to discuss this test choice with their physician	G1: 52 G2: 49 (NS)
Pignone, M(2000)[59]	Video, chart reminder	Trans-theoretical model	Attention control	249	G1: Viewed a video on car safety, seat belt use, and airbags and received a brochure on automobile safety G2: Viewed an educational video on CRC and CRCS and then chose one of three color-coded brochures that best reflected their readiness to be screened. A matching laminated card was attached to the patient's chart before the provider visit	G1: 23 G2: 37[b]
Thompson, B(2006)[85]	Mostly in person	Community organization principles	Survey-only	20 communities/ 1863 people	G1: No activities G2: Community organization principles with activities directed at the community (e.g., health fairs), organizational (awareness efforts through clinics, churches, worksites, etc.), small group (e.g., home health parties), and individual (e.g., promotoras) levels	FOBT[f] Hispanic G1: 53 G2: 70 NH White G1: 49 G2: 48
Zapka, J(2004)[98]	Video	Precede/proceed model; social cognitive theory	Survey-only	938	G1: Usual care G2: Viewed a video that encouraged patients to discuss CRCS, particularly SIG, with their physician at their upcoming appointment	G1: 55 G2: 55[c]

Patient navigator

Primary author	Delivery channel(s)	Theoretical framework	Control group	Final sample	Intervention description	% CRCS[a]
Christie, J(2008)[86]	Telephone	None reported	Usual care	21	G1: Patients were referred for COL by the primary care provider. A medical assistant faxed the referral form to the GI scheduler who called the patient to schedule COL and discuss the preparation. Patients were called 2 days before the COL G2: Patients were referred for COL by the primary care provider. A navigator reviewed the referral form and faxed it to the GI scheduler. The navigator facilitated all aspects of scheduling and completing COL	G1: 13 G2: 54 (NS)
Dietrich, A(2006)[89]	Telephone	None reported but could infer TTM based on evaluation measures	Active	1413	G1: A single telephone call during which staff answered questions about preventive care, advised women to obtain needed preventive care G2: A series of telephone support calls from a trained prevention care manager who facilitated the screening process by addressing barriers All women received the publication *Put prevention into practice personal health guide* which contained information about recommended preventive services	G1: 50 G2: 63[b]

(Continued)

Table 9–3. Continued

Primary author	Delivery channel(s)	Theoretical framework	Control group	Final sample	Intervention description	% CRCS[a]
Dietrich, A(2007)[90]	Telephone	None reported but based on clinical outreach program	Active	1316	G1: Modification of an existing mammography outreach program to include mailed educational materials on breast, cervical, and CRCS and a brief telephone call to recommend that they discuss cervical and CRCS with their provider G2: Modified outreach program but the telephone call included a detailed assessment of barriers to screening, assistance to overcome barriers, scheduling assistance, and appointment reminders	G1: 25 G2: 32 (NS)
Jandorf, L(2005)[93]	Mail and telephone	Precede/proceed model	Usual care	78	G1: FOBT cards were placed in the charts of all participants to serve as a cue to the physician to recommend CRCS. Physicians were encouraged to recommend FOBT completion and endoscopy G2: In addition to usual care, a navigator provided assistance to complete CRCS using written reminders, telephone calls, scheduling assistance, and encouragement	FOBT G1: 25 G2: 42 (NS) Endoscopy G1: 5 G2: 24[b]
Physician-directed interventions						
Ferreira, MR(2005)[91]	In person	None reported	Usual care	2 clinics/ 1978 patient charts	G1: Usual care was not described G2: A 2-hr workshop on rationale and guidelines for CRCS and on improving communication with patients with low-literacy skills. Every 4–6 months, during the study, providers were invited to attend 1-hr sessions to receive feedback on their own and the clinic's performance. Small group discussions and role-playing sessions focused on empowering providers to effectively recommend CRCS	G1: 32 G2: 41[b]
Ganz, P(2006)[92]	In person with telephone support	Cyclical model for practice change based on Dietrich's work	Usual care	36 clinics/ 1850 patient charts	G1: Usual care varied in the control group clinics G2: Quality-improvement program focused on CRCS that used the existing structure of the provider organizations and QI staff to implement multiple strategies over a 2-year period including the identification of organizational opinion leaders, enhancement of provider self-efficacy, and adherence to CRCS guidelines	G1: 26 G2: 26 (NS)
Lane, DS (2008)[94]	In person	Health belief model; trans-theoretical model; social cognitive theory; precaution adoption process model	Usual care/ attention control	8 clinics/ 2224 patient charts	G1: Usual care varied in the control group clinics. Providers in the control group received a CME on obesity G2: 1-hr CME session for providers at each clinic that included a brief description of four theories of health behavior that could be used to address common barriers to CRCS and facilitate risk communication and informed and shared decision making. This session was followed by a 1-hr facilitated strategic planning session with the entire health center staff using a strengths, weaknesses, opportunities, and threats (SWOT) analysis to identify ways to improve CRCS	G1: 41 G2: 61[b,g]

Primary author	Delivery channel(s)	Theoretical framework	Control group	Final sample	Intervention description	% CRCS[a]
Ruffin, M(2004)[96]	Prevention flow sheet with cues (providers) Wallet-size card (patients)	None reported	Usual care	22 clinics/ 17,215 patient charts	G1: Usual care varied in the control group clinics G2: *Provider intervention:* The goal of the office intervention was to provide to all staff members at every patient encounter the patient's screening history and current CRCS recommendations. Implementation varied based on the resources and organizational issues in the practice. The most common method was some type of prevention flow sheet with cues. *Patient intervention:* The goal was to provide patients with a record of their past screening and cues to future screening that was durable and portable	NS[h]
Walsh, J(2005)[97]	In person (providers) Mail (patients)	Principles of academic detailing	Usual care	94 providers/ 7993 patient charts	G1: Usual care varied by setting G2: *Provider intervention:* Educational seminars and academic detailing. Seminars were offered to all physicians in the IPA, whether they were participating in the study and whether they were in the intervention or the control group. Academic detailing involved a one-on-one interaction with each physician in the intervention group. "Principles of academic detailing include investigating knowledge and motivations, defining clear educational and behavioral objectives, presenting both sides of controversial issues, and stimulating active physician participation in interactions" (p. 1098) *Patient intervention:* Included a personalized letter, an educational brochure, and an FOBT kit. The letter was from the patient's physician, indicated CRCS was due, stated the importance of CRCS, and encouraged patients to discuss SIG or COL with their physician. The brochure addressed commonly asked questions about CRCS	Provider rates (patients enrolled 2 years): [i] G1: 79 G2: 75 (5 years): G1: 87 G2: 77 Patient rates (2 years): G1: 78 G2: 77 (5 years): G1: 80 G2: 84

ABBREVIATIONS: COL, colonoscopy; CRC, colorectal cancer; CRCS, colorectal cancer screening; FOBT, fecal occult blood test; GI, gastrointestinal; IQI, interquartile interval; NS, not significant; SIG, sigmoidoscopy; TTM, trans-theoretical model.

NOTE: [a]Percentages are for any recommended CRCS test unless otherwise noted.

[b]Statistically significant.

[c]No statistically significant difference for a combined measure of any CRCS test or for any of the separate tests studied; data for separate tests are not shown in the table.

[d]At 6-month follow-up there was no statistically significant difference between G1 vs. G2–4 combined (data not shown). At 14-month follow-up the only significant pairwise difference was between G1 vs. G3.

[e]The difference between G1 and each of the other three groups was statistically significant. The three intervention groups did not differ statistically from each other.

[f]Thompson et al. calculated rates of FOBT and SIG separately for Hispanic and non-Hispanic whites. Only FOBT comparisons are shown in the table. Rates of SIG for Hispanics were G1: 70 vs. G2: 84; for non-Hispanic whites they were G1: 80 vs. G2: 77. None of the comparisons was statistically significant.

[g]Because screening rates differed across groups at baseline, the outcome measure was calculated as the percentage change from baseline. There was no statistically main effect of the patient-directed, provider-directed, or combined intervention.

[h]Walsh et al. calculated CRCS rates for providers and for patients among patients enrolled 2 and 5 years. Rates were calculated for any CRCS test (shown in the table) and for FOBT, SIG, and COL. For physician rates, none of the comparisons was statistically significant. For patient rates, rates of SIG were significantly higher in the intervention group and rates of FOBT were significantly lower in the intervention group; all other comparisons were not significant.

[i]The outcome measured was CRCS completion, referral for screening SIG or COL, or dispensing an FOBT kit.

Walsh et al.[97] conducted educational seminars and academic detailing with one-on-one interaction with intervention group physicians to educate and motivate them to discuss and offer patients CRCS. The patient-directed intervention involved a personalized letter, an educational brochure, and an FOBT kit. Neither intervention was statistically different from the control group for any CRCS test use. Ruffin and Gorenflo[96] randomized practices to one of four groups: control, practice-based intervention, patient-based intervention, or both. The practice-based intervention consisted of changing the organizational structure so that at every patient encounter, the patient's screening history and current screening recommendations were available to all staff members. The patient intervention consisted of a wallet-sized card listing past screening status and providing cues to future screening. There was no statistically significant effect for any of the three intervention conditions.

DISCUSSION AND DIRECTIONS FOR FUTURE RESEARCH

Systematic reviews identified several effective strategies for promoting FOBT including minimal interventions such as patient and provider reminders, education, and organizational changes that reduced structural barriers.[78–80] More recently, health promotion interventions for CRCS in the United States have focused on CRCS by any recommended test. We found limited and inconsistent support for the approaches used in recent studies that targeted CRCS behaviors other than or in addition to FOBT. While navigation strategies that involved reducing barriers to CRCS appear promising, with the exception of the work by Dietrich et al.,[89,90] the studies were small-scale, pilot studies. Dietrich et al. studied only women; thus, the generalizability of their results to men is unknown. Support for other patient-directed approaches including tailoring and education/motivation was mixed, as was the evidence for provider-directed interventions. Many of the tailoring and education/ motivation interventions were based on approaches demonstrated to be effective in promoting mammography; however, the greater complexity associated with CRCS (e.g., multiple test options, multiple steps to complete the testing process) may introduce barriers that are not easily overcome by strategies that seek to educate and motivate patients and providers. For the foreseeable future, the guidelines will continue to recommend multiple CRCS options, and it is likely that new tests will be added to the menu of options. Further, the U.S. Preventive Services Task Force recommends that a decision about which test to do be made between patients and providers based on factors such as patient preferences, physician recommendation, and insurance coverage.[108] We know very little about whether or not, and if so how, patient and physician preferences, and their congruence or lack thereof, affect test completion. We also know very little about whether patients and providers are engaging in IDM and shared decision making and what the outcome of that process is.

There is a large body of cross-sectional research on sociodemographic, access, and psychosocial correlates of CRCS. There are far fewer prospective studies of predictors and almost no research on mediating and moderating factors. None of the intervention studies reviewed here conducted mediation analyses. Such analyses can help us better understand what works and why interventions fail. Additional research is needed to understand the effect of potential moderators of intervention effects or moderators of associations between psychosocial predictors of CRCS. Potential moderators that need to be more carefully examined include gender, prior CRCS test use, indicators of objective (e.g., family history) or perceived CRC risk, and the possible disagreement between patients and providers about test preferences.

In addition to achieving a better understanding of the mechanisms through which constructs from behavior change theories affect CRCS, we need to look beyond individual-level determinants and conceptualize screening behavior in the larger context in which the process of cancer screening occurs.[11,109] Further exploration of area-level factors such as neighborhood characteristics may increase our understanding of where and how to intervene to promote CRCS. Use of alternative paradigms such as organization and systems theories also may lead to new insights

into how to conceptualize behavior change for cancer screening.[110] New conceptualizations may require a different approach to study design. A number of recent authors have called for alternatives to the randomized controlled trial in order to increase the external validity of study results (e.g., see reference 111).

To date, most studies of CRCS have focused on promoting one-time or recent screening among people who have never been screened or are overdue. Considering the cancer-screening continuum, attention to adherence to follow-up of abnormal screening tests is important.[112,113] Promoting repeat or regular CRCS is likely to be even more challenging than for mammography because there are different test options with different time intervals for repeat screening. On the basis of their experience with one test, a patient may decide to try a different test option the next time. Longer time intervals for some CRCS tests require systems that can track patients' screening histories to identify patients who are due and to avoid overuse of resources.

Since we lack a national healthcare system through which screening programs can be conducted and the screening status of the population monitored, most screening programs in the United States are characterized as opportunistic, although some health plans systematically provide CRCS to eligible members. This circumstance limits our ability to conduct population-based intervention research in the United States that may have broader applicability. In contrast, countries with universal healthcare are able to enumerate the eligible population and offer screening systematically to average-risk people as is being done in a number of countries.[114] Some of these programs have nested behavioral interventions designed to increase screening in efficacy trials of the procedure (e.g., see reference 115) or evaluated the acceptability of different contact strategies and test regimens (e.g., see reference 116).

The low prevalence of CRCS relative to breast and cervical cancer remains a concern. The most recent national data continue to show that lack of awareness is a frequently cited reason for not being screened, suggesting that media coverage continues to be a reasonable population-level strategy. However, because obtaining CRCS requires contact with the healthcare system, primary care likely will continue to be the gateway for CRCS, and so there is a need to develop effective approaches to facilitate CRCS through primary care settings.[117,118] Both cervical and breast cancer screening have become a routine part of primary care, largely through changing office systems. One CRCS system barrier that has been removed in some settings is the need for a referral and a preliminary visit to a gastroenterologist before COL.[87]

As we identify effective strategies for increasing CRCS uptake, we will need to find ways to disseminate these strategies into practice. Ultimately, our success will depend on how internally and externally valid our intervention studies are. Application of frameworks for assessing internal[119,120] and external validity[121,122] in the implementation and evaluation of CRCS interventions will enable us to learn from our successes as well as our failures.

ACKNOWLEDGMENTS

This work was supported in part by R01 CA97263 (Drs. Vernon and McQueen), R01 CA112223 (Dr. Vernon), and American Cancer Society MSRG-08–222-01-CPPB (Dr. McQueen).

REFERENCES

1. Jemal A, Siegel R, Ward E, et al. Cancer statistics, 2008. *CA: Cancer J Clin.* 2008;58(2):71–96.

2. American Cancer Society. Cancer facts & figures 2008. http://www.cancer.org/docroot/STT/stt_0_2008.asp?sitearea=STT&level=1. Accessed August 11, 2008.

3. Hardcastle JD, Chamberlain JO, Robinson MHE, et al. Randomized controlled trial of fecal-occult-blood screening for colorectal cancer. *Lancet.* 1996;348(9040):1472–1477.

4. Kronborg O, Fenger C, Olsen J, Jorgensen OD, Sondergaard O. Randomized study of screening for colorectal cancer with fecal-occult-blood test. *Lancet.* 1996;348:1467–1471.

5. Mandel JS, Bond JH, Church TR, et al. Reducing mortality from colorectal cancer by screening for fecal occult blood. Minnesota Colon Cancer Control Study. *N Engl J Med.* 1993;328(19):1365–1371.

6. Newcomb PA, Norfleet RG, Storer BE, Surawicz TS, Marcus PM. Screening sigmoidoscopy and colorectal cancer mortality. *J Natl Cancer Inst.* 1992;84(20):1572–1575.

7. Selby JV, Friedman GD, Quesenberry CP Jr, Weiss NS. A case-control study of screening sigmoidoscopy and mortality from colorectal cancer. *N Engl J Med.* 1992;326(10):653–657.

8. Winawer SJ, Zauber AG, Ho MN, et al. Prevention of colorectal cancer by colonoscopic polypectomy. The National Polyp Study Workgroup. *N Engl J Med.* 1993;329:1977–1981.

9. Winawer S, Fletcher RH, Rex DK, et al. Colorectal cancer screening and surveillance: clinical guidelines and rationale-update based on new evidence. *Gastroenterology.* 2003;124(2):544–560.

10. Levin B, Lieberman DA, McFarland B, et al. Screening and surveillance for the early detection of colorectal cancer and adenomatous polyps, 2008: a joint guideline from the American Cancer Society, the US Multi-Society Task Force on colorectal cancer, and the American College of Radiology. *CA: Cancer J Clin.* 2008;58(3):130–160.

11. Meissner HI, Vernon SW, Rimer BK, et al. The future of research that promotes cancer screening. *Cancer.* 2004;101(Suppl 5):1251–1259.

12. Centers for Disease Control and prevention. Use of colorectal cancer tests—United States, 2002, 2004, and 2006. *MMWR Morb Mortal Wkly Rep.* 2008;57(10):253–258.

13. Meissner HI, Breen NL, Klabunde CN, Vernon SW. Patterns of colorectal cancer screening uptake among men and women in the US. *Cancer Epidemiol Biomarkers Prev.* 2006;15(2):389–394.

14. Vernon SW. Participation in colorectal cancer screening: a review. *J Natl Cancer Inst.* 1997;89(19):1406–1422.

15. Peterson SK, Vernon SW. A review of patient and physician adherence to colorectal cancer screening guidelines. *Semin Colon Rectal Surg.* 2000;11(1):58–72.

16. Jepson R, Clegg A, Forbes C, Lewis R, Sowden AJ, Kleijnen J. The determinants of screening uptake and interventions for increasing uptake: a systematic review. *Health Technol Assess.* 2000;4(14).

17. Vernon SW, Myers RE, Tilley BC. Development and validation of an instrument to measure factors related to colorectal cancer screening adherence. *Cancer Epidemiol Biomarkers Prev.* 1997;6(10):825–832.

18. Hiatt RA, Klabunde CN, Breen NL, Swan J, Ballard-Barbash R. Cancer screening practices from National Health Interview Surveys: past, present, and future. *J Natl Cancer Inst.* 2002;94(24):1837–1846.

19. Shapiro JA, Seeff LC, Thompson TD, Nadel MR, Klabunde CN, Vernon SW. Colorectal cancer test use from the 2005 National Health Interview Survey. *Cancer Epidemiol Biomarkers Prev.* 2008;17(7):1623–1630.

20. Cokkinides VE, Chao A, Smith RA, Vernon SW, Thun MJ. Correlates of underutilization of colorectal cancer screening among U.S. adults, age 50 years and older. *Prev Med.* 2003;36(1):85–91.

21. Seeff LC, Nadel MR, Klabunde CN, et al. Patterns and predictors of colorectal cancer test use in the adult US population: results from the 2000 National Health Interview Survey. *Cancer.* 2004;100(10):2093–2103.

22. Shapiro JA, Seeff LC, Nadel MR. Colorectal cancer-screening tests and associated health behaviors. *Am J Prev Med.* 2001;21(2):132–137.

23. McQueen A, Vernon SW, Meissner HI, Klabunde CN, Rakowski W. Are there gender differences in colorectal cancer test use prevalence and correlates. *Cancer Epidemiol Biomarkers Prev.* 2006;15(4):782–791.

24. Liang S-Y, Phillips KA, Nagamine M, Ladabaum U, Haas JS. Rates and predictors of colorectal cancer screening. *Prev Chronic Dis [serial online].* 2006. www.cdc.gov/pcd/issues/2006/oct/06_0010.htm. Accessed July 23, 2008.

25. Subramanian S, Amonkar MM, Hunt TL. Use of colonoscopy for colorectal cancer screening: evidence from the 2000 National Health Interview Survey. *Cancer Epidemiol Biomarkers Prev.* 2005;14(2):409–416

26. Wee CC, McCarthy EP, Phillips RS. Factors associated with colon cancer screening: the role of patient factors and physician counseling. *Prev Med.* 2005;41(1):23–29.

27. Klabunde CN, Schenck AP, Davis WW. Barriers to colorectal cancer screening among medicare consumers. *Am J Prev Med.* 2006;30(4):313–319.

28. Lafata JE, Divine G, Moon C, Williams LK. Patient-physician colorectal cancer screening discussions and screening use. *Am J Prev Med.* 2006;31(3):202–209.

29. Denberg TD, Melhado TV, Coombes JM, et al. Predictors of nonadherence to screening colonoscopy. *J Gen Intern Med.* 2005;20(11):989–995.

30. Janz NK, Becker MH. The health belief model: a decade later. *Health Educ Quart.* 1984;11(1):1–47.

31. Prochaska JO, Velicer WF, Rossi JS, et al. Stages of change and decisional balance for 12 problem behaviors. *Health Psychol.* 1994;13(1):39–46.

32. McQueen A, Tiro JA, Vernon SW. Construct validity and invariance of four factors associated with colorectal cancer screening across gender, race, and prior screening. *Cancer Epidemiol Biomarkers Prev.* 2008;17(9):2231–2237.

33. Hay JL, Coups EJ, Ford JS. Predictors of perceived risk for colon cancer in a national probability sample in the United States. *J Health Commun.* 2006;11(Suppl 1):71–92.

34. Consedine NS, Magai C, Krivoshekova YS, Ryzewicz L, Neugut AI. Fear, anxiety, worry, and breast cancer screening behavior: a critical review. *Cancer Epidemiol Biomarkers Prev.* 2004;13(4):501–510.

35. McQueen A, Vernon SW, Myers RE, Watts BG, Lee ES, Tilley BC. Correlates and predictors of colorectal cancer screening among male automotive workers. *Cancer Epidemiol Biomarkers Prev.* 2007;16(3):500–509.

36. Brown ML, Potosky AL, Thompson GB, Kessler LG. The knowledge and use of screening tests for colorectal and prostate cancer: data from the 1987 National Health Interview Survey. *Prev Med.* 1990;19(5):562–574.

37. Price JH. Perceptions of colorectal cancer in a socioeconomically disadvantaged population. *J Community Health.* 1993;18(6):347–362.

38. Wardle J, Sutton SR, Williamson S, et al. Psychosocial influences on older adults' interest in participating in bowel cancer screening. *Prev Med.* 2000;31(4):323–334.

39. Wackerbarth SB, Peters JC, Haist SA. Modeling the decision to undergo colorectal cancer screening: insights on patient preventive decision-making. *Med Care.* 2008;46(9 Suppl 1):S17–S22.

40. McCaffery KJ, Borril J, Williamson S, et al. Declining the offer of flexible sigmoidoscopy for bowel cancer: a qualitative investigation of the decision-making process. *Soc Sci Med.* 2001;53(5):679–691.

41. Weitzman ER, Zapka JG, Estabrook B, Goins KV. Risk and reluctance: understanding impediments to colorectal screening. *Prev Med.* 2001;32(6):502–513.

42. Tiro JA, Vernon SW, Hyslop T, Myers RE. Factorial validity and invariance of a survey measuring psychosocial correlates of colorectal cancer screening among African Americans and Caucasians. *Cancer Epidemiol Biomarkers Prev.* 2005;14(12):2855–2861.

43. Rawl SR, Champion VL, Menon U, Loehrer PJ, Vance GH, Skinner CS. Validation of scales to measure benefits and barriers to colorectal cancer screening. *J Psychosocial Oncol.* 2001;19(3/4):47–63.

44. Manne SL, Markowitz A, Winawer SJ, et al. Understanding intention to undergo colonoscopy among intermediate risk siblings of colorectal cancer patients: a test of a meditational model. *Prev Med.* 2003;36:71–84.

45. Hay JL, Ford JS, Klein D. Adherence to colorectal cancer screening in mammography-adherent older women. *J Behav Med.* 2003;26(6):553–576.

46. Fishbein M, Hennessy M, Yzer M, Douglas J. Can we explain why some people do and some people do not act on their intentions? *Psychol Health Med.* 2003;8(1):3.

47. Weinstein ND. The precaution adoption process. *Health Psychol.* 1988;7:355–386.

48. Lipkus IM, Skinner CS, Dement J, et al. Increasing colorectal cancer screening among individuals in the carpentry trade: test of risk communication interventions. *Prev Med.* 2005;40(5):489–501.

49. Williamson S, Wardle J. Increasing participation with colorectal cancer screening: the development of a psycho-educational intervention. In: Rutter D, Quine L, eds. *Changing health behaviour: intervention and research with social cognition models.* Buckingham, England: Open University Press; 2002:105–122.

50. Menon U, Szalacha LA, Belue R, Powell K, Martin KR. Interactive, culturally sensitive education on colorectal cancer screening. *Med Care.* 2008; 46(9 Suppl 1):S44–S50.

51. de Nooijer J, Lechner L, Candel M, de Vries H. Short- and long-term effects of tailored information versus general information on determinants and intentions related to early detection of cancer. *Prev Med.* 2004;38:694–703.

52. Kim J, Whitney A, Hayter S, Lewis C, Campbell M, Sutherland L. Development and initial testing of computer-based patient decision aid to promote colorectal cancer screening for primary care practice. *BMC Med Inform Decis Mak.* 2005;5:36.

53. Jorgensen CM, Gelb CA, Merritt TL, Seeff LC. Observations from the CDC: CDC's screen for life: a national colorectal cancer action campaign. *J Womens Health Gend Based Med.* 2001;10(5):417–423.

54. Geller BM, Skelly JM, Dorwaldt AL, Howe KD, Dana GS, Flynn BS. Increasing patient/physician communications about colorectal cancer. *Med Care.* 2008;46(9 Suppl 1):S36–S43.

55. Weinstein ND, Atwood K, Puleo E, Fletcher RH, Colditz GA, Emmons KM. Colon cancer: risk perceptions and risk communication. *J Health Commun.* 2004;9:53–65.

56. Lipkus IM, Skinner CS, Green LG, Dement J, Samsa GP, Ransohoff DF. Modifying attributions of colorectal cancer risk. *Cancer Epidemiol Biomarkers Prev.* 2004;13(4):560–566.

57. Lipkus IM, Green LG, Marcus AC. Manipulating perceptions of colorectal cancer threat: implications for screening intentions and behaviors. *J Health Commun.* 2003;8(3):213–228.

58. Dolan JG. Randomized controlled trial of a patient decision aid for colorectal cancer screening. *Med Decis Making*. 2002;22(2):125–139.

59. Pignone MP, Harris RP, Kinsinger LS. Videotape-based decision aid for colon cancer screening: a randomized, controlled trial. *Ann Intern Med*. 2000;133(10):761–769.

60. Ling BS, Moskowitz MA, Wachs D, Pearson B, Schroy PC III. Attitudes toward colorectal cancer screening tests. *J Gen Intern Med*. 2001;16(12):822–830.

61. Schroy PC III, Heeren TC. Patient perceptions of stool-based DNA testing for colorectal cancer screening. *Am J Prev Med*. 2005;28(2):208–214.

62. Hawley ST, Volk RJ, Krishnamurthy P, Jibaja-Weiss M, Vernon SW, Kneuper S. Preferences for colorectal cancer screening among racial/ethnically diverse primary care patients. *Med Care*. 2008;46(9 Suppl 1):S10–S16.

63. DeBourcy AC, Lichtenberger S, Felton S, Butterfield KT, Ahnen DJ, Denberg TD. Community-based preferences for stool cards versus colonoscopy in colorectal cancer screening. *J Gen Intern Med*. 2008;23(2):169–174.

64. Wolf RL, Basch CE, Brouse CH, Shmukler C, Shea S. Patient preferences and adherence to colorectal cancer screening in an urban population. *Am J Public Health*. 2006;96(5):809–811.

65. Braddock CH, Edwards KA, Hasenberg NM, Laidley TL, Levinson W. Informed decision making in outpatient practice: time to get back to basics. *JAMA*. 1999;282(24):2313–2320.

66. Wackerbarth SB, Tarasenko YN, Joyce JM, Haist SA. Physician colorectal cancer screening recommendations: an examination based on informed decision making. *Patient Educ Couns*. 2007;66(1):43–50.

67. Ling BS, Trauth JM, Fine MJ, et al. Informed decision-making and colorectal cancer screening: is it occurring in primary care? *Med Care*. 2008;46(9 Suppl 1):S23–S29.

68. Kahana E, Kahana B. Patient proactivity enhancing doctor-patient-family communication in cancer prevention and care among the aged. *Patient Educ Couns*. 2003;50(1):67–73.

69. Roter DL, Hall JA. Studies of doctor-patient interaction. *Annu Rev Public Health*. 1989;10:163–180.

70. Pruitt SL, Shim MJ, Mullen PD, Vernon SW, Amick BC 3rd. Association of area socioeconomic status and breast, cervical, and colorectal cancer screening: a systematic review. *Cancer Epidemiol Biomarkers Prev*. 2009;18(10):2579–2599.

71. Ponce NA, Huh S, Bastani R. Do HMO market level factors lead to racial/ethnic disparities in colorectal cancer screening? A comparison between high-risk Asian and Pacific islanders Americans and high-risk whites. *Med Care*. 2005;43(11):1101–1108.

72. Lian M, Jeffe DB, Schootman M. Racial and geographic differences in mammography screening in St. Louis City: a multilevel study. *J Urban Health*. 2008;85(5):677–692.

73. Frank LD, Kerr J, Sallis JF, Miles R, Chapman J. A hierarchy of sociodemographic and environmental correlates of walking and obesity. *Prev Med*. 2008;47(2):172–178.

74. Hamilton WL, Biener L, Brennan RT. Do local tobacco regulations influence perceived smoking norms? Evidence from adult and youth surveys in Massachusetts. *Health Educ Res*. 2008;23(4):709–722.

75. Biener L, Glanz K, McLerran D, et al. Impact of the working well trial on the worksite smoking and nutrition environment. *Health Educ Behav*. 1999;26(4):478–494.

76. Winawer SJ, Fletcher RH, Miller L, et al. Colorectal cancer screening: clinical guidelines and rationale. *Gastroenterology*. 1997;112(2):594–642.

77. Snell JL, Buck EL. Increasing cancer screening: a meta-analysis. *Prev Med*. 1996;25(6):702–707.

78. Stone EG, Morton SC, Hulscher MEJL, et al. Interventions that increase use of adult immunization and cancer screening services: a meta-analysis. *Ann Intern Med*. 2002;136(9):641–651.

79. Baron RC, Rimer BK, Breslow RA, et al. Client-directed interventions to increase community demand for breast, cervical, and colorectal cancer screening. *Am J Prev Med*. 2008;35(1S):S34–S55.

80. Baron RC, Rimer BK, Coates RC, et al. Client-directed interventions to increase community access to breast, cervical, and colorectal cancer screening. *Am J Prev Med*. 2008;35(1S):S56–S66.

81. Sabatino SA, Habarta N, Baron RC, et al. Interventions to increase recommendation and delivery of screening for breast, cervical, and colorectal cancers by healthcare providers: systematic reviews of provider assessment and feedback and provider incentives. *Am J Prev Med*. 2008;35(1 Suppl):S67–S74.

82. Marcus AC, Mason M, Wolfe P, Rimer BK, Lipkus IM. The efficacy of tailored print materials in promoting colorectal cancer screening: results from a randomized trial involving callers to the National Cancer Institute's Cancer Information Service. *J Health Commun*. 2005;10(Suppl 1):83–104.

83. Basch CE, Wolf RL, Brouse CH, et al. Telephone outreach to increase colorectal cancer screening in an urban minority population. *Am J Public Health*. 2006;96(12):2246–2253.

84. Rawl SM, Champion VL, Scott LL, et al. A randomized trial of two print interventions to increase colon cancer screening among first-degree relatives. *Patient Educ Couns*. 2008;71(2):215–227.

85. Thompson B, Coronado GD, Chen L, Islas I. Celebremos La Salud! A community randomized trial of cancer prevention (United States). *Cancer Causes Control*. 2006;17(5):733–746.

86. Christie J, Itzkowitz SH, Lihau-Nkanza I, Castillo A, Redd WH, Jandorf L. A randomized controlled trial using patient navigation to increase colonoscopy screening among low-income minorities. *J Natl Med Assoc*. 2008;100(3):278–284.

87. Denberg TD, Coombes JM, Byers TE, et al. Effect of a mailed brochure on appointment-keeping for screening colonoscopy. *Ann Intern Med*. 2006;145(12):895–900.

88. Costanza ME, Luckmann R, Stoddard AM, White MJ, Stark JR, Avrunin JS. Using tailored telephone counseling to accelerate the adoption of colorectal cancer screening. *Cancer Detect Prev*. 2007;31(3):191–198.

89. Dietrich AJ, Tobin JN, Cassels A, et al. Telephone care management to improve cancer screening among low-income women: a randomized controlled trial. *Ann Intern Med*. 2006;144(8):563–571.

90. Dietrich AJ, Tobin JN, Cassellss A, Robin CM, Reh M, Romero KA. Translation of a efficacious cancer-screening intervention to women enrolled in a medicaid managed care organization. *Ann Fam Med*. 2007;5(4):320–327.

91. Ferreira MR, Dolan NC, Fitzgibbon ML, et al. Health care provider-directed intervention to increase colorectal cancer screening among veterans: results of a randomized controlled trial. *J Clin Oncol*. 2005;23(7):1548–1554.

92. Ganz PA, Farmer MM, Belman MJ, et al. Results of a randomized controlled trial to increase colorectal cancer screening in a managed care health plan. *Cancer*. 2005;104(10):2072–2083.

93. Jandorf L, Gutierrez Y, Lopez J, Christie J, Itzkowitz SH. Use of a patient navigator to increase colorectal cancer screening in an urban neighborhood health clinic. *J Urban Health*. 2005;82(2):216–224.

94. Lane DS, Messina CR, Cavanagh MF, Chen JJ. A provider intervention to improve colorectal cancer screening in county health centers. *Med Care*; 2008;46(9 Suppl):S109–S116.

95. Myers RE, Sifri R, Hyslop T, et al. A randomized controlled trial of the impact of targeted and tailored interventions on colorectal cancer screening. *Cancer*. 2007;110(9):2083–2091.

96. Ruffin MT, Gorenflo DW. Interventions fail to increase cancer screening rates in community-based primary care practices. *Prev Med*. 2004; 39(3):435–440.

97. Walsh JME, Salazar R, Terdiman JP, Gildengorin G, Perez-Stable EJ. Promoting use of colorectal cancer screening tests: can we change physician behavior? *J Gen Intern Med*. 2005;20(12):1097–1101.

98. Zapka JG, Lemon SC, Puleo E, Estabrook B, Luvkmann R, Erban S. Patient education for colon cancer screening: a randomized trial of a video mailed before a physical examination. *Ann Intern Med*. 2004;141(9):683–692.

99. Kreuter MW, Strecher VJ, Glassman B. One size does not fit all: the case for tailoring print materials. *Ann Behav Med*. 1999;21(4):276–283.

100. Abrams DB, Milne BJ, Bulger D. Challenges and future directions for tailored communication research. *Ann Behav Med*. 1999;21(4):299–306.

101. Myers RE, Ross EA, Jepson C, et al. Modeling adherence to colorectal cancer screening. *Prev Med*. 1994;23(2):142–151.

102. Weinstein ND, Sandman PM. The precaution adoption process model. In: Glanz K, Rimer BK, Lewis FM, eds. *Health Behavior and Health Education*. 3rd ed. San Francisco, CA: Jossey-Bass; 2003:144–160.

103. Green LW, Kreuter MW. *Health promotion planning: an educational and ecological approach*. 3rd ed. Mountain View, CA: Mayfield; 1999.

104. Bandura A. *Social foundations of thought and action: a social cognitive theory*. Englewood Cliffs, NJ: Prentice Hall; 1986.

105. Dohan D, Schrag D. Using navigators to improve care of underserved patients: current practices and approaches. *Cancer*. 2005;104(4):848–855.

106. Chen LA, Santos S, Jandorf L, et al. A program to enhance completion of screening colonoscopy among urban minorities. *Clin Gastroenterol Hepatol*. 2008;6:443–450.

107. Myers RE, Hyslop T, Sifri R, et al. Tailored navigation in colorectal cancer screening. *Med Care*. 2008;46(9 Suppl):S1–S9.

108. U.S. Preventive Services Task Force. Screening for colorectal cancer: recommendations and rationale. *Ann Intern Med*. 2002;137(2):129–131.

109. Fisher EB. The importance of context in understanding behavior and promoting health. *Ann Behav Med*. 2008;35(1):3–18.

110. Resnicow K, Page SE. Embracing chaos and complexity: a quantum change for public health. *Am J Public Health*. 2008;98(8):1382–1389.

111. Glasgow RE. What types of evidence are most needed to advance behavioral medicine? *Ann Behav Med*. 2008;35(1):19–25.

112. Yabroff KR, Leader A, Mandelblatt JS. Is the promise of cancer-screening programs being compromised? Quality of follow-up care after abnormal screening results. *Med Care Res Rev*. 2003;60(1):1–39.

113. Bastani R, Yabroff KR, Myers RE, Glenn B. Interventions to improve follow-up of abnormal findings in cancer screening. *Cancer.* 2004;101(Suppl 5): 1188–1200.

114. Benson VS, Patnick J, Davies AK, et al. Colorectal cancer screening: a comparison of 35 initiatives in 17 countries. *Int J Cancer.* 2008;122(6):1357–1367.

115. Wardle J, Williamson S, McCaffery KJ, et al. Increasing attendance at colorectal cancer screening: testing the efficacy of a mailed, psychoeducational intervention in a community sample of older adults. *Health Psychol.* 2003;22(1):99–105.

116. Segnan N, Senore C, Andreoni B, et al. Randomized trial of different screening strategies for colorectal cancer: patient response and detection rates. *J Natl Cancer Inst.* 2005;97(5):347–357.

117. Klabunde C, Lanier D, Breslau ES, et al. Improving colorectal cancer screening in primary care practice: innovative strategies and future directions. *J Gen Intern Med.* 2007;22(8):1195–1205.

118. Klabunde CN, Lanier D, Meissner HI, Breslau ES, Brown ML. Improving colorectal cancer screening through research in primary care settings. *Med Care.* 2008;46(9 Suppl 1):S1-S4.

119. Davidson KW, Goldstein MG, Kaplan RM, et al. Evidence-based behavioral medicine: what is it and how do we achieve it? *Ann Behav Med.* 2003;26(3):161–171.

120. Kaplan RM, Trudeau KJ, Davidson KW. New policy on reports of randomized clinical trials [editorial]. *Ann Behav Med.* 2004;81.

121. Glasgow RE, Vogt TM, Boles SM. Evaluating the public health impact of health promotion interventions: the RE-AIM framework. *Am J Public Health.* 1999;89(9):1322–1327.

122. Green LW, Glasgow RE. Evaluating the relevance, generalization, and applicability of research: issues in external validation and translation methodology. *Eval Health Prof.* 2006;29(1):126–153.

CHAPTER 10

Cervical Cancer Screening

Suzanne M. Miller and Pagona Roussi

CERVICAL CANCER

Worldwide, cervical cancer is the second most common cancer among women, accounting for 10% of all female cancers, and the second most common cause of death from cancer, after breast cancer.[1] Each year almost 500,000 new cases are diagnosed and 230,000 cervical cancer deaths occur, over 75% of them in less-developed countries.[2] Cervical cancer is the 13th most common cancer overall in the United States,[3] and an estimated 11,070 new cases and 3870 deaths due to this disease are projected for 2008.[4] Screening for cervical cancer in the United States using the Papanicolaou (Pap) test, which allows for the detection of precancerous lesions, began in the 1950s. The introduction of early detection programs in unscreened populations, combined with effective and relatively inexpensive outpatient treatments for detected lesions, has resulted in a significant reduction in invasive cervical cancer rates.[1] Further, tests are now available to detect human papillomavirus (HPV), various subtypes of which have been causally associated with most forms of cervical cancer. These tests can be used as a primary screening tool or as an adjunct to Pap smear testing.[5] Perhaps most encouragingly, prophylactic vaccination for HPV types with high oncogenic potential (types 6, 11, 16, and 18) have recently been developed in an effort to prevent the occurrence of the sexually transmitted infection altogether.[6]

Despite the overall decline in cervical cancer incidence in the developed world, and of mortality rates in general, marked disparities in these rates still persist. For example, incidence rates in less-developed countries are almost twofold higher than those in more-developed countries.[1] Incidence is highest in Africa and Central/South America and lowest in North America and Oceania (Australia and New Zealand).[1] Mortality rates vary more than 10-fold across continents, with the ratio of mortality to incidence ranging from 0.27 in Oceania to 0.79 in Africa.[1] In the United States, Hispanics and older African Americans assume a disproportionate share of the cervical cancer burden.[7,8] Compared with non-Hispanic white women, average annual incidence rates from 2000 to 2004 are almost twice as high for Hispanic women, more than one-and-a-half times as high for African American women, and slightly higher for Asian American/Pacific Islander women.[8] Contributing to these disparities are lower rates of screening, more inadequate medical follow-up of abnormal screening results, and differences in medical treatment for identified lesions or abnormalities.[8,9]

This chapter provides an overview of the barriers to routine cervical cancer screening, as well as barriers to recommended follow-up if an abnormality is detected, with a focus on minorities and other underserved populations. It also reviews the literature on the development and evaluation of interventions designed to overcome these barriers. The Cognitive-Social Health Information Processing (C-SHIP) model is used as the integrative framework for the review of the existing literature.[10,11] Finally, the psychosocial implications of HPV testing and vaccination are discussed.

ACCESS TO CARE BARRIERS

Although cervical screening can successfully prevent the development of cancer, access to care barriers significantly undermine participation in routine screening and to recommended follow-up regimens among underserved minority women; these disparities become more pronounced as age increases.[7,8] Factors that have been associated with lower adherence include demographics (less education, low income, low acculturation levels, and unemployment), as well as lack of insurance.[7-9] Perhaps most noteworthy, underserved minority women are less likely to have a usual source of health care or to receive a recommendation to be tested or treated, both of which are strong predictors of screening barriers.[7-9] Other access barriers that have been reported by minority women, and women of low socioeconomic status (SES), include distance from the clinic, lack of transportation, long waiting hours, lack of child care, and lack of money to pay for the tests and treatment.[8,11] The importance of equal access to the system is highlighted by the findings of one study among 1553 African American and white military women where cost, health insurance, and other health disparities among the two ethnic groups were not a factor.[8] In this case, survival rates for cervical carcinomas were equivalent between the two groups.

THE COGNITIVE SOCIAL INFORMATION PROCESSING MODEL

In addition to access to care, women are characterized by well-defined psychosocial barriers to screening. The C-SHIP model[10-12] provides an integrative framework for identifying the key factors that influence the uptake and maintenance of health-related behaviors. This approach highlights the role of five main cognitive-affective processing units which interact in a complex and personal, but predictable, way for individuals undergoing health threats.[10-12] In particular, on the basis of the relevant literature and findings,[10-12] the theory holds that individuals' encodings (self-construals of risk), beliefs and expectancies about screening and treatment outcomes, health-related values and goals, screening- and cancer-related affects, and self-regulatory competencies combine in a dynamic way to produce a multifactorial response to the health challenge (see Table 10–1).[13]

PSYCHOSOCIAL BARRIERS TO ROUTINE CERVICAL CANCER SCREENING

First, with regard to cervical cancer-relevant encodings, low perceived risk for cervical cancer is common and is associated with nonadherence to routine screening.[8,9] Studies with both Dutch and British women, and with U.S. minority women, have shown that nonresponders are more likely to think that they are at low risk for cervical cancer.[9,14,15] From the C-SHIP perspective, encoding variables such as inadequate risk-related knowledge is also a key factor. Health literacy, which is "the degree to which individuals have the capacity to obtain, process and understand basic health information and services needed to make appropriate health decisions,"[7] has been found to be low among minority women populations.[7] In turn, low health literacy has been associated with low adherence to screening, even when other demographic factors are taken into account.[7,8] Language skills, which are poorer among immigrants and women with low acculturation levels, have been associated not only with low health literacy, but also with nonadherence to screening in the United States.[8] However, this finding is not universal, as studies conducted in the Netherlands and Sweden show similar levels of adherence between women born in these countries and immigrants to these countries,[15,16] possibly reflecting differences in ease of access to the U.S. and European health systems.

Second, beliefs and expectancies held by women contribute to differences in screening. In both the general population and among

Table 10-1. Key psychosocial mediators of behavioral and emotional responses to health threats

1. *Health-relevant encodings/self-construals:* Refers to appraisals regarding one's own health, personal health risks and vulnerabilities, and illness and disease. Includes appraisals of incoming threat and risk-relevant information (e.g., cancer risk feedback)
2. *Health-related beliefs and expectancies:* Specific beliefs and expectations activated in health information processing. Includes expectancies about potential outcomes of behavioral courses of actions (e.g., getting a pap test will reduce my chances of getting cervical cancer) and self-efficacy beliefs (e.g., "I am able to go for my visits for cancer screening when I am supposed to")
3. *Health-related values and goals:* Personal goals and values regarding health and issues that arise from health problems (e.g., importance of body image and child bearing; trusting in the healthcare system.)
4. *Healthcare affective processes:* Emotional states activated in health information processing (e.g., cancer risk-related worries and anxieties, negative feelings about the self; embarrassment)
5. *Health-related self-regulatory coping strategies and competencies:* Knowledge and action strategies for dealing with barriers to disease prevention and control behaviors and for the construction and maintenance of effective behavioral scripts over time. Includes coping skills for executing, maintaining, and adhering to long-term health protective behavioral and medical regimens (e.g., coping with practical barriers to risk-reduction and surveillance behaviors, coping with the social stigma of contracting a sexually-transmitted disease)

Adapted from Miller SM, Fang CY, Manne SL, Engstrom PE, Daly MB. Decision making about prophylactic oophorectomy among at-risk women: psychological influences and implications. Gynecol Oncol. 1999;75:406-412.

underserved minority women, mistrust in the medical benefits of screening and fatalistic beliefs regarding the incurability of cervical cancer have been associated with lower screening rates.[7-9,14,15] Other beliefs that appear to act as a barrier among underserved minority women include the idea that it is better not to know, to consider the test bad luck, to consider that the treatment for cancer is worse than the disease itself, to think that a health preventive action is not necessary unless symptoms are present, and to believe that "cutting" the cancer will lead to its spreading.[7,9]

Third, values and goals are reflected in how the individual weighs the "pros" and "cons" of screening, both of which have been found to influence adherence behaviors. Among the cons of screening are the perception of the examination as an intimate and vulnerable situation which causes embarrassment, fear, and pain,[7,14] and the potential social stigma associated with a diagnosis of cervical cancer because it is a sexually transmitted disease.[8,9] Among African American women, the mistrust of governmental agencies has been reported as a further con to screening.[8] In contrast, a sense that one has a moral responsibility toward sexual partners to be tested is considered a benefit of screening and has been associated with higher adherence.[15]

Finally, in order to be able to participate in screening, individuals must be able to develop specific action plans not only for managing practical and access barriers (e.g., strategies for dealing with the tendency to forget the appointment, lack of transportation, cost of care, family and work responsibilities), but also for managing the negative affects that can be activated by the screening process.[7,9,14] Indeed, negative reactions for some women start with the receipt of a notification to be screened, as it is interpreted as an indication that they have cancer.[17] Several studies have shown that women express concern about their ability to cope with the negative emotions expected to arise from the procedure[7,9,18] and the anxiety anticipated while waiting for the results,[14,18] both of which may act as barriers to screening.

PSYCHOSOCIAL BARRIERS TO FOLLOW-UP CARE TO AN ABNORMAL PAP TEST

The findings reported above indicate that a combination of access barriers and psychosocial factors work to undermine participation in routine screening. We now consider the psychosocial impact of an abnormal Pap test result and the barriers profile that emerges in this context. Following an abnormal Pap test result, a woman is recommended one of several courses of actions for medical follow-up, including having more frequent Pap screenings, undergoing a colposcopy (microscopic inspection of the cervix), which in turn may be followed by repeat screening.[19] Yet, not all women undergo follow-up of an abnormal Pap smear, with some

studies showing adherence rates to be as low as 40%.[20] According to the C-SHIP model, the impact of a positive Pap smear test result depends on how it is interpreted (encoded) and the affects/emotions, expectancies/beliefs, and health goals and values that become activated during cognitive-affective processing of this type of feedback.[12] Further, how a woman deals with the health problem long term depends importantly on her competencies and self-regulatory skills available to cope with the situation.

Encoding (in terms of increased perceptions of risk and vulnerability) seems to be a critical factor in the psychological response, especially in terms of the affects that become primed in response to an abnormal Pap test. Because of the lack of information related to health literacy level and cultural perspective, particularly for urban, minority women, a recommendation that a follow-up is needed is often misinterpreted as an indication that they have cancer.[21-24] Even mildly abnormal test results, with a recommendation for early repeat Pap screening, cause concerns about having cancer.[24] A positive Pap smear has also been associated with fears that it cannot be treated, concerns about the treatment, negative feelings about the self (such as feeling less attractive and more tarnished), fears about not being able to have children in the future, as well as concerns about relationships, lower interest in sex, and more negative attitudes toward sex.[14,22-24] Lack of knowledge about the implications of the abnormal Pap result and low understanding of the reasons for the follow-up appointment are some of the main barriers reported as responsible for delayed care and nonadherence.[13]

These exaggerated interpretations and beliefs about the meaning of an abnormal test result can lead to high levels of anxiety. In comparison with women who receive a negative test result, who report relief,[25] those who receive an abnormal result experience significant mood changes and heightened distress, including elevated levels of anxiety, depression, and intrusive ideation.[14,24] Even among women who report that they understand the meaning and consequences of having mild dysplasia, a considerable percentage report feelings of worry, anxiety, and daily distress, especially in the short-term.[14] Elevated levels of distress have been associated with lack of adherence to recommended follow-up.[14] Other work has found that the negative emotional responses are especially associated with the treatment experience.[13] Women referred for colposcopy report higher distress than women with mild abnormalities referred for early repeat testing,[14] and the levels of distress associated with the colposcopic examination are comparable to those of women about to undergo surgery.[24] Women also report that the colposcopic examination itself is uncomfortable, undignified, an invasion of the body, and engenders feelings of vulnerability and helplessness.[21]

Beliefs and expectancies have also been found to predict compliance, with fatalistic beliefs undermining adherence,[20,26] and the expectancy that one will be able to attend the appointments and control the health problem increasing adherence.[14] In addition, values and goals (reflected in the perceived pros and cons of adhering to the recommended follow-up care) are also linked to attendance rates and type of treatment chosen. For example, African American women are more likely to refuse treatment because they believe that it will negatively affect their fertility and are more likely to choose fertility sparing treatments compared to other groups.[7]

A basic premise of the C-SHIP model is that individuals are characterized by distinctive processing profiles in how they select, encode, and manage health risk–related information and how they react to it emotionally.[10–12] High monitoring, which involves attention to and scanning for threatening cues, and low monitoring, which involves distraction from and minimization of threat-relevant cues, are two characteristic cognitive-affective signature styles for processing health threats.[10–12] The monitoring signature style is not only associated with high attention to health threats, but is also linked to a cognition-emotion pattern involving heightened risk perceptions, lowered control expectations, and high health-related anxiety.[10,12] Studies of cervical cancer screening show that high monitors interpret their condition as more serious, worry more about it, and are more concerned about feeling greater pain, embarrassment, and discomfort during the colposcopy.[23] Monitors are also more likely to blame themselves and to experience higher levels of distress with respect to their health problem, putting them at risk not only for exaggerated emotional reactions but also for future nonadherence.[23]

INTERVENTIONS AIMED AT INCREASING ROUTINE CERVICAL CANCER SCREENING

Several systematic reviews have recently been conducted regarding the effectiveness of interventions to address barriers to routine screening adherence.[27–30] The interventions that have been developed are twofold. The first type aims at improving access to the healthcare system. The basic premise is that by reducing practical barriers (time, distance, transportation, dependent care, and administrative procedures), as well as economic barriers (out of pocket expenses for screening), uptake will be increased.[27] These interventions seem to be most effective for specific subgroups, such as women from low SES groups and those at high risk for cervical cancer.[29]

A subtype of this approach are interventions directed at the provider level, which entail assessment of physician services provided to women, in terms of offering and/or delivering screening, and feedback about how to improve the service care environment. Feedback can include a comparison of actual performance with a goal or a standard. In general, this type of intervention has been found to be effective in increasing screening rates.[30] In addition, economic incentives to providers have been used to improve educational efforts directed at clients, as well as direct recommendations to get screened. To date, there is insufficient evidence that this type of intervention is effective in increasing screening rates, probably because of the limited nature of the incentives used.[30]

The second type of intervention focuses on assessing and addressing psychosocial barriers of the women in need of testing.[27,29] These interventions involve such strategies as invitations to participate in screening and reminder postcards, letters, and calls, with a view to increasing the personal relevance of the test and knowledge about the need for screening.[27,29] Different variants of this approach have all been found to be effective, including open letters of invitation, letters with a specific appointment date, and telephone invitation.[27] With regard to educational interventions, the results show that one-on-one education increases adherence, especially when the information is delivered by lay people and is culturally targeted (e.g., framing the health information in a culturally relevant fashion, so that it appeals to individuals of a specific ethnic group).[27,29]

Given the concerns often raised by women that the examination situation itself is difficult, some studies have explored the possibility that female providers will lead to higher screening rates. In one of these studies, the findings showed that the increase in uptake was high when the first access was to a lay health worker, followed by screening with a female nurse practitioner; this effect was most pronounced (up to 25% increase) among minority women with greater need to be tested (e.g.,

older Native American and African American women).[31] Another study showed that when the invitation letter stated that the person performing the Pap smear was female, adherence was higher.[32]

INTERVENTIONS AIMED AT INCREASING ADHERENCE FOLLOWING AN ABNORMAL CERVICAL CANCER SCREENING RESULT

Interventions designed to improve access to the healthcare system (e.g., use of transportation and payment vouchers) generally have been found to be effective.[13,33] Interventions designed to overcome psychosocial barriers (e.g., increasing knowledge, increasing the perceived relevance of the test, raising perceived risk, reducing anticipatory distress, and enhancing self-regulatory skills)[34–37] have utilized a variety of channels to reach women, including personalized letters, telephone reminders, educational brochures, and/or counseling. These strategies significantly improve adherence rates, although the exclusive use of external prompts (e.g., reminders in letter form only) result in the smallest increases.[38]

Several studies show the potential for tailored interventions (assessment-based interventions that vary according to individual-level characteristics) to increase follow-up adherence among low-income, underserved women after receipt of an abnormal Pap smear test result.[39] Using a randomized controlled design, two studies examined the effects of tailored telephone counseling—designed to assess and address cognitive, affective, and self-regulatory barriers to adherence—on adherence to colposcopy among low SES women, primarily African American.[34,35] Both found the intervention to be highly effective in improving adherence to the scheduled colposcopy in comparison with standard care (scheduling call); further, adherence rates among the group that received the original telephone barriers counseling intervention remained high over time.[34] In a recent study, targeted to minority, low-income women, a community outreach approach was used which combined tailored counseling with a computerized tracking follow-up system (scheduling, tracking of, and appointment reminders).[36] The counseling was provided by a community health advisor matched to the ethnic identity of the target population (African American and Hispanic), and was tailored to barriers related to knowledge, beliefs, self-regulatory skills, as well as access to the healthcare system. In comparison with usual care, the combination of tailored barriers-based counseling and targeted community outreach was highly effective in increasing follow-up adherence after a positive Pap test result.[36] A case management approach targeted to low-income, predominantly foreign-born Latinas,[37] and designed to assess for, and intervene with, psychosocial and healthcare access barriers to follow-up adherence has also been found to increase follow-up in comparison with usual care.

As discussed earlier, the C-SHIP model proposes that individuals are characterized by distinctive processing profiles in how they select, encode, and manage health risk–related information and how they react to it affectively.[10–12] One study examined the interacting effects of monitoring style with the framing of informational messages on the responses of women scheduled for colposcopy.[40] Low monitors (women who distract from medical threats and feel less vulnerable to them) who received an educational intervention which emphasized the cost of nonadherence to screening recommendations (e.g., "late detection of precancerous conditions can decrease the chance that your treatment will be effective") 2 weeks before their scheduled appointment for colposcopy were less likely to cancel or postpone it.

HPV TESTING

Recently, it has been proposed that HPV DNA testing be incorporated both in primary screening for cervical cancer, as well as used to aid in the management of abnormal Pap test results.[41] Qualitative studies show that young women consider HPV feedback to be empowering in that it increases their perceived ability to prevent cervical cancer, even though they experience anxiety and distress when they test positive.[42,43] They also report positive behavioral intentions, in terms of changing their sexual and smoking behaviors.[42] At the same time, being HPV positive can engender feelings, such as stigmatization, since it is indicative of having a sexually transmitted infection. Young women who test positive for HPV express shame, feel stigmatized, and are concerned about social rejection.[43] In the same study, women who tested negative linked HPV positive status to issues of morality, and used terms such as "dirty" and "nasty" to describe women who test positive.[43]

Similar findings have been reported with adult women.[44] In a study with adult British women, a positive HPV test result was associated with increased distress, anxiety, and confusion, particularly when the HPV positive status was replicated 12 months later.[44] After the first positive test result, elevated levels of anxiety persisted among women who had several unanswered questions and poorer understanding of the test result. This subgroup also felt "unclean" and expressed concern about fertility and sexual relationships.[44]

Given that there is a relationship between education, level of understanding of the test result, and psychosocial outcomes, it is of concern that one U.S. survey found that fewer than 50% of women in the general population had heard of HPV and, of those, fewer than 50% knew that it was linked to cervical cancer.[41] Women who were young, educated, and non-Hispanic white were more likely to have heard about HPV, whereas being a minority was associated with low knowledge levels.[8] In a systematic review, only 21% of respondents (men and women) knew that HPV infection is common.[45]

The acceptance of HPV testing appears to be higher than expected, perhaps because women find it convenient and less intrusive than the Pap smear test. In a study with Mexican women, participants were trained to self-collect vaginal samples for HPV testing.[46] They preferred this approach to Pap smear testing, which they found to be embarrassing and uncomfortable. In non-Western cultures, where the nature of the exam can act as a barrier to cervical cancer control, HPV testing may be a way of increasing screening if women are properly trained to collect the samples on their own. Women of higher SES were especially likely to prefer self-collection of the HPV sample.[46] Negative psychosocial consequences of HPV testing (e.g., feelings of stigmatization) may be moderated by educating women about the meaning of the test result, cautioning health educators not to be judgmental when disclosing the results, and normalizing the situation by emphasizing the prevalence of the virus among sexually active women.

HPV VACCINATION

As indicated, two vaccines have been developed to prevent HPV infection, introduced to the United States in June 2006.[6] Current recommendations by the Advisory Committee on Immunization Practices include routine vaccination with the quadrivalent vaccine of all 11- to 12-year-old girls and vaccination of all 13- to 26-year-old females not previously vaccinated.[47] A recent systematic review of research conducted before the licensure of the vaccine showed that the majority of parents were willing to vaccinate their adolescent children if it were to be made available to them.[45] Fewer studies have investigated attitudes of adolescents themselves, but the findings indicate that acceptance rates are also high among this group.[45] The impact of sociodemographic variables, such as ethnicity, education, and income, in parents' and adults' acceptance rates has been explored but the findings are mixed.[45] High acceptance rates among parents and adults are associated with increased knowledge, high perceived risk, and beliefs that the vaccine is effective with regard to preventing cervical cancer.[45] In contrast, concerns about the long-term safety of the vaccine, and that the vaccination might be painful and uncomfortable act as barriers. Value-related issues, such as the concern that the vaccination will disinhibit the sexual behavior of adolescents, have been suggested as a potential barrier to uptake. However, few parents (6%–12%) actually express such concerns.[45] Finally, parents state that their physician's attitudes weigh in their decision, with those who are more accepting of the vaccine being more likely to be influenced by their physician than those who are not inclined to vaccinate their children.[45] The few studies that have been conducted in developing countries show similar trends in parents' attitudes.[47] Studies that have looked at the attitudes of healthcare providers found that they are positive toward vaccination but express reluctance to vaccinate very young adolescents. They also expressed reservations about raising this topic with parents since they view it as a culturally and religiously sensitive issue.[47]

Two recent studies examined the actual uptake of vaccination. The first, conducted in the United States, examined uptake in a group of 13- to 26-year-old women, the majority of whom were African American.[48] Five percent had received at least one vaccine shot and 66% intended to get vaccinated. However, practical issues, particularly cost, were an important barrier to uptake.[48] Risky sexual behavior was another factor associated with low intention to get vaccinated. In contrast, high knowledge about HPV, higher perceived severity of HPV infection, higher perceived benefits of HPV vaccination related to its safety and protection potential, and beliefs that important people in the woman's life would approve of vaccination were associated with high intentions.[48]

A second study, conducted in the United Kingdom, investigated the feasibility and acceptability of delivering the first two doses (out of three recommended) of the bivalent HPV vaccination to adolescent girls in the school setting, in anticipation of the implementation of a national HPV immunization program.[49] Program uptake for the first dose of the vaccine was 70.6%, with a small drop to 68.5% for the second dose. Vaccine uptake was lower in schools with higher proportions of minority ethnic groups and among girls who received free meals at school. The main reason for withholding parental consent was insufficient information about the vaccine and concerns about its long-term safety. Almost no parents mentioned the age of their daughter or the potential effect of the vaccine on adolescent sexual behavior as the reason for refusing consent. Two out of thirty-eight schools refused to participate on religious grounds.[49]

CONCLUSIONS AND FUTURE DIRECTIONS

There have been exciting recent advances in prevention, screening, and management technologies for cervical cancer.[1] Yet, a proportion of women do not get screened and/or, when faced with an abnormal Pap smear test, do not adhere to follow-up diagnostic, repeat screening, and treatment recommendations.[1,15–18] This is particularly true for low SES and minority women, indicating that there are still important barriers that need to be addressed, including healthcare access barriers such as the cost of screening and the lack of provider recommendations to get screened. In addition, significant psychosocial barriers have been identified, including lack of knowledge, low perceived personal relevance, fatalistic beliefs, and distress.[7–9,14,24] Psychosocial barriers, particularly at the emotional level, are of concern for women who receive an abnormal Pap smear test result or test HPV positive, since they are more likely to experience elevated anxiety, depression, and feelings of shame.[14,24,34]

Substantial research has been conducted to test the effectiveness of interventions aimed at healthcare access barriers and psychosocial barriers in order to increase adherence to routine cervical cancer screening and treatment recommendations. Interventions that target access barriers seem to be particularly effective for low SES and minority women.[28,30,38] With regard to psychosocial barriers, interventions developed to increase routine cervical cancer screening and recommended follow-up have focused on assessing and addressing lack of knowledge.[27,29,38] In addition, there is evidence to indicate that interventions targeted to specific minority groups and tailored to the individual's psychosocial profile (including emotional barriers) are effective.[36,37] In the future, it will be important to design and evaluate multicomponent interventions that comprehensively address access to care, while simultaneously being targeted to specific subgroups and tailored to psychosocial factors, and that can be readily disseminated within the healthcare system. In addition, programs developed in the future should more comprehensively address not only adherence to scheduled appointments, but also the promotion of less risky sexual behavior.[12]

With regard to the recognition of the role of HPV in cervical cancer risk, the evidence is encouraging: HPV knowledge has been shown to increase with the year a study was conducted.[50] Still, the low percentage of women who are aware of HPV[41] is indicative of the fact that more effort is needed in this area. One concern is that the higher awareness of the association between cervical cancer and HPV infection will lead to affected women experiencing greater stigma and possibly distress. Therefore, in the future, it may be important to educate women about

HPV in a nonevaluating and normalizing manner, with emphasis on the fact that HPV infection is a common problem.

This state of affairs may be changing drastically with the introduction of the HPV vaccine. The preliminary evidence regarding vaccination acceptance is promising and initial concerns that the majority of parents might oppose vaccination because of its potential to disinhibit adolescent sexual behavior have thus far proven unfounded.[45] However, the two studies that looked at actual uptake in England and the United States found disparities among ethnic groups.[48,49] The limited evidence available so far shows that providers might also play a key role in vaccine acceptance, at least until it is more widely accepted by parents.[45,47] As with cervical risk screening and follow-up testing, it will be important to develop interventions that address both access and psychosocial barriers to participation.

ACKNOWLEDGMENTS

This work was supported in part by NIH grants R01 CA104979 and 5P01 CA057586, the Fox Chase Cancer Center Behavioral Research Core Facility P30 CA06927, Department of Defense grants DAMD 17–01-01-1-0238 and DAMD 17–02-1-0382, and a Lance Armstrong grant 3600101. We are indebted to Drs. Amy Lazev and Pamela Shapiro for their feedback, to John Scarpato for his valuable insights, and to Mary Anne Ryan and Jennifer Lyle for technical assistance.

REFERENCES

1. Kamangar F, Dores GM, Anderson WF. Patterns of cancer incidence, mortality, and prevalence across five continents: defining priorities to reduce cancer disparities in different geographic regions of the world. *J Clin Oncol.* 2006;24(14):2137–2150.

2. Waggoner SE. Cervical cancer. *Lancet.* 2003;361(9376):2217–2225.

3. Espey DK, Wu XC, Swan J, et al. Annual report to the nation on the status of cancer, 1975–2004, featuring cancer in American Indians and Alaska Natives. *Cancer.* 2007;110(10):2119–2152.

4. American Cancer Society. *Cancer facts & figures 2008.* Atlanta: American Cancer Society; 2008.

5. Khan MJ, Castle PE, Lorincz AT, et al. The elevated 10-year risk of cervical precancer and cancer in women with human papillomavirus (HPV) type 16 or 18 and the possible utility of type-specific HPV testing in clinical practice. *J Natl Cancer Inst.* 2005;97(14):1072–1079.

6. Villa LL, Costa RL, Petta CA, et al. Prophylactic quadrivalent human papillomavirus (types 6, 11, 16, and 18) L1 virus-like particle vaccine in young women: a randomised double-blind placebo-controlled multicentre phase II efficacy trial. *Lancet Oncol.* 2005;6(5):271–278.

7. Akers AY, Newmann SJ, Smith JS. Factors underlying disparities in cervical cancer incidence, screening, and treatment in the United States. *Curr Probl Cancer.* 2007;31(3):157–181.

8. Downs LS, Smith JS, Scarinci I, Flowers L, Parham G. The disparity of cervical cancer in diverse populations. *Gynecol Oncol.* 2008;109(suppl 2):S22-S30.

9. Ackerson K, Gretebeck K. Factors influencing cancer screening practices of underserved women. *J Am Acad Nurse Pract.* 2007;19(11):591–601.

10. Diefenbach MA, Miller SM, Porter M, Peters E, Stefanek M, Leventhal H. Emotions and health behavior: a self-regulation perspective. In: Lewis M, Haviland-Jones JM, Barrett FL (eds). *Handbook of emotions,* 3rd ed. New York, NY: Guilford Press, 2008:645–660.

11. Khanna N, Phillips MD. Adherence to care plan in women with abnormal Papanicolaou smears: a review of barriers and interventions. *J Am Board Fam Pract.* 2001;14(2):123–130.

12. Miller SM, Mischel W, O'Leary A, Mills M. From human papillomavirus (HPV) to cervical cancer: psychosocial processes in infection, detection, and control. *Ann Behav Med.* 1996;18(4):219–228.

13. Miller SM, Shoda Y, Hurley K. Applying cognitive-social theory to health-protective behavior: breast self-examination in cancer screening. *Psychol Bull.* 1996;119(1):70–94.

14. Fylan F. Screening for cervical cancer: a review of women's attitudes, knowledge, and behaviour. *Br J Gen Pract.* 1998;48(433):1509–1514.

15. Tacken MA, Braspenning JC, Hermens RP, et al. Uptake of cervical cancer screening in The Netherlands is mainly influenced by women's beliefs about the screening and by the inviting organization. *Eur J Public Health.* 2007;17(2):178–185.

16. Rodvall Y, Kemetli L, Tishelman C, Tornberg S. Factors related to participation in a cervical cancer screening programme in urban Sweden. *Eur J Cancer Prev.* 2005;14(5):459–466.

17. Nathoo V. Investigation of non-responders at a cervical cancer screening clinic in Manchester. *Br Med J (Clin Res Ed).* 1988;296(6628):1041–1042.

18. Knops-Dullens T, de Vries N, de Vries H. Reasons for non-attendance in cervical cancer screening programmes: an application of the Integrated Model for Behavioural Change. *Eur J Cancer Prev.* 2007;16(5):436–445.

19. ACOG Practice Bulletin: clinical management guidelines for obstetrician-gynecologists. Number 45, August 2003. Cervical cytology screening (replaces committee opinion 152, March 1995). *Obstet Gynecol.* 2003;102(2):417–427.

20. Eggleston KS, Coker AL, Das IP, Cordray ST, Luchok KJ. Understanding barriers for adherence to follow-up care for abnormal pap tests. *J Womens Health (Larchmt).* 2007;16(3):311–330.

21. Bennetts A, Irwig L, Oldenburg B, et al. PEAPS-Q: a questionnaire to measure the psychosocial effects of having an abnormal pap smear. Psychosocial effects of abnormal pap smears questionnaire. *J Clin Epidemiol.* 1995;48(10):1235–1243.

22. Lerman C, Miller SM, Scarborough R, Hanjani P, Nolte S, Smith D. Adverse psychologic consequences of positive cytologic cervical screening. *Am J Obstet Gynecol.* 1991;165(3):658–662.

23. Miller SM, Roussi P, Altman D, Helm W, Steinberg A. Effects of coping style on psychological reactions of low-income, minority women to colposcopy. *J Reprod Med.* 1994;39(9):711–718.

24. Rogstad KE. The psychological impact of abnormal cytology and colposcopy. *BJOG.* 2002;109(4):364–368.

25. Wardle J, Pernet A, Stephens D. Psychological consequences of positive results in cervical cancer screening. *Psychol Health.* 1995;10(3):185–194.

26. Nelson K, Geiger AM, Mangione CM. Effect of health beliefs on delays in care for abnormal cervical cytology in a multi-ethnic population. *J Gen Intern Med.* 2002;17(9):709–716.

27. Baron RC, Rimer BK, Breslow RA, et al. Client-directed interventions to increase community demand for breast, cervical, and colorectal cancer screening: a systematic review. *Am J Prev Med.* 2008;35(suppl 1):S34-S55.

28. Baron RC, Rimer BK, Coates RJ, et al. Task Force on Community Preventive Services, Client-directed interventions to increase community access to breast, cervical, and colorectal cancer screening: a systematic review. *Am J Prev Med.* 2008 Jul;35(1 Suppl):S56–66.

29. Forbes C, Jepson R, Martin-Hirsch P. Interventions targeted at women to encourage the uptake of cervical screening. *Cochrane Database Syst Rev.* 2002;(3):1–55.

30. Sabatino SA, Habarta N, Baron RC, et al. Interventions to increase recommendation and delivery of screening for breast, cervical, and colorectal cancers by healthcare providers systematic reviews of provider assessment and feedback and provider incentives. *Am J Prev Med.* 2008;35(suppl 1):S67-S74.

31. Margolis KL, Lurie N, McGovern PG, Tyrrell M, Slater JS. Increasing breast and cervical cancer screening in low-income women. *J Gen Intern Med.* 1998;13(8):515–521.

32. Hicks C, Robinson K. Cervical screening: the impact of the gender of the smear-taker on service uptake. *Health Serv Manage Res.* 1997;10(3):187–189.

33. Marcus AC, Kaplan CP, Crane LA, et al. Reducing loss-to-follow-up among women with abnormal Pap smears. Results from a randomized trial testing an intensive follow-up protocol and economic incentives. *Med Care.* 1998;36(3):397–410.

34. Miller SM, Siejak KK, Schroeder CM, Lerman C, Hernandez E, Helm CW. Enhancing adherence following abnormal Pap smears among low-income minority women: a preventive telephone counseling strategy. *J Natl Cancer Inst.* 1997;89(10):703–708.

35. Lerman C, Hanjani P, Caputo C, et al. Telephone counseling improves adherence to colposcopy among lower-income minority women. *J Clin Oncol.* 1992;10(2):330–333.

36. Engelstad LP, Stewart S, Otero-Sabogal R, Leung MS, Davis PI, Pasick RJ. The effectiveness of a community outreach intervention to improve follow-up among underserved women at highest risk for cervical cancer. *Prev Med.* 2005;41(3–4):741–748.

37. Ell K, Vourlekis B, Muderspach L, et al. Abnormal cervical screen follow-up among low-income Latinas: Project SAFe. *J Womens Health Gend Based Med.* 2002;11(7):639–651.

38. Yabroff KR, Kerner JF, Mandelblatt JS. Effectiveness of interventions to improve follow-up after abnormal cervical cancer screening. *Prev Med.* 2000;31:429–439.

39. Miller S, Bowen D, Campbell MK, et al. Current research promises and challenges in behavioral oncology: report from the American Society of Preventive Oncology Annual Meeting, 2002. *Cancer Epidemiol Biomarkers Prev.* 2004;13:171–180.

40. Miller SM, Buzaglo JS, Simms S, et al. Monitoring styles in women at risk for cervical cancer: Implications for the framing of health-relevant messages. *Ann Behav Med.* 1999;21:27–34.

41. Tiro JA, Meissner HI, Kobrin S, Chollette V. What do women in the U.S. know about human papillomavirus and cervical cancer? *Cancer Epidemiol Biomarkers Prev.* 2007;16(2):288–294.

42. Kahn JA, Slap GB, Bernstein DI, et al. Psychological, behavioral, and interpersonal impact of human papillomavirus and Pap test results. *J Womens Health (Larchmt).* 2005;14(7):650–659.

43. Kahn JA, Slap GB, Bernstein DI, et al. Personal meaning of human papillomavirus and Pap test results in adolescent and young adult women. *Health Psychol.* 2007;26(2):192–200.

44. Waller J, McCaffery K, Kitchener H, Nazroo J, Wardle J. Women's experiences of repeated HPV testing in the context of cervical cancer screening: a qualitative study. *Psycho-Oncology.* 2007;16(3):196–204.

45. Brewer NT, Fazekas KI. Predictors of HPV vaccine acceptability: a theory-informed, systematic review. *Prev Med.* 2007;45(2–3):107–114.

46. Dzuba IG, Diaz EY, Allen B, et al. The acceptability of self-collected samples for HPV testing vs. the pap test as alternatives in cervical cancer screening. *J Womens Health Gend Based Med.* 2002;11(3):265–275.

47. Zimet GD, Shew ML, Kahn JA. Appropriate use of cervical cancer vaccine. *Annu Rev Med.* 2008;59:223–236.

48. Kahn JA, Rosenthal SL, Jin Y, Huang B, Namakydoust A, Zimet GD. Rates of human papillomavirus vaccination, attitudes about vaccination, and human papillomavirus prevalence in young women. *Obstet Gynecol.* 2008;111(5):1103–1110.

49. Brabin L, Roberts SA, Stretch R, et al. Uptake of first two doses of human papillomavirus vaccine by adolescent schoolgirls in Manchester: prospective cohort study. *BMJ.* 2008;336(7652):1056–1058.

50. Klug S, Hukelmann M, Blettner M. Knowledge about infection with human papillomavirus: a systematic review. *Prev Med.* 2008;46:87–98.

Breast Cancer Screening

Electra D. Paskett and John M. McLaughlin

OVERVIEW

Breast cancer is a leading cause of morbidity and mortality among women. Although screening offers the potential for earlier detection of tumors, resulting in better outcomes; many issues exist with screening modalities and ensuring optimal utilization of breast cancer screening tests by all women. This chapter describes the risk factors for breast cancer, validated early detection methods, screening patterns, predictors of screening, the role of screening in breast cancer survivors, psychosocial issues and anxiety in screening, and interventions that have been implemented to improve screening rates. Suggestions for future work to address unresolved issues and improve screening rates are also presented.

BACKGROUND: BREAST CANCER

Breast cancer is the most common non-skin cancer among women in the United States and in many other countries.[1] The chance of a woman developing some form of invasive breast cancer is about one in eight, and women living in North America have the highest rate of breast cancer in the world. In 2009, an estimated 192,370 new cases of invasive breast caner and 67,770 new cases of in situ breast cancer are expected to occur among women in the United States.[2] These deaths make breast cancer the second leading cause of cancer death in women, after only cancer of the lung.[1]

BREAST CANCER SCREENING GUIDELINES

General screening guidelines. Women are advised to get a mammogram every 1–2 years, starting at age 40.[3,4] Screening before this age is typically reserved for women with a higher than average risk for breast cancer (e.g., those who have already had the disease, or who have a family history of breast cancer, or with a genetic mutation that greatly increases their risk of developing breast cancer) because 95% of these cancers occur in women aged 40 and over.[3,4] In addition, women in their 20s and 30s should have a clinical breast examination (CBE) as part of a regular examination by a health expert, preferably every 3 years.[3,4] After age 40, women should have a breast examination by a health expert every year. Generally, it is recommended to have the CBE shortly before the mammogram.

Screening guidelines for women at high risk. Under previous American Cancer Society (ACS) guidelines, high-risk women were advised to discuss screening with their doctor. Updated ACS guidelines, however, are more specific about who is at increased risk and their options for screening. Now, women and their doctors are encouraged to discuss the possibility of beginning screening with CBE and mammography earlier (at age 30, or in rare cases, even younger). Another option is to consider screening with breast ultrasound or magnetic resonance imaging (MRI) in addition to a regular mammogram.[2]

Risk factors for developing breast cancer. Table 11–1 lists the risk factors for breast cancer established to date. Risk factors may be unrelated to an individual's lifestyle and essentially unchangeable (e.g., age, gender, genetics, family, or personal history) or related to lifestyle, allowing the potential for modification (e.g., alcohol consumption, diet, level of physical activity).[3,4] Among lifestyle factors, age and gender are the most straightforward and strongest predictors of developing cancer. A woman's chance of developing breast cancer is approximately 100 times higher than that of a man's. Men represent only 1% of all breast cancer cases and there are no data on the benefits or risks of screening males. Also, as with most cancers, a woman's chance of developing breast cancer increases with increasing age.[3,4]

In addition, between 5% and 10% of incident breast cancer cases are due to genetic mutations, typically of the *BRCA1* and *BRCA2* genes.[5] Breast cancers caused by *BRCA1/2* mutations generally occur at an earlier age than sporadic breast cancers, prompting the need for earlier screening in this group.[6] Other hereditary risk factors include having a family history of breast cancer in first degree relatives (approximately doubles the risk of developing breast cancer) or having a personal history of breast cancer. Breast cancer survivors have an increased risk of primary cancer in the contralateral breast.[3] However, most women who develop breast cancer do not develop a second primary cancer in the contralateral breast.[7]

Although risk for developing breast cancer is highest among women with a personal or family history, most women who are diagnosed with breast cancer do not have a personal or family history of the disease.[8] Thus, in addition to closely monitoring women at high risk for the disease and urging women to make healthy lifestyle choices, promoting regular screening to *all* eligible women is of utmost importance.

Race is also a noteworthy non-lifestyle-related risk factor for breast cancer mortality. While white women are slightly (yet, statistically) more likely to develop breast cancer than African American women, African American women are more likely to die of the disease.[9] This disparity in survival persists even after adjusting for socioeconomic status, age, and disease stage.[10] The disproportionately higher breast cancer-specific mortality in African American women is attributed, in part, to more aggressive tumors among blacks, and, in part, to health disparities in access to proper care.[4] African American women also develop breast cancer approximately a decade earlier than white women on average, and approximately 30%–40% of African American women with breast cancer are diagnosed before age 50, compared to 20% of white women.[5,10]

Women whose mothers were given diethylstilbestrol (DES) during pregnancy, who have a long menstrual history (women who were younger than age 12 at menarche or who went through menopause after age 55), or who as children or young adults had radiation treatment to the chest for another type of cancer or medical condition have increased risk of developing breast cancer.[3]

In contrast, lifestyle-related factors include a higher risk of developing breast cancer among women who do not engage in physical activity in the form of exercise, who are overweight or obese (after menopause),[11] who consume high-fat diets,[12] and who drink at least one alcoholic beverage per day.[13] In addition, long-term postmenopausal hormone therapy (PHT), especially combined estrogen and progestin therapy, is associated with increased breast cancer risk.[14] Evidence on the causative nature of estrogens, however, is unclear and this association is not fully understood.[15] Other lifestyle-related factors that result in a slightly higher risk of developing the disease include women who have had no children or who had their first child after age 30, who have recently used oral contraceptives, and who have never breastfed or who have breastfed less than 1.5 years are at a slightly higher risk of developing the disease.[3]

Table 11–1. Groups at higher risk for breast cancer as described by the American Cancer Society (ACS), 2008

Risk factors by type

Non-lifestyle–related risk factors for breast cancer

Age: 95% of breast cancers occur in women aged 40 and older

Gender: while men can get breast cancer, it is 100 times more common among women

Genetic risk factors: approximately 5%–10% of breast cancer cases are hereditary and result from gene mutations, most commonly mutations of the *BRCA1* and *BRCA2* genes

Family history: having one or more first-degree relatives—mother, sister, or daughter—diagnosed with breast cancer approximately doubles the risk

Personal history: women surviving breast cancer have an increased risk of primary cancer in the contralateral breast and have an increased risk of being diagnosed with another cancer compared to women never treated for breast cancer

Race: white women are slightly more likely to develop breast cancer than are African American women, but African American women are more likely to die of this cancer, due in part to more aggressive tumors among African American women

Previous breast radiation: women who as children or young adults had radiation therapy to the chest area as treatment for another cancer (e.g., lymphoma) or other medical condition have increased risk

Long menstrual history: women who started menstruating before 12 or who went through menopause after 55 have a slightly higher risk

Diethylstilbestrol (DES): women whose mothers were given DES during pregnancy have slightly higher risk

Lifestyle-related risk factors for breast cancer

Not having children: women who have had no children or who had their first child after age 30 have slightly higher risk

Oral contraceptive use: women who have recently used oral contraceptives have a slightly increased risk compared with women who have never used them

Postmenopausal hormone therapy (PHT): long-term use (several years) of PHT (especially combined estrogen and progestin therapy) is associated with increased risk

Not breast-feeding: women who have never nursed or who have nursed less than 1.5 years have a slightly increased risk compared to mothers who nurse 1.5–2 years

Overweight/obesity and high-fat diet: overweight/obese women and those who consume a high-fat diet have an increased risk, especially after menopause

Alcohol: women who drink one alcoholic beverage per day have a slight increased risk. Women who drink 2–5 alcoholic beverages daily have 1.5 times the risk of a nondrinker

Physical inactivity: those who do not engage in physical activity in the form of exercise have higher risk than those who do

See reference 2.

BREAST CANCER SCREENING MODALITIES

Mammography. Mammography uses ionizing radiation, specifically X-rays, to image breast tissue. This technology allows radiologists to identify breast cancers that are too small to detect upon physical examination and noninvasive forms of ductal carcinoma in situ. Numerous uncontrolled trials and retrospective analysis have shown mammography as an effective tool to diagnose small, early-stage breast cancers and that cancer-related survival is better in screened women than in non-screened women.[16] It should be noted, however, that such studies are susceptible to a number of biases, namely lead-time bias, length bias, overdiagnosis bias, and healthy volunteer bias.[17]

In spite of these potential biases in studies evaluating screening mammography, mammography remains a widely accepted tool for detecting breast cancers earlier and decreasing breast cancer mortality, especially for older women. A meta-analysis of data from four randomized controlled trials demonstrated that relative, breast cancer-specific mortality is decreased between 15% and 20% with screening mammography in women aged 40–70.[18] Absolute mortality benefit for women screened annually starting at age 40 and at age 50 are 4 per 10,000[19] and 5 per 1,000,[4] respectively.

The effectiveness of mammography lies largely in the extent of its sensitivity (the proportion of breast cancer detected when breast cancer is present). Sensitivity of the test depends on many factors, including lesion size, lesion conspicuity, breast tissue density, patient age, the hormone status of the tumor, overall image quality, and the interpretive skill of the radiologist. Overall sensitivity is approximately 75%[20] but ranges from 54% to 58% in women younger than 40 years to 81% and 94% in those older than 65 years.[21, 22] Studies have demonstrated that greater breast density explains most of the decreased mammographic sensitivity in younger women. High breast density is associated with 10%–29% lower sensitivity, and can be familial or may be affected by endogenous and exogenous hormones, selective estrogen receptor modulators such as tamoxifen, and diet, in addition to age.[23] Decreased mammographic sensitivity in younger women, however, has also been explained by the fact that younger women tend to have more rapid tumor growth.[23]

Failure to diagnose breast cancer is the most common cause of medical malpractice litigation. Half of the cases resulting in payment to the claimant had false-negative mammograms.[24] Studies have shown substantial variability in the interpretational skill of radiologists. In general, studies suggest that sensitivity, specificity, or both increase with higher volume of mammograms read by a radiologist.[25-27]

Clinical breast examination. No randomized trials of CBE as a sole screening modality have ever been done, for obvious ethical reasons. Sensitivity for CBE has been estimated to range from approximately 60% to 80% and specificity from 88% to 96%.[28] Predictive value positive (the proportion of cancers detected per abnormal examination) was estimated between 2% and 4%.[28,29] Other studies have demonstrated added usefulness of adding CBE to screening mammography, showing increases in both sensitivity and specificity, especially in older women.[30]

Breast self-examination. Monthly breast self-examination (BSE) is often advocated by various providers, organizations, and researchers; however, evidence for its effectiveness is weak or mixed, at best.[31] The largest randomized clinical trial of BSE, conducted in Shanghai, showed no reduction in breast cancer-specific mortality; however, it did demonstrate an increase in breast biopsies and diagnosis of benign lesions.[32] Most studies evaluating BSE, however, are subject to selection and recall bias and are difficult to interpret. Furthermore, BSE proficiency is often low among women.

Ultrasonography. Although some professionals advocate using ultrasound to evaluate palpable or mammagraphically identified abnormalities, there has been little evidence to support its use in population screening of women in any age group or risk status.[33]

Magnetic resonance imaging. Breast MRI, though less specific, is a more sensitive modality for breast cancer detection compared to screening mammography.[34,35] Thus, debate continues because even though studies of young high-risk women report MRI sensitivities ranging from 71% to 100% compared to 20% to 50% for mammography, women screened with MRI have more negative surgical biopsies.[36] As such, it is difficult to determine whether MRI screening is worthwhile with such high false-positive rates. Studies investigating this role for MRI are ongoing.

CURRENT AND PAST BREAST CANCER SCREENING PATTERNS

Although screening mammography compliance has generally increased over the last decade (Fig. 11–1), data from the Behavioral Risk Factor Surveillance System (BRFSS) indicate a statistically significant decline in the proportion of women aged 40 years or older during 2000–2005 who reported having had a mammogram in the preceding 2 years. The proportion decreased from 76.4% (75.8%, 76.9%) in 2000 to 74.6% (73.8%, 75.4%) in 2005 (test for trend, $p < 0.001$). This slight decline, though above the *Healthy people 2010* objective of 70%, suggests a need to monitor mammography screening more carefully.[37]

The reason for the apparent decline in screening mammography is unclear and might be attributable to a combination of factors. One study indicated that breast-imaging facilities face barriers including shortages of key personnel, malpractice concerns, and financial constraints.[38] Others have posited that there may be an insufficient number of specialists and available facilities to meet the needs of an expanding population—in the United States between 1990 and 2000, the number of women aged 40 years or older increased by more than 24 million.[39] Previously, low mammography use has been associated with not having a usual source of healthcare, not having health insurance, and being a recent immigrant.[40] However, determining the direct causes of this apparent decline in mammography use is difficult, and future studies need to confirm the decreasing trend. It is also worth noting that mammography

estimates using BRFSS data may overestimate the proportion of women who reported having had a mammogram in the preceding 2 years because of bias in who participates in BRFSS.[17]

PREDICTORS OF AND BARRIERS TO BREAST CANCER SCREENING

Socioeconomic status and demographic background. Prior studies have documented factors associated with receiving breast cancer screening examinations. These factors fall into categories of age,[41–43] income,[41–44] level of education,[41,43,45] type of health insurance,[44,46–48] race/ethnicity,[41,43,49,50] and geographic barriers.[41,43,45,47] In general, younger women are more likely to adhere to screening guidelines.[41,42] In one study, stratifying by age showed that of women aged 40–49 years, 83% had a mammogram in the previous year, and 90% a CBE; where only 68% of women 50 years and older had a mammogram in the previous year, and only 80% had a CBE. Of women aged 30–39, 49% had a mammogram in the previous year, and 85% had a CBE.[41]

Income is also a significant predictor of screening behavior. In the same study, the percentages of women receiving mammography and CBE in the previous year were 55% and 80%, respectively, for women with a combined household income less than $50,000 annually. For those with a household income more than $50,000 annually the percentages were 73% and 88%, respectively.[42] Another study showed that for each increasing quintile of socioeconomic status, the odds ratio of women receiving two or more preventive breast cancer services was 1.08 (1.04, 1.12).[41]

In addition, level of education attainment predicts screening behavior.[41,45] In one study of Australian women, the odds ratios for a woman in the low education strata compared to the high education strata for never having a mammogram, not having a recent mammogram, never having a CBE, not having a regular CBE, and not regularly performing a BSE were 1.55 (1.30, 1.85), 1.36 (1.13, 1.64), 1.91 (1.54, 2.36), 1.40 (1.18–1.67), and 1.28 (1.10, 1.50), respectively.[45]

Having health insurance[44,46–48] and the type of health insurance an individual has[44,48] are important predictors of screening behavior as well. One study showed that uninsured women were 64% less likely to be screened than those who had insurance.[46] Another study by Potosky et al.[48] showed that people aged 40–64 years with Medicaid coverage were 70% more likely to be screened in six different types of cancer prevention tests (mammography, CBE, Pap smear, fecal occult blood test, digital rectal examination, and proctosigmoidoscopy) than those who had no coverage. In addition, people 65 years and older who had supplemental private fee-for-service insurance, in addition to Medicare, were significantly more likely to receive five of the six major cancer screening tests than those who had only Medicare and Medicaid or Medicare only.[48]

Race/ethnicity is also a significant predictor of screening behavior. In a multivariate analysis, African American women had 0.59 (0.49, 0.71)

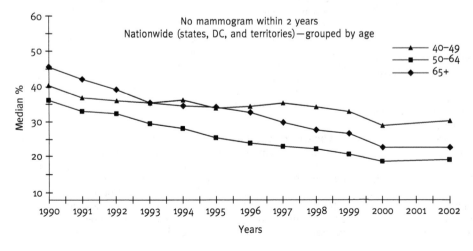

Fig. 11–1. Percentage of women reporting having had no mammogram within the past 2 years by age according to BRFSS. ABBREVIATION: BRFSS, Behavioral Risk Factor Surveillance System.

times the odds of having received two or more breast cancer preventive services when compared to white women.[41] While BRFSS data suggest that African American women aged 40 or older are more likely to report having had a mammogram within the past 2 years,[37] a study that controlled for age, race, and propensity to die (as a proxy for health status) showed that white women were 1.38 times more likely to receive mammograms than African American women.[51]

Other studies have shown knowledge of screening guidelines for Hispanics diagnosed with cancer was low,[49,52,53] and that Middle Eastern women have low levels of screening adherence.[45] Studies have also shown that removing economic and cultural barriers can be effective in increasing screening rates.[53,54]

Geographic barriers. Geographic barriers to breast cancer screening exist as well. Women who live in rural areas or disadvantaged areas are less likely to have proper uptake of cancer screening procedures.[41,45,47] Another study showed that women who live outside of metropolitan statistical areas (MSAs) are significantly less likely to adhere to screening guidelines.[43] These barriers, compounded by previously listed economic concerns, include lack of transportation,[47] poor access to healthcare facilities,[43] and an insufficient number of specialists.[55] One study by Freeman and Chu[56] showed that patient navigation systems can be effective in reducing these barriers—pairing underserved patients with appropriate treatment programs, specialists, and clinics.

The importance of physician referral. The best predictor of screening behavior is healthcare provider recommendation.[43,46] In one study, uninsured patients lacking provider recommendation were 98.5% less likely to be screened than a patient without insurance who had a physician referral.[46] Thus, lack of inquiry about family history and the lack of information provided by medical professionals prevents women from making well-informed decisions about breast cancer screening practices. Another study suggested that primary care physicians (general practitioners [GPs]) need to be better informed about cancer risk and screening. Specifically, the study showed that women seen regularly by obstetrician/gynecologists or internists were more likely to have annual mammograms than women usually seen by GPs.[57]

THE IMPORTANCE OF SCREENING AND HEALTH MAINTENANCE IN BREAST CANCER SURVIVORS

As grave as many of the statistics describing breast cancer are, another reality of breast cancer is that recent advances in early detection and in new types of therapies and their application have resulted in prolonged survival among women diagnosed with breast cancer. Although the breast cancer diagnosis rate has increased, the overall breast cancer death rate has dropped steadily since the early 1990s.[58] As a result, it is estimated that the current population of breast cancer survivors in the United States exceeds 2.3 million.[58] As technology aids early detection, this population is expected to grow,[1] and as it does, information related to health maintenance, screening practices, and emotional effects of cancer treatment related to anxiety, depression, and stress will become increasingly important. Women surviving breast cancer have an increased risk of a primary cancer in the contralateral breast and have an increased risk of being diagnosed with another cancer compared to women never treated for breast cancer.[58] It is important then, that this "high risk" group of survivors continues to maintain regular screening, complete necessary tests within recommended guidelines, and heed physician referrals and recommendations. Currently, few studies examine this growing survivor demographic and little is known about survivor compliance and adherence to health professionals' recommended courses of action. Moreover, there are many areas that need to be explored regarding how survivors' understanding of associated risks, perception of anxiety, and socioeconomic and cultural beliefs factor into associated rates of adherence to breast cancer screening recommendations. In a study of 241 long-term breast cancer survivors, 107 (44%) reported completing breast cancer surveillance (mammography and CBE) within recommended National Comprehensive Cancer Network (NCCN) guidelines, 102 (42%) completed more surveillance, and 32

(13%) completed less surveillance than is recommended.[59] Further studies are needed to look beyond recovery, at survivorship and the facets of remaining healthy through adherence to current screening guidelines, and the factors that influence adherence.

PSYCHOSOCIAL ISSUES IN BREAST CANCER SCREENING

Research that attempts to determine why certain individuals do or do not comply with screening recommendations suggests that psychosocial factors play an important role. When examining psychosocial issues that may influence an individual's screening adherence, researchers often conceptualize psychosocial processes into multilevel frameworks. The most widely used and researched theoretical model for the study of behavior changed in relation to breast cancer screening practices is the Health Belief Model (HBM).[60-62] This model focuses on four components: perceived susceptibility, perceived severity, perceived barriers, and perceived benefits.[63]

According to the HBM, increased knowledge of perceived severity and perceived benefits of screening procedures should be related to increased cancer screening practice. Indeed, knowledge about cancer and screening procedures has been found to be a significant facilitator of cancer screening behavior for breast cancer.[64] In many cases, some of the reasons reported for noncompliance for breast cancer screening represent a lack of appreciation for the concept of *asymptomatic illness*; that is, many people report not getting screening because they "felt healthy" and did not see the need to be screened.[65] Not surprisingly, income and education have been found to be related to the level of knowledge about cancer and cancer screening behaviors.[64]

In addition, on the basis of the HBM, a person's perception of susceptibility, or their perceived risk of developing a disease, is also important in determining health-related behaviors. Thus, the greater an individual believes their risk is of developing breast cancer, the more likely that individual should be to participate in screening.[66] Yet, this assumption is somewhat problematic. While research, in general, indicates that those who have a greater perceived risk for cancer are more likely to have undergone screening for breast cancer,[66] exaggeration of risk may create unnecessary anxiety and actually act as a barrier to breast cancer screening for some women.[67]

THE ROLE OF ANXIETY ON BREAST SCREENING PATTERNS

In a meta-analysis, Hay et al.[68] found there were over 60 studies that tested the relationship between cancer worry and cancer screening, yet these 60 studies were all cross-sectional studies and could not determine whether cancer anxiety influenced screening practices, or whether completion of screening influenced cancer worry, or whether both occurred at the same time. In short, a cross-sectional study is ineffective at measuring cause and effect.

Hay et al., however, analyzed 12 prospective studies that included a cancer screening measure and also measures of worry or anxiety about cancer. This meta-analysis had the power to examine more predictive relationships and supported the contention that breast cancer worry is associated with a stronger likelihood of screening, regardless of the method in which cancer worry was measured, and regardless of the type of screening (mammography or BSE).[68]

Prospective data from other studies also supports this finding showing that worry predicts adherence to fecal occult blood testing for colorectal screening,[69] ultrasound testing for ovarian cancer,[70] genetic testing for breast cancer,[71] and screening for melanoma.[72] Although anxiety about breast cancer is a meaningful predictor of screening behavior, high levels of breast cancer worry, however, are uncommon, and overall worry levels are low.[73,74] Therefore, as Hay et al. suggested, "the scenario of frightened, screening avoidant women is unfounded, perpetuated more by the media than by adequate empirical evidence."[68] Nonetheless, anxiety still seems to motivate women to get screened for breast cancer, and may play a central role in the fact that the odds of receiving appropriate screening for breast cancer is higher in breast cancer survivors than women in the general population controlling for compliance with mammography and CBEs.[44]

INTERVENTIONS INVOLVING BREAST CANCER SCREENING

Community-based breast cancer screening interventions largely use the HBM as a template for research design, but they may also incorporate components of the Theory of Reasoned Action (TRA). At the basis of the TRA is the idea that attitudes about health behavior and an individual's own idea of norms influence behavioral intentions. These intentions then influence whether certain behaviors (e.g., mammography) are adopted. In this way, TRA adds an element of social approval not addressed by the HBM.[63]

Thus, to be successful, community-based breast cancer screening interventions must be multifaceted. They should not only improve overall community knowledge of breast cancer screening recommendations, but also work to remove barriers—at the level of the patient, the provider, the surrounding environment (i.e., community), and the healthcare system. Furthermore, as explained by the TRA, to maintain these habits, the intervention must work to establish guidelines and recommendations that are achievable and socially acceptable.

Often in the most general sense, community-based interventions focus on removing barriers to receiving proper/standard care. Patient barriers include out-of-pocket costs, lack of health insurance, cultural and language differences, lack of information, and logistical challenges including lack of adequate transportation, childcare, or time off of work. Provider barriers include time and financial constraints, lack of staff support, staff turnover, language and cultural differences, forgetfulness, and bias. Barriers at the healthcare system level include communication issues between administrative or office staff and the patient, difficulty in arranging screening appointments, or inconvenient locations of facilities.[75] Interventions can focus, in the most general sense, on removing one of these barriers, or focus instead on removing multiple barriers at the patient, provider, or healthcare system level, or any combination of the three. Table 11–2 lists various intervention strategies for overcoming barriers at the patient-, provider-, and healthcare system-level and possible locations for their implementation.

The majority of community-based interventions have focused on populations of underserved groups that are disproportionately affected by breast cancer and are more likely to fall outside of screening guidelines. Patient-focused interventions typically have focused on patient reminders, culturally tailored messages and treatments, or providing multifaceted interventions that encompass a variety of both patient- and provider-level interventions to influence behavior change.[75] In general, while patient-targeted screening interventions using reminder letters and phone calls have increased mammography among women with high educational attainment or previous mammography, this approach has been less successful among women with lower educational attainment or no history of mammography. Thus, in such groups, removing cultural barriers (i.e., native language education, classroom instruction for patients, and culturally sensitive training for providers) has proven useful.[75] Researchers have suggested that health education materials must be relative to a patient's individual situation and culture. Removing financial barriers, including providing vouchers and free clinic service, have also proven important in populations that were diverse in race, ethnicity, and insurance status.

Yet, while removal of patient barriers is important, in studies with low-income and underinsured populations, provider targeted interventions have led to the greatest increases in screening mammography. Physicians that treat underserved populations typically face language barriers and have fewer resources, greater time pressure, and patient populations with more comorbidities.[75] In these settings, interventions utilizing "natural helpers," known over the years as case managers, lay health advisors, community health workers, outreach workers, promoters, or most recently, patient navigators,[76] have proven successful in increasing mammographic screening.[77]

Overall, studies have demonstrated a beneficial effect for "natural helpers" in increasing the use of mammography,[77] the promptness of diagnosis of breast cancer following an abnormal mammography, and the likelihood of receiving proper and timely treatment for breast

Table 11–2. Intervention strategies for overcoming barriers at the patient-, provider-, and healthcare system-level and possible locations for their implementation

Level of community-based intervention	Intervention types	Possible locations
Patient-level	Invitation letter	Individual homes
	Mailed patient educational material	College campuses
	Invitation phone calls	Community centers
	Home visits	Churches
	Training activities	Social organizations, groups, or networks
	Language translation	Workplace
	Financial incentives	
	Culturally sensitive patient educational patient training sessions	
Provider-level	Organizational change	Hospitals
	Mailed provider educational material	Private practices
	Language translation services	Clinics
	Use of natural helpers/patient navigators	
	Provider feedback	
	Provider reminder	
	Communication training among secretarial and office staff	
Healthcare system-level	Care vouchers	Hospitals
	Parking vouchers	Clinics
	Transportation vouchers	Emergency departments
	Organizational change	
	Relocation of facilities	
	Language translation services	
	Communication training among administrative and office staff	

cancer.[76] Most of these studies have been conducted in underserved or minority populations with the goal of identifying patient-level barriers to the specific health maintenance action, and then helping the participant resolve barriers in order to promote adherence to a required behavior.[76] These "natural helpers" could be of use in decreasing health disparities in underserved and minority populations if ways to integrate them into the healthcare system were possible, including reimbursement and funding. Thus, improving access to care for underserved patients is important, but ensuring that there exists an adequate number of well-trained providers with adequate facilities and funding in areas with underserved populations may be even more important.

SUMMARY

Breast cancer screening, though not perfect, is a necessary tool for reducing mortality among women in the United States and throughout the world. Screening for breast cancer is largely effective because breast cancer is a serious public health problem, affecting a large proportion of the population, which has detectible preclinical phases. Furthermore, the risks associated with the actual screening procedures are low, today's screening practices are reliable, and breast cancer screening is generally accepted by its target population.[78] In addition, past epidemiological studies have identified groups at increased risk for breast cancer and helped develop rigid guidelines for general screening and screening among women at higher risk of developing the disease.

In spite of this, there are still women who fail to adhere to recommended screening guidelines. The reasons for this are multifaceted and include issues at the patient-, provider-, and healthcare system level. Patient-level issues include psychosocial barriers including lack of knowledge, inappropriate perception of risk, embarrassment, anxiety, or fear; economic barriers such as high out-of-pocket expense or lack of health insurance; and logistical barriers including lack of transportation, childcare, or time off of work. Provider barriers include time and financial constraints, lack of staff support, staff turnover, language and cultural differences, forgetfulness, and bias. Barriers at the healthcare system level consist of communication problems, difficulty in arranging screening appointments, or inconvenient locations of facilities. Furthermore, it is often the case that racially diverse groups, poorer groups, and groups in remote, rural areas are disproportionately noncompliant with breast cancer screening recommendations and face more barriers at each level.

To combat these barriers, researchers have developed a wide range of breast cancer screening interventions. While some are highly targeted and focus on removing one specific barrier to screening, others are multilevel and incorporate multiple approaches, either simultaneously or sequentially. General research findings suggest that individuals who are racial or ethnic minorities, who are of low socioeconomic status, or who live in rural areas face a greater number of barriers, have lower knowledge of screening guidelines, and are generally less compliant with screening recommendations. Thus, the majority of community-based interventions focus on populations of underserved groups that are disproportionately affected by breast cancer and are more likely to fall outside of screening guidelines.

Generally, although simple, reminder-based patient-targeted screening interventions increase breast cancer screening compliance among better educated women with previous mammography, this approach is less successful among women with lower educational attainment or no history of mammography. In these women, removing cultural and financial barriers with more involved, service-based interventions is important. In addition, in underserved areas, ensuring there exists an adequate number of well-trained providers with adequate facilities is equally important, because physician recommendation is the strongest predictor of screening adherence.

Lastly, moving into the future, the role of "natural helpers," most recently referred to as patient navigators, in increasing screening compliance and timely diagnosis and treatment following an abnormal screening result must be continually evaluated. Decreasing barriers to breast cancer screening, with the ultimate goal of increasing screening compliance to reduce unnecessary breast cancer deaths, typically involves a multifaceted approach. Natural helpers are specifically trained to meet the unique needs of various populations serving as a bridge between patient-, provider-, and healthcare system-level gaps in breast cancer screening and care.

REFERENCES

1. Surveillance Epidemiology and End Results (SEER) Program. *Breast cancer incidence and mortality data.* Bethesda, MD: National Cancer Institute; 2006.

2. American Cancer Society. *Cancer facts & figures* 2009. Atlanta, GA: American Cancer Society, Inc.; 2009.

3. American Cancer Society. Detailed Guide: *Breast cancer.* American Cancer Society; 2008. http://www.cancer.org/docroot/CRI/content/CRI_2_4_3X_Can_breast_cancer_be_found_early_5.asp?sitearea=. Accessed August 2008.

4. National Cancer Institute. Breast cancer screening (PDQ): Health professional version. Bethesda, MD: National Cancer Institute, US National Institutes of Health; 2008. http://www.cancer.gov/cancertopics/pdq/screening/breast/healthprofessional. Accessed August 2008.

5. Aziz H, Hussain F, Sohn C, et al. Early onset of breast carcinoma in African American women with poor prognostic factors. *Am J Clin Oncol.* 1999;22(5):436–440.

6. Couch FJ, DeShano ML, Blackwood MA, et al. BRCA1 mutations in women attending clinics that evaluate the risk of breast cancer. *N Engl J Med.* 1997;336(20):1409–1415.

7. Horn PL, Thompson WD. Risk of contralateral breast cancer: associations with factors related to initial breast cancer. *Am J Epidemiol.* 1988; 128(2):309–323.

8. Colditz GA, Willett WC, Hunter DJ, et al. Family history, age, and risk of breast cancer. Prospective data from the Nurses' Health Study. *JAMA.* 1993;270(3):338–343.

9. American Cancer Society. *Cancer facts & figures 2006.* Atlanta, GA: American Cancer Society, Inc.; 2006.

10. Newman LA. Breast cancer in African-American women. *Oncologist.* 2005;10(1):1–14.

11. Reeves GK, Pirie K, Beral V, Green J, Spencer E, Bull D. Cancer incidence and mortality in relation to body mass index in the Million Women Study: cohort study. *BMJ.* 2007;335(7630):1134.

12. Wang J, John EM, Horn-Ross PL, Ingles SA. Dietary fat, cooking fat, and breast cancer risk in a multiethnic population. *Nutr Cancer.* 2008;60(4):492–504.

13. Smith-Warner SA, Spiegelman D, Yaun SS, et al. Alcohol and breast cancer in women: a pooled analysis of cohort studies. *JAMA.* 1998;279(7):535–540.

14. Rossouw JE, Anderson GL, Prentice RL, et al. Risks and benefits of estrogen plus progestin in healthy postmenopausal women: principal results From the Women's Health Initiative randomized controlled trial. *JAMA.* 2002;288(3):321–333.

15. Wiseman RA. Breast cancer: critical data analysis concludes that estrogens are not the cause, however lifestyle changes can alter risk rapidly. *J Clin Epidemiol.* 2004;57(8):766–772.

16. Moody-Ayers SY, Wells CK, Feinstein AR. "Benign" tumors and "early detection" in mammography-screened patients of a natural cohort with breast cancer. *Arch Intern Med.* 2000;160(8):1109–1115.

17. Centers for Disease Control. *BRFSS user's guide.* Atlanta, GA: Centers for Disease Control; 2008. ftp://ftp.cdc.gov/pub/Data/Brfss/userguide.pdf. Accessed August 2008.

18. Nystrom L, Andersson I, Bjurstam N, Frisell J, Nordenskjold B, Rutqvist LE. Long-term effects of mammography screening: updated overview of the Swedish randomised trials. *Lancet.* 2002;359(9310):909–919.

19. Moss SM, Cuckle H, Evans A, Johns L, Waller M, Bobrow L. Effect of mammographic screening from age 40 years on breast cancer mortality at 10 years' follow-up: a randomised controlled trial. *Lancet.* 2006;368(9552):2053–2060.

20. Carney PA, Miglioretti DL, Yankaskas BC, et al. Individual and combined effects of age, breast density, and hormone replacement therapy use on the accuracy of screening mammography. *Ann Intern Med.* 2003;138(3):168–175.

21. Rosenberg RD, Hunt WC, Williamson MR, et al. Effects of age, breast density, ethnicity, and estrogen replacement therapy on screening mammographic sensitivity and cancer stage at diagnosis: review of 183,134 screening mammograms in Albuquerque, New Mexico. *Radiology.* 1998;209(2):511–518.

22. Kerlikowske K, Grady D, Barclay J, Sickles EA, Ernster V. Likelihood ratios for modern screening mammography. Risk of breast cancer based on age and mammographic interpretation. *JAMA.* 1996;276(1):39–43.

23. Buist DS, Porter PL, Lehman C, Taplin SH, White E. Factors contributing to mammography failure in women aged 40–49 years. *J Natl Cancer Inst.* 2004;96(19):1432–1440.

24. Physician Insurers Association of America. *Breast cancer study.* Washington, DC: Physician Insurers Association of America; 1995.

25. Kerlikowske K, Grady D, Barclay J, et al. Variability and accuracy in mammographic interpretation using the American College of Radiology Breast Imaging Reporting and Data System. *J Natl Cancer Inst.* 1998;90(23):1801–1809.

26. Elmore JG, Wells CK, Lee CH, Howard DH, Feinstein AR. Variability in radiologists' interpretations of mammograms. *N Engl J Med.* 1994;331(22):1493–1499.

27. Smith-Bindman R, Chu P, Miglioretti DL, et al. Physician predictors of mammographic accuracy. *J Natl Cancer Inst.* 2005;97(5):358–367.

28. Baines CJ, Miller AB, Bassett AA. Physical examination. Its role as a single screening modality in the Canadian National Breast Screening Study. *Cancer.* 1989;63(9):1816–1822.

29. Bobo JK, Lee NC, Thames SF. Findings from 752,081 clinical breast examinations reported to a national screening program from 1995 through 1998. *J Natl Cancer Inst.* 2000;92(12):971–976.

30. Oestreicher N, Lehman CD, Seger DJ, Buist DS, White E. The incremental contribution of clinical breast examination to invasive cancer detection in a mammography screening program. *AJR Am J Roentgenol.* 2005;184(2):428–432.

31. Humphrey LL, Helfand M, Chan BK, Woolf SH. Breast cancer screening: a summary of the evidence for the U.S. Preventive Services Task Force. *Ann Intern Med.* 2002;137(5 pt 1):347–360.

32. Thomas DB, Gao DL, Ray RM, et al. Randomized trial of breast self-examination in Shanghai: final results. *J Natl Cancer Inst.* 2002;94(19):1445–1457.

33. Teh W, Wilson AR. The role of ultrasound in breast cancer screening. A consensus statement by the European Group for Breast Cancer Screening. *Eur J Cancer.* 1998;34(4):449–450.

34. Lehman CD, Gatsonis C, Kuhl CK, et al. MRI evaluation of the contralateral breast in women with recently diagnosed breast cancer. *N Engl J Med.* 2007;356(13):1295–1303.

35. Lord SJ, Lei W, Craft P, et al. A systematic review of the effectiveness of magnetic resonance imaging (MRI) as an addition to mammography and ultrasound in screening young women at high risk of breast cancer. *Eur J Cancer.* 2007;43(13):1905–1917.

36. Lawrence WF, Liang W, Mandelblatt JS, et al. Serendipity in diagnostic imaging: magnetic resonance imaging of the breast. *J Natl Cancer Inst.* 1998;90(23):1792–1800.

37. Centers for Disease Control. *Behavior risk factor surveillance system prevalence and trends data: Women's health, 2006.* Atlanta, GA: Centers for Disease Control; 2006. http://apps.nccd.cdc.gov/brfss/. Accessed August 2008.

38. Farria DM, Schmidt ME, Monsees BS, et al. Professional and economic factors affecting access to mammography: a crisis today, or tomorrow? Results from a national survey. *Cancer.* 2005;104(3):491–498.

39. Mills N, Donovan JL, Smith M, Jacoby A, Neal DE, Hamdy FC. Perceptions of equipoise are crucial to trial participation: a qualitative study of men in the ProtecT study. *Control Clin Trials.* 2003;24(3):272–282.

40. Agency on Healthcare Research and Quality (AHRQ). *National healthcare disparities report.* Rockville, MD: Agency on Healthcare Research and Quality; 2008.

41. Earle CC, Burstein HJ, Winer EP, Weeks JC. Quality of non-breast cancer health maintenance among elderly breast cancer survivors. *J Clin Oncol.* 2003;21(8):1447–1451.

42. Isaacs C, Peshkin BN, Schwartz M, Demarco TA, Main D, Lerman C. Breast and ovarian cancer screening practices in healthy women with a strong family history of breast or ovarian cancer. *Breast Cancer Res Treat.* 2002;71(2):103–112.

43. Meissner HI, Breen N, Taubman ML, Vernon SW, Graubard BI. Which women aren't getting mammograms and why? (United States). *Cancer Causes Control.* 2007;18(1):61–70.

44. Duffy CM, Clark MA, Allsworth JE. Health maintenance and screening in breast cancer survivors in the United States. *Cancer Detect Prev.* 2006;30(1):52–57.

45. Siahpush M, Singh GK. Sociodemographic variations in breast cancer screening behavior among Australian women: results from the 1995 National Health Survey. *Prev Med.* 2002;35(2):174–180.

46. Cairns CP, Viswanath K. Communication and colorectal cancer screening among the uninsured: data from the Health Information National Trends Survey (United States). *Cancer Causes Control.* 2006;17(9):1115–1125.

47. Coughlin SS, Wilson KM. Breast and cervical cancer screening among migrant and seasonal farmworkers: a review. *Cancer Detect Prev.* 2002;26(3):203–209.

48. Potosky AL, Breen N, Graubard BI, Parsons PE. The association between health care coverage and the use of cancer screening tests. Results from the 1992 National Health Interview Survey. *Med Care.* 1998;36(3):257–270.

49. Aparicio-Ting F, Ramirez AG. Breast and cervical cancer knowledge, attitudes, and screening practices of Hispanic women diagnosed with cancer. *J Cancer Educ.* 2003;18(4):230–236.

50. Finney Rutten LJ, Iannotti RJ. Health beliefs, salience of breast cancer family history, and involvement with breast cancer issues: adherence to annual mammography screening recommendations. *Cancer Detect Prev.* 2003;27(5):353–359.

51. Bynum JP, Braunstein JB, Sharkey P, Haddad K, Wu AW. The influence of health status, age, and race on screening mammography in elderly women. *Arch Intern Med.* 2005;165(18):2083–2088.

52. Durvasula RS, Regan PC, Ureno O, Howell L. Frequency of cervical and breast cancer screening rates in a multi-ethnic female college sample. *Psychol Rep.* 2006;99(2):418–420.

53. Warren AG, Londono GE, Wessel LA, Warren RD. Breaking down barriers to breast and cervical cancer screening: a university-based prevention program for Latinas. *J Health Care Poor Underserved.* 2006;17(3):512–521.

54. Freeman HP. Patient navigation: a community based strategy to reduce cancer disparities. *J Urban Health.* 2006;83(2):139–141.

55. Bazargan M, Lindstrom RW, Dakak A, Ani C, Wolf KE, Edelstein RA. Impact of desire to work in underserved communities on selection of specialty among fourth-year medical students. *J Natl Med Assoc.* 2006;98(9):1460–1465.

56. Freeman HP, Chu KC. Determinants of cancer disparities: barriers to cancer screening, diagnosis, and treatment. *Surg Oncol Clin N Am.* 2005;14(4):655–669, v.

57. Kaplan KM, Weinberg GB, Small A, Herndon JL. Breast cancer screening among relatives of women with breast cancer. *Am J Public Health.* 1991;81(9):1174–1179.

58. American Cancer Society. *Cancer facts & figures 2007.* Atlanta, GA: American Cancer Society, Inc.; 2007.

59. Katz ML, Donahue KA, Alfano CM, Day JM, Herndon JE II, Paskett ED. Cancer surveillance behaviors and psychosocial factors among long-term survivors of breast cancer. Cancer and Leukemia Group B 79804. *Cancer.* 2009;115(3):480–488.

60. Aiken LS, West SG, Woodward CK, Reno RR. Health beliefs and compliance with mammography-screening recommendations in asymptomatic women. *Health Psychol.* 1994;13(2):122–129.

61. Champion VL. The relationship of breast self-examination to health belief model variables. *Res Nurs Health.* 1987;10(6):375–382.

62. Stein JA, Fox SA, Murata PJ, Morisky DE. Mammography usage and the health belief model. *Health Educ Q.* 1992;19(4):447–462.

63. Janz NK, Becker MH. The health belief model: a decade later. *Health Educ Q.* 1984;11(1):1–47.

64. Lantz PM, Stencil D, Lippert MT, Beversdorf S, Jaros L, Remington PL. Breast and cervical cancer screening in a low-income managed care sample: the efficacy of physician letters and phone calls. *Am J Public Health.* 1995;85(6):834–836.

65. Weinrich SP, Weinrich MC. Cancer knowledge among elderly individuals. *Cancer Nurs.* 1986;9(6):301–307.

66. Vernon SW, Vogel VG, Halabi S, Bondy ML. Factors associated with perceived risk of breast cancer among women attending a screening program. *Breast Cancer Res Treat.* 1993;28(2):137–144.

67. Black WC, Nease RF Jr, Tosteson AN. Perceptions of breast cancer risk and screening effectiveness in women younger than 50 years of age. *J Natl Cancer Inst.* 1995;87(10):720–731.

68. Hay JL, McCaul KD, Magnan RE. Does worry about breast cancer predict screening behaviors? A meta-analysis of the prospective evidence. *Prev Med.* 2006;42(6):401–408.

69. Myers RE, Ross E, Jepson C, et al. Modeling adherence to colorectal cancer screening. *Prev Med.* 1994;23(2):142–151.

70. Schwartz M, Lerman C, Daly M, Audrain J, Masny A, Griffith K. Utilization of ovarian cancer screening by women at increased risk. *Cancer Epidemiol Biomarkers Prev.* 1995;4(3):269–273.

71. Lerman C, Hughes C, Benkendorf JL, et al. Racial differences in testing motivation and psychological distress following pretest education for BRCA1 gene testing. *Cancer Epidemiol Biomarkers Prev.* 1999;8(4 pt 2):361–367.

72. de Rooij MJ, Rampen FH, Schouten LJ, Neumann HA. Factors influencing participation among melanoma screening attenders. *Acta Derm Venereol.* 1997;77(6):467–470.

73. Burgess C, Cornelius V, Love S, Graham J, Richards M, Ramirez A. Depression and anxiety in women with early breast cancer: five year observational cohort study. *BMJ.* 2005;330(7493):702.

74. Carver CS, Antoni MH. Finding benefit in breast cancer during the year after diagnosis predicts better adjustment 5 to 8 years after diagnosis. *Health Psychol.* 2004;23(6):595–598.

75. Masi CM, Blackman DJ, Peek ME. Interventions to enhance breast cancer screening, diagnosis, and treatment among racial and ethnic minority women. *Med Care Res Rev.* 2007;64(suppl 5):195S–242S.

76. Wells KJ, Battaglia TA, Dudley DJ, et al. Patient navigation: state of the art or is it science? *Cancer.* 2008;113(8):1999–2010.

77. Freeman HP. Patient navigation: a community centered approach to reducing cancer mortality. *J Cancer Educ.* 2006;21(Suppl 1):S11–S14.

78. Shapiro S, Venet W, Strax P, Venet L, Roeser R. Ten- to fourteen-year effect of screening on breast cancer mortality. *J Natl Cancer Inst.* 1982;69(2):349–355.

Prostate Cancer Screening

Ronald E. Myers

INTRODUCTION

Prostate cancer is a worldwide public health problem. It is a greater problem in the United States and in Western European countries than in other parts of the world. Prostate cancer screening, which is used to find early-stage, treatable disease, is more commonly offered to men in the United States than in most other countries. Results of recent randomized trials have increased controversy about whether prostate cancer screening should be offered routinely to asymptomatic older adult men. However, there is consensus that adult men and their healthcare providers should discuss the pros and cons of screening and make an informed, shared decision about testing for the disease. A number of patient, provider, and practice factors have made it difficult to achieve this ideal. Current research on decision aids may help to increase informed decision making about screening and may have implications for related areas of concern, such as screening for prostate cancer risk, adherence to recommended follow-up of abnormal findings, and the uptake of protective health behaviors. This chapter discusses these issues and suggests future directions for work that is needed to advance the field of prostate cancer prevention and control.

VITAL STATISTICS AND SCREENING

In 2007, there were an estimated 254,000 deaths worldwide from prostate cancer, making this disease the sixth leading cause of cancer deaths among men.[1] Death rates for prostate cancer have declined in the United States and some Western European countries, including the United Kingdom, and Canada. Prostate cancer mortality rates are relatively low in Asia and North Africa, but are likely to increase.[2]

In the United States, prostate cancer is the most frequently diagnosed type of male cancer and the second leading cause of cancer-related death for men. It is estimated that in 2009 a total of 192,280 new cases of prostate cancer will be diagnosed, and 27,360 men will die from the disease.[3]

Approximately one in seven men in the United States will be diagnosed with prostate cancer during their lifetimes.[4] Among men in the general population, the risk for being diagnosed with prostate cancer increases with age, particularly after age 50. Almost two-thirds of prostate cancer cases are diagnosed in men who are 65 years of age or older. Prostate cancer incidence and mortality rates are substantially higher among African Americans and Caribbean American males, as compared to Caucasian males. Rates are also significantly higher among men who have an affected first-degree relative, as compared to men who do not have a family history.

Prostate cancer is most often detected using the digital rectal examination (DRE) and prostate-specific antigen (PSA) testing. Although other procedures have been advanced for use in screening (e.g., PSA velocity, PSA density, age-specific PSA range, and free PSA), the combined use of PSA testing and DRE is the most commonly recommended screening method.

Prostate cancer incidence rates in the United States increased dramatically from 1988 to 1992, and subsequently declined from 1992 to 1995. These trends may be attributed to the introduction of PSA testing as a prostate cancer screening method in the late 1980s and to the rapid uptake of this screening modality in primary care practice. Since 1995, prostate cancer incidence rates have remained relatively stable. The overwhelming majority of newly diagnosed prostate cancer cases are found at an early stage. Survival following treatment is high, with rates for localized prostate cancer approaching 100%.[3]

PSA testing has become part of routine care in the United States. Among men aged 50 or more, PSA testing has been performed for 55% of white non-Hispanic men and for 50% of black non-Hispanic men.[5] Use of this screening modality has been accompanied by a dramatic reduction in prostate cancer mortality. The uptake of PSA testing has not been as great in the United Kingdom as in the United States; and, it is interesting to note that while both countries have experienced declining prostate cancer mortality rates, the reduction in mortality has been more dramatic in the United States than in the United Kingdom.[6]

CONTROVERSY AND CONSENSUS

The routine practice of performing prostate cancer screening for older men has sparked substantial controversy between proponents and opponents of this practice. Proponents of prostate cancer screening take the position that epidemiologic data indicate screening is an effective method for identifying men with early prostate cancer. Further, those in favor of routine screening argue that men who are diagnosed with and treated aggressively for localized prostate cancer have higher survival rates as compared to men diagnosed with late-stage disease. International comparisons of mortality rates in the United States and other countries are also used to support the case for routine screening. The American Cancer Society and the American Urological Association recommend the routine use of combined DRE and PSA testing for men who have a reasonable life expectancy, particularly men who are at increased risk on the basis of race and family history.[3,7] Specifically, the organizations recommend that healthcare providers should offer annual DRE and PSA testing routinely for men aged 50 or more, and that screening should be initiated earlier for African American men and those who have a family history of prostate cancer.

Debate about prostate cancer screening has been spurred by findings from recently-reported randomized trials. Data from the trial conducted in the United States indicates that prostate cancer screening does not save lives,[8] while data from the European trial suggests that screening may produce a modest reduction in mortality.[9] Both trials concluded, however, that mass screening with PSA results in substantial overdiagnosis and related morbidity. In addition, it is not currently possible to determine whether a given screening-detected prostate cancer is indolent and may not present as a health problem, or if the lesion is aggressive and lethal. Thus, some men with a screening-detected prostate cancer will undergo invasive treatment for an indolent cancer that may not have caused any health problems. Routine screening has also been challenged, because the sensitivity and specificity of PSA testing and DRE are relatively low, even when combined. This situation can lead to false negative results that may provide unwarranted reassurance, or false positive results that may lead to unnecessary diagnostic procedures, including having a prostate biopsy. As a result, men who have an abnormal screening test result may needlessly experience anxiety, exposure to medical risks associated with diagnostic evaluation procedures, and side effects of treatment (e.g., bowel problems, incontinence, and impotence).[10] These concerns have led the United States Preventive Services Task Force (USPSTF) to conclude that there is not enough evidence to recommend for or against routine screening for prostate cancer.[11] It is important to point out, however, that the American Cancer Society, American Urological Association, the USPSTF, and other organizations the United States have recommended that men should discuss the pros and cons of prostate cancer screening with a healthcare provider before screening, and that men should make an informed, shared decision together with their providers as to whether to undergo testing.

FACTORS ASSOCIATED WITH SCREENING USE

Survey data collected in research studies suggest that most American men eligible for screening are aware of prostate cancer screening.[12] In fact, it has been reported that up to 75% of men aged 50 and older have had a PSA test and 65% expect that they will have a PSA test as part of a routine physical examination.[13–15] Chan and colleagues[16–18] have discovered, however, that most older adult men do not know important facts about prostate cancer screening that may influence decision making about screening use, including that it is not known whether screening reduces mortality and that screening produces false positive and false negative results. Further, it appears that most older men have few worries and concerns about having a prostate cancer-screening test and view screening as a normal part of routine care (RE Myers, unpublished data, 2006).[19,20] In general, men tend to view prostate cancer screening uncritically as a recommended preventive healthcare service.

A number of studies have reported on characteristics of men who are likely to undergo prostate cancer screening. Findings from these studies indicate that men likely to report having had a prostate cancer-screening test include those who are older, are white, are married, are nonsmokers, and have a higher level of formal education. Men who have had a screening examination are also likely to have a medical home, have insurance, perceive their risk for prostate cancer to be high, view screening as a beneficial preventive health procedure, and believe that healthcare providers support screening.[19,21–32]

Important disparities related to prostate cancer screening knowledge and use have been reported in the literature. Specifically, it has been reported that African American men are less likely to be knowledgeable about prostate cancer screening than white men.[19,26,33,34] In an analysis of Medicare claims data, Etzioni et al.[10] also found that African American men are also less likely to have prostate cancer screening than white men. In a more recent study, Gilligan et al.[35] examined data for a random sample of 69,968 anonymous Medicare beneficiaries 65 years of age and older, controlling for possible confounders. Results of multivariable analyses involving age, race, socioeconomic status, comorbidities, and PSA test use showed that African American men were half as likely as white men to undergo screening. Factors that have been found to predict prostate cancer screening among African American men include older age, being married, belief that screening should be done in the absence of prostate cancer symptoms, intention to screen, and support from a primary care provider.[36,37]

Little is known about factors that explain screening use in another high-risk segment of the population, men with a family history of prostate cancer. A study conducted by Beebe-Dimer et al.[38] involved 111 men, each of whom had one or more brothers diagnosed with prostate cancer. Analyses of survey data showed that the majority of the men perceived their risk for developing prostate cancer to be greater than or equal to 50% and expressed heightened concern about being diagnosed with the disease in the future. These findings are consistent with other reports on the association between family history and perceived risk for prostate cancer.[39,40] Jacobsen and colleagues[41] conducted a study designed to assess the relationship between family history of prostate cancer, perceived vulnerability, and participant use of prostate cancer screening. This investigation involved 83 men with a positive family history

of prostate cancer and 83 men with a negative family history of prostate cancer. The authors found that men with a positive family history reported greater perceived vulnerability to developing prostate cancer and a stronger intention to undergo screening. From their analyses, the authors also found that heightened concern about developing prostate cancer served to motivate screening use among men with a family history. In a study that focused on the impact of both race and family history, Bloom et al.[25] interviewed 88 African American men with a family history of prostate cancer and 120 with no family history of the disease. Men who had a family history of prostate cancer were more likely than those who did not have a family history to report having had recent PSA screening. It is interesting to note, however, that African American men in these two groups did not differ significantly in terms of their perceived risk, perhaps due to a shared perception of being at increased risk for prostate cancer on the basis of race.

FOLLOW-UP OF ABNORMAL SCREENING RESULTS

The response of patients to having an abnormal prostate cancer-screening test is relatively unexplored. Many men who have an abnormal prostate cancer screening result and receive a recommendation to have a prostate biopsy do not follow through. In one study, Krongrad et al.[42] showed that out of 76 patients with an abnormal PSA and/or DRE, only 43 (57%) pursued prostate biopsy. Several patient-level factors have been found to be associated with diagnostic evaluation after an abnormal cancer-screening result, including the lack of insurance coverage, not knowing about the abnormal finding, lack of understanding about follow-up procedures, worry about being diagnosed with cancer, concern about specific diagnostic procedures, and perceived lack of social support for follow-up.[43] In a study involving 413 asymptomatic African American men,[44] participants were asked to assume the following: they had undergone prostate cancer screening, were informed that they had an abnormal screening result, and were advised to have a prostate biopsy. In response to this scenario, participants were asked about their intention to adhere to the recommended follow-up. Of the 413 participants, 77% indicated that they intended to have the biopsy. Intention was positively and significantly associated with education, the belief that prostate cancer can be cured, self-efficacy, and physician support.

SCREENING FOR RISK

The Human Genome Project has catalyzed growth in research on genetic and epigenetic factors that confer increased risk for different cancers, including prostate cancer.[45,46] The project has focused increased attention to the problem of clarifying circumstances under which testing may be offered in clinical settings.[47,48]

Several studies have reported on interest among men in being screened for genetic risk. Bratt et al.[49] asked 101 unaffected sons of men diagnosed with prostate cancer about their interest in having a genetic testing for disease risk. Over 90% stated that they would have such testing if it were available. Miesfeldt et al.[50] asked a similar question to 342 men who were aged 50 or more and presented for prostate cancer screening at a medical clinic. Eighty-nine percent of the respondents stated that they would undergo genetic testing to determine their prostate cancer risk. Myers et al.[27] surveyed African American men aged 40–70 to assess their intention to have a genetic test for the purpose of determining their personal risk for developing prostate cancer in the future. Of these men, 86% stated that they intended to be tested, when such testing becomes available.

The reported strong interest in genetic risk assessment in different population groups is consistent with findings from earlier studies on cancer genetic risk assessment reported in the literature.[51–60] While further research in this area is needed before genetic testing for prostate cancer risk can be made available to men as part of routine care, it is important to anticipate this eventuality and learn how providers and patients can address the matter of informed decision making about having such testing. It is also important to determine what impact the results of risk assessment have on emotional well-being, social relationships, and lifestyle modifications in everyday life.

MAKING AN INFORMED, SHARED DECISION

As mentioned earlier, current prostate cancer screening guidelines recommend that healthcare providers make men who are eligible for prostate cancer screening aware of the pros and cons associated with screening and engage in shared decision making to facilitate patient informed decision making about prostate cancer screening. It seems, however, that this practice has not yet been adopted as part of routine care. In a national survey, Han et al.[61] reported that physicians often order PSA testing without discussing the pros and cons of screening with the patient. There are a variety of reasons for noncompliance with guidelines that recommend shared decision making in physician–patient encounters, including the need to attend to existing comorbidities, physician reluctance to address the issue of screening with patients who are perceived of as uninterested in screening, physician forgetfulness, physician belief that patients will not understand informational details, and physician lack of time.[62] Clearly, there is a need for methods that can be used in primary care practice settings to facilitate informed decision making about prostate cancer screening.[63] Decision aids may be useful tools to help address this problem. A number of studies have been conducted to determine the impact of decision aids (e.g., informational brochures, educational videotapes, interactive videodiscs, and websites), as well as formatted print material and decision boards (i.e., charts showing the likelihood of different events) related to a variety of health decisions.[64,65] Research on the use of decision aids in prostate cancer screening has been informative.

INTERVENTIONS TO FACILITATE INFORMED AND SHARED DECISION MAKING

In a review of the literature on the use of decision aids related to prostate cancer screening, Volk et al.[66] reported on 18 trials involving a total of 6221 trial participants that evaluated prostate cancer screening decision aids. The majority of the studies (n = 16) involved patients who visited primary care practices. The remaining two studies included individuals who attended community sites where access to screening was provided. In 10 of the studies, a videotape was used to prepare men for decision making about screening. One study combined a videotape and discussion. The remaining studies used scripted overviews, print materials, print materials combined with educational sessions, and Internet-based materials. Decision aids provided to participants in selected studies were designed as information delivery tools. Only two of the studies presented theory-based conceptual models that guided intervention delivery and evaluation. The authors found that exposure to decision aids served to increase participant knowledge and confidence in decision making about prostate cancer screening. Among individuals who presented for routine health care, exposure to decision aids tended to decrease participant enthusiasm for screening. Interestingly, decision aid use did not reduce screening if the opportunity to have screening were offered in the practice setting. When considered together, these observations suggest that perceptions about screening and actual screening use can be influenced both by exposure to information decision aids and by the nature of physician-patient encounters that take place in the practice setting.

Other reports suggest that the use of decision aids in clinic settings may serve to increase prostate cancer screening among African American patients and decrease screening among white patients.[36,67,68] A possible explanation for this phenomenon is the fact that risk factor information included in prostate cancer-screening decision aids may have the effect of raising awareness that being African American is a significant and substantial prostate cancer risk factor. It is reasonable to believe that for African Americans, exposure to such information may operate as a potent behavioral prompt.

As noted above, most studies on the use of decision aids to promote informed decision making about prostate cancer screening have not used theoretical models to guide intervention development or evaluation. In one study, however, Partin et al.[69] developed an informational pamphlet and related content designed to increase patient knowledge about prostate cancer and influence decision making about screening. Intervention development and outcomes analyses were grounded in social cognitive theory.[70] This framework reflects the view that background characteristics, cognitive processes, and environmental factors shape behavior and experienced consequences, which, in turn, influence cognitive and environmental processes. Myers and colleagues[71-73] have studied decision counseling as a mediated decision support method to increase informed and shared decision making about prostate cancer screening. Decision counseling is grounded in the Preventive Health Model (PHM), an explanatory framework that integrates self-regulation theory and analytic hierarchy processing theory.[73] In brief, the PHM assumes that informed decision making can be facilitated by assuring that the individual understands his decision situation and available decision alternatives (e.g., to have or not to have a screening examination), undergoes a systematic process of identifying and weighing of personal "pros" and "cons" related to the decision alternatives, and clarifies personal preference related to the alternatives. Decision counseling is a process that makes these concepts operational in the context of a mediated exchange involving a trained provider and patient who is asked to consider whether to have screening. The decision counseling session is concluded with the generation of a summary report that specifies the client's preferred decision alternative, the strength of the decision preference, and those factors that account for preference. This report is reviewed with the client by a healthcare provider to reach an informed shared decision that is consistent with the patient's personal values.[74] Research is needed to assess the impact of this approach on patient perceptions, provider-patient interactions, and behavioral outcomes.

FUTURE DIRECTIONS

Prostate cancer is a worldwide problem for older men. It is especially prevalent in developed countries and is an emerging public health issue in developing countries, where populations are adopting Western lifestyles and dietary patterns. While it is possible to find and treat early prostate cancer through the use of PSA testing and DRE, there is a substantial amount of controversy about the routine use of these modalities as part of primary care in the United States and in other countries. As mentioned earlier, the results of recent randomized prostate cancer screening trials have fueled the debate about whether prostate cancer screening should be part of routine care.

Since the controversy about prostate cancer screening is likely to persist, it is important to advance research on informed and shared decision making about prostate cancer screening in the context of primary care practice. It is necessary to conduct research that will help to identify effective theory-based methods for preparing men and their supportive others to clarify personal preferences related to screening and the follow-up of abnormal screening test findings. It is also critically important to develop approaches that enable patients to play an active role in deciding whether to be tested for risk and whether to be tested for prostate cancer. Findings from a recent report by Cegala, Street, and Clinch show that primary care patients who are active participants in the physician–patient encounter receive more information overall and obtain more thorough and complete answers to their questions.[75] These effects were especially pronounced in relation to medical tests and treatment procedures. The work of Greenfield, Kaplan, and Ware on the value of patient coaching indicates that substantial gains may be achieved in increasing patient participation in such discussions.[76,77] As research in this area proceeds, particular attention should be paid to the literacy and cultural sensitivity needs of men at average and increased risk for prostate cancer.

To achieve the goal of increasing the level of informed and shared decision making about prostate cancer screening and other important health decision situations that are characterized by uncertainty, there is a pressing need for studies that apply behavioral theory and decision theory to intervention development and evaluation. Insights related to patient behavior, provider behavior, and patient–provider interactions related to screening for prostate risk and early detection can help to inform the development of effective decision aids that may be used successfully in healthcare settings.[12]

Finally, research is being conducted in the area of prostate cancer prevention. Strategies that include reducing dietary fat and increasing the intake of various dietary supplements (e.g., selenium and vitamins D and E), soy, green tea, and lycopene are being explored.[4] Further, data from the recently concluded Prostate Cancer Prevention Trial support the use of finasteride as a chemopreventive agent. It is hopeful to note that many older adult men have reported that they engage in conventional or self-care activities (screening, lifestyle modification, dietary supplement use), which they believe may protect them from developing prostate cancer.[78] If, indeed, men are receptive to the notion of taking action to prevent prostate cancer, it is important for healthcare providers to be trained in the use of "best practice" interventions that serve to engage men in decision making about prostate cancer prevention and screening. Theory-based research is needed to develop, assess, and disseminate cost-effective methods that can be used at the individual and population level.

ACKNOWLEDGMENTS

I would like to express my sincere appreciation to Martha Kasper-Keintz, ScM, Heidi Swan, BA, and Almeta Mathis for providing administrative assistance in preparing this chapter.

REFERENCES

1. Garcia M, Jemal A, Ward EM, et al. *Global cancer facts & figures 2007*. Atlanta, GA: American Cancer Society; 2007:16.

2. Nelen V. Epidemiology of prostate cancer. In: Ramon J, Denis LJ, eds. *Prostate cancer*. Vol. 175. Berlin, Heidelberg: Springer-Verlag; 2007;1:1-7.

3. American Cancer Society. *Cancer facts & figures* 2009. Atlanta, GA: American Cancer Society; 2009.

4. Fleshner N, Zlotta AR. Prostate cancer prevention: past, present, and future. *Cancer*. 2007;110:1889–1899.

5. Behavioral Risk Factor Surveillance System. Public use data file, 2004. National Center for Chronic Disease Prevention and Health Promotion, Centers for Disease Control and Prevention; 2005.

6. Collin SM, Martin RM, Metcalfe C, et al. Prostate-cancer mortality in the USA and UK in 1975–2004: an ecological study. *Lancet Oncol*. 2008;9: 445–452.

7. American Urological Association. AUANet | About AUA | Policy Statements | Urological Services. http://www.auanet.org/about/policy/services. cfm#detection. Accessed June 9, 2008.

8. Andriole GL, Crawford D, Grubb RL, et al. Mortality results from a randomized prostate- cancer screening trial. *New Eng J Med*. 2009;360:1310–1319.

9. Schroeder FH, Hugosson J, Roobol MJ, et al. Screening and prostate-cancer mortality in a European randomised trial. *New Eng JfMed*. 2009;360: 1320–1328.

10. Etzioni R, Penson DF, Legler JM, et al. Overdiagnosis due to prostate-specific antigen screening: lessons from U.S. prostate cancer incidence trends. *J Natl Cancer Inst*. 2002;94:981–990.

11. U.S. Preventive Services Task Force. *Screening for prostate cancer: What's new from the USPSTF?* http://www.ahrq.gov/clinic/3rduspstf/prostatescr/prostatwh.htm. Accessed June 5, 2008.

12. Woolf SH, Krist AH, Johnson RE, Stenborg PS. Unwanted control: how patients in the primary care setting decide about screening for prostate cancer. *Patient Educ Couns*. 2005;56:116–124.

13. Sirovich BE, Schwartz LM, Woloshin S. Screening men for prostate and colorectal cancer in the united states: does practice reflect the evidence? *JAMA*. 2003;289:1414–1420.

14. Oboler SK, Prochazka AV, Gonzales R, Xu S, Anderson RJ. Public expectations and attitudes for annual physical examinations and testing. *Ann Intern Med*. 2002;136:652-659.

15. Voss JD, Schectman JM. Prostate cancer screening practices and beliefs. *J Gen Intern Med*. 2001;16:831–837.

16. Chan EC, Barry MJ, Vernon SW, Ahn C. Brief report: physicians and their personal prostate cancer-screening practices with prostate-specific antigen. A national survey. *J Gen Intern Med*. 2006;21:257–259.

17. Chan EC, Haynes MC, O'Donnell FT, Bachino C, Vernon SW. Cultural sensitivity and informed decision making about prostate cancer screening. *J Community Health*. 2003;28:393–405.

18. Chan EC, Vernon SW, Ahn C, Greisinger A. Do men know that they have had a prostate-specific antigen test? Accuracy of self-reports of testing at 2 sites. *Am J Public Health*. 2004;94:1336–1338.

19. Steele CB, Miller DS, Maylahn C, Uhler RJ, Baker CT. Knowledge, attitudes, and screening practices among older men regarding prostate cancer. *Am J Public Health*. 2000;90:1595–1600.

20. Steginga SK, Occhipinti S, McCaffrey J, Dunn J. Men's attitudes toward prostate cancer and seeking prostate-specific antigen testing. *J Cancer Educ*. 2001;16:42–45.

21. Eisen SA, Waterman B, Skinner CS, et al. Sociodemographic and health status characteristics with prostate cancer screening in a national cohort of middle-aged male veterans. *Urology*. 1999;53:516–522.

22. Tingen MS, Weinrich SP, Heydt DD, Boyd MD, Weinrich MC. Perceived benefits: a predictor of participation in prostate cancer screening. *Cancer Nurs*. 1998;21:349–357.

23. Moran WP, Cohen SJ, Preisser JS, et al. Factors influencing use of the prostate-specific antigen screening test in primary care. *Am J Manage Care*. 2000;6:315–324.

24. Calsoyas I, Stratton MS. Prostate cancer screening: a racial dichotomy. *Arch Intern Med*. 2004;164:1830–1832.

25. Bloom JR, Stewart SL, Oakley-Girvans I, et al. Family history, perceived risk, and prostate cancer screening among African American men. *Cancer Epidemiol Biomarkers Prev*. 2006;15:2167–2173.

26. Consedine NS, Morgenstern AH, Kudadjie-Gyamfi E, Magai C, Neugut AI. Prostate cancer screening behavior in men from seven ethnic groups: the fear factor. *Cancer Epidemiol Biomarkers Prev*. 2006;15:228–237.

27. Myers RE, Hyslop T, Jennings-Dozier K, et al. Intention to be tested for prostate cancer risk among African-American men. *Cancer Epidemiol Biomarkers Prev*. 2000;9:1323–1328.

28. Demark-Wahnefried W, Strigo T, Catoe K, et al. Knowledge, beliefs, and prior screening behavior among blacks and whites reporting for prostate cancer screening. *Urology*. 1995;46:346–351.

29. Roetzheim RG, Pal N, Tennant C, et al. Effects of health insurance and race on early detection of cancer. *J Natl Cancer Inst*. 1999;91:1409–1415.

30. Merrill RM. Demographics and health-related factors of men receiving prostate-specific antigen screening in Utah. *Prev Med*. 2001;33:646–652.

31. Boyd MD, Weinrich SP, Weinrich M, Norton A. Obstacles to prostate cancer screening in African-American men. *J Natl Black Nurses Assoc*. 2001;12:1–5.

32. Clarke-Tasker VA, Wade R. What we thought we knew: African American males' perceptions of prostate cancer and screening methods. *ABNF J*. 2002;13:56–60.

33. Barber KR, Shaw R, Folts M, et al. Differences between African American and Caucasian men participating in a community-based prostate cancer screening program. *J Community Health*. 1998;23:441–451.

34. Gwede CK, McDermott RJ. Prostate cancer screening decision making under controversy: implications for health promotion practice. *Health Promot Pract*. 2006;7:134–146.

35. Gilligan T, Wang PS, Levin R, Kantoff PW, Avorn J. Racial differences in screening for prostate cancer in the elderly. *Arch Intern Med*. 2004;164:1858–1864.

36. Myers RE, Chodak GW, Wolf TA, et al. Adherence by African American men to prostate cancer education and early detection. *Cancer*. 1999;86:88–104.

37. Myers RE, Daskalakis C, Cocroft J, et al. Preparing African-American men in community primary care practices to decide whether or not to have prostate cancer screening. *J Natl Med Assoc*. 2005;97:1143–1154.

38. Beebe-Dimmer JL, Wood DP Jr, Gruber SB, et al. Risk perception and concern among brothers of men with prostate carcinoma. *Cancer*. 2004;100:1537–1544.

39. Cormier L, Kwan L, Reid K, Litwin MS. Knowledge and beliefs among brothers and sons of men with prostate cancer. *Urology*. 2002;59:895–900.

40. Miller SM, Diefenbach MA, Kruus LK, Watkins-Bruner D, Hanks GE, Engstrom PF. Psychological and screening profiles of first-degree relatives of prostate cancer patients. *J Behav Med*. 2001;24:247–258.

41. Jacobsen PB, Lamonde LA, Honour M, Kash K, Hudson PB, Pow-Sang J. Relation of family history of prostate cancer to perceived vulnerability and screening behavior. *Psycho-Oncology*. 2004;13:80–85.

42. Krongrad A, Kim CO, Burke MA, Granville LJ. Not all patients pursue prostate biopsy after abnormal prostate specific antigen results. *Urol Oncol Semin Orig Invest*. 1996;2:35–39.

43. Bastani R, Yabroff KR, Myers RE, Glenn B. Interventions to improve follow-up of abnormal findings in cancer screening. *Cancer*. 2004;101:1188–1200.

44. Myers RE, Hyslop T, Wolf TA, et al. African-American men and intention to adhere to recommended follow-up for an abnormal prostate cancer early detection examination result. *Urology*. 2000;55:716–720.

45. Tabori U, Malkin D. Risk stratification in cancer predisposition syndromes: lessons learned from novel molecular developments in Li-Fraumeni syndrome. *Cancer Res*. 2008;68:2053–2057.

46. Ioannidis JP, Boffetta P, Little J, et al. Assessment of cumulative evidence on genetic associations: interim guidelines. *Int J Epidemiol*. 2008;37:120–132.

47. Rebbeck TR, Martinez ME, Sellers TA, Shields PG, Wild CP, Potter JD. Genetic variation and cancer: improving the environment for publication of association studies. *Cancer Epidemiol Biomarkers Prev*. 2004;13:1985–1986.

48. Rebbeck TR, Khoury MJ, Potter JD. Genetic association studies of cancer: where do we go from here? *Cancer Epidemiol Biomarkers Prev.* 2007;16:864–865.

49. Bratt O, Kristoffersson U, Lundgren R, Olsson H. Sons of men with prostate cancer: their attitudes regarding possible inheritance of prostate cancer, screening, and genetic testing. *Urology.* 1997;50:360–365.

50. Miesfeldt S, Jones SM, Cohn W, et al. Men's attitudes regarding genetic testing for hereditary prostate cancer risk. *Urology.* 2000;55:46–50.

51. Croyle RT, Lerman C. Interest in genetic testing for colon cancer susceptibility: cognitive and emotional correlates. *Prev Med.* 1993;22:284–292.

52. Lerman C, Daly M, Masny A, Balshem A. Attitudes about genetic testing for breast-ovarian cancer susceptibility. *J Clin Oncol.* 1994;12:843–850.

53. Lerman C, Seay J, Balshem A, Audrain J. Interest in genetic testing among first-degree relatives of breast cancer patients. *Am J Med Genet.* 1995;57:385–392.

54. Chaliki H, Loader S, Levenkron JC, Logan-Young W, Hall WJ, Rowley PT. Women's receptivity to testing for a genetic susceptibility to breast cancer. *Am J Public Health.* 1995;85:1133–1135.

55. Andrykowski MA, Munn RK, Studts JL. Interest in learning of personal genetic risk for cancer: a general population survey. *Prev Med.* 1996;25:527–536.

56. Tambor ES, Rimer BK, Strigo TS. Genetic testing for breast cancer susceptibility: awareness and interest among women in the general population. *Am J Med Genet.* 1997;68:43–49.

57. Jacobsen PB, Valdimarsdottier HB, Brown KL, Offit K. Decision-making about genetic testing among women at familial risk for breast cancer. *Psychosom Med.* 1997;59:459–466.

58. Loader S, Levenkron JC, Rowley PT. Genetic testing for breast-ovarian cancer susceptibility: a regional trial. *Genet Test.* 1998;2:305–313.

59. Bluman LG, Rimer BK, Berry DA, et al. Attitudes, knowledge, and risk perceptions of women with breast and/or ovarian cancer considering testing for BRCA1 and BRCA2. *J Clin Oncol.* 1999;17:1040–1046.

60. Durfy SJ, Bowen DJ, McTiernan A, Sporleder J, Burke W. Attitudes and interest in genetic testing for breast and ovarian cancer susceptibility in diverse groups of women in western Washington. *Cancer Epidemiol Biomarkers Prev.* 1999;8:369–375.

61. Han PK, Coates RJ, Uhler RJ, Breen N. Decision making in prostate-specific antigen screening National Health Interview Survey, 2000. *Am J Prev Med.* 2006;30:394–404.

62. Guerra CE, Jacobs SE, Holmes JH, Shea JA. Are physicians discussing prostate cancer screening with their patients and why or why not? A pilot study. *J Gen Intern Med.* 2007;22:901–907.

63. Hoffman RM, Helitzer DL. Moving towards shared decision making in prostate cancer screening. *J Gen Intern Med.* 2007;22:1056–1057.

64. O'Connor AM, Rostom A, Fiset V, et al. Decision aids for patients facing health treatment or screening decisions: systematic review. *BMJ.* 1999;319:731–734.

65. O'Connor AM, Stacey D, Entwistle V, et al. Decision aids for people facing health treatment or screening decisions [update of *Cochrane Database Syst Rev.* 2001;(3):CD001431; PMID: 11686990]. *Cochrane Database Syst Rev.* 2003:001431.

66. Volk RJ, Hawley ST, Kneuper S, et al. Trials of decision aids for prostate cancer screening: a systematic review. *Am J Prev Med.* 2007;33:428–434.

67. Volk RJ, Spann SJ, Cass AR, Hawley ST. Patient education for informed decision making about prostate cancer screening: a randomized controlled trial with 1-year follow-up. *Ann Fam Med.* 2003;1:22–28.

68. Kripalani S, Sharma J, Justice E, et al. Low-literacy interventions to promote discussion of prostate cancer: a randomized controlled trial. *Am J Prev Med.* 2007;33:83–90.

69. Partin MR, Nelson D, Radosevich D, et al. Randomized trial examining the effect of two prostate cancer screening educational interventions on patient knowledge, preferences, and behaviors. *J Gen Intern Med.* 2004;19:835–842.

70. Bandura A. *Social learning theory.* Englewood Cliffs, NJ: Prentice Hall; 1977.

71. Myers RE, Kunkel EJ. Preparatory education for informed decision-making in prostate cancer early detection and treatment. *Semin Urol Oncol.* 2000;18:172–177.

72. Liberatore MJ, Myers RE, Nydick RL, et al. Decision counseling for men considering prostate cancer screening. *Comput Oper Res.* 2003;30:1421–1434.

73. Myers RE. Self regulation and decision-making about cancer screening. In: Cameron LD, Leventhal H, eds. *Self-regulation of health and illness behaviour.* London and New York: Routledge; 2003:297–313.

74. Myers RE. Decision counseling in cancer prevention and control. *Health Psychol.* 2005;24:S71–S77.

75. Cegala DJ, Street RL Jr, Clinch CR. The impact of patient participation on physicians' information provision during a primary care medical interview. *Health Commun.* 2007;21:177–185.

76. Greenfield S, Kaplan S, Ware JE. Expanding patient involvement in care. Effects on patient outcomes. *Ann Intern Med.* 1985;102:520–528.

77. Kaplan SH, Greenfield S, Ware JE. Assessing the effects of physician-patient interactions on the outcomes of chronic disease. *Med Care.* 1989;27:S110–S127.

78. Kunkel EJS, Meyer B, Daskalakis C, et al. Behaviors used by men to protect themselves against prostate cancer. Cancer epidemiol biomakers prev. 2004;13:78–86.

PART IV

Screening and Testing for Genetic Susceptibility to Cancer

Paul B. Jacobsen, ED

CHAPTER 13

Genetic Susceptibility to Breast/Ovarian Cancer

Penelope Hopwood and Maggie Watson

BACKGROUND

More than a decade after the characterization of two highly penetrant breast/ovarian cancer predisposition genes *BRCA1/2*,[1,2] genetic counseling and testing, where there is a family history of hereditary breast or ovarian cancer (HBOC), has been developed into routine clinical practice. This translation of genetic knowledge into clinical practice has provided an opportunity for understanding: (1) how genetic information is disseminated through families, and understanding of cancer risk; (2) the impact of genetic testing on anxiety about cancer; and (3) how decisions are made relating to risk management.

The aim of genetic counseling and testing is to provide information which allows those at risk to make judgments about how they choose to manage this risk. Ultimately, genetic information needs to provide benefits in terms of lives saved and it will likely take at least a further decade before there is sufficient evidence on survival benefits.

Psychosocial research on the impact of testing for *BRCA1/2* genes has proliferated over the past decade and provides substantial knowledge which can be used to guide and support patients and families through the minefield of genetic testing.

FAMILY DISSEMINATION OF GENETIC INFORMATION AND UNDERSTANDING OF CANCER RISK

Logistics of *BRCA1/2* testing usually starts with the mutation search: the identification of a genetic fault not previously known within the family. The mutation search usually (although not always) begins in affecteds (a living family member with diagnosed cancer). It is not unusual for an uninformative result to be found in this process as there is likely a number of moderately penetrant predisposition genes, as yet unidentified, contributing to familial cancer cases. Women (occasionally men, although less frequently) receiving an uninformative result from the mutation search have often failed to understand this information and emotional reactions varied from disbelief about the reliability of the findings to elation that a gene had not been confirmed thus freeing them (mistakenly) from the burden of risk.[3] Often there was anger that genetic technology had failed them. Most patients receiving uninformative results, however, did not experience difficulty in disseminating this information to their family unlike those with a confirmed gene mutation. Those with a confirmed gene mutation often reported several difficulties.

These patients essentially were thrust into the role of gatekeepers or portal key holders of genetic information. They, and they alone, held this knowledge as the first in the family to be tested and a mantle of responsibility to disseminate the test results had to be assumed. They became the bearers of complex and emotionally challenging knowledge which was primarily of benefit if it could be passed on as family information and then used to guide risk management. We have used the term "cancer burden" to describe the conglomerate of difficult emotions placed on these family portal key holders who have had to share this genetic information with others in the families.[4] For example:

"I've talked to my brother and have tried to persuade him to have it [genetic testing] done because he has got two daughters and so I've suggested that it's a good idea and he said it was too much trouble and he couldn't be bothered" [Pamela]

"I suppose it's in the back of the mind, if people talk about it then it comes up and if people talk about it I do get upset over my sister and my mum [who died]..."
[Jane]

"My sister can't deal with it [genetic risk in the family], internalises it. You know..."
[Kathleen]

"I don't want to overload somebody else with this confusing issue..."
[Denise]

The doctor–patient confidentiality contract[5] prevents dissemination by the physician of information about gene carrier status in those receiving a positive mutation search result.

This dilemma has contributed to a move toward the notion of the "family covenant" which "offers a more explicit accounting for the concerns of third parties, while not violating individual rights (as all parties freely consent to the agreement)."[6] This health care agreement between physician and patient aims to treat the family as the "unit of care" and constitutes an agreement among family members that information affecting the family as a unit can be shared. This is not binding on all parties who do not consent to the covenant. When it works effectively, however, it allows the physician and all consenting family members to have access to information, obtained from the individual patients, which has known family health consequences and therefore belongs in the broader arena of family information. This approach may prove particularly effective for mutation search portal key holders who can then have their physician aligned with them and collaborating in the dissemination process. This may effectively reduce some of the psychosocial problems for the patients which have contributed to cancer burden. Factors mentioned by portal key holder patients include concerns about who to inform in the family because genetic inheritance is sometimes not well understood, and when to inform: patients often have to deal with family rifts. Most family members are willing to disseminate genetic information to close and distant relatives motivated by a sense of duty[7,8]; however, divorce, family rifts, and having little regular contact with relatives all act to limit dissemination to those who might benefit from the offer of genetic testing.[9,10] Where relationships were strained, information about genetic issues was often difficult to discuss with at-risk family members.[11]

These communication difficulties are not confined to the mutation search stage but also when it comes to passing information along once genetic testing becomes more widely available to family members unaffected (undiagnosed) by cancer. Understanding these communication difficulties will help to set in place clinical services aimed at supporting families through a difficult process.

As a result of psychosocial research it has now become common practice in cancer genetics to provide counseling before, and after, genetic testing for both affecteds and unaffecteds to ensure they understand what they are taking on in terms of communication needs in the family. The provision of information packs has also helped improve individual knowledge about hereditary cancers making it easier to understand who and how to disseminate information.[12]

Communication issues for men are often more complex for what are usually perceived to be female cancers. Less is known about male *BRCA1/2* carriers. Male uptake rates for genetic testing tend to be lower[13,14] and are often motivated by obligations to females in the family, especially their children. However, it has also been observed that decisions about genetic testing in men present conflict for some between the need to provide information to their children about risk and their duty to avoid harm by causing emotional distress.[15]

"I was a little hesitant about whether it was a good idea or a bad idea, because it seemed to me you could argue that if it turned out bad, that would simply increase the sort of level of worry for my children…."
[John]

Men likely need support services to help them with these issues.

"Someone's put a curse on this family. And it was quite terrifying….we were brought up with this terror of cancer. I've been living with it since I must have been four, knowing people are dying of this terrible Big C…"
[Alan]

However, there is little information as yet about how to pitch this support or what might be effective. In relation to family communication and genetic information dissemination, it is clear that families need support structures that will help them understand the biology of inheritance, the processes of cancer genetic counseling and testing, the implications of genetic information for family relationships, and the decision making that follows both the identification of a gene mutation in the family and the need to manage cancer risk in gene mutation carriers both unaffected and already affected by cancer. For identified noncarriers there is also the burden of "survivor guilt" and their anxieties about being denied the level of cancer screening offered to gene carriers.

THE IMPACT OF GENETIC TESTING ON ANXIETY ABOUT CANCER

During the period following on closely from the first characterization of the *BRCA1/2* gene mutations, it was not clear whether genetic testing would raise anxieties in those found to be carriers. It was recognized that women from families with high rates of HBOC might bear a heavy emotional burden due to their familial experiences of cancer including high bereavement rates, loss of their mother during childhood or adolescence, and their own fears of developing cancer. For women from high-risk families, where genetic testing was not yet available, high rates of distress were reported.[16] Whether the move to develop genetic testing for *BRCA*, once it became available, would increase or reduce anxiety was the focus of a number of investigations.

Generally, the evidence shows that genetic counseling and testing leads to significant decreases in anxiety across time[17,18] and does not lead to serious chronic psychological distress.[19] While genetic testing in a large U.K. cohort indicated an increase in cancer-related anxiety immediately following disclosure of a positive result in younger women, this reduced over the following 12-month period as risk management strategies were introduced.[20]

RISK MANAGEMENT

This section will consider the psychological aspects of options available to women who are mutation carriers and those at high risk. These options include preventive surgery and chemoprevention (primary prevention strategies) and breast screening (secondary prevention).

Bilateral prophylactic mastectomy. Bilateral prophylactic mastectomy (and to a lesser extent bilateral salpingo-oophorectomy) has been a controversial method of risk management and whilst protagonists supported women's choice, concerns were raised about potential complications and lack of knowledge of long-term benefit, as well as the risk of cancer occurring in residual breast tissue following mastectomy or preserved nipple and areola. Yet many women with a family history of breast-ovarian cancer, who have witnessed multiple deaths and disease episodes in their close relatives, see surgery as a chance to change the course of the family history for themselves and their offspring. Over the past decade, evidence has emerged of a high level of reduction in breast cancer incidence conferred by preventive mastectomies,[21,22] providing a basis for women to gain greater control over the disease compared with

previous generations. However, further long-term survival data following bilateral prophylactic mastectomy (BPM) are needed. For preventive oophorectomy, data are more limited but a reduction of ovarian cancers has also been reported.[23]

Eligibility criteria for undergoing preventive surgery have been clarified over recent years through ongoing research and the development of consensus statements, published protocols, and national guidelines. There is wide variation by country together with cultural differences in the acceptability and uptake of surgery[24,25] but causal factors for these differences are difficult to attribute. Psychological and sociodemographic predictors of uptake are similar across some countries in terms of high perceived risk, high breast cancer anxiety and having children. Research into factors affecting decision making has been a growing area of interest, especially where genetic testing is already available and being a *BRCA1/2* gene carrier is the most consistent factor associated with surgical decisions. However, available information is focused on Western countries and an understanding is needed in non-Western countries, where culture and beliefs may have different influences on decision-making.

Preoperative psychological counseling. Elective surgery offers the opportunity for unhurried decision making and consideration of surgical options, facilitating preoperative counseling to ensure that consent is fully informed and that expectations of risk reduction and breast reconstruction are realistic in the short and longer term.[26–29] It is a very personal decision, but having insufficient information has been shown to increase dissatisfaction rates with outcomes.[30,31] Counseling can include the woman's awareness of other risk management options, address her motivation for surgery (to ensure that she is not under pressure to please someone else), and explore the pros and cons of different reconstructive alternatives and associated complications.[32–34] The potential impact of surgery on body image, sexual functioning, cancer worry, mental health, and interpersonal relationships should also be considered in the context of the value placed on these aspects and women's existing expectations. However, women are often preoccupied with the family history and fears of cancer and appearance issues may not be a priority at this time. They should be advised that psychological adjustment postoperatively may be a long process. Given family bereavements and early life disruption due to the family history of cancer, women may have increased psychological vulnerability; this warrants review and discussion of social support and coping strategies.

Studies show that preoperatively, women often overestimate their risk of breast cancer and report a high level of cancer worry[35,36]; in comparison to those who decline surgery, they are also more likely to have had benign breast biopsies or carry a genetic mutation. A multidisciplinary team approach is needed to ensure that an optimal level of information on surgical and psychological issues is provided, with time for reflection and opportunity for the woman to ask questions and discuss uncertainties. Partners may also be involved in preoperative consultations so that their expectations are also realistic and postoperative adjustment better facilitated. Psychosexual problems are relevant to these discussions, together with future implications for breast-feeding.

Patient-reported outcomes. The potential was raised for disappointment with the cosmetic outcome or regret about undergoing the procedure but evidence of satisfaction has been reported in respect of decision making, emotional and physical recovery, and body image,[30,35,37–41] although the number of prospective longitudinal studies is small and there is a need for long-term follow-up. Recent studies have been consistent in reporting favorable results for the majority, with overall satisfaction with the decision, absence of significant impairment of quality of life and no increase in mental health problems (for a review, see reference 26). For the majority of women, psychological benefit is achieved through reduction of cancer worry and intrusive thoughts about cancer. Minor body image concerns are quite frequent, but this may be in keeping with the extent of expected changes following major breast surgery.[33,40] However, significant surgical complications can lead to poor body image outcomes and associated distress and access to postoperative support is needed. Some studies report that surgery can be achieved without overall detriment to sexual functioning, whilst others raise concerns. Preoperative sexual problems may be aggravated by the impact of surgery, which in turn can be blamed for deterioration. Little is known about the impact of preventive mastectomies on partners or adolescent daughters, who should form a focus for future research.

Prophylactic oophorectomy and ovarian surveillance. Although the risk of ovarian cancer is lower than that of breast cancer in the familial cancer setting, screening options are less reliable and the majority of ovarian cancers are detected at an advanced stage. Both pelvic ultrasound and CA 125 estimation currently lack the sensitivity and specificity needed for a reliable and cost-effective screening program. In most studies, uptake of bilateral prophylactic oophorectomy (BPO) has been shown to be higher than that of BPM.[42] There have been a number of reports of primary peritoneal cancer after bilateral prophylactic oophorectomy (BPO)[43] but the procedure has also been shown to effectively reduce the risk of breast cancer in premenopausal women with BRCA mutations.[44]

Many women who undertake BPO do so considerably before the natural menopause and a large proportion of these women can potentially suffer menopausal symptoms such as hot flushes, vaginal dryness, loss of libido, and tiredness and are at risk of other adverse effects on health such as osteoporosis.[45] Whilst women entering the natural menopause also suffer from these symptoms, it is likely that a surgically induced early menopause will produce more rapid, and in some cases, more severe symptoms; women in the general population could consider using hormone replacement therapy (HRT), but those with a genetic risk are concerned about potentially increasing their risk of breast cancer. A recent review of studies has provided additional information on the risk benefit trade off of HRT in this context[46] and will facilitate women's informed decision making.

Whilst the option of ovarian screening preserves ovarian function, there may be false positive results with associated surgical intervention. Psychosocial studies have addressed the respective psychosocial outcomes of surgery and screening[47-51] and recent research indicates a trade off between risk reduction and reduced cancer worry, at the cost of worse menopausal symptoms and sexual functioning in the surgical group, compared with screening, where preservation of fertility is balanced against continued cancer worry and cancer risk in premenopausal women.[52] Moreover, the benefit of HRT was found to be less than anticipated with respect to sexual dysfunction[53] in the surgical group, endorsing the need to discuss quality-of-life issues at the time of decision making for screening or surgery.

Chemoprevention. Chemoprevention using selective estrogen receptor modulators (SERMs) continues to be evaluated in randomized clinical trials but use of these agents is still not routine in clinical practice, because of possible adverse effects.[54] To date no long term differences have been found between tamoxifen and placebo drug treatment side effects that impair psychosocial or sexual functioning,[55,56] but differences in side effect profiles were noticed between tamoxifen and raloxifene.[57] Evidence of risk reduction has been found in postmenopausal women and quality-of-life data are accumulating[58] so that in the future informed choices will be available to women at risk. Currently, uptake and acceptability of chemoprevention remains low in the clinical trials setting.[59-61]

Breast cancer screening. Recommendations for surveillance of women at high risk vary across countries, both in terms of age at first screen and screening interval. However, in a review of the psychological impact of screening in women with a family history[62] findings indicated that most women do not appear to experience high levels of anxiety associated with screening. Those who are recalled for further tests do have raised anxiety, but no more than women without a family history. A recent evaluation of mammographic screening in the United Kingdom for women at moderate risk aged 40–45 reported that those who were recalled had a small increase in psychological consequences 6 months later compared with those with a clear screen, but the recalled group were more positive about the benefits of screening.[63] A number

of predictive factors for increased psychological vulnerability were identified, including recent death of a relative from breast cancer, high perceived risk and negative appraisals of the threat, and specific coping strategies. A false positive result had only a short-term negative effect.[64,65] Evaluation of magnetic resonance imaging for breast cancer screening is now emerging with favorable short-term quality-of-life effects reported[66] but long-term psychosocial outcomes are needed.

In conclusion, risk management options are often psychologically beneficial, but access and uptake are variable. Women make risk management decisions at different stages of life and require tailored information and the opportunity to discuss their options with a multidisciplinary team. In parallel, there is a need for more long-term prospective studies to clarify the psychosocial and behavioral consequences of different risk management options.

Ethical issues. The ethical issues are complex and wide-ranging. Who owns genetic information? How should genetic risk information be disseminated in families so that maleficence is avoided? What rights to privacy do gene mutation carriers have when the information they hold may benefit others in the family? How can this genetic technology be used so that it does not increase distress in families? How can genetic discrimination be prevented especially in those who seek health and life insurance?

The American Society of Clinical Oncology[67] recommends that federal laws prohibit insurance discrimination on the grounds of genetic risk and that providers protect confidentiality of individual genetic information while at the same time emphasizing the importance of sharing this information with family members. The provision of clear ethical, medical, and legal guidelines will provide families with the structures that will help them to cope with genetic risk.

In relation to physician–patient confidentiality issues, there clearly needs to be a family approach and the "family covenant" may provide a method to help patients disseminate genetic information in a way that avoids distress to themselves and those to whom the information may be passed. The family member's right not to know must be respected even though this may have adverse health consequences in the longer term. Families will benefit from good information to aid their decision making and future health behavior. Access to prophylactic surgery should be the patient's choice; equally patients with significant anxiety should be protected from major surgery if the benefit to future health is not clear. Future generations of gene carriers may seek cancer control for their offspring through techniques such as pre-implantation genetic diagnosis (PGD) and will need to be supported in this difficult and ethically challenging process.

Psychosocial research has helped over the past decade or so in our understanding of the emotional challenges of genetic testing, how best to provide information to families and how and when to provide emotional support.

CLINICAL SERVICE IMPLICATIONS

Within genetic services there should be provision of good psychosocial care with the same principles that are being applied to all cancer patients in supportive care guidelines, such as those developed in Europe and North America also being applied within the genetic context. Genetic specialists should be able to communicate effectively any bad news and provide at least some basic level of psychological care. There should be access to more specialist psychological care services across the whole genetic testing trajectory.

The following case* illustrates some of the complex clinical psychosocial issues:

Mary had lived most of her adult life feeling that she had no future due to the family history of cancer. She had never bothered to take out a pension plan nor thought about the fact that she might need to make longer term financial plans as, for her, there had seemed no point. The threat of cancer had sat "like a black dog" on her shoulders for years. At the age of 46 she was able to have a genetic test which confirmed that she carried the BRCA1 gene mutation. She went on to have a bilateral mastectomy without reconstruction. She shed tears of joy when telling her psychologist how she had been released of the burden of breast cancer, then tears of distress when telling her how difficult it had been to tell her two daughters about her genetic test results. Her mother, a breast cancer survivor who had refused genetic testing, forbade Mary disseminating the genetic information to her younger sister and brother. Later she came back to tell her psychologist how difficult it had been to get her husband's support and how sexual intimacy had disappeared from her life; she felt that she had both gained and lost in this "genetics game". However across a series of individual counseling sessions she began to use her substantial emotional and intellectual resources to heal and regain her view of the life she wanted and knew she now could have.

* Some details have been changed to protect patient anonymity.

CONCLUSION

In the year or so following the characterization of the first common cancer predisposition genes, the medical community attempted to take charge of this highly sensitive information so that it could be used for patients' good; both medical and emotional.

The American Society of Clinical Oncology, for instance, set out a defining statement for the future which was adopted on February 20, 1996[67]:

ASCO recognizes that cancer specialists must be fully informed of the range of issues involved in genetic testing for cancer risk. The newly discovered and still developing ability to identify individuals at highest risk for cancer holds the promise of improved prevention and early detection of cancers. It also poses potential medical, psychological, and other personal risks that must be addressed in the context of informed consent for genetic testing.... ASCO endorses continued support of patient-oriented research to analyze the psychological impact of genetic testing of at-risk populations.

More than a decade later the research community has made many efforts to fulfill the requirements of this statement and we are able to say that, not only are we now well informed by psychological research, but also we continue to integrate this knowledge into clinical care of patients and their families to support them in living with their increased risk of cancer.

REFERENCES

1. Miki Y, Swensen J, Shattuck Eidens D, et al. A strong candidate for the breast and ovarian cancer susceptibility gene BRCA1. *Science*. 1994;266:66–71.

2. Wooster R, Bignell G, Lancaster J, et al. Identification of the breast susceptibility gene *BRCA2*. *Nature*. 1995;378:789–791.

3. Hallowell N, Foster C, Eeles R, Murday V, Watson M. Genetic testing for women previously diagnosed with breast/ovarian cancer: examining the impact of BRCA1 and BRCA2 mutation searching. *Genetic Testing*. 2002;6:79–87.

4. Foster C, Watson M, Moynihan C, Ardern-Jones S, Eeles R. Genetic testing for breast and ovarian cancer predisposition: cancer burden and responsibility. *J Health Psychol*. 2002;7:469–484.

5. General Medical Council. Confidentiality: protecting and providing information. www.gmc-uk.org/guidance/confidentiality. Accessed November 2, 2009.

6. Doukas DJ, Berg JW. The family covenant and genetic testing. *Am J Bioeth*. 2001;1:2–9.

7. Foster C, Eeles R, Ardern-Jones A, Moynihan C, Watson M. Juggling roles and expectations: dilemmas faced by women talking to relatives about cancer and genetic testing. *Psychol Health*. 2004;19:1–17.

8. McGiven B, Everett J, Yager GG, Baumiller RC, Hafertepen A, Saal HM. Family communication about positive BRCA1 and BRCA2 genetic test results. *Genet Med*. 2004;6:503–509.

9. Hughes C, Lerman C, Schwartz M, et al. All in the family: evaluation of the process and content of sisters' communicating about BRCA1 and BRCA2 genetic test results. *Am J Med Genet*. 2002;107:143–150.

10. Julian-Reynier C, Eisinger F, Cabal F, et al. Disclosure to the family of breast/ovarian cancer genetic test results: patient's willingness and associated factors. *Am J Med Genet*. 2000;94:13–18.

11. Ormondroyd E, Moynihan C, Ardern-Jones A, et al. Communicating genetic research results to families: problems arising when the patient participant is deceased. *Psycho-Oncology*. 2008;17:804–811.

12. Appleton S, Watson M, Rush R, et al. A randomised controlled trial of a psycho-educational intervention for women at increased risk of breast cancer. *Br J Cancer*. 2004;90:41–47.

13. Julian- Reynier C, Sobol H, Sevilla C, Nogues C, Bourret P; French Cancer Genetic Network. Uptake of hereditary breast/ovarian cancer genetic testing in a French national sample of BRCA1 families. The French Cancer Genetic Network. *Psycho-Oncology*. 2000;9:504–510.

14. Foster C, Evans DGR, Eeles R, et al. Predictive testing for BRCA1/2: attributes, risk perception and management in a multi-centre cohort. *Br J Cancer*. 2002;86:1209–1216.

15. Hallowell N, Ardern-Jones A, Eeles R, et al. Men's decision-making about predictive BRCA1/2 testing: the role of family. *J Genet Couns*. 2005;14:207–217.

16. Lloyd S, Watson M, Waites B, et al. Familial breast cancer: a controlled study of risk perception, psychological morbidity and health beliefs in women attending for genetic counselling. *Br J Cancer*. 1996;74:482–487.

17. Meiser B, Halliday JL. What is the impact of genetic counselling in women at increased risk of developing hereditary breast cancer? A meta-analytic review. *Soc Sci Med*. 2002;54:1463–1470.

18. Braithwaite D, Emery J, Walter F, Prevost AT. Sutton S. Psychological impact of genetic counselling for familial cancer: a systematic review and meta-analysis. *J Natl Cancer Inst*. 2004;96:122–133.

19. Schilich-Bakker KJ, ten Kroode HF, Warlam-Rodenhuis CC, van den Bout J, Ausems MG. Barriers to participating in genetic counselling and BRCA testing during primary treatment for breast cancer. *Genet Med*. 2007;9:766–777.

20. Watson M, Foster C, Eeles R, et al. Psychosocial impact of breast/ovarian (BRCA1/2) cancer-predictive genetic testing in a UK multi-centre clinical cohort. *Br J Cancer*. 2004;91:1787–1794.

21. Hartmann LC, Schaid DJ, Woods JE, et al. Efficacy of bilateral prophylactic mastectomy in women with a family history of breast cancer. *N Engl J Med*. 1999;340:77–84.

22. Rebbeck TR, Friebel T, Lynch HT, et al. Bilateral prophylactic mastectomy reduces breast cancer risk in BRCA1 and BRCA2 mutation carriers: the PROSE Study Group. *J Clin Oncol*. 2004;6:1055–1062.

23. Finch A, Beiner M, Lubinski J, et al.; Hereditary Ovarian Cancer Clinical Study Group. Salpingo-oophorectomy and the risk of ovarian, fallopian tube, and peritoneal cancers in women with a BRCA1 or BRCA2 Mutation. *J Am Med Assoc*. 2006;296:185–192.

24. Meiser B, Gaff C, Julian-Reynier C, et al. International perspectives on genetic counselling and testing for breast cancer risk. *Breast Dis*. 2006–2007;27L:109–125.

25. Metcalfe KA, Birenbaum-Carmeli D, Lubinski J, et al. International variation in rates of uptake of preventive options in BRCA1 and BRCA2 mutation carriers. *Int J Cancer*. 2008;122:2017–2022.

26. Lostumbo L, Carbine N, Wallace J, Ezzo J. Prophylactic mastectomy for the prevention of breast cancer [Review]. *Cochrane Database Syst Rev*. 2004;(4):CD002748.

27. Lalloo F, Bailden A, Brain A, Hopwood P, Evans DGR, Howell A. A protocol for preventative mastectomy in women with an increased lifetime risk of breast cancer. *Eur J Surg Oncol*. 2000;26:711–713.

28. Josephson U, Wickman M, Sandelin K. Initial experiences of women from hereditary breast cancer families after bilateral prophylactic mastectomy: a retrospective study. *Eur J Surg Oncol*. 2000;26:351–356.

29. Petit JY, Greco M; on behalf of EUSOMA. Quality control in prophylactic mastectomy for women at high risk of breast cancer. *Eur J Cancer*. 2002;38:23–26.

30. Bresser PJ, Seynaeve C, van Gool AR, et al. Satisfaction with prophylactic mastectomy and breast reconstruction in genetically predisposed women. *Plast Reconstr Surg*. 2006;117L:1675–1682.

31. Altschuler A, Nekhlyudov L, Rolnick SJ, et al. Positive, negative and disparate—women's differing long-term psychosocial experiences of bilateral or contralateral mastectomy. *Breast J*. 2008;14:25–32.

32. Barton MB, West CN, Liu IL, et al. Complications following bilateral prophylactic mastectomy. *Natl Cancer Inst Monogr*. 2005;35:61–66.

33. Contant CM, Menke-Pluijmers MB, Seynaeve C, et al. Clinical experience of prophylactic mastectomy followed by immediate breast reconstruction in women at hereditary risk of breast cancer (HB(O)C) or a proven BRCA1 and BRCA2 germ-line mutation. *Eur J Surg Oncol*. 2002;28:627–632.

34. Zion SM, Slezak JM, Sellers TA, et al. Re-operations after prophylactic mastectomy with or without implant reconstruction. *Cancer*. 2003;98:52–60.

35. Hatcher MB, Fallowfield L, A'Hern R. The psychosocial impact of bilateral prophylactic mastectomy: prospective study using questionnaires and semi-structured interviews. *BMJ*. 2001;322:76–79.

36. Metcalfe KA, Narod SA. Breast cancer risk perception among women who have undergone bilateral prophylactic mastectomy. *J Natl Cancer Inst*. 2002;94:1564–1567.

37. Brandberg Y, Sandelin K, Erikson S, et al. Psychological reactions, quality of life and body image after bilateral prophylactic mastectomy in women at

high risk for breast cancer: a prospective 1-year follow-up study. *J Clin Oncol.* 2008;26:3943–3949.

38. Hopwood P, Lee A, Shenton A, et al. Clinical follow-up after bilateral risk reducing ('prophylactic') mastectomy: mental health and body image outcomes. *Psycho-Oncology.* 2000;9:462–472.

39. Metcalfe KA, Esplen MJ, Goel V, Narod SA. Psychosocial functioning in women who have undergone bilateral prophylactic mastectomy. *Psycho-Oncology.* 2004;13:14–25.

40. van Oostrom I, Meijers-Heijboer H, Lodder L, et al. Long-term psychological impact of carrying a BRCA1/2 mutation and prophylactic surgery: a 5-year follow-up study. *J Clin Oncol.* 2003;21:3867–3874.

41. Stefanek ME, Helzlsouer KJ, Wilcox PM, Houn F. Predictors of and satisfaction with bilateral prophylactic mastectomy. *Prev Med.* 2005;24:412–419.

42. Friebel TM, Domchek SM, Neuhausen SL, et al. Bilateral prophylactic oophorectomy and bilateral prophylactic mastectomy in a prospective cohort of unaffected BRCA1 and BRCA2 carriers. *Clin Breast Cancer.* 2007;7:875–882.

43. Bermejo-Pérez MJ, Márquez-Calderón S, Llanos-Méndez A. Effectiveness of preventive interventions in BRCA1/2 gene mutation carriers: a systematic review. *Intl J Cancer.* 2007;121:225–231.

44. Rebbeck TR, Lunch HT, Neuhausen SL, et al. Prevention and Observation of Surgical Endpoints Study Group. Prophylactic oophorectomy in carriers of BRCA1 or BRCA2 mutations. *N Engl J Med.* 2002;346:1616–1622.

45. Shuster LT, Gostout BS, Grossardt BR, Rocca WA. Prophylactic oophorectomy in premenopausal women and long term health. *Menopause Int.* 2008;14:111–116.

46. Domchek SM, Rebbeck TR. Prophylactic oophorectomy in women at increased cancer risk. *Curr Opin Obstet Gynecol.* 2007;19:27–30.

47. Elit L, Esplen MJ, Butler K, Narod S. Quality of life and psychosexual adjustment after prophylactic oophorectomy for a family history of ovarian cancer. *Fam Cancer.* 2001;1:149–156.

48. Fry A, Busby-Earle C, Rush R, Cull A. Prophylactic oophorectomy versus screening: psychosocial outcomes in women at increased risk of ovarian cancer. *Psycho-Oncology.* 2001;10:231–241.

49. Hallowell N. A qualitative study of the information needs of high-risk women undergoing prophylactic oophorectomy. *Psycho-Oncology.* 2000;9:486–495.

50. Meiser B, Tiller K, Gleeson MA, Andrews L, Robertson G, Tucker KM. Psychological impact of prophylactic oophorectomy in women at increased risk of ovarian cancer. *Psycho-Oncology.* 2000;9:496–503.

51. Tiller K, Meiser B, Butow P, et al. Psychological impact of prophylactic oophorectomy in women at increased risk of developing ovarian cancer: a prospective study. *Gynecol Oncol.* 2002;86:212–219.

52. Madalinska JB, Hoellenstein J, Bleiker E, et al. Quality-of-life effects of prophylactic salpingo-oophorectomy versus gynaecologic screening among women at increased risk of hereditary ovarian cancer. *J Clin Oncol.* 2005;**23**:6890–6898.

53. Madalinska JB, van Beurden M, Bleiker EM, et al. The impact of hormone replacement therapy on menopausal symptoms in younger high-risk women after prophylactic salpingo-oophorectomy. *J Clin Oncol.* 2006;24:3576–3582.

54. Reeder JG, Vogel VG. Breast cancer risk management. *Clin Breast Cancer.* 2007;7:833–840.

55. Fallowfield L, Fleissig A, Edwards R, et al. Tamoxifen for the prevention of breast cancer: psychosocial impact on women participating in tow randomised controlled trials. *J Clin Oncol.* 2001;19:1885–1892.

56. Cullen J, Schwartz MD, Lawrence WF, Selby JV, Mandelblaatt JS. Short-term impact of cancer prevention and screening activities on quality of life. *J Clin Oncol.* 2004;22:943–952.

57. Land SR, Wickerham DL, Constantineo JP, et al. Patient-reported symptoms and quality of life during treatment with Tamoxifen or Raloxifene for breast cancer prevention: the NSABP Study of Tamoxifen and Raloxifene (STAR) P-2 trial. *J Am Med Assoc.* 2006;295:2742–2751.

58. Ganz PA, Land SR. Risks, benefits, and effects on quality of life of selective estrogen-receptor modulator therapy in postmenopausal women at increased risk of breast cancer. *Menopause.* 2008;15:797–803.

59. Bober SL, HokE LA, Duda RB, Regan MM, Tung NM. Decision-making about tamoxifen for high risk women. *J Clin Oncol.* 2004;22:4951–4957.

60. Taylor R, Taguchi K. Tamoxifen for breast cancer chemoprevention: low uptake by high risk women after evaluation of a breast lump. *Ann Fam Med.* 2005;3:242–247.

61. Evans D, Lalloo F, Shenton A, Boggis C, Howell A. Uptake of screening and prevention in women at very high risk of breast cancer. *Lancet.* 2001;358:889–890.

62. Watson EK, Henderson BJ, Brett J, Bankhead C, Austoker J. The psychological impact of mammographic screening on women with a family history of breast cancer—a systematic review. *Psycho-Oncology.* 2005;14:939–948.

63. Tyndel S, Austoker J, Henderson BJ. What is the psychological impact of mammographic screening on younger women with a family history of breast cancer? Findings from a prospective cohort study by the PIMMS Management Group, Duffy S, Evans G, Fielder H, Gray J, Mackay J, Macmillan D. *J Clin Oncol.* 2007; 25:3823–3830.

64. Brain K, Henderson BJ, Tyndel S, et al. Predictors of breast cancer related distress following mammography screening in younger women on a family history breast screening programme. *Psycho-Oncology.* 2008;17:1180–1188.

65. Henderson BJ, Tyndel S, Brain K, et al. Factors associated with breast cancer-specific distress in younger women participating in a family history mammography screening programme. *Psycho-Oncology.* 2008;17:74–82.

66. Rijnsburger AJ, Essink-Bot ML, van Dooren S, et al. Impact of screening for breast cancer in high risk women on health-related quality of life. *Br J Cancer.* 2004;91:69–76.

67. Statement of the American Society of Clinical Oncology: genetic testing for cancer susceptibility, Adopted on February 20, 1996. *J Clin Oncol.* 1996;14 (5)1730–1736.

CHAPTER 14

Psychosocial Issues in Genetic Testing for Hereditary Colorectal Cancer

Andrea Farkas Patenaude and Susan K. Peterson

INTRODUCTION

Genetic testing for hereditary colorectal cancer (CRC) syndromes is increasingly used in clinical practice to ascertain inherited disease susceptibility or genetic etiology. A primary benefit of genetic testing is the ability to offer targeted options for cancer risk reduction and risk management to people at increased cancer risk due to an inherited susceptibility. Since genetic testing for hereditary CRC syndromes became clinically available over a decade ago, psychosocial research has focused on understanding individuals' motivations and decisions regarding genetic testing, the psychological impact of genetic risk notification, effects on family and interpersonal relationships, and factors that influence the uptake of risk-reduction options (e.g., screening, risk-reducing surgery, or chemoprevention). While more has been studied about the impact of genetic testing on families with hereditary breast-ovarian cancer, there is a growing literature addressing psychosocial issues for individuals at risk for hereditary colon cancers. We will review the literature on the impact of genetic counseling and testing on individuals at risk for two common hereditary CRC syndromes, Lynch syndrome (also referred to as hereditary nonpolyposis colon cancer or HNPCC) and familial adenomatous polyposis (FAP). Findings from these studies can guide clinicians in understanding why people seek genetic counseling and testing, how they cope with the results of testing, and how they subsequently integrate that information into cancer prevention and treatment decisions.

LYNCH SYNDROME

Medical implications for mutation carriers. It is estimated that 2%–5% of all CRCs are due to germline mutations associated with Lynch syndrome, a hereditary CRC condition.[1,2] Lynch syndrome is an autosomal dominant condition characterized by predisposition to early (adult) onset colorectal, endometrial, ovarian, stomach, small bowel, hepatobiliary tract, pancreatic, urinary tract, brain, and skin cancers.[3,4] The term "Lynch syndrome" is increasingly preferred to describe this condition, rather than HNPCC, in part because it emphasizes the risk for all associated cancers, reflecting the need for comprehensive cancer screening.[1,2]

Deleterious germline mutations in several mismatch repair genes (including *MLH1, MSH2, MLH6, PMS2*) are responsible for inherited susceptibility to Lynch syndrome. Identification of a familial mutation allows for targeted risk-reduction strategies in mutation carriers and for notification of risk to relatives who may also be carriers. Children of carriers have a 50% risk of carrying the deleterious mutation. In general, genetic testing for hereditary cancer syndromes is considered most informative when testing is initiated in a family member with a syndrome-specific cancer.[5] Genetic testing for Lynch syndrome optimally begins with preliminary microsatellite instability testing of a Lynch syndrome-associated cancer tumor (preferably, a CRC tumor) from a patient with a Lynch syndrome-associated cancer whose clinical characteristics and/or family cancer history are consistent with this condition.[1] High levels of microsatellite instability are associated with, but not diagnostic of, Lynch syndrome.[1] Suggestive family history, clinical characteristics, and high microsatellite instability levels increase the likelihood that a deleterious mismatch repair mutation will be identified through genetic testing.

Lifetime CRC risk in Lynch syndrome vary for men and women. Risks of developing CRC for male mismatch repair mutation carriers have been reported ranging from 74% to 82%, while CRC risks for women are 30%–54%.[6,7] Age of CRC onset in Lynch syndrome is younger than in the general population and has varied across study samples. For patients who are part of high-risk clinic populations, mean age of diagnosis of a first CRC has been reported in the mid-forties (compared to age 64 in the general population).[4,8] Some studies have suggested that in population-based (rather than high-risk clinic-based) samples of carriers of particularly *MLH1* and *MSH2* mutations, cancers occur somewhat later, around age 54 for men and age 60 for women.[9] Cancer risks may vary depending on the specific mismatch repair gene mutation that causes Lynch syndrome, but there is not yet definitive information available.[1] Because the majority of Lynch syndrome-related CRCs occur in the ascending colon, colonoscopy is the preferred screening modality. Recommended screening for those with known or suspected Lynch syndrome-associated mutations includes colonoscopy every 1–2 years beginning between ages 20–25 for most at-risk individuals and somewhat later, age 30, for members of families with *MSH6* mutations.[1]

Female mismatch repair mutation carriers also have significant risks (40%–60%) for endometrial adenocarcinoma, with age of onset occurring around age 50 (vs. population means around age 60) and a 12% risk for ovarian cancer.[6,10] More than 75% of the endometrial cancer associated with Lynch syndrome is diagnosed at the earliest stage, and one study showed a 5-year survival rate of 88%.[11] At present, data are lacking regarding the efficacy of endometrial or ovarian cancer screening for women at risk for Lynch syndrome and it is unclear whether endometrial screening reduces mortality.[1,2] However, because early signs of endometrial cancer (i.e., vaginal bleeding) might be missed in premenopausal women at risk, women with Lynch syndrome are advised to undergo annual transvaginal ultrasound for possible detection of ovarian cancer and annual endometrial biopsy, beginning at age 30–35 years.[1] Evidence supports the efficacy of prophylactic hysterectomy and oophorectomy for reducing gynecologic cancer risk in Lynch syndrome,[12] and women are advised to consider risk-reducing surgery after completion of childbearing.[1,13,14]

Modestly increased rates of cancer occurrence are reported for other Lynch syndrome-associated cancers.[6,7,15] There are no standard screening tests for these cancers, given the lower rates of occurrence, but some do recommend upper gastrointestinal tract (GI) endoscopy or imaging of the upper abdomen to detect cancers in those regions. These recommendations remain controversial,[1] but regular primary care visits and follow-up of symptoms is recommended for mutation carriers.

Psychosocial issues

Uptake. The extent to which genetic testing is embraced by individuals at risk for hereditary CRC is critical. It is only through genetic testing that those members of high-risk families who carry cancer-predisposing mutations and who are truly at increased hereditary risk for colorectal and associated cancers can be distinguished from those who do not carry familial mutations who are only at general population risk. Reported uptake of genetic testing for Lynch syndrome varies from 14% to 75% across studies,[16–18] reflecting possible cultural and sample selection biases. More recently, the optimal approach to genetic testing for Lynch syndrome has been considered to begin with microsatellite instability (MSI) testing in tumors of CRC patients who meet the revised Bethesda guidelines for this syndrome.[1,19] However, little is known about uptake and preferences for MSI testing. A single study has reported low levels of knowledge and awareness of MSI testing among a sample of patients who met the revised Bethesda criteria and who were offered MSI testing.[20] Patients generally held positive attitudes regarding the benefits of MSI testing; however, those with higher levels of cancer-specific distress perceived a greater number of barriers to having MSI testing. These findings suggest that colorectal cancer patients may benefit from improved education about MSI testing in order to improve understanding and facilitate informed decision making about the test.

Motivation. Factors positively affecting uptake of genetic testing for Lynch syndrome include having a personal history of cancer, having more relatives with Lynch syndrome-related cancers, higher perceived risk of colorectal and related cancers, stronger beliefs that hereditary CRC would influence one's life and that of one's offspring, and more intrusive thoughts about CRC.[16,18,21–23] Uptake of genetic testing did not differ by gender, but higher educational level, having a spouse or partner and being employed correlated positively with uptake.[18,16,21] Both men and women appear motivated to seek testing to determine whether offspring are at increased cancer risk. Women may be more likely than men to want testing to determine whether they require enhanced cancer screening and to undergo testing as a response to recommendations of a physician or genetic counselor.[24] Decliners of genetic testing for Lynch syndrome were more likely to report depressive symptoms, to be nonadherent to colorectal screening recommendations, to have less confidence they could cope with a positive test result, to be concerned about insurability, and to worry about the emotional impact of genetic testing on self and family.[16,21,23]

Risk Perception. Decision making for genetic testing assumes an accurate understanding of the, admittedly complex, risks involved. However, studies indicate that while accuracy of risk perception regarding Lynch syndrome-associated cancers among at-risk individuals increases following genetic counseling,[25] even counseled individuals often do not accurately report their cancer risks. Psychological factors, such as having lost a parent to Lynch syndrome early in life, were associated with higher perceived risks. Inaccurate cancer risk perceptions among individuals undergoing genetic counseling for Lynch syndrome encompass both over- and underestimation of risk, with only one-third to one-half of participants in one study accurately reporting the levels of risk conveyed in the genetic counseling they attended.[26] Understanding risk perception for Lynch syndrome is complicated by the fact that there are multiple cancer risks to consider; however, one study showed that mismatch mutation carriers' understanding about risks for extracolonic cancers were significantly improved following genetic counseling and testing.[25]

Decision aid for Lynch syndrome genetic counseling and testing. Given the complexity of the decision to undergo genetic testing, researchers have begun to test innovative strategies to facilitate education and decision making about inherited cancer risk and genetic testing. To help at-risk individuals with decision making about whether to undergo genetic testing, an Australian group developed and tested a targeted print decision aid.[27] Participants (n = 153) were randomized to receive the decision aid or a standard pamphlet (control group). Those who used the decision aid had less decisional conflict regarding genetic testing and were more likely to be classified as having made an informed choice compared to control group participants, though the decision aid did not influence the genetic testing decision or subsequent regret. Among men, but not women, use of the decision aid was associated with greater cancer genetics knowledge. Decision making about genetic testing for Lynch syndrome is a multistep process and decision aids may be particularly useful in this context.

Distress. Genetic counseling is highly recommended before genetic testing for Lynch syndrome and has been shown to reduce distress of affected and unaffected at-risk individuals.[28] Most studies of psychosocial outcomes of genetic testing focus on short-term outcomes (up to 12 months). Research suggests that individuals who have received test results for Lynch syndrome-related mutations experienced immediate increased general distress,[29,30] cancer-specific distress,[31] and worry about cancer,[30] but that the mean increases did not raise scores above normal levels. Generally, distress receded over the first year following genetic testing[28,30] and were at pretest levels by 12 months.[31,32] One study of follow-up 3 years after disclosure of test result showed scores similar to those before genetic testing, except that noncarriers' cancer-specific distress was significantly lower than baseline scores.[32]

Research has shown, however, that there are subgroups of tested individuals who are at greater than average risk of psychological distress following testing, especially those at higher baseline levels of anxiety or depression.[24,30,33–35] Women, younger people, nonwhites, and individuals with less satisfactory social support and lower educational levels had higher levels of general and cancer-specific distress, regardless of mutation status, in the 12 months following testing.[30] Other studies have reported that individuals with a prior history of major or minor depression or those with more affected first-degree relatives or those reporting more intense grief reactions had greater distress 1–6 months after disclosure.[34,36] A recent study showed that reductions in distress over the first 6 months following disclosure for Lynch syndrome-genetic testing was moderated by the individual's style of coping with information about health. Those with high-monitoring coping styles were generally more distressed than low monitors, especially if they had indeterminate or positive test results.[37]

Generally, individuals testing negative experienced relief and decreased distress, which was long-lasting.[29–32] Such individuals are advised that they no longer require enhanced screening and can return to following general population guidelines for colonoscopy screening.[38] It has been found, however, that some at-risk individuals testing negative for Lynch syndrome-related mutations evidence distrust of the test result to the extent that they do not give up colorectal screening,[39,40] although this has not been found in all studies.[25]

Screening. An important determinant of the success of genetic counseling and testing is the degree to which at-risk individuals who are found to be mutation carriers alter their behavior to try to prevent the cancers they are at risk for. Among unaffected carriers, one study found almost 80% had a colonoscopy within 2 years of receiving their test result.[41] In another study, carriers reported significant increases in screening behavior following disclosure. Within 6–12 months following disclosure, 61% were compliant with colonoscopy recommendations and 54% had undergone extracolonic screening.[2] Noncarriers showed decreases in their screening behavior, although 11% had undergone colonoscopy and 14% had had extracolonic screening. In that study increased age and mutation status significantly predicted colonoscopy uptake and perceived likelihood of being a carrier and discussion with physician about mutation status were associated with extracolonic screening. Hadley (2008) reported that 71% of carriers and 49% of noncarriers had shared their genetic test result with their physician by 12 months. Reports of prophylactic hysterectomy and oophorectomy remain rare.[25]

Family Communication. Communication among family members about the presence of a deleterious mutation for hereditary CRC is important to accomplish one of the aims of cancer genetic testing, the early identification of family members, especially unaffected family members, who are at high risk of carrying the deleterious mutation. This identification makes possible initiation of early detection or prevention strategies. Lacking such communication, the at-risk individuals may not be aware of the hereditary etiology of the cancers which have occurred, of their own risks, or of the options available for genetic counseling/testing and targeted screening. It has been the decision of most professional medical and ethical groups that such communication should be the province of the relatives who have been tested or their surrogates[42] to protect the privacy of family members. It has been recognized, however, that there are barriers to such communication which could mean that some family members are not informed in a timely way about the options for genetic testing or targeted screening.[43]

Several quantitative and qualitative studies address attitudes in high-risk Lynch syndrome families regarding how information about familial disease should be conveyed to family members. Peterson et al. (2003) report that family members highly value dissemination of information. In a Canadian study, 93% of CRC patients in a cancer registry thought it was their duty to tell all at-risk relatives about a hereditary mutation.[44] In that study, however, subjects reported that difficult relationships (18.5%) and lack of contact with relatives (30%) would prevent them from telling some family members. Being informed by a proband is a powerful incentive to undergo genetic counseling and testing, though not all individuals so informed sought these services.[17] Family members in another study believed if parents of at-risk individuals failed to discuss the hereditary risks with their children, other relatives should intervene to provide that information.[45] Sharing of information decreased with distance from the nuclear family.[46–48] Mothers were seen as most influential in spreading information about familial mutations within the family network.[47] Motivations for and against informing of relatives was explored in a Dutch study which showed that presence of a fatal case of CRC within the family and encouragement from professionals spurred communication.[46] Disrupted or suboptimal family relationships or initial difficulty in contacting or speaking with relatives markedly hindered sharing of information about hereditary risk.[48] Information sharing in some families took years.[46] An Italian study found significant psychological barriers to the spread of information within hereditary CRC families. Ponz de Leon et al. (2004) found that among 292 first-degree relatives of affected individuals identified through a population-based cancer registry, 66% did not undergo genetic testing. The major reasons for this were failure of tested individuals to contact their relatives, lack of helpful collaboration from local family doctors, and a fatalistic approach on the part of family members about cancer, which led them, when informed, to feel uninterested in genetic counseling and testing.[41]

Concern about preventable cancers occurring in uninformed relatives of mutation carriers led Finnish researchers to pilot a program in which medical professionals directly contacted 286 uninformed relatives at 50% risk of carrying a familial mismatch-repair mutation conveying high risk for colorectal and associated cancers.[49] A letter to the at-risk individuals asked for consent to receive a telephone call from a research nurse. Those consenting learned about the possibility of hereditary cancer in their family and were offered genetic counseling and testing. A questionnaire was completed before testing. Of the 286 participants, 51% consented. While the attrition before testing was higher in the direct contact study than in a prior study where two-thirds of the at-risk relatives had had prior contact with the HNPCC surgeons and received the same information in a letter identifying that the family carried a deleterious mutation, there was little adverse reaction to the direct contact among the relatives. Among the 34 directly contacted relatives who proved to be mutation carriers, 34% (n = 11) were found on the first posttest colonoscopy to have colorectal neoplasia, two with locally advanced cancers. This supported the views of the researchers about the importance of early information about hereditary CRC risk.[49]

FAMILIAL ADENOMATOUS POLYPOSIS

Medical implications for mutation carriers. Familial adenomatous polyposis is a rare (1 in 5–10,000 births) genetic condition which predisposes mutation carriers to early CRC, preceded by the development of hundreds of colonic polyps and to a range of extraintestinal manifestations, some of which can also be life-threatening.[50] Approximately 60%–70% of cases are traceable to familial mutations present in parents; others appear to be new mutations. FAP is a dominant, autosomal disorder with a penetrance of 100%, meaning that cancer develops universally in mutation carriers, rarely before age 20, but typically decades earlier than CRC in the general population.[51] FAP is due to mutations in the *APC* gene on chromosome 5 which can be identified by genetic testing. Because the polyps associated with FAP develop as early as the teens or twenties, annual colonoscopic screening is initiated in those suspected or known to be mutation carriers by age 10–12[52] Genetic testing is often initiated around puberty or mid-adolescence (and, with suggestive symptoms, even earlier).[50] Prophylactic colectomy (i.e., removal of part of the colon) is the ultimate treatment for FAP and surgery is often completed in young adulthood to try to prevent development of CRC. There are two

standard surgeries which are done; each surgery is typically completed in two stages, with an intermediate ileostomy. The two surgeries, ileorectal anastomosis (IRA) or ileal pouch-anal anastomosis (IPAA), have ramifications in terms of increased numbers of daily bowel movements (3–4 for IRA and 4–5 for IPAA) and continence (72%–98 % for IRA and 60%–98% for IPAA), which, in turn, affect psychosocial functioning.[53]

APC genetic testing is often viewed as a medical management decision, since there is clear and immediate benefit to the testing, and, hence, it is one of the few circumstances where the genetic testing of children is advised as standard of care. The identification of those found not to be mutation carriers, that is, those found through genetic testing not to carry the familial mutation, ends the need for annual colonoscopic screening for those individuals and also ends worry about future surgery, with consequent cost savings and avoidance of psychosocial harms. Confirmation of the diagnosis can initiate surgical planning.

Psychosocial issues

Uptake. The question asked about APC testing is typically, "When?" rather than "Whether?," due to the medical and psychosocial benefits for children and adolescents of learning whether they are *APC* mutation carriers. There are data suggesting that uptake of genetic testing for FAP is higher than that for Lynch syndrome and may be above 80% among asymptomatic at-risk adults[54–56] and 96% for children ages 10–16.[57]

The optimal timing of APC testing occurs when the individual being tested is of sufficient age, maturity, and psychological stability to understand the reasons why testing is being offered and the implications of the test result.[50] In an Australian study of young adults with FAP, however, 61% had a preference to test their children at birth or very early in life (before age 10), before any such understanding could occur.[56] Genetic counseling and follow-up along the life span, in recognition of the lifelong issues raised by FAP, is recommended.[50,56]

Distress. Several studies have investigated the distress of children tested for *APC* mutations. Mean scores for individuals in these studies remain in the normal range on measures of anxiety, depression, and behavioral functioning following disclosure of test result.[53,58] However, the scores in a study of 43 children from 23 families in which one parent had FAP did indicate the interdependence of emotional reactions within families affected by FAP.[58] Having an ill mother was associated with significantly higher depression scores in children who were themselves mutation carriers, with the authors suggesting that mothers' reactions to their own illness may color the children's reactions more than paternal feelings. In families where some children tested positive and others negative, parents who were not FAP mutation carriers had significantly increased depression scores after disclosure of their children's results.

In a long-term follow-up study (23–55 months) of 48 tested child FAP patients and their parents, the interdependence of reactions of family members was also noted. Mutation carriers who had a sibling who was also a mutation carrier had significantly higher depression scores at 1 year postdisclosure. Mutation-positive children with no siblings who were mutation positive had significantly decreased depression scores at 1 year. Among parents, depression at 1 year was significantly higher for those with children who had mixed test results (some positive and some negative). Such families were recommended for additional support for both children and parents.[59]

While mean scores of distress in studies of the impact of genetic testing for hereditary CRC are not above norms, subsets of individuals with greater distress have been found in all studies. In a cross-sectional study of adults who had previously undergone APC genetic testing, the mutation carriers had higher levels of state anxiety than noncarriers and were more likely to have clinically significant anxiety levels.[60] Lower optimism and lower self-esteem were associated with higher anxiety in this study,[60] and FAP-related distress, perceived seriousness of FAP, and belief in the accuracy of genetic testing were associated with more state anxiety among carriers.[61]

Individuals testing negative for APC mutations, while relieved of much of the medical burden of the disease, often experience guilt about avoiding the lifelong worry and need for intervention which their parents and/or siblings often share.[59,62] Anxiety may be high in these children as well and their need for support should be considered in any plan to offer emotional counseling to FAP family members.

A more recent Australian study of 18- to 35-year-old young adults with or at-risk for FAP which utilized FAP-specific measures of distress suggested that unmarried (i.e., single) individuals and those who had had more extensive initial surgery had greater distress.[53] In that study 20%–30% of subjects reported negative impact on aspects of body image and sexual functioning; over half were dissatisfied with their bodies and 30% of women had pain on intercourse. Ten percent of subjects had scores consistent with significant stress response on the impact of event avoidance scale. Avoidance of FAP-related information was greater among single participants. Negative impacts regarding life choices and relationships were reported by 10%–20% of subjects. Twenty-two to thirty percent of subjects felt FAP made them less or not at all willing to have children, with the highest percentage among unmarried participants. Psychological functioning was highest among subjects who had not yet had any surgery, with more negative outcomes related to body image, sexual functioning, and affect reported by those who had had IPAA surgery. Having such intrusive surgery during the period of young adulthood when sexual identity and sexual relationships are being established is, the authors believe, highly problematic. They advise that when medically feasible, psychosocial factors should be incorporated into surgical decision making. In some cases, especially those where patients are not yet in stable relationships, it may be advisable to consider less extensive surgery, with further surgery later in life.[53] The findings in this report are supported by another study showing higher health-related quality of life among married patients with FAP or related desmoids tumors.[24]

Screening. Less is known about psychological aspects of screening for FAP than about Lynch syndrome screening after genetic testing. One study of a small number of individuals (aged 17–53 years) with a family history of FAP, who were offered participation in a genetic counseling and testing protocol, found that among those who were asymptomatic, all reported undergoing at least one endoscopic surveillance before participation in the study.[63] Only 33% (2 of 6 patients) reported continuing screening at the recommended interval. Of the affected people who had undergone colectomy, 92% (11 of 12 patients) were adherent to recommended colorectal surveillance. In another cross-sectional study of 150 people with a clinical or genetic diagnosis of classic FAP or attenuated FAP and at-risk relatives, 52% of those with FAP and 46% of relatives at risk for FAP had undergone recommended endoscopic screening.[64] Among people who had or were at risk for attenuated FAP, 58% and 33%, respectively, had undergone screening. Compared with people who had undergone screening within the recommended time interval, those who had not screened were less likely to recall provider recommendations for screening and were more likely to lack health insurance or insurance reimbursement for screening and more likely to believe that they were not at increased risk for CRC. Only 42% of the study population had ever undergone genetic counseling. A small percentage of participants (14%–19%) described screening as a "necessary evil," indicating a dislike for the bowel preparation, or experienced pain and discomfort. Nineteen percent reported that these issues might pose barriers to undergoing future endoscopies. Nineteen percent reported that improved techniques and the use of anesthesia have improved tolerance for screening procedures.

Family Communication. There are no studies of family communication in FAP families.

DISCUSSION

The literature on psychosocial aspects of hereditary CRC is considerably more limited than that on psychosocial aspects of genetic counseling and testing for hereditary breast-ovarian cancer. Lynch syndrome and FAP studies are often based on relatively small samples and are difficult to compare because of differences in the nature of the samples surveyed (e.g., population vs. high-risk clinical registry samples, affected vs. unaffected individuals, Lynch syndrome vs. FAP, after genetic counseling vs.

after genetic testing, age range), the time frame (e.g., longitudinal vs. cross-sectional studies), and varying follow-up periods (6 months vs. 12 months or longer). It is difficult to calculate adherence, since colonoscopies may be recommended to occur every 1–2 years, so figures for colonoscopy use in the first 12 months following disclosure may not clearly indicate if the individual is adherent or not. Since there is varying enthusiasm for transvaginal ultrasound and endometrial biopsy, adherence rates may be related to physician recommendation more explicitly than for other recommended screening behaviors.

Nonetheless, it appears that some facts are emerging about the impact of genetic testing on individuals at high risk for hereditary cancers. In general, mean distress scores for individuals undergoing genetic testing for hereditary CRC, as for hereditary *BRCA1/2* testing,[65] are not above population norms. There are, however, subsets of subjects, sometimes up to a quarter of the sample, who do experience significant disease or testing-related distress. Distress may be related to the intensity of recommended screening, single marital status, the test results of other family members, or the impact of the surgery. These factors, many tied to psychological rather than medical variables, suggest that counseling, both genetic and psychological, is important for individuals dealing with hereditary disease, not just at the time of testing, but at many other points along the trajectory of patient care for these diseases. One of the differentiating features of hereditary disease is that, as patients have said, "It's never over." As such, support services must be geared to the on-going needs of those who continue to face genetic risk for serious diseases. Future research will help to define the best ways to provide such services.

The issue of how best to inform relatives about familial mutations predisposing to markedly elevated, early cancer risks and the definition of duty to warn in the context of genetic testing for diseases where potentially life-saving interventions exist raise interesting and challenging questions. The Finnish findings supporting the detection of additional cases of CRC in directly contacted relatives of mutation carriers[49] is supported by findings from Australia where a similar rate of participation (40%) was observed among directly contacted relatives who had not previously been contacted by the probands who carried *BRCA1/2* mutations.[66] Attitudes may be changing about the relative value of confidentiality and privacy and the need to inform at-risk relatives about their high levels of cancer risk and about options to detect or prevent cancer.

Recognizing that there are some families where certain people do not correspond in any fashion puts the onus on medical professionals to communicate with such members…To save lives, all family members of someone having the HNPCC mutation must be informed by whoever is able to do so (family member, physician, or genetic counselor). Being notified of the possibility TWICE, in lieu of not being notified at all, is a much better solution to this problem.[44]

We do not yet fully understand how broadly the availability of genetic testing for hereditary disease might affect family relationships.[67]

It is clear that psychosocial factors play a large role in the impact of cancer genetic testing for CRC. Uptake of testing, adherence to screening recommendations, surgical choice, and family communication are likely to be influenced by the individual's experience of hereditary illness in their family, their affective style and information preferences, as well as other little-studied social factors, such as socioeconomic status and access to genetic health services. Such factors will impact the ultimate integration of genetic testing into general medical practice. Hereditary CRC offers a model illustrating the potentially life-saving value of genetic testing where critical attention to psychological issues and support needs may optimize utilization.

REFERENCES

1. Lindor NM, Petersen GM, Hadley DW, et al. Recommendations for the care of individuals with an inherited predisposition to Lynch Syndrome. *JAMA.* 2006;296:1507–1517.

2. Hadley DW, Jenkins JF, Steinberg SM, et al. Perceptions of cancer risks and predictors of colon and endometrial cancer screening in women undergoing genetic testing for Lynch Syndrome. *J Clin Oncol.* 2008;26:948–954.

3. Watson P, Riley B. The tumor spectrum in Lynch Syndrome. *Fam Cancer.* 2005;4:245–248.

4. Lynch HT, de la Chapelle A. Hereditary colorectal cancer. *N Engl J Med.* 2003;348:919–932.

5. National Comprehensive Cancer Network. *NCCN clinical practice guidelines in oncology: colorectal cancer screening version 1.* Rockledge, PA: National Comprehensive Cancer Network; 2007.

6. Dunlop MG, Farrington SM, Carothers AD, et al. Cancer risk associated with germline DNA mismatch repair gene mutations. *Hum Mol Genet.* 1997;6: 105–110.

7. Aarnio M, Sankila R, Pukkula E, et al. Cancer risk in mutation carriers of DNA-mismatch-repair genes. *Int J Cancer.* 1999;81:214–218.

8. Gruber SB. New developments in Lynch Syndrome (hereditary nonpolyposis colorectal cancer) and mismatch repair gene testing. *Gastroenterology.* 2006;130:577–587.

9. Hampel H, Stephens J, Pukkala E, et al. Cancer risk in hereditary nonpolyposis colorectal cancer syndrome. *Gastroenterology.* 2005;129:415–421.

10. Aarnio M, Mecklin J, Aaltonen L, Nystrom-Lahti M, Jarvinen H. Life-time risk of different cancers in hereditary non-polyposis colorectal cancer (HNPCC) syndrome. *Int J Cancer.* 1995;64:430–433.

11. Boks DE, Trujillo AP, Voogd AC, Morreau H, Kenter GG, Vasen HF. Survival analysis of endometrial carcinoma associated with hereditary nonpolyposis colorectal cancer. *Int J Cancer.* 2002;102:198–200.

12. Schmeler KM, Lynch HT, Chen LM, et al. Prophylactic surgery to reduce the risk of gynecologic cancers in the Lynch Syndrome. *N Engl J Med.* 2006;354:261–269.

13. Lu KH, Kinh M, Kohlmann W, et al. Gynecologic cancer as a 'sentinel cancer' for women with hereditary nonpolyposis colorectal cancer syndrome. *Obstet Gynecol.* 2005;105:569–574.

14. Engstrom P. Update: NCCN colon cancer clinical practice guidelines. *J Natl Compr Canc Netw.* 2005;3:S25-S28.

15. Lin KM, Shashidharan M, Ternent CA, et al. Colorectal and extracolonic cancer variations in MLH1/MSH2 hereditary nonpolyposis colorectal cancer kindreds and the general population. *Dis Colon Rectum.* 1998;41:428–433.

16. Lerman A, Hughes C, Trock BJ, et al. Genetic testing in families with hereditary nonpolyposis colon cancer. *JAMA.* 1999;281:1618–1622.

17. Peterson SK, Watts BG, Koehly LM, et al. How families communicate about HNPCC genetic testing: findings from a qualitative study. *Am J Med Genet C Semin Med Genet.* 2003;119C:78–86.

18. Atkan-Collan K, Mecklin J-P, Jarvinen H, et al. Predictive genetic testing for hereditary non-polyposis colorectal cancer: uptake and long-term satisfaction. *Int. J Cancer (Pred Onc).* 2000;89:44–50.

19. Umar A. Boland CR, Terdiman JP, et al. Revised Bethesda Guidelines for hereditary nonpolyposis colorectal cancer (Lynch syndrome) and microsatellite instability. *J Natl Cancer Inst.* 2004;96(4):261–268.

20. Manne SL, Chung DC, Weinberg DS, et al. Knowledge and attitudes about microsatellite instability testing among high-risk individuals diagnosed with colorectal cancer. *Cancer Epidemiol Biomarkers Prev.* 2007;16:2110–2117.

21. Codori AM, Petersen GM, Miglioretti DL, et al. Attitudes toward colon cancer gene testing: factors predicting test uptake. Cancer Epidemiol Biomarkers Prev. 1999;8:345–51.

22. Balmana J, Stoffel EM, Emmons KM, Garber JE, Syngal S. Comparison of motivations and concerns for genetic testing in hereditary colorectal and breast cancer syndromes. *J Med Genet.* 2004;41:e44.

23. Hadley DW, Jenkins JF, Dimond E, de Carvalho M, Kirsch I, Palmer CG. Genetic counseling and testing in families with hereditary nonpolyposis colorectal cancer. *Arch Intern Med.* 2003;163:573–582.

24. Esplen MJ, Berk T, Butler K, Gallinger S, Cohen Z, Trinkhaus M. Quality of life in adults diagnosed with familial adenomatous polyposis and desmoids tumour. *Dis Colon Rectum.* 2004;47:687–696.

25. Claes E, Denayer L, Evers-Kiebooms G, et al. Predictive testing for hereditary nonpolyposis colorectal cancer: subjective perception regarding colorectal and endometrial cancer, distress, and health-related behavior at one year posttest. *Genet Test.* 2005;9:54–65.

26. Domanska N, Nilbert M, Siller M, Silfverberg B, Carlsson C. Discrepancies between estimated and perceived risk of cancer among individuals with hereditary nonpolyposis colorectal cancer. *Genet Test.* 2007;11:183–186.

27. Wakefield CE, Meiser B, Homewood J, Ward R, O'Donnell S, Kirk J. Australian Genetic Testing Decision Aid Collaborative Group. Randomized trial of a decision aid for individuals considering genetic testing for hereditary nonpolyposis colorectal cancer risk. *Cancer.* 2008;113:956–965.

28. Keller M, Jost R, Haunstetter C, et al. Psychosocial outcome following genetic risk counseling for familial colorectal cancer: a comparison of affected patients and family members. *Clin Genet.* 2008;74:414–424.

29. Aktan-Collan K, Haukkala A, Mecklin JP, Uutela A, Kääriäinen H. Psychological consequences predictive genetic testing for hereditary non-

polyposis colorectal cancer (HNPCC): a prospective follow-up study. Int J Cancer. 2001;93:608–11.

30. Gritz ER, Peterson SK, Vernon SW, et al. Psychological impact of genetic testing for hereditary nonpolyposis colorectal cancer. J Clin Oncol. 2005;23: 1902–10

31. Meiser B, Collins V, Warren R, et al. Psychological impact of genetic testing for hereditary non-polyposis colorectal cancer. *Clin Genet.* 2004;66:502–511.

32. Collins VR, Meiser B, Ukoumunne OC, Gaff C, St John DJ, Halliday JL. The impact of predictive genetic testing for hereditary non-polyposis colorectal cancer: three years after testing. *Genet Med.* 2007;9:290–297.

33. Vernon SW, Gritz ER, Peterson SK, et al. Intention to learn results of genetic testing for hereditary colon cancer. *Cancer Epidemiol Biomarkers Prev.* 1999;8:353–360.

34. Van Oostrom I, Meijers-Heijboer H, Duivenvoorden HJ, et al. Experience of parental cancer in childhood is a risk factor for psychological distress during genetic cancer susceptibility testing. *Ann Oncol.* 2006;17:1090–1095.

35. Vernon SW, Gritz ER, Peterson SK, et al. Correlates of psychologic distress in colorectal cancer patients undergoing genetic testing for hereditary colon cancer. *Health Psychol.* 1997;16:73–86.

36. Murakami Y, Okamura H, Sugano K, et al. Psychologic distress after disclosure of genetic test results regarding hereditary nonpolyposis colorectal carcinoma. *Cancer.* 2004;101:395–403.

37. Shiloh S, Koehly L, Jenkins J, Martin J, Hadley D. Monitoring coping style moderates emotional reactions to genetic testing for hereditary nonpolyposis colorectal cancer: a longitudinal study. *Psycho-Oncology.* 2008;17:746–755.

38. Burke W, Petersen G, Lynch P, et al. Cancer Genetics Studies Consortium. Recommendations for follow-up care of individuals with an inherited predisposition to cancer, I. *JAMA.* 1997;277:915–919.

39. Michie S, Collins V, Halliday J, Marteau T. Likelihood of attending for bowel screening after a negative genetic test result: the possible influence of health professionals. *Genet Test.* 2002;6:307–311.

40. Halbert CH, Lynch H, Lynch J, et al. Colon cancer screening practices following genetic testing for hereditary nonpolyposis colon cancer (HNPCC) mutations. *Arch Intern Med.* 2004;164:1881–1887.

41. Ponz de Leon M, Benatti P, DiGregorio C, et al. Genetic testing among high-risk individuals in families with hereditary nonpolyposis colorectal cancer. *Brit J Cancer.* 2004;90:882–887.

42. American Society of Human Genetics Social Issues Subcommittee on Familial Disclosure. ASHG statement: professional disclosure of familial genetic information. *Am J Hum Genet.* 1998;62:474–483.

43. Gaff CL, Clarke AJ, Atkinson P, et al. Process and outcome in communication of genetic information within families: a systematic review. *Eur J Hum Genet.* 2007;15:999–1011.

44. Kohut K, Manno M, Gallinger S, Esplen MJ. Should healthcare providers have a duty to warn family members of individuals with an HNPCC-causing mutation? A survey of patients from the Ontario Familial Colon Cancer Registry. *J Med Genet.* 2008;44:404–407.

45. Pentz RD, Peterson SK, Watts B, et al. Hereditary nonpolyposis colorectal cancer family members' perceptions about the duty to inform and health professionals' role in disseminating genetic information. *Genet Test.* 2005;9:261–268.

46. Mesters I, Ausems M, Eichorn S, Vasen H. Informing one's family about genetic testing for hereditary non-polyposis colorectal cancer (HNPCC): a retrospective exploratory study. *Fam Cancer.* 2005;4:163–167.

47. Koehly LM, Peterson SK, Watts BG, Kempf KK, Vernon SW, Gritz ER. A social network analysis of communication about hereditary non-polyposis colorectal cancer genetic testing and family functioning. *Cancer Epidemiol Biomarkers Prev.* 2003;12:304–313.

48. Stoeffel EM, Ford B, Mercado RC, et al. Sharing genetic test results in Lynch Syndrome: communication with close and distant relatives. *Clin Gaestroenterol Hepatol.* 2008;6:333–338.

49. Atkan-Collan K, Haukkala A, Pylvanainen K, et al. Direct contact in inviting high-risk members of hereditary colon cancer families to genetic counseling and DNA testing. *J Med Genet.* 2007;44:732–738.

50. Rozen P, Macrae F. Familial adenomatous polyposis: the practical applications of clinical and molecular screening. *Fam Cancer.* 2006;5:227–235.

51. Bulow S. Familial adenomatous polyposis. *Ann Med.* 1989;21:299–307.

52. Douma KFL, Aaronson NK, Vasen HFA, Bleiker EMA. Psychosocial issues in genetic testing for familial adenomatous polyposis. A review of the literature. *Psycho-Oncology.*2008;17:737–745.

53. Andrews L, Mireskandari S, Jessen J, et al. Impact of familial adenomatous polyposis on young adults: quality of life outcomes. *Dis Colon Rectum.* 2007;50:1306–1315.

54. Petersen GM, Boyd PA. Gene tests and counseling for colorectal cancer risk: lessons from familial polyposis. *J Natl Cancer Inst Monogr.* 1995;17:67–71.

55. Whitelaw S, Northover JM, Hodgson SV. Attitudes to predictive DNA testing in familial adenomatous polyposis. *J Med Genet.* 1996;33:540–543.

56. Andrews L, Mireskandari S, Jessen J, et al. Impact of familial adenomatous polyposis on young adults: attitudes toward genetic testing, support, and information needs. *Genet Med.* 2006;8(11):697–703.

57. Evans DG, Maher ER, Macleod R, Davies DR, Craufurd D. Uptake of genetic testing for cancer predisposition. *J Med Genet.* 1997;34:746–748.

58. Codori AM, Petersen G, Boyd P, Brandt J, Giardello FM. Genetic testing for cancer in children: short term psychological effect. *Arch Pediatr Adolesc Med.*1996;150:1131–1138.

59. Codori AM, Zawacki KL, Petersen GM, et al. Genetic testing for hereditary colorectal cancer in children: long-term psychological effects. *Am J Med Genet.* 2003;116A:117–128.

60. Michie S, Bobrow M, Marteau TM. Predictive genetic testing in children and adults: a study of emotional impact. *J Med Genet.* 2001;38:519–526.

61. Michie S, Weinman J, Miller J, Collins V, Halliday J, Marteau TM. Predictive genetic testing: high risk expectations in the face of low risk information. *J Behav Med.* 2002;25:33–50.

62. Duncan RE, Gillam L, Savulescu J, Williamson R, Rogers JG, Delatycki MB. "You're one of us now": young people describe their experience of predictive genetic testing for Huntington Disease (HD) and familial adenomatous polyposis (FAP). *Am J Med Genet C Semin Med Genet.* 2008;148C:47–55.

63. Stoffel EM, Garber JE, Grover S, Russo L, Johnson J, Syngal S. Cancer surveillance is often inadequate in people at high risk for colorectal cancer. *J Med Genet.* 2003;40:e54.

64. Kinney AY, Hicken B, Simonsen SE, et al. Colorectal cancer surveillance behaviors among members of typical and attenuated FAP families. *Am J Gastroenterol.* 2007;102:153–162.

65. Meiser B. Psychological impact of genetic testing for cancer susceptibility: an update of the literature. *Psycho-Oncology.* 2005;14:1060–1074.

66. Suthers G, Armstrong J, McCormack J, Trott D. Letting the family know: balancing ethics and effectiveness when notifying relatives about genetic testing for a familial disorder. *J Med Genet.* 2006;43:665–670.

67. Finkler K, Skrzynia C, Evans JP. The new genetics and its consequences for family, kinship, medicine and medical genetics. *Soc Sci Med.* 2003;57:403–412.

PART V

Psychological Issues Related to Site of Cancer

Ruth McCorkle, ED

CHAPTER 15

Instruments in Psycho-Oncology

William F. Pirl

INTRODUCTION

Many instruments are available to measure the psychosocial health of individuals with cancer. Although these instruments have typically been utilized more in research, there is growing interest in incorporating them into clinical care as standardized assessments. These assessments could be used to screen for psychosocial distress or measure the performance of care.

The wide variety of existing instruments can often make choosing one a difficult decision. On the surface, a particular instrument may seem like it could be used in all types of settings, but it could be inappropriate for some purposes. Unfortunately, there is no clear consensus on which specific instruments are the "best" for specific purposes. Most of the time a choice has to be made on the basis of the intended goal of measurement.

Although this chapter is not an exhaustive or comprehensive review of instruments, it will attempt to provide an introductory guide to the use of instruments in psycho-oncology. It will first present a framework for selecting and interpreting instruments and then describe some of the most commonly used instruments.

While general quality-of-life instruments will often contain domains for emotional and social well-being, this chapter is limited to more specific instruments. With the exceptions of cognition and substance abuse, most of these instruments are self-report and can be completed by patients on their own. Clinician-administered instruments that require training in their administration and scoring to ensure reliability, such as the Structured Clinical Interview for DSM Disorders (SCID) and the Hamilton Depression Rating Scale for Depression, are not presented.

INSTRUMENT SELECTION

The choice of an instrument should be on the basis of the following seven considerations:

1. *Goal of using the instrument*: Is the instrument being used to assess the level of symptoms or to identify a diagnostic category? Instruments can be scales for symptoms, diagnostic checklists, or both. Is it being used in research or clinical care? More detailed and rigorous assessments might be important for research, whereas patient acceptability and brevity may be critical in clinical care.
2. *Population*: To whom will the instrument be administered? The same instrument may not be appropriate for all groups: the general population, people being treated for cancer, certain types of cancers, and long-term cancer survivors. Some items in an instrument may not be relevant to the intended population. Examine the content of the instrument and investigate what instruments have been used in that population.
3. *Psychometrics*: Has the instrument been rigorously developed so that there is evidence that it actually measures the intended attribute (validity) and is consistent in its measurement (reliability)? Is there data on using the instrument in the specific intended population? The creation of a new instrument requires testing its properties, such as validation and reliability, before using it in a research or clinical setting. Because the research on the validity and reliability of an instrument usually only exist on using the instrument as a whole, modifying an instrument in any way may change its properties and limit the inferences that can be drawn. A more detailed presentation of

psychometrics can be found in the textbook, *Health Measurement Scales*, by Streiner and Norman.[1]
4. *Sensitivity/specificity*: In screening, there is often a trade off between how well the instrument can identify all cases (sensitivity) and how well it can limit those identified to only be cases (specificity). In a particular situation, would you rather err on the side of overidentifying many people so that you will not miss anyone (high sensitivity and low specificity) or risk missing some people because you want to make sure those who are identified really have it (low specificity and high sensitivity). Review published studies using the instrument, including the primary paper on its development, for these data.
5. *Sensitivity to change*: If you are following a symptom over time, will the instrument be able to detect meaningful differences? These data can often be found in papers on the psychometrics of an instrument.
6. *Burden of the instrument*: How long does it take to complete? Instruments that require 20 minutes to complete may not be compatible with screening in a busy clinic. How is the instrument administered? Is it a straight-forward self-report instrument or will a staff person be required to aid in its completion? Is the instrument in the public domain for use at no cost or will it have to be purchased for each patient?
7. *Ease of scoring*: Some instruments can be quickly scored by hand so that the results can be used in real time. Others may require more elaborate scoring algorithms or even computer assistance.

INSTRUMENTS

General distress. Because psychosocial health covers many areas including psychological, social, and practical needs, a general instrument that includes assessment beyond psychological symptoms is necessary.

1. *Distress Thermometer* (www.nccn.org): Developed by the NCCN as a screening instrument, the Distress Thermometer can be downloaded as part of the Distress Guidelines. Although it can be thought of as a one-item scale assessing the level of distress, it also contains a problem list in which sources of distress can be identified by the completer. It appears to correlate well with other longer instruments such as the Hospital Anxiety and Depression Scale (HADS) and Brief Symptom Inventory (BSI)[2] and scores of 4 and above are suggestive of clinically meaningful levels of distress warranting further evaluation. It appears to be sensitive to changes over time.[3] Although it may be a reasonable screen for distress, it performs less well for identifying specific psychiatric disorders such as major depressive disorder.[4] It takes only a few minutes to complete, which makes it feasible to use in busy clinical settings.

   In clinical care, the Distress Thermometer's problem list can be used to guide further assessment. If a patient checked, "yes," to an item under "Emotional Problems," you could consider giving them one of the instruments described later for emotional problems, such as the HADS and/or Patient Health questionnaire (PHQ). If a patient checked, "yes," to an item under "Spiritual/Religious Concerns," you could consider evaluating this further by taking a spiritual history with the FICA questions described later or even quantifying spiritual well-being with the FACIT-Sp. If a patient checked, "yes," to problems with "memory/concentration" under "Physical Problems," consider further assessment with the Mini Mental Status Examination (MMSE).

Some forms of distress may not be readily identified by the Distress Thermometer, such as substance abuse, dementia, and delirium. On the basis of the patient's history and clinical presentation, other assessments should be done for further evaluation. For substance abuse, consider the CAGE questions or Alcohol Use Disorders Identification Test (AUDIT) described under the heading, "Substance Abuse." If there is concern about possible dementia, tests under the heading, "Cognition," the MMSE, and the Clock Drawing Test should be considered. If there is concern about delirium, the tests under the "Cognition" heading and an instrument more specific for delirium such as the Confusion Assessment Method (CAM) should be considered.

2. *Psychosocial Screen for Cancer (PSCAN)*[5]: The PSCAN is a more extensive assessment of general distress. This 21-item self-report instrument assesses social support and psychological symptoms, mainly depressive and anxiety symptoms. It has been relatively recently developed and at the time of writing this chapter, only preliminary psychometrics are available. It appears to correlate well with measures on depression, anxiety, and social support. However, there is little data about its sensitivity to change over time and accuracy of measurements for research.

Emotional problems. When overall emotional functioning is the focus of assessment, instruments that measure different types of psychological symptoms are needed. All of these instruments assess depressive and anxiety symptoms, and some include other symptoms. This category contains two types of instruments: diagnostic and symptom scales.

Diagnostic.

1. *PHQ*[6]: This self-report instrument was developed to screen for psychiatric disorders in primary care and assesses eight specific psychiatric disorders based on DSM-IV criteria. While the 9 items for depression, referred to as the PHQ-9, and 22 items for anxiety disorders may easily translate into oncology settings, the modules for somatoform disorder and eating disorders may not be appropriate. The instrument can be scored to see if someone meets diagnostic criteria for the disorders, but also can provide a continuous score to measure levels of symptoms. It was validated in primary care patients, but has been used in studies with cancer patients.[6,7] The depression and anxiety modules take about 5 minutes to complete.

Scales

1. *BSI*[8]: This instrument has 53 items covering nine dimensions: anxiety, depression, hostility, interpersonal sensitivity, obsessive compulsive, paranoid ideation, phobic anxiety, psychoticism, and somatization. It also comes in a brief form, the 18-item BSI-18 that covers three dimensions: anxiety, depression, and somatization. It has been validated in a wide range of patient populations including cancer patients.[9] The BSI-18 takes about 10 minutes to complete but requires purchasing either computer software or hand-scoring kits for scoring.

2. *PHQ*[6]: As mentioned earlier, the PHQ can be scored both categorically to give likely diagnoses and continuously to give level of symptoms.

3. *HADS*[10]: This 14-item scale was developed to minimize the contribution of physical symptoms in the assessment of anxiety and depression in medically ill patients. It has been widely used in cancer patients and has been found to correlates at .70 with a clinician-administered assessment of depressive symptoms.[11] (Razavi et al., 1990) The HADS has depression and anxiety subscales, each 7 items, and can be scored separately or together for a total distress score. It has two cut offs: 8 and 11. Using 8 there is greater sensitivity, but greater likelihood over overidentifying possible cases. Using 11, there is greater sensitivity but lower specificity (Fig. 15–1).

Depression

Diagnostic. *Patient Health Questionnaire-9 (PHQ-9)*[6]: The PHQ-9 consists of the nine depression items on the PHQ. To meet criteria for a probable diagnosis of major depression, patients must endorse having the two items for low mood and anhedonia and at least five other symptoms for "at least half of the time" or more, consistent with the DSM-IV criteria. Lesser criteria exist as well for "other depressive syndromes."

Hospital Anxiety and Depression Scale (HADS)

Patients are asked to choose one response from the four given for each Interview. They should give an immediate response and be dissuaded from thinking too long about their answers. The question relating to anxiety are marked "A", and to depression "D". The score for each answer is given in the right column. Instruct the patient to answer how it currently describes their feelings.

A	I feel tense or 'wound up':	
	Most of the time	3
	A lot of the time	2
	From time to time, occasionally	1
	Not at all	0

Fig. 15–1. Hospital Anxiety and Depression Scale (HADS).
SOURCE : Reprinted from Zigmond AS, Snaith RP. The hospital anxiety and depression scale. *Acta Psychiatr Scand.* 1983;67:361–370.

D	I still enjoy the things I used to enjoy:	
	Definitely as much	0
	Not quite so much	1
	Only a little	2
	Hardly at all	3

A	I GET A SORT OF FRIGHTENED FEELING AS IF SOMETHING AWFUL IS ABOUT TO HAPPEN:	
	Very definitely and quite badly	3
	Yes, but not too badly	2
	A little, but it doesn't worry me	1
	Not at all	0

D	I can laugh and see the funny side of things:	
	As much as I always could	0
	Not quite as much now	1
	Definitely not so much now	2
	Not at all	3

A	Worrying thoughts go through my mind:	
	A great deal of the time	3
	A lot of the time	2
	From time to time but not too often	1
	Only occasionally	0

D	I feel cheerful:	
	Not at all	3
	Not often	2
	Sometimes	1
	Most of the time	0

Fig. 15–1. Continued.

A	I can sit at ease and feel relaxed:	
	Definitely	0
	Usually	1
	Not often	2
	Not at all	3

D	I feel as if I am slowed down:	
	Nearly all the time	3
	Very often	2
	Sometimes	1
	Not at all	0

A	I get a sort of frightened feeling like 'butterflies' in the stomach:	
	Not at all	0
	Occasionally	1
	Quite often	2
	Very often	3

D	I have lost interest in my appearance:	
	Definitely	3
	I don't take so much care as I should	2
	I may not take quite as much care	1
	I take just as much care as ever	0

A	I feel restless as if I have to be on the move:	
	Very much indeed	3
	Quite a lot	2
	Not very much	1
	Not at all	0

Fig. 15–1. Continued.

D	I look forward with enjoyment to things:	
	As much as ever I did	0
	Rather less than I used to	1
	Definitely less than I used to	2
	Hardly at all	3

A	I get sudden feelings of panic:	
	Very often indeed	3
	Quite often	2
	Not very often	1
	Not at all	0

D	I can enjoy a good book or radio or TV programme:	
	Often	0
	Sometimes	1
	Not often	2
	Very seldom	3

D	Scoring (add the As = Anxiety. Add the Ds = Depression). The norms below will give you an idea of the level of Anxiety and Depression.	
	0-7 = Normal	
	8-10 = Borderline abnormal	
	11-21 = Abnormal	

Reference:

Zigmond and Snaith (1983)

Fig. 15–1. Continued.

Scales

1. *Beck Depression Inventory (BDI)*[12]: This 21-item instrument is one of the most widely used self-report scales for depression in general populations, but it contains a number of somatic items that may result in elevated scores based on medical illness—especially fatigue, appetite, and so on. However, it has been used in a number of studies of cancer patients. Scores can range from 0 to 63, with 10 or greater suggesting at least mild major depression. To better reflect DSM-IV criteria, the BDI was revised to the BDI-II. The BDI-II has less emphasis on somatic symptoms and has been validated in primary care patients.[13] (Arnau et al., 2001) It too has good performance in cancer patients.[14] These scales are easy to use and take approximately 5–10 minutes to complete.

2. *Center for Epidemiologic Studies Depression Scale (CES-D)*[15]: The use of this 20-item scale has been growing in popularity over the past several years in oncology. Although one reason often cited for its popularity is its minimal focus on somatic symptoms, some of its items assess physical symptoms similar to other depression scales. Its validity and reliability has been demonstrated in specific groups of cancer patients such as breast cancer patients.[16] It takes less than 5 minutes to complete. Scores can range from 0 to 60, with scores of 16 or greater suggesting a probable case of major depression. It is free to use without permission (Fig. 15–2).

3. *HADS*[10]: While the CES-D may be gaining in popularity over the HADS, it remains the instrument with the least focus on somatic symptoms. However, the BDI, CES-D, and HADS may all be reasonable screening instruments for depression in ambulatory cancer patients without statistical differences in their performances.[17] Scores on the 7-item depression subscale can range from 0 to 21, with 8 being the lowest threshold for a probable case of major depression.

4. *PHQ-9*[6]: As a continuous scale, scores on the PHQ-9 can range from 0 to 27, with scores greater than 15 suggesting a depressive disorder.

Anxiety
Diagnostic

1. *PHQ*[6]: The PHQ contains 22 items on anxiety that evaluate diagnoses of panic disorder and generalized anxiety disorder. Although there is some data on the PHQ-9 for depression in patients with cancer, there is little data on its utility for anxiety disorders in this population.

Center for Epidemiologic Studies Depression Scale (CES-D), NIMH

Below is a list of the ways you might have felt or behaved. Please tell me how often you have felt this way during the past week.

	During the Past Week			
	Rarely or none of the time (less than 1 day)	Some or a little of the time (1-2 days)	Occasionally or a moderate amount of time (3-4 days)	Most or all of the time (5-7 days)
1. I was bothered by things that usually don't bother me.	❑	❑	❑	❑
2. I did not feel like eating; my appetite was poor.	❑	❑	❑	❑
3. I felt that I could not shake off the blues even with help from my family or friends.	❑	❑	❑	❑
4. I felt I was just as good as other people.	❑	❑	❑	❑
5. I had trouble keeping my mind on what I was doing.	❑	❑	❑	❑
6. I felt depressed.	❑	❑	❑	❑
7. I felt that everything I did was an effort.	❑	❑	❑	❑
8. I felt hopeful about the future.	❑	❑	❑	❑
9. I thought my life had been a failure.	❑	❑	❑	❑
10. I felt fearful.	❑	❑	❑	❑
11. My sleep was restless.	❑	❑	❑	❑
12. I was happy.	❑	❑	❑	❑
13. I talked less than usual.	❑	❑	❑	❑
14. I felt lonely.	❑	❑	❑	❑
15. People were unfriendly.	❑	❑	❑	❑
16. I enjoyed life.	❑	❑	❑	❑
17. I had crying spells.	❑	❑	❑	❑
18. I felt sad.	❑	❑	❑	❑
19. I felt that people dislike me.	❑	❑	❑	❑
20. I could not get "going."	❑	❑	❑	❑

SCORING: zero for answers in the first column, 1 for answers in the second column, 2 for answers in the third column, 3 for answers in the fourth column. The scoring of positive items is reversed. Possible range of scores is zero to 60, with the higher scores indicating the presence of more symptomatology.

Fig. 15–2. Center for Epidemiologic Studies Depression Scale (CES-D), NIMH.

SOURCE: Reprinted from Radloff LS. *Applied psychological measurement.* Vol. 1, No. 3. pp. 385–401, Copyright 1977 by Lenore Sawyer Radloff by permission of SAGE Publications.

Scales

1. *HADS*[10]: Similar to the depression subscale, there are seven items on anxiety symptoms and scores can range from 0 to 21 with 8 or greater being the cut off for probable cases of anxiety.
2. *Beck Anxiety Inventory (BAI)*[18]: Although this may be one of the most widely used scales for anxiety in general populations, it does contain somatic items that may be present in people with cancer regardless of anxiety. It is not commonly used in cancer populations, but it has been used in medically ill populations.[19] It has 21 items and takes about 5 minutes to complete. Scores can range from 0 to 63 and scores of 10 or greater are suggestive of at least mild anxiety.
3. *State Trait Anxiety Inventory (STAI)*[20]: This 40-item scale is widely used in general populations and, along with the HADS, is one of the most frequently used anxiety scales in studies of people with cancer. It attempts to measure both temporary "state" anxiety and long-standing "trait" anxiety. It has been normed in several specific populations, including male medical patients. Although there are not cancer-specific norms, it has been used in cancer patients.[21] It takes approximately 10 minutes to complete.
4. *Impact of Events Scale (IES)*[22]: The IES is a 15-item scale that is designed to assess psychological symptoms after a particular negative event. In medical settings, it can be useful to measure distress from a specific event, such as receiving bad news or having a traumatic medical experience. It has been widely used in cancer patients and is commonly used in studies of genetic counseling for cancer risk.[23,24] It has subscales for two classes of posttraumatic stress disorder symptoms, intrusion (7 items), and avoidance (8 items). It takes 5–10 minutes to complete. There is also a revised version of the IES (IES-R) that contains an additional 7 items on another class of posttraumatic stress disorder symptoms, hyperarousal.

Cognition

General cognition. In contrast to the other instruments presented so far, assessments of cognition are typically clinician administered.

1. *MMSE*[25]: The MMSE is a 14-item clinician-administered instrument to assess cognition, regardless of cause. It contains items on orientation, attention, recall, visual-spatial construction, and language abilities. Scores of 24 or less suggest severe impairment. Further neuropsychological assessment is often needed for dementia, particularly assessments that include tests of frontal lobe functioning. The MMSE can be used to serially follow patients at risk for developing cognitive impairment or patients who have had alterations in their cognition particularly by delirium (Fig. 15–3).
2. *Clock Drawing Test*: The Clock Drawing Test is a pen-and-paper test that assesses several cognitive abilities. It is a good adjuvant test of executive functioning when given with the MMSE and is often a favorite of psychiatry consultation-liaison services. Patients are asked to draw a clock on a piece of paper, putting the numbers on the face, and making the hands on the clock designate a specific time, such as 10 minutes before 2. This task tests patients' ability to follow complex commands, sequence and plan their actions, and visual-spatial ability. The drawn clock can be objectively scored by a validated scoring system. There are two scoring systems, each of which has reasonable sensitivity and specificity in identifying cognitive dysfunction[26] (Juby, Tench, and Baker, 2002)[27,28] (Fig. 15–4).

Delirium

1. *CAM*[29]: The CAM is a 9-item scale that can be used to recognize and diagnose delirium. The scale is designed to be completed after a clinical interview and a review of the patient's medical record. It takes 10–20 minutes to complete and is probably the most widely used instrument for delirium (Fig. 15–5).
2. *Delirium Rating Scale (DRS)*[30]: The DRS is a 10-item scale that can be used to measure the severity of delirium, follow its clinical course, and assess responses to treatment. The scoring is based on clinical information such as a mental status examination, history, and laboratory findings. It takes at least 30–45 minutes to collect all of the information needed for the scale. Score of 10 or greater are suggestive of delirium. There is also a revised version that contains 16 items, the DRS-R-98.
3. *Memorial Delirium Assessment Scale (MDAS)*[31]: The MDAS is a 10-item clinician-administered assessment that evaluates the areas of cognition most sensitive to impairment with delirium: arousal, level of consciousness, memory, attention, orientation, disturbances in thinking, and psychomotor activity. It can take approximately 20 minutes to complete. Scores range from 0 to 30. A score of 13 or above suggests delirium. This scale, used to serially, can monitor changes in function (Fig. 15–6).

MMSE Sample Items

Orientation to Time
  "What is the date?"

Registration
  "Listen carefully. I am going to say three words. You say them back after I stop.
  Ready? Here they are...
  APPLE (pause), PENNY (pause), TABLE (pause). Now repeat those words back to me." [Repeat up to 5 times, but score only the first trial.]

Naming
  "What is this?" [Point to a pencil or pen.]

Reading
  "Please read this and do what it says." [Show examinee the words on the stimulus form.]
  CLOSE YOUR EYES

"Reproduced by special permission of the Publisher, Psychological Assessment Resources, Inc., 16204 North Florida Avenue, Lutz, Florida 3549, from the Mini Mental State Examination, by Marshal Folstein and Susan Folstein, Copyright 1975, 1998, 2001 by Mini Mental LLC, Inc. Published 2001 by Psychological Assessment Resources, Inc. Further reproduction is prohibited without permission of PAR, Inc. The MMSE can be purchased from PAR, Inc. by calling (813) 968–3003."

Fig. 15–3. Mini Mental Status Examination.
SOURCE: Reproduced by special permission of the Publisher, Psychological Assessment Resources, Inc., 16204 North Florida Avenue, Lutz, FL 33549, from the Mini Mental State Examination, by Marshal Folstein and Susan Folstein, Copyright 1975, 1998, 2001 by Mini Mental LLC, Inc. Published 2001 by Psychological Assessment Resources, Inc. Further reproduction is prohibited without permission of PAR, Inc. The MMSE can be purchased from PAR, Inc. by calling (813) 968–3003.

Watson Method (Watson, et al., 1993)
1. Divide the circle into 4 equal quadrants by drawing one line through the center of the circle and the number 12 (or a mark that best corresponds to the 12) and a second line perpendicular to and bisecting the first.
2. Count the number of digits in each quadrant in the clockwise direction, beginning with the digit corresponding to the number 12. Each digit is counted only once. If a digit falls on one of the reference lines, it is included in the quadrant that is clockwise to the line. A total of 3 digits in a quadrant is considered to be correct.
3. For any error in the number of digits in the first, second, or third quadrants assign a score of 1. For any error in the number of digits in the fourth quadrant assign a score of 4.
4. Normal range of score is 0–3. Abnormal (demented) range of score is 4–7.

Sutherland Method (Sutherland, et al., 1989)
Scores are assigned based on specific criteria.
Score Criterion
10–6 Drawing clock face with circle and number is general intact.
10 Hands are in correct position.
9 Slight errors in placement of the hands.
8 More noticeable errors in the placement of hour and minute hands.
7 Placement of the hands is significantly off course
6 Inappropriate use of the clock hands (such as use of digital display or circling numbers despite repeated instructions.)
5–1 Drawing of clock face with a circle and numbers is not intact.
5 Crowding of numbers at one end of the clock or reversal or numbers. Hands may still be present in some fashion.
4 Further distortion of number sequence. Integrity of clock face is now gone (numbers missing or placed at outside the boundaries of the clock face).
3 Numbers and clock face no longer obviously connected in the drawing. Hands are not present.
2 Drawing reveals some evidence of instructions being received but only a vague representation of a clock.
1 Either no attempt or an uninterpretable effort is made.
Scores of 6 or more are considered normal.

Fig. 15–4. Scoring of clock drawing test.

SCREENING TOOLS FOR MEASURING DISTRESS

Instructions: First please circle the number (0-10) that best describes how much distress you have been experiencing in the past week including today.

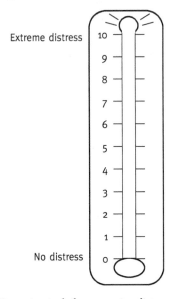

Extreme distress   10

No distress   0

Second, please indicate if any of the following has been a problem for you in the past week including today. Be sure to check YES or NO for each.

YES NO **Practical Problems**
☐ ☐ Child care
☐ ☐ Housing
☐ ☐ Insurance/financial
☐ ☐ Transportation
☐ ☐ Work/school

Family Problems
☐ ☐ Dealing with children
☐ ☐ Dealing with partner

Emotional Problems
☐ ☐ Depression
☐ ☐ Fears
☐ ☐ Nervousness
☐ ☐ Sadness
☐ ☐ Worry
☐ ☐ Loss of interest in usual activities

☐ ☐ **Spiritual/religious concerns**

Other Problems:_____

YES NO **Physical Problems**
☐ ☐ Appearance
☐ ☐ Bathing/dressing
☐ ☐ Breathing
☐ ☐ Changes in urination
☐ ☐ Constipation
☐ ☐ Diarrhea
☐ ☐ Eating
☐ ☐ Fatigue
☐ ☐ Feeling Swollen
☐ ☐ Fevers
☐ ☐ Getting around
☐ ☐ Indigestion
☐ ☐ Memory/concentration
☐ ☐ Mouth sores
☐ ☐ Nausea
☐ ☐ Nose dry/congested
☐ ☐ Pain
☐ ☐ Sexual
☐ ☐ Skin dry/itchy
☐ ☐ Sleep
☐ ☐ Tingling in hands/feet

Fig. 15–5. Screening tools for measuring distress.
SOURCE: Reproduced with permission from The NCCN 1.2008 Distress Management Clinical Practice Guidelines in Oncology. ©National Comprehensive Cancer Network, 2008. http://www.nccn.org. Accessed September 24, 2008. To view the most recent and complete version of the guidelines, go online to www.nccn.org.

Substance abuse (alcohol abuse)

1. *CAGE*[32]: One of the most commonly used assessments for substance abuse is the set of CAGE questions for alcohol abuse. These questions have been widely used to assess alcohol abuse in patients with, both medical illnesses and cancer.[33-35] CAGE is an acronym for the four questions:

1. Have you ever felt the need to CUT DOWN?
2. Do you get ANNOYED when other people are critical of your drinking?

3. Do you feel GUILTY about using?
4. Have you ever needed an EYE-OPENER in the morning?

A "yes" answer to at least two of these questions suggests alcohol abuse or dependence. (Please see Chapter 46 on Substance abuse.)

2. *AUDIT*[36]: The AUDIT is a 10-item self-report or clinician-administered instrument to assess alcohol abuse in terms of quantity, dependence, and adverse consequences of drinking. It takes approximately

INSTRUCTIONS: Rate the severity of the following symptoms of delirium based on current interaction with subject or assessment of his/her behavior or experience over past several hours (as indicated in each item.)

ITEM 1-REDUCED LEVEL OF CONSCIOUSNESS (AWARENESS): Rate the patient's current awareness of and interaction with the environment (interviewer, other people/objects in the room; for example, ask patients to describe their surroundings).

- ❑ 0: none   (patient spontaneously fully aware of environment and interacts appropriately)
- ❑ 1: mild   (patient is unaware of some elements in the environment, or not spontaneously interacting appropriately with the interviewer; becomes fully aware and appropriately interactive when prodded strongly; interview is prolonged but not seriously disrupted)
- ❑ 2: moderate   (patient is unaware of some or all elements in the environment, or not spontaneously interacting with the interviewer; becomes incompletely aware and inappropriately interactive when prodded strongly; interview is prolonged but not seriously disrupted)
- ❑ 3: severe   (patient is unaware of all elements in the environment with no spontaneous interaction or awareness of the interviewer, so that the interview is difficult-to-impossible, even with maximal prodding)

ITEM 2-DISORIENTATION: Rate current state by asking the following 10 orientation items: date, month, day, year, season, floor, name of hospital, city, state, and country.

- ❑ 0: none   (patient knows 9-10 items)
- ❑ 1: mild   (patient knows 7-8 items)
- ❑ 2: moderate   (patient knows 5-6 items)
- ❑ 3: severe   (patient knows no more than 4 items)

ITEM 3-SHORT-TERM MEMORY IMPAIRMENT: Rate current state by using repetition and delayed recall of 3 words [patient must immediately repeat and recall words 5 min later after an intervening task. Use alternate sets of 3 words for successive evaluations (for example, apple, table, tomorrow, sky, cigar, justice)].

- ❑ 0: none   (all 3 words repeated and recalled)
- ❑ 1: mild   (all 3 repeated, patient fails to recall 1)
- ❑ 2: moderate   (all 3 repeated, patient fails to recall 2-3)
- ❑ 3: severe   (patient fails to repeat 1 or more words)

ITEM 4-IMPAIRED DIGIT SPAN: Rate current performance by asking subjects to repeat first 3, 4, then 5 digits forward and then 3, then 4 backwards; continue to the next step only if patient succeeds at the previous one.

- ❑ 0: none   (patient can do at least 5 numbers forward and 4 backward)
- ❑ 1: mild   (patient can do at least 5 numbers forward, 3 backward)
- ❑ 2: moderate   (patient can do 4-5 numbers forward, cannot do 3 backward)
- ❑ 3: severe   (patient can do no more than 3 numbers forward)

Breitbart W et al. The Memorial Delirium Assessment Scale. J Pain Symptom Manage. 1997 Mar;13(3):128–37.

Fig. 15–6. Memorial Delirium Assessment Scale (MDAS) ©1996.

SOURCE: Reprinted from *Journal of Pain and Symptom Management*, Volume 13, Issue 3, William Breitbart, Barry Rosenfeld, Andrew Roth, Mark J. Smith, Ken Cohen, Steven Passik, The Memorial Delirium Assessment Scale, pp. 128–137, Copyright 1997, with permission from Elsevier.

ITEM 5-REDUCED ABILITY TO MAINTAIN AND SHIFT ATTENTION: As indicated during the interview by questions needing to be rephrased and/or repeated because patient's attention wanders, patient loses track, patient is distracted by outside stimuli or over-absorbed in a task.

❑ 0: none   (none of the above; patient maintains and shifts attention normally)

❑ 1: mild   (above attentional problems occur once or twice without prolonging the interview)

❑ 2: moderate   (above attentional problems occur often, prolonging the interview without seriously disrupting it)

❑ 3: severe   (above attentional problems occur constantly, disrupting and making the interview difficult-to-impossible)

ITEM 6-DISORGANIZED THINKING: As indicated during the interview by rambling, irrelevant, or incoherent speech, or by tangential, circumstantial, or faulty reasoning. Ask patient a somewhat complex question (for example, "Describe your current medical condition.").

❑ 0: none   (patient's speech is coherent and goal-directed)

❑ 1: mild   (patient's speech is slightly difficult to follow; responses to questions are slightly off target but not so much as to prolong the interview)

❑ 2: moderate   (disorganized thoughts or speech are clearly present, such that interview is prolonged but not disrupted)

❑ 3: severe   (examination is very difficult or impossible due to disorganized thinking or speech)

ITEM 7-PERCEPTUAL DISTURBANCE: Misperceptions, illusions, hallucinations inferred from inappropriate behavior during the interview or admitted by subject, as well as those elicited from nurse/family/chart accounts of the past several hours or of the time since last examination.

❑ 0: none   (no misperceptions, illusions, or hallucinations)

❑ 1: mild   (misperceptions or illusions related to sleep, fleeting hallucinations on 1-2 occasions without inappropriate behavior)

❑ 2: moderate   (hallucinations or frequent illusions on several occasions with minimal inappropriate behavior that does not disrupt the interview)

❑ 3: severe   (frequent or intense illusions or hallucinations with persistent inappropriate behavior that disrupts the interview or interferes with medical care)

ITEM 8-DELUSIONS: Rate delusions inferred from inappropriate behavior during the interview or admitted by the patient, as well as delusions elicited from nurse/family/chart accounts of the past several hours or of the time since the previous examination.

❑ 0: none   (no evidence of misinterpretations or delusions)

❑ 1: mild   (misinterpretations or suspiciousness without clear delusional ideas or inappropriate behavior)

❑ 2: moderate   (delusions admitted by the patient or evidenced by his/her behavior that do not or only marginally disrupt the interview or interfere with medical care)

❑ 3: severe   (persistent and/or intense delusions resulting in inappropriate behavior, disrupting the interview or seriously interfering with medical care)

Breitbart W et al. The Memorial Delirium Assessment Scale. J Pain Symptom Manage. 1997 Mar;13(3):128-37.

Fig. 15–6. Continued.

ITEM 9-DECREASED OR INCREASED PSYCHOMOTOR ACTIVITY: Rate activity over past several hours, as well as activity during interview, by circling (a) hypoactive, (b) hyperactive, or (c) elements of both present.

❑ 0: none   (normal psychomotor activity)

❑ a b c 1: mild   (hypoactivity is barely noticeable, expressed as slightly slowing of movement. Hyperactivity is barely noticeable or appears as simple restlessness.)

❑ a b c 2: moderate   (hypoactivity is undeniable, with marked reduction in the number of movements or marked slowness of movement; subject rarely spontaneously moves or speaks. Hyperactivity is undeniable, subject moves almost constantly; in both cases, exam is prolonged as a consequence.)

❑ a b c 3: severe   (hypoactivity is severe; patient does not move or speak without prodding or is catatonic. Hyperactivity is severe; patient is constantly moving, overreacts to stimuli, requires surveillance and/or restraint; getting through the exam is difficult or impossible.)

ITEM 10-SLEEP-WAKE CYCLE DISTURBANCE (DISORDER OF AROUSAL): Rate patient's ability to either sleep or stay awake at the appropriate times. Utilize direct observation during the interview, as well as reports from nurses, family, patient, or charts describing sleep-wake cycle disturbance over the past several hours or since last examination. Use observations of the previous night for morning evaluations only.

❑ 0: none   (at night, sleeps well; during the day, has no trouble staying awake)

❑ 1: mild   (mild deviation from appropriate sleepfulness and wakefulness states: at night, difficulty falling asleep or transient night awakenings, needs medication to sleep well; during the day, reports periods of drowsiness or, during the interview, is drowsy but can easily fully awaken him/herself)

❑ 2: moderate   (moderate deviations from appropriate sleepfulness and wakefulness states: at night, repeated and prolonged night awakening; during the day, reports of frequent and prolonged napping or, during the interview, can only be roused to complete wakefulness by strong stimuli)

❑ 3: severe   (severe deviations from appropriate sleepfulness and wakefulness states: at night, sleeplessness; during the day, patient spends most of the time sleeping or, during the interview, cannot be roused to full wakefulness by any stimuli)

Breitbart W et al. The Memorial Delirium Assessment Scale. J Pain Symptom Manage. 1997 Mar;13(3):128-37.

Fig. 15–6. Continued.

3 minutes to administer and scores 8 or greater are suggestive of alcohol use disorders. While there have not been comparison studies in cancer patients, the AUDIT may identify drinking problem better than the CAGE in some populations.[37]

Spirituality

1. *FICA Questions*[38]: A spiritual assessment can be organized around four main themes to give a sense of the patient's dependence on spirituality in coping with illness. These themes are not quantitatively scored and focus on strengths. They can be remembered using the acronym, FICA.

1. FAITH AND BELIEF: "Do you consider yourself spiritual or religious?" "Do you have spiritual beliefs that help you cope with stress" "What gives your life meaning?"
2. IMPORTANCE: "What importance does your faith or belief have in your life?" "Have your beliefs influenced how you take care of yourself in this illness?" "What role do your beliefs play in regard to your health?"
3. COMMUNITY: "Are you part of a spiritual or religious community? Is this of support to you and how?" "Is there a group of people that you really love or who are important to you?"

4. ADDRESS IN CARE: "How would you like me, your healthcare provider, to address these issues in your healthcare?"
Copyright 2000 by Christina M. Puchalski, MD, FACP

2. *FACIT-Sp* (www.facit.org): The FACIT-Sp is a quantitative measure of spiritual well-being and is part of the FACIT quality-of-life assessment system. It contains 12 items specific to spiritual well-being. It has been studied in cancer patients and appears to be sensitive to change.[39] While 3 of the 12 items specifically reference "faith or spiritual beliefs," there are no questions about "religion" and the majority of items appear to assess a sense of peace or meaning.

REFERENCES

1. Streiner DL, Norman GR. *Health measurement scales: a practical guide to their development and use.* 3rd ed. Oxford University Press: New York; 2003.

2. Jacobsen PB, Donovan KA, Trask PC, et al. Screening for psychologic distress in ambulatory cancer patients. *Cancer.* 2005;103:1494–1502.

3. Gessler S, Low J, Daniells E, et al. Screening for distress in cancer patients: is the distress thermometer a valid measure in the UK and does it measure change over time? A prospective validation study. *Psycho-Oncology.* 2008;17(6):538–547.

4. Mitchell A. Pooled results from 38 analyses of the accuracy of distress thermometer and other ultra-short methods of detecting cancer-related mood disorders. *J Clin Oncol.* 2007;25:4670–4681.

5. Linden W, Yi D, Barroetavena MC, MacKenzie R, Doll R. Development and validation of a psychosocial screening instrument for cancer. *Health Qual Life Outcomes.* 2005;3:54–61.

6. Spitzer RL, Kroenke K, Williams JBW. Validation and utility of a self-report version of PRIME-MD: the PHQ primary care study-Primary Care Evaluation of Mental Disorders, Patient Health Questionnaire. *JAMA.* 1999;282:1737–1744.

7. Ell K, Quon B, Quinn DI, et al. Improving treatment for depression among low-income patients with cancer: the design of the ADAPt-C study. *Gen Hosp Psychiatry.* 2007;29:223–231.

8. Derogatis LR, Melisaratos N. The Brief Symptom Inventory: an introductory report. *Psychol Med.* 1983;13:595–605.

9. Zabora J, BrintzwnhofeSzoc K, Jacobsen P, et al. A new psychosocial screening instrument for use with cancer patients. *Psychosomatics.* 2001;42:241–246.

10. Zigmond AS, Snaith RP. The hospital anxiety and depression scale. *Acta Psychiatr Scand.* 1983;67:361–370.

11. Razavi D, Delvaux N, Farvacques C, Robaye E. Screening for adjustment disorders and major depressive disorders in cancer in-patients. *Br J Psychiatry.* 1990;156:79–83.

12. Beck AT, Ward CH, Mendelson M, Mock J, Erbaugh J. An inventory of measuring depression. *Arch Gen Psychiatry.* 1961;4:53–63.

13. Arnau RC, Meagher MW, Norris MP, Bramson R. Psychometric evaluation of the Beck Depression Inventory-II with primary care medical patients. *Health Psychol.* 2001;20:112–119.

14. Hopko DR, Bell JL, Armento ME, et al. The phenomenology and screening of clinical depression in cancer patients. *J Psychosoc Oncol.* 2001;6:31–51.

15. Radloff LS. The CES-D Scale: a self-report depression scale for research in the general population. *Appl Psychol Meas.* 1977;1:385–401.

16. Hann D, Winter K, Jacobsen PB. Measurement of depressive symptoms in cancer patients: evaluation of the Center for Epidemiological Studies Depression Scale (CES-D). *J Psychosom Res.* 1999;46:437–443.

17. Katz MR, Kopek N, Waldron J, Devins GM, Tomlinson G. Screening for depression in head and neck cancer. *Psycho-Oncology.* 2004;13:269–280.

18. Beck AT, Epstein N, Brown G, et al. An inventory of measuring clinical anxiety: psychometric properties. *J Consult Clin Psychol.* 1988;56:893–897.

19. Wetherell JL, Arean PA. Psychometric evaluation of the Beck Anxiety Inventory with older medical patients. *Psychol Assess.* 1997;2:136–144.

20. Spielberger CD. *Manual for the State-Trait Anxiety Inventory (STAI).* PaloAlto, CA: Consulting Psychologists Press; 1983.

21. Ransom S, Jacobsen PB, Booth-Jones M. Validation of the Distress Thermometer with bone marrow transplant patients. *Psycho-Oncology.* 2006;15:604–612.

22. Horowitz MJ, Wilner N, Alvarez W. Impact of Event Scale: a measure of subjective distress. *Psychosom Med.* 1979;41:209–218.

23. Schlich-Bakker KJ, Warlam-Rodenhuis CC, van Echtelt J, van den Bout J, Ausems MG, ten Kroode HF. Short term psychological distress in patients actively approached for genetic counseling after diagnosis of breast cancer. *Eur J Cancer.* 2006;42:2722–2728.

24. Mehnert A, Koch U. Prevalence of acute and post-traumatic stress disorder and comorbid mental disorders in breast cancer patients during primary cancer care: a prospective study. *Psycho-Oncology.* 2007;16:181–188.

25. Folstein MF, Folstein SE, McHugh PR. "Mini-mental state." A practical method for grading cognitive state for the clinician. *J Psychiatr Res.* 1975;12:189–198.

26. Juby A, Tench S, Baker V. The value of clock drawing in identifying executive cognitive dysfunction in people with a normal Mini-Mental State Examination score. *Can Med Assoc J.* 2002;167:859–864.

27. Sutherland T, Hill JL, Mellow AM, et al. Clock drawing in Alzheimer's disease: a novel measure of dementia severity. *J Am Geriatr Soc.* 1989;37:725–729.

28. Watson YI, Arfken CL, Birge SJ. Clock completion: an objective screening test for dementia. *J Am Geriatr Soc.* 1993;41:1235–1240.

29. Inouye SK, van Dyck CH, Alessi CA, Balkin S, Siegal AP, Horwitz RI. Clarifying confusion: The Confusion Assessment Method. A new method for the detection of delirium. *Ann Intern Med.* 1990;113:941–948.

30. Trzepacz PT, Baker RW, Greenhouse J. A symptom rating scale for delirium. *Psychiatry Res.* 1988;23:89–97.

31. Breitbart W, Rosenfeld B, Roth A, Smith MJ, Cohen K, Passik S. The Memorial Delirium Assessment Scale. *J Pain Symptom Manage.* 1997;13:128–137.

32. Ewing JA. Detecting alcoholism: the CAGE Questionnaire. *JAMA.* 1984;252:1905–1907.

33. Bruera E, Moyano J, Seifert L, Fainsinger RL, Hanson J, Suarez-Almazor M. The frequency of alcoholism among patients with pain due to terminal cancer. *J Pain Symptom Manage.* 1995;10:599–603.

34. Bradley KA, Kivlahan DR, Bush KR, McDonell And MB, Fihn SD. Ambulatory Care Quality Improvement Project Investigators. Variations on the CAGE alcohol screening questionnaire: strengths and limitations in VA medical populations. *Alcohol Clin Exp Res.* 2001;25:1472–1478.

35. Chow E, Connolly R, Wong R, et al. Use of the CAGE questionnaire for screening problem drinking in an out-patient palliative radiotherapy clinic. *J Pain Symptom Manage.* 2001;21:491–497.

36. Barbor TF, Bohn MJ, Kranzler HR. The Alcohol Use Disorders Identification Test (AUDIT): validation of a screening instrument for use in medical settings. *J Stud Alcohol.* 1995;56:423–432.

37. Bradley KA, Bush KR, McDonnell MB, Malone T, Finn SD. Screening for problem drinking: comparison of CAGE and AUDIT. Ambulatory Care Quality Improvement Project (ACQUIP). Alcohol Use Disorders Identification Test. *J Gen Intern Med.* 1998;13:379–388.

38. Puchalski CM, Romer AL. Taking a spiritual history allows clinicians to understand patients more fully. *J Pall Med.* 2000;3:129–137.

39. Johnson ME, Piderman KM, Sloan JA, et al. Measuring spiritual quality of life in patients with cancer. *J Support Oncol.* 2007;5:437–442.

CHAPTER 16

Central Nervous System Tumors

Alan D. Valentine

INTRODUCTION

Central nervous system (CNS) tumors, whether of primary or metastatic origin, are among the most challenging forms of cancer with which patients and caregivers must contend. Vulnerable to the many psychosocial stresses associated with cancer diagnosis and treatment, brain tumor patients in particular (often if not always) face progressive compromise of peripheral neurological function, subtle and overt cognitive dysfunction, and widely variable changes of mood and affect. Treatment of CNS cancer (e.g., surgery, chemotherapy, radiation therapy [XRT]) is itself actively or potentially neurotoxic. Associated loss of independence and ability to function safely and effectively at home and in the workplace often places physical, emotional, and financial hardships on patients and caregivers. The fact that many primary malignant brain tumors are associated with poor outcomes and that progression of systemic cancers into the CNS is an ominous indicator of disease trajectory makes CNS cancer especially emotionally burdensome from the time it is detected. Finally, the common western association of "brain" with "mind" means that CNS cancer, more than any other form of malignancy, may constitute a threat to an individual's sense of self and personal integrity.

Primary brain and CNS tumors are relatively uncommon, accounting for approximately 21,810 (1.5%) of new cancer diagnoses, and 13,070 (2.3%) cancer-related deaths annually.[1] Meningiomas, which are usually nonmalignant, are the most common tumor type. Glioblastomas are the most common primary malignant brain tumors, accounting for approximately 19% of all new cases.[2] Unfortunately they are generally associated with dismal prognoses, with 5-year survival rates of <5%.[2] An estimated 51,410 new cases of primary malignant and benign brain tumors were diagnosed in 2007. Central nervous system tumors, which are usually benign (i.e., meningiomas, craniopharyngiomas), can cause significant neuropsychiatric and emotional morbidity because of mass effect, disruption of endocrine function, and recurrence.

Metastatic tumors are by far the most common form of intracranial brain neoplasm in adults.[3] The true incidence and prevalence of metastatic brain tumors is not known, but is thought to be increasing, with rates 10 times that of primary brain tumors, and 150,000–200,000 new cases detected annually.[4,5] Brain metastases are expected to become even more common as treatment of many cancers improves and patients live longer. Several primary cancers have a high likelihood of metastasis to the brain. In general, descending order of these include lung (especially small cell and adenocarcinoma), breast, melanoma, renal cell, and colon.[6] These primary tumors account for 85% of metastases.[7] It is unclear whether primary and metastatic brain tumors are routinely associated with distinctly different neuropsychiatric sequelae and from a clinical standpoint it may be best to consider the issue as one of brain injury, regardless of cause.

Leptomeningeal spread of cancer occurs in 5% of patients with systemic cancers, including solid tumors (especially lung cancer, breast cancer, and melanoma), and also lymphomas and leukemias.[8,9] Patients with leptomeningeal metastasis are likely to develop diffuse neurological deficits (including slowed cognition) and usually require treatment associated with neuropsychiatric side effects (i.e., brain radiation, intrathecal chemotherapy).

COGNITIVE AND BEHAVIORAL DYSFUNCTION

Cognitive dysfunction is encountered in at least 70% of cases of CNS malignancy.[10] It is a leading, if not primary, variable affecting quality of life (QOL) for brain tumor patients and caregivers[11,12] and often precedes or predicts radiographic disease progression.[13] Virtually all common disorders of memory, attention, arousal and perception, and many unique presentations, have been described in brain tumor patients. In the absence of focal neurological findings or symptoms, there is nothing that reliably points to brain tumors as causes of such cognitive impairment, though presence of focal neurological signs and symptoms and presentations in certain settings (i.e., patients with known malignancy, long-term smokers, acute behavior changes) will raise the index of suspicion.

Several factors are of potential influence. These include lesion location, rate of tumor growth, number of tumor foci, patient age, secondary effects of tumor or treatment, and diaschisis effects.

With notable possible exceptions, the following general observations can be made: Rapidly growing tumors are more likely to cause acute altered mental status (e.g., delirium) or sudden loss of cognitive ability. Slow growing benign or malignant tumors are likely to cause insidious changes of cognition, consistent with the early stages of primary dementias. Clinical scenarios associated with multiple tumor foci increase the likelihood of involvement of critical CNS structures or neurotransmitter pathways and consequently increase risk for altered cognition. The elderly and patients with premorbid cognitive impairment may have diminished cognitive reserve at baseline and are thus more vulnerable to new or progressing CNS insults than younger or very high functioning patients.

Because of the routine availability of neuroimaging modalities, the association of behavioral changes or cognitive deficits and lesion location is of decreased importance for diagnostic purposes, and a brain tumor's anatomical location is likely of less influence than other cited factors as a cause for a presentation.[14] However, lesion location may be useful to clinicians and caregivers regarding expected difficulties in the disease trajectory. Dominant hemisphere lesions (or effects of their treatment) may be associated with loss of verbal or written language function. Nondominant hemisphere disease may be associated with impairment of visual-spatial processing ability. Frontal and temporal lesions of either hemisphere can cause memory dysfunction and more posterior-located disease may be associated with inability to process visual cues resulting in various agnosias.[15] Treatment effects, including anatomic damage caused by surgery or XRT, may also cause cognitive dysfunction.

Cognitive dysfunction with slowing and/or decreased level of arousal may also be due to drug side effects, especially anticonvulsants at high serum levels, analgesics, and anxiolytics.

Frontal lobe tumors. Frontal lobe tumors are frequently, if not always, associated with cognitive dysfunction.[16] While the term "frontal lobe syndrome" is widely accepted in clinical practice, it must be kept in mind that distant pathology can cause presentations identical to that associated with frontal lesions. Descriptions of frontal and prefrontal syndromes are relevant to problems routinely associated with management of CNS cancer.[17,18]

Frontal lobe pathology associated with tumor or treatment is likely to result in compromised higher executive function. In this dorsolateral prefrontal/*dysexecutive syndrome*, patients develop psychomotor slowing. They loose the ability to switch cognitive sets, perseverate, and have difficulty taking on new tasks. They may develop diminished attention to self-care and flattening of affect. Quite often they appear to be depressed. The constellation of symptoms also suggests progression of subcortical dementia.

Patients may also develop an orbitofrontal/*disinhibited type syndrome*. Such individuals are emotionally labile, demonstrate poor social judgment, and have little insight into their behavior. Others may develop a mesial frontal/*apathetic syndrome*, with verbal and motor slowing, and eventually urinary incontinence, and lower extremity weakness.[17] Though these syndromes have not been well studied in patients with brain tumors, it is likely that dysexecutive syndromes are most common. Mixed presentations should be expected.

Temporal lobe tumors. Cognitive dysfunction associated with temporal lobe tumors may be a function of direct damage to dominant/nondominant sites resulting in impairment of verbal and nonverbal memory as well as receptive and/or expressive language function. Physical or physiological disruption of neurotransmitter pathways to and from the frontal lobes can also result in frontal/prefrontal lobe syndromes characteristic of damage to anterior structures. Seizure activity may also cause transient cognitive dysfunction and associated pharmacotherapy (especially the older, more sedating anticonvulsants) may contribute to ongoing dysfunction.

Diencephalon tumors. These tumors are often associated with memory dysfunction. Compromise of frontal-subcortical circuits in diencephalic structures would also predispose to the development of frontal lobe syndromes. *Parietal lobe tumors* are more likely to be associated with sensory disturbances (i.e., agnosias) and neglect syndromes than frank memory dysfunction. *Pituitary tumors* (i.e., adenomas, craniopharyngiomas) with adverse effects on endocrine function can cause depressive syndromes.[14,19,20]

PERSONALITY, BEHAVIOR, PSYCHOSIS

Besides cognitive impairment consistent with dementia, presentations consistent with almost all primary psychiatric disorders have been described in patients with primary and metastatic brain tumors. The same is true of rare neuropsychiatric syndromes. At first glance and absent physical examination and work-up, there is little if anything that distinguishes psychopathology due to brain tumors from primary psychiatric disorders.

Changes in personality are often associated with frontal lobe (up to 70%) and temporal lobe (>50%) tumors and may (e.g., lung cancer) be the first sign of an occult carcinoma.[14] Often the presentation involves "coarsening" or exaggeration of premorbid personality traits. Changes are usually subtle early on and become more pronounced with disease progression. On occasion there is a marked, fairly dramatic change that brings the patient to evaluation.

Disinhibition presenting as paroxysmal rage, sudden violence, and impulsivity may be encountered, and may require environmental changes or antipsychotics and mood stabilizers to protect the patient and others. These behaviors typically resolve gradually as an unintended consequence of disease progression.

Anxiety and "schizophrenia" have traditionally been associated with temporal lobe tumors. The former association is probably more appropriate. Psychosis manifesting as hallucinations and/or delusions can be a function of delirium, seizure, and drug side effects.

Mood disorders. Rates of depression in primary brain tumor patients vary greatly, depending on diagnostic criteria and the setting of the evaluation, with incidence of 25%–30% in ambulatory settings using strict criteria, and much higher estimates in perioperative populations.[21,22] There is at least a suggestion that depression predicts decreased length of survival in this setting.[22,23]

Mood disorders including depression and mania have been most often associated with frontal and temporal lobe lesions, and have also been reported with lesions in other locations.[24-26] Again, because of

diaschisis, tumors in other locations could easily cause the same presentations. Pituitary tumors (e.g., craniopharyngiomas) or the effects of their treatment may disrupt the hypothalamic-pituitary-end organs axis and render a patient hormone-dependent, with adverse effects on mood, energy level, sexual function, and motivation, in addition to metabolic dysregulation.[20] Drug side effects, notably those of corticosteroids and anticonvulsants, are common causes of mood disorders in this setting.

Adjustment disorders or "reactive" depressions in patients trying to cope with loss of independence, cognitive ability, physical function, and disease poorly responsive to treatment are to be expected.

Anxiety. Rates of anxiety in patients with primary brain tumors have recently been reported to vary from 13% to 75%, with differences attributable to different detection methods and points of assessment.[27-29] Some investigators have found that right hemisphere tumors are more likely to be associated with anxiety.[30] There is a tendency for rates of anxiety to trend downward after treatment (radiation or surgery), possibly reflecting the reactive nature of initial symptomatology[27,31] and the subsequent physical and psychological benefits of treatment.

ADVERSE EFFECTS OF THERAPY

Treatments of primary and metastatic brain tumors are themselves potential causes of psychiatric morbidity.

Radiation therapy. Radiation therapy is integral to management of known primary and metastatic CNS tumors, and as prophylaxis against leptomeningeal metastasis to the CNS. Brain XRT is associated with three major neurotoxicity syndromes.[32,33] *Acute radiation syndrome* usually occurs during or shortly after completion of XRT, and is characterized by delirium, nausea, and vomiting. It is thought to be associated with cerebral edema and raised intracranial pressure. Patients undergoing cranial XRT are usually treated with corticosteroids to prevent or minimize raised intracranial pressure and so the acute radiation syndrome is infrequently encountered. *Early delayed radiation syndrome* is thought due to temporary demyelination and is characterized by reemergence of neurological symptoms and sometimes a "somnolence syndrome." It usually resolves over days or weeks and again, steroids are protective. *Late delayed radiation syndrome* develops months or years after completion of XRT and involves progressive, often irreversible, cognitive impairment. Radiation necrosis and progressive leukoencephalopathy are implicated as primary causes of the late delayed syndrome. Several other XRT-associated disorders of cognitive function have been described in children and adults.[34] Factors that influence XRT-induced neurotoxicity include age, cumulative radiation dose, concomitant chemotherapy, and length of survival post-XRT.[32]

Chemotherapy. The blood-brain barrier prevents passage of many chemotherapy and other antineoplastic agents into the CNS. Several antineoplastic drugs are associated with neuropsychiatric side effects when delivered to the CNS by intravenous or intrathecal routes. Acute encephalopathy is seen with the administration of methotrexate, which may also cause a permanent leukoencephalopathy. Cytosine arabinoside is associated with acute encephalopathy, which usually resolves, and cerebellar syndrome, which may resolve or persist indefinitely. The interferons are associated with variable degrees of cognitive dysfunction. Procarbazine is a weak monoamine oxidase inhibitor which occasionally causes anxiety and must be used cautiously, if at all, with most antipsychotic and antidepressant drugs.[35]

Surgery. Surgical resection of primary and metastatic brain tumors is often tolerated remarkably well. However, perioperative delirium is common. Patients with lesions in sensitive areas may experience temporary (sometimes permanent) language or motor deficits that result in problematic anxiety and depression.

Corticosteroids, analgesics, anticonvulsants. Steroids are ubiquitous in cancer care. Patients with primary or metastatic brain tumors are likely to be treated with corticosteroids at various points in the disease process, especially during and after XRT and after surgery. In some cases the patient is obligated to treatment with steroids indefinitely. While steroids are generally protective against vasogenic edema and raised intracranial pressure, the drugs can cause psychosis, mania, and, especially with long-term use, depressive symptoms. Dose decrease or discontinuation is often helpful. When that is not possible, symptomatic treatment with psychotropic medications is appropriate.

Patients treated for primary or metastatic brain tumors may be more vulnerable to sedating effects of opioid analgesics. Anticonvulsants, especially but not exclusively older drugs including phenobarbital, phenytoin, and carbamazepine, may cause sedation and confusion at therapeutic or high levels.

ASSESSMENT

Assessment of psychiatric symptoms in patients with brain tumors can be challenging. The overlap between primary or reactive mood, anxiety, and thought disorders and those caused by tumor or treatment is considerable. Patients are often poor historians.

The evaluation process is fairly straightforward, if not always revealing. A thorough history should be obtained with attention to premorbid symptomatology. Especially in cases of cognitive impairment, it is helpful and often necessary to rely on family members or other caregivers for aspects of the history. Because of the great emotional and prognostic significance of cancer in the nervous system, it is important to ask anxious and depressed patients about reactions to diagnosis, understanding of clinical status, and perceptions of the future.

A search for reversible and treatable causes of symptoms should be commenced. This includes review of medications as well as laboratory, electrophysiological, and neuroimaging studies. Patients followed in academic and large community cancer centers are followed closely and it is unlikely that psycho-oncologists who practice in those settings will be required to make a diagnosis of cancer in the nervous system. However, an index of suspicion is always warranted and, especially in the setting of co-existent focal neurological signs and symptoms (e.g., headache, seizure, gait disturbance, sensory-motor impairment), the possibility of new or progressive CNS disease should be considered.

Neuropsychological assessment is invaluable in evaluation of the brain tumor patient with behavioral symptoms.[15] In major medical centers such assessment is a routine component of treatment planning before surgery or XRT. Especially in early stages of disease, neuropsychological test batteries can detect and characterize subtle cognitive deficits. Serial tests help track the rate of recovery or decline. Characterization of impairment (deficit vs. handicap) is useful for posttreatment rehabilitation and mobilization of appropriate support resources.[15]

MANAGEMENT

Pharmacotherapy. Little data is available from clinical trials to guide the use of psychotropic drugs in patients with brain tumors. With a few significant exceptions, the guidelines for use of antidepressants, anxiolytics, and antipsychotics in cancer patients are applicable (See Chapter 51). The general recommendation to "start low and go slow" is especially applicable to treatment of patients with cancer in the CNS.

Antidepressants. Most antidepressants can be used safely in brain tumor patients. *Tricyclic antidepressants* may not be well tolerated because of sedative and anticholinergic effects. Use of *bupropion* is not recommended in any patient with past history of seizures or current seizure risk. Drug–drug interactions should be considered. Concomitant use of selective serotonin-reuptake inhibitors and some anticonvulsants (i.e., carbamazepine, phenytoin) can increase levels of the latter.

Anxiolytics. Brain tumor patients may be especially sensitive to sedative effects of benzodiazepines (BZPs). The use of shorter half-life drugs (i.e., alprazolam, lorazepam) is preferred. BZPs may also cause disinhibition or agitation in patients with significant cognitive impairment. In such cases low-dose antipsychotics may be used for the same purpose. Buspirone metabolism may be altered by some anticonvulsants.

Antipsychotics. These medications are generally safe in patients with CNS cancer. Many if not all patients with CNS disease are on anticonvulsants, minimizing the problem of lowered seizure threshold associated with phenothiazine and butyrophenone antipsychotics.

A typical antipsychotics (i.e., quetiapine, olanzapine) are associated with metabolic syndrome; attention to serum glucose levels is appropriate, especially in patients treated with corticosteroids.

Psychostimulants. These medications, including methylphenidate, D-amphetamine, and possibly modafinil, may be very effective in palliation of psychomotor slowing, depression, and cognitive impairment associated with treatment of brain tumors.[36] The drugs are generally well tolerated, but can cause anxiety and insomnia and are problematic in patients with unstable blood pressure.

Psychotherapy. Psychotherapy in the setting of CNS cancer is usually supportive, using crisis intervention and psychoeducational techniques.[37] A primary goal is to provide accurate information, and decrease uncertainty and fear to the degree possible. Relaxation training can be very useful for patients without major cognitive impairment. Patients and caregivers may benefit from participation in support groups. National advocacy organizations such as the National Brain Tumor Foundation (http://www.braintumor.org/) and the American Brain Tumor Foundation (http://hope.abta.org/) can provide other valuable resources for the supportive care of patients with CNS cancer.

Cognitive and vocational rehabilitation. Patients with benign and malignant brain tumors may benefit greatly from cognitive and vocational rehabilitation where such services are available. Neuropsychological and vocational testing can identify potentially remediable deficits and help patients and caregivers develop realistic goals regarding education, employment, and independence and safety in the home.[15]

FAMILIES, CAREGIVERS, AND STAFF

Families and caregivers of patients with cancer in the nervous system face all the problems of families of patients with nonneurological cancer and often the added burden of dealing with progressive cognitive decline and poor prognosis.[37] Rates of psychiatric morbidity are higher in caregivers than in the general population. There is potential for adversely affected physical and emotional health, family and vocational function, and care of the identified patient. Ongoing medical and psychosocial care of the patient with CNS cancer should include assessment of caregiver support. Families and caregivers can benefit from many of the supportive techniques used to help patients. Support groups and education can be especially helpful. In some cases it may be necessary to identify or provide resources for individual therapy or pharmacotherapy for depression.

Neuro-oncology staff members may also be especially vulnerable to distress, as they will work with highly complex patients in a setting where loss or the prospect is a part of daily practice. Structured group support rounds and individual supervision of trainees are among techniques that can be used to mitigate stress associated with this specialized practice.[37,38]

CONCLUSION

Since the publication of the first edition of this text, progress has been made in some areas of psycho-oncology research related to CNS cancer. This is especially true regarding QOL assessment. Validated assessment scales have been developed[39,40] and common, potentially treatable symptoms (i.e., depression, fatigue) and symptom clusters have been identified as adverse influences on QOL and survival in this setting.[11,41–43] It is expected that QOL and symptom research will be refined in this complex setting. Research into new pharmacological interventions to ease symptom burden is underway and much more is required.[44,45]

Patients with CNS cancer and their caregivers are uniquely vulnerable to distress and dysfunction in all domains of psychosocial oncology. While this presents many challenges, it also affords clinicians and researchers in the field many opportunities to be of service to this special patient population.

REFERENCES

1. Jemal A, Siegel R, Ward E, et al. Cancer statistics, 2008. *CA Cancer J Clin.* 2008;58(2):71–96.
2. CBTRUS. *Supplement report: primary brain tumors in the United States, 2004.* Hinsdale, IL: Central Brain Tumor Registry of the United States; 2008.
3. Sul J, Posner JB. Brain metastases: epidemiology and pathophysiology [Review]. *Cancer Treat Res.* 2007;136:1–21.
4. Klos KJ, O'Neill BP. Brain metastases [Review]. *Neurologist.* 2004;10(1):31–46.
5. Gavrilovic IT, Posner JB. Brain metastases: epidemiology and pathophysiology [Review]. *J Neurooncol.* 2005;75(1):5–14.
6. Yung WK, Kunschner LJ, Sawaya R, Chang CL, Fuller GM. Intracranial metastases. In: Levin VA, ed. *Cancer in the nervous system.* 2nd ed. Washington, DC: Oxford University Press; 2002:321–340.
7. Delattre JY, Krol G, Thaler HT, Posner JB. Distribution of brain metastases. *Arch Neurol.* 1988;45(7):741–744.
8. Grossman SA, Krabak MJ. Leptomeningeal carcinomatosis [Review]. *Cancer Treat Rev.* 1999;25(2):103–119.
9. Demopoulus A, DeAngelis LM. Neurologic complications of leukemia [Review]. *Curr Opin Neurol.* 2002;15(6):691–699.
10. Tucha O, Smely C, Preier M, Lang K. Cognitive deficits before treatment among patients with brain tumors. *Neurosurgery.* 2000;47(2):324–333.
11. Meyers CA, Hess KR, Yung WK, Levin VL. Cognitive function as a predictor of survival in patients with recurrent malignant glioma. *J Clin Oncol.* 2000;18(3):646–650.
12. Weitzner MA, Meyers CA. Cognitive functioning and quality of life in malignant glioma patients: a review of the literature [Review]. *Psycho-Oncology.* 1997;6(3):169–177.
13. Meyers CA, Hess KR. Multifaceted end points in brain tumor clinical trials: cognitive deterioration precedes MRI progression. *Neuro-Oncology.* 2003;5(2):89–95.
14. Price TRP, Goetz KL, Lovell MR. Neuropsychiatric aspects of brain tumors. In: Yudofsky SC, Hales RE, eds. *The American psychiatric publishing textbook of neuropsychiatry and clinical neurosciences.* 4th ed. Washington, DC: American Psychiatric Publishing, Inc.; 2002:753–781.
15. Meyers CA, Kayl AE. Neurocognitive dysfunction. In: Levin VA, ed. *Cancer in the nervous system.* Washington, DC: Oxford University Press; 2002:557–571.
16. Botez MI. *Handbook of clinical neurology.* New York; Elsevier; 1974;17:234–280.
17. Duffy JD, Campbell JJ III. The regional prefrontal syndromes: a theoretical and clinical overview. *J Neuropsychiatr.* 1994;6(4):379–387.
18. Chow TW, Cummings JL. Frontal-subcortical circuits. In: Miller BL, Cummings JL, eds. *The human frontal lobes.* New York, NY: The Guilford Press; 1999:3–26.
19. Meyers CA. Neurobehavioral functioning of adults with pituitary disease [Review]. *Psychother Psychosom.* 1988;67(3):168–172.
20. Weitzner MA. Neuropsychiatry and pituitary disease: an overview [Review]. *Psychother Psychosom.* 1998;67(3):125–132.
21. Wellisch DK, Kaleita TA, Freeman D, Cloughesy T, Goldman J. Predicting major depression in brain tumor patients. *Psycho-Oncology.* 2002;11(3):230–238.
22. Litofsky NS, Farace E, Anderson F Jr, et al. Depression in patients with high-grade glioma: results of the Glioma Outcomes Project. *Neurosurgery.* 2004;54(2):358–366.
23. Mainio A, Tuunanen S, Hakko H, Asko N, Koivukangas J, Pirrka R. Decreased quality of life and depression as predictors for shorter survival among patients with low-grade gliomas: a follow-up from 1990 to 2003. *Eur Arch Psychiatry Clin Neurosci.* 2006;256(8):516–521.

24. Starkstein SE, Boston JD, Robinson RG. Mechanisms of mania after brain injury. 12 case reports and review of the literature [Review]. *J Nerv Ment Dis.* 1988;176(2):87–100.
25. Madhusoodanan S, Danan D, Moise D. Psychiatric manifestations of brain tumors: diagnostic implications [Review]. *Expert Rev Neurother.* 2007;7(4):343–349.
26. Greenberg DB, Brown GL. Mania resulting from brain stem tumor. *J Nerv Ment Dis.* 1985;173(7):434–436.
27. Pringle AM, Taylor R, Whittle IR. Anxiety and depression in patients with an intracranial neoplasm before and after tumour surgery. *Br J Neurosurg.* 1999;13(1):46–51.
28. Arnold SD, Forman LM, Brigidi BD, et al. Evaluation and characterization of generalized anxiety and depression in patients with primary brain tumors. *Neuro-Oncology.* 2008;10(2):171–181.
29. D'Angelo C, Mirijello A, Leggio L, et al. State and trait anxiety and depression in patients with primary brain tumors before and after surgery: 1-year longitudinal study. *J Neurosurg.* 2008;108(2):281–286.
30. Mainio A, Hakko H, Tuurinkoski T, Koivukangas J, Rasanen P. The effect of brain tumour laterality on anxiety levels among neurosurgical patients. *J Neurol Neurosurg Psychiatry.* 2003;74(9):1278–1282.
31. Kilbride L, Smith G, Grant R, Kilbride L, Smith G, Grant R. The frequency and cause of anxiety and depression amongst patients with malignant brain tumours between surgery and radiotherapy. *J Neurooncol.* 2007;84(3):297–304.
32. New P. Radiation injury to the nervous system [Review]. *Curr Opin Neurol.* 2001;14(6):725–734.
33. Posner JB. Side effects of radiation therapy. In: Rottenberg, DA ed. *Neurologic complications of cancer.* Philadelphia, PA: FA Davis; 1995:311–337.
34. Keime-Guibert F, Napolitano M, Delattre JY. Neurological complications of radiotherapy and chemotherapy [Review]. *J Neurol.* 1998;245(11):695–708.
35. Warren KE, Fine HA. Systemic chemotherapy of central nervous system tumors. In: Prados M, ed. *Brain cancer.* Hamilton, Ontario: BC Decker, Inc.; 2002:193–210.
36. Meyers CA, Weitzner MA, Valentine AD, Levin VA. Methylphenidate therapy improves cognition, mood, and function of brain tumor patients. *J Clin Oncol.* 1998;16(7):2522–2527.
37. Valentine AD, Passik SD, Massie MJ. Psychiatric and psychosocial issues. In: Levin VA, ed. *Cancer in the nervous system.* New York, NY: Oxford University Press; 2005:572–590.
38. Passik SD, Ricketts PL. Central nervous system tumors. In: Holland JC, ed. *Psycho-oncology.* New York, NY: Oxford University Press; 1998:303–313.
39. Weitzner MA, Meyers CA, Gelke CK, Byrne KS, Cella D, Levin VA. The functional assessment of cancer therapy (FACT) scale. Development of a brain subscale and revalidation of the general version (FACT-G) in patients with primary brain tumors. *Cancer.* 1995;75(5):1151–1161.
40. Gilbert M, Armstrong T, Meyers C. Issues in assessing and interpreting quality of life in patients with malignant glioma. *Semin Oncol.* 2000;27(3 Suppl 6):20–26.
41. Pelletier G, Verhoef MJ, Khatri N, Hagen N. Quality of life in brain tumor patients: the relative contributions of depression fatigue, emotional distress, and existential issues. *J Neurooncol.* 2002;57(1):41–49.
42. Brown PD, Ballman KV, Rummans TA, et al. Prospective study of quality of life in adults with newly diagnosed high-grade gliomas. *J Neurooncol.* 2006;76(3):283–291.
43. Armstrong TS, Cohen MZ, Eriksen LR, Hickey JV. Symptom clusters in oncology patients and implications for symptom research in people with primary brain tumors [Review]. *J Nurs Scholarsh.* 2004;36(3):197–206.
44. Shaw EG, Rosdhal R, D'Agostino RB Jr, et al. Phase II study of donepezil in irradiated brain tumor patients: effect on cognitive function, mood, and quality of life. *J Clin Oncol.* 2008;24(9):1415–1420.
45. Gehring K, Sitskoorn MM, Aaronson NK, Taphoorn MJB. Interventions for cognitive deficits in adults with brain tumors [Review]. *Lancet Neurol.* 2008;7(6):548–560.

CHAPTER 17

Head and Neck Cancer

Gerald M. Devins, Kristen J. Otto, Jonathan C. Irish, and Gary M. Rodin

Head and neck cancer includes malignancies that arise on the lips and in the mouth, pharynx (including the nasopharynx, oropharynx, and hypopharynx), larynx, salivary glands, paranasal sinuses, and skin of the head and neck. It is the sixth most common cancer worldwide, accounting for approximately 5% of all new cancers. Squamous cell carcinoma, by far the most common of the head and neck malignancies, accounts for approximately 250,000 annual deaths worldwide. The mean age at diagnosis of those who develop squamous cell carcinomas of the upper aerodigestive tract is 60 years.[1] Head and neck cancer introduces significant and unique psychosocial challenges and adaptive demands. Moadel, Ostroff, and Schantz provide an excellent review of this subject in the first edition of this textbook.[2] This chapter is intended to complement its predecessor with a focus on intervening developments.

BEHAVIORAL RISK FACTORS FOR HEAD AND NECK CANCER

Behavioral and lifestyle factors play an important role in the etiology of head and neck cancer. Tobacco use, the most important risk factor for squamous cell carcinomas of the head and neck, has been linked to approximately 85% of cases.[3] Other specific associations include betel-nut chewing with oral squamous cell carcinoma and wood or nickel-dust inhalation with paranasal sinus cancers. Unprotected sun exposure is an important risk factor for squamous cell carcinomas of the lips and skin. Sexual activity and the number of sexual partners have been associated with human papillomavirus (HPV) infection and with squamous cell carcinomas of both the oral cavity and oropharynx. HPV-associated cancers tend to occur in people who are younger than the average person with head and neck cancer and have an overall better response to treatment and prognosis.[4]

MEDICAL AND SURGICAL TREATMENT

Treatment varies by subsite, but the best oncologic control must be balanced against the preservation of form and function. Organ preservation strategies include the use of radiation (or radiation with concurrent chemotherapy) to treat cancers of the pharynx and larynx. Surgical treatment in these subsites is often reserved as salvage therapy for nonsurgical treatment failures. For subsites, such as the oral cavity, salivary glands, and sinuses, surgery is often first-line treatment, with radiation given postoperatively to optimize tumor control. Although treatment varies by subsite, the goal of "organ preservation" is always important because crucial functions, such as speech and swallowing, are often at risk. Indeed, these effects may be as important as the cancer itself in terms of their impact on quality of life (QOL). Advances in surgical reconstructive techniques over the past 30 years, including microvascular free tissue transfer, have enabled enormous improvements in postoperative functional and cosmetic outcomes. They have established surgical therapy as a mainstay in the treatment of squamous cell carcinomas of many subsites.

PROGNOSIS

Overall, 5-year survival rates for head and neck cancer have been stable over the past two decades. In general, a 50% 5-year survival rate is anticipated, although individual survival is influenced substantially by tumor stage and subsite, comorbid medical conditions, ability to tolerate optimal treatment regimens, continued tobacco and alcohol exposure, and second primary malignancies.

SYMPTOMS AND FUNCTIONAL IMPAIRMENT

The symptoms of head and neck cancer are often multiple and vary by the site of origin. Pain, difficulties swallowing (dysphagia), painful swallowing (odynophagia), hoarse voice (dysphonia), earache (otalgia), weight loss, and shortness of breath are among the most common presenting symptoms. Symptom distress is often severe and significantly compromises QOL. All who present with new squamous cell carcinoma of the head and neck warrant comprehensive investigation, including adjacent subsites, due to the propensity for multiple or metachronous primaries. Second lesions within the head and neck occur in 3%–5% of cases.[5] Primary lung cancers are found in approximately 6%.[6] Ongoing clinical surveillance is crucial because people with a significant history of tobacco and alcohol exposure often have "field cancerization" that places them at long-term risk for new primary development due to carcinogen exposure along the entire upper aerodigestive tract.

"Organ preservation" regimens (radiation therapy or concurrent radiation and chemotherapy) are now the standard of care, but long-term side effects of treatment can still compromise organ function. Advances in targeted-radiation delivery, with the use of intensity-modulated radiation therapy, reduce collateral damage to normal, surrounding tissue while maximizing dosage to the tumor volume. Despite these advances, treatment side effects are often significant and life-changing. Radiation to the head and neck often causes a substantial permanent reduction in saliva production, leading to chronic dry mouth (xerostomia). It also leads to chronic fibrosis of the subcutaneous tissues, as well as of the pharyngeal and esophageal musculature, causing dysphagia, and, occasionally, stricture formation. Radiation-related edema and fibrosis can cause airway problems necessitating chronic tracheostomy dependence. Altered or diminished taste (dysgeusia), decreased neck and shoulder range of motion, and chronic pain can occur following treatment.

The interaction of certain factors may amplify adverse effects of treatment. For example, side effects can intensify and persist for long durations when chemotherapy is delivered concurrently with radiation. Long-term gastrostomy-tube dependence occurs in as many as one-third of people. Surgical therapy imposes its own long-term problems. In particular, profound alterations in QOL often result from undesirable cosmetic outcomes related to chronic tracheostomy or tracheostoma dependence, incisions on the face and neck, and extirpation of whole organs (i.e., eyes, nose, larynx, tongue, and mandible). Facial disfigurement can lead to shame and social avoidance, thereby compromising QOL.

PSYCHOSOCIAL STRESSORS

A burgeoning literature documents multiple stressors and adaptive challenges associated with head and neck cancer.[7] Many are common across all cancers, including uncertainty about disease progression, the threat of death, treatment side effects, enforced dependency, disabling symptoms, and disruption of lifestyles, activities, and interests. Head and neck cancer introduces incremental stressors such as the functional difficulties related to swallowing, chewing, eating, and speech, physical symptoms such as chronic pain, and psychosocial stressors including disfigurement and stigma.

Disfigurement. Facial disfigurement, largely attributable to surgery, has long been considered among the most disturbing stressors associated with head and neck cancer. This is expected since the face is highly visible and is of vital importance to the sense of self, interpersonal relationships, and communication. In that regard, research has confirmed that disfigurement is associated with negative effects on self-image, romantic, family, and other relationships,[8] and mood.[9] Sometimes distress is even greater in marital partners than in patients.[10] Fortunately, recent developments in surgical reconstructive techniques significantly reduce residual disfigurement, which may ameliorate some of these adverse psychosocial effects.[9]

Recent studies indicate that both individual characteristics and the social environment may moderate the effect of disfigurement following head and neck surgery. Social support, for example, may buffer the impact of disfigurement, particularly among women surgically treated for head and neck cancer. [11] "Social self-efficacy" (i.e., the belief that one can exercise control over the reactions and openness of other people)[12] may also moderate the psychosocial impact of disfigurement. Some authors speculate that cancer-related dysfunctions (e.g., difficulties with speech, chewing, or swallowing) and disfigurement interact synergistically to compromise the sense of bodily integrity.[13] Measures of disfigurement are available, rated by physicians, patients, or by objective scales, but it is not yet clear how discrepant findings should be interpreted. The use of different measures of disfigurement may account for some of the inconsistencies in the research literature.

Illness intrusiveness. Illness intrusiveness entails the disruption of lifestyles, valued activities, and interests due to disease and/or treatment.[14] It is an intervening variable that mediates the effects of disease and treatment on subjective well-being and QOL. Illness intrusiveness exerts its effects in chronic, disabling and life-threatening conditions by reducing pleasure and satisfaction derived from valued activities, and by diminishing personal control over the ability to obtain positive, and/or avoid negative, outcomes. Illness intrusiveness in head and neck cancer, as in other chronic, disabling, or life-threatening conditions is consistently associated with decreased psychological well-being and increased emotional distress. It is likely that symptom burden contributes importantly to illness intrusiveness in head and neck cancer, but this remains to be tested.

Psychological, social, and contextual factors modify the level of illness intrusiveness that results from the circumstances of disease and treatment.[14] Individual characteristics associated with high illness intrusiveness include young age and low annual family income. Advanced education is also associated with high illness intrusiveness in relation to the instrumental domains of life (e.g., work, financial situation), social relationships but not in intimate relationships. Research, to date, identifies five factors that modify the psychosocial impact of illness intrusiveness: stigma, self-concept, gender, age, and culture. These factors are discussed below in relation to head and neck cancer.

Stigma. Stigma is characterized by exclusion, rejection, blame, or devaluation due to experienced or anticipated adverse social judgment based on an enduring feature of identity.[15] Stigma has long been associated with cancer, dating back to early beliefs in its origins as a sexually transmitted disease.[16] Although most cancers are no longer believed to derive from such etiologies, cancers believed attributable to one's own actions are more highly stigmatized than those believed to be independent of lifestyle or behavior.[17]

Cancer-related stigma is associated with compromised psychosocial well-being, constrained interpersonal relationships, limited financial opportunities, and reduced access to treatment and care.[17] It often leads people to delay seeking medical attention and can complicate treatment and compromise prognosis. It is associated with risk-inducing health behaviors (e.g., smoking and alcohol abuse) and with prominent disfigurement, and therefore may be expected in cancers of the head and neck. Surprisingly, however, stigma has rarely been evaluated in psychosocial studies of head and neck cancer. In the only reported study of stigma in this context, long-term laryngeal cancer survivors reported that stigma attributable to laryngectomy and the stoma correlated with reduced life happiness and increased depressive symptoms.[18]

PSYCHOSOCIAL AND PSYCHIATRIC OUTCOMES

Distress is common in people with cancer and most often represents a final common pathway through which multiple risk and protective factors exert their effects.[19] Anxiety, depression, suicide, and impaired marital functioning are the most widely studied psychosocial consequences of head and neck cancer. Symptoms of depression most often reflect a cumulative, delayed response to multiple stressors and burdens associated with cancer and its treatment.[19] Clinically significant depressive symptoms occur 2–3 times more frequently in people affected by cancer or other major medical conditions compared to the general population.[20] Systematic studies of people with head and neck cancer indicate that 16%–20% meet criteria for adjustment disorder, minor depression, or major depression, similar to the rates found in other medical conditions.[21,22]

Recent research confirms that physical distress and dysfunction are among the strongest predictors of depressive symptoms.[23] A variety of individual, social, and contextual factors, however, codetermine this outcome in cancer patients. These include social support, attachment security, low spiritual well-being, and young age.[19,24] In contrast to the gender differences reported in the general population,[25] no consistent gender differences in emotional distress or depressive symptoms have been found in head and neck cancer (or, indeed, in other cancers). Tumor stage, number of physical symptoms, pretreatment depression, and avoidant coping are associated with depression in head and neck cancer when people are treated with radiotherapy and surgery.[26]

Symptoms of anxiety may be as common as symptoms of depression in individuals with head and neck cancer. Anxiety symptoms may be triggered by a variety of disease- and treatment-related threats and concerns. One that is specific to head and neck cancer is the use of facemasks in the delivery of radiation treatment, which may trigger anxiety or panic attacks associated with claustrophobia in some patients. Such symptoms may require treatment with anxiolytic medication or relaxation techniques for the treatment to proceed.

The prevalence of psychological distress in head and neck cancer may be affected by individual premorbid behaviors and characteristics and by the effects of disease and treatment. Contrary to expectation, disfigurement is not consistently associated with distress in head and neck cancer.[9,10] However, an adverse emotional impact due to disfigurement appears most likely to occur in individuals who have little social support,[9] and high levels of stigma and cancer-induced illness intrusiveness.[18] Alcohol and tobacco use, common in individuals with head and neck cancer, increase the risk of depression.[27,28] Suicide rates are mildly elevated in individuals with cancer, but occur more often in association with head and neck cancer than with many other cancer types. In that regard, a review of 1572 suicides in people with cancer indicated that increased risk is associated with head and neck cancer, myeloma, advanced disease, low social or cultural support, and limited treatment options.[27]

The high prevalence of distress and suicide among people with head and neck cancer supports calls for routine screening for distress in this population. A number of brief, psychometrically sound, self-report instruments can be routinely integrated into clinical practice, although this strategy is unlikely to improve psychosocial outcomes unless test results activate specific psychosocial interventions.

Impact on couples. Spouses and partners of people with head and neck cancer are often profoundly affected by the disease and its treatment. The literature indicates relatively high levels of health-related QOL, overall, for both patients and their partners, although partners typically report lower QOL and more frequent psychiatric problems. Research to date confounds gender with patient–partner status since almost all of the "partners" involved in these studies are female. Compared to men with head and neck cancer, their wives report greater distress[10] and more frequent anxiety disorders.[29] The role of marital satisfaction, too, appears to differ between male patients and their wives. Whereas the quality of the marital relationship is a more powerful determinant of QOL for wives, physical complaints influence QOL more powerfully for their husbands with head and neck cancer.[30] In part, this reflects the greater tendency of women to assume the psychosocial burden of their partner's ill health.

However, at least one study in head and neck cancer indicates that both husbands and wives experience a change in the marital relationship such that it becomes increasingly characterized by the suspension of personal pursuits and increased adoption of a "supportive caregiver" role.[31] Future research is needed to replicate these observations and to disentangle the relative contributions of gender and patient–partner status.

QUALITY OF LIFE AND HEALTH-RELATED QUALITY OF LIFE

A growing literature addresses QOL and the ways in which this is affected by head and neck cancer and its treatment. In this section, we describe some of the recent research and relevant constructs.

Quality of life. Quality of life is a global concept, conceived to reflect the totality of human well-being, including (but not limited to) physical, psychological, social, economic, and spiritual domains. The notion of *health-related quality of life* (HRQOL) addresses QOL as it is affected by disease and treatment. When oncology treatment is curative in intent, preservation of HRQOL is fundamental to success because such interventions aim to restore health. Protection of HRQOL is also central when the treatment aim is palliative because this outcome cannot be achieved without satisfactory QOL. The study of HRQOL can also inform treatment selection, decision making, and health policy.

Measuring quality of life in head and neck cancer. Psychometrically sound instruments are available to measure HRQOL among people affected by head and neck cancer. Generic instruments tap domains of experience that are relevant across the spectrum of cancer diagnoses. In some cases, complementary modules assess HRQOL elements that are unique to head and neck cancer. (See reference 32 for a useful review of instruments specific to head and neck cancer.)

Descriptive studies. Numerous studies have described HRQOL among people affected by head and neck cancer. Many are retrospective and their validity is threatened by the lack of randomization and experimental control. A number of studies, however, involve more rigorous, prospective-longitudinal experimental designs in which a cohort, diagnosed with and treated for specific head and neck cancer diagnoses, is identified (typically at diagnosis or pretreatment) and followed over the course of treatment, in some cases, long after active treatment has ended. Prospective, longitudinal studies provide useful descriptions of the course of psychosocial adjustment in head and neck cancer that can inform the types and timing of psychosocial interventions.

Retrospective studies. Retrospective studies typically focus on homogeneous patient samples with regard to cancer site, but usually combine cases across stages of disease and durations of treatment. These studies indicate generally positive HRQOL following treatment for head and neck cancer. Generic instruments demonstrate positive psychosocial outcomes, but disease-specific measures (e.g., emphasizing physical function) indicate modest deterioration. Low HRQOL has been associated with fear of recurrence.[33] A number of authors speculate that people with laryngeal cancer may be at increased risk for compromised QOL due to the extent and severity of side effects, most notably the loss of natural speech and disfigurement (e.g., visible stoma following successful surgery). Although such speculations are credible, available evidence does not substantiate them.

Prospective studies. Prospective studies offer a more rigorous description of the "natural history" of HRQOL over the course of head and neck cancer and its treatment because participants serve as their own controls. Despite daunting logistical challenges and intensive resource requirements, a number of such studies have been reported. Many track HRQOL over the first year of treatment whereas others provide longer posttreatment follow-up, extending as long as 5 years.[34] Overall, results indicate that HRQOL deteriorates during the first 3 months following diagnosis while people undergo treatment.[35] Negative effects are limited largely to the domains of physical symptoms and treatment side effects, but these often lead to corresponding psychosocial changes. In most cases, HRQOL returns to or approximates (albeit at a slightly lower level than) pretreatment levels by the 1-year milestone[36] and remains stable thereafter in most cases.[37] In at least one study, HRQOL at diagnosis significantly predicted survival and HRQOL 5 years posttreatment.[37]

Determinants. A growing literature examines a wide range of factors that appear to shape HRQOL among people treated for head and neck cancer. Factors identified, to date, as determinants of HRQOL include (1) premorbid characteristics, including HRQOL, socioeconomic status, functional status, and dispositional optimism; (2) tumor stage; (3) functionally disabling treatment side effects (including difficulties in speech, swallowing, chewing, and eating as well as dry mouth and taste disturbances); (4) smoking and "problem [alcohol] drinking"; (5) pain; (6) depression; and (7) fear of recurrence.

Evaluating treatment outcome and comparing alternative treatments. Many funding agencies require cancer-treatment trials to include HRQOL as an outcome of interest, stimulating research about the effects of cancer treatment on HRQOL and comparing outcomes across therapies. Many of the reported studies are randomized controlled trials, the evidence from which should be compelling. Most of these studies, however, employ HRQOL instruments that are specific to head and neck cancer and are heavily weighted with items that tap common symptoms and/or treatment side effects. More generic clinimetric HRQOL instruments provide a more balanced assessment of overall life functioning, but do not indicate the more specific effects of the disease on HRQOL.

The vast majority of head and neck cancer patients achieve good long-term psychosocial adaptation, with no discernable HRQOL impairment.[38] However, impairment is most often observed during the period of active treatment, particularly related to the physical side effects and associated functional limitations.[39] It is not clear, however, whether or to what extent these results are determined by the effects of response shift or personal development stimulated by crisis, a phenomenon commonly referred to as "posttraumatic growth."

QOL and survival. Considerable debate addresses the relation between QOL and survival. At least four studies examine this issue in head and neck cancer. Results have been inconsistent. Some studies have documented a statistically significant predictive relation between premorbid HRQOL and survival, but have not controlled effectively for important prognostic factors (e.g., comorbid conditions).

PSYCHOSOCIAL INTERVENTIONS

Head and neck cancer requires a coordinated, multidisciplinary treatment approach that optimally includes specialists in oncology, radiation, psychosocial care, speech and language pathology, occupational therapy, physiotherapy, nutrition, and dentistry.[40] Psychological support should be provided, along with attention to all of the physical and functional problems that may occur as a result of the disease and its treatment. Coordination of care amongst the health professionals involved may be an important factor in achieving the best possible patient outcomes. Preparation of the patient with information about the symptoms and limitations that may occur and help in developing strategies to overcome them may be crucial to facilitate recovery and restore QOL. This can include providing information about communication options, swallowing and oral motor exercises, nutritional intake, and measures to diminish lymphedema and functional limitations. Long-term recovery and reduction of illness intrusiveness may also require ongoing education and support.

The literature on the evaluation of psychosocial interventions for people with head and neck cancer is still relatively small, compared to that for other cancers, and has largely focused on psychoeducational interventions and cognitive-behavior therapy (CBT). *Psychoeducation* refers to the provision of information about the disease and its treatment in a therapeutic context and the ways in which affected individuals can manage these challenges. *CBT* addresses irrational assumptions, self-defeating appraisals, and other cognitive errors as well as maladaptive coping responses that compromise psychological well-being. *Supportive-expressive therapy* and specific treatments for symptoms of anxiety and depression are commonly provided, but their impact has not yet been subject to systematic study in this population. Screening for distress and referral for psychosocial care have been recommended for all patients with cancer, but the effectiveness of this strategy has not been demonstrated for people with head and neck cancer.

One recent study[41] evaluated the impact of regular support provided by nurses and dieticians in the form of "head and neck cancer conferences" held throughout active treatment and for up to 3 years postdiagnosis. The primary focus of the intervention was on the disease, its treatment, treatment side effects, and providing information and emotional support to patients and their families to decrease treatment side effects and improve nutritional status. Compared to usual care, however, few HRQOL benefits were evident for the experimental support program. Another study evaluated a two-step, multidimensional psychoeducational intervention delivered by a trained health educator immediately before hospitalization for surgery and during short-term recovery.[42] In this intervention, two 60–90-minute, one-on-one instructional sessions, are supplemented by a booklet that includes information about preparing for surgery and the postoperative course and for their return home. Evaluation to date is limited to a single, randomized controlled pilot study, but results are encouraging. All participants considered the treatment helpful and highly satisfactory; none withdrew prematurely. At follow-up (3-months postdischarge), the intervention group demonstrated increased knowledge, less body-image disturbance, lower anxiety, and a trend toward higher well-being relative to usual-care controls.

"Nucare" is a psychoeducational coping intervention[43] that was developed to teach people to cope with cancer by emphasizing personal control, introducing new emotional and instrumental coping responses, and stressing a collaborative partnership between nurses and patients (and their families). Modules address problem solving, relaxation techniques, cognitive coping skills, goal setting, communication, social support, and lifestyle (summarized in supplementary workbook and audio cassette or CD). A recent controlled study in head and neck cancer[44] found better QOL and lower levels of depressive symptoms in those who received the intervention as compared to those who received usual care. Results also indicated that head and neck cancer participants in this study strongly preferred a traditional, one-on-one therapeutic format or a self-administered format that can be completed at home, rather than group therapy.[45] At least one study has reported improved QOL in people with head and neck cancer as a result of both supportive group therapy and education.[46]

A promising new CBT intervention focused specifically on head and neck cancer comprises a 9-week program of telephone-based, nurse-administered CBT plus prescription medications that targets problems involving smoking, alcohol use, and/or depression.[47] The intervention is intended to help people with head and neck cancer access and apply health-related information adaptively to contend with disease- and treatment-related stressors. Outcomes at 6-month follow-up in a randomized controlled trial indicate significant improvements in smoking, drinking, and depression, although CBT-group superiority is limited to smoking cessation. *Telemedicine* programs are relevant to all affected by head and neck cancer, but they are especially valuable when people reside at considerable distances from a major cancer center. An initial randomized controlled trial indicates partial support for its effectiveness.[48] *Social-skills training* can also facilitate long-term adaptation by promoting effective interaction with others in those whose illness or treatment has caused them to withdraw from social relationships.

CONCLUSION

Head and neck cancer imposes significant adaptive challenges and coping demands, both for patients and for their loved ones. The threat and burden associated with many other cancers is compounded in this disease by the unique demands of treatment, the disturbing psychological effects that result from disfigurement of the face, head, and neck region, and the troublesome functional limitations associated with disturbances in speech and swallowing. Improvements in medical, surgical, and radiation treatments have significantly diminished treatment-related side effects, but have not improved survival rates over the past few decades. Emotional distress, anxiety, and depression occur in a substantial minority of people with head and neck cancer, adverse effects on spouses and marital relationships can be substantial, and suicide rates are higher than in many other cancers. An active approach to multidisciplinary care, routine screening for distress, and referral of those in need for specialized psychosocial care may improve outcomes.

Research suggests that HRQOL is often restored to pretreatment levels by the end of the first year posttreatment. Further research is needed, however, to determine whether and to what extent these positive findings reflect a return to premorbid states, response shift, posttraumatic growth, or methodologic artifacts. Symptom burden, disfigurement, illness intrusiveness, and stigma continue to impose significant psychosocial strain on many affected people. Unfortunately, there remains a dearth of empirically tested interventions that are specific to or have been evaluated in people with head and neck cancer. The relative neglect of the psychosocial research in head and neck cancer is an important gap that must be addressed. In the meantime, it is clear that people with head and neck cancer face unique and substantial physical and psychosocial challenges and that the active support of a multidisciplinary team is essential to their recovery and rehabilitation.

REFERENCES

1. Davies L, Welch HG. Epidemiology of head and neck cancer in the United States. *Otolaryngol Head Neck Surg.* 2006;135(3):451–457.

2. Moadel AB, Ostroff JS, Schantz SP. Head and neck cancer. In: Holland JC, ed. *Psycho-oncology.* New York, NY: Oxford University Press; 1998:314–323.

3. Licitra L, Rossini C, Bossi P. Advances in the changing patterns of aetiology of head and neck cancers. *Curr Opinion Otolaryngol Head Neck Surg.* 2006;14(2):95–99.

4. Schantz SP, Yu GP. Head and neck cancer incidence trends in young Americans, 1973–1997, with a special analysis for tongue cancer. *Arch Otolaryngol Head Neck Surg.* 2002;128(3):268–274.

5. Dhooge IJ, De Vos M, Van Cauwenberge PB. Multiple primary malignant tumors in patients with head and neck cancer: results of a prospective study and future perspectives. *Laryngoscope.* 1998;108(2):250–256.

6. Deleyiannis FWB, Thomas DB. Risk of lung cancer among patients with head and neck cancer. *Otolaryngol Head Neck Surg.* 1997;116:630–636.

7. Rogers SN, Ahad SA, Murphy AP. A structured review and theme analysis of papers published on 'quality of life' in head and neck cancer: 2000–2005. *Oral Oncol.* 2007;43(9):843–868.

8. Gamba A, Romano M, Grosso IM, et al. Psychosocial adjustment of patients surgically treated for head and neck cancer. *Head & Neck.* 1992;14(3):218–223.

9. Katz MR, Irish JC, Devins GM, Rodin GM, Gullane PJ. Psychosocial adjustment in head and neck cancer: the impact of disfigurement, gender and social support. *Head & Neck.* 2003;25:103–112.

10. Vickery LE, Latchford G, Hewison J, Bellew M, Feber T. The impact of head and neck cancer and facial disfigurement on the quality of life of patients and their partners. *Head & Neck.* 2003;25(4):289–296.

11. Taylor SE, Klein LC, Lewis BP, Gruenewald TL, Gurung RAR, Updegraff JA. Biobehavioral responses to stress in females: tend-and-befriend, not fight-or-flight. *Psychol Rev.* 2000;107(3):411–429.

12. Hagedoorn M, Molleman E. Facial disfigurement in patients with head and neck cancer: the role of social self-efficacy. *Health Psychol.* 2006;25(5):643–647.

13. Callahan C. Facial disfigurement and sense of self in head and neck cancer. *Soc Work Health Care.* 2004;40(2):73–87.

14. Devins GM, Bezjak A, Mah K, Loblaw DA, Gotowiec AP. Context moderates illness-induced lifestyle disruptions across life domains: a test of the illness intrusiveness theoretical framework in six common cancers. *Psycho-Oncology.* 2006;15(3):221–233.

15. Weiss MG, Ramakrishna J, Somma D. Health-related stigma: rethinking concepts and interventions. *Psychol Health Med.* 2006;11(3):277–287.

16. Patterson JT. *The dread disease: cancer and modern American culture.* Cambridge, MA: Harvard University Press; 1987.

17. Lebel S, Devins GM. Stigma in cancer patients whose behavior may have contributed to their disease. *Future Oncol.* 2008;4(5):717–733.

18. Devins GM, Stam HJ, Koopmans JP. Psychosocial impact of laryngectomy mediated by perceived stigma and illness intrusiveness. *Can J Psychiatry.* 1994;39(10):608–616.

19. Rodin G, Lo C, Mikulincer M, Donner A, Gagliese L, Zimmermann C. Pathways to distress: the multiple determinants of depression, hopelessness, and the desire for death in metastatic cancer patients. *Soc Sci Med.* 2009;68(3):562–569.

20. Peveler R, Carson A, Rodin G. Depression in medical populations. *BMJ.* 2002;325:149–152.

21. Katz MR, Kopek N, Waldron J, Devins GM, Tomlinson G. Screening for depression in head and neck cancer. *Psycho-Oncology.* 2004;13:269–280.

22. Kugaya A, Akechi T, Okuyama T, et al. Prevalence, predictive factors, and screening for psychologic distress in patients with newly diagnosed head and neck cancer. *Cancer.* 2000;88(12):2817–2823.

23. Rodin G, Lloyd N, Katz M, et al. The treatment of depression in cancer patients: a systematic review. *Support Care Cancer.* 2007;15(2):123–136.

24. Koenig HG, George LK, Siegler IC. The use of religion and other emotion-regulating coping strategies among older adults. *Gerontologist.* 1988;28:303–310.

25. Weissman MM, Bland RC, Canino GJ, et al. Cross-national epidemiology of major depression and bipolar disorder. *JAMA.* 1996;276(4):293–299.

26. de Leeuw JRJ, De Graeff A, Ros WJG, Blijham GH, Hordijk GJ, Winnubst JAM. Prediction of depressive symptomatology after treatment of head and neck cancer: the influence of pre-treatment physical and depressive symptoms, coping, and social support. *Head & Neck.* 2000;22(8):799–807.

27. Kendall WS. Suicide and cancer: a gender-comparative study. *Ann Oncol.* 2007;18:381–387.

28. Rodin G, Nolan RP, Katz MR. Depression (in the medically ill). In: Levenson J, ed. *APPI textbook of psychosomatic medicine.* Washington, DC: American Psychiatric Press, Inc.; 2004:113–217.

29. Zwahlen RA, Dannermann C, Grätz KW, et al. Quality of life and psychiatric morbidity in patients successfully treated for oral cavity squamous cell cancer and their wives. *J Oral Maxillofac Surg.* 2008;66(6):1125–1132.

30. Jenewein J, Zwahlen RA, Zwahlen D, Drabe N, Moergeli H, Büchi S. Quality of life and dyadic adjustment in oral cancer patients and their female partners. *Eur J Cancer Care.* 2008;17(2):127–135.

31. Röing M, Hirsch JM, Holmström I. Living in a state of suspension—a phenomenological approach to the spouse's experience of oral cancer. *Scand J Caring Sci.* 2008;22(1):40–47.

32. Ringash J, Bezjak A. A structured review of quality of life instruments for head and neck cancer patients. *Head & Neck.* 2001;23(3):201–213.

33. Smith GI, Yeo D, Clark J, et al. Measures of health-related quality of life and functional status in survivors of oral cavity cancer who have had defects reconstructed with radial forearm free flaps. *Br J Oral Maxillofac Surg.* 2006;44(3):187–192.

34. Nordgren M, Jannert M, Boysen M, et al. Health-related quality of life in patients with pharyngeal carcinoma: a five-year follow-up. *Head & Neck.* 2006;28(4):339–349.

35. Kelly C, Paleri V, Downs C, Shah R. Deterioration in quality of life and depressive symptoms during radiation therapy for head and neck cancer. *Otolaryngol Head Neck Surg.* 2007;136(1):108–111.

36. De Graeff A, de Leeuw JRJ, Ros WJG, Hordijk GJ, Blijham GH, Winnubst JAM. Long-term quality of life of patients with head and neck cancer. *Laryngoscope.* 2000;110(1):98–106.

37. Nordgren M, Abendstein H, Jannert M, et al. Health-related quality of life five years after diagnosis of laryngeal carcinoma. *Int J Radiat Oncol Biol Phys.* 2003;56(5):1333–1343.

38. Griffiths G, Parmar MKB, Bailey AJ. Physical and psychological symptoms of quality of life in the CHART randomized trial in head and neck cancer: short-term and long-term patient reported symptoms. CHART Steering Committee. Continuous hyperfractionated accelerated radiotherapy. *Br J Cancer.* 1999;81(7):1196–1205.

39. Tschudi D, Stoeckli S, Schmid S. Quality of life after different treatment modalities for carcinoma of the oropharynx. *Laryngoscope.* 2003;113(11): 1949–1954.

40. Dingman C, Hegedus PD, Likes C, McDowell P, McCarthy E, Zwilling C. A coordinated multidisciplinary approach to caring for the patient with head and neck cancer. *J Support Oncol.* 2008;6:125–131.

41. Petruson KM, Silander EM, Hammerlid EB. Effects of psychosocial intervention on quality of life in patients with head and neck cancer. *Head & Neck.* 2003;25(576):584.

42. Katz MR, Irish JC, Devins GM. Development and pilot testing of a psychoeducational intervention for oral cancer patients. *Psycho-Oncology.* 2004;13:642–653.

43. Edgar L, Rosberger Z, Nowlis D. Coping with cancer during the first year after diagnosis. *Cancer.* 1992;69:817–828.

44. Vilela LD, Nicolau B, Mahmud S, et al. Comparison of psychosocial outcomes in head and neck cancer patients receiving a coping strategies intervention and control subjects receiving no intervention. *J Otolaryngol.* 2006;35(2):88–96.

45. Allison PJ, Edgar L, Nicolau B, Archer J, Black M, Hier M. Results of a feasibility study for a psycho-educational intervention in head and neck cancer. *Psycho-Oncology.* 2004;13(7):482–485.

46. Hammerlid E, Persson LO, Sullivan M, Westin T. Quality-of-life effects of psychosocial intervention in patients with head and neck cancer. *Otolaryngol Head Neck Surg.* 1999;120(4):507–516.

47. Duffy SA, Ronis DL, Valenstein M, et al. A tailored smoking, alcohol, and depression intervention for head and neck cancer patients. *Cancer Epidemiol Biomarkers Prev.* 2006;15(11):2203–2208.

48. van den Brink JL, Moorman PW, de Boer MF, et al. Impact on quality of life of a telemedicine system supporting head and neck cancer patients: a controlled trial during the postoperative period at home. *J Am Med Inform Assoc.* 2007;14(2):198–205.

CHAPTER 18

Gastrointestinal Cancer

Robert S. Krouse

The most common new cases of gastrointestinal (GI) cancers in the United States are colorectal cancer (CRC) (148,810), followed by gastroesophageal (GE) (37,970) and pancreas (37,680).[1] Colorectal cancer typically presents earlier and has greater survival, while other GI tumors are more insidious in presentation and carry a worse prognosis. As with all cancers, there is great stress associated with diagnosis. For GI cancers, this will be greatly associated with the site of tumor, as well as the histological type and stage.

Special health-related quality of life (HR-QOL) issues and psychosocial adjustment due to impairment of GI function must be considered with tumors of the GI tract. This may impact the patient as well as his family and other social circles, and can lead to isolation, depression, anxiety, and an alteration in family dynamics around mealtime, which is integral to normal familial functioning.[2] Thus, the social and cultural context in which patients and their families must cope with GI cancer is of psychosocial relevance.

Other issues that may lead to patient and familial concern include pain, fatigue, and significant weight loss, although this is true for all cancer patients. The symptom cluster of pain, depression, and fatigue is common with many cancers,[3] and is clearly true for many GI malignancies. Symptoms more commonly associated with GI cancers such as nausea and vomiting, abdominal distention, diarrhea, or constipation will lead to great distress. Interdisciplinary care is imperative to ensure the best outcome.

CANCER OF THE ESOPHAGUS AND STOMACH

Overview of symptoms, treatment, and survival. Tumors of the esophagus and stomach can be grouped together in consideration of HR-QOL and psychosocial implications for several reasons, including (1) poor prognosis, (2) anatomic proximity, and (3) relationship to the ability to eat and its repercussions on HR-QOL. In the United States, the incidence of esophageal (16,470) and gastric (21,500)[1] cancer may be less common than in other parts of the world, but adenocarcinomas of the esophagus and proximal stomach are rapidly increasing, especially among white males.[4,5] Esophageal cancer is more common in men (ratio 3.7:1), as is gastric cancer (ratio 1.6:1).[1] Gastrointestinal stromal tumors (GIST) have gained recent prominence, and the stomach is by far the most common site of these tumors.[6]

Common symptoms and signs related to GE tumors are often nonspecific and may lead to a long prodrome before diagnosis. They may include weight loss, difficulty swallowing (especially with esophageal and GE junction tumors), GE reflux, chest and upper abdominal pain, anemia, fatigue, and early satiety. Treatment options will revolve around the extent and the site of disease. If metastasis or invasion of local structures is noted, surgical extirpation is unlikely. While detailed descriptions of operative approaches are beyond the scope of this chapter, they include a major abdominal procedure, and esophageal cancers will frequently necessitate incisions in the chest or neck. The addition of chemotherapy and radiation may provide an improvement in local recurrence and survival for GE cancers.

As GE tumors are frequently diagnosed late, long-term survival is frequently poor. No matter what the treatment offered, recurrence rates are high (up to 66% for esophageal cancer; 80% for gastric cancer),[7–10]

and 5-year survival is low (15.8% for esophageal cancer; 24.7% for gastric cancer).[11]

For gastric GIST tumors, wide margins or extensive lymphadenectomy is unnecessary. Therefore, unless the tumor is quite large necessitating removal of a majority of the stomach, the long-term sequelae of a gastric procedure is usually minimal. Chemotherapy is more tolerable and often prolonged, and radiation is unlikely to be offered.

HR-QOL and psychosocial implications. The major goal in the treatment of GE cancers is to enable the patient to eat. In esophageal and GE junction tumors, surgery can lead to long-term ability to eat and improved HR-QOL, even in the setting of palliative resection,[12] but may not be offered due to bulk of disease at presentation or progression on preoperative therapy. In an unresectable gastric cancer, a bypass procedure may not lead to the intended goal of prolonged ability to eat.[13]

While the type of surgical procedure does not appear to impact HR-QOL, different types of gastric resection may affect eating behavior and physical and emotional functioning.[14] For example, dumping syndrome is more common with a distal gastrectomy, and reflux is more common if the GE junction is included in the specimen. These problems may lead to depression and other HR-QOL problems. Especially in the elderly, a usually reduced-performance status after gastrectomy needs to be considered.[15]

The complication of leak is more common for esophageal resections (14%–16%)[16] than gastric resections (0%–12.7%).[17,18] This will typically resolve with drainage and jejunostomy feeding. If no complications arise, patients may go home soon after they begin to eat if there is appropriate home support. As with all major procedures, the presence of diminished stamina for some time is an expected consequence for many patients, especially as many are elderly. The most common long-term problem after esophageal resection, especially if there is a leak, is an esophageal stricture. As local recurrence will also cause similar symptoms related to blockage while swallowing, this may lead to anxiety until the etiology is confirmed. In addition, persistent postoperative pain syndromes will require careful consideration and possible work-up to rule out cancer recurrence. The most common treatment for benign stricture is dilatation, which will be uncomfortable and will produce anxiety. If a prolonged problem, depression may also occur. Endoscopic stenting in esophageal cancer may lead to long-term treatment of benign or malignant strictures, depending on location of the blockage. If it is too proximal or distal, this treatment might not be available.

The benefits of chemotherapy are less clear with metastatic disease than in the adjuvant setting, and this may affect a patient's psychological status, especially if there were issues before diagnosis. In addition, alcohol dependence, which is a risk factor for esophageal cancer, must be considered by clinicians related to potential postoperative withdrawal.[19] Excessive drinking or drug use can occur after diagnosis for those with dependence problems. It will complicate follow-up and palliative care. A responsible family member or friend may be absent, making matters even more difficult.[19]

Short- and long-term follow-up is imperative, especially for patients who have had major resections of their esophagus or stomach. This will allow patients and family members to ask questions that arise or were not asked previously. In addition, long-term complications can be addressed promptly to avoid inability to sleep, weight loss, anxiety, and depression. Frequently problems such as reflux can be managed simply with antacids, positional changes when sleeping, or sedatives.

Enlisting the support of the family is crucial in all phases of treatment in assisting the patient's emotional and social rehabilitation as well as the family's adjustment to rapid and fundamental changes in everyday life. In the case of severe emotional distress, psychiatric consultation is warranted to provide diagnosis and management by psychotherapeutic and pharmacological intervention. Behavioral means are helpful at times for control of nausea and anorexia, particularly when it is related to anxiety. Rehabilitation is often fully achieved within a few months, but the return to work may take longer.

As survival is frequently limited, hospice care should be anticipated for all patients with GE tumors. Palliative care in gastric cancer is commonly related to obstruction and bleeding. Interdisciplinary approaches should be considered in both of these instances. Related to obstruction, a bypass may not provide optimal results.[13] Endoscopic metallic stents is an effective and feasible method of palliation for both gastric and esophageal tumors.[20] For bleeding, there are also several alternative approaches to an operation, including radiation therapy and angiography with embolization.[21] Relatively low doses of radiation will often eliminate bleeding for the life of the patient.[22] Finally, one may consider an endoscopic approach. While this may not be practical or useful, it may slow or stop bleeding at least temporarily.[21]

CANCER OF THE COLON AND RECTUM

Overview of symptoms, treatment, and survival. Colorectal cancer is the most common site of GI tumors. The incidence in the United States is 108,070 for colon and 40,740 for rectal cancer.[1] Overall occurrence of CRC is nearly equal for men and women.[1] Owing to common early detection measures, many of these tumors present in early, curable stages. Signs and symptoms include change in bowel habits, rectal bleeding, anorexia, weight loss, and abdominal pain. Adenocarcinoma is the most common histological type of CRC. Other types of CRC, such as carcinoid or GIST tumors, are comparatively rare, and focus is almost exclusively on adenocarcinoma.

Treatment approaches to CRC depends primarily on the site of the tumor. If the tumor is at the rectosigmoid junction or proximal, surgical approaches are the initial and possibly only treatment. Postoperative chemotherapy is dependent on the stage of tumor. Typically, patients with stages I and II tumors will not receive chemotherapy, while patients that are stage III will receive chemotherapy.

Rectal cancer will often involve chemoradiation therapy as well as resection. Neoadjuvant chemoradiation will be advised for T3 or N1 tumors to help preserve anal sphincters and lower local recurrence. If a patient does not have adequate anal sphincter function preoperatively, no attempt is made to save the sphincters. Postoperative radiation still has utility in efforts to minimize local recurrence.

The two most common surgical treatments for rectal cancer include abdominoperineal resection (APR) (resection of the rectum and anus with permanent ostomy) and low anterior resection (LAR) (anastomosis of bowel with or without a temporary "protective" ostomy). If the tumor involves adjacent (e.g., bladder) organs, partial or total resection of these organs may be indicated. If tumors are a very early stage (T1), local excision may be offered. The recurrence rates may be as high as 17%,[23] but it is reasonable to consider as the morbidity is much less and long-term HR-QOL better.

Advances in sphincter-preserving techniques are also allowing more patients to avoid a permanent ostomy.[24] There are variations of approaches to attempt to minimize bowel movements and improve function after a low anastomosis. The treatment approach is tailored on the basis of multiple factors, including site, depth of invasion, and size of tumor, the surgeon's training and experience, anal tone, and patient health status; the major consideration being the distance from the tumor to the anal verge. Surgery on the sigmoid colon may carry some of the risks of LAR as procedures (dissection, resection, and anastomoses) frequently enter the rectum.

Rectal cancer patients requiring a permanent ostomy is 10%–35% (Mark C. Hornbrook and Lisa J. Herrinton, personal communication, 2008).[25,26] Temporary stomas are not well reported, and may be 8%–33% of those that undergo anastamosis (Mark C. Hornbrook and Lisa J. Herrinton, personal communication, 2008).[27] There is a population of patients whose anastomoses fail and go on to get a permanent ostomy. This is most likely due to poor anal function, anastomotic leak, stricture, fistula, or recurrence. While a known issue, this is not well described in the literature.[28] In one report, 8% of patients who had temporary ostomy did not have their ostomy reversed.[29]

The overall 5-year survival of CRC is 64.4%, which is nearly identical for colon (63.9%) and rectal (65.6%) cancers.[11] The approximate 5-year survival with appropriate treatments for stage I is 93.2%, stage II is 82.5%, stage III is 59.5%, and stage IV is 8.1%.[30] While treatments for CRC have rapidly improved, advanced stage disease still portends a poor survival.

HR-QOL and psychosocial implications. HR-QOL issues for patients with CRC depend greatly on the stage of cancer and site of tumor. Therefore, it is important to consider colon cancer and rectal cancers separately.

For colon cancer, site of tumor, amount of colon excised, urgency of procedure, and stage all play a role in HR-QOL issues. Right-sided tumors will mandate the removal of the ileocecal valve which limits effluent into the colon. Therefore, removal of this structure may lead to watery to soft bowel movements. This will typically resolve with time, but not for all patients. Excision of other sites of colon will less frequently lead to such problems. If a total or near total colectomy or proctocolectomy is mandated, there will be less water absorption capacity, leading to multiple loose bowel movements per day. While this may resolve partially or totally with time, it is often long lasting or permanent. An urgent operation, such as with obstruction, perforation, or bleeding, may have dramatic effects on the nature of the procedure carried out and HR-QOL and survival outcomes. For example, the likelihood of a temporary or permanent ostomy will be greater. In emergency settings, the hospital course is usually more difficult leading to further rehabilitation issues. Overall for most patients with colon cancer, HR-QOL will be similar to the general population after recovery from treatments.[31]

Rectal cancer is much more likely to have long-term functional and HR-QOL effects due to the anatomic location of these tumors and the differences in treatment approaches. Among rectal cancer patients, there is a commonly held conviction that patient HR-QOL is improved with anastomosis versus permanent ostomy. One study showed that patients undergoing both LAR and APR experienced frequent or irregular bowel movements and diarrhea, which often prevent patients from leaving their home.[32] Stoma patients reported higher level of psychological distress (e.g., low self-esteem), including a more negative body image. In general, younger female patients showed more impairment than older male patients; however, there was a broad spectrum in all age groups. Both groups showed impairment in social functioning (e.g., leisure activities) but this was more prevalent in stoma patients. A Cochrane review examined all controlled or observational clinical trials in which a well-known, validated, reliable multidimensional quality of life (QOL) instrument was used.[33] Six studies found that ostomy patients did not have a worse QOL, one found slightly worse QOL, and four found a significantly worse QOL. The authors concluded that existing observational studies do not allow firm conclusions as to the question of whether the QOL of people after anterior resection [rectal-sparing surgery] is superior to that of people after abdominoperineal excision [ostomy]. The included studies challenged the assumption that anterior resection patients fare better.[33]

More recently, a meta-analysis of QOL for patients undergoing major rectal procedures found that there were no differences in general QOL, although there were differences in several dimensions that make up HR-QOL. They conclude that an APR, which includes a colostomy, cannot be justified on the grounds of QOL alone.[34] This has been disputed in the long-term (>5 years) rectal cancer population, where multiple dimensions of HR-QOL were worse for survivors with ostomies. Importantly, most differences were not highly significant and global HR-QOL was not reported.[35]

For patients who are able to have an anastamosis, functional issues are often a significant problem,[25,26] most commonly related to multiple bowel movements per day. Patients who have poor control of their bowel function may need adult diapers. This can be a great stress for many patients, and lead to changes in eating habits, along with isolation and fear of travel. Some patients may have strictures, which lead to problems with constipation and may ultimately necessitate an ostomy.

Sexuality is an issue that may affect all rectal cancer patients. While it is much more studied in men, it clearly affects women related to libido and potentially anatomic problems such as vaginal stricture.[36] One study described decreased libido, vaginal lubrication, and frequency of orgasm after APR for rectal cancer[37]; others reported dyspareunia, diminished orgasm, and less frequent or cessation of intercourse in more than half of the patients.[32] While in a combined population of cancer and noncancer patients, females have displayed less sexual concerns than men; this was more of a problem for younger women.[38] For males, sexuality was impaired regardless of age. Age, tumor size, location and spread, surgical damage of pelvic nerves,[39] as well as the patient's and the partner's emotional coping are the most important factors that contribute to the large range of dysfunction reported across all studies.

Impotence rates vary from 15% to 92%.[39] While the incidence of impotence is less with newer surgical techniques, it is still significant.[40] In addition, adjuvant therapies will increase sexual dysfunction.[41] In fact, it has been shown that the preoperative ability to have orgasm was eliminated in 50% of both men and women with multimodality rectal cancer treatment.[41]

Patients that are diagnosed with CRC at a younger age warrant special attention as more feelings of stigmatization are noted.[42] For patients with ulcerative colitis, it must be considered that they frequently have psychological problems due to the emotional effects of a long-standing chronic illness. Patients with polyposis syndromes or other genetic predispositions to CRC may require surgery at an early age, and consideration of their psychological needs is imperative.

Patients with ostomies. Cohen et al. notes that for patients with cancer "concern about a colostomy frequently supersedes all other considerations of the patient."[43] The patient who is unable to decide to undergo surgery may be helped by meeting and talking with an ostomate.[44,45] The postoperative period is smoother and emotionally less distressing when it follows adequate preoperative preparation.[46] An individual assessment (e.g., misconceptions) and teaching on practical issues are important.[47] Equipment options must be discussed. In addition, the placement of the stoma is given attention to take into account skinfolds and patient preference (e.g., with regard to clothing).[48] Importantly, comorbidities may actually have a greater impact on HR-QOL than ostomies, though.[49]

An early study, Sutherland,[50] showed ostomy patients who had survived disease-free from rectal cancer for 5 or more years showed considerable impairment in both social (work, community, and family) and sexual (of both neurologic and psychological origin) function. Depression, chronic anxiety, and a sense of social isolation were frequently observed. Patients also had difficulties in the practical management of the colostomy associated with the use of inferior equipment at that time. Significant problems occurred with spillage and odor despite lengthy irrigation procedures. Ostomies have since been shown to be associated with multiple HR-QOL difficulties irrespective of the type or reason for the ostomy,[48] including: problems with appearance; difficulty paying for supplies[51]; skin or leakage complications[52]; psychological problems; and interference with work, recreational, and sporting activities.[32,28] Twenty-six percent of ostomates experience high degrees of embarrassment due to issues such as leakage, odor, and noise.[53] This may lead to greater levels of depression and anxiety, along with greater problems with intimacy and isolation. Spirituality, which is closely aligned with the psychological domain, is likely influenced by a stoma,[54] and thus must be considered for patients having psychological problems postoperatively.

Thomas and colleagues[55] reported approximately 20% of stoma patients (mixed diagnoses) experience a serious level of psychiatric disturbance during the first year. The vast majority occurred during postoperative recovery. A recent report comparing veterans with stomas to those who had similar procedures but did not require an ostomy found more patients with stomas felt depressed (52% vs. 36%) or suicidal (12% vs. 5%) in the postoperative period.[48] Although this was not only CRC survivors (approximately 50%), this finding does further highlight the problem.

Difficulty coping with the stoma initially and at 3 months after surgery was a greater determinant of psychiatric disturbance over the first year than difficulty in coping with the illness.[56,57] Factors associated with increased risk of psychiatric disturbance were past psychiatric history, postoperative physical symptoms and complications, perceived inadequate advice after surgery regarding the stoma and its functioning, as well as traits of neuroticism, anxiety, and obsessionality.[58] Patients' physical state (e.g., fatigue, pain, smell) may also be closely related to the prevalence of anxiety and depression.[59] For long-term CRC survivors (>5 years since diagnosis), living with an ostomy is common with other chronic care issues related to cancer's effects and are broad and pervasive.[45]

Enterostomal nurses can have great impact on preoperative understanding of stomas and postoperative rehabilitation. Preoperative psychological preparation may reduce anxiety and stress to aid recovery.[46] Nurses and patients meeting before the operation may also increase trust and cooperation.[46] In addition to this goal, preoperative ostomy site marking can eliminate problems related to clothing and care that will lead to poor psychosocial outcomes. In the postoperative setting, ensuring patients feel comfortable with self-care will lead to independence and reduce stress.[46] Improved self-efficacy may ease the burden of ostomy.[60] The goal is early postoperative management of stomas for both patients leading to greater independence and psychological health.

Spouses and significant others are often the most helpful for coping with an ostomy.[57] For the first 2 months, concerns about the stoma may be the main issue for patients and families.[61] Life and death concerns begin to surface later, when the patient has mastered the stoma management.

As stated previously, sexuality and sexual dysfunction can play a large role in the psychosocial health of CRC survivors. This can be especially important for ostomy survivors. The presence of an ostomy for males may be associated with lower rates of sexual activity and higher erectile dysfunction.[62] In addition, lower rates of sexual activity and satisfaction significantly correlated with social and psychological dimensions of HR-QOL. Men may be more likely to feel isolated and rate intimacy very low.[48] In addition, patients with ostomy are more likely to have negative feelings about their body appearance,[63] which can lead to diminished intimacy and greater isolation.

Intimacy concerns are not only related to the patients, but ostomies also affect spouses and other partners. Persson et al.[64] conducted focus groups to study spouses' reactions to their partner's ostomy and found that spouses (1) had difficulty with the partner's altered body, (2) reported feeling distant from their partners because of the distress caused by the stoma surgery, (3) reported difficulty looking at the stoma, and (4) struggled to hide feelings of disgust. Twenty-three percent indicated their partner responded negatively during the first sexual experience after ostomy surgery, and 30% stated their partner reacted with much caution, fearing they would hurt the stoma.[65] People with ostomies who remain sexually active report that anxiety about a physical relationship was primarily overcome with the supportive and positive attitude of their partner.[66] For others, the fear of rejection caused them to conceal their ostomy from their partners for many years and to decrease attempts to have a sexual relationship.[66]

PANCREATIC CANCER

Overview of symptoms, treatment, and survival. The pancreas is the second most common site of GI tumors and the fourth leading cause of cancer death in adults in the United States.[1] The overall male to female ratio is equal.[1] Frequent presentations include jaundice, pain, and weight loss. The most common type of pancreatic cancer is ductal adenocarcinomas. Even with improved surgical techniques, the median survival is still only between 4 and 6 months[67]; overall survival is less than 5% at 5 years. This is largely because a majority of patients have locally advanced or metastatic disease at diagnosis; only a minority of patients are candidates for "curative" resection. Patients with one of the rare endocrine tumors have a much better outlook.

The only treatment with a curative intent includes surgical resection. The indicated procedure is based on the location of the tumor. Most commonly, this will entail a pancreaticoduodenectomy (the Whipple procedure) which includes resection of the duodenum, head of pancreas, common bile duct, gallbladder, and frequently the distal stomach. If the tumor is in the distal or body of the pancreas, the most common procedure is a distal pancreatectomy, often including the spleen in the resection specimen.

Morbidity from pancreatic procedures is common. Early complications include wound problems and leaks, most frequently from the pancreatic anastomosis. Later complications include delayed gastric emptying, diabetes, and difficulty digesting foods, especially fats. While diabetes can be controlled with medications and oral pancreatic enzyme replacement manages digestion problems, delayed gastric emptying may be quite distressing and unlikely to respond to medicines. It is imperative to not eat near bedtime and be erect at all times when eating.

There are multiple palliative procedures for pancreatic cancer. Currently, biliary stenting is the primary treatment for obstruction. While it has greater recurrence rates than surgical bypass, stenting has less morbidity.[68] Stenting can also be used for gastric outlet obstructions with great efficacy.[69] If an operation for curative intent is aborted due to determinations of unresectability, a biliary bypass may be undertaken at that time. As late gastric outlet obstructions may occur if a patient has either a stent placed or a bypass in 8%–41.4% of patients,[68,70,71] it should also be considered if a patient is undergoing a biliary bypass.[70,71]

Five-year survival with pancreaticoduodenectomy also is 0%–11% (73). Multiple adjuvant chemoradiation have been noted to improve survival to 10%–19%, and 45% in one series.[72] They often carry a great burden of treatment-related morbidity. Aggressive treatments are clearly not indicted for many patients and in centers that do not have extensive experience with such regimens.

HR-QOL and psychosocial implications. Depression has been associated with pancreatic cancer before diagnosis and reported for many years.[73–78] Early clinical case reports described a triad of depression, anxiety, and premonition of impending doom.[74] Depression and other psychological difficulties have since been confirmed to be more common in pancreatic cancer than other GI malignancies.[79–81] Owing to the other constellation of problems related to pancreatic cancer, depression may be overlooked.[82] The range of depression in pancreatic cancer patients is 25%–75%, depending on scales used and when evaluation occurs during the course of disease.[78] Suicidal ideation may be up to 17%.[83] Symptoms such as persistent dysphoric mood, hopelessness, anhedonia, and suicidal ideation are clear markers of depression. Previous history, drug history, and family history increase the risk of depression. While depression is common, it does not appear to affect survival.[84]

Symptoms of psychological distress are confounded by pain, which clearly affects HR-QOL and function. Most studies reported pain at diagnosis in at least 80% of the patients.[85] Overall, pain prevalence increased by up to 97% during disease course.

While chemotherapy may have a limited role in the treatment of pancreatic cancer to augment survival, there may be a role for the improvement of pain and performance status.[86] In the setting of unresectable pancreatic cancer, gemcitabine alone or with other chemotherapies has been reported to improve pain in up to 57% of patients. This has been confirmed via decreased analgesic consumption and pain severity scores.[87–89] The use of chemotherapy with the goal of improving pain or other symptoms must be carefully weighed against the burden of this treatment. In addition, it must be clear to the patient and family the intent of treatment so that miscommunications do not arise.

As 80% present with metastatic disease at diagnosis[67] palliative care is of primary importance. Interestingly, those that survive a pancreaticoduodenectomy have similar HR-QOL as normal subjects, indicating that for those who do survive, long-term HR-QOL is acceptable.[90]

Diagnosis and management of depression in pancreatic cancer. It is imperative for practitioners to look for symptoms of depression and refer quickly to those with expertise in treating these patients. It has been recommended that psycho-oncologists, or psychiatrists who focus on cancer patients, should be involved to help distinguish normal emotional reactions from those patients with a true psychiatric illness needing more extensive treatment.[82] These may include psychotherapy, cognitive-behavioral techniques, and psychopharmaceutical agents.

Tricyclic antidepressants are used most frequently to treat depression in pancreatic cancer patients.[91] These medications may also help with pain control. Dosing should start low and increase slowly due to sensitivity in this population. Nortriptyline should be used if there is hepatic dysfunction. Selective serotonin-reuptake inhibitors are typically also well tolerated and may have fewer toxicities. Psychostimulants can also be used if it is also desired to address fatigue.

A common situation is one in which a patient shows depression and distress in the context of increasing pain. Pain clearly impacts on depression and adequate pain control is mandatory in treating depression in the pancreatic cancer patient.[92] Although opioid analgesics in most cases are effective, underdosing still is common.[93] Nerve blocks of the celiac plexus may be required and give good relief in most patients.[94] It can also decrease opioid use and disturbing constipation.[95] Celiac plexus block may lead to longer survival for some patients,[96] although this has been disputed.[95]

In addition to tumor-related pain, GI symptoms, including anorexia, nausea, and vomiting, as well as narcotic-induced constipation and fatigue, have a major impact on patients' psychological well-being. Given the poor outlook in terms of survival and the burden of increasing symptoms, management should focus on maximum comfort and symptom control. The need for a multidisciplinary approach is highlighted by the fact that physical and emotional components of psychological burden are inextricably mingled in these patients.

CONCLUSIONS

GI cancers, while heterogeneous in presentation and treatment, have a commonality regarding impact related to nutritional status, eating, and bowel function. The social and psychological implications of these functions are all-encompassing and it is paramount to focus on these issues as a priority toward mental health. In addition, treatments often leave patients scarred and disfigured, which carries added psychosocial burdens. Finally, as these diseases frequently present in an advanced stage, palliative care issues are often important to consider.

Importantly, an interdisciplinary approach to GI cancers is imperative to recognize and address all symptoms, including those related to psychological difficulties, throughout treatment and long-term follow-up. This includes surgeons, medical oncologists, radiation oncologists, and other specialists such as gastroenterologists and interventional radiologists. Pain and palliative care specialists are often necessary. Finally, the importance of the psychological specialist must not be ignored.

ACKNOWLEDGMENT

The author thanks Mary Wagner for her insightful edits and comments.

REFERENCES

1. Jemal A, Siegel R, Ward E, et al. Cancer statistics, 2008. *CA Cancer J Clin.* 2008; 58:71–96.

2. Price BS, Levine EL. Permanent total parenteral nutrition: psychological and social responses of the early stages. *J Parenteral Ext Nutr.* 1979;3:48–52.

3. Fleishman SB. Treatment of symptom clusters: pain, depression, and fatigue. *J Natl Cancer Inst Monogr.* 2004;32:119–123.

4. Brown LM, Devesa SS, Chow WH. Incidence of adenocarcinomas of the esophagus among white Americans by sex, stage, and age. *J Natl Cancer Inst.* 2008;100:1184–1187.

5. Kubo A, Corley DA. Marked regional variation in adenocarcinomas of the esophagus and the gastric cardia in the United States. *Cancer.* 2002;95:2096–2102.

6. Katz SC, DeMatteo RP. Gastrointestinal stromal tumors and leiomyosarcomas. *J Surg Oncol.* 2008;97:350–359.

7. van Lanschot JJB, Tilanus HW, Voormolen MHJ, van Deelen RAJ. Recurrence pattern of oesophageal carcinoma after limited resection does not support wide local excision with extensive lymph node dissection. *Br J Surg.* 1994;81:1320–1323.

8. Kelsen DP, Ginsberg R, Pajak TF, et al. Chemotherapy followed by surgery compared with surgery alone for localized esophageal cancer. *N Engl J Med.* 1998;339:1979–1984.

9. Mariette C, Balon J, Piessen G, Fabre S, Van Seuningen I, Triboulet J. Pattern of recurrence following complete resection of esophageal carcinoma and factors predictive of recurrent disease. *Cancer.* 2003;97:1616–1623.

10. Lacueva FJ, Calpena R. Gastric cancer recurrence: clues for future approaches to avoiding an old problem. *J Clin Gastroenterol.* 2001;32:3–4.

11. Ries LAG, Young JL, Keel GE, Lin YD, Horner M-J, eds. SEER Survival Monograph: cancer survival among adults: US SEER program, 1988–2001, Patient and Tumor Characteristics. NIH Pub. No. 07-6215. Bethesda, MD: National Cancer Institute, SEER Program; 2007.

12. Branicki FJ, Law SY, Fok M, Poon RT, Chu KM, Wong J. Quality of life in patients with cancer of the esophagus and gastric cardia: a case for palliative resection. *Arch Surg.* 1998;133:316–322.

13. Kikuchi S, Tsutsumi O, Kobayashi N, et al. Does gastrojejunostomy for unresectable cancer of the gastric antrum offer satisfactory palliation? *Hepato-Gastroenterology.* 1999;46:584–587.

14. Buhl K, Schlag P, Herfarth C. Quality of life and functional results following different types of resection for gastric carcinoma. *Eur J Surg Oncol.* 1990;16:404–409.

15. Habu H, Saito N, Sato Y, Takeshita K, Sunagawa M, Endo M. Quality of postoperative life in gastric cancer patients seventy years of age and over. *Int Surg.* 1988;73:82–86.

16. Hulscher JBF, van Sandick JW, de Boer AGEM, et al. Extended transthoracic resection compared with limited transhiatal resection for adenocarcinomas of the esophagus. *N Engl J Med.* 2002;347:1662–1669.

17. Kono K, Iizuka H, Sekikawa T, et al. Improved quality of life with jejunal pouch reconstruction after total gastrectomy. *Am J Surg.* 2003;185:150–154.

18. Doglietto GB, Pacelli F, Caprino P, et al. Palliative surgery for far-advanced gastric cancer: a retrospective study on 305 consecutive patients. *Am Surg.* 1999;65:352–355.

19. Breeden JH. Alcohol, alcoholism, and cancer. *Med Clin N Am.* 1984;68:163–177.

20. Joeng JY, Kim YJ, Han JK, et al. Palliation of anastomotic obstructions in recurrent gastric carcinoma with the use of covered metallic stents: clinical results in 25 patients. *Surgery.* 2004;135:171–177.

21. Imbesi JJ, Kurtz RC. A multidisciplinary approach to gastrointestinal bleeding in cancer patients. J Supp Oncol. 2005;3:101–110.

22. Coia LR. The role of radiation therapy in gastrointestinal bleeding. *J Support Oncol.* 2005;3:111–112.

23. Paty PB, Nash GM, Baron P, et al. Long-term results of local excision for rectal cancer. *Ann Surg.* 2002;236:522–530.

24. Tytherleigh MG, Mortensen NJ. Options for sphincter preservation in surgery for low rectal cancer. *Br J Surg.* 2003;90:922–933.

25. Schmidt CE, Bestmann B, Kuchler T, Longo WE, Kremer B. Prospective evaluation of quality of life of patients receiving either abdominoperineal resection or sphincter-preserving procedure for rectal cancer. *Ann Surg Oncol.* 2005;12:117–123.

26. Jess P, Christiansen J, Bech P. Quality of life after anterior resection versus abdominoperineal extirpation for rectal cancer. *Scand J Gastroenterol.* 2002;37:1201–1204.

27. Gastinger I, Marusch F, Steinert R, et al. Protective defunctioning stoma in low anterior resection for rectal carcinoma. *Br J Surg.* 2005; 92:1137–1142.

28. Matthiessen P, Hallböök O, Rutegård J, Simert G, Sjödahl R. Defunctioning stoma reduces symptomatic anastomotic leakage after low anterior resection of the rectum for cancer. *Ann Surg.* 2007;246:207–214.

29. Bailey CMH, Wheeler JMD, Birks M, Farouk R. The incidence and causes of permanent stoma after anterior resection. *Colorectal Dis.* 2003;5:331–334.

30. O'Connell JB, Maggard MA, Ko CY. Colon cancer survival rates with the new American Joint Committee on Cancer sixth edition staging. *J Natl Cancer Inst.* 2004;96:1420–1425.

31. Gall CA, Weller D, Esterman A, et al. Patient satisfaction and health-related quality of life after treatment for colon cancer. *Dis Colon Rectum.* 2007;50:801–809.

32. Sprangers MAG, Taal BG, Aaronson NK, te Velde A. Quality of life in colorectal cancer: stoma vs. non stoma patients. *Dis Colon Rectum.* 1995;38:361–369.

33. Pachler J, Wille-Jørgensen P. Quality of life after rectal resection for cancer, with or without permanent colostomy. *Cochrane Database Syst Rev.* 2005;(2):CD004323.

34. Cornish JA, Tilney HS, Heriot AG, Lavery IC, Fazio VW, Tekkis PP. A meta-analysis of quality of life for abdominoperineal excision of rectum versus anterior resection for rectal cancer. *Ann Surg Oncol.* 2007;14:2056–2068.

35. Fucini C, Gattai R, Urena C, Bandettini L, Elbetti C. Quality of life among five-year survivors after treatment for very low rectal cancer with or without a permanent abdominal stoma. *Ann Surg Oncol.* 2008;15:1099–1106.

36. Zippe C, Nandipati K, Agarwal A, Raina R. Sexual dysfunction after pelvic surgery. *Int J Impot Res.* 2006;18:1–18.

37. Bergman B, Nilsson S, Petersen I. The effect on erection and orgasm of cystectomy, prostatectomy and vesiculectomy of cancer of the bladder: a clinical and electromyography study. *Br J Urol.* 1979;51:114–120.

38. Schmidt C, Bestmann B, Kuchler T, Longo WE, Kremer B. Ten-year historic cohort of quality of life and sexuality in patients with rectal cancer. *Dis Colon Rectum.* 2005;48:483–492.

39. Keating JP. Sexual function after rectal excision. *Aust NZ J Surg.* 2004;74:248–259.

40. Enker WE, Havenga K, Polyak T, Thaler H, Cranor M. Abdominoperineal resection via total mesorectal excision and autonomic nerve preservation for low rectal cancer. *World J Surg.* 1997;21:715–720.

41. Mannaerts GH, Schijven MP, Hendrikx A, Martijn H, Rutten HJ, Wiggers T. Urologic and sexual morbidity following multimodality treatment for locally advanced primary and locally recurrent rectal cancer. *Eur J Surg Oncol.* 2001;27:265–272.

42. MacDonald LD, Anderson HR. Stigma in patients with rectal cancer: a community study. *J Epidemiol Community Health.* 1984;38:284–290.

43. Cohen AM, Minsky BD, Schilsky RL. Cancer of the colon. In: Devita LT, Hellman S, Rosenberg SA, eds. *Cancer: principles and practice of oncology.* 5th ed. Philadelphia, PA: Lippincott; 1997:1163.

44. Genzdilov AV, Alexandrin GP, Simonov NN, Evtjuhin AI, Bobrov UF. The role of stress factors in the postoperative course of patients with rectal cancer. *J Surg Oncol.* 1977;9:517–523.

45. McMullen CK, Hornbrook MC, Grant, M, et al. The greatest challenges reported by long-term colorectal cancer survivors with stomas. *J Support Oncol.* 2008;6:175–182.

46. Rust J. Care of patients with stomas: the pouch change procedure. *Nurs Stand.* 2007;22:43–47.

47. Jeter K. Perioperative teaching and counseling. *Cancer.* 1992;70:1346–1349.

48. Krouse RS, Grant M, Wendel CS, et al. A mixed-methods evaluation of health-related quality of life for male veterans with and without intestinal stomas. *Dis Colon Rectum.* 2007;50:2054–2066.

49. Jain S, McGory ML, Ko CY, et al. Comorbidities play a larger role in predicting quality of life compared to having an ostomy. *Am J Surg.* 2007;194:774–779.

50. Sutherland AM, Orbach CE, Dyk RB, Bard M. The psychological impact of cancer and cancer surgery: I. Adaptation to the dry colostomy: preliminary report and summary of findings. *Cancer.* 1952;5:857–872.

51. Coons SJ, Chongpison Y, Wendel CS, Grant M, Krouse RS. Overall quality of life and difficulty paying for ostomy supplies in the VA ostomy health-related quality of life study: an exploratory analysis. *Med Care.* 2007;45:891–895.

52. Pittman J, Rawl SM, Schmidt CM, et al. Demographic and clinical factors related to ostomy complications and quality of life in veterans with an ostomy. *J Wound Ostomy Continence Nurs.* 2008;35:493–503.

53. Mitchell KA, Rawl SM, Schmidt CM, et al. Demographic, clinical, and quality of life variables related to embarrassment in veterans living with an intestinal stoma. *J Wound Ostomy continence Nurs.* 2007;34:524–532.

54. Baldwin CM, Grant M, Wendel CS, et al. Influence of intestinal stoma on spiritual quality of life of U.S. veterans. *J Holist Nurs.* 2008;26:185–194.

55. Thomas C, Madden F, Jehu D. Psychological effects of stomas—I. Psychosocial morbidity one year after surgery. *J Psychosom Res.* 1987;3l:311–316.

56. Thomas C, Turner P, Madden F. Coping and the outcome of stoma surgery. *J Psychosom Res.* 1988;32:457–467.

57. Krouse RS, Grant M, Rawl SM, et al. Coping and acceptance: the greatest challenge for veterans with intestinal stomas. *J Psychosom Res.* 2009;66:227–233.

58. Thomas C, Madden F, Jehu D. Psychological effects of stomas—II. Factors influencing outcome. *J Psychosom Res.* 1987;31:317–323.

59. Wade BE. Colostomy patients: psychological adjustment I at l0 weeks and I year after surgery in districts which employed stoma-care nurses and districts which did not. *J Adv Nurs.* 1990;15:1297–1304.

60. Bekkers MJTM, van Knippenberg FCE, van den Borne HW, van Berge-Henegouwen GP. Prospective evaluation of psychological adaptation to stoma surgery: the role of self-efficacy. *Psychosomatic Med.* 1996;58:183–191.

61. Oberst MT, James RH. Going home: patient and spouse adjustment following cancer surgery. *Top Clin Nurs.* 1985;7:46–57.

62. Symms MR, Rawl SM, Grant M, et al. Sexual health and quality of life among male veterans with intestinal ostomies. *Clin Nurs Spec.* 2008;22:30–40.

63. Schneider EC, Malin JL, Kahn KL, Ko CY, Adams J, Epstein AM. Surviving colorectal cancer. *Cancer.* 2007;110:2075–2082.

64. Persson E, Severinsson E, Hellstrom A. Spouses' perceptions of and reactions to living with a partner who has undergone surgery for rectal cancer resulting in a stoma. *Cancer Nurs.* 2004;27:85–90.

65. Gloeckner M. Perceptions of sexuality after ostomy surgery. *J Enteros Ther.* 1991;18:36–38.

66. Rozmovits L, Ziebland S. Expressions of loss of adulthood in the narratives of people with colorectal cancer. *Qual Health Res.* 2004;14:187–203.

67. Yeo CJ, Yeo TP, Hruban RH, et al. Cancer of the pancreas. In: DeVita VT, Hellman S, Rosenberg SA, eds. *Cancer. Principles and practice of oncology.* 7th ed. Philadelphia, PA: Lippincott Williams & Wilkins; 2005:945–986.

68. Smith AC, Dowsett JF, Russell RCG, Hatfield ARW, Cotton PB. Randomised trial of endoscopic stenting versus surgical bypass in malignant low bileduct obstruction. *Lancet.* 1994;344:1655–1660.

69. Telford JJ, Carr-Locke DL, Baron TH, et al. Palliation of patients with malignant gastric outlet obstruction with the enteral Wallstent: outcomes from a multicenter study. *Gastrointest Endosc.* 2004;60:916–920.

70. Van Heek NT, DeCastro SMM, van Eijck CH, et al. The need for a prophylactic gastrojejunostomy for unresectable periampullary cancer. *Ann Surg.* 2003;238:894–905.

71. Lillemoe KD, Cameron JL, Hardacre JM, et al. Is prophylactic gastrojejunostomy indicated for unresectable periampullary cancer? *Ann Surg.* 1999;230:322–330.

72. Picozzi VJ, Traverso LW. The Virginia Mason approach to localized pancreatic cancer. *Surg Oncol Clin N Am.* 2004;13:663–674.

73. Yaskin JD. Nervous symptoms at earliest manifestations of carcinoma of the pancreas. *J Am Med Assoc.* 1931;96:1664–1668.

74. Savage C, Butcher W, Noble D. Psychiatric manifestations in pancreatic disease. *J Clin Psychopathol.* 1952;13:9–16.

75. Latter KA, Wilbur DL. Psychic and neurological manifestations of carcinoma of the pancreas. *Mayo Clinic Proc.* 1937;12:457–462.

76. Karliner W. Psychiatric manifestations of cancer of the pancreas. *N Engl J Med.* 1967;56:2251–2252.

77. Arbitman R. Psychiatric manifestations of carcinoma of the pancreas. *Psychosomatics.* 1972;13:269–271.

78. Boyd AD, Riba M. Depression and pancreatic cancer. *J Natl Compr Canc Netw.* 2007;5:113–116.

79. Holland JC, Hughes AH, Tross S, et al. Comparative psychological disturbance in patients with pancreatic and gastric cancer. *Am J Psychiatry.* 1986;143:982–986.

80. Joffe RT, Rubinow DR, Denicoff KD, Maher M, Sindelar WF. Depression and carcinoma of the pancreas. *Gen Hosp Psychiatry.* 1986;8:241–245.

81. Carney CP, Jones L, Woolson RF, Noyes R, Doebbeling BN. Relationship between depression and pancreatic cancer in the general population. *Psychosom Med.* 2003;65:884–888.

82. Passik SD. Supportive care of the patient with pancreatic cancer: role of the psycho-oncologist. *Oncology.* 1996;10(suppl):33–34.

83. Passik SD, Breitbart WS. Depression in patients with pancreatic carcinoma. *Cancer.* 1996;78:615–626.

84. Sheibani-Rad S, Velanovich V. Effects of depression on the survival of pancreatic adenocarcinomas. *Pancreas.* 2006;32:58–61.

85. Saltzburg D, Foley KM. Management of pain in pancreatic cancer. *Surg Clin North Am.* 1989;69:629–649.

86. Koeppler H, Duru M, Grundheber M, et al. Palliative treatment of advanced pancreatic carcinoma in community-based oncology group practices. *J Support Oncol.* 2004;2:159–163.

87. Burris HA, Moore MJ, Andersen J, et al. Improvements in survival and clinical benefit with gemcitabine as first-line therapy for patients with advanced pancreas cancer: a randomized trial. *J Clin Oncol.* 1997;15:2403–2413.

88. Feliu J, Mel R, Borrega P, et al. Phase II study of a fixed dose-rate infusion of gemcitabine associated with uracil/tegafur in advanced carcinoma of the pancreas. *Ann Oncol.* 2002;13:1756–1762.

89. Ulrich-Pur H, Kornek GV, Raderer M, et al. A phase II trial of biweekly high dose gemcitabine for patients with metastatic pancreatic adenocarcinomas. *Cancer.* 2000;88:2505–2511.

90. Huang JJ, Yeo CJ, Sohn TA, et al. Quality of life and outcomes after pancreaticoduodenectomy. *Ann Surg.* 2000;231:890–898.

91. Ellison NM, Chevlen E, Still CD, Dubagunta S. Supportive care for patients with pancreatic adenocarcinoma: symptom control and nutrition. *Hematol Oncol Clin N Am.* 2002;16:105–121.

92. Shakin EJ, Holland J. Depression and pancreatic cancer. *J Pain Symptom Manage.* 1988;3:194–198.

93. Kelsen DP, Portenoy RK, Thaler HT, et al. Pain and depression in patients with newly diagnosed pancreas cancer. *J Clin Oncol.* 1995;13:748–755.

94. Sharp KW, Stevens EJ. Improving palliation in pancreatic cancer. *South Med J.* 1991;84:469–471.

95. Yan BY, Myers RP. Neurolytic celiac plexus block for pain control in unresectable pancreatic cancer. *Am J Gastroenterol.* 2007;102:430–438.

96. Lillemoe KD, Brigham RA, Harmon JW, Feaster MM, Saunders JR, d'Avis JA. Surgical management of small-bowel radiation enteritis. *Arch Surg.* 1983;118:905–907.

CHAPTER 19

Hepatobiliary Cancer

Richard Fielding

INTRODUCTION

Definitions. Hepatobiliary cancers (HBC) comprise two main types: cancers of the hepatocytes, hepatocellular carcinoma (HCC), and cancer of the epithelial cells of the intrahepatic bile ducts, cholangiocarcinoma (CAC). A combination of these types (HCC/CAC) occurs rarely. The liver is also preferentially invaded by secondary metastases, usually from digestive tract primaries. These are not discussed here.

The hepatobiliary system comprises the liver and contiguous bile ducts and gall-bladder which collect and store, respectively, bile from the liver. Functionally, the liver fulfills a complex range of roles: synthesis (coagulation and anticoagulation factors, albumen, cholesterol, bile); storage (vitamins, glycogen, minerals); metabolism (carbohydrate, protein, lipids, hormones); detoxification (metabolites, drug metabolism); immune (reticuloendothelial system); and secretory (bile, clotting factors) functions. Liver dysfunction generates complex pathologies affecting digestion, metabolism, weight, fluid-balance, and vasculature, amongst others.

Chronic inflammation of the liver arising from immunological or toxicological causes results in the diffuse scaring and other fibrotic changes known as cirrhosis that destroy the functional capacity of the liver, and underlies primary liver cancer (HCC). The consequence of this loss of function is a range of symptoms that may be the first signs of cirrhosis, including the sudden onset of abdominal fluid retention (ascites) or vascular symptoms, such as portal hypertension or eosophageal varices, leading to the discovery of HCC. More commonly, the first signs of HCC are abdominal pain or discomfort, jaundice, or weight loss and wasting. Any of these symptoms signal advanced disease. In CAC, a less common form of HBC, chronic inflammation of the bile duct generates a glandular tissue cancer (adenocarcinoma,) which usually presents with symptoms of bile-duct blockage (obstructive jaundice) characterized by yellowing of the skin and sclera, pale stools, itching, and back pain.

EPIDEMIOLOGY

Etiology and prevalence. Hepatobiliary cancer epidemiology varies by gender, ethnic group, and geographical regions (Table 19–1). Worldwide, HBC incidence is increasing. Currently, incidence is highest in eastern and South east Asia and sub-Saharan Africa. More males than females have HBC, partly because cirrhotic (fibrotic) HCC primarily affects older men. The HCC sex ratio is greater in high-incidence countries.[1] HCC is the most common form of liver cancer, the fifth most common cancer worldwide in terms of incidence, and the fourth in terms of annual mortality rate.[2] The high seroprevalence of Hepatitis B surface antigen (HBsAg) across Asia reflects widespread chronic Hepatitis B infection, the predominant cause of HCC in Asia, accounting for 52.3% of HCC cases worldwide. Korea, Japan, Italy, and Spain all have high HCsAg seroprevalence, reflecting widespread chronic Hepatitis C infection, which predominates as a cause in those countries, accounting for a further 25% of HCC cases worldwide.[3] Alcoholic cirrhosis and food contamination account for most of the remaining cases. Alcohol-related damage exacerbates viral hepatitis-induced cirrhosis, primarily in developed countries.[3] In Africa, HCC seems to be primarily linked to aflatoxin contamination of food. Consequently, while some national rates of HB/CsAg are low in absolute terms, pockets within the community may have very high rates; such is the case for Koreans living in the United States, for example.

Cholangiocarcinoma is primarily prevalent in South East Asia, particularly northern Thailand and Northern Laos, where it maps the endemic distribution of the liver flukes *Opisthorchis viverrini* and *Clonorchis sinensis*, the principal etiological agents. Chronic liver fluke infestation accounts for approximately 60% of HBC in northeastern Thailand and 7.7% of HBC in the United States.[4] In both locations viral hepatitis also remains an important cause of HCC.

Control. Estimates of new cases vary from 372,000[2] to between 500,000[3] and 564,000 (398,000 males, 166,000 females)[5] per annum. An annual incidence comprising 2.5%–7% of all cirrhotic patients[3] suggests that HBC constitutes 4.6% of all new cancers.[2] The annual mortality rate approximates to the incidence[2] and this implies that curative effectiveness is extremely limited once symptoms emerge. Eighty percent of the burden is in Asia and sub-Saharan Africa.[6] Vertical transmission from infected mother to baby during birth is an important mode of transmission in Asia, so vaccination at birth of all neonates is a highly effective preventive strategy against Hepatitis B virus (HBV) and hence HCC. Even where the mother is not HBV positive, neonatal immunization confers lifelong protection. Universal neonatal vaccination has reduced HBsAg prevalence significantly and will continue to do so in Taiwan, China, and Hong Kong. In Japan, Korea, Europe, and North America HCC rates are rising as Hepatitis C prevalence compounded by growing alcohol consumption increases. Hepatitis C vaccine development is in its early stages. In Europe and North and South America, Caucasian populations are less affected by HCC than Africans, who in turn are less affected than Asians, Pacific Islanders, and Native Americans.[7] This changing causal pattern is producing a downward shift in age of presentation of HCC toward 40–60 years.[7] In high-risk countries, onset can occur as early as 20 years of age. Because the ~5% survival rate of HCC is dismal, prevention of infection and cirrhosis, and screening of all high-risk groups are key strategies for disease control.

Cholangiocarcinoma occurs most often in the 50–70 year age range and is equally common in males and females. Control involves breaking the reproductive cycle of liver fluke and this is related to both education and development, but is compromised by the growing influence of other factors that influence etiology. Once symptoms appear prognosis for both HCC and CAC is poor.

Screening, diagnosis, and prognosis. Screening by ultrasound and blood alpha fetal protein (AFP) determination detects early disease (tumor size exceeding 2–3 cm), but is only cost-effective in high-risk populations where the incidence is high. Cost/tumor detected is inversely proportional to the tumor incidence,[8] especially when directed at older patients. Adjusting for lead-time bias (earlier detection of untreatable disease), initial studies of screening failed to show any benefit in survival but more recent studies demonstrate some improved outcomes in early-detected cases.[8] The time for tumors to reach detectable size (~2 cm) is 4–12 months,[3] so screening of high-risk individuals should therefore be performed about every 6 months.[3,9] In Japan, survival rates improved somewhat between 1991 and 1995, but have remained flat thereafter, probably due to greater detection of early-stage disease by screening which, as with almost all cancers, improves probability of

Table 19-1. Age-standardized (world population) liver cancer rate/100,000, top and bottom 10 countries by incidence

Location	ASR (W)—male	Location	ASR (W)—female
Korea	44.9	Thailand, Lampang	14.8
China, Guangzhou	42.5	Zimbabwe, Harare	12.7
Japan, Hiroshima	39.8	China, Jiashan	12.6
Italy, Naples	34.8	Korea	12.0
Thailand, Lampang	32.3	Japan, Hiroshima	11.9
Egypt, Gharbia	21.9	Italy, Naples	10.2
Philippines, Manila	21.7	Philippines, Manila	7.0
Singapore	18.8	Singapore	4.8
France, Calvados	15.2	Egypt, Gharbia	4.5
Switzerland, Ticino	16.3	French Polynesia	4.4
Peru, Trujilo	2.4	Cyprus	1.1
United Kingdom[a]	2.3	Canada	1.1
Tunisia, Sous	2.2	Norway	1.1
Norway	2.1	Australia, south	0.9
Canada	1.9	India, Karunagapaly	0.8
The Netherlands	1.8	Algeria, Setif	0.7
Iceland	1.8	The Netherlands	0.7
India, Nagpur	1.6	Tunisia, Sous	0.7
Belgium, Antwerp	1.2	Iceland	0.6
Algeria, Setif	1.1	Belgium, Antwerp	0.6

IARC data include national, regional, and city cancer registries. Some countries have multiple urban registries. Other urban registries in the same country may have higher rates than the next ranked country. For example, the top 20 registries ranked for female liver cancer incidence comprise nine Korean, four Chinese, two Japanese, two Italian, one Thai, one Zimbabwean, and a U.S. Los Angeles Korean registry. To give a broader international picture, only the registry reporting the highest incidence. Data were selected by priority: national, regional, urban.
[a]National rate estimated from provincial rates.
SOURCE: www.iarc.fr/

good outcomes.[10] The possibilities for early detection of both HCC and CAC, allowing significantly improved survival have been enhanced by identification of high-risk groups, closer monitoring, better imaging, and improved diagnostic and operative techniques.

Physical status, baseline liver function, ascites, bilirubin, and portal vein thromboembolism independently predict HCC outcome.[11,12] Tumor stage and liver function remain the most important prognostic features, with early-stage disease, enabling lower operative trauma, offering the best options for successful outcome. However, staging systems for HCC are varied, and have until recently been unclear and hence of uncertain utility.[13,14] In CAC, improved endoscopic investigation now enables earlier surgery, and this can double mean survival time to around 3 years.[15] For inoperable disease, radiotherapy offers the best intervention outcomes, though benefits are limited.[16]

MANAGEMENT

Cure versus disease control. Curative therapeutic approaches in HCC and CAC primarily depend on surgical resection or transplantation. For inoperable tumors, maintenance of liver function and palliative symptomatic treatment remain the only viable options for treatment. Surgical resection can temporarily improve quality of life (QOL) in the physical, social, and emotional well-being domains. However, because recurrence within 2–3 years is likely, a subsequent deterioration in QOL will be seen.[17] The surgery itself is major and can leave patients in a significantly weakened state if remaining liver function is compromised through cirrhosis. This brings problems associated with dependency and adjusting to life with often severely impaired functional status. The liver is, however, unique in that it is the only body organ that can fully regenerate if in a healthy state, though whole lobes once removed do not regrow.

Transplantation raises challenges, not only among the 5% or so who will receive it. There is the uncertainty and the wait: will there be a suitable cadaveric donor and will it come in time? For most this does not happen. The possibility of a live related donor, such as a sibling donating part of their liver is tantalizing and this might bring potential conflicts of interest and potentially pressure on one family member from others. There is not the space to explore these ethics here, but they do have a significant bearing as the recognition of what living with chronic viral hepatitis infection means. While transplants can be life saving, they bring with them the possibility of new problems. Other treatment approaches include chemoembolization, radioimplantation, and external beam radiation. A number of chemotherapy regimens have been used for HBC, including platinum compounds in combination with gemcitabine,[18] but until recently no agent was approved specifically for use in HBC and most reports suggest little long-term curative activity from chemotherapy. New monoclonal antibodies, such as multikinase and vascular endothelial growth factor (VEGF) inhibitors may offer some improvement but the evidence is not yet robust. Consequently, the HBC patient may face extreme helplessness. Transarterial chemoembolization (TACE) offers some palliative relief and can extend survival somewhat.[19] The patient with more advanced or recurrent disease is almost certainly facing a dire prognosis and will therefore need palliative care.

PSYCHO-ONCOLOGY

Clinical and research work on the roles of psychosocial factors in HBC progression is very limited, but increasing. Research to date has tended to focus on QOL, depression, and prognosis in those with HCC and is beginning to document the nature and extent of problems faced by patients with HBC.

Impact of Diagnosis. Many high-risk communities face significant barriers in accessing screening and early-diagnostic facilities.[20] Consequently, most cases of HCC and CAC are detected when patients seek assistance for symptoms, by which time disease is well advanced and treatment options are very limited. The diagnosis is effectively, though not always a confirmation of impending death and the impact on patient and family is significant. Where the patient is the breadwinner in a younger family, the implications for the family are severe. Older adult patients may have wider support networks of younger working adult children. Sensitive and supportive exploration of the family's situation is mandatory to determine likely impact. Families may seek expensive or traditional remedies to effect a cure but they may provide benefit only in the same way that many complimentary therapies do; by giving families some sense of control over the remorseless deterioration that can occur. Without treatment death usually occurs within 3–6 months.[10–13]

HCC prognosis: The roles of depression and quality of life. To date only one study has examined the prognostic role of psychological depression in HBC. Steel and colleagues[21] at Pittsburgh, United States, studied 101 HBC patients, noting that vascular invasion and Centre for Epidemiological Surveys Depression (CES-D) scale score independently predicted survival. In patients with vascular invasion, higher CES-D scores (≥16, clinical depression range) were associated with a significantly shorter median survival time of 5.2 months compared with a median of 11.2 months among patients with lower (<16) CES-D scores. In patients without vascular invasion, high CES-D scores were associated with a median survival of 17 months, while those with low CES-D scores survived for a median of 26.6 months. Initially, these results look very promising. However, confounding remains a possible explanation. Despite extensive efforts to adjust for potential contamination, including a binary adjustment for presence/absence of cirrhosis, patients with a history of heavy alcohol use had a lower natural killer cell (NKC) count, and low NKC count was also associated with higher CES-D scores. Inclusion of the NKC count in subsequent Cox's Regression and mediational models ejected CES-D scores from the equation. This suggests that confounding best explains the data: poor liver function follows alcohol use and also causes low NKC activity.[22,23] A causal association between depression and alcohol use would not be unusual: many people who abuse alcohol are depressed, and excess alcohol consumption increases rates of depressions.[24] Hence, depression might predate the declining liver function responsible for low NKC activity. Another study by the same group suggests that this is the most likely explanation.[25] More careful recent studies of women with advanced breast cancer have failed to confirm earlier claims of survival benefits from interventions that reduced distress and depression: declines in depression had no effect on survival.[26]

The link between alcohol use and depressive disorder indicates a potential point of psychological intervention. Programs targeting chronic drinking should also consider the co-occurrence of depressive disorders as treatment for these disorders might help to significantly improve recovery rates from drinking. Appropriate psychotherapeutic and antidepressant use are likely to make potentially important contributions to managing patients with known cirrhosis.

The role of health-related quality of life (HRQOL) as an independent prognostic indicator in HCC remains equivocal, facing as it does the difficult methodological problem of excluding reverse causality in any apparent relationship between QOL and outcomes. In a study of newly diagnosed Chinese HCC (n = 253) and lung cancer (n = 358) patients recruited between 1995 and 1997, QOL as measured by the Functional Assessment of Cancer Therapy-General (Chinese) (FACT-G Ch) scale[27] showed significant univariate associations between a number of dimensions of HRQOL, including functional, physical, and total FACT-G (Ch) scores; eating ability, eating appetite, and eating enjoyment; self-care ability; and survival. Cox models, fully adjusted for a wide range of clinical variables including disease stage (operable/inoperable), pain, mood, and prior treatment, showed no QOL predictors for either HCC or lung cancer patients. Only disease stage and eating appetite predicted survival in HCC, with earlier-stage patients, and those with better appetite surviving longer.[28] On a comparable sample of 233 Chinese patients with inoperable liver cancer, the EORTC QLQ-C30, another global QOL measure, was used to predict survival in a two-arm trial of palliative chemotherapy versus hormonal therapy.

Cox's models were again used to determine predictors of survival after adjustment for other independent influences. Poorer liver function, poorer appetite and being in the chemotherapy arm, and having higher physical domain and role domain QOL scores were associated with significantly longer survival.[29] While it is tempting to suggest that appetite loss, the consistent finding in both studies, reflects a QOL dimension, it could possibly reflect decline in liver function, a consistent predictor of outcome. These data suggest that lead-time bias accounts for the apparent survival effects associated with better QOL scores. We have to await clarification of this. The recent development of specific hepatic subscales for some of the generic QOL instruments may help to provide more resolution of these questions.[30,31] Considerable potential lies in using such targeted instruments to evaluate what interventions make a difference to HBC patients.

Since the predictive power of HRQOL may vary as a function of disease type, diseases that have better prognoses may show more sensitivity to HRQOL, hence conferring greater predictive power to HRQOL scores. In other words, the limited number of studies that have shown effects of HRQOL on outcomes may suffer from reverse causality. All QOL studies must effectively eliminate this problem if they hope to convincingly demonstrate a causal role for QOL on prognosis, irrespective of the disease involved.

Distress. There is a dearth of data on the prevalence of distress in non-Western cancer populations and HBC patients specifically. In 253 Hong Kong Chinese HCC patients, completing a simple 5-point visual analogue measure of "depression" at diagnosis 32% (95% confidence interval = 26.2%–37.7%) scored above 2 (mean 2.92). Six weeks later, among 203 survivors, fewer respondents 17% (11.8%–22.2%) scored above 2 (mean 2.98), and at 3 months after diagnosis of the 127 surviving patients, 15% (8.8%–23.2%) scored above 2 (mean 3.12). Among a comparison group of 377 Hong Kong Chinese lung cancer patients, who faced a similar prognostic outlook to that of HCC patients, 28% (23.5%–32.5%) scored above 2 (mean 3.03) on a 5-point VA measure of depression at diagnosis; at 3 months post diagnosis, of 302 survivors, 28% (23%–33%) scored above 2 (mean 3.0), and at 6 months post diagnosis, of 186 survivors, 27% (20.6%–33.4%) scored above 2 (mean 3.06). In contrast, a sample of 303 Hong Kong Chinese women with early-stage breast cancer completed the Chinese Health Questionnaire, a sinocized version of the General Health Questionnaire with 78% (73%–83%) achieving scores above the clinical cut-off in the moderate-to-severe range 1 week after surgery, to 64% (59%–69%) at 8 months postoperatively. A sample of 100 Mainland Chinese patients with HCC were examined using the CES-D scale and 49% (39%–59%) were found to have "possible depressive symptoms."[32] Akechi et al.[33] have reported that one in five of a sample of Japanese patients with advanced lung cancer experience clinical levels of depression, which persisted throughout the illness in 35%. This limited literature suggests that levels of distress and depression in HCC may not be particularly widespread relative to lung and breast cancer patients. However, mood and other emotional disturbances appear to be present at quite high levels in those affected.

Transitions to palliative care. Because the prognosis for HBC remains poor, most patients will face the need to accept transition from curative to palliative care with the attendant difficulties that this may raise. Highly integrated multidisciplinary team approaches to care of HBC patients are therefore most desirable, with palliative specialists involved from the beginning. Pain is a significant symptom following resection, or in the case of inoperable disease, from disease progress and fatigue from declining liver function. Pain significantly impairs QOL and has major interactions with depressive disorders, with the result that both pain and depression are amplified. Effective management of pain is therefore critical and screening for depressive disorders is warranted in all patients, with treatment as required. Pain is generally well controlled with natural and synthetic opiates and nonsteroidal drugs, and antidepressant medication may also be beneficial, while radionucleotides and radiotherapy are effective adjuncts, and depression responds well to psychotherapy.[34] However, a significant barrier to effective pain control using opiates is anxiety; among health professionals about the possibility of respiratory suppression and accidental overdosing, and among patients from fears of addiction.[35,36] These anxieties can be largely avoided among staff by involving the palliative physician or pain control team including anesthetists from the earliest stages following diagnosis as specialists in symptom management, and among patients by regular discussions with the patient to elicit any anxieties, and reassurance about addiction fears: opiate use in this context seldom induces dependency. In this way, abrupt change in the team or management orientation signaling a move from "cure" to "abandonment" can be minimized if not avoided all together.

Practitioner–patient interactions. Most HBC occurs in countries that may have few if any psycho-oncology resources, and interactions may be subject to traditional patterns of practitioner–patient relationships. Many Asian countries retain paternalistic attitudes to doctor–patient relationships and this restricts the open communication awareness necessary for effective western-style psychosocial care. There has been little investigation of this in Asia. Of 87 male terminal Japanese HBC patients 67% died without knowing their diagnosis, yet all knew and accepted their impending death.[37] Such observations are characteristic of strongly paternalistic values. Patient satisfaction among 222 Chinese HCC patients, measured by a indigenously developed and validated instrument, the nine-item Patient Satisfaction Questionnaire,[38] was strongly linked to doctors' expressions of caring. General emotional support from the doctor was a better predictor of patients' QOL than was informational support.[39] The desire for different types of communication (care vs. information) varies. HBC patients in Asia may at times prioritize feeling cared for over needing information. In many Asian communities, withholding bad news is considered to be a compassionate act and a doctor is expected to demonstrate caring though professional action. Communicating care is therefore beneficial and a critical skill in many communities. Younger patients tend to have more international values and may differ from older patients, desiring more precise information to manage their responsibilities, whereas older patients may be more fatalistic, relinquishing control, and expecting to be taken care of because of this tradition. This is sometimes difficult to understand in western cultures advocating individualized choice and responsibility, and risks being overlooked by contemporary medical school graduates used to algorithmic approaches to practice. Among 1136 Hong Kong adults more younger than older people expressed a desire to know their diagnosis and prognosis if they were to have cancer.[40] Hence, the need to assess each patient's communication needs remains central to effective care. Transitions from curative to palliative care may need to be carried out differently in Asian than in western cultures, but again, the integrated team approach offers greatest flexibility and can help minimize difficult discontinuities in supportive care.

Given that so many HBC patients are non-Caucasian, it is important for western trained and practicing health workers to consider these issues in their professional interactions with those from cultural minorities. Communicating care can take many forms: in the west, we may reach out to touch the patient; in Asia, giving the patient a glass of warm water can, for some, communicate the same concern. The evidence base for optimal communications practices awaits development in Asian contexts.

PREVENTION

HCC is one of the few cancers in which the causes are well known and highly preventable. Preventive strategies all have major psychosocial components and should be at the forefront of intervention efforts.

Primary prevention. Primary preventive strategies include advocacy to leverage attitude change and action for development strategies to improve food and water sanitation in Africa (prevention of aflatoxin contamination of food). Prevention of food contamination is important and relies on development aid being specifically targeted to rural communities for varieties of staples, such a groundnuts and corn with low susceptibility to *Aspergillus flavus* and *Aspergillus parasiticus*, the principal sources of aflatoxins and enhanced food storage facilities, such as grain silos to keep harvests dry, and the importance of safe handling in the retail chain. The extensive development needs of Africa and parts of Asia demand a broad-spectrum strategy. Providing a safe food supply is comparable to the need to provide clean drinking water as a basic developmental priority. In North East Thailand, health education on effective food hygiene and avoidance of eating uncooked animal products and provision of latrines are important strategies to control liver fluke infestation. Extensive efforts to prevent nematode infestation are already implemented, but face significant barriers in the form of traditional food practices. Raw cyprinoid river fish consumption is particularly problematic being a traditional food in this part of Thailand and a critical link in the life cycle of liver flukes. There is evidence that, despite widespread *O. viverrini* infestation, "only" approximately 10% of the population of North east Thailand develop CAC.[41] This implicates other lifestyle factors, including alcohol, salted-fish consumption, and smoking in CAC,[41] presenting an opportunity for lifestyle reeducation.

Hepatitis transmission is a major problem. Promoting neonatal vaccination against Hepatitis B in high prevalence areas to prevent vertical transmission where this is not already performed is a core strategy. The WHO advocated that Hepatitis B vaccination should be universal for all neonates and adolescents by 1997 and by 2003 151 countries had followed this recommendation.[42] Uptake of hepatitis B vaccination during adolescence is generally high, often exceeding 90%.[43] There is currently no vaccine against Hepatitis C, so transmission prevention remains the most important strategy. Psychosocial inputs have important roles in enhancing HBC prevention. Reducing transmission of hepatitis can be facilitated by risk behavior prevention and alcohol abuse education, possibly by way of substance abuse programs, needle replacement programs, and health awareness campaigns defining transmission routes (unprotected intercourse; injecting drug use; sharing eating, shaving, teeth-cleaning utensils; group eating habits that transmit saliva to and from shared dishes at meal times). Internet-based education is increasing but is less accessible in the poorer communities where need is usually greatest. Promoting taxation and other controls on alcohol, the primary noninfectious cause of cirrhosis, is a key strategy and public policy advocacy is a critical component of this. Non-hepatitis cirrhosis increases with the growing availability of cheap alcohol.[44] A study of Japanese men attributes 71% of deaths due to cirrhosis and 77% of deaths from HCC to alcohol abuse. In older age groups, the risk for HCC attributable to alcohol was much lower than for other cancers.[45] This suggests that as HBV and HBC decline as causes of HCC in Japan and elsewhere due to vaccination and other policies, alcohol becomes an increasingly important cause of HCC. Public policies, such as in Hong Kong where alcohol tax has recently been removed all together, can upregulate alcohol consumption and are detrimental for control of HBC. Taxation policies to control pricing are therefore likely to be crucial elements in helping to prevent alcoholic cirrhosis, particularly by limiting consumption amongst younger and teenage drinker. Though these areas are not part of the traditional domain of psycho-oncology, they nonetheless represent an important branch of the discipline that awaits development or convergence with other disciplines such as public health and health promotion: cancer control increasingly relies upon behavioral interventions because lifestyle factors are so important. Cancer control efforts extend from population to individual interventions and there is growing recognition of the need for multidisciplinary interventions. In this regard psycho-oncology has important contributions to offer.

Secondary prevention. Secondary prevention activities include detection-related issues, enhancing understanding and facilitating responses, and adherence to screening programs for at-risk populations or early-detection strategies in high-risk communities, facilitating adherence to antiviral medication which can reduce subsequent cancer rates by up to 40% in HBsAg- or HCsAg-positive groups, and provision of advice for personal health enhancement and to limit onward transmission. Secondary prevention strategies need to target at-risk groups and, as these are traditionally harder to reach groups (injecting drug users, commercial sex clients and providers), strategies need to be innovative. Several studies have looked at both knowledge of risk and screening uptake in high-risk populations. Ma and colleagues[46] explored knowledge, attitudes, and behavior surrounding HBV screening among 256 Vietnamese-Americans living in the United States. While 46% of the respondents had heard of HBV, 33% knew about HBV screening and 35% had taken vaccination. However, uptake levels were low, with only 7.5% screened and 6% vaccinated.[46] An earlier study examined the same questions among 715 Vietnamese-Americans, and found that 81% had heard of HBV, and 67% had been screened for HBV, but again, despite large differences in prevalence, knowledge deficits were apparent, particularly regarding transmission pathways.[47] Among a sample of 320 Cambodian immigrant women living in the eastern United States, 56% had heard of HBV and only 38% had been screened.[48] Again knowledge deficits were identified.

Treatment of people chronically infected with HBV or HCV can reduce the risk of cirrhosis. Around one-third of chronically infected HBV patients show signs of liver fibrosis.[49] Long-term antiviral treatment is effective in preventing development of fibrosis and HCC in chronic HBV carriers.[50] Long-term interferon therapy for chronic HCV infection seems to cause depressive responses in recipient[51] affecting willingness to continue treatment.

Tertiary prevention. Tertiary prevention interventions include needs assessment, understanding of emotional impacts, and counseling among people and families diagnosed with cancer. In particular, helping patients for whom there is a possibility of related-donor transplantation is an area that has been little explored. A Japanese study examined the impact of liver resection for treatment of HCC and concluded that "depression and anxiety were not very strong" following surgery, but found a close interaction between QOL and symptoms of depression and anxiety. The authors interpreted their results to indicate that improving QOL through debulking or removal of the tumors was a significant influence on helping to resolve symptoms of depression and anxiety.[52] Facilitating communications awareness and optimization in clinicians working with such patients, and identifying the impacts of diagnosis are other important areas. Finally, very few evaluations of interventions to address HBC patients' psychosocial needs are to be found. One small trial of 28 HBC patients randomized to receive either psychosocial counseling or attention control concluded that such interventions were feasible, but lacked statistical power to show any effects from the intervention.[53] Tertiary prevention areas are the traditional focus of psycho-oncology, but in the case of HBC, because these diseases are well understood and preventable, psycho-oncologists can play a major role in contributing to primary and secondary prevention.

CONCLUDING COMMENTS

Hepatobiliary cancers are widespread and important cancers. The pattern of incidence is changing, patients are becoming younger and as HBV vaccination becomes more widespread, HCV and alcoholic cirrhosis will become more prevalent as causes. Being relatively well understood and preventable, focus on preventive efforts in these cancers is urgently needed. It is a major public health challenge to reach those usually poor or marginalized communities with the highest risk prevalence. The high incidence of HBC means that there is a large unmet need among this group of patients for more traditional psycho-oncology services, but many poor communities may have limited access to medical care and many affected patients do not come to the attention of those regional centers that tend to have specialist counseling or psycho-oncology services. In most developed countries, the incidence of HBC is currently lower but will rise with the growing consumption of alcohol. Often there is a limited range of expertise other than in one or two regional centers, and immigrant groups most affected may find themselves facing several barriers to diagnostic, physical or support and counseling services. Reasons include consultation patterns, low index of clinical suspicion, less onward referral to specialists, and linguistic, geographical, and financial barriers to care. Cultural patterns of care which keep disease "in the family" to avoid stigmatization are also issues to address. Finding ways to overcome these challenges is

important if psycho-oncological care is to be effectively implemented for these patients.

REFERENCES

1. Yu MC, Yuan JM, Govindarajan S, Ross RK. Epidemiology of hepatocellular carcinoma. *Can J Gastroenterol*. 2000;14:703–709.
2. Kew MC. Epidemiology of hepatocellular carcinoma. *Toxicology*. 2002;181–182:35–38.
3. Montalto G, Cervello M, Giannitrapani L, Dantona F, Terranova A, Castagnetta LA. Epidemiology, risk factors, and natural history of hepatocellular carcinoma. *Ann NY Acad Sci USA*. 2002;963:13–20.
4. Srivatanakul P, Sriplung H, Deerasamee S. Epidemiology of liver cancer: an overview. *Asian Pac J Cancer Prev*. 2004;5:118–125.
5. Bosch FX, Ribes J, Cléries R, Díaz M. Epidemiology of hepatocellular carcinoma. *Clin Liver Dis*. 2005;9:191–211.
6. McGlynn KA, London WT. Epidemiology and natural history of hepatocellular carcinoma. *Best Pract Res Clin Gastroenterol*. 2005;19:3–23.
7. El-Serag HB. Hepatocellular carcinoma: an epidemiologic view. *J Clin Gastroenterol*. 2002;35:s72-s78.
8. Yuen MF, Lai CL. Screening for hepatocellular carcinoma: survival benefits and cost-effectiveness. *Ann Oncol*. 2003;14:1463–1467.
9. Sherman H. Hepatocellular carcinoma: epidemiology, risk factors, and screening. *Semin Liver Dis*. 2005;25:143–154.
10. Toyoda H, Kumada T, Kiriyama S, et al. Changes in the characteristics and survival rate of hepatocellular carcinoma from 1976 to 2000: analysis of 1,365 patients in a single institution in Japan. *Cancer*. 2004;100:2415–2421.
11. Martins A, Cortez-Pinto H, Marquez-Vidal P, et al. Treatment and prognostic factors in patients with hepatocellular carcinoma. *Liver Int*. 2006;26:680–687.
12. Taura N, Hamasaki K, Nakao K, et al. The impact of newer treatment modalities on survival in patients with hepatocellular carcinoma. *Clin Gastroenterol Hepatol*. 2006;4:1177–1183.
13. Sala M, Forner A, Varela M, Bruix J. Prognostic prediction in patients with hepatocellular carcinoma. *Semin Liver Dis*. 2005;25:171–180.
14. Kung JW, MacDougall M, Madhavan KK, Garden OJ, Parkes RW. Predicting survival in patients with hepatocellular carcinoma: a UK perspective. *Eur J Surg Oncol*. 2007;33:188–194.
15. Yang WL, Zhang XC, Zhang DW, Tong BF. Diagnosis and surgical treatment of hepatic hilar cholangiocarcinoma. *Hepatobiliary Pancreat Dis Int*. 2007;6:631–635.
16. Petera J, Papik Z, Zouhar M, Jansa J, Odrazka K, Dvorak J. The technique of intensity-modulated radiotherapy in the treatment of cholangiocarcinoma. *Tumori*. 2007;93:257–263.
17. Blazeby JM, Currie E, Zee BC, et al. Quality of life in patients with hepatocellular carcinoma, the EORTC QLQ-HCC18. *Eur J Cancer*. 2004;40:2439–2444.
18. Verderame F, Russo A, Di Leo R, et al. Gemcitabine and oxaliplatin combination chemotherapy in advanced biliary tract cancers. *Ann Oncol*. 2006;17:68–72.
19. Wang YB, Chen MH, Yan K, Yang W, Dai Y, Yin SS. Quality of life after radiofrequency ablation combined with transcatheter arterial chemoembolization for hepatocellular carcinoma: comparison with transcatheter arterial chemoembolization alone. *Qual Life Res*. 2007;16:389–397.
20. Mann AG, Trotter CL, Adekoyejo Balogun M, Ramsey ME. Hepatitis C in ethnic minority populations in England. *J Viral Hepatitis*. 2008;15:421–426.
21. Steel JL, Geller DA, Gamblin TC, Olek MC, Carr BI. Depression, immunity, and survival in patients with hepatobiliary carcinoma. *J Clin Oncol*. 2007;25:2343–2344.
22. Hirofuji H, Kakumu S, Fuji A, Ohtani Y, Murase K, Tahara H. Natural killer and activated killer activities in chronic liver disease and hepatocellular carcinoma: evidence for a decreased lymphokine-induced activity of effector cells. *Clin Exp Immunol*. 1987;68:348–356.
23. Hirata M, Harihara Y, Kita Y, et al. Immunosuppressive effect of chenodeoxycholic acid on natural killer cell activity in patients with biliary atresia and Hepatitis C virus-related liver cirrhosis. *Dig Dis Sci*. 2002;47:1100–1106.
24. Conway KP, Compton W, Stinson FS, Grant BF. Lifetime comorbidity of DSM-IV mood and anxiety disorders and specific drug use disorders: results from the National Epidemiologic Survey on Alcohol and Related Conditions. *J Clin Psychiatry*. 2006;67:247–257.
25. Steel JL, Chopra K, Olek MC, Carr BI. Health-related quality of life: hepatocellular carcinoma, chronic liver disease, and the general population. *Qual Life Res*. 2007;16:203–215.
26. Kissane DW, Grabsch B, Clarke DM, et al. Supportive-expressive group therapy for women with metastatic breast cancer: survival and psychosocial outcome from a randomized controlled trial. *Psycho-Oncology*. 2007;16:277–286.

27. Yu CLM, Fielding R, Chan CLW, et al. Measuring quality of life in Chinese cancer patients: a validation of the Chinese version of the Functional Assessment of Cancer Therapy General (FACT-G) scale. *Cancer*. 2000;88:1715–1727.

28. Fielding R, Wong WS. Quality of life as a predictor of cancer survival among Chinese liver and lung cancer patients. *Eur J Cancer*. 2007;43:1723–1730.

29. Yeo W, Mo FK, Koh J, et al. Quality of life is predictive of survival in patients with unresectable hepatocellular carcinoma. *Ann Oncol*. 2006;17:1037–1038.

30. Heffernan N, Cella D, Webster K, et al. Measuring health-related quality of life in patients with hepatobiliary cancers: the functional assessment of cancer therapy-hepatobiliary questionnaire. *J Clin Oncol*. 2002;20:2215–2239.

31. Poon RT, Fan ST, Yu WC, Lam BK, Chan FY, Wong J. A prospective longitudinal study of quality of life after resection of hepatocellular carcinoma. *Arch Surg*. 2001;136:693–699.

32. Wan LH, Gong ME, Liu M, Chen Y, Long T. The relationship between depressive symptom and immature defense mechanism in patients with primary liver cancer. *Chin Mental Health J*. 2003;17:153–156.

33. Akechi T, Okamura H, Nishiwaki Y, et al. Psychiatric disorders and associated and predictive factors in patients with unresectable non-small cell lung carcinoma: a longitudinal study. *Cancer*. 2001;92:2609–2622.

34. Lorenz KA, Lynn J, Dy SM, et al. Evidence for improving palliative care at the end of life: a systematic review. *Ann Intern Med*. 2008;148:147–159.

35. Fielding R. Discrepancies between patient and nurses' perception of post-operative pain: shortcomings in pain control. *J HK Med Assoc*. 1994;46:142–146.

36. Fielding R, Irwin MG. The knowledge and perceptions of nurses and interns regarding acute pain and post-operative pain control. *HK Med J*. 2006;12:31–34.

37. Maeda Y, Hagihara A, Kobori E, Nakayama T. Psychological process from hospitalization to death among uninformed terminal liver cancer patients in Japan. *BMC Palliat Care*. 2006;5:6.

38. Wong WS, Fielding R, Wong CM, Hedley AJ. Psychometric properties of the 9-item Chinese Patient Satisfaction Questionnaire (ChPSQ-9) in Chinese patients with hepatocellular carcinoma. *Psycho-Oncology*. 2008;17:292–300.

39. Wong WS, Fielding R. The association between patient satisfaction and quality of life in Chinese lung and liver cancer patients. *Med Care*. 2008;46:293–302.

40. Fielding R, Hung J. Preference for information and treatment-decision involvement in cancer care among a Hong Kong Chinese population. *Psycho-Oncology*. 1996;5:321–329.

41. Honjo S, Srivatanakul P, Sriplung H, et al. Genetic and environmental determinants of risk for cholangiocarcinoma via *Opisthorchis viverrini* in a densely infested area in Nakhon Phanom, northeast Thailand. *Int J Cancer*. 2005;117:854–860.

42. Centre for Disease Control and Prevention. Global progress toward universal childhood hepatitis B vaccination, 2003. *MMWR Morb Mortal Wkly Rep*. 2003;52:868–870.

43. Wallace LA, Bramley JC, Ahmed S, et al. Determinants of universal adolescent hepatitis B vaccine uptake. *Arch Dis Child*. 2004;89:1041–1042.

44. Xie X, Mann RE, Smart RG. The direct and indirect relationships between alcohol prevention measures and alcoholic liver cirrhosis mortality. *J Stud Alcohol*. 2000;61:499–506.

45. Makimoto K, Oda H, Higuchi S. Is heavy alcohol consumption an attributable risk factor for cancer-related deaths among Japanese men? *Alcohol Clin Exp Res*. 2000;24:382–385.

46. Ma GX, Shive SE, Fang CY, et al. Knowledge, attitudes, and behaviors of hepatitis B screening and vaccination and liver cancer risks among Vietnamese Americans. *J Health Care Poor Underserv*. 2007;18:62–73.

47. Taylor VM, Choe JH, Yasui Y, Li L, Burke N, Jackson JC. Hepatitis B awareness, testing, and knowledge among Vietnamese American men and women. *J Community Health*. 2005;30:477–490.

48. Taylor VM, Jackson JC, Chan N, Kuniyuki A, Yasui Y. Hepatitis B knowledge and practices among Cambodian American women in Seattle, Washington. *J Community Health*. 2002;27:151–163.

49. Fung J, Lai CL, But D, Wong D, Cheung TK, Yuen MF. Prevalence of fibrosis and cirrhosis in chronic hepatitis B: implications for treatment and management. *Am J Gastroenterol*. 2008;103:1421–1426.

50. Yuen MF, Seto WK, Chow DH, et al. Long-term lamivudine therapy reduces the risk of long-term complications of chronic hepatitis B infection even in patients without advanced disease. *Antivir Ther*. 2007;12:1295–1303.

51. Moore SM. Concurrent and longitudinal relations between interferon alpha treatment for remediation of Hepatitis C and depression in a sample of incarcerated male adults. *Diss Abs Int A Hum Soc Sci*. 2004;64:3963.

52. Koyama K, Fukunishi I, Kudo M, Sugawara Y, Makuuchi M. Psychiatric symptoms after hepatic resection. *Psychosomatics*. 2003;44:86–87.

53. Steel JL, Nadeau K, Olek M, Carr BI. Preliminary results of an individually-tailored psychosocial intervention for patients with advanced heapatobiliary carcinoma. *J Psychosocial Oncol*. 2007;25:19–42.

CHAPTER 20

Lung Cancer

Mary E. Cooley, Julie Lynch, Kilah Fox, and Linda Sarna

OVERVIEW OF LUNG CANCER

People with lung cancer are acknowledged to have more unmet psychosocial needs and greater distress than people with other cancers. In part, this is because, as yet, there is no effective method for the early detection of lung cancer and the majority of people are diagnosed with advanced stage disease. Numerous studies have delineated the array of psychosocial consequences associated with lung cancer. The purposes of this chapter are to review the literature on the psychosocial needs of people with lung cancer across the disease and treatment trajectory, including the emerging literature on the psychosocial concerns of those undergoing experimental lung cancer screening and lung cancer survivors, to suggest evidence-based strategies to address the needs of this population and identify gaps in the literature.

Tobacco and the legacy of lung cancer. To have a context for understanding the psychosocial consequences of lung cancer, it is important to address the enormity of the lung cancer problem both in the United States (US) and worldwide. Lung cancer emerged in the twentieth century as the leading cause of cancer-related mortality both in the United States and worldwide. The primary reasons for this high mortality are the lack of effective methods for early diagnosis and the minimal efficacy of current treatments for advanced stage disease.

There are nearly 1.2 million deaths per year worldwide with 49% or 574,000 of these deaths occurring in Asian countries, 28% or 342,000 deaths in Europe, and 15% or 178,000 deaths in North America.[1] In the United States in 2008, approximately 162,000 people died from lung cancer, which accounted for 29% of all cancer deaths and resulted in 2,700,000 person-years of life lost. In the United States, although the four major cancer sites have seen significant decreases in mortality rates from 1995 through 2004, lung cancer in females has continued to increase at a rate of 0.2% per year.[2]

The incidence of lung cancer worldwide reflects a pattern similar to the mortality rate. In 2004, there were 1.35 million newly diagnosed cases of lung cancer with 49% or 661,000 of these in Asia, 28% or 375,000 in Europe, and 17% or 226,000 in North America. In the twenty-first century, 70% of lung cancers are projected to occur in developing countries.[1] Yet, the age-standardized incidence rates per 100,000 vary widely across different countries. In most countries, including the United States, lung cancer is one of the most common cancers, representing 15% of all newly diagnosed cancers.[1,2] Lung cancer incidence and mortality rates vary by race/ethnicity, age, and gender. Lung cancer incidence and mortality rates are highest among African Americans. Moreover, disparity rates are highest among African American male patients. Although reasons for these disparities are not entirely clear, differences in access to care, quality of health care delivery, and/or having an increased number of comorbidities may play a role.[3]

The rise and slight decline in United States in lung cancer incidence and mortality has paralleled trends of cigarette smoking. It is now widely acknowledged that cigarette smoking causes 85%–90% of lung cancers.[4] The risk of death from smoking-related lung cancer is correlated with age of initiation, the number of packs smoked, and the total number of years smoking persists. However, even nonsmokers are diagnosed with lung cancer, especially women. Other risk factors for lung cancer include exposure to environmental tobacco smoke, occupational exposures such as radon, and genetics.

Understanding the epidemiology of lung cancer is important in addressing one of the unique psychosocial concerns of people with lung cancer, the stigma and blame due to the link with tobacco use.[5] It is important to remember that most smokers begin smoking in their early youth, before they were legally able to purchase cigarettes. Ample evidence supports that smoking is not just a "habit."[6] Nicotine is very addictive as only 5 out of 100 smokers who make a quit attempt are able to quit smoking 1-year later without assistance. As tobacco control policy efforts in the United States have increased and smoking has declined, the social unacceptability of smoking[7] has contributed to a unique situation for people with lung cancer, as compared to patients diagnosed with other types of cancer. Patients with lung cancer with a smoking history report fear of poorer health care.[5] Conversely, some healthcare providers (HCP) may be reluctant to even address tobacco status with patients with lung cancer because they do not want them to experience distress. This of course prevents smokers from getting tobacco dependence treatment or former-smokers from getting the support needed to prevent relapse.

Overview of lung cancer and its treatments. Psychosocial concerns can vary according to the type of histology of lung cancer and the stage of disease as this affects the type of cancer treatment and prognosis. Two major types of lung cancer exist: non-small cell lung cancer (NSCLC) and small cell lung cancer (SCLC). NSCLC is the major type of lung cancer, comprising approximately 80%–85% of all lung cancers, whereas SCLC makes up the remaining 15%–20% of cases. NSCLC consists of several histological types; the most common include squamous cell carcinoma, adenocarcinoma, bronchoalveolar carcinoma, and large cell carcinoma. Patients with NSCLC may experience metastasis to the brain which can cause a full range of psychological consequences, including alterations in cognitive function. As the majority of patients with SCLC present with widely metastatic disease, central nervous system involvement is common. Early stage NSCLC (stage I and II) is treated with surgery as the primary modality. When surgery is not an option, radiation therapy is used for control of the primary tumor and chemotherapy is used for advanced locoregional and metastatic disease.[8] The use of combined modalities has become more common to enhance survival rates. Five-year survival rates for those with early stage NSCLC can be as high as 70%, whereas survival rates for those with locoregional disease range from 10% to 30% and survival rates for those with metastatic disease are less than 5%.[8]

A two-stage system is usually used for SCLC: limited and extensive disease. Limited stage disease is treated with chemotherapy and radiation, whereas extensive stage is treated with chemotherapy alone. In contrast to NSCLC, surgery plays a limited role in the treatment of SCLC. Limited stage SCLC is treated with curative intent, with approximately 20% of patients achieving a cure. Although 20%–30% of patients with extensive stage SCLC may experience complete response to initial treatment with chemotherapy, the response duration is usually short with a median survival of 4 months.[8]

LUNG CANCER PREVENTION AND EARLY DETECTION

Eliminating uptake of smoking, exposure to secondhand smoke, and promoting smoking cessation are essential for preventing the majority of lung cancers. Even after diagnosis, smoking cessation remains an important way to improve clinical outcomes (i.e., health-related quality of life, response to cancer treatment, risk of cancer recurrence, and survival) after the diagnosis of lung cancer.[9-11] Further information about smoking cessation and cancer is found in Chapter 2.

Currently, there is no recommended screening test for the early detection of lung cancer. Risk for developing lung cancer remains elevated among former-smokers for many years after smoking cessation. In fact, 50% of all ever-smokers are former-smokers,[12] thus, there has been a tremendous interest in finding ways to detect lung cancer at earlier stages among those who are at high risk for developing lung cancer.

In the past, randomized trials evaluated chest x-ray and sputum cytology as an early detection test but did not find evidence that these tests were effective in decreasing lung cancer mortality.[13] A new imaging technology, low-dose computed tomography (CT) or helical CT, has emerged as a potential screening test for lung cancer. Helical CT can detect tumors well under 1 cm in size as compared to x-ray which can detect tumors approximately 1–2 cm in size. A large randomized screening trial, the National Lung Cancer Screening Trial sponsored by the National Cancer Institute, for individuals at risk for developing lung cancer is underway (http://www.cancer.gov/clinicaltrials/NCI-NLST). Preliminary results are promising, but final results of this trial are expected in 2010.

Identification of an effective screening tool for lung cancer has enormous implications for future treatment and care of those at risk for developing lung cancer. Several studies have examined psychological and behavioral issues surrounding the use of helical CT for lung cancer screening, especially decisions around quitting smoking. Schnoll and colleagues[14] examined interest in and awareness of helical CT for lung cancer screening, correlates of participation in screening, and potential reactions to screening results among high-risk individuals. A total of 172 current- or former-smokers with no personal history of lung cancer completed a survey. Results of the study indicated that 77% of responders were unaware of screening for lung cancer and 62% were highly interested in screening for lung cancer. Interest in screening was positively related to higher screening self-efficacy, higher knowledge of asymptomatic illness, and greater perceived cancer risk. In the face of a positive scan, 52% of smokers indicated that they would quit smoking, whereas 43% would consider quitting and less than 3% would continue smoking. In the face of a negative scan, 19% of smokers indicated that they would quit smoking, whereas 61% would consider quitting and 20% would continue smoking. Fifty-nine percent of smokers indicated that they were highly interested in smoking cessation counseling along with lung cancer screening.

Several other studies have examined smoking cessation rates among high-risk individuals who underwent helical CT screening and found that notification of abnormal test results yielded smoking abstinence rates between 7% and 42%.[15,16] Townsend and colleagues[15] examined the relationship between smoking cessation and receiving results from three annual helical CT scans for screening. Among current-smokers at baseline, smoking abstinence during the 3-year follow-up was associated with older age, worse pulmonary function, and having an abnormal CT finding the previous year requiring interim follow-up. Results from this study indicated that smokers with abnormal CT findings from multiple CT screens were more likely to be abstinent at the 3-year follow-up (19.8% abstinence with no abnormal CT screen, 19.8% with one abnormal CT screen, 28% with two abnormal CT screens, and 42% with three abnormal CT screens). Taylor and colleagues[16] examined the impact of lung cancer screening on smoking cessation and motivational readiness to quit smoking among 313 high-risk individuals undergoing helical CT screening. Before receiving the helical CT, 20% of participants indicated that they were ready to stop smoking in the next 30 days, 45% were ready to stop smoking within the next 6 months, and 35% were not thinking about quitting smoking. At 1 month after the helical CT scan was completed, 7% of smokers indicated that they had quit smoking and 4% of former-smokers had relapsed back to smoking. Among younger smokers (≤64 years), an abnormal helical CT result was associated with an increased readiness to quit smoking, whereas a normal result was associated with becoming less ready to quit smoking. Schnoll and colleagues[17] also examined smoking cessation rates and correlates of

motivational readiness to quit smoking among 55 female smokers who underwent helical CT screening for lung cancer. Following lung cancer screening and meeting with an oncologist to discuss smoking cessation, 16% of women quit smoking. Greater motivation to quit smoking was associated with older age, lower nicotine addiction, fewer lung cancer symptoms, higher quitting self-efficacy, and acknowledgment of the advantages of quitting smoking.

Although the data are encouraging, CT screening for lung cancer is still experimental. Taken together, these studies of patients undergoing helical CT screening indicate that the experience of screening provides an opportunity to enhance treatment for tobacco dependence. These findings also indicate that more intensive interventions are needed to address the powerful addictive properties of nicotine that makes quitting smoking a difficult task even among people who view themselves as vulnerable to lung cancer.

PSYCHOSOCIAL AND BEHAVIORAL ISSUES AND LUNG CANCER

The illness trajectory extends from prevention and early detection of lung cancer to diagnosis, active treatment, surveillance, survivorship, recurrence, and end-of-life. The following section of this chapter will review common lung cancer symptoms that patients and their families may experience during various phases of the illness trajectory as these are often inextricably tied to psychosocial distress and management.

LUNG CANCER SYMPTOMS

At the time of diagnosis, most patients experience a range of symptoms that are related to location and size of the primary tumor and sites of metastases. Symptoms, including those influencing mental status, also may be influenced by the biochemical impact of the tumor (e.g., altered calcium levels). These symptoms change over time, influenced by different treatment options, and often influence psychosocial concerns.

The most common symptoms in newly diagnosed lung cancer patients are fatigue, pain, insomnia, and depression. Cooley and colleagues[18] examined the prevalence of symptoms over time in 117 patients receiving treatment for lung cancer and noted that fatigue and pain were the most common symptoms for all treatment groups at entry to the study and these symptoms continued to be the most common symptoms at 3 and 6 months. However, difficulty in breathing and coughing become problematic at 3 and 6 months for approximately one-third of patients. Altogether, patients were noted to experience an average of four symptoms at entry to the study, three symptoms at 3 months and three symptoms at 6 months. Wang and colleagues[19] reported the prevalence and severity of symptoms during treatment with chemotherapy and radiation treatments in 64 patients with NSCLC and found that 25% of the sample had fatigue and 20% had pain, insomnia, or dyspnea at moderate to severe levels before starting treatment. By the end of treatment, 63% of patients reported two or more moderate to severe symptoms with fatigue being the most severe throughout the course of treatment.

Similarly, high rates of emotional distress have been identified among patients with lung cancer. Graves and colleagues[20] examined the rates and predictors of emotional distress in lung cancer patients being seen in an outpatient setting. A total of 333 patients completed the distress thermometer. Over half (62%) of the patients reported distress at a significant level; predictors of distress included younger age, pain, fatigue, anxiety, and depression. Hopwood and Stephens[21] examined self-reported rates of depression in patients with inoperable disease and examined correlates associated with depression to help identify at-risk patients. A total of 987 patients with NSCLC and SCLC completed the Hospital Anxiety and Depression Scale (HADS) and the Rotterdam Symptom Checklist. Depression was self-rated in 322 patients (33%) before treatment and persisted in more than 50% of patients. SCLC patients had a threefold higher prevalence of case depression than those with NSCLC (25% vs. 9%, $p < 0.0001$). Multivariate analysis showed that functional impairment was the most important risk factor for depression. Pretreatment physical symptom burden, fatigue, and clinician-rated performance status were also independent predictors, but cell type was not.

CURATIVE TREATMENT AND LUNG CANCER SURVIVORSHIP

Surgical resection (e.g., pneumonectomy, lobectomy) is the treatment of choice for patients who have potentially curable disease. Few studies have explored the psychosocial consequences in this population during the postoperative recovery period or among long-term survivors. Sarna et al.[22] found that severe symptoms, including fatigue, dyspnea, and pain, continued months after thoracotomy. Depression and the number of comorbid diseases contributed to symptom severity. The presence and importance of depressed mood in this patient population has been reported by others. Uchitomi and colleagues[23] examined the clinical course of depression for 1 year after curative resection among 212 patients with NSCLC. The frequency of depression was 5%–8% after curative resection and did not change over the year. Predictors of psychological outcome at 1 year included an episode of depression after the diagnosis or at 1 month after surgery and lower educational level. As depression is treatable, the need for early diagnosis and intervention, even among lung cancer survivors, is essential.

Recent studies have monitored health-related quality of life (HRQOL) during recovery. Barlesi et al.[24] report that preoperative HRQOL was important in identifying those at risk for postoperative problems with those living alone being at increased risk. Surgical approaches to lung cancer are changing with increased use of less invasive video-assisted thoracoscopy, limited data suggest that this approach is associated with fewer disruptions in HRQOL.

Research in lung cancer survivorship is emerging.[25] The majority of studies focused on HRQOL and symptoms have focused on patients with advanced stage disease. However, several studies have indicated that some survivors experience ongoing symptoms, especially dyspnea related to the extent of surgical resection. Many who received a pneumonectomy had permanent reductions in functional status although reductions in pulmonary impairment are not directly related to dyspnea. For others, chronic postthoracotomy pain or pain associated with postoperative complications such as frozen shoulder can be a lingering issue, impacting recovery and overall HRQOL. Altered functional status and fatigue have also been reported among survivors. The anxiety and fear of recurrence is not unexpected among this population where long-term survivors are so few.

PALLIATIVE AND END-OF-LIFE CARE

A diagnosis of lung cancer is often complicated by the fact that the disease is usually diagnosed after it has spread beyond the lungs; thus, palliative treatment, including symptom management, and maintaining HRQOL are important foci for care. Of all the patients who develop NCLC each year, 55% are diagnosed with advanced disease at stage IIIB or stage IV that is not amenable to curative treatment.[26] Thus, palliative care is an essential part of care for lung cancer patients and their families and should ideally begin at diagnosis and continue throughout the illness trajectory.

Palliative care is interdisciplinary care that is provided to relieve suffering and improve HRQOL for patients with advanced illness and their families.[27] The use of palliative care programs has been associated with a decrease in the severity of symptoms, improved patient and family satisfaction, lower rates of in-hospital deaths, and shorter hospital length of stay.[27] The American College of Chest Physicians (AACP) has published evidence-based guidelines for the care of lung cancer patients and their families, which include topics such as palliative care consultation, HRQOL measurement, communication issues between patients and HCPs, advanced directives, the role of ethics committees in resolving end-of-life problems, and providing bereavement care to family members after the death of their loved one.[27,28] Tables 20–1 and 20–2 provide the specific recommendations provided by the ACCP to enhance care for patients with advanced lung cancer and their families.

In a comprehensive review of noninvasive interventions delivered by HCP for improving HRQOL in patients with lung cancer, the use of nurse follow-up programs and nursing interventions to manage breathlessness showed benefit in improving symptoms, emotional status, and functional status.[29] Another study by McCorkle and colleagues[30] found that follow-up care provided by oncology specialist nurses to terminally ill lung cancer patients resulted in less spousal psychological distress during bereavement as compared to those who did not receive the specialized nurse intervention.

Spirituality is being recognized as an important domain of HRQOL especially among those with advanced illness. Meraviglia[31] examined the effects of spirituality on the sense of well-being in 60 patients with lung cancer. Results from this study found that higher meaning in life scores were associated with higher psychological well-being scores. Prayer mediated the relationship between current physical health and psychological well-being. In another study, Wells and colleagues[32] identified the widespread use of prayer as a self-management strategy for symptom management in women with lung cancer. A total of 188 women with NSCLC completed a survey about their use of complementary and alternative therapies that they used for symptom control. Results of this study found that prayer (35%) and meditation (12%) were among the most commonly used strategies for self-management of distressing symptoms.

As the above section illustrates, lung cancer patients are at risk for multiple problems that influence HRQOL. Ostlund and colleagues[33] explored what dimensions of HRQOL predict global HRQOL in lung cancer patients and found that emotional functioning and fatigue were significant predictors of overall HRQOL. In another study, Sarna and colleagues[34] examined the relationship between demographic, clinical, health status, and meaning of illness to HRQOL in 217 women with lung cancer. Results from this study indicated that depressed mood, negative conceptualizations of the meaning of illness, and younger age were associated with global HRQOL and were correlated with poorer physical, psychological, and social dimensions of HRQOL. In summary, these findings highlight the multiple problems (severe symptom burden, high levels of psychological distress, and poor functional status) that lung cancer patients often experience during their illness and underscore the importance of ongoing assessment of HRQOL.

ASSESSMENT OF PSYCHOSOCIAL DISTRESS

The identification of psychosocial concerns among patients with lung cancer is essential to initiate appropriate treatment. Multiple studies have identified that high levels of symptom distress as well as lower levels of global HRQOL are associated with length of survival in lung cancer patients.[35,36] In addition, a recent study examined the relationship between symptom change, objective tumor measurements, and performance status in advanced lung cancer and found that disease progression and declining functional status were associated with worsening symptoms (i.e., pain, dyspnea, and cough), suggesting that symptom self-reports could be used by HCP to monitor patient status and inform treatment modification.[37]

A variety of valid and reliable assessment tools are available to monitor and to identify psychosocial concerns during lung cancer treatment and care. Chapter 2 discussed the use of these assessment tools in psycho-oncology. The potential utility of using standardized and ongoing HRQOL assessment in the clinical setting during lung cancer care as opposed to only during clinical trials is starting to be recognized. Use of these questionnaires in the clinical setting may be used to enhance communication between patients and their HCPs, promote early recognition of impaired HRQOL that require intervention, or identify changes in symptoms over time in response to medical treatments. Table 20–3 provides a list of the most commonly used HRQOL questionnaires used in the care of lung cancer patients.[38–41]

Functional status is an important aspect of HRQOL and a construct in the clinical care of cancer patients. The level of physical compromise is used to guide decisions about patient participation in clinical trials and is strongly related to length of survival.[42] A recent study examined the prevalence of poor functional status among lung cancer patients and the concordance of patient and HCP ratings of functional status.[43] Results of the study showed that the prevalence of poor functional status (defined as performance status 2–4 on a 0–4 scale) was quite high and HCPs tend to underestimate poor performance status as compared to patients; 34% of HCPs identified patients had poor functional status versus 48% of patients reported that they had poor functional status.

Table 20–1. ACCP-2003 evidence-based guidelines for end-of-life care

1. It is recommended that clinicians increase their focus on the patient's experience of illness to improve congruence of treatment with patient goals and preferences: (a) be realistic, practical, sensitive, and compassionate; (b) listen; (c) allow/invite the patient to express his or her reaction to the situation; (d) provide a contact person; (e) and continually reassess the patient's goals of therapy as part of treatment planning
2. End-of-life planning should be integrated as a component of assessment of goals of treatment and treatment planning
3. An experienced clinician should inform the patient of the diagnosis and its meaning. The day-to-day contact person should also be present at this meeting and should coordinate care
4. Clinicians treating patients with lung cancer should avail themselves of the increasing body of educational resources to improve communication at the end of life
5. Hospice and/or the palliative care service should be involved early in the patient's treatment, as part of the team
6. Each patient with lung cancer should be asked if he or she has an advance directive, and the clinician should assume responsibility for placing it in the chart
7. With patients for whom there are questions about the validity or interpretation of an advance directive, seek guidance from the hospital legal counsel or ethics committee
8. In making end-of-life decisions for patients with lung cancer, ethics consultation by Hospital Ethics Committees should be requested when assistance is needed in clarifying applicable law and policy related to patient autonomy and competence, informed consent, withholding life-prolonging treatments, surrogate preferences, decision making for patients without family, and resource allocation, as well as determining how ethical norms should be interpreted, or negotiating interpersonal conflicts among patients, families, and physicians
9. Given the potential variations in ethics consultations, the requesting party and the consultant should clarify beforehand the specific objectives of the consultation, the selection of participants, the process to be used in deliberation or negotiation, and the manner in which results will be disclosed and recorded
10. Decision making about intensive care unit treatment should incorporate available knowledge about prognosis, including the use of a cancer-specific outcome prediction model to complement clinical judgment, and weigh reasonably expected benefits of critical care against potential burdens, including distressing physical and psychological symptoms
11. In the inoperable or unresectable patient with lung cancer, prolonged mechanical ventilation is discouraged in view of dismal reported outcomes
12. In the critically ill patient with lung cancer, palliative care, including expert management of symptoms and effective communication about appropriate goals of treatment, should not be postponed until death is imminent, but should be an integral component of the diagnostic and treatment plan for all patients, including those still pursuing life-prolonging therapies as well as those more obviously at the end of life
13. The goal of palliative care should be to achieve the best quality of life for the patients and their families
14. Multimodality palliative care teams should be developed and encouraged to participate in patient management

See reference 28.

Table 20–2. ACCP-2007 evidence-based guidelines for palliative care

1. Palliative care should be integrated into the treatment of patients with advanced lung cancer, including those pursuing curative or life-prolonging therapies
2. It is recommended that palliative and end-of-life care include involvement of a palliative care consultation team, which should be made available to all patients with advanced stage lung cancer
3. Standardized evaluations with symptom assessment and abbreviated disease-specific HRQOL questionnaires should be administered by the responsible member of the healthcare team at the appropriate frequency
4. Clinicians of patients who die from lung cancer should extend communication with the bereaved family and friends after death
5. Proactive interventions, such as those listed below, are recommended to improve grief outcomes: (a) informing the patient and family of foreseeable death within weeks; (b) forewarning the family of impending death; and (c) enabling effective palliative care, focused on spiritual, existential, physical, and practical concerns
6. It is recommended that clinicians of dying patients with lung cancer encourage caregivers to maintain a healthy lifestyle during the period of caregiver burden, as well as during bereavement
7. It is recommended that clinicians of patients dying from lung cancer honor rituals of death and mourning in a culturally sensitive manner

ABBREVIATION: HRQOL, health-related quality of life.

Functional decline is particularly important for older adults with lung cancer. For example, Kurtz and colleagues[44] examined the predictors of depressive symptomatology in 211 geriatric patients with lung cancer. Significant predictors of depressive symptoms were decreased social functioning and increased symptom severity. In addition, patients who had not received radiation therapy were more depressed than those who had received treatment within the last 40 days.

The use of a comprehensive geriatric assessment can be useful in caring for older adults with lung cancer. The emergence of geriatric assessment screening tools, such as the Vulnerable Elders-13 Survey, will help address this issue.[45] Areas for assessment that have been identified as essential in the elderly include evaluation of functional status, assessment of comorbidities, altered cognition, increased risk of depression, diminished social support, and altered nutritional status.[45]

Table 20-3. Health-related quality of life questionnaires used in lung cancer settings

Instrument	No. of items	Dimensions measured	Time	Reliability	Validity	Languages
European Organization for Research and Treatment of Cancer (EORTC-QLQ-30)[38]	30	5 functional scales, 3 symptom scales, global health status/QoL scale, additional single items	10–15 minutes	Cronbach's α = 0.79	Construct	Translated into 81 languages
Lung Cancer Symptom Scale (LCSS)[40]	Patient scale = 9 Observer scale = 6	Physical, functional, social, psychological, spiritual QOL	10–15 minutes	Cronbach's α = 0.86	Construct discriminant	Translated into 47 languages
Functional Assessment of Chronic Illness Therapy Measurement System (FACIT)[41]	27	Physical (7) Social (7) Emotional (6) Functional well-being (7) Additional (9) for FACT-L	5 minutes	Cronbach's α = 0.89 Test-retest correlation coefficient = 0.92	Discriminant	Translated into 53 languages
Medical Outcome Study Short Form (MOS-SF-36)[39]	36 items, 2 scales, 8 subscales	General health (5), mental health (5), physical functioning (10), limits due to emotional problems (3), limits due to health problems (2), vitality (4), body pain (2), social functioning (2)	5–10 minutes	Cronbach's α = 0.80	Content Criterion Concurrent Construct Predictive	Translated into 110 languages

FAMILY IMPACT AND PSYCHOSOCIAL CONCERNS

Given the shift in the delivery of cancer care to the outpatient setting, family members have assumed an increased responsibility in providing clinical care to their family members diagnosed with lung cancer. Although family caregiving can provide many rewards, it can also be associated with caregiver strain or burden. Caregiver strain occurs when caregivers perceive difficulty performing roles or feel overwhelmed by their tasks. Caregiver burden may be less apparent and refers to caregiver emotional reactions to the caregiving situation such as worry, anxiety, frustration, or fatigue.[46] As families assume the role of caregiver for patients with lung cancer, they often provide multidimensional assistance with managing day-to-day symptoms, providing emotional support, assisting in activities of daily living, and providing transportation to healthcare visits. Without adequate support or knowledge, these day-to-day responsibilities in managing health and household tasks can make caregiving a difficult and challenging role. Porter and colleagues[47] examined self-efficacy for managing pain, symptoms, and function in 152 patients with lung cancer and their caregivers, and the associations between self-efficacy and patient and caregiver adjustment. Patients low in self-efficacy reported significantly higher levels of pain, fatigue, symptoms, depression, anxiety, and worse physical and functional well-being as did patients whose caregivers were low in self-efficacy. There were also significant associations between patient and caregiver adjustment, with lower levels of self-efficacy associated with higher levels of caregiver strain and psychological distress.

Two other studies examined distress and quality of life among lung cancer patients and family members.[48,49] Carmack-Taylor and colleagues[49] examined the prevalence of patient and spousal distress and predictors of psychological distress. Results indicated that 35% of patients and 36% of spouses were distressed. Patient and spousal distress was correlated. Predictors for patient distress were less positive social interaction support, more behavioral disengagement, self-distraction coping, and spouses using less humor as a coping mechanism. Predictors for spousal distress were more behavioral disengagement, substance use coping, and blaming the patient for causing their cancer. In another study, Sarna and colleagues[48] found that poorer physical HRQOL of family members was associated with older age, comorbid conditions, less education, and alcohol use. Poorer emotional HRQOL of family members was associated with younger age, depressed mood, and not being a spouse.

Unfortunately, few intervention studies have been conducted among lung cancer patients and their families. This is an important area for future research. Honea and colleagues[46] conducted a review of interventions to reduce caregivers strain and support healthy outcomes for family caregivers in cancer and suggested that education, support, psychotherapy, and respite interventions have demonstrated the greatest effect in reducing caregiver strain. Table 20–4 provides a list of resources for education and support to lung cancer patients and their families.

FUTURE DIRECTIONS

As reviewed in this chapter, persons with lung cancer are at risk for a range of psychosocial issues and may experience psychosocial comorbidity. Despite declines in smoking in the United States population, lung cancer will remain a major cause of death and misery in future decades. Encouraging preliminary results of early detection of lung cancer also brings new challenges that require ongoing investigation. However, as the majority will have incurable disease at the time of diagnosis, continued efforts are needed to monitor symptoms and HRQOL so that concerns can be identified quickly and appropriate treatment delivered.

Further investigations of the need for cultural tailoring of psychosocial interventions is paramount as the face of lung cancer changes with

Table 20–4. Education and support resources for patients with lung cancer

Organization name	Address/phone	Website	Description
American Cancer Society	12 Regional Offices across the United States Headquarters located in Atlanta, GA 1·800·ACS·2345	http://www.cancer.org	A nationwide community-based organization dedicated to eliminating cancer through advocacy, education, research sponsorship, and service. Patient education material available in several different languages, including Asian languages
American Society of Clinical Oncology	1900 Duke Street, Ste. 200, Alexandria, VA 22314	http://www.cancer.net/patient/Cancer+Types/Lung+Cancer	The philanthropic arm of the ASCO, an international organization composed of more than 25,000 oncology health professionals. Offers comprehensive patient education material on disease and treatment options
The CHEST Foundation	3300 Dundee Road, Northbrook, IL 60062 Phone: (800) 343–2227 Phone: (847) 498–1400	http://www.chestnet.org/downloads/patients/guides/lung-Cancer5048.pdf	The philanthropic arm of American College of Physicians. Creates educational programs, supports research, and raises public awareness about diseases of the chest and prevention. Link to a patient education brochure for advanced lung cancer. It discusses palliative care, symptoms, and pain management
CancerCare National Office	275 Seventh Ave, Flr. 22, New York, NY 10001 Phone: 212–712–8400	www.lungcancer.org	Program of CancerCare, a nonprofit organization that provides free, professional support services to anyone affected by cancer
Journal of American Medical Association	AMA P.O. Box 10946, Chicago, IL 60610–0946 Phone: 1–800–262–2350	http://jama.ama-assn.org/cgi/reprint/297/9/1022.pdf	Information sheet developed by JAMA to educate patients about lung cancer. Also available in Spanish
Lung Cancer Alliance	888 16th St., NW, Ste. 800, Washington, DC 20006 Phone: 800–298–2436 (US) Phone: 202–463–2080	www.lungcanceralliance.org	U.S.-based nonprofit organization dedicated to lung cancer patient support and advocacy. Patient support programs include a toll-free hotline, Phone Buddy program, online support community, and a Clinical trials matching service
Mesothelioma Applied Research Foundation	3944 State Street, Ste. 340, Santa Barbara, CA 93105 (877) 363–6376	www.curemeso.org	Nonprofit collaboration of patients and families, physicians, advocates, and researchers dedicated to eradicating mesothelioma
National Coalition for Cancer Survivorship	1010 Wayne Avenue, Silver Spring, MD 20910 Phone: 301–650–9127 Phone: 888–650–9127	www.canceradvocacy.org	Survivor-led cancer advocacy organization focused on advocating for quality cancer care and patient education
National Institute of Health, Senior Health	9000 Rockville Pike, Bethesda, Maryland 20892 Phone: 301–496–4000	http://nihseniorhealth.gov/lungcancer/toc.html	NIH Senior Health offers online tutorials (both audio and print) customized to educate aging patients about lung cancer
National Lung Cancer Partnership	222 N. Midvale Blvd. Ste. 6, Madison, WI 53705 Phone: 608–233–7905	www.nationallungcancerpartnership.org	U.S. lung cancer advocacy organization founded by physicians and researchers and focused on understanding how the disease affects women and men differently
US National Library of Medicine	8600 Rockville Pike, Bethesda, MD 20894	http://www.nlm.nih.gov/medlineplus/lungcancer.html	Website offering comprehensive information about lung cancer, treatment options, and links to patient education. Available in 12 languages.
		http://www.nlm.nih.gov/medlineplus/tutorials/lungcancer/htm/lesson.htm	Medline Plus offers on online audio- and text-based tutorial to educated patients about lung cancer. Also available in Spanish

expected increases in poor, less educated, and some ethnic minorities due to patterns of tobacco use. As lung cancer is primarily a disease of older adults, special consideration of the aging process, including the presence of comorbid diseases and the impact that this may have on the ability of family members to provide ongoing care for their loved ones, is needed. Significant strides have been made in understanding the molecular biology of lung cancer and how this can be harnessed to enhance treatment of patients with advanced stage disease. The use of targeted agents, such as the epidermal growth factor receptor-tyrosine kinase inhibitors, has resulted in monumental changes in the treatment of patients in the advanced stages of their disease. A small but significant number of patients have received tremendous benefit from the use of these agents. However, the toxicities associated with these agents are different from other modalities (i.e., facial rash) and have significant psychosocial impact, which have not been studied as yet.[50,51]

Although there is a growing literature providing evidence about the psychosocial consequences of lung cancer at all phases of the disease, intervention studies are still relatively limited given the vast burden of the disease. The need for adequate symptom management of disease symptoms and treatment, along with psychosocial care requires an interdisciplinary approach that can uncover innovative strategies to enhance the quality of care for lung cancer patients and their families.

ACKNOWLEDGMENTS

This work was supported by grants from the National Cancer Institute (Grant no. 1K07-CA92692, Principal Investigator, Mary E. Cooley and 1 U56 CA11863502, Principal Investigators Karen M. Emmons and Adam Colon-Carmona, Julie Lynch, Predoctoral Fellow, University of Massachusetts-Boston, PhD Program in Health Policy, Cancer Nursing and Health Disparities).

REFERENCES

1. Ferlay J, Bray F, Pisani P, Parkin D. *GLOBOCAN 2002: Cancer incidence. Mortality and prevalence worldwide*. IARC CancerBase No. 5, version 2.0, Lyon: IARC Press; 2004.

2. Jemal A, Siegel R, Ward E, et al. Cancer statistics, 2008. *CA Cancer J Clin.* Mar-Apr 2008;58(2):71–96.

3. Abidoye O, Ferguson MK, Salgia R. Lung carcinoma in African Americans. *Nat Clin Pract Oncol.* 2007;4(2):118–129.

4. U.S. Department of Health and Human Services. *The health consequences of smoking: a report of the surgeon general*. Atlanta, GA: U.S. Department of Health and Human Services, Centers for Disease Control and Prevention, National Center for Chronic Disease Prevention and Health Promotion, Office on Smoking and Health; 2004.

5. Chapple A, Ziebland S, McPherson A. Stigma, shame, and blame experienced by patients with lung cancer: qualitative study. *BMJ.* 2004; 328(7454):1470.

6. U.S. Department of Health and Human Services. *Reducing the health consequences of smoking—25 years of progress*. Atlanta, GA: Centers for Disease Control, National Center for Chronic Disease Prevention and Health Promotion, Office on Smoking and Health; 1989.

7. Stuber J, Galea S, Link BG. Smoking and the emergence of a stigmatized social status. *Soc Sci Med.* 2008;67(3):420–430.

8. DeVita VT Jr, Hellman S, Rosenberg SA. *Cancer: principles & practice of oncology*. 8th ed. Philadelphia, PA: Lippincott, Williams & Wilkins; 2008.

9. Johnston-Early A, Cohen MH, Minna JD, et al. Smoking abstinence and small cell lung cancer survival: an association. *J Am Med Assoc.* 1980;244:2175–2179.

10. Richardson GE, Tucker MA, Venzon DJ, et al. Smoking cessation after successful treatment of small-cell lung cancer is associated with fewer smoking-related second primary cancers. *Ann Intern Med.* 1993;119(5):383–390.

11. Garces YI, Yang P, Parkinson J, et al. The relationship between cigarette smoking and quality of life after lung cancer diagnosis. *Chest.* 2004;126(6):1733–1741.

12. Rock VJ, Malarcher A, Kahende JW, Asman K, Husten C, Caraballo R. *Cigarette smoking among adults—Unites States 2006*. Atlanta, GA: Centers for Disease Control and Prevention; Nov 9, 2007.

13. Manser RL, Irving LB, Stone C, Byrnes G, Abramson M, Campbell D. Screening for lung cancer. *Cochrane Database Syst Rev.* 2004(1):CD001991.

14. Schnoll RA, Bradley P, Miller SM, Unger M, Babb J, Cornfeld M. Psychological issues related to the use of spiral CT for lung cancer early detection. *Lung Cancer.* 2003;39(3):315–325.

15. Townsend CO, Clark MM, Jett JR, et al. Relation between smoking cessation and receiving results from three annual spiral chest computed tomography scans for lung carcinoma screening. *Cancer.* 2005;103(10):2154–2162.

16. Taylor KL, Cox LS, Zincke N, Mehta L, McGuire C, Gelmann E. Lung cancer screening as a teachable moment for smoking cessation. *Lung Cancer.* 2007;56(1):125–134.

17. Schnoll RA, Miller SM, Unger M, McAleer C, Halbherr T, Bradley P. Characteristics of female smokers attending a lung cancer screening program: a pilot study with implications for program development. *Lung Cancer.* 2002;37(3):257–265.

18. Cooley ME, Short T, Moriarty H. Symptom prevalence, distress, and change over time in adults receiving treatment for lung cancer. *Psycho-Oncology.* 2003;12(7):694–708.

19. Wang XS, Fairclough DL, Liao Z, et al. Longitudinal study of the relationship between chemoradiation therapy for non-small-cell lung cancer and patient symptoms. *J Clin Oncol.* 2006;24(27):4485–4491.

20. Graves KD, Arnold SM, Love CL, Kirsh KL, Moore PG, Passik SD. Distress screening in a multidisciplinary lung cancer clinic: prevalence and predictors of clinically significant distress. *Lung Cancer.* 2007;55(2):215–224.

21. Hopwood P, Stephens RJ. Depression in patients with lung cancer: prevalence and risk factors derived from quality-of-life data. *J Clin Oncol.* 2000;18(4):893–903.

22. Sarna L, Cooley ME, Brown JK, Chernecky C, Elashoff D, Kotlerman J. Symptom severity one to four months post-thoracotomy for lung cancer. *Am J Crit Care.* 2008;17(5):455–467.

23. Uchitomi Y, Mikami I, Nagai K, Nishiwaki Y, Akechi T, Okamura H. Depression and psychological distress in patients during the year after curative resection of non-small-cell lung cancer. *J Clin Oncol.* 2003;21(1):69–77.

24. Barlési F, Doddoli C, Loundou A, Pillet E, Thomas P, Auquier P. Preoperative psychological global well being index (PGWBI) predicts postoperative quality of life for patients with non-small cell lung cancer manages with thoracic surgery. *Eur J Cardiothorac Surg.* 2006;30:548–553.

25. Sarna L GJF, Coscarelly A. Physical and psychosocial issues in lung cancer survivors. In: Chang AE, Hayes DF, Kinsella TJ, Pass HI, Schiller JH, Stone RM, Strecher VJ, eds. *Oncology: an evidence-based approach*. New York, NY: Springer; 2006:1871–1890.

26. Ries L, Young J, Keel G, Eisner M, Lin Y, Horner M-J. *SEER Survival Monograph: cancer survival among adults: U.S. SEER Program, 1988–2001, Patient and Tumor Characteristics*. SEER Program, NIH Pub. No. 07-6215. Bethesda, MD: National Cancer Institute; 2007.

27. Griffin JP, Koch KA, Nelson JE, Cooley ME. Palliative care consultation, quality-of-life measurements, and bereavement for end-of-life care in patients with lung cancer: ACCP evidence-based clinical practice guidelines (2nd edition). *Chest.* 2007;132(Suppl 3):404S-422S.

28. Griffin JP, Nelson JE, Koch KA, et al. End-of-life care in patients with lung cancer. *Chest.* 2003;123:312–331.

29. Sola I, Thompson E, Subirama M, Lopez C, Pascual A. Non-invasive interventions for improving well-being and quality if life in patients with lung cancer. *Cochrane Database Syst Rev.* 2004;18(4):CD004282.

30. McCorkle R, Robinson L, Nuamah I, Lev E, Benoliel JQ. The effects of home nursing care for patients during terminal illness on the bereaved's psychological distress. *Nurs Res.* 1998;47(1):2–10.

31. Meraviglia M. The effects of spirituality on well-being of people with lung cancer. *Oncol Nurs Forum.* 2004;31(1):89–94.

32. Wells M, Sarna L, Cooley ME, et al. Use of complementary and alternative medicine therapies to control symptoms in women living with lung cancer. *Cancer Nurs.* 2007;30(1):45–55.

33. Ostlund U, Wennman-Larsen A, Gustavsson P, Wengstrom Y. What symptom and functional dimensions can be predictors for global ratings of overall quality of life in lung cancer patients? *Support Care Cancer.* 2007;15(10):1199–1205.

34. Sarna L, Brown JK, Cooley ME, Williams RD, Chernecky C, Padilla G & Danao LL. Quality of life and meaning of illness of women with lung cancer. *Oncol Nurs Forum.* 2005;32(1):E9-E19.

35. Degner LF, Sloan JA. Symptom distress in newly diagnosed ambulatory cancer patients and as a predictor of survival in lung cancer. *J Pain Symptom Manage.* 1995;10(6):423–431.

36. Dharma-Wardene M, Au HJ, Hanson J, Dupere D, Hewitt J, Feeny D. Baseline FACT-G score is a predictor of survival for advanced lung cancer. *Qual Life Res.* 2004;13(7):1209–1216.

37. Cella D, Eton D, Hensing TA, Masters GA, Parasuraman B. Relationship between symptom change, objective tumor measurements, and performance status during chemotherapy for advanced lung cancer. *Clin Lung Cancer.* 2008;9(1):51–58.

38. Aaronson N, Ahmedzai S, Bergman B, Bullinger M, Cull A, Duez N. The European Organization for Research and Treatment of Cancer QLQ-C30: a quality of life instrument for use in international clinical trials in oncology. *J Natl Cancer Inst.* 1993;85:365–376.

39. Ware J, Kosinski M. *SF-36 Physical and mental health summary scales: a manual for users of version 1*. Lincoln, RI: QualityMetric Incorporated; 2001.

40. Hollen P, Gralla R. Comparison of instruments to measure quality of life in lung cancer. *Semin Oncol.* 1996;23:31–40.

41. Cella DF, Bonomi AE, Lloyd SR, Tulsky DS, Kaplan E, Bonomi P. Reliability and validity of the Functional Assessment of Cancer Therapy-Lung (FACT-L) quality of life instrument. *Lung Cancer.* 1995;12(3):199–220.

42. Dacjzman E, Kasymjanova G, Kreisman H, Swinton N, Pepe C, Small D. Should patient-rated performance status affect treatment decisions in advanced lung cancer? *J Thorac Oncol.* 2008;3:1133–1136.

43. Lilenbaum RC, Cashy J, Hensing TA, Young S, Cella D. Prevalence of poor performance status in lung cancer patients: implications for research. *J Thorac Oncol.* 2008;3(2):125–129.

44. Kurtz M, Kurtz J, Stommel M, Given C, Given B. Predictors of depressive symptomatology of geriatric patients with lung cancer: a longitudinal study. *Psycho-Oncology.* 2002;11(1):12–22.

45. Mohile SG, Bylow K, Dale W, et al. A pilot study of the vulnerable elders survey-13 compared with the comprehensive geriatric assessment for identifying disability in older patients with prostate cancer who receive androgen ablation. *Cancer.* 2007;109(4):802–810.

46. Honea NJ, Brintnall R, Given B, et al. Putting evidence into practice: nursing assessment and interventions to reduce family caregiver strain and burden. *Clin J Oncol Nurs.* 2008;12(3):507–516.

47. Porter LS, Keefe FJ, Garst J, McBride CM, Baucom D. Self-efficacy for managing pain, symptoms, and function in patients with lung cancer and their informal caregivers: associations with symptoms and distress. *Pain.* 2008;137(2):306–315.

48. Sarna L, Cooley ME, Brown JK, et al. Quality of life and health status of dyads of women with lung cancer and family members. *Oncol Nurs Forum.* 2006;33(6):1109–1116.

49. Carmack-Taylor CL, Badr H, Lee JH, Fossella F, Pisters K, Gritz ER & Schover L. Lung cancer patients and their spouses: psychological and relationship functioning within 1 month of treatment initiation. *Ann Behav Med.* 2008;36:129–140.

50. Lynch TJ Jr, Kim ES, Eaby B, Garey J, West DP, Lacouture ME. Epidermal growth factor receptor inhibitor-associated cutaneous toxicities: an evolving paradigm in clinical management. *Oncologist.* 2007;12(5):610–621.

51. Sequist LV, Lynch TJ. EGFR tyrosine kinase inhibitors in lung cancer: an evolving story. *Annu Rev Med.* 2008;59:429–442.

Genitourinary Malignancies

Andrew J. Roth and Alejandro González-Restrepo

Genitourinary (GU) cancers are common and represent a frequent cause of cancer death.[1] With the exception of testicular cancer, the incidence of GU cancers (e.g., prostate, bladder, renal and penile cancers) increases with advancing age. Thus, understanding coincident life phase characteristics is important in optimizing the ability of each patient to cope with his illness. The effect of treatment on the quality of life (QOL) of patients has become more significant as survival has improved for many GU cancers. QOL areas of concern include coping with body image and integrity changes, varying degrees of sexual and physical intimacy dysfunction, and infertility. These issues compound the generic difficulties of coping with cancer, such as dealing with pain, fatigue, and other complications of treatment, including interruption of daily functioning, and career uncertainty. These issues also complicate primary treatment decisions as patients are often weighing curability and longevity potential of different options against possible posttreatment QOL concerns. This chapter gives an overview of medical and psychosocial issues as well as their management in patients and their families.

PROSTATE CANCER

Epidemiology. Prostate cancer is the most common non-skin cancer in males in the United States, with an estimated 186,320 new cases in 2008. Approximately 65% of these new cases occur in men over the age of 65.[1] It is also the second leading cause of cancer death in men. Incidence and mortality rates are more than twice as high in men of African descent.[2] This generally older population of men has particular needs influenced by their generational and developmental phase of life. Psychological reactions are influenced by psychiatric history and other significant life changes or events such as recent widowhood, recent or impending retirement, available supports and loss of friends or family, in particular from cancer or prostate cancer. Five to ten percent of all prostate cancers are believed to be of familial predisposition. Some nutritional factors, such as diets high in saturated fat, have been correlated with increased incidence of prostate cancer.[3]

Screening guidelines. American Cancer Society guidelines recommend a yearly digital rectal examination (DRE) for men 50 years of age and older, along with an annual prostate-specific antigen (PSA) test. Men who are at high risk, such as African Americans or those with a strong family history of prostate cancer, are advised to begin PSA testing starting at age 45.[1] Other than self-examination for testicular cancer, prostate cancer is the only GU cancer that has a reliable tool for early detection.

Diagnosis and medical work-up. It is unclear whether early detection by PSA testing and treatment of indolent forms of prostate cancer is beneficial when the distress and impairment of QOL from the primary treatments of surgery or radiotherapy is taken into account.[4] These uncertainties have implications for the psychological well-being of men and their families. However, it is difficult to distinguish more lethal from more benign varieties of prostate cancer before men receive primary treatment. In the past many men would die of another cause, never knowing they had prostate cancer, with detection only occurring at autopsy. Those who were diagnosed with the disease often presented with signs of metastatic disease, such as pain and urinary problems.

A PSA level can be normal even in the presence of cancer. It is also not cancer specific. False positive results can be seen with prostatitis, benign prostatic hypertrophy, and after manipulation of the prostate as with transrectal ultrasound and needle biopsies or DRE. Improvement in the specificity of this test has helped rule out many false positives. However, PSA levels may vary with the age of the patient as well as other medical factors. One of the psychological distresses oncologists have noted in patients is the degree of anxiety surrounding each PSA test, and the anticipation before getting the results. This has been termed "PSA anxiety," "PSA-itis," and "PSA-dynia."[5–7] Some men put great significance on each test and even on minuscule changes within the normal range, leading themselves and their families to excessive worry. Level of worry about a current result may be related to the trend of recent test results—in one study[8] men with stable PSA levels had less anxiety than those whose scores were either going up or going down. Men apparently are looking for good news only and "seeking peace of mind,"[9] and feel devastated and angry by unwanted or unexpected increases.

Management/treatment. To date there has not been a definitive comparative analysis of the major primary treatment options for prostate cancer. Thus, there is still legitimate professional disagreement and controversy about selection of primary treatments.[10] Though overall QOL may not be significantly different with the primary treatment options, there may be compromises when considering specific treatment side effects and long-term complications.[11,12] Primary treatment options vary from "watchful waiting," also described as "expectant monitoring," and "active surveillance" to surgery, radiation, and cryotherapy. Watchful waiting (deferred therapy) is often recommended for those with significant comorbid illness, low-grade indolent cancers, and less than 10 years life expectancy. Active surveillance is suggested for younger men with early-stage disease who get more frequent follow-up and observation. Though promising to prevent unnecessary compromise to QOL with treatment complications, further study is still needed to observe long-term medical and psychological benefits and complications.[13,14] The definitive treatment choice in the past was surgery, the open radical prostatectomy. Not all urologists perform the newer "nerve sparing" procedure that has decreased the rate of complications of impotence and urinary incontinence. Today, surgical treatment options include laparoscopic and robotic prostatectomies which claim less bleeding, less chance of infection, and less time in the hospital after the procedure.[15]

Radiation therapy, either conventional *intensity-modulated radiation therapy* (IMRT) or by seed implants often in combination with external beam radiotherapy, may yield decreased, though delayed incidence of impotence than surgery; however, there are increased difficulties with bowel function. Postradiation treatment PSA levels take a variable amount of time to reach a nadir of undetectable PSA that would indicate likely cure from the cancer; this can lead to prolonged anxiety.

For more advanced prostate cancer, hormonal manipulation is used to decrease the synthesis of testosterone or its action on prostate cancer cell growth. This can be done with gonadotropin releasing hormone (GnRH) agonists such as leuprolide or goserelin, estrogenic substances such as diethylstilbestrol, peripheral antiandrogenic agents, such as flutamide, or bicalutamide, or by orchiectomy, or surgical castration. Hormonal therapy at this stage of disease is not curative. Equally effective in slowing tumor growth with similar side effect profiles, medical hormonal therapy may be preferred over orchiectomy by patients because of improved body image and therefore improved QOL; however, it is an expensive treatment. Side effects of androgen ablation may include erectile dysfunction (ED), loss of libido, hot flashes, gynecomastia, irritability, anxiety, and depression. Pirl and colleagues[16] found that men most at risk for depression while on hormonal therapy were those who had histories significant for major depression. If side effects to anti-androgens become too bothersome, oncologists often consider intermittent therapy, with some time off of hormones. Chemotherapeutic agents are used for more advanced tumors—they too are not curative.

Management of psychological distress. Uncertainty about choice of treatment options and related outcomes including potential sexual dysfunction, urinary incontinence, weakness, fatigue, pain, and other side effects of the disease or treatment can have profound effects on mood, irritability, and anxiety, especially for those men who are used to feeling that they control their fates. Many men entertain multiple second opinions regarding their primary therapy. Some spend multiple hours on the Internet and in libraries attempting to "leave no stone unturned" by gathering enough information to find the perfect treatment for them. They can quickly reach a level of "information overload" that adds to anxiety and frustration. Treatment choices and decisions may vary based on the extent of disease, age of patient, life expectancy, specialty bias of physician, side effect risk profile acceptable to a patient, expense, and geography.[17] Personality factors and coping strategies may influence a man's satisfaction with his treatment.[18] Some men choose surgery to quell anxiety, knowing that there will be a second, direct look at their tumor and extent of disease. Others choose radiation because of the fear of general anesthesia. An example of a helpful "take control" attitude is the man who changes his diet to what is thought of as a prostate friendly diet with low fat, high soy, fish oil, selenium and other nutrients, and begins or continues a regular exercise program. Hormonal therapies can be particularly distressing because of sexual, energy, or concentration side effects.

In general, men with prostate cancer respond to education and various types of brief psychotherapy, including supportive, cognitive-behaviorally oriented, and insight-oriented therapies. However, some men are reluctant to participate in therapy, particularly older men who have never done so previously. Support groups are available specifically for men with prostate cancer. Two of the national support groups available to men are "Us Too" and "Man to Man."

Difficulties with sexual functioning occur from aging, the cancer itself and from surgery, radiation, and hormonal therapy.[19,20] Hormonal therapy, in particular, eliminates libido which often decreases distress about ED; however, decreased desire for any physical intimacy can be harmful to a relationship. Coupled with ED, feelings of being emasculated occur. An honest or realistic assessment of sexual functioning before primary treatment may assist a man in choosing a more appropriate treatment option for him. Therapies to improve ED include phosphodiesterase-5 (PDE-5) inhibitors such as sildenafil, tadalafil and vardenafil, penile injections, vacuum erection devices, and penile prostheses. However, most men are not initially comfortable with non-pill forms of treatment. For those men who are particularly bothered by sexual dysfunction, sex therapy with a trained therapist familiar with cancer issues can help them express the feelings engendered by this dysfunction, and also help a couple learn alternative ways of sharing sexual intimacy.

Urinary incontinence occurs as a complication of surgery and radiation. Loss of urinary continence leads men to shun social engagements. The fear of urine leaking, of smelling of urine, and of having to use diapers feels regressive and is humiliating. Urologists and their staffs can work with patients to identify etiologies of incontinence, to educate patients and families about the incontinence, and to offer suggestions to alleviate or reduce symptoms. Interventions for urinary incontinence include pelvic muscle reeducation, bladder training, and anticholinergic medications. Artificial urinary sphincter implantation appears to be a durable treatment when needed after prostatectomy or radiation therapy.[21] Psycho-oncologists can help with support-, cognitive-, and behaviorally oriented strategies to cope with incontinence and sometimes with antidepressants or anxiolytics to treat psychiatric barriers to better coping.

Pain is often a symptom of advanced prostate cancer which can be difficult to control. Pain syndromes result from local expansion and inflammation of the prostate gland, from local tumor growth, and from distant long bone, vertebral, and skull metastases. Pain not only impairs mobility but also accompanies neurologic impairments such as cranial nerve deficits, paralysis, incontinence of bowel and bladder, and impotence.[22] Patients with pain are significantly more depressed or anxious when compared with patients without pain; these mood changes may not be related to the extent of disease.[23,24] However, older men are often reluctant to take pain medications or dosages adequate to truly help.

Weakness and fatigue are particularly upsetting symptoms to men who have led active and independent lives and who are now more dependent on family or friends. Fatigue and weakness can be caused by the illness, hormonal or radiation therapy, pain medication, steroids, and other factors. Helping the patient to reorganize his schedule and set realistic goals may result in less distress. A psychostimulant, such as modafinil or methylphenidate, may counter the sedating effects of opioids, increase motivation, enhance appetite, and elevate a patient's mood. Roth and colleagues[25] found that methylphenidate may be an effective treatment for fatigue even in older men with prostate cancer, as long as they are monitored by their physicians for possible tachycardia and increases in blood pressure. An activating antidepressant such as bupropion, which will not compromise sexual functioning, or fluoxetine can be used to increase energy.

Hot flashes in men with prostate cancer are caused by medical and surgical androgen ablation. They are the result of increased vasomotor activity, possibly related to increased noradrenergic activity and decreased serotonergic activity that leads to diaphoresis, feelings of intense heat, and chills, similar to symptoms that women have during menopause. At times hormonal therapy must be stopped because of the effect these flashes cause in terms of drenching sweat and discomfort. Antidepressants like the selective serotonin reuptake inhibitors (SSRIs), such as sertraline and paroxetine; serotonin-norepinephrine reuptake inhibitors (SNRIs), such as venlafaxine; and antiepileptic medications, such as gabapentin, have been reported to reduce the frequency and intensity of hot flashes.[26-28] Teaching men to change habits such as decreasing caffeine, alcohol, and hot fluid intake may be useful to prevent or decrease the frequency or extent of the hot flashes.

Couples and intimate relationships are vulnerable in the context of prostate cancer. At a time when a couple's communication needs to be at its best, it is often at its worst because of the stress of the situation. Older men tend to be uncomfortable sharing emotions. They often have a need to be seen as the protector and provider for the family, however, incompatible this is with the reality of their current physical deterioration. Studies have shown that spouses and partners have even more distress than patients.[24,29] Couple's counseling can improve the ability of spouses and partners to cope with the cancer together. These options are also useful for those with other GU cancers that affect sexuality.

TESTICULAR CANCER

Epidemiology. Testicular cancer is the most common cancer in American men between the ages of 20 and 40 accounting for 46% of all cancers in this age range, though it accounts for only about 1% of all male cancers.[21] It is considerably more common in Caucasian than African American men, with intermediate rates for Hispanics, Native Americans, and Asians. Distinct geographical and racial variations suggest both genetic and environmental factors promoting the development of testicular cancer.[30] One major risk factor is cryptorchidism, the congenital failure of one or both testes to descend into the scrotal sac.[31] Patients with Klinefelter syndrome have a higher risk for germ cell tumors (GCT) located outside of the gonads. There is also evidence of increased risk in men infected with human immunodeficiency virus/acquired immunodeficiency syndrome (HIV/AIDS) and in those having a prior testicular cancer.

Diagnosis and medical work-up. Testicular self-examination is the most common form of detection of this cancer, usually with the presence of a small, hard lump in either testicle, an enlarged testicle, a collection of fluid, or unusual pain. However, most patients will first seek medical attention because of development of a painless, swollen testis. In approximately 25% of patients the first symptoms will be related to metastatic disease, back pain being the most common from tumor in the retroperitoneum. Pulmonary symptoms such as shortness of breath, chest pain, or hemoptysis occur due to advanced lung metastases.[32]

The standard diagnostic procedure, after ruling out infection or other disease by urinalysis, urine culture, and a testicular ultrasound, is to remove the affected testis via inguinal orchiectomy. Biopsy is not possible in this disease because the cancer cells may spread during the procedure. Orchiectomy also prevents further growth of the primary tumor. Ninety percent of testicular cancers are GCT, which are subdivided into seminomas and nonseminomas. Lymphoma is the second most common tumor of the testis and should be suspected in men over age 50. Staging of the extent of disease to develop a treatment plan is accomplished by computed tomography (CT) or magnetic resonance imaging (MRI). The tumor markers α-fetoprotein (AFP), β-human chorionic gonadotropin (β-HCG), and lactate dehydrogenase (LDH) are used for the detection of small tumors and for comparison over time to evaluate response to treatment. Retroperitoneal lymph node dissection (RPLND) is critical to stage nonseminomatous GCT and must always be performed with curative intent. This procedure is often associated with ejaculatory dysfunction and secondary infertility, though newer nerve sparing procedures may preserve normal ejaculation.

Medical management and treatment. Survival in this population has significantly improved in recent years owing to improved diagnostic and treatment techniques, with over 95% of patients expected to be cured. Cure rates depend on the stage of disease, approaching 100% for early-stage seminomas and nearly 100% overall survival for stage I nonseminomatous GCT. Approximately 85% of men with advanced testicular cancer will be cured with a combination of chemotherapy and surgery.

The effects on fertility and the possibility of storing sperm should be discussed with all patients undergoing chemotherapy or radiotherapy.[30] Treatment differs for seminomatous and nonseminomatous tumors, as well as stage of disease. Early-stage seminomatous disease is treated with orchiectomy and radiation therapy; chemotherapy with the drug carboplatin has proved as effective as radiation. Treatment of moderate disease will combine orchiectomy with either radiation or chemotherapy. More advanced disease is treated with orchiectomy and multidrug chemotherapy. Common regimens of chemotherapies include bleomycin, etoposide, and cisplatin (BEP).

Nonseminomas have often metastasized at the time of clinical presentation. Early and moderate stage disease can be treated with orchiectomy alone, or followed by either RPLND, observation with frequent follow-ups, or chemotherapy. Chemotherapy regimens similar to those used in seminoma tumors may be used in advanced-stage nonseminoma treatment. High-dose chemotherapy with peripheral blood stem cell transplantation is used for metastatic refractory germ cell cancer and has been found to improve survival for some patients.[33]

Management of psychosocial issues. Many psychosocial stressors are related to coping with side effects of the cancer therapy. However, this tumor occurs in young men when sexuality, fertility, and intimacy are critically important. Although unilateral orchiectomy does not lead to infertility or sexual dysfunction, men are often concerned about their appearance. Artificial testicular implants have been successful in helping men cope with this issue. RPLND can lead to infertility by causing retrograde ejaculation, though sexual desire and ability to have erections and orgasms are not affected. However, a pattern of sexual avoidance and decreased sexual interest can develop related to the distress of the cancer treatment in general. Although there is substantial recovery in sexual life after treatment,[34] a significant number of men will have long-term sexual dysfunction.[35] Couple's therapy can address these issues and help the couple gain some perspective on how their relationship has been changed by cancer. Occupational performance does not seem to be affected long term.[34]

Infertility can be related to surgery, with RPLND posing the greatest threat by interfering with ejaculation. Infertility can also be due to radiotherapy or chemotherapy. Sperm production can be affected by radiation therapy and infertility from this degree of radiation is temporary in most patients. Many men with testicular cancer have been found to have low sperm counts even before diagnosis, perhaps due to an autoimmune process probably confined to the few months before diagnosis. Unfortunately, this can limit the usefulness of sperm banking at the time of diagnosis. Antegrade ejaculation may return spontaneously over the months or years following surgery, and the administration of sympathomimetic drugs can convert retrograde to antegrade ejaculation. Whether due to acquired infertility or because of decreased desire of having children, paternity rates are 15%–30% lower than in the general population.[36]

Chemotherapeutic agents such as cyclophosphamide can also cause infertility, though this may last for a transient period of 2–3 years after completing chemotherapy. Trask and colleagues[37] found no significant difference among 16 study subjects in distress and QOL measured before, during, and after chemotherapy. Anticipatory anxiety and fear of the chemotherapy side effects decreased over time. The most disruptive symptoms noted were fatigue and changes in sleep, mood, and appetite. A study of cured testicular cancer patients found a progressive worsening in QOL among patients in the surveillance or watchful waiting group when compared to those who had undergone chemotherapy with or without RPLND, or radiotherapy. These latter groups incidentally had better working ability and greater satisfaction with life. Suggested explanations include having a greater appreciation of life and relationships in cancer survivors as well as having suffered from a life-threatening disease and having coped with it gives patients a positive view of life. The surveillance group was worried about not receiving treatment despite reassurance about their prognosis.[38] Patients in a wait-and-see or surveillance group also have lower rates of paternity and lower satisfaction with sexual relationships.[34]

Psychologically, the impact of this illness can affect key aspects of a young man's life or a young couple's relationship. Its presentation at the peak of a young male adult's development leads to heightened risk of depression, anxiety, anticipation of pain, bodily trauma, and death. Apart from infertility, fears about the effects on sexual functioning need to be addressed, especially before a young man has been involved in a long-term sexual relationship. Thorough sexual histories should include questions about frequency and intensity of sexual activity including masturbation, desire, erection, orgasm, and satisfaction. Approximately 10% of patients will have long-term psychological problems.[35] A large study in a Norwegian population reported a greater prevalence of anxiety disorders in long-term testicular cancer survivors when compared to a matched healthy population, with no differences observed in depression measures.[39] Surviving patients have to be concerned with late complications of curative therapy, as is seen in other malignancies, as well as fears of recurrence. For these reasons, it is thought that supportive and educational counseling should be offered before and after cancer treatment.

Long-term effects from chemotherapy can lead to other QOL problems; for instance, compromised renal function from cisplatin, Reynaud's phenomenon following combinations of vinblastine and bleomycin, pulmonary toxicity with bleomycin, and neuropathy and ototoxicity attributable to cisplatin and vinblastine leave patients with secondary deficits that challenge their daily living. Short- and long-term consequences are also seen with the use of radiotherapy in the form of erectile and ejaculation disorders and secondary tumors.[33]

BLADDER CANCER

Epidemiology. There will be an estimated 68,810 new cases of bladder cancer diagnosed in 2008[1]; the majority of these cases will occur in men (51,230). The incidence is greater in whites who almost double that of blacks, followed by Hispanics and Asians who have the lowest incidence. The largest known risk factor is tobacco smoking, leading to twice the number of cases relative to those who do not smoke. Risk increases with age as 70% of cases are diagnosed after age 65. Certain cancer treatments such as high-dose cyclophosphamide or ifosfamide and radiation treatment to the pelvis may increase the risk of developing bladder cancer. Only about 1% of all cases can be attributed to an inherited cause from a reduced ability to break down harmful chemicals. People at high risk due to exposure or selected bladder birth defects may benefit from screening with urine cytology and cystoscopy. Currently, there are no good tests for early detection and widespread screening of bladder cancer. Most are detected because they cause grossly visible or microscopic hematuria. Over 90% of bladder cancers are transitional cell carcinomas (TCC). Bladder cancer is unlikely to be found incidentally at autopsy, indicating that it is expected to cause symptoms or other significant problems at some time during a patient's life. Disease stage has been shown to be the single best predictor of outcome for TCC of the bladder.[40]

Diagnosis and management. There is more of a consensus about the diagnostic work-up and treatment plan for bladder cancer than for other GU cancers. Cystoscopy is the basis for diagnosis and monitoring of bladder cancer.[41] If detected at an early stage (0–I), the 5-year survival rate is 85%–95%. For more advanced disease (II–IV), the survival rates are between 16% and 55%, depending on extent of disease.[1] Categorizing cases into superficial bladder cancer or muscle-invasive bladder cancer is a useful way to describe treatment and the multiple effects on QOL.

Superficial bladder cancer. Transurethral resection of the bladder (TURB) is the primary modality for diagnosis of these tumors and is also the definitive treatment for low-grade and superficial tumors, with perioperative bladder instillation of chemotherapy recommended for most patients.[42] Agents used for this local treatment are the immune modulator *Bacillus* Calmette-Guerin (BCG) and chemotherapeutic agents, such as mitomycin and thiotepa usually given by the intravesical route. Cystitis is often an uncomfortable side effect of these treatments; cutaneous complications from intravesical instillations may be quite severe.[43] Attempts to avoid or postpone cystectomy for localized, superficial bladder cancers may require long-term follow-up with repeated cystoscopies which can have negative psychological effects. However, for high-risk noninvasive bladder cancers or those not responding to bladder instillation, a cystectomy is recommended by many specialists.[44,45] It remains to be seen what effect the presence of genetic markers such as the p53 gene or mutations of the fibroblast growth factor receptor 3 (FGFR3) will have upon treatment options. Studies focusing on the impact of transurethral resection followed by bladder instillation found the initial therapy period producing the greatest amount of symptoms with over 80% of patients reporting problems such as burning on urination, gross hematuria, and urinary frequency, yet less than half of patients reported reduced physical activity. During maintenance therapy the previous symptoms decreased significantly. Despite being informed of the good prognosis of their illness, there was a strong negative psychological impact, with most patients feeling that their lives would be negatively disrupted.[46]

Men receiving treatment for early-stage bladder cancer generally do not have sexual dysfunction. However, there have been reports of men developing penile curvature after frequent cystoscopy. The overall impact on sexual activity is independent of age and gender.[47] Complaints of decreased sexual desire, feelings of contamination by the cancer, painful intercourse, and other urethral symptoms are reported.

Muscle-invasive bladder cancer. Radical cystectomy (bladder removal) remains the standard procedure for muscle-invasive bladder carcinoma. Surgery alone, or in combination with other treatments, is used in over 90% of cases. Precystectomy chemotherapy alone or with radiation has improved some treatment results for more advanced tumors. Studies suggest a window of opportunity of less than 12 weeks from diagnosis of invasive disease to radical cystectomy to improve prognosis.[48]

Radiation therapy alone is controversial in some patients with bladder cancer. Compared with cystectomy, radiation treatment provides better short-term QOL in the physical, psychological, and sexual domains, although one study found no difference in the QOL between both treatments after 18 months.[49] Frequent symptoms affecting QOL postradiotherapy include frequency, nocturia, urgency, and reduced bladder capacity. Surrounding organs are frequently affected and the dose and volume of radiation is correlated with the more unpleasant symptoms of fecal leakage and urgency, and diarrhea with blood and mucus.[50] Significant gastrointestinal symptoms may persist 2–3 years after pelvic radiotherapy, including the development of proctitis.[51] Modern radiation therapy techniques offer the potential to improve cure rates and reduce adverse effects.[52] Radical cystectomy impacts sexual and urinary functioning in men in a fashion similar to radical prostatectomy. A large proportion of men suffer erectile dysfunction, though the incidence is decreasing with nerve and seminal vesicle sparing techniques. Testosterone secretion is unimpaired, so sexual desire remains unchanged in the long term. Prostate-sparing cystectomy is still to show oncologic efficacy despite its functional advantages.[53]

With cystectomy, many patients have been helped by the internal development of urinary reservoirs constructed from bowel (see Fig. 21–1).[54] These can be anastomosed to either the skin or urethra. When attached to the urethra, continence can be maintained. This has permitted the creation of the neobladder, with which almost all patients achieve daytime urinary continence.[40] Although complications are higher than with the conduit, these procedures obviate the need for an appliance, and are welcomed psychologically.

Women make a better adjustment to the presence of a urinary diversion than men do; this is perhaps related to their being more independent in their stoma care than men. Radical cystectomy in women also includes hysterectomy and oophorectomy and resection of the anterior wall of the vagina. The major sexual side effect for women is genital pain, particularly during intercourse. Decreased sexual arousal, desire, and loss of sexual attractiveness are frequently reported. Surgical modifications to preserve internal genitalia have been suggested as long as cancer control is not compromised.[55] Use of vaginal dilators, lubricants, and estrogen creams can help women become more comfortable during sexual activity by overcoming the consequences of scarring and premature menopause.[56]

Advanced-disease TCC is usually treated with systemic chemotherapy: usually a combination of methotrexate, cisplatin, and vinblastine (MCV) with or without Adriamycin (M-VAC); a combination of

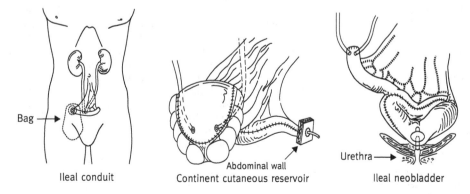

Fig. 21–1. Options for urinary tract reconstruction (diversion) with cystectomy.

Bag → Ileal conduit

Abdominal wall → Continent cutaneous reservoir

Urethra → Ileal neobladder

SOURCE: Reprinted from Seminars in Oncology, Vol. 34 No. 2, Parekh DJ and Donat SM, Urinary diversion: options, patient selection, and outcomes, Pages No. 98–109, Copyright (2007), with permission from Elsevier.

gemcitabine and cisplatin (GemCIS); cyclophosphamide or a taxol-based combination.[57,58]

Urinary tract reconstruction procedures affect overall QOL, mostly in the sexual and urinary spheres. Symptoms vary with the type of reconstruction. Patients with ileal conduits report impaired body image, increased self-consciousness, and decreases in travel and activity level likely related to urinary leakage, odor, and skin irritation at the stoma site. Those with continent diversion report symptoms related to having to use a catheter, while neobladder patients report nighttime leakage. Almost all populations, regardless of reconstruction technique, have sexual dysfunction related to negative physical or psychological effects of the procedure.[59] A sound strategy to achieve greater QOL after radical cystectomy is thorough and active counseling on the various reconstructive alternatives before the surgery that allows choice of the type of urinary diversion on the basis of patient preference, anatomy, and tumor status.[60,61]

KIDNEY CANCER

Epidemiology. Approximately 54,000 patients will be diagnosed with this cancer in 2008, and more than 13,000 will die of the disease.[1] The incidence rises with age, as with TCC of the bladder and prostate cancer. Renal cell carcinoma is the most common neoplastic lesion of the kidney and is almost twice as common in men as in women. Often the diagnosis is made incidentally at the time of radiographic procedures such as ultrasonography or a CT scan for nonurologic problems. There has been some association with cigarette smoking, obesity, and exposure to lead phosphate, dimethyl nitrosamine, and aflatoxins. In addition, obesity, exposure to asbestos, cadmium, and trichloroethylene have been implicated in the development of some kidney cancers.[62] A large percentage of these cancers may remain undiagnosed during life as for prostate cancer; however, with renal cancers a significant proportion of those found incidentally at autopsy actually caused death.[1] A significant number of new cases have overt metastatic disease at the time of diagnosis. Prognosis of these patients is bleak, with a median survival of less than 1 year. The increased use of ultrasound has resulted in a higher detection rate of lower stage tumors.

Diagnosis and management. Patients' presentations may range from the triad of hematuria, pain, and palpable renal mass to more obscure paraneoplastic syndromes, fever, anemia, or polycythemia. Diagnosis is made by intravenous pyelography (IVP), ultrasound, renal arteriography, CT scans, and MRI. Initial evaluations include chest x-rays to evaluate potential sites of pulmonary metastases. Pathologic staging is the most important determinant of prognosis.

The treatment of choice for localized disease is surgical removal of the affected kidney, with regional lymphadenectomy. Five year survival for stage I disease ranges from 60% to 75%, and from 40% to 65% in those with stage II disease. Renal preservation with only partial excision of renal tissue by open surgical or laparoscopic procedures has become more widely accepted, though there is still uncertainty about long-term prognosis. Treatment can provide challenges because of compromised renal function. Most survivors of localized kidney cancer have normal physical and mental health regardless of the type of nephrectomy performed, though QOL is better for patients with more renal parenchyma remaining after surgery.[63]

To date, chemotherapeutic agents have not demonstrated sufficient antitumor activity to prolong the survival of patients with metastatic disease. Sorafenib is a new chemotherapeutic agent that has shown promise in older as well as younger patients.[64] Another agent, sunitinib, was found to provide better QOL to patients with metastatic disease than interferon alpha.[65]

Immunotherapy, autolymphocyte therapy, vaccines, and nonspecific immunomodulators may prolong survival for patients with metastatic renal disease. Interferon and high-dose interleukin-2, used with some success in treating advanced renal cancer, can cause depression and anxiety, which may be mediated through cytokines with physical or somatic side effects such as fatigue and fever. It is possible that patients most at risk of developing significant depression on these drugs are those who have higher baseline depressive symptom scores.[66] An important

study found that those patients who were to get treated with high-dose interferon alpha and who received prophylactic treatment of an SSRI antidepressant had less depression than those who did not get the antidepressant; and for many, major depression onset was delayed.[67] Delirium and cognitive deficits may also be seen as an independent effect of interferon and interleukin on the central nervous system.

The poor prognosis for this illness is the cause for much psychological distress experienced by many patients and their families after diagnosis and treatment. Later stages of disease are highlighted by metastases to bone, lungs, and brain, and necessitates coping with pain, shortness of breath, concentration deficits, and other cognitive difficulties. Distress is caused by periods when the person is free of disease after surgery but has the knowledge that recurrence is likely. The conflict of maintaining hope for successful treatment, in the context of discouraging odds, can be burdensome and can lead to various degrees of anxiety and depression. As with other GU cancers, many patients with renal cancer report worse sexual functioning than in comparable chronically ill populations.[68]

PENILE CANCER

Epidemiology. Penile cancer occurs in about 1 in 100,000 men in the United States; about 1250 new cases of penile cancer will be diagnosed and approximately 290 men will die of it in 2008. Despite its low incidence in the United States, it is much more common in some parts of Africa and South America, accounting for up to 10% of cancers in men. Squamous cell carcinoma accounts for approximately 95% of penile cancers. Most are found in the foreskin or on the glans, but it may develop in any area. Known risk factors include human papilloma virus (HPV) infection, found in about half of cases. Smoking, AIDS, and exposure to ultraviolet (UV) light treatment increase the risk as well.[1]

Diagnosis, management, and quality of life. Ulceration and fissures are the most common initial symptoms[69] and 15%–50% of patients delay seeking treatment for 6 months to a year despite clear symptoms in most cases. Suggested explanations for this delay include "psychological reasons," fear, and anxiety which lead to neglect, minimization, or denial of the symptoms.[70]

Radical surgery is the most effective approach to management of stage II and more advanced cases, with total amputation being preferred in patients with involvement of the proximal third of the penis or in urethra-infiltrating tumors.[71] However, this intervention carries serious anatomical and functional limitations as well as psychological and sexual morbidity; alternative treatments such as partial penectomy and organ preserving treatments are often considered. Compromise of psychological well-being is reported more often in patients who underwent a total penectomy compared to those who underwent a partial amputation, whereas social life problems were not significantly changed.[71] Similar to other amputations, the phenomenon of phantom penis has been described, curiously occurring only in the erect state.[72]

Psychological adjustment to the diagnosis and anticipation of partial penectomy elicits fears of mutilation and loss of sexual pleasure as well as the fear of dying and consequences to the family. After surgery, the most frequent difficulties include resuming sexual activity and the discomfort of having to sit to urinate. Encouragement from wives and families were significant factors in the recovery of some patients.[73] No significant levels of anxiety or depression were noted. No changes were observed with respect to family life or interactions with other people. Most patients reported changes in their sexual activity, although overall functioning, sexual interest, and satisfaction was normal or slightly decreased in a majority of patients. There were no problems in the relationship with their partners and masculine self-image remained mostly normal or only slightly affected. The frequency of coitus was unchanged or only slightly decreased in most cases.

The objective of conservative treatments is complete tumor removal with complete penile preservation. These procedures have increased incidence of recurrence and progression of disease, which emphasizes the importance of appropriate patient selection. Recent surgical approaches to preserve penile tissue and functional integrity without compromising oncologic control are helping to minimize the impact of disease on

QOL. Alternative procedures include reconstruction of the glans using skin from the thigh, rectus abdominal muscles, and glanuloplasty with distal urethra among others.[74-76]

Potential late complications after radiotherapy include penile urethra and external meatus strictures and penile necrosis. Approximately 50% of patients with penile necrosis usually undergo amputation of the penis.[71] Nonetheless, a study comparing sexuality after successful treatment regimens suggested radiotherapy as the treatment of choice when preservation of sexuality is a major objective.[77]

As with other GU cancers the evaluation of sexuality before recommendation of different treatment alternatives is important. Clinicians must be aware of psychological symptoms. Before treatment, physicians must comprehensively discuss the different treatment options including expected results and possible consequences. No assumptions should be made about the importance of sexuality in a patient's life. It has been shown that physicians evaluate posttreatment sexuality to be more impaired than that experienced by patients.[77-79] Arriving at a therapeutic choice must be a joint effort between the patient, the physician, and the partner if appropriate.

SUMMARY

The GU neoplasms are affecting a larger proportion of our population as detection methods are improving. The illnesses and treatments affect patients' QOL in multiple domains. Most prominent QOL issues include coping with changes in sexuality, bladder and bowel function, body image, relationships, fatigue and pain in later stages of disease, and lifestyle. Assessment of these problems is not easy, particularly in distinguishing between physical and psychological etiologies of distress. Discomfort and beliefs about stigma on the part of the patient, the family, and the healthcare provider in discussing these issues provide formidable barriers to evaluation and resolution of distress. Although there are fears that acknowledging and addressing psychological issues will make these symptoms worse, psychological interventions provide avenues for decreased stress and improved quality of living. Not addressing these issues often leads to increased suffering, major psychiatric disorders and feelings of despair, demoralization, isolation, hopelessness, and suicidal ideation.

Medical caregivers should have a low threshold for assessment of patients' distress as well as referral to mental health practitioners. Once assessed, management of these areas includes a spectrum of psychological and psychiatric interventions that includes education, individual and group psychotherapy, couples therapy, cognitive- and behaviorally oriented interventions, and medications. These referrals may be facilitated by increased knowledge on the part of the mental health practitioner about the illness and treatment-specific stressors, as well as a closer liaison with the GU oncology staff.

ACKNOWLEDGMENTS

The authors would like to acknowledge the contribution of Dr. Howard Scher, co-author of the chapter for the last edition of this book who has supported and inspired expertise in clinical care and research about the psychosocial needs of men with prostate cancer and other genitourinary cancers. We also want to acknowledge Dr. Christian Nelson, who has contributed greatly to the research on quality of life in men with genitourinary cancers, in particular regarding sexual functioning and cognitive problems after treatment. We also wish to acknowledge the financial support of the PepsiCo Company, the T. J. Martell Foundation, and the NIH for support of the work of Dr. Roth.

REFERENCES

1. American Cancer Society. *Cancer facts & figures, 2008*. Atlanta, GA: American Cancer Society; 2008.

2. Ries L, Melbert D, Krapcho M, Mariotto A, Miller BA, Feuer EJ, et al. (eds.), *SEER cancer statistics review, 1975–2004*. National Cancer Institute. Bethesda, MD 2007. www.seer.cancer.gov/csr/1975_2004/. Accessed August 3 2009.

3. Wang Y, Corr JG, Thaler HT, et al. Decreased growth of established human prostate LNCaP tumors in nude mice fed a low-fat diet. *J Natl Cancer Inst.* 1995;87:1456–1462.

4. Mokulis J, Thompson I. Screening for prostate cancer: pros, cons, and reality. *Cancer Control.* 1995;(Jan/Feb):15–21.

5. Roth AJ, Rosenfeld B, Kornblith AB, et al. The memorial anxiety scale for prostate cancer: validation of a new scale to measure anxiety in men with prostate cancer. *Cancer.* 2003;97:2910–2918.

6. Lofters A, Juffs HG, Pond GR, Tannock IF. "PSA-itis": knowledge of serum prostate specific antigen and other causes of anxiety in men with metastatic prostate cancer. *J Urol.* 2002;168(6):2516–2520.

7. Klotz L. PSAdynia and other PSA-related syndromes: a new epidemic—a case history and taxonomy. *Urology.* 1997;50:831–832.

8. Roth A, Nelson CJ, Rosenfeld B, et al. Assessing anxiety in men with prostate cancer: further data on the reliability and validity of the Memorial Anxiety Scale for Prostate Cancer (MAX-PC) *Psychosomatics.* 2006;47:340–347.

9. Dale W, Bilir P, Han M, Meltzer D. The role of anxiety in prostate carcinoma. *Cancer.* 2005;104:467–478.

10. Wilt T, MacDonald R, Rutks I, Shamliyan TA, Taylor BC, Kane RL. Systematic review: comparative effectiveness and harms of treatments for clinically localized prostate cancer. *Ann Intern Med.* 2008;148:435–448.

11. Eton D, Lepore SJ. Prostate cancer and health-related quality of life: a review of the literature. *Psycho-Oncology.* 2002;11:307–326.

12. Sanda M, Dunn RL, Michaleski J, et al. Quality of life and satisfaction with outcome among prostate-cancer survivors. *N Engl J Med.* 2008;358:1250–1261.

13. Klotz L. Active surveillance for prostate cancer: trials and tribulations. *World J Urol.* 2008;26:437–442.

14. Johansson B, Holmberg L, Onelov E, Johansson JE, Steinenck G. Time, symptom burden, androgen deprivation, and self-assessed quality of life after radical prostatectomy or watchful waiting: the Randomized Scandinavian Prostate Cancer Group Study Number 4 (SPCG-4) Clinical Trial. *Eur Urol.* 2009 Feb;55(2):261–532.

15. Hakimi A, Feder M, Ghavamian R. Minimally invasive approaches to prostate cancer: a review of the current literature. *Urol J.* 2007;4:130–137.

16. Pirl W, Siegel GI, Good R. Depression in men receiving androgen deprivation therapy for prostate cancer: a pilot study. *Psycho-Oncology.* 2002;11: 519–523.

17. Harlan L, Brawley O, Pommerenke F, Wali P, Kramer B. Geographic, age, and racial variation in the treatment of local/regional carcinoma of the prostate. *J Clin Oncol.* 1995;13:93–100.

18. Blank T, Bellizzi KM. After prostate cancer: predictors of well-being among long term prostate cancer survivors. *Cancer.* 2006;106:2128–2135.

19. Ofman U. Sexual quality of life in men with prostate cancer. *Cancer (Suppl).* 1994;75:1949–1953.

20. Steginga S, Occhipinti S, Dunn J, Gardiner RA, Heathcote P, Yaxley J. The supportive care needs of men with prostate cancer. *Psycho-Oncology.* 2000;10:66–75.

21. Lai H, Hsu EI, Teh BS, Butler EB, Boone TB. 13 years of experience with artificial urinary sphincter implantation at Baylor College of Medicine. *J Urol.* 2007;177:1021–1025.

22. Payne R. Pain management in the patient with prostate cancer. *Cancer.* 1993;71(Suppl 3):11131–11137.

23. Heim H, Oei TPS. Comparison of prostate cancer patients with and without pain. *Pain.* 1993;53:159–162.

24. Kornblith A, Herr HW, Ofman US, Scher HI, Holland JC. Quality of life of patients with prostate cancer and their spouses. The value of a data base in clinical care. *Cancer.* 1994;73:2791–2802.

25. Roth A, Nelson CJ, Rosenfeld B, et al. Psychostimulants for fatigue in men with prostate cancer. *ASCO Prostate Cancer Symposium.* February 2006:275.

26. Roth A, Scher HI. Sertraline relieves hot flashes secondary to medical castration as treatment of advanced prostate cancer. *Psycho-Oncology.* 1998;7:129–132.

27. Loprinzi C, Barton DL, Carpenter LA, et al. Pilot evaluation of paroxetine for treating hot flashes in men. *Mayo Clin Proc.* 2004;79:1247–1251.

28. Adelson K, Loprinzi CL, Hershman DL. Treatment of hot flushes in breast and prostate cancer. *Expert Opin Pharmacother.* 2005;6:1095–1106.

29. Couper J, Bloch S, Love A, Duchesne G, Macvean M, Kissane DW. The psychosocial impact of prostate cancer on patients and their partners. *Med J.* 2006;16(185):428–432.

30. Dearnaley D, Huddart R, Horwich A. Regular review: managing testicular cancer. *BMJ.* 2001;322(7302):1583–1588.

31. Bosl G, Bajorin DF, Sheinfeld J, Motzer J. Cancer of the testis. In: DeVita V, Lawrence TS, Rosenberg SA (eds.), *Cancer: Principles and practice of oncology.* 8th ed. Philadephia, PA: Lippincott; 2008:1465–1483.

32. Nichols C, Timmerman R, Foster RS, Roth BJ, Einhorn LH. Neoplasms of the testis. In: Bast RJ, Kufe DW, Pollock RE, et al. (eds.), *Cancer medicine.* 5th ed. Hamilton: BC Decker Inc; 2000.

33. Kollmannsberger C, Kuzcyk M, Mayer F, Hartmann JT, Kanz L, Bokemeyer C. Late toxicity following curative treatment of testicular cancer. *Semin Surg Oncol.* 1999;17(4):275–281.

34. Ozen H SA, Toklu C, Rastadoskouee M, Kilic C, Gogus A, Kendi S. Psychosocial adjustment after testicular cancer treatment. *J Urol.* 1998;159(6): 1947–1950.

35. Heidenreich A, Hofmann R. Quality-of-life issues in the treatment of testicular cancer. *World J Urol.* 1999;17(4):230–238.

36. Bertetto O, Bracarda S, Tamburini M, Cortesi E. Quality of life studies and genito-urinary tumors. *Ann Oncol.* 2001;12(Suppl 3):S43-S48.

37. Trask P, Paterson AG, Fardig J, Smith DC. Course of distress and quality of life in testicular cancer patients before, during, and after chemotherapy: results of a pilot study. *Psycho-Oncology.* 2003;12(8):814–820.

38. Arai Y, Kawakita M, Hida S, Terachi T, Okada Y, Yoshida O. Psychosocial aspects in long-term survivors of testicular cancer. *J Urol.* 1996;155(2): 574–578.

39. Dahl A, Haaland CF, Mykletun A, et al. Study of anxiety disorder and depression in long-term survivors of testicular cancer. *J Clin Oncol.* 2005;23(10): 2389–2395.

40. McDougal W, Shipley WU, Kaufman DS, Dahl DM, Michaelson MD, Zietman AL. Cancer of the bladder, ureter, and renal pelvis. In: DeVita V, Lawrence TS, Rosenberg SA (eds), *Cancer: Principles and practice of oncology.* 8th ed. Philadelphia, PA: Lippincott; 2008:1358–1361.

41. Barocas D, Clark PE. Bladder cancer. *Curr Opin Oncol.* 2008;20: 307–314.

42. Clarke P. Bladder cancer. *Curr Opin Oncol.* 2007;19:241–247.

43. Kureshi F, Kalaaji AN, Halvorson L, Pittelkow MR, Davis MDP. Cutaneous complications of intravesical treatments for bladder cancer: granulomatous inflammation of the penis following BCG therapy and penile gangrene following mitomycin therapy. *J Am Acad Dermatol.* 2006;55:328–331.

44. Oosterlinck W, Witjes F, Sylvester R. Diagnostic and prognostic factors in non-muscle-invasive bladder cancer and their influence on treatment and outcomes. *Eur Urol Suppl.* 2008;7:516–523.

45. Skinner E. The best treatment for high-grade T1 bladder cancer is cystectomy. *Urol Oncol.* 2007;25:523–525.

46. Bohle A, Balck F, von Weitersheim J, Jocham D. The quality of life during intravesical bacillus Calmette-Guerin therapy. *J Urol.* 1996;155(4):1221–1226.

47. Mack D, Frick J. Quality of life in patients undergoing bacille Calmette-Guerin therapy for superficial bladder cancer. *Br J Urol.* 1996;78(3):369–371.

48. Fahmy N, Mahmud S, Aprikian AG. Delay in the surgical treatment of bladder cancer and survival: systematic review of the literature. *Eur Urol.* 2006;50:1176–1182.

49. Lynch W, Jenkins BJ, Fowler CG, Hope-Stone HF, Blandy JP. The quality of life after radical radiotherapy for bladder cancer. *Br J Urol.* 1992;70: 519–521.

50. Henningsohn L. Quality of life after therapy for muscle-invasive bladder cancer. *Curr Opin Urol* 2006;16:356–360.

51. Andreyev H, Vlavianos P, Blake P, Dearnaley D, Norman AR, Tait D. Gastrointestinal symptoms after pelvic radiotherapy: role for the gastroenterologist? *Int J Radiat Oncol Biol Phys.* 2005;62:1464–1471.

52. Milosevic M, Gospodarowicz M, Zietman A, et al. Radiotherapy for bladder cancer. *Urology.* 2007;69:80–92.

53. Kefer J, Cherullo EE, Jones JS, Gong MC, Campbell SC. Prostate-sparing cystectomy: has Pandora's box been opened? *Expert Rev Anticancer Ther.* 2007;13:179–187.

54. Parekh D, Donat SM. Urinary diversion: options, patient selection, and outcomes. *Semin Oncol.* 2007;34:98–109.

55. Miranda-Sousa A, Davila HH, Lockhart JL, Ordorica RC, Carrion RE. Sexual function after surgery for prostate or bladder cancer. *Cancer Control.* 2006;13:179–187.

56. Ofman U, Kingsberg SA, Nelson CJ. Sexual problems. In: DeVita V, Lawrence TS, Rosenberg SA (eds.), *Cancer: Principles and practice of oncology.* 8th ed. Philadelphia, PA: Lippincott; 2008:2804–2809.

57. Von der Maase H, Hansen SW, Roberts JT, et al. Gemcitabine and cisplatin versus methotrexate, vinblastine, doxorubicin, and cisplatin in advanced

or metastatic bladder cancer: results of a large, randomized, multinational, multicenter, phase III study. *J Clin Oncol.* 2000;18(7):3068–3077.

58. Albers P, Siener R, Perabo FG, et al. Gemcitabine monotherapy as 2nd-line treatment in cisplatin refractory transitional cell carcinoma. Paper presented at American Society of Clinical Oncology; 2000.

59. Botteman M, Pashos C, Hauser R, Laskin B, Redaelli A. Quality of life aspects of bladder cancer: a review of the literature. *Qual Life Res.* 2003;12:675–688.

60. Wright J, Porter MP. Quality-of-life assessment in patients with bladder cancer. *Natl Clin Pract Urol* 2007;4:147–154.

61. Davidsson T, Wullt B, Konyves J, Mansson A, Mansson W. Urinary diversion and bladder substitution in patients with bladder cancer. *Urol Oncol.* 2007;5(5):224–231.

62. Linehan W, Schmidt LS. *Cancers of the genitourinary system in DeVita, Hellman and Rosenberg's cancer: Principles and practice of oncology.* 8th ed. Philadephphia, PA: Lippincott, Williams and Wilkens; 2008.

63. Clarke P, Schover LR, Uzzo RG, Hafez KS, Rybicki LA, Novick AC. Quality of life and psychological adaptation after surgical treatment for localized renal cell carcinoma: impact of the amount of remaining renal tissue. *Urology.* 2001;57:252–256.

64. Eisen T, Oudard S, Szcylik C, et al. Sorafenib for older patients with renal cell carcinoma: subset analysis from a randomized trial. *J Natl Cancer Inst.* 2008. Oct 15;100(20):1454–63.

65. Cella D, Li JZ, Cappalleri JC, et al. Quality of life in patients with metastatic renal cell carcinoma treated with sunitinib or interferon alfa: results from a phase III randomized trial. *J Clin Oncol.* 2008;26:3763–3769.

66. Capuron L, Ravaud A, Miller AH, Dantzer R. Baseline mood and psychosocial characteristics of patients developing depressive symptoms during interleukin-2 and/or interferon-alpha cancer therapy. *Brain Behav Immun.* 2004;18:205–213.

67. Musselman D, Lawson DH, Gumnick JF, et al. Paroxetine for the prevention of depression induced by high-dose interferon alfa. *N Engl J Med.* 2001;344(13):961–966.

68. Anastasiadis A, Davis AR, Sawczuk IS, et al. Quality of life aspects in kidney cancer patients: data from a national registry. *Cancer.* 2003;11:700–706.

69. Skeppner E, Windahl T, Andersson SO, Fugl-Meyer KS. Treatment-seeking, aspects of sexual activity and life satisfaction in men with laser-treated penile carcinoma. *Eur Urol.* 2008;54:631–639.

70. Misra S, Chaturvedi A, Misra NC. Penile carcinoma: a challenge for the developing world. *Lancet Oncol.* 2004;5:240–247.

71. Ficarra V, Maffei N, Piacentini I, Al Rabi N, Cerruto MA, Artibani W. Local treatment of penile squamous cell carcinoma. *Urol Int.* 2002;69:169–173.

72. Fisher C. Phantom erection after amputation of penis. Case description and review of the relevant literature on phantoms. *Can J Neurol Sci.* 1999;26:53–56.

73. D'Ancona C, Botega NJ, De Moraes C, Lavoura NS Jr, Santos JK, Rodrigues Netto N. Quality of life after partial penectomy for penile carcinoma. *Urology.* 1997;50:593–596.

74. Palminteri E, Berdondini E, Lazzeri M, Mirri F, Barbagli G. Resurfacing and reconstruction of the glans penis. *Eur Urol.* 2007;52:893–898.

75. Kayes O, Durrant CA, Ralph D, Floyd D, Withey S, Minhas S. Vertical rectus abdominis flap reconstruction in patients with advanced penile squamous cell carcinoma. *BJU Int.* 2007;178:941–944.

76. Gulino G, Sasso F, Falabella R, Bassi PF. Distal urethral reconstruction of the glans for penile carcinoma: results of a novel technique at 1-year of followup. *J Urol.* 2007;73:554–560.

77. Opjordsmoen S, Waehre H, Aass N, Fossa SD. Sexuality in patients treated for penile carcinoma: patients' experience and doctors' judgement. *Br J Urol.* 1994;73:554–560.

78. Wise T, Boland R. Psychosocial consequences of penectomy following carcinoma of the penis. *J Sex Educ Ther.* 1997;22:39–41.

79. Witkin M, Kaplan HS. Sex therapy and penectomy. *J Sex Marital Ther.* 1982;8:209–221.

CHAPTER 22

Gynecologic Cancers

Margaret I. Fitch

INTRODUCTION

In 2006, there were 71,090 cases of gynecologic cancer and 26,360 deaths in the United States.[1] Gynecologic cancers include ovarian, cervical, endometrial, vulvar, and vaginal types. Each differs in terms of risk factors, median age at diagnosis, ethnic distribution, type of treatment, and survival probability.

Endometrial cancer, the most common gynecologic cancer, is the fifth most common cancer in women worldwide. Cervical cancer is the second most common cancer among women worldwide and is the third most common cause of all cancer deaths.[2] Ovarian cancer is the fourth leading cause of cancer-related deaths in women but the number one killer in gynecologic malignancies.[3] Vulvar cancer represents less than 4% of all gynecologic cancers and vaginal cancer less than 1%. As with other cancers, prognosis from gynecologic cancer is linked to the stage of disease and grade of tumor at diagnosis.

Treatment for gynecologic cancers includes surgery followed by chemotherapy and/or radiation.[4–7] Each has the potential for major side effects during the primary treatment interval and significant late and long-term effects. In particular, surgery for gynecologic cancer results in extensive body and functional changes while the chemotherapeutic agents of choice have high toxicity burdens. Recent advances in treatment have resulted in a growing cadre of women who can anticipate a good outcome from their treatments.[8] These women are in an excellent position to identify where improvements can be made in psychosocial care.

Gynecologic cancers and their treatments have more than a physical impact. There are emotional, psychological, social, spiritual, and practical consequences as well. For each woman, the cancer journey is a unique experience and each will cope in her own fashion.[9,10] Understanding the individual's unique perspective is a critical step in being able to provide effective psychosocial interventions.

HOW WOMEN EXPERIENCE GYNECOLOGIC CANCERS

This chapter focuses on the perspectives of women who have experienced a gynecologic cancer. Seeing the cancer journey through the eyes of women who have lived through the events and understanding their views about key challenges are important steps in providing psychosocial care. Research is relatively scant regarding quality of life and the psychosocial challenges faced by women living with a gynecologic cancer. However, the past decade has seen an increasing interest in the needs of this population.

The narratives women tell about their experiences with a gynecological cancer are often descriptions about a journey of transition and change.[11] The meaningful points of transition along this journey are moments when change is significant and fundamental decisions are required; where life alters irrevocably, yet still moves on.

The cancer journey for women is lived in a connected and continuous fashion, yet all too often the journey feels fragmented. The complexity of cancer care requires women to move through different settings and see different providers who may pay little attention to what has happened before. Women feel they are starting over with each new provider and each new request for information. They often feel challenged finding their way to resources and support.

The description below, drawn from research concerning women's experiences with gynecologic cancers, contains commonly identified perspectives within qualitative work supported by observations from a broader literature. The description is organized to reflect the steps in the cancer journey identified as significant transitions by the women. The challenges highlighted are the ones women described as key themes across each phase and are supported by exemplars portraying the women's voices. As much as possible, the words and the language are theirs.

Finding an abnormality. The cancer journey begins with finding an abnormality and wondering whether something might be seriously wrong. Unless there is a distressing symptom for which urgent help is needed, symptoms associated with gynecologic cancers can go unrecognized as signs for cancer.[11] Women often confuse symptoms with normal body changes related to menopause or the aftermath of childbearing.

Looking back I would say, yes, there were symptoms there. But had I realized that this could be a warning sign of cancer I certainly would have done something about it. But I just thought they were annoyances or things that changed as a result of having children or things that were changing as a result of aging ... (Sally)

Assigning meaning to the symptom and deciding what action is needed are critical aspects at this stage of the cancer journey. Whether a symptom is recognized as serious and knowing where to go to access medical advice can be complex in light of the uncertainty surrounding symptoms of gynecologic cancers.

Appraisal of symptoms or the interpretation of their importance accounts for the major portion of patient delay.[12] What eventually sends patients to seek help is pain, incapacity, fear, advice or encouragement from a friend or relative, or time for a routine medical check-up.[13]

Undergoing tests. In the case where symptoms are vague, women find it difficult to describe clearly what is happening to them. They believe something about their bodies is different, but find it hard to find the words to describe it to the physician.

I had symptoms for...like at least two years. I complained to my GP...sexual intercourse was painful. I complained to her about being tired all the time, having no energy...why do I feel sick all the time? ... Finally the pain got so bad...(Gail)

Given this situation, women can feel others do not believe them or their concerns are being dismissed.[11] Yet, when symptoms mimic common inflammatory gastrointestinal disease, the diagnostic process is somewhat complex.[14] Particularly in the case of ovarian cancer, women can be dismayed at the length of time they feel it takes physicians to focus on ovarian cancer as a possible explanation for their symptoms and feel valuable time has been lost.[15] When a definitive diagnosis is made following a seemingly protracted period of investigation, women may feel anger toward their physicians for what they believe is a missed diagnosis or may hold a sense of regret for not acting assertively in their own interest.[15]

Another challenge for women is preparing for tests. Many describe access to information about tests and what to expect as not being easy.

Having this type of information allows women to feel prepared and better able to get through the procedures.[16–18] Particularly in light of the invasive nature of pelvic examinations, emotional and mental preparation is important.

Mentally I feel like I have to prepare myself…I have to relax…I have to consciously think about what's going on…once they decided to do a Pap smear and everything but I didn't even know that that was going to happen. I wasn't prepared for that and I was pretty uncomfortable. (Susan)

Waiting for results is another major issue for women. Dealing with the uncertainty while waiting for the answers is one of the greatest challenges for patients.[19] Many feel they have lost control at this point and cannot influence what will happen.

Hearing the diagnosis. To hear one has cancer evokes shock, numbness, and disbelief. It is a moment when life is irrevocably changed, regardless of the cancer type. Some women recall this period as the beginning of an emotional roller coaster.

It was devastating, just devastating. There is no other word for it…so overwhelming…I felt helpless to do anything. I didn't know what to do. (Meg)

For many, telling others about the cancer diagnosis is challenging. Women often feel overwhelmed and not in possession of enough information to tell others. In particular, telling children is a source of distress.[20] There are fears about frightening the child, yet not wanting to exclude the child. Adolescents describe wanting to know at least the basics about their mother's situation.[21]

Women worry particularly about children in light of the emotional impact and change that has entered into their children's lives. They also worry whether they passed cancer on to the children, especially their daughters. Women with young children are particularly fearful about what life will be like for their children should they die.[20,22]

Making a decision about treatment. Once the diagnosis has been made, women are anxious to begin treatment but want to learn about treatment options and prognosis. However, accessing understandable, relevant information is a challenge.[23] Many struggle with the medical terminology and language of statistics,[24] feeling overwhelmed with what they learn and the decisions to be made.

Once I heard, then everything was happening so fast…I had less than 3 days. And all I could think of in that three days was, who's going to wash the clothes? Who's going to do the cooking? Who's going to take my boy to school? If I don't have any income, who's going to pay the mortgage? What will happen to the house? (Marta)

In our work with ovarian cancer patients, many women reported that they felt very little or no involvement in decision making regarding the initial treatment. Some were simply too ill at the time while others felt inadequately prepared to be involved.[25] They felt they did not have enough information about ovarian cancer, yet were being pressured to decide about treatment. Some felt they were *"on an assembly line"* with little control over events and being rushed into starting treatment. When faced with this situation, they elected to follow the recommendations of their doctors.

One key issue women face as they make the decision about treatment is fertility. Having to consider this issue when feeling vulnerable and overwhelmed adds considerable distress to the situation and challenge to decision making. Feelings of unfairness about the situation overwhelm many.

Receiving treatment. Receiving treatment can be conceptualized as having three phases: starting, getting through, and finishing.

Starting treatment is often associated with concerns about what is ahead. Questions about the treatment, side effects, and expected course of events are on many women's minds.[26] Obtaining information about their specific situation often remains an issue. The information they receive is perceived as too general. Many are concerned about managing the side effects and organizing their lives.

Getting through treatment takes considerable effort. Each treatment has side effects that create demands. Surgery means a loss of body organs steeped in meanings about being a woman and femininity. Postoperatively there is pain, limited mobility, and fatigue. Chemotherapy is described by some as "using the big guns." The regimes are relatively toxic and can cause nausea, vomiting, fatigue, neuropathy, cognitive changes, and hair loss. Pelvic radiation can cause changes in bowel and bladder function, fatigue, and skin irritation. Dealing with side effects is a major issue during this period.[27,28]

It's treatment non-stop, non-stop. Very little reprieve…there's ups and downs…when you are actively being treated, it's your whole life. (Donna)

During treatment, most women are unable to carry on with their usual work and household activities. Life takes on a cyclical pattern of feeling unwell, gradually regaining some capacity to function, and then facing the same thing over again with the next treatment. Repeatedly women talk about the challenge of looking after themselves as well as their families and their frustration at not being able to do what they usually do.[20,22] They often see themselves as being centrally responsible for the maintenance of the family and household and struggle with letting this responsibility go or others taking it over. Partners and children may have to assume new responsibilities and career-related activities may have to be put on hold.

Studies have reported changes in quality of life for women receiving treatment for gynecological cancers.[29–35] These studies document how fatigue and high rates of anxiety and depression have impacted women's daily lives. Those who lived with pain and fatigue lost the ability to enjoy life, engage in normal activities, and maintain employment status.

Finishing treatment is often a time of mixed emotions. On one hand, women are relieved to complete the arduous treatment and begin to focus on recovery. On the other hand, there is fear about the future. Some women regret there will be fewer visits to the cancer centre and have feelings of abandonment and being "cut adrift."

Finding a "new" normal. As women leave their primary treatment behind, they embark on various survivorship pathways. Some are cured, but have lingering side effects such as fatigue; some have a period of remission, followed by recurrence; others continue to fight the disease on a daily basis.

When women start to feel physically stronger, they begin to reflect about what has happened and what lies ahead. They are challenged to come to terms with what their "new life" will be to manage the emotional reactions they experience.

Women will engage in the process of reestablishing their roles within their families and their workplaces. But at the same time, they may need to adapt to changes in their capacity to work and perform activities of daily living.

I have been forced to acknowledge the impact of chemotherapy, radiation and surgery to my body and my spirit. It is not any single one of them, but all of them together that has been so physically and emotionally devastating. …. It's a double or triple whammy! (Lila)

Part of this reestablishment process involves identifying what is important and whether lifestyle changes are needed. Issues may emerge because of changes in relationships, roles, and attitudes about life priorities. Howell and colleagues[22] described the challenges women had to master following ovarian cancer as living with uncertainty and lack of control, confronting fear of the unknown and the stigma of having cancer, and facing the possibility of recurrence and death.

The challenge is to accept…I have cancer and I have to bear with this for the rest of my life…like you can live normally, like you can drive, you can still work, you can take your son to school, then you have to consider that as a cure. But it's a bomb; it's like a time bomb in your body. It could blow up any time if you don't take care of yourself. (Mandy)

Women describe this process of reflection as an opportunity to clarify beliefs, identify new priorities, or reaffirm what is important to them. Work regarding posttraumatic growth after cancer has emphasized the value of this reflection for cancer survivors.[36,37]

The growing cadre of survivors who have been treated for gynecologic cancer describe coping with many issues shared by other cancer survivors.[38–40] Recently, more research has focused on gynecologic cancer survivors and reports have appeared describing the needs of this population.[41–48] Reports cite more issues related to being younger, less educated, un-partnered, and living with more extensive disease.[49,50]

In addition, there are unique issues for those who have experienced gynecologic cancer. The changes in body structure and function following gynecologic cancer treatment create physical and psychosexual changes for most women. Whether these become challenges depends on the support they receive and the importance of sexuality in their lives.[51–53] Some women will experience a greater sense of intimacy with their partners despite not having sexual intercourse any more, while others will struggle to regain a measure of sexual satisfaction and self-esteem.

Losing bowel and bladder function as well as sexual sensation rocked my whole sense of self—as a woman and in my world. I am still struggling to maintain my dignity in the face of the shame these physical losses bring me. I am better now than four years ago when I was filled with despair. It has taken me this long to learn to live positively despite my disabilities. (Karen)

Fertility can be an issue for younger women when the treatment has rendered them infertile.[22] Infertility brings forth an acute sense of loss and missed opportunity. When the supportive care needs of younger women are compared against those of older women, issues of fertility, treatment-induced menopause, and sexuality are cited as concerns for a larger proportion of the younger women.[54–56] With treatment-induced menopause, the intensity of the symptoms can be heightened in contrast to those of a naturally occurring menopause. Also, younger women may experience a sense of isolation as they undergo menopause. Because none of their peers are experiencing it, their access to a supportive network can be compromised.

Finally, the majority of survivors talk about the fear of recurrence as a primary challenge. Although it may lessen over time, the fear never entirely vanishes. New aches or pains evoke the idea cancer could be back.

We make plans for the future now like we normally did before. We talk about when the kids graduate; when they move out, we're going to sell the house. We make all these plans. But in my mind I still have this, "yeah, if I am still here." (Helen)

Hearing there is a recurrence. To hear there is recurrent disease is a very difficult moment. This is a message that signals women's entry into the world of metastatic disease.

Women describe a sense of disillusionment and discouragement that the disease is back. They must face decision making about treatment again and the reality of more treatment side effects. Once again access to information becomes of paramount importance. However, there is a fundamental difference for these women. They possess a good deal of information from their previous experiences and may want a different decision-making role than at the onset of their cancer experience. This can be a time when women become more assertive, pushing for information, seeking second opinions, exploring complementary and alternative therapies, and attempting to regain a measure of control over their lives.

The time of recurrence is a particularly vulnerable point in the process of communication between healthcare providers and women. In one report,[57] women described a sense of hopelessness emerging from the healthcare team as they talked about plans for managing symptoms rather than treating the recurrence. At a time when the women felt especially vulnerable, they perceived health professionals turning away.

Living with metastatic or advancing disease is a time when symptoms reappear, progress, and need to be managed well. Of frequent concern in this population is the prevention and management of pain, ascites, and malignant bowel obstructions.[58] This is also a time when women are trying to balance living with dying. Questions arise about what the future holds, the expected course of events, what will happen to family members, and what will happen at the point of death.

This disease has completely eroded almost all future dreams and hopes of mine. Due to the lack of adequate treatment for this disease, my life expectancy is extremely short. I will not see my children mature into adulthood. I will not share the years ahead with my husband. I am not able to do physically taxing activities with my friends and family. This is particularly difficult because my children are still young. I am not able to work any more—which changes our financial picture somewhat. But the most difficult aspect for me is knowing that my children won't have a mother for much longer. (Sarah)

As symptoms progress and mobility becomes more limited, women face the challenges around loss of independence and having to turn to others for help. They feel their world is closing in and becoming more constricted. Yet for many, hope remains a constant companion. Focusing on what is important and what is still achievable is a source of comfort.

Living with metastatic disease involves living with a heightened sense of uncertainty and a need to focus on priorities. There may be unfinished "life business" women want to complete and a desire to plan for events such as funerals and distribution of belongings while there is still energy to engage in the process.

Facing the end of life and last days of living. As the end of life approaches with greater certainty, several decisions ought to be made: Will the last days be spent at home or in a palliative care setting? What is the plan about resuscitation? What care responsibilities are the family willing and able to perform? These are challenging questions and require conversations that can be difficult. Not everyone in the family may be at the same point in coping with the reality of the impending death.

The last days of living require excellent symptom management for the patient and strong emotional support for the family. The major concern for the family is to know the patient is not in pain. All are anticipating the impending loss and will respond accordingly. Family members are uncertain about what to do and may feel helpless. Providing information about what to expect can be beneficial for them.

PROVIDING PSYCHOSOCIAL CARE FOR WOMEN WITH GYNECOLOGIC CANCER

Women living through an experience with gynecologic cancer face many challenges and must cope with a myriad of changes. The experience can be a cascade of unfolding events that leave the woman feeling much like she is on a roller coaster, catapulting along without much control. Although feeling emotional distress is part of this journey it needs to be mitigated early in the course of the illness.[59–61] At present, many women and their family members remain uncertain where they can turn for help regarding the distress they feel. Intentional efforts are required to identify women's concerns and the ones who are at high risk for psychosocial distress. Efforts are needed in cancer settings to inform women about available services and resources.

Standards and guidelines regarding psychosocial care for adult cancer patients have been published.[11] These guidelines emphasize the need for structures and processes to be established within cancer facilities to ensure all patients to have regular comprehensive assessment, good symptom management, effective communication with the healthcare team, tailored or individualized support from their principal cancer care team, as well as timely and relevant referral to psychosocial experts when needed (e.g., social workers, psychologists, psychiatrists, chaplains, dieticians, physiotherapists, occupational therapists, etc.). Screening for emotional distress as the sixth vital sign, using a standardized measure, needs to be a standard of practice early in the course of the illness.

To date, there has been little research testing psychosocial interventions specifically designed for women with gynecologic cancers. Much of the program development for this population has had to depend on work drawn from other disease populations (i.e., breast). Recently, some attention is being paid to the psychosocial care of women with gynecologic cancers. Reports have emphasized the need for interventions that incorporate all domains of quality of life.[62,63]

A significant development over the past decade has been the growth in peer and survivor organizations. In particular, ovarian cancer groups have been strong advocates for education about early detection and support women who have been diagnosed with the disease (www.ovariancanada.org). Innovative programs for medical and nursing students have been mounted with survivors teaching students about what it is like to live with the illness.[64] Survivorship workshops have been designed for ovarian cancer survivors to help women pick up the pieces of their lives after their treatment. Evaluation of the program has shown women finding the information and the interaction with other survivors to be most helpful.[65]

CONCLUSION

Work is needed both in understanding the specific needs of women who have been diagnosed with a gynecologic cancer and in understanding what interventions will be most useful to support them throughout their cancer journey. Advances in treatment have resulted in a growing cadre of women who can anticipate a good outcome from their treatment. However, they will still face change and challenge as they move through the arduous course of treatment and coping with the lingering side effects. A priority for the coming years must be to find effective approaches for providing psychosocial care for this population across the cancer journey.

REFERENCES

1. American Cancer Society. *Cancer: facts and figures, 2006*. American Cancer Society; 2006.
2. Jemal A, Siegel R, Ward E, et al. Cancer statistics 2008. *CA: Cancer J Clin*. 2008;58(2):71–96.
3. National Cancer Institute of Canada. *Cancer statistics 2008*. Toronto: Author; 2008.
4. Brisw RE, Tomacruz RS, Armstrong DK, Trimble EL, Montz FJ. Survival effects of maximal cytoreductive surgery for advanced ovarian carcinoma during the platinum era: a meta-analysis. *J Clin Oncol*. 2002;20:1248–1259.
5. Ledermann JA, Wheeler S. How should we manage patients with platinum-sensitive recurrent ovarian cancer? *Cancer Invest*. 2004;22(Suppl 2):2–10.
6. Bordurka DC, Bevers MW. Preinvasive disease of the lower female genital track. In: Barakat RR, et al. (eds.), *Handbook of gynecologic oncology*. 2nd ed. London: Martin Dunitz; 2002.
7. Hatch KD, Berek JS. Intraepithelial disease of the cervix, vagina and vulva. In: Berek JS (ed.), *Novak's gynecology*. 13th ed. Philadelphia, PA: Lippincott, Williams & Watkins; 2002:471–503.
8. Berkenblit A, Cannistra SA. Advances in the management of epithelial ovarian cancer. *J Reprod Med*. 2005;50(6):426–438.
9. Fitch MI, Porter HB, Page BD. *Supportive care framework: a foundation for person-centred care*. Pembroke, ON: Pappin Communications; 2008.
10. Lazarus R, Folkman S. *Stress, appraisal and coping*. New York: Springer; 1984.
11. Fitch MI, Deane K, Howell D, Gray RE. Women's experiences with ovarian cancer: reflections on being diagnosed. *Can Oncol Nurs J*. 2002;12(3):152–159.
12. Andersen BL, Cacioppo JT, Roberts DC. (1995) Delay in seeking a cancer diagnosis delay stages and psychophysiology comparison processes. *Br J Soc Psychol*. 1995;34:33–52.
13. Hackett T, Cassem N, Raker T. Patient delay in cancer. *New Engl J Med*. 1973;289:14–20.
14. Wikborn C, Pettersson F, Moberg PJ. Delay in diagnosis of epithelial ovarian cancer. *Int J Gynecol Obstet*. 1996;52(3):263–267.
15. Smith A. Whisperings of ovarian cancer: acknowledging women's voices. *Clin J Oncol Nurs*. 2008;12(6):913–920.
16. Mulcahy V. Women's experiences with pelvic examinations: a phenomenological study. Unpublished Master's Thesis, University of Toronto; 1995.
17. Velji K, Fitch MI. The experience of women receiving brachytherapy for gynecologic cancer. *Oncol Nurs Forum*. 2001;28(4):743–751.
18. Carr E, Brockbank K, Allen S, Strike P. Patterns and frequency of anxiety in women undergoing gynecological surgery. *J Clin Nurs*. 2006;15:341–352.
19. Power J, Brown L, Ritvo P. A qualitative study examining psychosocial distress, coping, and social support across the stages and phases of epithelial ovarian cancer. *Health Care Women Int*. 2008;29(4):366–383.
20. Fitch MI, Bunston T, Elliot M. When Mom's sick: changes in a mother's role and in the family after her diagnosis of cancer. *Cancer Nurs*. 1999;22(1):58–63.
21. Fitch MI, Abramson T. Information needs of adolescents when a mother is diagnosed with breast cancer. *Can Oncol Nurs J*. 2007;17(1):16–20.
22. Howell D, Fitch MI, Deane KA. Impact of ovarian cancer perceived by women. *Cancer Nurs*. 2003;26(1):1–9.
23. Manderson L, Markovic M, Quinn M. "Like roulette": Australian women's explanations of gynecologic cancers. *Soc Sci Med*. 2005;61:323–332.
24. Jefferies H. Ovarian cancer patients: are their informational and emotional needs being met? *J Clin Nurs*. 2002;11:41–47.
25. Fitch MI, Deane K, Howell D. Living with ovarian cancer: women's perspectives on treatment and treatment decision-making. *Can Oncol Nurs J*. 2003;13(1):8–13.
26. Browall M, Carlsson M, Horvath G. Information needs of women with recently diagnosed ovarian cancer: a longitudinal study. *Eur J Oncol Nurs*. 2004;8:200–207.
27. Steele R, Fitch MI. Supportive care needs of gynecologic cancer patients. *Cancer Nurs*. 2008;31(4):284–291.
28. Ferrell B, Smith S, Cullinane C, Melancon C. Symptom concerns of women with ovarian cancer. *J Pain Symptom Manage*. 2003;25(6):528–538.
29. Kornblith AB, Thaler HT, Wong G, et al. Quality of life of women with ovarian cancer. *Gynecol Oncol*. 1995;59:231–242.
30. Ersek M, Ferrel BR, Hassey Dow K, Melancon CH. Quality of life in women with ovarian cancer. *West J Nurs Res*. 1997;19(3):334–350.
31. Montazeri A, McEwen J, Gillis CR. Quality of life in patients with ovarian cancer: current state of research. *Support Care Cancer*. 1996;4(3):169–179.
32. Lakusta CM, Atkinson MJ, Robinson JW, Nation J, Taenzer P, Campo MG. Quality of life in ovarian cancer patients receiving chemotherapy. *Gynecol Oncol*. 2001;81:490–495.
33. Guidozzi F. Living with ovarian cancer. *Gynecol Oncol*. 1993;50(2):202–207.
34. Jenkins B. Patients reports of sexual changes after treatment for gynecological cancer. *Oncol Nurs Forum*. 1998;15(3):231–242.
35. Ferrell B, Cullinane CA, Ervin K, Melancon C, Uman GC, Juarez G. Perspectives on the impact of ovarian cancer: women's views on quality of life. *Oncol Nurs Forum*. 2005;32(6):1143–1149.
36. Magee S, Skalzo K. *Picking up the pieces: moving forward after surviving cancer*. Vancouver: Raincoast; 2006.
37. Clemmens DA, Knafl K, Lev EL, McCorkle R. Cervical cancer: patterns of long-term survival. *Oncol Nurs Forum*. 2008;35(6):897–903.
38. Ganz PA. Menopause and breast cancer: symptoms, late effects, and their management. *Semin Oncol*. 2001;28(3):274–283.
39. Aziz NM, Rowland JH. Trends and advances in cancer survivorship research: challenge and opportunity. *Semin Radiat Oncol*. 2003;13(3):248–266.
40. Denmark, Aziz M, Rowland JH, et al. 2005. Riding the crest of the teachable moment: promoting long term health after the diagnosis of cancer. *J Clin Oncol*. 2005;23(24):5814–5830.
41. Vistad I, Fossa SD, Dahl AA. A critical review of patient-rated quality of life studies of long-term survivors of cervical cancer. *Gynecol Oncol*. 2006;102(3):563–572.
42. Ferrell B, Cullinane CA, Ervin K, Melancon C, Uman GC, Juarez G. Perspectives on the impact of ovarian cancer: women's views on quality of life. *Oncol Nurs Forum*. 2005;32(6):1143–1149.
43. Pignata S, Ballatori E, Favalli G, Scambia G. Quality of life: gynecological cancers. *Ann Oncol*. 2001;12(3):37–42.
44. Tabano M, Condosta D, Coons M. Symptoms affecting the quality of life in women with gynecologic cancer. *Semin Oncol Nurs*. 2002;18(3):223–230.
45. Constanzo E, Lutgendorf S, Rothrock N, Andersen B. Coping and quality of life among women extensively treated for gynecological cancer. *Psycho-Oncology*. 2006;15:132–142.
46. Petersen R, Graham G, Quinlivan J. Psychologic changes after a gynecologic cancer. *J Obstet Gynaecol Res*. 2005;31(2):152–157.
47. Lockwood-Rayermann S. Survivorship issues in ovarian cancer: a review. *Oncol Nurs Forum*. 2006;33(3):553–562.
48. Clemmens DA, Knafl K, Lev EL, McCorkle R. Cervical cancer: patterns of long term survival. *Oncology Nurs Forum*. 2008;35(6):897–903.
49. Schulman-Green D, Ercolano E, Dowd M, Schwartz P, McCorkle R. Quality of life among women after surgery for ovarian cancer. *Palliat Support Care*. 2008;6(3):239–247.
50. Gil KM, Gibbons HE, Jenison EL, Hopkins MP, von Gruenigen VE. Baseline characteristics influencing quality of life in women undergoing gynecologic oncology surgery. *Health Qual Life Outcomes*. 2007;5:25.
51. Grimel ER, Winter R, Kapp K, Haas J. Quality of life and sexual functioning after cervical cancer treatment: a long-term follow-up study. *Psycho-Oncology*. 2008;Aug 13 (Epub ahead of print).
52. Amsterdam A, Krychman ML. Sexual dysfunction in patients with gynecologic neoplasms: a retrospective pilot study. *J Sex Med*. 2006;3(4):646–649.

53. Lagana L, Classen C, Caldwell R, et al. Sexual difficulties of patients with gynecological cancer. *Prof Psychol Res Pr.* 2005;36(4):391–399.

54. Fitch MI, Gray RE, Franssen E. Perspectives on ovarian cancer: young women's views. *Can Oncol Nurs J.* 2000;10(3):101–108.

55. Fitch MI, Gray RE, Franssen E. Perspectives on living with ovarian cancer: older women's views. *Oncol Nurs Forum.* 2001;28(9):1433–1442.

56. Davis C, Zinkand J, Fitch MI. Treatment induced menopause for breast and gynecological survivors. *Can Oncol Nurs J.* 2000;10(1):14–21.

57. Fitch MI. Psychosocial management of patients with recurrent ovarian cancer: treating the whole patient to improve quality of life. *Semin Oncol Nurs.* 2003;19(3):40–53.

58. Moretti R, Pizzi B, Colizza MT, Carta G. Symptom management in a patient with end-stage ovarian cancer: case report. *Eur J Gynaecol Oncol.* 2007;28(4):25–27.

59. Lauver D, Connolly-Nelson K, Vang P. Stressors and coping strategies among female cancer survivors after treatments. *Cancer Nurs.* 2007;30(2):101–111.

60. Sukegawa A, Miyagi E, Suzuki R, et al. Post traumatic stress disorder in patients with gynecologic cancers. *J Obstet Gynaecol Res.* 2006;32(3):349–353.

61. Zabora J, Brintzenhofeszoc K, Curbow B, Hooker C, Piantadosi S. The prevalence of psychological distress by cancer site. *Psycho-Oncology*, 2001;10:19–28.

62. Otis-Green S, Ferrell B, Sun V, Spolum M, Morgan R, MacDonald D. Feasibility of an ovarian cancer quality-of-life psychoeducational intervention. *J Cancer Educ.* 2008;23(4):214–221.

63. McCorkle R, Dowd M, Ercolano E, et al. Effects of a nursing intervention on quality of life outcomes in post-surgical women with gynecologic cancers. *Psycho-Oncology.* 2008;Jun 20 (Epub ahead of print).

64. Fitch ML, McAndrew A, Ross E, Turner F. Survivors teaching students. *Oncol Nurs Forum.* 2008;35(3):556. (Abstract 3112).

65. Fitch M, Turner F, Magee S, McAndrew, Ross E. Picking up the pieces: moving forward after surviving cancer. *Eur J Cancer.* 2007;5(4):453 (Abstract 8152).

CHAPTER 23

Skin Neoplasms and Malignant Melanoma

Peter C. Trask and Phyllis Butow

Skin neoplasms continue to be one of the more common forms of cancer while also being one of the most curable. Skin neoplasms can occur in the flat squamous cells of the outermost layer of the skin, or in the basal or melanocyte cells of the lower skin layer. These three types of skin cancer are subsequently classified into two categories: (1) keratinocytic or nonmelanoma skin cancer which includes basal cell carcinoma (BCC) and squamous cell carcinoma (SCC), and (2) melanoma. BCC and SCC are common, easily treatable, and highly curable, whereas melanoma is less common, yet often easily treatable if caught early.

BASAL CELL AND SQUAMOUS CELL CARCINOMA

Incidence and mortality. Over 1 million cases of nonmelanoma skin cancer are expected in 2009,[1] with BCC and SCC accounting for over 90% of all skin cancers.[2] BCCs occur approximately four times more than SCCs and account for more than 75% of nonmelanoma skin cancer. The incidence of BCC and SCC varies by geographic region and race, with higher incidences reported in areas of high sun concentration, and in whites. The relationship between cumulative sun exposure and SCC is higher than that for BCC. Incidences of both cancers are also higher in individuals over 40 years of age, and are slightly more frequent in males. Although almost 100% curable if diagnosed and treated early, approximately 2780 people will die of nonmelanoma skin cancer in the United States each year. Like the incidence, the mortality rates are higher in males than in females.[2]

Description. Basal cell carcinoma tends to grow slowly over months to years, rarely metastasizes, and tends to occur most frequently in areas that are regularly exposed to the sun such as the face, upper trunk, and neck. Early BCC presents as pink to red, pale or waxy, round to oval nodules which may occasionally bleed when ulcerated. If untreated, BCC can spread locally to both surrounding tissue and bone. SCC is also most often observed on areas of the body that have been exposed to sun, including the nose, ears, and lower lip of the face, as well as the back of the hands. SCC presents as a scaly, red, irregularly shaped patch of skin often in damaged (e.g., within scars) or chronically irritated skin which can ulcerate and bleed. They occasionally occur in the genital area. SCC frequently grows faster than BCC and can increase in both depth and diameter with time.[3]

Etiology. The occurrence of BCC is correlated with sun exposure. This relationship appears stronger for exposure that occurred early in life and at intense, intermittent (i.e., recreational) duration than for cumulative lifetime exposure. Other factors that increase the likelihood of BCC include exposure to inorganic arsenic, ionizing radiation, and immunosuppression. As an example of the latter, there is an increased incidence of BCC in individuals who have undergone organ transplant. Sun exposure and being immunosuppressed also contribute to the development of SCC. In addition, SCC is increased in individuals who have been treated with phototherapy, and in those who have mutations in the *p53* tumor-suppressor gene.[3]

Prevention. Given the link between sun exposure and both BCC and SCC, it is not surprising that the prevention of both includes reducing sun exposure through the use of sun-protective clothing, broad spectrum (i.e., ultraviolet A and B [UVA and UVB] blocking of at least sun-protection factor 15 [SPF-15]) sunscreens, and limited sun exposure during periods of the days with the highest concentrations of UVA and UVB radiation (usually between the hours of 11 a.m. and 3 p.m.). In addition, individuals should limit their exposure to occupational hazards.[3]

Diagnosis. As with some other types of cancer (e.g., breast, testicular), BCC and SCC are frequently self-diagnosed. The regular practice of a thorough skin self-examination once a month can increase the likelihood that any skin cancers are found early. As part of this examination, individuals should pay particular attention to any new growths or sudden or progressive changes in growths that are already present. To increase the likelihood of lesions being diagnosed in an early stage, suspicious growths should be evaluated with minimal delay; an evaluation which would likely involve an excisional biopsy and pathological tissue examination.[3]

Treatment. For the vast majority of BCC and SCC diagnoses (approximately 90%), treatment is limited to surgical excision. In the minority of cases where the cancer is more advanced, radiation, electrodessication, cryosurgery, or more radical surgeries may be necessary. Subsequent plastic surgery may be needed to reduce the disfigurement resulting from the surgery.[3,4]

Prognosis. Given that the majority of these cancers are found early, they are almost 100% curable.[3]

MALIGNANT MELANOMA

Incidence and mortality. Approximately 62,480 individuals are expected to be diagnosed with melanoma, the most common serious form of skin cancer, in 2009 (American Cancer Society [ACS]). In the United States, melanoma of the skin constitutes 5% (approximately n = 34,950) of the new cancers in men and 4% (approximately n = 27,530) of the new cases in women, making it the sixth and seventh most common cancer, respectively. The lifetime probability of developing melanoma is 1 in 41 for men and 1 in 63 for women, an incidence that has remained relatively stable since 2000. The 5-year survival rates for all stages of melanoma are 91.1%; however, this is primarily a reflection of the high rates of survival for melanoma found in the local stage (98.5%). When melanoma has either regional or distant spread, the 5-year survival rates are considerably lower; 65.2% and 15.3%, respectively. Although approximately 8420 individuals will die from melanoma in 2009, the death rates have remained stable in women and men over age 50 since 1990 and 1998, respectively, and have been decreasing in those younger than 50. As with the other forms of skin cancer, melanoma affects whites more than other races, occurring at a rate more than 10 times higher than that observed in African Americans. Like other skin cancers, melanoma is most common in areas with high sun concentration, with Australia and New Zealand having the world's highest incidence rates.[2,5]

Description. In general, melanoma is characterized by changes in the ABCDs (asymmetry, border, color, and dimension) of a pigmented lesion. Lesions that exhibit any of these signs should be examined. There are five different types of melanoma according to the American Joint Committee on Cancer (AJCC): lentigo maligna melanoma, superficial spreading melanoma, nodular melanoma, acral-lentiginous melanoma, and mucosal lentiginous melanoma. The first three types comprise between 80% and 85% of all diagnosed melanomas. Superficial spreading melanoma, comprising 70% of all melanomas, may take a long time to develop; are usually composed of many shades of brown, black, tan, red, and white; and usually appear flat with irregular borders. They are most common on the head, neck, trunk, and extremities of individuals between 40 and 50 years of age. Approximately 10% of all melanomas are classified as lentigo maligna. These melanomas are most common on sun-exposed areas of the skin and are most common in individuals over the age of 70 years. Commonly large, tan to dark brown, with irregular borders, these lesions may have been present for 5–15 years before becoming invasive. Ten to fifteen percent of melanomas are nodular malignant. Unlike the two previous forms which may take years to develop, nodular malignant melanoma demonstrates rapid vertical growth, are dark and uniform in color, and may develop on any bodily surface. It also occurs more often in individuals between the ages of 40 and 50. The final two forms of melanoma, acral and mucosal lentiginous, occurs on the palms, soles, subungual, or mucosal (i.e., mouth, throat, anus, vagina, or conjunctiva) areas of the body. These occur more often in individuals with dark skin, are large, and are often seen in individuals over 59 years.[4]

Etiology. Ultraviolet light appears to be important in the development of melanoma.[6] Although melanoma can occur in as little as 2 years between sun exposure and the development of melanoma, studies of the incidence of melanoma in individuals who moved to a sunny climate and those who have lived there all of their lives suggest that the chronic duration of the exposure is important. Individuals with fair skin, with red or blond hair, freckles, who burn easily or have had severe sunburns are at increased risk of developing melanoma. For these individuals in particular, acute, intense, and intermittent exposure which increases the likelihood of a blistering sunburn increases the likelihood of melanoma. There may also be a relationship between hormones and genetics and melanoma. In particular, melanoma is more common in women, is rare before puberty, and may change after pregnancy. In addition, individuals in families with various genetic abnormalities are at greater risk of developing melanoma.[6]

Prevention. As with the nonmelanoma skin cancers, staying out of the sun during periods of high sun intensity, wearing UVA- and UVB-protecting sunscreen, as well as sun-protective clothing can help reduce the risk of melanoma.

Diagnosis. The majority of melanomas are diagnosed after observation of changes in an existing lesion or the development of a new lesion. To further define the ABCDs noted earlier, the following changes warrant further attention. (1) Asymmetry: if one side of the lesion is not identical to the other side; (2) Border: an irregular border or notching; (3) Color: darkening, multiple colors, or spread of color; (4) Dimension: a sudden or continuous enlargement in either size or elevation. In addition to these, five other changes can be a warning sign of a potential melanoma. These include (5) Characteristics of the surface: scaling or crusting, oozing, or bleeding; (6) Appearance of surrounding skin: redness, swelling, or inflammation; (7) Consistency of the mole; (8) Sensation: itching, tenderness, or pain; and (9) Sudden appearance of a new mole.[7]

Once diagnosed, staging of melanomas occur through the AJCC Staging System.[8] They are also measured by Clark's Level and Breslow Depth.[9,10] The AJCC staging is provided in Table 23–1. Both Clark's Level and Breslow Depth describe the degree of invasion of the tumor through the skin. Whereas Clark's Levels are classified based on which portions of the skin the tumor has passed through (i.e., from the epidermis to the subcutaneous fat), Breslow depth uses an ocular micrometer to measure the tumor from the base of the tumor to the deepest melanoma cell. In each case, greater invasion is associated with poorer prognosis.

Treatment. Surgical excision is usually sufficient if the melanoma is diagnosed in an early stage; the key being to remove the tumor with sufficient margins to ensure excision of cancerous cells. For more advanced tumors, however, radiation, limb perfusion, lymph node dissections, adjuvant therapy with either interferon or dacarbazine, or human monoclonal antibodies are utilized. Side effects from these additional therapies can be significant and affect patients' quality of life.[7]

Prognosis. The prognosis for early-stage melanomas is excellent with between a 95% and 100% cure rate. As the stage of the melanoma increases, however, the 5-year survival rates drop dramatically, with survival for distant stage disease being approximately 65%, whereas advanced stage survival is only 15%.[2]

BEHAVIORAL/PSYCHOSOCIAL FACTORS AND SKIN CANCER

Sun exposure. The fact that one of the primary causes of skin cancer is sun exposure makes it an important public health issue. Of greatest concern is how to educate the public, especially in areas of greater sun concentration, on how to minimize the exposure and hence the risk of developing skin cancer. As one of the highest sun concentration countries, Australia has led the way in education campaigns, focusing on increasing sunscreen use and wearing sun-protective clothing (e.g., shirts, hats), as well as minimizing exposure during times of greatest sun concentration. They have also developed playgrounds for children that have covered areas and adopted "no hat, no play" policies for school children, a policy that increased the use of sun-protective hats in all but one school studied.[11] For public health interventions such as Australia's "slip, slop, slap" campaign, one that was also adopted by the ACS, to be effective, however, fundamental sun exposure behaviors such as tanning and not wearing sunscreen or protective clothing need to be changed.

In a U.S. study from 2003, Demko and colleagues[12] estimated that between 11% and 37% of white adolescents had used a tanning bed. More recently, Haas[13] noted that although teenagers are well-informed about the risks of skin cancer from sun exposure, they continue to have pro-tanning attitudes, with at least a quarter of adolescents in one study thinking that if one had to burn to get a tan it would be worth it.[14] Thus, although they know that staying out of the sun, wearing sunscreen and clothes which cover areas at risk such as the arms and face, would help reduce the risk of skin cancer, very few of them actually engage in these behaviors. Indeed, over two-thirds of adolescents fail to practice effective sun protection.[15] Clearly, additional work is needed to change sun exposure behaviors.

Additional information on sun exposure can be found in Chapter 5 of the Behavioral and Psychological Factors in Cancer Risk section of this book.

Skin self-examination. Additionally important is educating the public on the signs and symptoms of skin cancer. Apparent changes on the skin can be observed early if individuals are encouraged to thoroughly look at their skin, and for areas that are harder to see, have someone else do it for them. Early detection in one case-control study reduced melanoma mortality by 63%.[16] Unfortunately, thorough examination of the skin is rarely performed with several studies reporting that thorough examination is only done by 9%–18% of participants.[17,18] Interventions, such as the "Check-It-Out Project," have included cues, aids, and videos designed to help people see and recognize changes on their skin, with the goal being to increase skin self-examination and follow-up with physicians.[18] Although they have been successful at increasing self-examination in people who receive the intervention,[18] widespread dissemination to the general public has not occurred, with the result being that the majority of individuals do not thoroughly examine their skin.

Stress. There has been little research exploring the role of stress, attitude, and personality factors in the development of melanoma. Temoshok[19] has reported the largest series of studies investigating biopsychosocial aspects of cutaneous malignant melanoma. Two studies investigated the relationship of variables derived from a videotaped psychosocial interview and from self-report measures, and two histopathology indicators: tumor thickness and level of invasion. In a multiple

Table 23–1. AJCC staging system for melanoma

Stage	TNM	Criteria	Comments
0	Tis	Melanoma in situ	
IA	T1aN0M0	≤1.0 mm	Micrometastasis without ulceration based on elective lymph node dissection or sentinel node biopsy
IB	T1bN0M0	≤1.0 mm	Macrometastasis with ulceration or Clark level IV/V as detected clinically or via the presence of extracapsular extension of disease
	T2aN0M0	1.01–2.0 mm	Micrometastasis without ulceration based on elective lymph node dissection or sentinel node biopsy
IIA	T2bN0M0	2.01–4.0 mm	Macrometastasis with ulceration or Clark level IV/V as detected clinically or via the presence of extracapsular extension of disease
	T3aN0M0		
IIB	T3bN0M0	2.01–4.0 mm	
	T4aN0M0	>4.0 mm	
IIC	T4bN0M0	>4.0 mm	
IIIA	T1–4aN1aM0	1 lymph node	Micrometastasis based on elective lymph node dissection or sentinel node biopsy
			Macrometastasis as detected clinically or via the presence of extracapsular extension of disease
IIIB	T1–4aN2bM0	2–3 lymph nodes	Micrometastasis based on elective lymph node dissection or sentinel node biopsy
			Macrometastasis as detected clinically or via the presence of extracapsular extension of disease
			Intratransit or satellite metastasis without lymph nodes
IIIC	Any TN2cM0	≥4 lymph nodes, matted nodes or combination	
	Any TN3M0	of intratransit/satellite metastasis, ulcerated primary and lymph nodes	
IV	Any T any N M	M1a: distant skin, subcutaneous, lymph nodes	Normal LDH
		M1b: lung metastasis	Normal LDH
		M1c: all other sites	Elevated LDH

ABBREVIATIONS: LDH, low density lipopolysaccharide; TNM, tumor, node, metastasis.
SOURCE: Modification of Table 108–2; AJCC Staging manual criteria, from Chapter 108, Malignant melanoma by Morton DL, et al., in Holland and Frei (eds), *Cancer Medicine*, 7th ed.; 2006, BC Decker Inc., London. Reprinted with permission from the publisher.

regression analysis, patient delay in seeking medical attention emerged as the most significant variable predicting tumor thickness. Further analysis found longer delays in patients who had lesions on the back, less previous knowledge of melanoma, less understanding of its treatment, and less minimization of its seriousness.

Another study compared repressive coping reactions—defined as the discrepancy between reported anxiety and that reflected in electrodermal activity—in melanoma patients, cardiovascular disease patients, and disease-free controls. The melanoma group was significantly more "repressed" on the combined self-report/physiological measure, as well as on other self-report measures of repressiveness.[20]

Despite these findings, reviewers of the literature on the relationship between psychosocial factors and cancer overall have concluded that there is no consistent evidence for such a relationship.[21]

Distress, fear, pain, and disfigurement. Many people with melanoma and their carers face practical, emotional, and psychological demands in addition to the physical effects of the disease and treatment.[22] The impact on families of those with melanoma is also considerable, as they share in the fears of relapse, the traumas of treatment, and the sadness of late-stage disease. Challenges in melanoma include the existential fear faced by anyone with a diagnosis of a life-threatening disease, pain and discomfort associated with treatment, and body image changes associated with disfiguring surgery.[22] Patients with deeply indented scars, such as those that occur with skin grafting following removal of skin, subcutaneous and deep fascia, as well as those whose scars are longer than they anticipated, may be particularly distressed.[23]

While most studies have found that patients adjust well to melanoma in the long term, distress is common. In a prospective survey of 144 patients with stage I melanoma who did not relapse, 21% reported moderate to high levels of distress 3 months after excision, 26% at 7-month follow-up, and 29% at 13-month follow-up.[22]

Patients' psychosocial needs are significant, and frequently go undetected and unmet. Bonevski et al.[24] assessed the perceived needs of a sample of patients attending the Newcastle Melanoma Unit. Patients reported the most unmet needs in relationship to health information, psychological issues, and melanoma-specific issues. The authors recommended that patient needs should be monitored routinely in oncology care so that groups of patients with specific needs could be identified.[24]

Influence of psychosocial characteristics on prognosis. There has been a long-standing research interest in a potential relationship between patients' psychological characteristics and social support, and outcome. Nine prospective cohort studies have explored the impact of psychosocial characteristics on outcome in melanoma. Only one explored outcomes in patients with metastatic melanoma.

The results of these studies have been mixed. In early-stage melanoma, three studies reported a null effect.[25-27] In the largest of these studies, with the longest follow-up (to 11 years), Bergenmar et al.[25] followed 437 patients with localized cutaneous melanoma who had completed measures of anxiety and depression at their first follow-up after surgery. There was no relationship between baseline anxiety and depression and the time to recurrence. Three studies reported a weak effect.[28-30] Fawzy et al.,[30] for example, explored psychosocial predictors of time to recurrence in 68 patients with stage I or II malignant melanoma who had participated in a randomized controlled trial (RCT) of a psychiatric intervention. Controlling for group allocation, and disease and demographic prognostic variables, at 6-year follow-up higher baseline rates of total mood distress and higher baseline active-behavioral coping were associated with lower recurrence and death rates, and an increase in active-behavioral coping over the study period was related to better survival ($p = 0.03$), with a trend apparent for recurrence ($p = 0.06$). Fawzy et al.[30] posited that the more distressed patients and those who tended to cope by taking active steps to solve problems may have been more motivated to prevent recurrence by staying out of the sun and protecting their skin.

Finally, two studies reported larger effect sizes.[31,32] In a large prospective study, Brown et al.[31] followed 426 patients with locoregional melanomas >0.7 mm for 6 years who were assessed for a range of psychological variables at diagnosis. In an analysis that controlled for all other prognostic demographic and disease variables, patients who at baseline used less avoidance ($p = 0.03$) and were more concerned about their disease ($p = 0.008$) had a greater time to recurrence, and there was a trend for patients who perceived the aim of treatment as cure ($p = 0.06$) to have longer time until recurrence. As in Fawzy et al.,[30] these psychosocial variables might be related to active behaviors aimed at prevention, although this was not measured.

One study explored psychosocial predictors of time to death in late-stage melanoma. Butow et al.[33] followed 125 patients with metastatic melanoma for 6 years. Controlling for other prognostic factors, patients who perceived the aim of treatment to be cure ($p < 0.001$), minimized their illness ($p < 0.05$), were more angry ($p < 0.05$), were married ($p < 0.01$), and who reported better QOL ($p < 0.05$) survived longer. Patients who believed treatment would lead to cure survived about twice as long (10.6 months) as those who did not (5.6 months). As in all cohort studies, it is hard to interpret positive results as it is always possible that at baseline, patients were influenced by illness characteristics that were prognostic but not recorded in the traditional prognostic measures. Further research is required to establish if there is a link between psychosocial factors and outcome in melanoma.

Additional studies on the issues with which individuals with advanced or metastatic cancer are faced with, are discussed in the Palliative and Terminal Care section of this book.

PSYCHOSOCIAL INTERVENTIONS FOR SKIN CANCER

Interventions following diagnosis. A recent systematic review of the literature[34] revealed that only five RCTs have been conducted evaluating psychosocial interventions for patients with melanoma, but the findings of all five (one with four publications reporting follow-up results) suggest that psychological interventions *can* improve psychosocial outcomes for melanoma patients, including reducing general mood disturbance, distress, and anxiety.[30,35-41] These interventions were primarily cognitive-behavioral, incorporating health education, stress management, illness-related problem-solving skills, and psychological support. Two studies reported large effects[35,39] at 6 months although in the second study,[39] which evaluated long-term effects, differences between the groups had dissipated by 12 months, by which time most patients were feeling better. Two of the studies with smaller samples reported small short-term effects[38,41] and one reported large effects despite a small sample size.[40]

Three of the studies targeting coping[35,38,39] reported an increase in active coping or a reduction in passive coping in the intervention group, suggesting that these interventions can also help patients to take active steps to cope with their illness. Importantly, one study[40] demonstrated that psychosocial interventions cannot only reduce patients' distress, but also reduces in a cost-effective manner. In this study, a small RCT of cognitive-behavioral therapy (CBT) was conducted for patients with heterogeneous melanomas who were reporting clinically significant levels of distress. Only 38 patients participated in the study, which was nonetheless able to report a significant reduction of distress at 3 months after intervention for the CBT group ($p = 0.005$). CBT was marginally more expensive (49c per minute) than the cost to nursing staff of dealing with distress-driven phone calls during standard care (41c per minute). The cost/benefit ratio (total costs/change in distress), however, was significantly lower for CBT. The cost to change distress in standard care was >$402 for a one-point change in distress versus $7.66 for CBT. Including

reimbursement for service in the analysis, CBT would generate $1.16 per minute while standard care would cost the hospital $0.40. Thus CBT is cost-effective.

A qualitative study explored patient perceptions of psychological intervention to try and identify the active component of these interventions.[42] Twenty-six patients with metastatic melanoma who were participating in a RCT of individual CBT versus relaxation training were interviewed about the benefits of therapy by a researcher blinded to allocation. Patients reported similar benefits regardless of allocation, which pertained to receiving patient-centered care from someone outside their family who they trusted and to whom they could speak openly. Thus nonspecific therapist factors appeared to be more important than the actual therapy delivered. However, changes in coping style reported in other studies[30,35-39] suggest that skill development is also an important intervention component. This conclusion is supported by a cancer-wide systematic review of psychological interventions which suggested that structured interventions may offer more benefit than those of a purely supportive nature.[43]

The positive findings regarding efficacy of psychological intervention in melanoma patients reflects the wider findings found in heterogeneous cancers. The National Institute for Clinical Excellence (NICE) guidelines[44] recently reviewed evidence for the efficacy of psychosocial interventions in all cancer patients. Three systematic reviews or meta-analyses of good quality, four systematic reviews or meta-analyses of poor quality, four RCTs of poor quality, and one observational study of fair quality were identified. The majority of studies reported benefits, with few inconclusive studies. Benefits included both affective and physical improvements, improved coping, and better understanding. Most recent guidelines on cancer care recommend that psychosocial interventions be made available to all cancer patients.

Influence of psychosocial interventions on prognosis. Only one study has explored the impact of a psychosocial intervention on prognosis in patients with melanoma.[35,36] All patients were stage I, with a relatively good prognosis. Immediately after the intervention (primarily cognitive-behavioral, incorporating health education, stress management, illness-related problem-solving skills, and psychological support) there was a significant increase in one of the large granular lymphocyte subpopulations, CD8. At 6 months, the intervention group had an increased number of natural killer cells and an increased cytotoxicity, a decrease in a major T-cell subpopulation-CD4 helper/inducer cells, and some increases in the percentage of larger granular lymphocytes. This was correlated with change in depression and anxiety. At the 6-year follow-up, 10/34 in the control group had died and three had local recurrences. In the intervention group 3/34 had died and four had recurrences.[30] Participation in the intervention lowered the risk of recurrence by more than 2.5, and decreased the risk of death sevenfold. At 10-year follow-up, Fawzy et al.[37] reported that participation in the intervention did not lower the risk of recurrence but decreased the risk of death threefold.

Despite these promising findings, results of studies in cancer generally have been equivocal. A recent systematic review concluded that there was insufficient evidence for a relationship between psychosocial interventions and survival of cancer, given methodological flaws and contradictory findings.[45] Further research is required to establish the impact of psychosocial intervention on prognosis in patients with melanoma.

Additional information on psychological interventions can be found in the Interventions section of this book.

CONCLUSIONS

Although skin neoplasms and melanoma continue to be prevalent, the fact that almost all of them are 100% curable if diagnosed and treated early is extremely positive. Nevertheless, the fact that some melanomas are not diagnosed until they are in an advanced stage, and the increasing incidence in some age groups and geographic locations suggests that there continues to be a need for intervention on both group and individual levels.

On the individual level, monthly skin self-examination and physician examination as part of annual physical examinations could increase the likelihood of finding skin cancers in early stages. Currently, a thorough skin examination is not a consistent part of annual physical examinations. On a societal level, increasing awareness through public health campaigns, and the creation of sun-friendly playgrounds (i.e., those with areas of shade above the play equipment) and beaches (e.g., through provision of free umbrellas), would convey the importance of sun safety. The increase in SPF clothing lines, sunless tanning products, and availability of SPF sunscreens is a positive step, although the continued proliferation of indoor tanning salons potentially sends a mixed message that artificial "sun" is alright.

Finally, there is a continued need for the innovation of new treatments for advanced melanoma whose survival rates continue to be a meager 15%. It has been over 10 years since the Eastern Cooperative Oncology Group's protocol 1684 demonstrated some benefit in survival for adjuvant treatment with interferon -alpha (IFN-α).[46] Since then, various chemotherapeutic and biological combinations and single agents, vaccines, and gene therapies have been tried without any significant increase in overall survival. Ideally, the continued efforts of pharmaceutical companies will result in improved treatments for individuals with advanced stage disease. Until then, psychosocial interventions to deal with the side effects of an advanced cancer diagnosis and treatment will continue to be necessary.

REFERENCES

1. Jemal A, Siegel R, Ward E, et al. Cancer statistics, 2009. *CA: Cancer J Clin.* 2009;5:225–249.

2. American Cancer Society. *Cancer facts & figures—2008.* Atlanta, GA: American Cancer Society; 2008.

3. Neel VA, Sober AJ. Other skin cancers. In: Kufe DW, Bast RC, Hait WN, Hong WK, Pollock RE, Weichselbaum RR, et al. (eds). *Cancer medicine.* Ch. 109. London, ON: BC Decker; 2006:1663–1674.

4. Armstrong BK, Kricker A. Skin cancer. *Dermatol Clin.* 1995;13:583–594.

5. Morton DL, Essner R, Kirkwood JM, Wollman RC. Malignant melanoma. In: Kufe DW, Bast RC, Hait WN, Hong WK, Pollock RE, Weichselbaum RR, et al. (eds). *Cancer medicine.* 7th ed. Ch. 108. London, ON: BC Decker; 2006:1645–1662.

6. Manson JE, Rexrode KM, Garland FC, Garland CF, Weinstock MA. The case for a comprehensive national campaign to prevent melanoma and associated mortality. *Epidemiology.* 2000;11:728–734.

7. Jensen EH, Margolin KA, Sondak VK. Melanoma and other skin cancers. In: Pazdur R, Coia LR, Hoskins WJ, Wagman LD (eds). *Cancer management: A multidisciplinary approach.* 9th ed. Ch. 23. Lawrence, KS: CMP Media; 2005:531–572.

8. Balch CM, Buzaid AC, Soong SJ, et al. Final version of the American Joint Committee on Cancer staging system for cutaneous melanoma. *J Clin Oncol.* 2001;19:3635–3648.

9. Clark WH Jr, From L, Bernardino EA, Mihm MC Jr. The histogenesis and biologic behavior of primary human malignant melanoma of the skin. *Cancer Res.* 1969;29:705.

10. Breslow A. Prognostic factors in the treatment of cutaneous melanoma. *J Cutan Pathol.* 1979;6:208.

11. Giles-Corti B, English DR, Costa C, Milne E, Cross D, Johnston R. Creating SunSmart schools. *Health Educ Res.* 2004;19:98–109.

12. Demko CA, Borawski EA, Debanne SM, Cooper KD, Stange KC. Use of indoor tanning facilities by white adolescents in the United States. *Arch Pediatr Adolesc Med.* 2003;157:854–860.

13. Haas AF. Teens and tans: implementing behavioral change. *Arch Dermatol.* 2007;143:1058–1061.

14. Geller AC, Brooks DR, Colditz GA, Koh HK, Frazier AL. Sun protection practices among offspring of women with personal or family history of skin cancer. *Pediatrics.* 2006;117:e688–e694.

15. Cokkinides VE, Johnston-Davis K, Weinstock M, O'Connell MC. Sun exposure and sun-protection behaviors and attitudes among US youth 11 to 18 years of age. *Prev Med.* 2001;33:141.

16. Berwick M, Begg CB, Fine JA, Roush GC, Bernhill RL. Screening for cutaneous melanoma by skin self-examination. *J Natl Cancer Inst.* 1996;88:17–23.

17. Weinstock MA, Martin RA, Risica PM, et al. Thorough skin examination for the early detection of melanoma. *Am J Prevent Med.* 1999;17:169–175.

18. Weinstock MA, Risica PM, Martin RA, et al. Reliability of assessment and circumstances of performance of thorough skin self-examination for the early detection of melanoma in the Check-It-Out Project. *Prev Med.* 2004;38:761–765.

19. Temoshok L. Biopsychosocial studies on cutaneous malignant melanoma: psychosocial factors associated with prognostic indicators, progression, psychophysiology and tumor-host response. *Soc Sci Med.* 1985;20(8):833–840.

20. Kneier AW, Temoshok L. Repressive coping reactions in patients with malignant melanoma as compared to cardiovascular patients. *J Psychosom Res.* 1984;28:145–155.

21. Schwarz S, Messerschmidt H, Doren M. Psychosocial risk factors for cancer development. *Medizinische Klinik.* 2007;102(12):967–979.

22. Brandberg Y, Mansson-Brahme E, Ringborg U, Sjoden PO. Psychological reactions in patients with malignant melanoma. *Eur J Cancer.* 1995;31A(2):157–162.

23. Cassileth BR, Lusk EJ, Tenaglia AN. Patients' perceptions of the cosmetic impact of melanoma resection. *Plast Reconstr Surg.* 1983;71(1):73–75.

24. Bonevski B, Sanson-Fisher R, Hersey P, Paul C, Foot G. Assessing the perceived needs of patients attending an outpatient melanoma clinic. *J Psychosoc Oncol.* 1999;17:101–118.

25. Bergenmar M, Nilsson B, Hansson J, Brandberg Y. Anxiety and depressive symptoms measured by the Hospital Anxiety and Depression Scale as predictors of time to recurrence in localized cutaneous melanoma. *Acta Oncol.* 2004;43(2):161–168.

26. Canada AL, Fawzy NW, Fawzy FI. Personality and disease outcome in malignant melanoma. *J Psychosom Res.* 2005;58(1):19–27.

27. Gibertini M, Reintgen DS, Baile WF. Psychosocial aspects of melanoma. *Ann Plast Surg.* 1992;28(1):17–21.

28. Cassileth BR, Walsh WP, Lusk EJ. Psychosocial correlates of cancer survival: a subsequent report 3 to 8 years after cancer diagnosis. *J Clin Oncol.* 1988;6(11):1753–1759.

29. Brandberg Y, Mansson-Brahme E, Ringborg U, Sjoden PO. Psychological reactions in patients with malignant melanoma. *Eur J Cancer.* 1995;31A(2):157–162.

30. Fawzy FI, Fawzy NW, Hyun CS, et al. Malignant melanoma. Effects of an early structured psychiatric intervention, coping, and affective state on recurrence and survival 6 years later. *Arch Gen Psychiatry.* 1993;50(9):681–689.

31. Brown JE, Brown RF, Miller RM. Coping with metastatic melanoma: the last year of life. *Psycho-Oncology.* 2000;9(4):283–292.

32. Rogentine GN Jr, van Kammen DP, Fox BH, et al. Psychological factors in the prognosis of malignant melanoma: a prospective study. *Psychosom Med.* 1979;41(8):647–655.

33. Butow PN, Coates AS, Dunn SM. Psychosocial predictors of survival in metastatic melanoma. *J Clin Oncol.* 1999;17(7):2256–2263.

34. Butow P. Psychosocial issues in melanoma. In: *Clinical practice guidelines for the management of melanoma in Australia and New Zealand.* Cancer Council Australia and Australian Cancer Network, Sydney and New Zealand Guidelines Group, Wellington; 2008.

35. Fawzy FI, Cousins N, Fawzy NW, Kemeny ME, Elashoff R, Morton D. A structured psychiatric intervention for cancer patients. I. Changes over time in methods of coping and affective disturbance. *Arch Gen Psychiatry.* 1990;47(8):720–725.

36. Fawzy FI, Kemeny ME, Fawzy NW, et al. A structured psychiatric intervention for cancer patients. II. Changes over time in immunological measures. *Arch Gen Psychiatry.* 1990;47(8):729–735.

37. Fawzy FI, Canada AL, Fawzy NW. Malignant melanoma: effects of a brief, structured psychiatric intervention on survival and recurrence at 10-year follow-up. *Arch Gen Psychiatry.* 2003;60(1):100–103.

38. Fawzy NW. A psychoeducational nursing intervention to enhance coping and affective state in newly diagnosed malignant melanoma patients. *Cancer Nurs.* 1995;18(6):427–438.

39. Boesen EH, Ross L, Frederiksen K, et al. Psychoeducational intervention for patients with cutaneous malignant melanoma: a replication study. *J Clin Oncol.* 2005;23(6):1270–1277.

40. Bares C, Trask C, Schwartz S. An exercise in cost-effectiveness analysis: treating emotional distress in melanoma patients. *J Clin Psychol Med Settings.* 2002;9(3):193–199.

41. Trask PC, Paterson AG, Griffith KA, Riba MB, Schwartz JL. Cognitive-behavioral intervention for distress in patients with melanoma: comparison with standard medical care and impact on quality of life. *Cancer.* 2003;98(4):854–864.

42. MacCormack T, Simonian J, Lim J, et al. 'Someone who cares': a qualitative investigation of cancer patients' experiences of psychotherapy. *Psycho-Oncology.* 2001;10(1):52–65.

43. Bottomley A. Psychosocial problems in cancer care: a brief review of common problems. *J Psychiatr Ment Health Nurs.* 1997;4(5):323–331.

44. National Institute for Health and Clinical Excellence. *Guidance on cancer services—improving supportive and palliative care for adults with cancer. The Manual.* London: National Health Service; 2004.

45. Newell SA, Sanson-Fisher RW, Savolainen NJ. Systematic review of psychological therapies for cancer patients: overview and recommendations for future research. *J Natl Cancer Inst.* 2002;94(8):558–584.

46. Kirkwood JM, Strawderman MH, Ernstoff MS, Smith TJ, Borden EC, Blum RH. Interferon alfa-2b adjuvant therapy of high-risk resected cutaneous melanoma: the Eastern Cooperative Oncology Group Trial EST 1684. *J Clin Oncol.* 1996;**14**(1):7–17.

CHAPTER 24

Breast Cancer

Julia H. Rowland and Mary Jane Massie

Breast cancer remains the most widely studied type of cancer with respect to its psychosocial impact.[1] This is due in large measure to its high prevalence, but also reflects the fact that the disease affects women of all ages, involves complex care, and concerns a body part with great significance to women and their partners. In this chapter we review the physical, psychological, social, and economic impact of cancer on the lives of women and those who care for and about them, along with the diverse treatment modalities, some of which are evolving rapidly, used to cure or control the illness, and the common sequelae of these treatments.

Breast cancer, the most common form of cancer among American women, will be diagnosed in a projected 182,460 women in the year 2008. However, fewer than 41,000 women will die of the disease, and mortality rates continue to decline. Currently, there are 6.1 million women living with a history of cancer, of whom 43% had breast cancer.[2] Most women diagnosed with breast cancer can expect to be cured of or live for long periods with their disease. However, unlike treatment for other chronic diseases, treatments for cancer are often intensive and associated with short- and long-term side effects. Practice trends have moved toward the use of multidrug regimens delivered over shorter periods (dose intensity), sometimes in combination with higher drug doses (dose density), resulting in increasing demands on patients' physical, psychological, and social resources. Further, new developments in genetic testing and in surgical, radiotherapeutic, and medical treatments, along with the greater use of preoperative systemic therapy, now provide many women with a variety of treatment choices. With the publication in 2008 of the Institute of Medicine's report, *Cancer care for the whole patient: Meeting psychosocial health needs*, oncology practitioners acknowledge that the patient's needs, hopes, and desires are as important as, and at times more important than, the tumor in planning and delivering optimal care.[3]

Although breast cancer is a major stressor for any woman, there is great variability in women's psychological responses. This chapter outlines the pattern of responses to breast cancer during and after treatment, and factors that may increase a woman's risk for poor adaptation.

FACTORS THAT IMPACT PSYCHOLOGICAL RESPONSE

A woman's psychological response to her disease is affected by existing sociocultural and psychological factors, as well as the medical issues that she confronts (Table 24–1).

Comprehensive care requires assessing, and as needed addressing, each of these areas during the course of the patient's illness.

Sociocultural context and psychosocial issues in decision making. Current public attitudes toward cancer have resulted in (1) increasing the patient's role in decision making, and (2) a demand for continued investment in breast cancer research, including the psychosocial and behavioral aspects of cancer. Women today have a greater understanding of and more resources to manage their breast cancer illness and recovery than ever before, as well as more therapeutic options from which to choose. Nonetheless, the associated demand on complex decision making can be stressful.

Over the course of care, women face three major decision points, each of which precipitates its own set of related choices to be considered (Table 24–2).

The first is whether the initial discovery of a lump or symptom requires further evaluation. A woman's decision at this point is informed by her access to and the cost of specialized care; her age, level of education or knowledge, and attitudes and beliefs about cancer; her personality and coping style; and the nature of her relationship with her primary care provider.[4] Delays in seeking care have been attributed to age (e.g., >65 years), a symptom other than a breast lump, the woman's sense of privacy, a lack of trust or otherwise poor relationship with the primary care provider, a fear of cancer and of treatments for cancer, a low perception of risk, less spirituality, and willful ignorance of symptoms.[5] Language barriers, inadequate resources, and inaccurate beliefs may disproportionally affect the likelihood of seeking care among Latina and African-American women.[6,7] If a delay in seeking care has occurred, personal guilt or anger at her physician can interfere with a woman's acceptance of treatment. Focusing on the value of the care she will now be receiving rather than dwelling on the past can help mitigate this distress.

The second major set of decisions women confront involves identification and selection of a breast cancer treatment plan, often a complex process (see Table 24–2). Most women report having a choice in primary treatment between mastectomy and breast conservation. Regional variations in care as well as differences based on a woman's age, ethnicity, and culture can impact treatments offered or received. For example, black and Hispanic women appear less likely than white women to receive follow-up radiation after lumpectomy.[8]

The time between diagnosis and initiation of treatment is one of the most stressful periods, exceeded only by the period of waiting for surgical or other test results. Studies show that the quality of physician communication during this phase is a critical determinant of subsequent psychological well-being.[9] At this juncture, some women may consider whether to seek a second opinion about their treatment options or pursue care elsewhere. Motivation to seek second opinions may be driven by anxiety, an unsatisfactory experience with a provider, an insurance carrier mandate, a desire for a more active role in the process, or the desire to hear a different recommendation.[10] Support networks and online access to information about current standard therapies and clinical trials may help patients and families understand better the opinions they have received and even facilitate location of breast specialists in their region.

Many cancer centers offer multidisciplinary consultations after a breast cancer diagnosis is established. In these settings, women obtain treatment options from a surgeon, a medical oncologist, and a radiation oncologist. In some centers, the consultative team may have as members other specialists, including a pathologist, plastic surgeon, mental health professional, genetic counselor, clinical research nurse, or, increasingly, a patient navigator. Such programs can be helpful in reducing stress by providing information tailored to a woman's specific situation. In addition, a number of centers use instructional kits, audiotapes, videotapes, compact discs, and online educational tools designed to explain treatment options with easy-to-understand and even interactive communication formats. Research suggests that use of such decision aids can improve understanding of treatment options,[11] increase the likelihood that women with early-stage disease will consider breast-conserving surgery,[12] and reduce decisional conflict and induce greater satisfaction with decisions made.[13]

Oncology providers should attempt to understand the woman's physical and psychological needs so that the nature of the discussion and the treatment recommendations are consistent with those needs. Although their involvement in the process is important to improving breast cancer survivors' quality of life,[14] clinicians should be aware that not all women want to make the final decision about treatment. Further, desire for details

Table 24–1. Factors that contribute to the psychological responses of women to breast cancer

Current sociocultural context, treatment options, and decision making

a. Changes in surgical and medical management away from a uniform approach; introduction of sentinel node biopsies and neoadjuvant therapy; more therapeutic options and acknowledged uncertainty; introduction of novel-targeted and tailored therapies; more clinical trials
b. Social attitudes
c. Public figures openly sharing their breast cancer experience
d. Autobiographic accounts of and "how to" guides for dealing with and surviving breast cancer in the popular press
e. Ethical imperative for patient participation in treatment issues; legal imperative for knowledge of treatment options
f. Variations in care by ethnicity, location, age
g. Public awareness of treatment and research controversies; advocacy for more research funding and lay oversight

Psychological and psychosocial factors

a. Type and degree of disruption in life-cycle tasks caused by breast cancer (e.g., marital, childbearing, work)
b. Psychological stability and ability to cope with stress
c. Attitudes toward illness, breast cancer in particular
d. Prior psychiatric history
e. Availability of psychological and social support (partner, family, friends)

Medical factors

a. Stage of cancer at diagnosis
b. Treatment(s) received: mastectomy or lumpectomy with irradiation, neo-adjuvant and/or adjuvant chemotherapy, endocrine therapy, targeted treatment (e.g., Herceptin)
c. Availability of rehabilitation
   i. Psychological (for self, partner, and family)
   ii. Physical (cosmetic and functional)
d. Psychological support provided by physicians and staff

Table 24–2. Major decision points across the course of breast cancer care

Detection and diagnosis of a suspicious symptom

a. What constitutes a worrisome symptom
b. Whether to seek attention for or disclose a symptom (or delay)
c. Whom to consult
d. What type of procedure(s) to undergo to confirm cancer (e.g., MRI, type of biopsy, biomarkers, etc.)

Selection of treatment options

a. Local therapy
   i. How to treat the breast
     – Mastectomy with or without reconstruction, and if reconstruction, type and timing
     – Breast conservation, with or without irradiation
   ii. How to treat the axilla
     – Sentinel node biopsy
     – Full axillary dissection
     – No assessment
b. Systemic therapy
   i. Chemotherapy: type and duration; neo-adjuvant use or not
   ii. Endocrine therapy: type and duration
   iii. Molecularly targeted therapy: type and duration
c. Other considerations
   i. Clinical trial participation
   ii. Second opinions
   iii. Genetic testing with or without prophylactic surgery

Posttreatment follow-up care

a. Whether to seek follow-up care or follow recommendations
b. Who should perform follow-up
   i. Oncologist (medical, radiation, and/or surgical)
   ii. Primary care physician
   iii. Both
   iv. Other (e.g., oncology or primary care nurse practitioner)
c. How often follow-up should occur
d. What tests should be performed or services provided and with what periodicity, including plans to promote optimal psychosocial as well as physical recovery

ABBREVIATION: MRI, magnetic resonance imaging.

may vary over time. Uncomfortable with extensive details at the outset, a woman may later be more receptive to and even desire greater information about her own care, a change in attitude to which the physician should be alert. Although desire for unrealistic treatment might be discouraged, deferring final decisions can be supported. It is important for women to know that they have time to make a well-considered decision. Clinicians can help limit excessive information gathering; however, by setting a stop date to the search. In cases where a woman feels overwhelmed by the process, it can be helpful to have the emotional pressure temporarily removed by postponing surgery and reviewing the situation and possible treatments in a psychiatric consultation during which the woman can express her concerns and fears and identify the reasons for her emotional response. Throughout the decision-making process, it should be remembered that physician recommendation plays a critical role in women's choice of treatment and that central to a woman's successful adaptation is her relationship with her treating physicians and broader care team.

Psychological variables in adaptation. In 1980, Meyerowitz[15] identified three broad psychosocial responses to breast cancer: (1) psychological discomfort (anxiety, depression, or anger); (2) behavioral changes caused by physical discomfort, marital or sexual disruption, or altered activity level; and (3) fears and concerns related to body image, recurrence, or death. Although women, today, face very different treatment scenarios, the psychological concerns that affect adaptation remain the same. In addition to these variables, the age at which cancer occurs, the patient's existing emotional characteristics (personality and coping style), and the availability and extent of interpersonal support also affect her response to illness (Table 24–3).

The age when breast cancer occurs is of prime importance because younger women frequently have different concerns from older women.[16] Concerns about the threat to life and future health, as well as fears of potential disfigurement, loss of femininity, disability, and distress associated with treatment are common to all women diagnosed with breast cancer. These are often more pronounced, however, in younger women, who may perceive the cancer diagnosis as "off-timed" in the normal life course and that they have more to lose due to the threat to their future, such as a career or having and rearing offspring.[17] Feeling different or isolated is a theme also voiced by younger women. Research has not focused as much on older women, in particular those aged 65 and older, despite their representing almost half of current breast cancer survivors. It has been suggested that older patients may experience less distress because of greater life experience, including familiarity with medical settings, but this has not been clearly established. In fact, women older than age 80 with breast cancer may struggle with concurrent major losses, particularly of a spouse, and suffer the adverse effects of other, concurrent medical conditions. Older women with breast cancer are at risk for experiencing greater decrements in their health-related quality of life and lower psychosocial well-being than healthy peers.[18] They also may be at risk for significantly higher rates of decline in upper body function[19] and may be significantly less likely to receive appropriate surgical care or rehabilitation.

Table 24-3. Risk factors for poor adaptation

Medical

a. More advanced disease
b. More intense or aggressive treatment
c. Other/multiple comorbid medical conditions
d. Fewer rehabilitative options
e. Poor doctor–patient relationship or communication

Personal

a. Prior psychiatric history
b. Past trauma history (especially physical or sexual abuse)
c. Rigid or limited coping capacity
d. Helpless/hopeless outlook
e. Low income/education
f. Multiple competing demands (e.g., work, child or other family care, economic)
g. Poor marital/interpersonal relationship
h. Younger age (<40 years) or older age (>80 years)

Social

a. Lack of social support (and/or religious affiliation)
b. Limited access to service resources
c. Cultural biases
d. Social stigma or illness taboo

Breast cancer specific

a. Prior breast cancer experience
b. Recurrence or second breast cancer
c. Loss of family or friends to breast cancer
d. High investment in body image, in particular breasts

SOURCE: Adapted from Weisman D. Early diagnosis of vulnerability in cancer patients. *Am J Med Sci.* 1976;271:187.

Table 24-4. Women with breast cancer who should be considered for psychiatric evaluation

Those who present with current symptoms or a history of the following:
- depression or anxiety
- suicidal thinking (attempt)
- substance or alcohol abuse
- confusional state (delirium or encephalopathy)
- mood swings, insomnia, or irritability from steroids

Those who
- have a family history of breast cancer
- are very young, old, pregnant, nursing, single, or alone
- are adjusting to multiple losses and managing multiple life stresses
- seem paralyzed by cancer treatment decisions
- fear death during surgery or are terrified by loss of control under anesthesia
- request euthanasia
- seem unable to provide informed consent

Other variables affecting adaptation include the personality and unique coping patterns of the patient. Women who use active coping and problem-solving techniques report better mood and adaptation.[20] Being flexible in use of coping styles over time may be particularly helpful.[21] For example, the use of distraction, while helpful when waiting for test results or managing the stress of a chemotherapy infusion, is impractical when attention to changes in treatment details is needed. Further, women who are able to draw on and use available social resources and support adapt better and may even live longer than women who do not.[22] In contrast, women who are passive or feel hopeless or pessimistic are rigid in their coping style, or become isolated and reject help when it is offered adapt more poorly. Although prolonged anxiety or depression is not an expected reaction to a cancer diagnosis, women who become persistently depressed may be at risk of not only poor quality of life but also premature death,[23] and should be considered promptly for professional psychological assessment and support (Table 24-4). (See also chapters on anxiety and depression.) Prior trauma and current stressful life events can also adversely affect a woman's adaptation to breast cancer.[24]

An area of public interest and active research is the effect of a patient's attitude on her vulnerability to breast cancer and her survival. Many women express concern that they "brought it on themselves" or that their bad attitude or lifestyle may be making the cancer worse. Such beliefs can become an added psychological burden for many women with breast cancer, sometimes causing them to seek questionable and unproven therapies as primary treatment. Although epidemiologic studies have failed to confirm an association between stress and breast cancer development[25] or survival,[26] it is important to mitigate chronic stress when it occurs.

Additional important factors in adaptation are a patient's prior experiences with breast cancer and body image. Levels of psychological distress during and after treatment can be elevated by the memory of a friend's or family member's death from breast cancer. Some women cannot tolerate the idea of losing or damaging a breast, and may dangerously delay consultation for a symptom, particularly if their community views cancer as stigmatizing.

A woman's sociocultural background and ethnocultural affinity memberships can further influence her breast cancer experience. Although a growing area of research focus, interpreting between-group differences in studies involving diverse samples of women is complicated because ethnicity is frequently confounded with such variables as income, education, and treatment—factors known to be associated with quality of life.[27] Data from two historically understudied minority groups of women nevertheless are worth noting. Lesbian breast cancer survivors may be more comfortable with body image and perceive greater social support than their heterosexual peers. They also tend to experience more difficulty interacting with physicians, however.[28] Survivors in rural areas are at greater risk for relationship problems, lack of support, and feelings of isolation. They are particularly prone to develop concerns about how partners and family will cope during absences for treatment, the burden of running farms or property alone, and the financial strain of transportation and healthcare costs.[29]

Finally, adjustment depends on the response from other significant people, from spouse or partner, family and friends. The impact of these relationships on family as well as cancer patients' and survivors' outcomes is addressed at greater length in Part XI of this volume.

Medical variables in adaptation. The medical variables that influence psychological adaptation are the stage of breast cancer at diagnosis, the treatment required, the prognosis, and the available rehabilitative opportunities. The length and intensity of current treatments and the recognition that women treated for breast cancer must be followed for extended periods of time represent a growing challenge for healthcare providers and the broader healthcare delivery system.

Surgery

Mastectomy. Medical as well as psychosocial variables inform a woman's decision concerning mastectomy. The medical variables include tumor type, size, location, and aggressiveness. The psychosocial variables are equally complex. For some women, the thought of leaving tumor cells in the breast is intolerable, and they feel more secure with mastectomy. Others selecting mastectomy perceive the breast containing cancer as an offending part that should be removed. Still other women elect mastectomy because of the lack of geographically convenient high-quality irradiation, fear of irradiation and its side effects, or an inability to devote as much as 6 weeks to daily irradiation treatments because of family and work demands. Research suggests that several additional characteristics may distinguish women who elect to have mastectomy from those who elect breast-sparing surgery. These include older age, preferring to have no therapy beyond surgery, being black or Hispanic (or possibly low income), and among older women, living with extended or nonfamily members or in an assisted-living setting.[30]

Considerable literature exists documenting the physical, psychological, and social impact of loss of one or both breasts on women's health and function. Surgery can result in a sense of mutilation and diminished self-worth, the loss of a sense of femininity and sexual attractiveness, the loss of sexual function, anxiety, depression, hopelessness, guilt, shame, or fear of recurrence, abandonment, and death.[1,15] Nationally, fewer than half of women diagnosed with early-stage breast cancer elect to have a mastectomy. Of late, however, the number of women selecting ipsilateral mastectomy with contralateral prophylactic mastectomy has increased.[31] Part of this increase results from greater use of preoperative magnetic resonance imaging (MRI).[32] At the same time, more women are having breast reconstruction than previously, although as discussed later, a number of those undergoing mastectomy are not made aware of their reconstruction options. In general, women who are well adjusted before they have a mastectomy and whose disease is in an early stage can expect at 1 year to have a quality of life equal to that of their healthy peers. Today, there is less emphasis on the importance of the type of surgery performed to a woman's psychological health than in an earlier period, likely due to refinements in surgical techniques and more surgical options; rather, there is greater appreciation of the key role that personal and social characteristics and the adjuvant therapy given play in predicting women's adaptation.[33]

Breast-conserving therapy. Early studies showed that women having breast-conserving therapy (BCT) manifest somewhat better overall adjustment than those having mastectomy.[34] These early studies indicated that women who selected BCT over mastectomy were more concerned about insult to body image, were more dependent on their breasts for self-esteem, and believed they would have had difficulty adjusting to loss of the breast. Satisfaction with surgical results can have a marked bearing on psychosexual morbidity. Indeed, early studies showed that younger women, known to be at increased risk for psychosocial problems in adaptation to breast cancer, tended to elect BCT and some reported greater satisfaction with sexual activity. However, longer-term follow-up of more current cohorts of breast cancer survivors has failed to show differences in overall quality of life based on type of surgery alone.[35] In particular, research indicates that benefits to sexual function associated with BCT are less than previously believed.[36] This may be because adjuvant chemotherapy, particularly in younger women who may experience premature menopause, is known to have a significant negative impact on sexual functioning. What we have learned is that BCT is not a psychosocial panacea; rather, it is a surgical and cosmetic option that may facilitate good adaptation for some women.

Irradiation. It is important to note that women undergoing irradiation, whether as part of their breast-conserving management, or less commonly following mastectomy, are at risk for psychological disturbance, in particular depressive symptoms or persistent fears about their disease and the risk of recurrence.[1] Further, when discussing irradiation one additional factor should be considered—risk for lymphedema.

Lymphedema may be seen in association with irradiation. In particular, women undergoing resection of axillary lymph nodes followed by axillary irradiation are at increased risk of developing lymphedema. On the other hand, women receiving irradiation to the breast only can be reassured that this will not increase the risk of lymphedema. Women who go on to develop lymphedema are at high risk for problems in both psychological and social functioning, including difficulties with body image, depression, physical discomfort, and functional limitations.[37] Fortunately, the proportion of women affected by this condition has decreased with broader use of sentinel node biopsy. However, this latter tissue-sparing approach has not eliminated the problem.[38] Data from pilot studies suggest that an upper-body exercise program does not increase arm circumference or volume in women who already have lymphedema and may improve their quality of life.[39] Additional larger-scale studies are needed to confirm this effect and, importantly, to develop evidence-based guidelines for care that might benefit thousands of women.

Breast reconstruction. Postmastectomy breast reconstruction is an important rehabilitative option for women undergoing mastectomy. Rates of reconstruction are hard to come by but appear to be slowly rising.[40] However, there is increasing evidence that reconstruction is not being routinely addressed with patients. In their surveillance, epidemiology, and end results or SEER-based sample, Alderman and colleagues[41] found that only a third of mastectomy patients reported that their general surgeon discussed reconstruction with them before treatment. Reconstruction was more likely to be discussed with younger, more educated women with large tumors. Of note, when reconstruction was discussed, patients were found to be four times more likely to have a mastectomy.[41]

Relatively few studies have systematically examined the psychosocial impact of mastectomy alone compared with mastectomy plus reconstruction. Contemporary studies have sought to evaluate psychosocial and sexual results for women selecting one of three different surgical options: lumpectomy, mastectomy alone, or mastectomy with reconstruction. Parker and colleagues,[35] using a prospective longitudinal research design and examining early adaptation among women undergoing each of the three different procedures, found few differences in adaptation 2 years after treatment. In what remains the largest three-way comparison study, investigators found no differences in women's emotional, social, or role functions by type of surgery.[42] However, women in both mastectomy groups (with or without reconstruction) complained of more physical symptoms related to their surgeries than women undergoing lumpectomy. Further, 45.4% of women having mastectomy plus reconstruction reported a negative impact on their sex lives, while 41.3% of women having mastectomy alone and only 29.8% of women having lumpectomy reported this result from their treatment. Important factors in sexual outcome are that mastectomy with or without reconstruction results in permanent loss of sensation in the area, and postmastectomy irradiation decreases the cosmetic results of reconstruction, particularly with implants.

A number of sociodemographic differences have been observed between women who do and do not undergo postmastectomy reconstruction. Specifically, women who undergo reconstruction are generally younger, are better educated, have higher incomes, are more likely to be partnered, and have earlier stage of disease.[42,43] Women who are older, Hispanic, or born outside the United States are less likely to have reconstruction.[44] Fewer African-American women undergo reconstruction; this may be due to economic and access barriers (including lower rates of referral for these procedures) but may also be related to lower interest in having reconstruction. Asian women are also less likely than white women to undergo reconstruction.[45] Some data suggest that self-identified lesbian or bisexual women regret having chosen reconstruction versus mastectomy alone, leading to adjustment problems.[46]

Regrettably, few efforts have been made to understand the psychological variables associated with who does and does not seek reconstruction, in particular in the present era in which autologous tissue procedures and immediate reconstruction represent standard options for care. Further, additional research is needed on the impact on women's satisfaction and functioning related to the extent of surgery performed and procedures used to achieve symmetry between the breasts.

Timing of reconstruction: immediate versus delayed. Research with women undergoing immediate reconstruction has shown high levels of patient satisfaction with surgical results and less psychosocial morbidity than in those who undergo mastectomy alone, although these differences diminish over time.[47] Patients undergoing immediate reconstruction report being less depressed and anxious and experience less impairment of their sense of femininity, self-esteem, and sexual attractiveness than their peers who delay or do not seek reconstruction. Al-Ghazal et al.[48] reported that 76% of women who delayed surgery would have preferred immediate reconstruction, whereas only 5% of those electing immediate reconstruction wished they had delayed such surgery.

Type of reconstruction: implant versus transverse rectus abdominis myocutaneous flap. The research evaluating psychosocial outcomes for women undergoing reconstruction using transverse rectus abdominis myocutaneous flap (TRAM) surgery has also been an area of interest. In our own research, we looked at 146 women on average 3 years after undergoing reconstruction; 95 (65%) had an implant and 51 (35%) underwent TRAM surgery.[49] No differences were seen between groups in satisfaction with the appearance or feel of their breasts or the overall impact of breast cancer on their sex lives, although there was a consistent tendency for the women with TRAM reconstructions to report greater comfort and satisfaction. This pattern is consistent with others' findings and the observation that timing of reconstruction may be more important than procedure on women's long-term adaptation.[47] However, women who had an implant were significantly more worried about having a problem with their reconstruction; 25% of women with implants indicated they worried about the future versus only 8% of the TRAM group. Longer-term follow-up of cosmetic outcomes for implant recipients confirms these fears. Clough et al.[50] report that overall cosmetic outcome was rated as acceptable in 86% at 2 years but had declined to 54% by 5 years. A similar pattern was not observed among TRAM reconstructions, in which assessment of cosmetic outcome remained stable over time. Ongoing research is needed not only to document women's long-term psychosocial outcomes after reconstruction, including response to newer surgical flap techniques (e.g., deep inferior epigastric perforator), but also to help elucidate trends in and the interplay between type and timing of surgery.[47]

Regardless of the type of reconstructive surgery proposed or selected, women need to be well informed about what to expect. Key concerns of women about reconstruction include the cost of the surgery, the length of time under anesthesia, the number of procedures required, the cosmetic results achievable, and the safety of the techniques used, both in terms of potential for complications and in the case of implants, risk of masking recurrent cancer, or promoting autoimmune disease. Thorough review of the nature and timing of any planned symmetry and nipple-reconstruction procedures is also important.

Systematic therapy

Adjuvant chemotherapy. Use of adjuvant chemotherapy has been shown to reduce risk of recurrence and improve overall survival. Despite this vital benefit, systemic adjuvant treatment is also associated with acute and persistent adverse side effects including diminished physical activity and function, pain, and poorer general health.[51,52] Thus, a recommendation for adjuvant chemotherapy requires a woman to consider not only an additional demanding therapeutic modality and a lengthened treatment period, but also a potentially increased threat to health as a consequence of her breast cancer diagnosis. These issues, including which drugs or protocol to use, constitute a key component of treatment decision making (Table 24–2).

Anticipation of chemotherapy can be difficult. Women fear the transient acute effects of chemotherapy (e.g., nausea, hair loss, anemia) and, with greater public awareness and discussion of these, the potential for persistent effects such as fatigue, pain, memory problems, sexual dysfunction, weight gain, and depression.[53] It is essential to prepare a patient psychologically for chemotherapy with educational materials, nursing input, and an outline by the physician of the disease- and treatment-related expectations.

Most women cope with the short-term adverse psychological effects through reliance on reassurance that they have done everything possible to eradicate their disease. Clinicians need to be aware; however, that for some women declines in health-related quality of life during treatment increase risk for discontinuation of chemotherapy.[54] Monitoring for problems and addressing them promptly are important in ensuring adherence to the planned course of care.

Nausea and vomiting from adjuvant chemotherapy are normally well controlled with pharmacologic and behavioral interventions. Other side effects, however, such as hair loss, weight gain, problems with concentration, premature menopause, and fatigue, have psychological consequences that warrant special attention. Many women report that alopecia, a visible indicator of disease, was more distressing than their breast cancer diagnosis. Early discussion of hair loss and providing information about wigs, the cost of which is often reimbursed by insurers as prosthetic devices, together with a referral to the American Cancer Society's *Look Good…Feel Better* program, can help reduce distress about appearance.

The reason chemotherapy causes weight gain remains unclear. Abnormal weight gain can lead to diminished self-esteem and, more importantly, may be associated with a worse prognosis.[55] For these reasons, exercise programs have been introduced during chemotherapy and

have been found to be feasible, well tolerated, and a benefit to women in controlling weight gain, improving functional and cardiac status, and potentially enhancing quality of life.[56]

Many women undergoing chemotherapy report difficulty with attention, concentration, memory, and processing speed. These troubling neurocognitive effects that may also be related to type as well as dose of chemotherapy are the focus of active research[57] and are covered in detail in Chapter 34. It should be noted that women's complaints about cognitive compromise have not been consistently associated with neuropsychological test performance, and the incidence of complaints tends to be higher than the documented rate of cognitive deficits.[58] Nevertheless, if cognitive dysfunction is found to persist over time or, as some studies suggest, worsen,[59] this troubling side effect could become a dose-limiting factor in breast cancer treatment decisions and care.

A troublesome side effect of chemotherapy in premenopausal women is premature menopause[60] (see also Chapter 33 on Sexuality after Cancer). Threatened or actual loss of fertility and the acute onset of menopause often cause significant distress. The symptoms caused by chemotherapy-induced menopause (e.g., hot flashes, night sweats, and vaginal dryness and atrophy) can produce severe physical, and by consequence emotional, discomfort. Vaginal changes can result in dyspareunia and lead to disruption in desire for or ability to engage in intimate relationships. Topical vaginal estrogen (e.g., Estring, Vagifem) has been recommended for women experiencing severe dyspareunia but is avoided by many clinicians treating women with breast cancer due to fear of exacerbating underlying disease. Although vaginal lubricants and moisturizers can be helpful, thinning of the vaginal mucosa may still result in irritation during intercourse. Education about the nature and management of these troublesome side effects is critical, as is provision of emotional support in coping with them.

Hot flashes are among the most common acute and long-term side effects of chemotherapeutic breast cancer treatment. This symptom is seen secondary to chemotherapy-induced premature menopause, after exposure to endocrine therapy, or consequent to cessation of hormone replacement therapy following diagnosis.[61] Although new data suggest that they may be important indicators of therapeutic efficacy,[62] hot flashes, nonetheless, can be profoundly debilitating for some women. A variety of medications are used to address this problem, including antidepressants. However, there is an accumulating body of evidence that several selective serotonin-reuptake inhibitor (SSRI) antidepressant drugs, especially fluoxetine and paroxetine, might interfere with tamoxifen metabolism by inhibiting the CYP2D6 enzyme. Venlafaxine and mirtazapine are antidepressants that minimally affect CYP2D6 activity and are a reasonable consideration for depressed women taking tamoxifen.[63] A further difficult-to-treat sequela of chemotherapy is loss of libido that likely is associated with a reduction in circulating androgens.

Finally, increased use of multidrug, dose-dense, and intense chemotherapy is leading more women to complain of prolonged fatigue[64] (see Chapter 32). Longer follow-up studies of chemotherapy-exposed groups have shown that chemotherapy-related fatigue, that may last months to years after treatment,[65] is unrelated to anemia and is unrelieved by rest.[66] In a large prospective study, 20% of women, on average 7 years post-treatment, experienced persistent fatigue. This persistent effect was associated with depression, cardiovascular problems, and prior treatment with both radiation and chemotherapy.[65] At present, there is a limited evidence base for effective interventions to control fatigue.[67]

Since therapies for breast cancer are evolving so quickly, understanding persistent and late-occurring effects and addressing them with treated women are challenging. Adverse effects of newer therapies, such as neuropathies associated with taxanes or pain syndromes reported in association with granulocyte colony-stimulating factor exposure, need continued study. Introduction of arguably less toxic therapies including molecularly targeted agents, such as trastuzumab (Herceptin), increases the need for longitudinal outcome data, especially in light of early reports of troubling side effects.[68] Past and potential limitations on current findings need to be taken into account when counseling women about treatment choice, particularly when disease is limited.

There is growing recognition that as critical as it is to prepare women well for the commencement of treatment, it is equally important to prepare them for ending a lengthy course of radiation and/or chemotherapy,

Table 24–5. Challenges related to ending treatment

1. Fear that the cancer will return
2. Concern about ongoing monitoring (e.g., whom to call if a problem/symptom arises)
3. Loss of a supportive environment
4. Diminished sense of well-being due to treatment effects (often feeling less well than when treatment was initiated)
5. Social demands: "re-entry" problems (dealing with expectations of family and friends that the breast cancer patient will quickly be back to "normal" and resume full function equivalent to preillness levels)

as this is when fears of recurrence peak.[69] A number of other factors also contribute to anxiety at this pivotal time (Table 24–5). In recognition of the many persistent effects of treatment, some clinicians routinely advise women anticipating the end of treatment to allot as many months for their recovery as were spent being treated for their cancer. This may be particularly important advice to help women negotiate the "re-entry" phase of their recovery, as they struggle to regain a sense of what will be their "new normal" and constructively interact with family members, friends, and colleagues, who may expect everything to return to usual shortly after the termination of treatment. Developing and discussing a treatment summary and follow-up care plan (issues discussed in greater detail in the survivorship section later) can also help ease the distress of women as they make the transition to recovery. Two booklets that form part of the NCI's *Facing Forward* series, *Life after cancer treatment*, and *When someone you love has completed cancer treatment* provide useful information for the woman and her family about what to expect after initial therapy ends.

Adjuvant endocrine therapy. Women who go on to adjuvant endocrine therapies may gain a sense of relief knowing that they are still doing something active to prevent recurrence. Long-term treatment (e.g., beyond 5 years) with tamoxifen and aromatase inhibitors (AIs) has drawn growing attention to their latent psychological and sexual impact. Tamoxifen, while an antiestrogen, has weak estrogenic effects on the vaginal mucosa. Some older women find that the associated increase in hot flashes with tamoxifen (or an AI) is a limiting factor in its use. By contrast, some younger patients report that tamoxifen provides relief from the vaginal dryness that accompanies chemotherapy-induced premature menopause. A small subset of women become depressed with the use of tamoxifen that can require temporary or even permanent discontinuation of its use. The impact of tamoxifen exposure on brain function is also being studied.[70] It is worrisome that rates of discontinuation or inconsistent use of tamoxifen, potentially as a consequence of its adverse side effects, may be higher than previously believed.[71]

Information about the psychological and sexual impact of the AIs is still evolving.[72,73] These agents have been associated with joint and muscle pain.[74] One report found that as many as 10% of women had discontinued AI use because of these side effects.[75] The impact of these newer therapies on women's sense of well-being as well as adherence patterns are areas warranting future research.

RECURRENT AND ADVANCED DISEASE

The number of women facing recurrent local and distant disease has grown, as has research examining women's reactions to these events.[76] With advances in breast cancer treatment, women are living longer even in the context of metastatic disease. Diagnosis of a recurrence is often described as "devastating." Recovering overall quality of life is slower following a recurrence than after initial diagnosis. Despite the physical burden of recurrence, however, during the year after diagnosis women show steady improvement in psychological functioning, reflecting the adaptive capacity of survivors.[76] Compared with disease-free survivors, women with recurrent breast cancer report poorer physical functioning and perceived health, more impairment in emotional well-being, more problems in relationships with family and healthcare providers, and less

hope. Even when recurrent disease is localized, significant levels of psychiatric morbidity may occur.[76,77] Family members of these women also report high levels of emotional distress.[77] When psychological distress persists in the context of a recurrence, it may serve to drive away rather than elicit support from a social network. Women with recurrent disease and their family members represent vulnerable groups for whom more intensive psychosocial intervention is warranted.

INTERVENTIONS

Psychosocial and behavioral intervention research in cancer has a long history (see also Part IX in this volume), particularly that designed for and tested among women treated for breast cancer.[78] Interventions used in the context of breast cancer vary greatly by type (e.g., individual vs. group); orientation (e.g., behavioral vs. cognitive vs. supportive); mode of delivery (in person vs. remote, e.g., by phone, Internet, or teleconference); duration (time limited vs. open ended); and timing (e.g., before, during, or after treatment); as well as by target populations served (early vs. advanced, younger than age 40 vs. older, partnered vs. single, or mixed). Nevertheless, the fundamental purpose of these interventions has been the same: to provide each woman with the skills or resources necessary to cope with her illness and to improve the quality of her life and health. However, three points must be made regarding the use of such programs in the overall care of patients with breast cancer and their families.

First, taken as a whole, researchers have found that patients who received an intervention designed to improve knowledge or coping or to reduce distress do better than those who did not. Specifically, patients provided or randomized to some form of individual or group intervention experienced less anxiety and depression, had an increased sense of control, had improved body image and better sexual function, reported greater satisfaction with care, and exhibited improved medication adherence.[79,80] Studies have demonstrated that "usual" care is often inadequate for many women and that additional education and support have the potential to significantly enhance women's function and well-being. Significant attention needs to be brought to bear on the development and delivery of psychosocial care models to enhance understanding of who needs what, delivered by whom, and when in the course of care.[81] Further, understanding the economic impact of these programs or services in terms of delivery, changes in healthcare utilization, and out-of-pocket expenses may be critical if we are to expect broader uptake of these into routine practice.[82,83]

Second, use of psychosocial interventions with respect to breast cancer continues to grow. Use of these services reflect not only patient demand for supportive care but also growing recognition that addressing psychosocial issues may improve outcomes for patients.[3] The current consensus is that psychosocial interventions do not prolong survival[84] but help women "live better," although there are provocative data to suggest that women in the highest medical and psychological risk groups may realize a survival benefit.[85]

Third, although an individually tailored intervention should result in the best outcome for any given patient, this may not be feasible, suitable, or even desirable in all cases. Some patients with cancer resist being singled out for individual psychological therapy and feel burdened by any label that might suggest that they may be mentally ill. Furthermore, increasing evidence shows that participation in group activity offers a uniquely supportive and normalizing experience for many patients with cancer struggling to deal with the realities of their new or continued status as cancer survivors. In studies that have specifically compared use of individual interventions to group interventions, groups were as effective as individual counseling or support in reducing patient distress. Use of new communication technologies, in particular the Internet, but also established ones, such as teleconferencing and telephone, to provide group support represents the new frontier in intervention research. These technologies not only extend the capacity to reach women isolated by geography or physical limitations, but also (in the case of phone and Internet) permit some degree of anonymity and content control for those women more hesitant to engage in face-to-face programs. Indeed, the Internet may offer a unique vehicle to improve access to information and social support and reduce isolation.[86,87]

Research suggests that four key elements are vital to achieving optimal outcomes for all cancer survivors: (1) access to state-of-the-art cancer care; (2) active coping, in particular active participation or engagement in one's care, even if this means delegating decision making; (3) perceived availability, and if needed, use of social support; and (4) having a sense of meaning or purpose in life (this can include someone to live for, spiritual belief or connectedness, or a way to make sense of illness and health and one's place in the world). Many of the psychosocial and behavioral interventions developed in cancer are designed to foster or reinforce some or all of these core needs. However, access to these services remains a problem.

Clinician awareness about and referral of patients to even such well-established programs as the American Cancer Society's Reach to Recovery are variable.[88] Providers in one health maintenance organization reported referring 70% of their patients to system-provided services and estimated that 40% of patients used these, when in fact fewer than 10% of patients reported this was the case. Further, patient barriers to service use cited in this study were lack of awareness of the service and lack of provider referral.[89]

Key to the development of an effective intervention is the recognition that for many women, cancer represents a transitional event. As defined by Andrykowski et al.,[90] cancer is "a traumatic event that alters an individual's assumptive world with the potential to produce long-lasting changes of both a positive as well as negative nature." As such, the primary goal in any intervention is to use this shift in worldview to help minimize the negative and enhance the positive impact of illness on recovery and well-being.

BREAST CANCER SURVIVORS

Growing attention is being focused on cancer survivors and the experience of living through and beyond their illness and its treatment.[91] There are a number of reasons for this, the most obvious being the sheer number of survivors. Breast cancer survivors represent the largest constituent group (24%) of the current population of the almost 12 million cancer survivors in the United States. There are currently more than 2.5 million women with a history of breast cancer, of whom almost 343,000 were diagnosed 20 or more years ago.[2] A second reason for the increased attention to breast cancer's latent impact is the lengthening course of survival expected for most women. Although cancer survivorship is covered elsewhere in this volume (Part XII), summarized here are a few key points specific to breast cancer survivors' health and care.

Despite wide variability in adaptation to diagnosis and treatment, most women will return to lives that are as full as and often richer personally than before their illness; in many cases, survivors' social and emotional functioning is reported to be better than that of control or comparison samples of unaffected peers. Although some women leave jobs following a cancer diagnosis, either by choice or because of disability,[92] employment patterns show that breast cancer survivors who continue to work may work longer hours even than their unaffected peers.[93] Besides being a vital source of income and often of needed healthcare coverage, work can also be an important source of social support and self-esteem as well as distraction from illness during treatment. Most of those in manual labor jobs (which often includes women with lower education and income) find that employers are accommodating to their needs.[94] However, counseling around work-related issues and referral for help in negotiating workplace issues are important in aiding women's continued employment as desired.

In general, the current generation of studies has led clinicians to realize that concern about high rates of impairment in treated women may have been exaggerated. Breast cancer does not appear to lead to the development of posttraumatic stress disorder in significant numbers of women.[95] Indeed, the remarkable resilience of survivors and expression by many women that their illness was a special turning point has spawned an entire genre of studies examining what is referred to as posttraumatic growth or benefit-finding.[96] Also impressive has been the willingness of women to share important details about their cancer experience and recovery to improve the lives of women who will be diagnosed and treated after them. The growing interest in cancer

Table 24–6. Triggers for fear of recurrence

1. Routine follow-up visits and tests
2. Anniversary dates (e.g., date of diagnosis, end of cancer treatment, birthday)
3. Worrisome or "suspicious" symptoms
4. Persistent treatment-related side effects (especially fatigue or pain)
5. Change in health (e.g., weight loss, fatigue)
6. Illness in a family member
7. Death of a fellow survivor/prominent cancer survivor
8. Times of stress
9. Idiosyncratic triggers (e.g., "learned responses" such as the smell of alcohol due to association with receipt of chemotherapy; sight of the treatment center)

survivorship, as reflected in the number of programs designed specifically to address survivors' needs after treatment that are offered by the National Cancer Institute (NCI)-designated cancer centers, is testament that survivors' call to action is being heard. Services provided at these and other centers focus on two main areas: (1) surveillance and (2) health and well-being after treatment.

Follow-up care after breast cancer. Although concern about disease recurrence may diminish over time, for most breast cancer survivors, it never fully goes away. Part of this persistent anxiety may be attributable to breast cancer survivors' understanding that their cancer could recur at any time after treatment and that medical follow-up must continue for life. In the context of this ongoing risk, many women reject calling themselves "survivors." Degree of worry may fluctuate and be triggered by a variety of sources including continuing physical problems after treatment[97] (Table 24-6). Fear may lead to frequent self-examination for signs and symptoms of recurrence, anxiety well in advance of a doctor visit, and worry about the future. In some women fear can cause severely disabling reactions including hypochondriac-like preoccupation with health at one extreme or avoidance and denial at the other, inability to plan for the future, and despair. At the same time, family members' fear of recurrence in the survivor can have a direct and adverse affect on family quality of life.[98] Surprisingly, despite its prevalence, relatively few interventions have been developed that specifically target this aspect of women's recovery. The one exception is work by Mishel and her colleagues,[99] who have developed interventions to help women successfully cope with uncertainty. Although other interventions that effectively reduce distress and improve a sense of well-being might be expected to result in decreased worry about disease recurrence, this remains to be tested.

Regardless of whether a woman sees or refers to herself as a survivor, it is important that treated women recognize a lifetime need for follow-up. Issues related to follow-up care constitute the third major set of decisions in the breast cancer patient's illness pathway (Table 24-2). In response to recommendations from both the President's Cancer Panel and the Institute of Medicine that survivors receive a treatment summary and plan for future care at the end of treatment, the American Society of Clinical Oncology has created electronic templates for the generation of this information specifically for use with breast cancer survivors. The status of and challenge to this new area of care are well described by Kattlove and Winn,[100] who note that optimal follow-up care must address women's needs with respect not only to surveillance, genetic counseling and testing, and detection and treatment of second primaries, but importantly also to treatment complications, physiologic alterations, and psychosocial problems. Ganz and Hahn[101] provide guidance on how to implement these more comprehensive care plans for breast cancer survivors transitioning to recovery.

An important take-home message in all of the research discussed is that a cancer diagnosis represents for many a "teachable moment" for healthcare providers along with breast cancer survivors themselves,[102] a moment currently being missed by many oncology practitioners.[103] The crisis of cancer often creates a window of receptivity during which healthcare professionals can provide patients with educational messages about and support for pursuing healthy lifestyle choices. Although these activities, if adopted, may not alter length of breast cancer survival, they do carry the potential to significantly reduce individual risk for treatment-related or other chronic illness-related morbidities and potentially other cancers. Encouraging breast cancer survivors to take control of what they can in their lives may enable them to live with better health in and less fear of the future.

Health behavior after breast cancer. An emerging focus of breast cancer follow-up care is the role of health promotion (see also Chapter 78). Attention to this topic is being spurred by survivors' interest in and growing demand for informed guidance about what they can do to reduce their risk of cancer-related morbidity and mortality. Many breast cancer survivors already report taking better care of themselves in the wake of cancer, with particular focus on adopting healthier lifestyles, reducing stress, eating better, and exercising regularly.[51] Two areas receiving significant research attention with respect to their impact on women's health outcomes are stress management and physical activity interventions. As noted earlier, many women believe the stress in their lives can precipitate or exacerbate breast disease. For these survivors, reducing stress is seen as potentially lifesaving. Researchers at the University of Miami's Mind Body Center have developed a standardized 10-week training program that equips women with the cognitive and behavioral skills necessary to identify, analyze, and manage stress.[104] A second avenue to stress reduction is staying active during or becoming physically active after cancer treatment.

One of the fastest-growing areas of behavioral research in general, and with respect to cancer in particular[105,106] is physical activity interventions. Research shows that physical activity can improve mood (reduce anxiety and depression), enhance cardiovascular function, control weight, improve body image and self-esteem, reduce nausea and fatigue, and potentially alter immune function.[107,108] Weight, diet, and to a more variable extent, exercise have been linked to both breast cancer risk and mortality.[109,110] To date, two observational studies[111,112] and one randomized clinical trial[113] have found a survival benefit for women who became or remained moderately physically active after breast cancer treatment. As the evidence of their benefits for survivors mounts, lifestyle changes (in particular physical activity, smoking cessation, weight control, and to some extent, lower fat and more fruit and vegetable consumption) are being recommended after treatment,[114–116] although it is expected that learning to tailor these recommendations to vulnerable subpopulations will be needed.[117]

Finally, use of complementary and alternative medicine (CAM), estimated as applied by one-third to over 80% of patients during active cancer treatment,[118,119] is also seen in the posttreatment setting.[120] In our own research,[51] most women reported using some form of vitamins (86.6%) and followed diets or took dietary supplements (60.7%). The most commonly used dietary practices were following a low-fat (48.4%), low-calorie (20.4%), or low-salt (18.6%) diet. Many also took herbal preparations (49.3%), often using more than one remedy (62%). Of note, women who reported using St. John's wort (9.8%) also reported significantly more symptoms of emotional distress than nonusers. This finding, similar to others' reports of poorer psychological functioning among patients using CAM remedies,[121] suggests that some women may be self-medicating depressive symptoms. Asking about what CAM practices or products a woman may be pursuing is important to guiding her care both during and after treatment.

CONCLUSION

Breast cancer, the most common cancer in women, has a unique and at times complex psychological impact, but one to which psychologically healthy women respond well without the development of serious psychological symptoms. Increased use of local treatment using breast-conserving and reconstructive procedures is reducing the negative effect on self-image and body image. Broader dissemination of information from psychological studies of adaptation to the available treatment options can help in efforts to determine the best treatment to meet patients' physical and emotional needs. Addressing the psychosocial and psychosexual needs of patients with breast cancer improves quality of survival and may even enhance length of survival from other, comorbid conditions and events, even if not from cancer. As newer therapies are introduced, such as the molecularly targeted treatments of the future, research on their immediate and delayed psychosocial impact is needed. With the increasing demand for their involvement in care, special attention must be directed to the psychological well-being of the immediate relatives of women with breast cancer, especially their partners and offspring. Finally, as women live longer with a history of breast cancer, attention to their evolving physical, psychological, and social needs must become an integral part of their comprehensive care.

REFERENCES

1. Rowland JH, Massie MJ. Psycho-social adaptation during and after breast cancer. In: Harris JR, Lippman ME, Morrow M, Osborne CE (eds). *Diseases of the breast*. Philadelphia, PA: Lippincott, Williams & Wilkins; 2009:1103–1123.

2. Ries LAG, Melbert D, Krapcho M, et al. (eds). SEER cancer statistics review, 1975–2005. 2008. Available at: http://seer.cancer.gov/csr/1975_2005/. Accessed August 12, 2009.

3. Adler NE, Page AEK (eds). *Cancer care for the whole patient: Meeting psychosocial health needs*. Washington, DC: National Academies Press; 2008.

4. Bish A, Ramirez A, Burgess C, Hunter M. Understanding why women delay in seeking help for breast cancer symptoms. *J Psychosom Res*. 2005;58:321–326.

5. Friedman LC, Kalidas M, Elledge R, et al. Medical and psychosocial predictors of delay in seeking medical consultation for breast symptoms in women in a public sector setting. *J Behav Med*. 2006;29:327–334.

6. Ashing-Giwa KT, Padilla GV, Bohorquez DE, Tejero JS, Garcia M. Understanding the breast cancer experience of Latina women. *J Psychosoc Oncol*. 2006;24:19–52.

7. Reifenstein K. Care-seeking behaviors of African American women with breast cancer symptoms. *Res Nurs Health*. 2007;30:542–557.

8. Freedman RA, He Y, Winer EP, Keating NL. Trends in racial and age disparities in definitive local therapy of early-stage breast cancer. *J Clin Oncol*. 2008 Dec 22. Epub ahead of print. 2009;27:713–719.

9. Epstein RM, Street RL Jr. *Patient-centered communication in cancer care: Promoting healing and reducing suffering*. Bethesda, MD: National Cancer Institute; 2007.

10. Mellink WA, Dulmen AM, Wiggers T, Spreeuwenberg PM, Eggermont AM, Bensing JM. Cancer patients seeking a second surgical opinion: results of a study on motives, needs, and expectations. *J Clin Oncol*. 2003;21:1492–1497.

11. Wise M, Han JY, Shaw B, McTavish F, Gustafson DH. Effects of using online narrative and didactic information on healthcare participation for breast cancer patients. *Patient Educ Couns*. 2008;70:348–356.

12. Waljee JF, Rogers MA, Alderman AK. Decision aids and breast cancer: do they influence choice for surgery and knowledge of treatment options? *J Clin Oncol*. 2007;25:1067–1073.

13. O'Leary KA, Estabrooks CA, Olson K, Cumming C. Information acquisition for women facing surgical treatment for breast cancer: influencing factors and selected outcomes. *Patient Educ Couns*. 2007;69:5–19.

14. Andersen MR, Bowen DJ, Morea J, Stein KD, Baker F. Involvement in decision-making and breast cancer survivor quality of life. *Health Psychol*. 2009;28:29–37.

15. Meyerowitz BE. Psychosocial correlates of breast cancer and its treatments. *Psychol Bull*. 1980;87:108–131.

16. Mosher CE, Danoff-Burg S. A review of age differences in psychological adjustment to breast cancer. *J Psychosoc Oncol*. 2005;23:101–114.

17. Avis NE, Crawford S, Manuel J. Quality of life among younger women with breast cancer. *J Clin Oncol*. 2005;23:3322–3330.

18. Robb C, Haley WE, Balducci L, et al. Impact of breast cancer survivorship on quality of life in older women. *Crit Rev Oncol Hematol*. 2007;62:84–91.

19. Westrup JL, Lash TL, Thwin SS, Silliman RA. Risk of decline in upper-body function and symptoms among older breast cancer patients. *J Gen Intern Med*. 2006;21:327–333.

20. Falagas ME, Zarkadoulia EA, Ioannidou EN, Peppas G, Christodoulou C, Rafailidis PI. The effect of psychosocial factors on breast cancer outcome: a systematic review. *Breast Cancer Res*. 2007;9:R44.

21. Manuel JC, Burwell SR, Crawford SL, et al. Younger women's perceptions of coping with breast cancer. *Cancer Nurs*. 2007;30:85–94.

22. Kroenke CH, Kubzansky LD, Schernhammer ES, Holmes MD, Kawachi I. Social networks, social support, and survival after breast cancer diagnosis. *J Clin Oncol*. 2006;24:1105–1111.

23. Groenvold M, Petersen MA, Idler E, Bjorner JB, Fayers PM, Mouridsen HT. Psychological distress and fatigue predicted recurrence and survival in primary breast cancer patients. *Breast Cancer Res Treat*. 2007;105:209–219.

24. Green BL, Krupnick JL, Rowland JH, et al. Trauma history as a predictor of psychologic symptoms in women with breast cancer. *J Clin Oncol.* 2000;18:1084–1093.

25. Garssen B. Psychological factors and cancer development: evidence after 30 years of research. *Clin Psychol Rev.* 2004;24:315–338.

26. Lillberg K, Verkasalo PK, Kaprio J, Teppo L, Helenius H, Koskenvuo M. Stressful life events and risk of breast cancer in 10,808 women: a cohort study. *Am J Epidemiol.* 2003;157:415–423.

27. Giedzinska AS, Meyerowitz BE, Ganz PA, Rowland JH. Health-related quality of life in a multiethnic sample of breast cancer survivors. *Ann Behav Med.* 2004;28:39–51.

28. Fobair P, O'Hanlan K, Koopman C, et al. Comparison of lesbian and heterosexual women's response to newly diagnosed breast cancer. *Psychooncology.* 2001;10:40–51.

29. Bettencourt BA, Schlegel RJ, Talley AE, Molix LA. The breast cancer experience of rural women: a literature review. *Psychooncology.* 2007;16:875–887.

30. Mandelblatt JS, Hadley J, Kerner JF, et al. Patterns of breast carcinoma treatment in older women: patient preference and clinical and physical influences. *Cancer.* 2000;89:561–573.

31. Tuttle TM, Habermann EB, Grund EH, Morris TJ, Virnig BA. Increasing use of contralateral prophylactic mastectomy for breast cancer patients: a trend toward more aggressive surgical treatment. *J Clin Oncol.* 2007;25:5203–5209.

32. Kuhl C, Kuhn W, Braun M, Schild H. Pre-operative staging of breast cancer with breast MRI: one step forward, two steps back? *Breast.* 2007;16(Suppl 2):S34–S44.

33. Carver CS, Smith RG, Petronis VM, Antoni MH. Quality of life among long-term survivors of breast cancer: different types of antecedents predict different classes of outcomes. *Psychooncology.* 2006;15:749–758.

34. Moyer A. Psychosocial outcomes of breast-conserving surgery versus mastectomy: a meta-analytic review. *Health Psychol.* 1997;16:284–298.

35. Parker PA, Youssef A, Walker S, et al. Short-term and long-term psychosocial adjustment and quality of life in women undergoing different surgical procedures for breast cancer. *Ann Surg Oncol.* 2007;14:3078–3089.

36. Thors CL, Broeckel JA, Jacobsen PB. Sexual functioning in breast cancer survivors. *Cancer Control.* 2001;8:442–448.

37. McWayne J, Heiney SP. Psychologic and social sequelae of secondary lymphedema: a review. *Cancer.* 2005;104:457–466.

38. McLaughlin SA, Wright MJ, Morris KT, et al. Prevalence of lymphedema in women with breast cancer 5 years after sentinel lymph node biopsy or axillary dissection: objective measurements. *J Clin Oncol.* 2008;26:5213–5219.

39. Ahmed RL, Thomas W, Yee D, Schmitz KH. Randomized controlled trial of weight training and lymphedema in breast cancer survivors. *J Clin Oncol.* 2006;24:2765–2772.

40. Stanton AL, Ganz PA, Kwan L, et al. Outcomes from the moving beyond cancer psychoeducational, randomized, controlled trial with breast cancer patients. *J Clin Oncol.* 2005;23:6009–6018.

41. Alderman AK, Hawley ST, Waljee J, Mujahid M, Morrow M, Katz SJ. Understanding the impact of breast reconstruction on the surgical decision-making process for breast cancer. *Cancer.* 2008;112:489–494.

42. Rowland JH, Desmond KA, Meyerowitz BE, Belin TR, Wyatt GE, Ganz PA. Role of breast reconstructive surgery in physical and emotional outcomes among breast cancer survivors. *J Natl Cancer Inst.* 2000;92:1422–1429.

43. Morrow M, Mujahid M, Lantz PM, et al. Correlates of breast reconstruction: results from a population-based study. *Cancer.* 2005;104:2340–2346.

44. Greenberg CC, Schneider EC, Lipsitz SR, et al. Do variations in provider discussions explain socioeconomic disparities in postmastectomy breast reconstruction? *J Am Coll Surg.* 2008;206:605–615.

45. Tseng JF, Kronowitz SJ, Sun CC, et al. The effect of ethnicity on immediate reconstruction rates after mastectomy for breast cancer. *Cancer.* 2004;101:1514–1523.

46. Boehmer U, Linde R, Freund KM. Breast reconstruction following mastectomy for breast cancer: the decisions of sexual minority women. *Plast Reconstr Surg.* 2007;119:464–472.

47. Atisha D, Alderman AK, Lowery JC, Kuhn LE, Davis J, Wilkins EG. Prospective analysis of long-term psychosocial outcomes in breast reconstruction: two-year postoperative results from the Michigan Breast Reconstruction Outcomes Study. *Ann Surg.* 2008;247:1019–1028.

48. Al-Ghazal SK, Fallowfield L, Blamey RW. Comparison of psychological aspects and patient satisfaction following breast conserving surgery, simple mastectomy and breast reconstruction. *Eur J Cancer.* 2000;36:1938–1943.

49. Rowland JH, Meyerowitz BE, Ganz PA, Wyatt G, Desmond K, Honig S. Body image and sexual functioning following reconstructive surgery in breast cancer survivors (BCS). *Proc Am Soc Clin Oncol.* 1996:124. Abstract 163.

50. Clough KB, O'Donoghue JM, Fitoussi AD, Vlastos G, Falcou MC. Prospective evaluation of late cosmetic results following breast reconstruction: II. TRAM flap reconstruction. *Plast Reconstr Surg.* 2001;107:1710–1716.

51. Ganz PA, Desmond KA, Leedham B, Rowland JH, Meyerowitz BE, Belin TR. Quality of life in long-term, disease-free survivors of breast cancer: a follow-up study. *J Natl Cancer Inst.* 2002;94:39–49.

52. Michael YL, Kawachi I, Berkman LF, Holmes MD, Colditz GA. The persistent impact of breast carcinoma on functional health status: prospective evidence from the Nurses' Health Study. *Cancer.* 2000;89:2176–2186.

53. Bower JE. Behavioral symptoms in patients with breast cancer and survivors. *J Clin Oncol.* 2008;26:768–777.

54. Richardson LC, Wang W, Hartzema AG, Wagner S. The role of health-related quality of life in early discontinuation of chemotherapy for breast cancer. *Breast J.* 2007;13:581–587.

55. Majed B, Moreau T, Senouci K, Salmon RJ, Fourquet A, Asselain B. Is obesity an independent prognosis factor in woman breast cancer? *Breast Cancer Res Treat.* 2007;111:329–342.

56. Schmitz KH, Ahmed RL, Hannan PJ, Yee D. Safety and efficacy of weight training in recent breast cancer survivors to alter body composition, insulin, and insulin-like growth factor axis proteins. *Cancer Epidemiol Biomarkers Prev.* 2005;14:1672–1680.

57. Ahles TA, Saykin AJ, McDonald BC, et al. Cognitive function in breast cancer patients prior to adjuvant treatment. *Breast Cancer Res Treat.* 2008;110:143–152.

58. Castellon SA, Ganz PA, Bower JE, Petersen L, Abraham L, Greendale GA. Neurocognitive performance in breast cancer survivors exposed to adjuvant chemotherapy and tamoxifen. *J Clin Exp Neuropsychol.* 2004;26:955–969.

59. Hermelink K, Untch M, Lux MP, et al. Cognitive function during neoadjuvant chemotherapy for breast cancer: results of a prospective, multicenter, longitudinal study. *Cancer.* 2007;109:1905–1913.

60. Schover LR. Premature ovarian failure and its consequences: vasomotor symptoms, sexuality, and fertility. *J Clin Oncol.* 2008;26:753–758.

61. Carpenter JS, Andrykowski MA, Cordova M, et al. Hot flashes in postmenopausal women treated for breast carcinoma: prevalence, severity, correlates, management, and relation to quality of life. *Cancer.* 1998;82:1682–1691.

62. Cuzick J, Sestak I, Cella D, Fallowfield L. Treatment-emergent endocrine symptoms and the risk of breast cancer recurrence: a retrospective analysis of the ATAC trial. *Lancet Oncol.* 2008;9:1143–1148.

63. Stearns V, Johnson MD, Rae JM, et al. Active tamoxifen metabolite plasma concentrations after coadministration of tamoxifen and the selective serotonin reuptake inhibitor paroxetine. *J Natl Cancer Inst.* 2003;95:1758–1764.

64. Minton O, Stone P. How common is fatigue in disease-free breast cancer survivors? A systematic review of the literature. *Breast Cancer Res Treat.* 2008;112:5–13.

65. Bower JE, Ganz PA, Desmond KA, et al. Fatigue in long-term breast carcinoma survivors: a longitudinal investigation. *Cancer.* 2006;106:751–758.

66. Bower JE. Prevalence and causes of fatigue after cancer treatment: the next generation of research. *J Clin Oncol.* 2005;23:8280–8282.

67. Mock V. Evidence-based treatment for cancer-related fatigue. *J Natl Cancer Inst Monogr.* 2004;32:112–118.

68. Bird BR, Swain SM. Cardiac toxicity in breast cancer survivors: review of potential cardiac problems. *Clin Cancer Res.* 2008;14:14–24.

69. McKinley ED. Under Toad days: surviving the uncertainty of cancer recurrence. *Ann Intern Med.* 2000;133:479–480.

70. Jenkins V, Shilling V, Fallowfield L, Howell A, Hutton S. Does hormone therapy for the treatment of breast cancer have a detrimental effect on memory and cognition? A pilot study. *Psychooncology.* 2004;13:61–66.

71. Barron TI, Connolly R, Bennett K, Feely J, Kennedy MJ. Early discontinuation of tamoxifen: a lesson for oncologists. *Cancer.* 2007;109:832–839.

72. Buijs C, de Vries EG, Mourits MJ, Willemse PH. The influence of endocrine treatments for breast cancer on health-related quality of life. *Cancer Treat Rev.* 2008;34:640–655.

73. Mok K, Juraskova I, Friedlander M. The impact of aromatase inhibitors on sexual functioning: current knowledge and future research directions. *Breast.* 2008;17:436–440.

74. Crew KD, Greenlee H, Capodice J, et al. Prevalence of joint symptoms in postmenopausal women taking aromatase inhibitors for early-stage breast cancer. *J Clin Oncol.* 2007;25:3877–3883.

75. Henry NL, Giles JT, Ang D, et al. Prospective characterization of musculoskeletal symptoms in early stage breast cancer patients treated with aromatase inhibitors. *Breast Cancer Res Treat.* 2007;111:365–372.

76. Yang HC, Thornton LM, Shapiro CL, Andersen BL. Surviving recurrence: psychological and quality-of-life recovery. *Cancer.* 2008;112:1178–1187.

77. Northouse LL, Mood D, Kershaw T, et al. Quality of life of women with recurrent breast cancer and their family members. *J Clin Oncol.* 2002;20:4050–4064.

78. Stanton AL. Psychosocial concerns and interventions for cancer survivors. *J Clin Oncol.* 2006;24:5132–5137.

79. Osborn RL, Demoncada AC, Feuerstein M. Psychosocial interventions for depression, anxiety, and quality of life in cancer survivors: meta-analyses. *Int J Psychiatry Med.* 2006;36:13–34.

80. Rehse B, Pukrop R. Effects of psychosocial interventions on quality of life in adult cancer patients: meta analysis of 37 published controlled outcome studies. *Patient Educ Couns.* 2003;50:179–186.

81. Zimmermann T, Heinrichs N, Baucom DH. "Does one size fit all?" moderators in psychosocial interventions for breast cancer patients: a meta-analysis. *Ann Behav Med.* 2007;34:225–239.

82. Carlson LE, Bultz BD. Benefits of psychosocial oncology care: improved quality of life and medical cost offset. *Health Qual Life Outcomes.* 2003;1:8.

83. Mandelblatt JS, Cullen J, Lawrence WF, et al. Economic evaluation alongside a clinical trial of psycho-educational interventions to improve adjustment to survivorship among patients with breast cancer. *J Clin Oncol.* 2008;26:1684–1690.

84. Smedslund G, Ringdal GI. Meta-analysis of the effects of psychosocial interventions on survival time in cancer patients. *J Psychosom Res.* 2004;57:123–135.

85. Andersen BL, Yang HC, Farrar WB, et al. Psychologic intervention improves survival for breast cancer patients: a randomized clinical trial. *Cancer.* 2008;113:3450–3458.

86. Gustafson DH, McTavish FM, Stengle W, et al. Reducing the digital divide for low-income women with breast cancer: a feasibility study of a population-based intervention. *J Health Commun.* 2005;10(Suppl 1):173–193.

87. Meier A, Lyons EJ, Frydman G, Forlenza M, Rimer BK. How cancer survivors provide support on cancer-related Internet mailing lists. *J Med Internet Res.* 2007;9:e12.

88. Fernandez BM, Crane LA, Baxter J, Gallagher K, McClung MW. Physician referral patterns to a breast cancer support program. *Cancer Pract.* 2001;9:169–175.

89. Eakin EG, Strycker LA. Awareness and barriers to use of cancer support and information resources by HMO patients with breast, prostate, or colon cancer: patient and provider perspectives. *Psychooncology.* 2001;10:103–113.

90. Andrykowski MA, Curran SL, Studts JL, et al. Psychosocial adjustment and quality of life in women with breast cancer and benign breast problems: a controlled comparison. *J Clin Epidemiol.* 1996;49:827–834.

91. Rowland JH, Bellizzi KM. Cancer survivors and survivorship research: a reflection on today's successes and tomorrow's challenges. *Hematol Oncol Clin North Am.* 2008;22:181–200.

92. Short PF, Vasey JJ, Belue R. Work disability associated with cancer survivorship and other chronic conditions. *Psychooncology.* 2008;17:91–97.

93. Bradley CJ, Bednarek HL, Neumark D. Breast cancer and women's labor supply. *Health Serv Res.* 2002;37:1309–1328.

94. Bouknight RR, Bradley CJ, Luo Z. Correlates of return to work for breast cancer survivors. *J Clin Oncol.* 2006;24:345–353.

95. Kornblith AB, Herndon JE, II, Weiss RB, et al. Long-term adjustment of survivors of early-stage breast carcinoma, 20 years after adjuvant chemotherapy. *Cancer.* 2003;98:679–689.

96. Bellizzi KM, Blank TO. Predicting posttraumatic growth in breast cancer survivors. *Health Psychol.* 2006;25:47–56.

97. Gill KM, Mishel M, Belyea M, et al. Triggers of uncertainty about recurrence and long-term treatment side effects in older African American and Caucasian breast cancer survivors. *Oncol Nurs Forum.* 2004;31:633–639.

98. Mellon S, Northouse LL, Weiss LK. A population-based study of the quality of life of cancer survivors and their family caregivers. *Cancer Nurs.* 2006;29:120–131.

99. Mishel MH, Germino BB, Gil KM, et al. Benefits from an uncertainty management intervention for African-American and Caucasian older long-term breast cancer survivors. *Psychooncology.* 2005;14:962–978.

100. Kattlove H, Winn RJ. Ongoing care of patients after primary treatment for their cancer. *CA Cancer J Clin.* 2003;53:172–196.

101. Ganz PA, Hahn EE. Implementing a survivorship care plan for patients with breast cancer. *J Clin Oncol.* 2008;26:759–767.

102. Ganz PA. A teachable moment for oncologists: cancer survivors, 10 million strong and growing! *J Clin Oncol.* 2005;23:5458–5460.

103. Sabatino SA, Coates RJ, Uhler RJ, Pollack LA, Alley LG, Zauderer LJ. Provider counseling about health behaviors among cancer survivors in the United States. *J Clin Oncol.* 2007;25:2100–2106.

104. Antoni MH, Lechner SC, Kazi A, et al. How stress management improves quality of life after treatment for breast cancer. *J Consult Clin Psychol.* 2006;74:1143–1152.

105. Courneya KS, Katzmarzyk PT, Bacon E. Physical activity and obesity in Canadian cancer survivors: population-based estimates from the 2005 Canadian Community Health Survey. *Cancer.* 2008;112:2475–2482.

106. Galvao DA, Newton RU. Review of exercise intervention studies in cancer patients. *J Clin Oncol.* 2005;23:899–909.

107. Schwartz AL. Physical activity after a cancer diagnosis: psychosocial outcomes. *Cancer Invest.* 2004;22:82–92.

108. McTiernan A. Physical activity after cancer: physiologic outcomes. *Cancer Invest.* 2004;22:68–81.

109. Pischon T, Nothlings U, Boeing H. Obesity and cancer. *Proc Nutr Soc.* 2008;67:128–145.

110. Murtaugh MA, Sweeney C, Giuliano AR, et al. Diet patterns and breast cancer risk in Hispanic and non-Hispanic white women: the Four-Corners Breast Cancer Study. *Am J Clin Nutr.* 2008;87:978–984.

111. Holmes MD, Chen WY, Feskanich D, Kroenke CH, Colditz GA. Physical activity and survival after breast cancer diagnosis. *JAMA.* 2005;293:2479–2486.

112. Holick CN, Newcomb PA, Trentham-Dietz A, et al. Physical activity and survival after diagnosis of invasive breast cancer. *Cancer Epidemiol Biomarkers Prev.* 2008;17:379–386.

113. Pierce JP, Stefanick ML, Flatt SW, et al. Greater survival after breast cancer in physically active women with high vegetable-fruit intake regardless of obesity. *J Clin Oncol.* 2007;25:2345–2351.

114. Mahon SM. Tertiary prevention: implications for improving the quality of life of long-term survivors of cancer. *Semin Oncol Nurs.* 2005;21:260–270.

115. Kellen E, Vansant G, Christiaens MR, Neven P, Van Limbergen E. Lifestyle changes and breast cancer prognosis: a review. *Breast Cancer Res Treat.* 2008 Apr 4. Epub ahead of print.

116. Doyle C, Kushi LH, Byers T, et al. Nutrition and physical activity during and after cancer treatment: an American Cancer Society guide for informed choices. *CA Cancer J Clin.* 2006;56:323–353.

117. Stull VB, Snyder DC, Demark-Wahnefried W. Lifestyle interventions in cancer survivors: designing programs that meet the needs of this vulnerable and growing population. *J Nutr.* 2007;137:243S–248S.

118. Goldstein MS, Lee JH, Ballard-Barbash R, Brown ER. The use and perceived benefit of complementary and alternative medicine among Californians with cancer. *Psychooncology.* 2008;17:19–25.

119. Velicer CM, Ulrich CM. Vitamin and mineral supplement use among US adults after cancer diagnosis: a systematic review. *J Clin Oncol.* 2008;26:665–673.

120. Matthews AK, Sellergren SA, Huo D, List M, Fleming G. Complementary and alternative medicine use among breast cancer survivors. *J Altern Complement Med.* 2007;13:555–562.

121. Montazeri A, Sajadian A, Ebrahimi M, Akbari ME. Depression and the use of complementary medicine among breast cancer patients. *Support Care Cancer.* 2005;13:339–342.

CHAPTER 25

Sarcoma

James L. Klosky and Sheri L. Spunt

Bone and soft tissue sarcomas are a heterogeneous group of cancers that arise from primitive mesenchymal cells throughout the body. Population-based data suggest that these cancers account for approximately 0.9% of cancer cases overall, but 13% of cancers in pediatric patients. Aggressive multimodality therapy, including various combinations of surgery, chemotherapy, and radiotherapy, is generally necessary for cure. Currently, the overall 5-year survival rate of patients with bone and soft tissue sarcomas is about two-thirds of that of the general population.[1] Thus, sarcomas produce considerable morbidity as well as mortality. This chapter reviews the major clinical features, treatment, and outcomes of bone and soft tissue sarcomas, and addresses the major psychological issues facing individuals affected by these rare tumors.

SOFT TISSUE SARCOMAS

Soft tissue sarcomas are about four times more common than bone sarcomas, and there are approximately 10,000 new cases in the United States annually.[1] At least 30 different histological subtypes exist. In pediatric patients, rhabdomyosarcoma is by far the most common subtype, whereas in adults there is no predominant histology.[2] Soft tissue sarcomas are somewhat more common in males than in females and are slightly less common in the Hispanic population.[1] The incidence of soft tissue sarcomas increases with increasing age.

Most soft tissue sarcomas are sporadic, although a small percentage of patients have an underlying risk factor. Known predisposing conditions include Li-Fraumeni syndrome (germline *p53* mutation),[3] hereditary retinoblastoma (germline *RB* mutation),[4] neurofibromatosis type I(NF-1),[5] HIV infection,[6] and radiation exposure.[7]

Soft tissue sarcomas usually present as a painless mass, although they may impinge on other normal structures, thereby producing other symptoms. These tumors may arise virtually anywhere in the body. Rhabdomyosarcoma, which occurs primarily in the pediatric age group, is most common in the head and neck region, in the genitourinary structures, and in the extremities. Other soft tissue sarcomas most often affect the extremities or body wall, although certain subtypes have an anatomic site predilection (e.g., uterine leiomyosarcoma). Among the small proportion of patients who present with metastatic disease, most have lung involvement. Lymph node, bone, and bone marrow disease is also relatively common in rhabdomyosarcoma.

The approach to treatment of soft tissue sarcomas depends on the histological subtype and grade of the tumor, its size, whether it is amenable to surgical removal, and the extent of the disease.[8,9] Surgery is the mainstay of treatment for patients with soft tissue sarcomas other than rhabdomyosarcoma, and may be curative in some cases. Radiotherapy is often needed if the tumor cannot be adequately excised; the dose required is relatively high. Chemotherapy is routinely used only for patients with rhabdomyosarcoma, where the standard regimen is vincristine and actinomycin D, with or without cyclophosphamide. The utility of chemotherapy in other histological subtypes is debatable, although it is most commonly used for patients with tumors not amenable to surgery and for those at high risk for the development of metastatic disease (principally those with large, high-grade tumors). The most active agents in the treatment of soft tissue sarcomas (other than rhabdomyosarcoma) are ifosfamide and doxorubicin, although various other regimens are used for specific histological subtypes.

Treatment of soft tissue sarcomas is associated with a variety of potential late effects.[10] Children and adolescents are at greater risk for certain complications because of their incomplete growth and development at the time of treatment. Young patients also have more time to develop late-occurring complications such as secondary neoplasia, which may develop many years after treatment. Surgery is often very aggressive, since for most histological subtypes cure depends to a significant extent on complete removal of the tumor. As a result, patients may lose expendable organs or experience functional impairment or physical deformity. Radiotherapy may contribute to organ dysfunction, functional difficulties, and cosmesis, particularly in young patients who have not yet completed their growth and development. Radiotherapy may also induce the development of second cancers. Long-term chemotherapy complications include cardiomyopathy (doxorubicin), infertility and gonadal hormone deficiency (cyclophosphamide, ifosfamide), renal insufficiency (ifosfamide), and secondary neoplasia (cyclophosphamide, ifosfamide, doxorubicin).

BONE SARCOMAS

Bone sarcomas are considerably less common than soft tissue sarcomas, with approximately 2400 patients diagnosed in the United States each year.[1] The most common bone sarcomas are osteosarcoma, chondrosarcoma, and Ewing sarcoma. Each is slightly more common in males than in females. Ewing sarcoma is particularly rare in black patients. Osteosarcoma and Ewing sarcoma are largely diseases of adolescents and young adults; 30% of osteosarcoma cases and 6% of Ewing sarcoma cases are reported in patients aged 40 years and older. Conversely, chondrosarcoma is typical in older patients, with over 70% of cases reported in patients aged 40 years and older.

As is the case with soft tissue sarcomas, most bone sarcomas are sporadic, although a small proportion of patients have an underlying predisposition. The major risk factors for osteosarcoma are hereditary retinoblastoma (germline *RB* mutation),[4] Li-Fraumeni syndrome (germline *p53* mutation),[3] Paget's disease,[11] and radiation exposure.[7] Approximately 10% of chondrosarcomas arise within a benign lesion, and this tumor also may occur after radiation exposure. There are no known risk factors for Ewing sarcoma.

Most bone tumors present with pain, swelling, and, in some cases, limited range of motion of the affected area. The most common sites of origin of osteosarcoma are in the bones around the knee and in the upper arm near the shoulder; it is often mistaken for an athletic injury because of its location and predilection for adolescents and young adults. Chondrosarcoma most often occurs in the pelvis and lower leg but can also affect the upper arm and ribs. Typical sites of Ewing sarcoma are the pelvis, long bones of the arms and legs, and the ribs. Tumors of the pelvis and ribs may grow very large before symptoms cause patients to seek medical attention. A small proportion of patients have metastatic disease at the time of initial presentation. The most common site of bone tumor metastases is the lung; spreading to other bones is less common. The bone marrow may also be involved in Ewing sarcoma.

Treatment of bone sarcomas depends on the anatomic location, tumor grade, and extent of disease.[9,12] Systemic chemotherapy is given to all patients with Ewing sarcoma, most of those with osteosarcoma, and few patients with chondrosarcoma; selected subtypes of osteosarcoma and most cases of chondrosarcoma do not require chemotherapy. Standard chemotherapy for Ewing sarcoma includes vincristine, doxorubicin, cyclophosphamide, ifosfamide, and etoposide. Agents typically used to treat osteosarcoma and chondrosarcoma include cisplatin, doxorubicin, high-dose methotrexate, ifosfamide, and etoposide. The mainstay of local tumor control for osteosarcoma and chondrosarcoma is surgical resection; radiotherapy is used only for tumors that are unresectable. Ewing sarcoma may be surgically excised, irradiated, or treated with a combination of surgery and radiotherapy. In recent years, limb-sparing procedures have limited the number of patients requiring amputation.[9]

The late effects of therapy for bone sarcomas depend on the site of the primary tumor and the treatment delivered.[10] Surgical complications related to limb-sparing procedures include prosthesis loosening/breakage/infection, bone fracture, limb length discrepancy with secondary scoliosis, and altered gait pattern. Amputees may require stump revisions due to various complications, may experience chronic phantom pain, and may have difficulty finding a comfortable, functional, and cosmetically appealing external prosthesis. Radiotherapy impairs bone and soft tissue growth, resulting in limb length discrepancies, and produces altered physical appearance and dysfunction of organs within the radiotherapy field. Radiotherapy carries a risk of inducing second cancers, and treatment of the gonads produces infertility and gonadal hormone insufficiency. Major long-term complications of chemotherapy include loss of hearing (cisplatin), cardiomyopathy (doxorubicin), renal insufficiency (ifosfamide, cisplatin), infertility and gonadal hormone insufficiency (cyclophosphamide, ifosfamide), and secondary neoplasia (cyclophosphamide, ifosfamide, etoposide, doxorubicin, cisplatin).

PSYCHOLOGICAL ISSUES

Patients with a history of sarcoma generally report global psychological functioning much like that of their healthy peers. These rates of psychological health are consistently robust across the sarcoma survivorship continuum ranging from pediatric to geriatric survivors. For example, children and adolescents 3–4 years posttreatment for bone sarcoma report favorable mental health and global functioning outcomes[13] that do not differ significantly from healthy controls.[14] As part of the Childhood Cancer Survivor Study,[15] adult survivors of childhood solid tumor (and their siblings) report lower levels of global distress (including depression, anxiety, and somatic distress) as compared to the standardized norms of the Brief Symptoms Inventory (BSI-18), with no differences existing across solid tumor type. Although the pretreatment mental heath scores of adults receiving treatment for soft tissue sarcoma were significantly lower than normative Canadian values, no differences were identified after 6 weeks or 12 months among those having received pre- or postoperative radiation therapy (RT), respectively.[16]

Despite these favorable mental health outcomes, many of the demographic and socioeconomic variables related to poorer psychological health in the general population also affect those with a history of sarcoma. Specifically, female gender and lower levels of income and education all associate with relatively poorer mental health outcomes in sarcoma patients.[13,15,17,18] Furthermore, these survivors are at risk for poor social competence outcomes including lower rates of employment and marriage, particularly among male survivors.[15,19] These findings suggests that the disruptions in childhood social development during pediatric sarcoma treatment may result in relatively poorer social outcomes in adulthood. With respect to the contribution of treatment-related and physical health-related variables to psychological outcomes, high-dose chemotherapy (particularly alkylating agents), cranial and/or chest irradiation, and poor health status along with current health problems all correlate with relatively adverse mental health outcomes.[13,15]

In summary, sarcoma survivors report favorable psychological outcomes, but sociodemographic, treatment and health-related factors place certain sarcoma subgroups at risk for impaired psychological functioning. Having reviewed the global mental health literature among sarcoma patients, the following discussion addresses late effects associated with sarcoma treatment which threaten the psychological health of sarcoma survivors. These include amputation/limb sparing, physical dysfunction and pain, infertility and impaired psychosexual functioning, and cancer recurrence.

LATE EFFECTS OF SARCOMA TREATMENT ASSOCIATED WITH ADVERSE PSYCHOLOGICAL OUTCOMES

Amputation and limb-sparing procedures. Much research has been conducted examining differences in mental health outcomes among sarcoma patients who have undergone either amputation or limb sparing as part of cancer treatment and in general, few differences have emerged. Among adolescents, for example, Ginsberg and colleagues[20] found no mental health differences across treatment procedure (amputation, limb-sparing surgery, rotationplasty) nor across amputation site (above or below knee amputation) as measured by the mental health component scales of the SF-36v.2. With the notable exception of the Zebrack et al.[15] study which found psychological benefit associated with amputation (presumably due to relief associated with a lower risk of local recurrence and fewer surgeries required for endoprosthesis revision/complication), current literature suggests no differences in mental health outcomes among adults surviving childhood cancer treated with amputation or limb-sparing surgery.[18,21,22] Similarly, a psychological advantage related to either limb sparing or amputation among those experiencing adult onset sarcoma has not been established.[23,24]

It is important to note that although there are many similarities between limb sparing and amputation, each treatment approach carries distinct treatment demands that should be considered by the patient and their family before consenting for treatment. One of the primary challenges related to limb sparing is the potential for many surgical procedures after the initial operation. These surgeries may be due to endoprosthetic malfunction, infection, nonunion of bones, fractures or contractures, correction of leg length discrepancy, or any number of related complications. In addition to surgery, patients undergoing limb sparing should also anticipate the need to expend significant time and effort participating in rehabilitation after each operation. Those undergoing amputation will also have surgery, but typically the postoperative demands are significantly reduced compared to limb-sparing procedures. Primary challenges for those undergoing amputation include adjusting to the permanent loss of their limb, coping with phantom pain, and adapting to the use of a prosthesis. Across both procedures, patients may be at increased risk for changes in body image. For those experiencing amputation, time to psychologically adjust to an artificial limb is often needed, whereas body image issues for limb-sparing patient typically relate to the potential for limb deformity and impaired function.

Physical dysfunction and pain. The associations between physical functioning, pain, and psychological outcomes have been well described in the sarcoma literature. Across age groups, inverse relationships exist between pain and physical functioning with both factors directly relating to mental health outcomes. Yet, sarcoma-related functional limitations and pain manifest differently based on patient age group and location of tumor. For example, among pediatric sarcoma patients, predictors of poorer mobility include increased pain, having a tumor greater than 8 cm, lower-extremity location of tumor, and poor quality of life.[14,25] In addition to functional limitation, predictors of pain in this group included retroperitoneal tumor origin and cancer recurrence.[13,26]

Functional limitations play a qualitatively different role in the psychological functioning of adult survivors of childhood sarcoma, particularly when one considers the length of time and the critical periods in which observable functional differences manifest between the sarcoma survivors and their peers. For example, adult survivors of childhood sarcoma may experience reduced range of motion in a treated extremity, chewing or swallowing problems among those who received radiation therapy for sarcomas of the head and neck, or bladder dysfunction related to pelvic sarcoma treatment. When one takes into account growth impairment or structural consequences of sarcoma treatment (including body dysmorphia), it is easy to understand how psychological distress may develop in these sarcoma survivors, particularly when their growth is complete and the late effects of cancer treatment have been fully realized. Although little research has been conducted examining perceptions of body dysmorphia and mental health among sarcoma survivors, relationships between functional limitation and emotional distress, poor self-image, and interpersonal/social problems have been found among adult survivors of childhood sarcoma.[27]

Although adult onset sarcoma patients do not have to contend with the developmental challenges associated with sarcoma treatment, they are not immune to treatment-related problems associated with physical functioning and pain. For example, Davis and colleagues[16] examined differences in functional and health status outcomes among adults with extremity soft tissue sarcoma who were randomized to either a pre- or a postoperative radiotherapy treatment group. Although short-term benefits related to function, disability, and pain outcomes were identified among those receiving postoperative radiation therapy, no differences remained across treatment groups after 6 weeks postoperatively. Predictors of poorer functional outcomes among all participants included increased tumor size, lower-extremity tumor, motor nerve sacrifice, and wound healing complications. Pain was primarily associated with lower-extremity tumor and prior tumor excision. Mental health scores among those receiving preoperative radiation therapy did not differ from normative values after surgery, whereas mental health reductions in the postoperative radiotherapy group resolved by 12 months after surgery.

Infertility and impaired psychosexual functioning.

One long-term sequela of sarcoma therapy that may impact quality of life is infertility. Alkylating agents like cyclophosphamide and ifosfamide, which are commonly used in the treatment of sarcomas, produce a dose-related risk of infertility with higher cumulative dose and longer length of treatment conferring the greatest risk for fertility problems.[28-30] This dose-dependent relationship remains true with regard to radiation therapy as higher doses translate to greater risk of gonadal dysfunction in both men and women and a risk of uterine vascular insufficiency in women.[29,31] In a recent study examining late effects in long-term survivors of pediatric sarcoma, Mansky and colleagues[17] report that 76% of men were infertile, whereas 49% of women experienced premature menopause. Despite the known risk of infertility after cancer treatment, only between 19% and 24% of young men at high risk for treatment-related infertility cryopreserve sperm before cancer treatment, with even fewer women undergoing fertility preserving procedures.[32,33] It is still unclear as to why these rates are so low, particularly in light of the high priority that survivors of childhood cancer place on fertility and the high psychological distress associated with infertility.[34]

Certain sarcoma survivors who retain their fertility will struggle with decision making with regard to procreation due to the increased risk of passing on a cancer predisposition to their offspring. This is the case in survivors of bilateral retinoblastoma, NF-1, and in those with Li-Fraumeni syndrome. These patients are regularly counseled regarding the risk of transmitting a cancer predisposition should they pursue biological children. Patients and families with familial cancer syndromes may experience psychological distress if these early messages are not recalled or considered, particularly if the now-adult patient is sexually active and in a committed relationship with the intention of producing biological children.

Another, but understudied, outcome of sarcoma treatment relates to problems associated with psychosexual functioning. Depending on the treatment, sarcoma survivors may be at high risk for psychosexual dysfunction resulting from physical discomfort, poor body image, emotional distress, negative sexual self-concept, or structural abnormalities. Although difficulties with psychosexual functioning have been reported among adults with reproductive cancers, fewer research studies exist substantiating psychosexual outcomes in those surviving sarcoma, despite our clinical experience which suggests otherwise. Much like those adult women who have been treated for gynecologic cancer, patients surviving childhood pelvic tumors (e.g., rhabdomyosarcoma of the genitourinary tract) may be at risk for sexual dissatisfaction and dysfunction, lower levels of sexual desire, and pain during vaginal intercourse.[35,36] Erectile dysfunction is the most commonly reported sexual problem experienced by men after prostate cancer treatment, although these men also report decreased sexual desire, difficulty reaching orgasm, and pain with ejaculation.[37] Similar symptoms have been observed among men with a history of treatment for pelvic sarcoma and those who have undergone retroperitoneal lymph node dissection for testicular and paratesticular tumors.

Adult patients receiving multimodality limb-sparing therapy for soft tissue sarcoma also report significant declines in pleasure from sex at 6 months after treatment with reductions in frequency of intercourse and libido extending 12 months after treatment.[38] These reductions were presumably due to testicular or ovarian dysfunction or radiation fibrosis, which may have affected normal sexual activity. Psychosexual functioning has direct implications for satisfaction with romantic relationships and overall quality of life. It is important to establish whether sarcoma survivors are at risk for problems related to psychosexual functioning, as beneficial psychological or behavioral interventions may result from routine screening during posttreatment follow-up visits.

Cancer recurrence.

Patients treated for sarcoma have a relatively high risk of experiencing tumor recurrence. Owing to the associations between cancer recurrence and relatively poorer psychological outcomes, there have been suggestions in the literature that parents and patients surviving pediatric sarcoma are at an increased risk for posttraumatic stress symptoms (PTSS) or posttraumatic stress disorder (PTSD), due to increased worry about experiencing an additional cancer event. Jurbergs and colleagues,[39] for example, found little evidence of PTSS or PTSD among children/adolescents and families on treatment and surviving pediatric cancer, except in cases where the child suffered cancer recurrence. Specifically, 28% of parents whose children's tumor had recurred reported symptoms consistent with a diagnosis of PTSD. This rate was significantly higher than those reported by parents of newly diagnosed, on-treatment children (10%), parents of children off treatment without tumor recurrence (10%), and parents of healthy children (10%). Although all pediatric cancer diagnoses were included in this study, it stands to reason that the subset of patients with sarcoma, with their high risk of tumor recurrence, are at increased risk for psychological distress. These families should therefore be appropriately screened for psychopathology and provided intervention if warranted.

CONCLUSION

Over the past few decades, treatment for sarcomas has become more effective and, in some cases, less toxic. Advances in surgical techniques have permitted limb-sparing procedures in many patients and more conformal radiotherapy approaches have maintained high rates of local tumor control with less exposure of normal tissues to the deleterious effects of radiation. However, successful treatment for sarcoma continues to require aggressive surgery and the use of relatively toxic chemotherapy and/or radiotherapy in many cases. It stands to reason that patients treated for sarcoma would have relatively poorer mental health outcomes due to the challenges posed by acute and chronic late effects associated with treatment along with the risks associated with cancer recurrence. Yet a review of the current literature does not substantiate this assumption. The psychological functioning of sarcoma survivors is much like that of the healthy U.S. population, and a similarity exists across both groups regarding sociodemographic and economic risk factors that may affect mental health outcomes. Although there are certainly premorbid factors (history of psychopathology, maladaptive coping, dysfunctional family system) and consequences of treatment (amputation/limb sparing, poor physical functioning, pain, infertility, recurrent disease) which may place patients at high risk for psychological problems post diagnosis, the prognosis for an adaptive psychological response to these challenges is generally favorable for the majority of patients surviving sarcoma.

REFERENCES

1. Ries L, Melbert D, Krapcho M, et al. SEER cancer statistics review, 1975–2005. National Cancer Institute; 2008.

2. Spunt SL, Pappo AS. Childhood nonrhabdomyosarcoma soft tissue sarcomas are not adult-type tumors. *J Clin Oncol.* 2006;24(12):1958–1959; Author reply 1959–1960.

3. Tabori U, Malkin D. Risk stratification in cancer predisposition syndromes: lessons learned from novel molecular developments in Li-Fraumeni syndrome. *Cancer Res.* 2008;68(7):2053–2057.

4. Acquaviva A, Ciccolallo L, Rondelli R, et al. Mortality from second tumour among long-term survivors of retinoblastoma: a retrospective analysis of the Italian retinoblastoma registry. *Oncogene.* 2006;25(38):5350–5357.

5. Sorensen SA, Mulvihill JJ, Nielsen A. Long-term follow-up of von Recklinghausen neurofibromatosis. Survival and malignant neoplasms. *N Engl J Med.* 1986;314(16):1010–1015.

6. McClain KL, Leach CT, Jenson HB, et al. Association of Epstein-Barr virus with leiomyosarcomas in children with AIDS. *N Engl J Med.* 1995;332(1):12–18.

7. Virtanen A, Pukkala E, Auvinen A. Incidence of bone and soft tissue sarcoma after radiotherapy: a cohort study of 295,712 Finnish cancer patients. *Int J Cancer.* 2006;118(4):1017–1021.

8. Meyer WH, Spunt SL. Soft tissue sarcomas of childhood. *Cancer Treat Rev.* 2004;30(3):269–280.

9. Wunder JS, Nielsen TO, Maki RG, O'Sullivan B, Alman BA. Opportunities for improving the therapeutic ratio for patients with sarcoma. *Lancet Oncol.* 2007;8(6):513–524.

10. Landier W, Bhatia S, Eshelman DA, et al. Development of risk-based guidelines for pediatric cancer survivors: the Children's Oncology Group long-term follow-up guidelines from the Children's Oncology Group Late Effects Committee and Nursing Discipline. *J Clin Oncol.* 2004;22(24):4979–4990.

11. Deyrup AT, Montag AG, Inwards CY, Xu Z, Swee RG, Krishnan Unni K. Sarcomas arising in Paget disease of bone: a clinicopathologic analysis of 70 cases. *Arch Pathol Lab Med.* 2007;131(6):942–946.

12. Arndt CA, Crist WM. Common musculoskeletal tumors of childhood and adolescence. *N Engl J Med.* 1999;341(5):342–352.

13. Tabone MD, Rodary C, Oberlin O, et al. Brief report: quality of life of patients treated during childhood for a bone tumor: assessment by the child health questionnaire. *Pediatr Blood Cancer.* 2005;45:207–211.

14. Frances JM, Morris CD, Arkader A, Nikolic ZG, Healey JH. What is quality of life in children with bone sarcoma? *Clin Orthop Relat R.* 2007;459:34–39.

15. Zebrack BJ, Zevon MA, Turk N. Psychological distress in long-term survivors of solid tumors diagnosed in childhood: a report from the childhood cancer survivor study. *Pediatr Blood Cancer.* 2007;49:47–51.

16. Davis AM, O'Sullivan B, Bell RS, et al. Function and health status outcomes in a randomized trial comparing preoperative and postoperative radiotherapy in extremity soft tissue sarcoma. *J Clin Oncol.* 2002;20:4472–4477.

17. Mansky P, Arai A, Stratton P. Treatment late effects in long-term survivors of pediatric sarcoma. *Pediatr Blood Cancer.* 2007;48:192–199.

18. Nagarajan R, Clohisy DR, Neglia JP, et al. Function and quality-of-life of survivors of pelvis and lower extremity osteosarcoma and Ewing's sarcoma: the childhood cancer survivor study. *Br J Cancer.* 2004;91:1858–1865.

19. Yonemoto T, Tatezaki S, Ishii T, Hagiwara Y. Marriage and fertility in long-term survivors of high grade osteosarcoma. *Am J Clin Oncol.* 2003;26(5):513–516.

20. Ginsberg JP, Rai SN, Carlson CA, et al. A comparative analysis of functional outcomes in adolescents and young adults with lower-extremity bone sarcoma. *Pediatr Blood Cancer.* 2007;49:964–969.

21. Lane JM, Christ GH, Khan SN, Backus SI. Rehabilitation for limb salvage patients: kinesiologic parameters and psychologic assessment. *Cancer.* 2001;92:1013–1019.

22. Christ GH, Lane JM, Marcove R. Psychosocial adaptation of long-term survivors of bone sarcoma. *J Psychosoc Oncol.* 1995;13(4):1–22.

23. Refaat Y, Gunnoe J, Hornicek FJ, Mankin HJ. Comparison of quality of life after amputation or limb salvage. *Clin Orthop Relat R.* 2002;297:298–305.

24. Weddington WW, Segraves KB, Simon MA. Psychological outcome of extremity sarcoma survivors undergoing amputation or limb salvage. *J Clin Oncol.* 1985;3:1393–1399.

25. Marchese VG, Spearing E, Callaway L. Relationships among range of motion, functional mobility, and quality of life in children and adolescents after limb-sparing surgery for lower-extremity sarcoma. *Pediatr Phys Ther.* 2006;18(4):238–244.

26. Pham TH, Iqbal CW, Zarroug AE, Donohue JH, Moir C. Retroperitoneal sarcomas in children: outcomes from an institution. *J Pediatr Surg.* 2007;42(5):829–833.

27. Hudson MM, Tyc VL, Cremer LK. Patient satisfaction after limb-sparing surgery and amputation for pediatric malignant bone tumors. *J Pediatr Oncol Nurs.* 1998;15(2):60–69.

28. Kenney LB, Laufer MR, Grant FD, Grier H, Diller L. High risk of infertility and long term gonadal damage in males treated with high dose cyclophosphamide for sarcoma during childhood. *Cancer.* 2001;91:613–621.

29. Bahadur G. Fertility issues for cancer patients. *Mol Cell Endocrinol.* 2000;169(1–2):117–122.

30. Meistrich ML, Wilson G, Brown BW, da Cunha MF, Lipshultz LI. Impact of cyclophosphamide on long-term reduction in sperm count in men treated with combination chemotherapy for Ewing and soft tissue sarcomas. *Cancer.* 1992;70(11):2703–2712.

31. Critchley HO, Wallace WH. Impact of cancer treatment on uterine function. *J Natl Cancer Inst Monogr.* 2005;34:64–68.

32. Schover LR, Rybicki LA, Martin BA, Bringelsen KA. Having children after cancer: a pilot survey of survivors' attitudes and experiences. *Cancer.* 1999;86:697–709.

33. Schover LR, Brey K, Lichtin A, Lipshultz LI, Jeha S. Knowledge and experience regarding cancer, infertility, and sperm banking in younger male survivors. *J Clin Oncol.* 2002;20:1880–1889.

34. Burns KC, Boudreau C, Panepinto JA. Attitudes regarding fertility preservation in female adolescent cancer patients. *J Pediatr Hematol Oncol.* 2006;28:350–354.

35. Carter J, Rowland K, Chi D, et al. Gynecologic cancer treatment and the impact of cancer-related infertility. *Gynecol Oncol.* 2005;97:90–95.

36. Gershenson DM, Miller AM, Champion VL, et al. Reproductive and sexual function after platinum-based chemotherapy in long-term ovarian germ cell tumor survivors: a gynaecologic oncology group study. *J Clin Oncol.* 2007;25:2792–2797.

37. Schover LR. Sexuality and fertility after cancer. *Hematology.* 2005;2005:523–527.

38. Chang AE, Steinberg SM, Culnane M. Functional and psychosocial effects of multimodality limb-sparing therapy in patients with soft tissue sarcomas. *J Clin Oncol.* 1989;7:1217–1228.

39. Jurbergs N, Long A, Ticona L, Phipps S. Symptoms of posttraumatic stress in parents of children with cancer: are they elevated relative to parents of healthy children? *J Pediatr Psychol.* Epub ahead of print.

CHAPTER 26

Hematopoietic Dyscrasias and Stem Cell/Bone Marrow Transplantation

Betsy L. Fife and Christopher A. Fausel

INTRODUCTION

Hematologic malignancies, that is, leukemia, lymphoma, and multiple myeloma (MM), have always been associated with a great deal of fear and uncertainty despite notable medical advances that have been made in recent years to significantly decrease mortality. It is not only the life-threatening nature of the diseases themselves, but also the highly challenging and life-threatening treatment often used to bring about remission that generates this response, specifically hematopoietic stem cell (HSCT)/bone marrow transplantation (BMT).

We begin this discussion with a description of major medical aspects of these hematologic malignancies and treatment by transplantation to provide a framework for understanding the psychological, emotional, and social impact of these illnesses. Because they involve all members of the family, ramifications of the illnesses and their treatment for the recipient, the family caregiver, and the family as a unit will be included. This discussion will be based on research findings from the literature with an emphasis on the past 15 years, and will conclude with a summary of recommendations for future research that will be needed if we are to provide the most effective interventions to prevent secondary psychosocial morbidity and promote the highest possible quality of life (QOL) for this population.

THE CLINICAL COURSE AND TREATMENT OF HEMATOLOGIC MALIGNANCIES

Hematologic malignancies account for approximately 15% of all cancers in adults and children. Acute myelogenous leukemia (AML) and acute lymphocytic leukemia (ALL) account for less than 3% of all cancers, but they are the leading cause of death due to cancer in the United States in people under 35 years of age, explaining the fear factor and stress with which they are associated. The causes of the leukemias are largely unknown; however, radiation, prior exposure to chemotherapy, exposure to certain chemicals, and genetic factors contribute to the incidence of these malignancies. Blood count and bone marrow are diagnostic with normal blood cells being replaced by abnormal leukemic cells.

Major advances in the treatment of these diseases have been made in the past decade, with more patients being cured or experiencing a prolonged life. Goals and principles of treatment for ALL include similar strategies for both adults and children with four components: remission induction, consolidation/intensification, maintenance, and central nervous system (CNS) prophylaxis. Although complete remission is seen in 65%–85% of adults only 20%–40% are cured, while children do much better with the majority being cured by chemotherapy alone. Two sanctuary sites require additional treatment, the CNS and the testes where leukemic cells are protected from the effects of systemic chemotherapy. If there is no additional treatment to eradicate cells in the CNS, 50% of those surviving 2 or more years will develop CNS involvement manifested as increased intracranial pressure.

Another major diagnostic category of hematologic malignancies is non-Hodgkin lymphoma (NHL) and Hodgkin lymphoma. The incidence of NHL is rising at a rate of 3%–4% a year, which is exceeded only by that of melanoma and lung cancer in women. The median age at diagnosis of NHL is 48 years, while Hodgkin lymphoma is the predominant form in children. Certain viruses have been implicated in the etiology of NHL, but that is not well established.

Multiple myeloma accounts for 1% of all cancers and 15% of hematologic malignancies. At this time it remains incurable; however, the median age at diagnosis is 71 years with the highest incidence in Caucasian males. Risk factors include exposure to radiation, pesticides, and herbicides. Approximately 70% of patients present with bone disease.

High-dose therapy (HDT) followed by HSCT/BMT is commonly employed in the treatment of MM as well as in the treatment of leukemias and lymphomas. This procedure involves the ablation of the recipient's bone marrow by the use of high doses of cytotoxic chemotherapy, sometimes in conjunction with total-body irradiation (TBI), which is then followed by replacement of the marrow with disease-free healthy bone marrow and/or harvested stem cells. Allogeneic transplantation using an HLA-matched donor is preferred in the treatment of leukemias with the goal being a cure and the prevention of recurrence. Best results are obtained when patients are transplanted during first remission, but the risk of treatment-related mortality is significant due primarily to infection or graft-versus-host disease which can become a chronic incurable condition. An alternative is autologous hematopoietic stem cell transplantation, which utilizes the patient's own stem cells harvested prior to the transplant. It is associated with a lower treatment-related mortality rate, but a higher rate of relapse. Recipients of both types of transplantation are discharged to the care of their families while their medical condition is still tenuous, and the risk of complications remains high. It is estimated that the recovery of normal immune functioning may require as long as 2 years.

People suffering from hematologic malignancies are expected to endure several months of treatment, with some experiencing a cure while others live with chronic illness or imminent death. Most of the treatments for these diseases are toxic and are associated with significant physical and emotional burdens for patients and their families, and a comprehensive approach to treatment is needed if they are to receive adequate support.

PSYCHOLOGICAL, EMOTIONAL, AND SOCIAL DIMENSIONS OF HSCT/BMT

The treatment decision and the consenting process. Transplantation holds hope for the treatment of malignant hematologic diseases that previously were incurable; however, it is an exceedingly intrusive therapy that continues to be associated with high levels of uncertainty, morbidity, and mortality. The opportunity this advancement in medical technology provides may actually increase the potential stress recipients and their families may experience due to the decisions that must now be made.[1] First, in the case of the allogeneic transplant, there is the issue of identifying a donor. Is there a family member who is a match, and does that family member wish to be a donor? If there is more than one family member who is a match, does the selection of the donor result in one member feeling unimportant if not selected, or guilty if s/he is the optimal match and is fearful of undergoing the donation process? If a search outside the family is necessary to find a donor, do the potential recipient and family believe they have gone far enough, not leaving any stone unturned if a donor is not found? Second, in the case of both allogeneic and autologous transplants there is the financial issue for all but the wealthiest of individuals. Does the family have insurance? Will this insurance, if available, cover enough of the cost to make a transplant feasible? Is a major financial move such as mortgaging or selling one's home required to obtain the resources necessary for the transplant? Third, what are the chances for success and a reasonable outcome—do they make the potential side effects as well as the necessary family sacrifices worthwhile, and are the expectations for the treatment realistic? The alternatives are a conventional therapy that does not hold the promise of a cure, but is associated with a relatively low risk of mortality, versus a high-risk treatment which holds greater promise for a cure of the disease. Central to the consenting process is the fact that potential recipients and their caregivers/family members often cannot adequately comprehend the full potential impact of the procedure when they are confronted with the choice between premature death and a high risk but potentially life-saving therapy; therefore, the ability to make a rational decision is seriously compromised.[2]

Impact of transplantation on the recipient. Greater numbers of recipients are surviving the most acute phase of transplantation; consequently, there has been increasing concern about the QOL for those individuals in this population both immediately following treatment and long-term. Multiple studies provide evidence that the quality of the outcome for transplant recipients is highly variable, with some individuals reporting an improved status while others report a decline.[2-5] The majority of studies focus on multidimensional aspects of QOL throughout the first year after treatment, with a few looking at long-term effects.

Assessment of the physical status of survivors and the symptomatology they experience immediately following transplant and throughout the first year indicates the severity of the impact of this therapy. Survivors frequently struggle with physically challenging problems that make it difficult to meet everyday expectations as they live in anticipation of a "cure" and strive to return to life as it was before cancer.

Immediately following high-dose chemotherapy, recipients frequently experience the pain of mucositis, and sometimes graft-versus-host disease if they are allogeneic recipients. All live with a temporary period of severe immunosuppression which restricts their social interaction and results in feelings of isolation and loneliness. Extreme fatigue and the loss of strength are also to be expected during this period in the trajectory; however, it becomes a particularly distressing symptom as it continues after hospitalization. Survivors through 1 year after transplant frequently report a significantly decreased level of energy, strength, and physical functioning compared to that experienced before transplant, with a frequency that may exceed 60% of study participants.[3] This prolonged fatigue and compromised physical status is often not anticipated by the recipient and may be particularly discouraging.[4-8]

Difficulty in sleeping; problems with nausea, anorexia, and eating; and a dissatisfaction with personal appearance have also been found to be common. Likely attributable to a lack of energy, the side effects of chemotherapy, and concern about appearance is the issue of sexual dysfunction in this population. This was reported as being a problem by 41% of men and 49% of women in one study,[9] with only 37% indicating "normal" sexual activity in another study.[10] Sexual problems such as a lack of desire and interest, impotence, and difficulty with intimacy and partner relationships were mentioned as being problematic in a number of studies concerned about QOL.[6,11,12] Similarly, 30% of women and 16% of men expressed concern regarding fertility and the possibility of being unable to have children.[9]

Unfortunately, neurologic complications are not an uncommon occurrence in people undergoing HSCT/BMT due to high-dose chemotherapy that may also be combined with TBI. Subjective perceptions including difficulty concentrating and memory problems are frequently mentioned by participants in QOL studies ranging from fewer than 15% of participants[6,10] to as high as 39%.[8] A recent study using neuropsychological tests evaluated the cognitive functioning of 40 BMT recipients at least 2 years after transplant, all of whom underwent TBI in addition to high-dose chemotherapy, and the results were compared with healthy population norms. Mild to moderate cognitive impairment was found in 60% of this sample.[13] Other studies have been performed that corroborate the potential for the occurrence of neurologic morbidity in this population.[14-16]

Associated with these physical complications are psychological and emotional issues that are detrimental to achieving a full recovery. A number of studies conducted over the past 15 years have been concerned with the adaptation of this population to the extreme levels of stress they experience. Constantly present is the uncertainty regarding the possibility of relapse and the tentative chances for long-term survival. There is never any reassurance that cancer will not return or that a new form of the disease will not appear; only the passing of time can provide some measure of comfort. Consequently, a substantial proportion of recipients experience significant levels of distress with anxiety and depression predominating that do not necessarily dissipate as the severity of physical symptoms decreases. In studies specifically evaluating the incidence of distress, the number of recipients reporting moderate to severe symptoms ranged from a low of 29% to a high of 93%.[5,9,17]

The protracted illness and treatment experience of the transplant recipient has social as well as psychological/emotional consequences, but they often are not as readily recognized. These individuals encounter major disruptions in social relationships and the roles they assume in everyday life, with 62% of participants in one study indicating this was a problem 6 months following hospital discharge, and 48% indicating it continued to be problematic 12 months following hospitalization.[9] At the outset of the treatment trajectory, recipients experience separation from family and friends during induction. Effort has been made to shorten the period of hospitalization, but it is a minimum of 2 to 3 weeks, and for many at a treatment center a long distance from home. Furthermore, recipients are severely immunologically compromised when they do return home, which necessarily results in limited social contact with the outside world and a feeling of isolation. Return to the hospital for the treatment of related problems (i.e., graft-versus-host disease, infection, etc.) is a frequent occurrence for a number of recipients. They must also cope with the stigmatizing effects of being a "cancer patient," perceived as less competent and unable to resume former roles both within and outside the family. Loss of employment and job discrimination are not uncommon, which affect their QOL as well as their financial status. All of these experiences contribute to the loss of a sense of personal control, so important to self-esteem and a feeling of general well-being.[18]

A more recent research focus has been the identification of those factors that may predict success or morbidity in adaptation to the overwhelming stress imposed by the experience of HSCT/BMT. This is crucial to treatment decision making as well as to the development of interventions which will be effective in minimizing psychosocial morbidity secondary to the transplant. The effects of demographic characteristics have been examined and have been inconclusive, although older patients, those with a lower level of education, and men have generally been found to be more vulnerable. While allogeneic recipients have greater physical challenges to contend with, the psychological adaptation of this group has not been found to be significantly different from those receiving autologous transplants.[7]

There is evidence that the choice of coping strategies has a significant impact on psychosocial well-being in this population. The availability of social support, particularly emotional support, has been consistently demonstrated to have a strong positive impact on well-being and positive adaptation, while the use of avoidance coping has had an equally robust negative effect on adjustment.[19-24] It may be that recipients who have an active coping style with adequate support comply more readily with health behaviors that have a vital influence on both their physical and mental health. There is also evidence that the level of psychosocial distress before transplant, as well as the sense of personal control the recipient is able to maintain throughout the trajectory may be predictive of long-term adaptation.[23,25,26]

As pointed out earlier, the consenting process is associated with considerable stress that can interfere with clear communication with the transplant team and result in deficient comprehension of vital information, and therefore interfere with rational consideration of the cost/benefit ratio for the treatment. Consequently, unrealistic expectations for the outcome of treatment may result in discordance between the hope of "returning to normal," as defined by the recipient, and the actual functional status that is achieved; subsequently, this has been found to result in increased distress that influences long-term adjustment.[27]

The family and HSCT/BMT. Regardless of whether the transplant recipient is an adult or a child, current understanding of the effects of this challenging treatment on the family and its individual members is limited. Owing to the critical nature of the transplant the primary focus has been on the life, the well-being, and the survival of the recipient; however, family members are the recipient's partners throughout the process, they are crucial to optimal recovery, and they must also cope with the impact.

Transplantation requires a prolonged hospital stay, often long distances from home, which severely disrupts everyday life for the entire family. It may require that children live with relatives while the well parent spends extended time with a critically ill partner/spouse, and the recipient may need to be rehospitalized for the treatment of severe complications. If the recipient is a child, most frequently one parent remains in the hospital with the child, while the second parent or relatives/friends care for the family at home. Effective communication within the family is difficult at best, and may leave those remaining at home concerned about how the transplant is progressing; are they being kept fully informed, or is there an effort to "protect" them from potentially disturbing information. Maintaining a sense of cohesiveness and stability within the family is challenging, role continuity and the assumption of responsibilities as usual becomes impossible under these circumstances, and consequently the possibility of the occurrence of secondary mental health problems within the family increases.

The family caregiver. The research which has been performed concerning the family of the recipient has focused primarily on family caregivers and the issues they confront. Most frequently, the recipient has been diagnosed as having a hematologic malignancy for some time before the transplant and it may be the last treatment option available, in which case the level of uncertainty and anxiety will have been elevated for the caregiver and other family members for a considerable period of time.

The trajectory post-HSCT/BMT presents a number of challenges for caregivers as insurance issues and financial constraints result in shorter periods of hospitalization for the recipient. It is mistakenly assumed that the intensity of care required following hospital discharge is considerably less than during the period of hospitalization; however, this frequently is not the case and the caregiver is not equipped with adequate knowledge and skill to comfortably and adequately manage caregiving requirements. Furthermore, there usually are not medically trained individuals readily available to provide support such as responding to questions as needed, or to provide assistance if an emergency should occur. This in turn leaves the family caregiver vulnerable to experiencing high levels of anxiety and potential feelings of guilt if serious complications occur during this period of time.[28,29] A focus group with these caregivers confirms they did not feel they had been adequately prepared to take on the level of responsibility they had to assume, and they had been unable to arrange for the homecare resources and backup support they would need in an emergency.[30]

In addition to these stressors imposed by the role itself, is the stress resulting from major role changes and the strain of additional responsibilities and disruption of activities that have been part of the caregiver's life. Employment often has to be curtailed adding additional financial concerns, and the recipient is at least temporarily unable to function as an equal partner sharing family responsibilities and providing mutual support. The caregiver takes on the role of the lone executive in a family that is experiencing high levels of threat and disorder, and is left to assist other family members as they struggle to cope with alternate periods of hope, fear, and depression.

Several studies have examined the effects of this stress on the emotional and psychological well-being of the caregiver. Generally, findings indicate that these caregivers experience levels of anxiety and depression exceeding that of recipients and also greater than that of "non-medical norms" when their data are included in the analyses.[28,31–34] It is particularly disturbing, and cause for concern, that one study found not only do caregivers experience greater distress than recipients and normal controls, but also are less likely to receive mental health intervention.

Outcomes in this study were obtained a mean of 7 years after transplant when it is presumed that active caregiving has long been over.[29]

Given the threat experienced by both the recipient and the caregiving partner, the level of satisfaction and cohesiveness within this relationship is a potential problem; however, little has been done to look at this important aspect of family adjustment. The findings of a single longitudinal study of 131 dyads, which includes before transplant to 1 year after transplant with three data points, indicate the reason for concern.[31] Particularly significant was a decline in the level of agreement within the dyad regarding the degree of relationship satisfaction each individual was experiencing. Couples were matched in their perceptions of the quality of the relationship before transplant, but by 6 months after transplant the satisfaction of the caregiver was significantly lower than that of the recipient. This trend continued to 1 year after transplant, with a total of 49% of the dyads expressing dissatisfaction. Factors associated with this finding were the gender of the caregiver with women being less satisfied than men, an elevated level of depression before the transplant, and an allogeneic transplant. It is also suggested that an additional contributor may be caregiver feelings of isolation, with many people focusing on the needs of the recipient while the caregiver is providing extensive support, but receiving little in return. An additional recent study also found marital distress to be a problem for these dyads.[29]

The focus in this discussion has been the family of the adult recipient; however, transplantation is also commonly used in the treatment of childhood cancers. Cancer during childhood is unexpected and is highly distressing and disruptive for all family members. It results in severe stress for parents, and it is suggested that the suffering parents' experience may exceed that experienced by their children. Parental distress may subsequently increase the likelihood and severity of problems developing in the child's emotional and psychological adjustment.[35] Treatment of childhood cancer by HSCT/BMT is associated with the variability of problems found in the adult population along with pain and discomfort for the child that the parent is unable to prevent or control.[36] This further increases parents' feelings of helplessness and distress. What's more, one parent must necessarily assume the primary care of this child, usually the mother, resulting in absences and less time for other children in the family. The remaining spouse must continue employment and concentrate on maintaining the home environment, meeting the needs of children who remain at home. Needless to say, this places challenging demands on the partner relationship, as well as on the maintenance of cohesiveness and stability within the family unit.[37]

Siblings of children undergoing transplantation are also vulnerable to the development of psychological and behavioral problems as a result of the interruption in family life, family instability, and separation from the caregiving parent as well as from the sibling recipient.[38] In addition, approximately 75% of the time a sibling is the donor for an allogeneic transplant, and therefore they too are subjected to invasive medical procedures.[39]

DIRECTIONS FOR FUTURE RESEARCH

Transplantation challenges the QOL of each family member as well as that of the recipient, as they are all confronted with a continuous assault of stressors. Furthermore, the use of both blood and marrow transplants is increasing dramatically, with over 53,000 performed worldwide in 2000 (International BMT/Autologous Blood and Marrow Transplant Registry). Therefore, we must understand the problems of family members and the family system as well as those of the recipient. At what points in the trajectory are problems most likely to occur, what factors are associated with adaptive coping, and what are the clinical markers indicating vulnerability to the development of psychosocial morbidity secondary to the transplant? Answers to these questions are fundamental to the development of effective interventions.

Understanding of the transplant experience for the recipient from making the decision to undergo treatment throughout the first critical year has been documented by a number of descriptive studies; however, knowledge of specific difficulties family members confront throughout this time period is more limited. Currently, research findings are not available that can provide a basis for identifying those families and individual members at high risk for the development of secondary morbidity. This is a significant issue for both the recipient and family members, as the family support system is considered to be an influential factor in determining the physical and emotional recovery of the recipient.[6,7,19,34,40,41] Moreover, if the recipient survives and the family is destroyed in the process what have we accomplished?

The use of several specific research strategies would increase our level of understanding regarding the psychological, emotional, and social outcomes in this population. First, there are indications that recovery is often not complete within 1 year after transplant, and if we are to evaluate the long-term outcome of transplantation longitudinal studies are essential that follow recipients and their families from before transplant for a period of several years after treatment. Long-term residual effects have been shown as far out as 7 years for both recipients and caregivers, and the majority of studies have been cross-sectional. Second, the use of multiple sites, large heterogeneous samples, the inclusion of variables indicating diagnoses and specific regimens in the analyses, as well as the consistent use of a limited number of selected reliable and valid measures would contribute significantly to the quality and generalizability of findings.

On the basis of available findings, interventions are sorely needed, even though increased knowledge and understanding regarding the problems this population experiences is necessary for maximum effectiveness. During the period before transplant, when treatment options are being explored and consenting takes place, discussion of potential sequelae and residual effects is imperative even if the prospective recipient may have difficulty giving them the necessary consideration. Support for caregivers as they confront the awesome responsibility of homecare for these critically ill family members is also essential, but seldom provided. Along with detailed instruction and information, is the need for frequent contacts by the transplant team to respond to questions and to assess any existing needs—care does not end at the time of hospital discharge.

Finally, psychosocial assessment of both the recipient and family, particularly the potential caregiver before transplant, could provide data important to the decision-making process; research has indicated that distress levels in the pretransplant period are associated with posttransplant adjustment as far out as 1 year. Continued long-term psychosocial assessment would then be important for those who are found to be most vulnerable.

REFERENCES

1. Patenaude AF. Psychological impact of bone marrow transplantation: current perspectives. *Yale J Biol Med.* 1990;63:515–519.

2. Andrykowski MA. Psychiatric and psychosocial aspects of bone marrow transplantation. *Psychosom.* 1994;35:13–24.

3. Baker F, Denniston M, Zabora JR, Marcellus C. Cancer problems in living and quality of life after bone marrow transplantation. *J Clin Psychol Med Settings.* 2003;10:27–34.

4. McQuellon RP, Russell GB, Rambo TD, Craven BL, Radford, J, Perry JJ. Quality of life and psychological distress of bone marrow transplant recipients: the 'time trajectory' to recovery over the first year. *Bone Marrow Transplant.* 1998;21:477–486.

5. Neitzert CS, Ritvo P, Dancey J, Weiser K, Murray C, Acery J. The psychosocial impact of bone marrow transplantation: a review of the literature. *Bone Marrow Transplant.* 1998;22:409–422.

6. Molassiotis A, van den Akker OBA, Milligan DW, Goldman JM, Boughton BJ, Holmes JA. Quality of life in long-term survivors of bone marrow transplantation: comparison with a matched group receiving maintenance chemotherapy. *Bone Marrow Transplant.* 1996;17:240–258.

7. Andrykowski MA, Greiner CB, Altmaier EM, Burish TG, Antin JH, McGarigle CM. Quality of life following bone marrow transplantation: findings from a multicentre study. *Br J Cancer.* 1995;71:1322–1329.

8. Bush NE, Haberman M, Donaldson G, Sullivan KM. Quality of life of 125 adults surviving 6–18 years after bone marrow transplantation. *Soc Sci Med.* 1995;40:479–490.

9. Baker F, Zabora JR, Polland A, Wingard J. Reintegration after bone marrow transplantation. *Cancer Pract.* 1999;7:190–197.

10. Andrykowski MA, Bruehl S, Brady MJ, Hemsley-Downey PJ. Physical and psychosocial status of adults one-year after bone marrow transplantation: a prospective study. *Bone Marrow Transplant.* 1995;15:837–844.

11. Vose JM, Kennedy BC, Bierman PJ, Kessinger A, Armitage JO. Long-term sequelae of autologous bone marrow or peripheral stem cell transplantation for lymphoid malignancies. *Cancer.* 1992;69:784–789.

12. Altmaier EM, Gingrich RD, Fyfe MA. Two-year adjustment of bone marrow transplant survivors. *Bone Marrow Transplant.* 1991;7:311–316.

13. Harder H, Cornelissen JJ, Van Gool AR, Duivenvoorden HJ. Cognitive functioning and quality of life in long-term adult survivors of bone marrow transplantation. *Cancer.* 2002;95:183–192.

14. Gallardo D, Ferra C, Berlanga J, de la Banda E, Ponce C, Salar A. Neurologic complications after allogeneic bone marrow transplantation. *Bone Marrow Transplant.* 1996:18:1135–1139.

15. Snider S, Bashir R, Bierman P. Neurologic complications after high-dose chemotherapy and autologous bone marrow transplantation for Hodgkins disease. *Neurology.* 1994;44:681–684.

16. Meyers C, Weitzner M, Byrne K, Valentine A, Champlin RE, Przepiorka D. Evaluation of the neurobehavioral functioning of patients before, during, and after bone marrow transplantation. *J Clin Oncol.* 1994;12:820–826.

17. Whedon M, Stearns D, Mills LE. Quality of life of long-term adult survivors of autologous bone marrow transplantation. *Oncol Nurs Forum.* 1995; 22:1527–1535.

18. Haberman M. The meaning of cancer therapy: bone marrow transplantation as an example of therapy. *Semin Oncol Nurs.* 1995;11:23–31.

19. Frick E, Ramm G, Bumeder I, Schulz-Kindermann F, Tryoller M, Fischer N. Social support and quality of life of patients prior to stem cell or bone marrow transplantation. *Br J Health Psychol.* 2006;11:451–462.

20. Grulke N, Bailer H, Hertenstein B, Kachele H, Arnold R, Tschuschke V. Coping and survival in patients with leukemia undergoing allogeneic bone marrow transplantation—long-term follow-up of a prospective study. *J Psychosom Res.* 2005;59:337–346.

21. Widows MR, Jacobsen PB, Booth-Jones M, Fields KK. Predictors of posttraumatic growth following bone marrow transplantation for cancer. *Health Psychol.* 2005;24:266–273.

22. Jacobsen PB, Sadler IJ, Booth-Jones M, Soety E, Weitzner MA, fields KK. Predictors of posttraumatic stress disorder symptomatology following bone marrow transplantation for cancer. *J Consult Clin Psychol.* 2002;0:235–240.

23. Fife BL, Huster GA, Cornetta KG. Longitudinal study of adaptation to the stress of bone marrow transplantation. *J Clin Oncol.* 2000;18:1539–1549.

24. Widows MR, Jacobsen PB, Fields KK. Relation of psychological vulnerability factors to posttraumatic stress disorder symptomatology in bone marrow transplant recipients. *Psychosom Med.* 2000;62:873–882.

25. Broers S, Kaptein AD, LeCessie S, Fibbe W, Hengeveld M. Psychological functioning and quality of life following bone marrow transplantation: a 3-year follow-up study. *J Psychosom Res.* 2000;48:11–21.

26. Keogh F, O'Riordan J, McNamara C, Duggan C, McCann SR. Psychosocial adaptation of patients and families following bone marrow transplantation: a prospective longitudinal study. *Bone Marrow Transplant.* 1998;22:905–911.

27. Andrykowski MA, Brady MJ, Greiner CB, Altmaier EM, Burish TG, Anin JH. 'Returning to normal' following bone marrow transplantation: outcomes, expectations, and informed consent. *Bone Marrow Transplant.* 1995; 15:573–581.

28. Boyle D, Blodgett L, Gnesdiloff S, White J, Bamford AM, Sheridan M. Caregiver quality of life after autologous bone marrow transplantation. *Cancer Nurs.* 2000;28:193–203.

29. Bishop, MM, Beaumont JL, Hahn EA, Cella D, Andrykowski M, Brady MJ. Late effects of cancer and hematopoietic stem-cell transplantation on spouses or partners compared with survivors and survivor-matched controls. *J Clin Oncol.* 2007;25:1403–1411.

30. Stetz KM, McDonald JC, Compton K. Needs and experiences of family caregivers during bone marrow transplantation. *Oncol Nurs Forum.* 1996;23:1442–1447.

31. Langer S, Abrams J, Syrjala K. Caregiver and patient marital satisfaction and affect following hematopoietic stem cell transplantation: a prospective longitudinal investigation. *Psychooncology.* 2003;12:239–253.

32. Siston AK. Patient and caregiver adaptation to allogeneic transplantation. *Dissertation Abstracts Int.* 1998;59:2436.

33. Sutherland HJ, Fyles GM, Adams G, Hao Y, Lipton JH, Minden MD. Quality of life following bone marrow transplantation: a comparison of patient reports with population norms. *Bone Marrow Transplant.* 1997; 19:1129–1136.

34. Syrjala KL, Chapko MK, Vitaliano PP, Cummings C, Sullivan KM. Recovery after allogeneic marrow transplantation: prospective study of predictors of long-term physical and psychosocial functioning. *Bone Marrow Transplant.* 1993;11:319–327.

35. Rabineau K, Mabe PA, Vega RA. Parenting stress in the pediatric oncology population. *J Pediatr Oncol.* 2008;30:358–365.

36. Streisand R, Rodrique JR, Houde C. Brief report: parents of children undergoing bone marrow transplantation. *J Pediatr Psychol*. 2000;25:331–337.

37. Phipps S, Mulhern RK. Family cohesion and expressiveness promote resilience to the stress of pediatric bone marrow transplant: a preliminary report. *J Dev Behav Pediatr*. 1995;16:257–263.

38. Wilkins KL, Woodgate RL. An interruption in family life: siblings' lived experience as they transition through the pediatric bone marrow transplant trajectory. *Oncol Nurs Forum*. 2007;34:E28-E35.

39. Packman WL. Psychosocial impact of pediatric BMT on siblings. *Bone Marrow Transplant*. 1999;24:701–702.

40. Rodrigue JR, Pearmen TP, Moreb J. Morbidity and mortality following bone marrow transplantation: predictive utility of pre-BMT affective functioning, compliance, and social support stability. *Int J Behav Med*. 1999;6:241–254.

41. Futterman AD, Wellisch DK, Bond G, Carr CR. The psychosocial levels system. A new rating scale to identify and assess emotional difficulties during bone marrow transplantation. *Psychosom*. 1991;37:177–186.

CHAPTER 27

HIV Infection and AIDS-Associated Neoplasms

Joanna S. Dognin and Peter A. Selwyn

Rates of human immunodeficiency virus (HIV), the virus leading to acquired immunodeficiency syndrome (AIDS), have reached pandemic proportions, resulting in 38.6 million people infected worldwide. First recognized as a syndrome in 1981,[1,2] the joint United Nation Programme on AIDS (UNAIDS) and the World Health Organization (WHO) estimate that HIV/AIDS has claimed the lives of 2.5 million people worldwide.[1] Hardest hit has been Africa, specifically sub-Saharan Africa where UNAIDS South Africa reports the prevalence rates of adults aged 15–49 to be 18.1%. Outside of Africa, global trends of HIV suggest that the incidence of infection has been stabilizing. Despite this, the numbers of people living with HIV continues to rise due to both population growth and the availability of life sustaining therapies. By the close of 2005, there were an estimated 4.1 million newly infected people.[1] The socio-political and psychosocial issues linked in the global HIV epidemic are massive and include gaining greater access to and adhering to antiretroviral treatments, behavior change efforts aimed at prevention, human rights and gender discrimination, children orphaned by AIDS, and co-occurring malignancies and infections. A proper description of these global issues is beyond the scope of this chapter. Instead this chapter will focus on recent trends in the epidemic within the United States, specifically on the co-occurrence of HIV and cancer, and the ways in which these malignancies impact the psychological functioning of those infected.

By the end of 2006, the Centers for Disease Control and Prevention (CDC) estimated that 491,727 people were living with HIV/AIDS in the United States.[2] These estimates are based on data from states with confidential name-based HIV reporting, and may be an underestimate, as UNAIDS estimates that 1.2 million people in the United States are currently living with HIV/AIDS.[1] Over the past decade or so, there have been tremendous changes in the face of the HIV/AIDS epidemic, both in the availability of more effective medical treatment options and in the epidemiological profile of those infected. The introduction of highly active anti-retroviral treatment (HAART) in 1996 revolutionized HIV treatment, transforming the course of HIV from a certain death to a potentially manageable, but unpredictable, future. The history of HIV treatment in the United States can be divided into two distinct phases: before the advent of HAART, "Pre-HAART era" (from 1981 to 1996), and since HAART, "HAART era" (from 1996 to present). This chapter will focus primarily on the ways in which the HIV/AIDS epidemic has changed in the HAART era, and will include recent demographic shifts among newly infected people; psychological issues connected to the ambiguity of an uncertain future; the development of co-occurring malignancies; and psychological issues associated with AIDS-related malignancies. We will use three case examples to illustrate how the psychological health of individuals and families are impacted by the unique interplay of HIV and cancer. Finally, we will discuss changes in palliative care and the need to combine curative therapies with palliative care in the third decade of HIV/AIDS.

DEMOGRAPHICS IN THE HAART ERA

The advent of HAART in 1996, along with other advances in HIV treatment, significantly extended the lives of HIV-infected individuals. In countries where access to HAART is readily available, the average death rate has decreased by 75%,[3] and between 1995 and 2002, antiretroviral treatment averted or delayed death for between 33,000 and 42,000 people within the United States.[4] As HIV-infected people are living longer and as HIV/AIDS shifts in the public perception, new challenges have emerged. Perhaps in part due to the growing notion that HIV has become a manageable or chronic disease, public health prevention campaigns have failed to slow the rate of new infections. In surveillance data from 38 areas (33 states and 5 U.S. dependent areas), the CDC estimates were approximately 35,000 new infections each year for the years 2003 through 2006.[2] Further, living longer with HIV is accompanied by serious morbidities as a myriad of new cancer diagnoses are being seen[3,5–10] and the incidence and prevalence of chronic liver disease, cardiovascular disease, and diabetes also continues to increase.[11,12]

Another major demographic shift has been in the epidemiological profile of HIV, which currently demonstrates significant racial and ethnic disparities. In the beginning of the epidemic, HIV/AIDS primarily affected the gay community; intravenous substance users; people who received tainted blood products; and perinatally infected children. In contrast, the demographic profile has shifted in recent years: male-to-male sexual contact and intravenous drug use continue to account for a substantial amount of new infections, while infections among children and those with blood transfusions have dropped precipitously[2] due, respectively, to the discoveries around HAART's ability to reduce mother–child transmission, and stricter governmental regulations around blood products. However, most notable in the current demographic profile of HIV is the rapidly increasing rate of new infections due to heterosexual contact, especially among young minority populations. Among areas with long-term, confidential name-based reporting, African Americans—who comprise just over 12% of the U.S. population—account for 50% of new HIV diagnoses, and Hispanics—who account for 14% of population—represent 18% of new infections.[1] As HIV/AIDS further spreads among disenfranchised populations, and as the HIV care shifts from preparing for death to coping for an uncertain future, numerous psychosocial issues occur.

PSYCHIATRIC AND PSYCHOLOGICAL ISSUES IN THE HAART ERA

HIV/AIDS has long been associated with a range of psychological and psychiatric issues, especially given that its major risk factors correspond with stigmatized societal behaviors (intravenous drug use, male-to-male sexual contact, risky sexual behaviors), and that infections have been increasing among already disenfranchised populations. Demographic groups with increased HIV risk tend to also have higher rates of psychiatric disorders and less access to mental health treatment. For example, African Americans and Hispanics are consistently found to be untreated, undertreated, or improperly diagnosed for mental health issues, alcoholism, and drug abuse.[13–15] Once infected, this picture is further complicated by the stress of living with a potentially life-threatening disease, leading to a cycle of increased social stressors and emotional distress, significant physical health concerns, and potentially further marginalization. To further compound these struggles, treatment for the disease itself requires remarkably high adherence (95%).[16] Given all of these factors, it is not surprising that being HIV positive is associated with significant psychiatric comorbidities.

Recent exploration of psychiatric diagnoses reveals significant amounts of distress. Tegger and colleagues[17] conducted a review of the electronic medical records of 1774 HIV-infected outpatients, and found that 63.0% met criteria for any psychiatric diagnosis, with 45.0% diagnosed as having dysthymia; 38.0% having bipolar disorder; 34.0% with substance use disorder; and 10.0% as having an anxiety disorder. Another prevalence study involving brief psychiatric interviews of 2864 HIV-positive outpatients found rates of any psychiatric disorder being 47.0%, with 36.0% having major depression; 26.5% having dysthymia; 15.8% having generalized anxiety disorder; 12.5% having drug dependence; and 10.5% having panic attacks.[18] Israelski et al.[19] found high rates of psychiatric distress in their standardized screening of 210 HIV outpatients, most notably documenting that 77.0% experienced symptoms related to recent or past experiences of trauma, with 34.0% meeting full criteria for posttraumatic stress disorder (PTSD) and another 43.0% having acute stress disorder. Finally, among vulnerable populations of incarcerated HIV-infected people, psychiatric distress is also significant. In a review of the electronic medical records of 6168 incarcerated men and women diagnosed with HIV, Baillargeon and colleagues[20] found that 16.7% had a documented psychiatric diagnosis, with the percentage increasing to 20.6% when studying prisoners co-infected with HIV and Hepatitis C, and 20.5% of prisoners with HIV and Hepatitis B, emphasizing that psychiatric distress is greater among those whose HIV is compounded by other diseases.

Despite the notion that HIV has become more of a potentially chronic and manageable disease, measures of "quality of life" clearly demonstrate that living with HIV is considerably more challenging than living with other "chronic" conditions. In 2000, one study used data from the HIV Cost and Services Utilization Study and found that physical and emotional well-being of patients with an AIDS diagnosis was significantly worse than both the general population and the patients afflicted with a variety of chronic diseases (epilepsy, gastroesophageal reflux disease, prostate cancer, diabetes, and depression).[21] While adults with asymptomatic HIV were found to have physical well-being similar to the general population, all adults with HIV/AIDS had significantly worse emotional functioning than all other chronic diseases, except depression.[22]

One model of conceptualizing the lower life satisfaction among HIV-infected people is the chronic illness quality of life model (CIQOL).[22] CIQOL purports that for those living with HIV, life satisfaction can be predicted by five variables: AIDS-related discrimination, barriers to healthcare and social services, physical well-being, social support, and engagement coping. Heckman[22] used data from 275 HIV-infected adults to evaluate this model, and found that AIDS-related discrimination lowered life satisfaction by impeding access to healthcare, social services, and social support services. In this sample, he also found that life satisfaction was positively linked to physical well-being, underscoring again the role of physical health in quality of life for HIV-infected people.

Perhaps one of the most psychologically challenging issues of the HAART era is coping with the tremendous psychological uncertainty of HIV treatment, given that the long-term effects of available treatments are still largely unknown. While an HIV diagnosis no longer requires one to prepare for imminent death, considering an antiretroviral regimen confronts one with the particular challenges of modern life with HIV: when to initiate treatment, how to maintain the high level of adherence necessary for optimal effect, and how to deal with the psychological meaning of daily medications. Patients on HAART may experience medication-related complications such as lipodystrophy, hypercholesterolemia, diabetes, and neuropsychiatric disorders,[12] which may decrease self-esteem and well-being. In addition to these potential complications, antiretrovirals (ARVs) may be seen as intrusions to daily life. They not only remind patients of their disease status but also risk exposing their status to others when faced with taking pills in public.[23] All of these factors contribute to the tremendous ambivalence experienced by many[12,23,24] around taking these medications. Psychologically, these conflictual internal experiences may compromise one's ability to adhere at the 95% level required for optimal effect.

Finally, the promise of new treatments gives hope, a sense of renewal and the opportunity to redefine what living with HIV means. In the HAART era, individuals with HIV have been able to develop families, return to work, become advocates, and lead meaningful and productive lives. For some who struggled with substance abuse, an HIV diagnosis may have forced them to care for themselves, and begin the recovery process. As the rate of new HIV infections continues to rise among young people, many other issues become apparent, including choosing sexual partners, disclosing one's status, handling the complications

Table 27–1. Types of AIDS-defining and non–AIDS-defining malignancies

AIDS-defining malignancies	Non–AIDS-defining malignancies
Kaposi sarcoma	Hodgkin disease
Non-Hodgkin lymphoma	Prostate cancer
Invasive cervical cancer	Anal cancer
	Lung cancer
	Testicular cancer
	Head and neck cancer
	Anorectal cancer
	Melanoma

ABBREVIATION: AIDS, acquired immunodeficiency syndrome.

of both serodiscordant and seroconcordant relationships, as well coping with the impact of HIV disease on childbearing. Underscoring these issues are constant uncertainty about the future, concerns about whether and for how long medications will continue to work, exacerbations and remissions in health, and fears about disclosure and stigma.

PSYCHOLOGICAL ISSUES ASSOCIATED WITH AIDS-RELATED MALIGNANCIES

One particular challenge in the era of HAART has been the development of co-occurring cancers, both ones known to be associated with an AIDS diagnosis (AIDS-defining malignancies or "ADMs"), as well as an array of cancers not specifically associated with HIV (Non–AIDS-defining malignancies or "Non-ADMs"). Approximately 30%–40% of HIV-infected patients are likely to develop malignancies.[3] Since the advent of HAART, the overall incidence of ADMs has been decreasing; yet as HIV-infected individuals live longer, new types of cancers are becoming more prevalent,[25] as listed in Table 27–1.

Overall, the availability of HAART has been particularly advantageous in lowering the rate of ADMs. For instance, Kaposi sarcoma (KS), the most common ADM, has significantly declined, with its incidence decreasing by 30%–50% in the United States and Europe since protease inhibitors have been used.[3,5,6] Similarly, the use of HAART has led to an overall reduction in the incidence of non-Hodgkin lymphoma and improved its outcomes.[6] In contrast, there has been an increase in cervical cancer diagnoses,[3] and HAART has had little impact on the incidence of human papillomavirus (HPV) associated tumors in HIV patients.[6]

While HAART has helped to reduce the overall impact of ADMs, a new array of cancers are on the rise[25]; a list of which can be found in Table 27–1. Of all those cancers, Hodgkin disease is the most common non-ADMs.[3,7] Anal cancers, which are similar to cervical cancer in that they are also related to HPV, have also been increasing. Unfortunately, the availability of HAART appears to have little effect on them.[3,26,27] Similarly, the incidence of lung cancer among HIV-positive people is also escalating. While HIV-infected patients smoke more than the general population, this alone does not appear to account for the observed disparity in lung cancer diagnoses.[8–10] The higher rate of lung cancer may be related to the aging of the HIV population as well as the effects of chronic immune suppression. The availability of HAART appears to have little effect on lung cancer. Patients with HIV and lung cancer usually have dismal outcomes compared to lung cancer in the general population.[8] Other malignancies have been observed to occur in the HIV-infected population. They include prostate cancer,[28–31] leukemias,[9] testicular cancer, and head and neck cancer.

The challenges of living with both HIV and cancer are substantially different from those before life-preserving HIV treatments were available. While the incidence of co-infection with HIV and cancer is well documented in the literature, there is a gap in understanding the psychological consequences of living with two potentially deadly and very different diseases. While there have been comparisons between psychosocial aspects

Table 27–2. Psychosocial typology of illness, HIV/AIDS versus cancer

Illness	HIV/AIDS		
Time phase	Pre-HAART	HAART era	Cancer
Onset	Gradual	Gradual	Gradual
Course	Progressive	Progressive	Progressive
		OR	OR
		Relapsing	Relapsing
Outcome	Fatal	Shortened life span	Nonfatal (benign)
		OR	OR
		Fatal	Fatal (malignant)
Incapacitation	Severe	Mild, moderate	Mild, moderate
		OR	OR
		Severe	Severe

ABBREVIATIONS: AIDS, acquired immunodeficiency syndrome; HAART, highly active retroviral treatment; HIV, human immunodeficiency virus.
SOURCE: Adapted from John Rolland's Illness Model.[33]

of cancer and HIV in terms of therapeutic interventions, perceptions of pain, and experiences of stigma,[32] the psycho-oncology literature and the literature on HIV mental health remain largely disparate. We will present one particular conceptual model[33] for understanding illness, family, and disease. Then we will present three case vignettes to demonstrate how such a model can guide our understanding of the unique psychological issues of living with both HIV and cancer.

FAMILY SYSTEMS ANALYSIS

The particular systemic analysis of disease and family that follows is grounded in John Rolland's integrative "family systems-illness model."[33] Living with a life-threatening illness does not occur in isolation—all individuals are members of family and social systems, which impact one's psychosocial functioning and the ability to cope with the adversity involved in chronic disease management. Owing to the specific psychosocial risk factors (substance abuse, homosexual activity) involved in contracting HIV, many HIV-infected individuals are strained from their families and develop outside communities of support. Nonetheless, when we say family, we are referring not only to one's traditional nuclear family, but also to one's close support network. Illness itself becomes like a family member, with each illness's "personality" being determined by the illness's psychosocial typology (or disease characteristics) and time phase.[33] The contextual understanding of one's family system combined with various disease factors shapes the experience one has of their illness.

The requirements of the family as a support system vary widely and can be understood in relation to the following factors[33]:

1. Disease psychosocial typology (onset, course, outcome, and incapacitation)
2. Disease time phase (crisis, chronic, or terminal)
3. Family functioning (structure, communication processes, life cycle, and belief systems)
4. Family's multigenerational experiences with illness, loss, and crisis
5. Individual's life cycle
6. Family's health and illness belief system
7. Amount of physical anticipatory loss.

Coping with chronic disease largely depends on the psychosocial meaning the disease has to the patient, society, and family; the time of life when it strikes; its intensity; and how long it is expected to persist. For a person living with HIV and then diagnosed with cancer, an even more complicated psychosocial picture unfolds where one's resources to deal with cancer may or may not differ from their ability to cope with HIV.

The "personality" or psychosocial typology of HIV/AIDS before the availability of HAART was dire (see Table 27–2). Then, the disease had a gradual symptomatic presentation, followed by a progressive course, a fatal outcome, and severe incapacitation, requiring individuals and families to cope with more short-term but severe health crises. Once HAART became readily available, the psychosocial typology of HIV/AIDS became less grim but more uncertain. While for some the disease course continues to be progressive, others experience long asymptomatic periods followed by severe exacerbations that are managed with different regimens. Also variable are the levels of incapacitation including not only physical but also emotional and societal factors. Comparing the typology of the HIV/AIDS in the HAART era with that of cancer depicts similar patterns. The course, outcome, and incapacitation of cancer largely depend on its particular type, location, and malignancy. To combine the profile of HIV/AIDS in the HAART era with that of cancer can only increase uncertainty for individuals and families. Three case examples will be discussed which depicts this profile.

CASE #1

"Maria" is a 37-year-old Latina female who contracted HIV 8 years ago from heterosexual contact with her husband. She was tested for HIV after her husband became mysteriously and gravely ill and subsequently died from an infection secondary to AIDS. After the death of her husband, the realization of his betrayal, and her subsequent HIV diagnosis, Maria found herself interpersonally isolated. She kept both her HIV status and the true cause of her husband's death hidden from her friends and family. She started ARVs 2 years ago, maintained adequate adherence, and has remained asymptomatic ever since. Around the same time, she met her current boyfriend and trusting that she had found love again, revealed her diagnosis to him. At first, he appeared incredibly supportive and took it upon himself to parcel out her daily medications. Over time, he became increasingly more controlling, and from time to time began withholding her medications. As she found herself more and more isolated, she was dealt another blow when she received a second diagnosis—cervical cancer.

As she began treatment for her cancer, her partner once again appeared the model boyfriend, caring for her through her chemotherapy, and impressing her medical providers with his constant attention toward her. Once the immediate crisis around her health again subsided, his controlling behavior increased, and soon erupted into physical violence. He threatened to expose her HIV status if she dared to leave him. He regularly reminded her that her diagnoses of HIV and cancer likely prevented her from having any children, and that she should feel fortunate that he remained willing to still be involved with her.

For Maria, the psychosocial meaning of HIV is intricately linked with her husband's betrayal. Her feelings around this are unresolved, and complicated by both grieving his death and the fact that he left her with the same disease that killed him. The legacy of secrets that began with her husband's indiscretions continues for Maria, as she begins to isolate herself from her support network. Her unresolved grief, anger, lowered feelings of self-worth, and isolation, combined with her desperate need to still relate set the perfect backdrop for her to become involved with an overcontrolling partner. The psychosocial impact of her cancer diagnosis is also great: both diseases are striking her during the life cycle phase when she would have considered having children. The combination of a sexually acquired, and socially stigmatized, disease and a cancer in the reproductive area symbolically seals the loss of this dream, which her partner uses to further shame, control, and isolate her.

This case illustrates the various ways in which the social stigma of HIV, combined with a second diagnosis of cancer, can disrupt individual and family functioning. While the potential for better health and longer lives brought on by HAART has lessened the physical incapacitation of HIV, the emotional and social incapacitation can still be severe. The choice of partners for people who are HIV-infected can be problematic especially when one is already disenfranchised and isolated by fears of disclosure and stigma. The context in which HIV often occurs—poverty, substance abuse, isolation, risky sexual behaviors, or having partners with high-risk behaviors—makes it no surprise that for HIV-positive women, intimate partner violence is more frequent, more severe, and associated with worse health outcomes.[34-37] Vulnerability toward abuse is heightened for the HIV-infected person when an abusive partner also retains the power to disclose one's status or withhold medication. Given this context, the addition of a cancer diagnosis to HIV can further stall a person's individual and family life cycle path and maintain a system of power inequity between partners that can, for some, contribute to partner abuse.

CASE #2

"Anton" is a 22-year-old White male of Italian descent admitted to the hospital with pneumonia. He is given an HIV test and is diagnosed with full-blown AIDS. Given his extremely low T-cell count, his providers hypothesize that he likely seroconverted as an adolescent. While Anton had never before been tested for HIV, he suspected he might be positive after a former male partner became sick. Anton lives with his parents and brothers, who are unaware of his sexual orientation—they are Catholic and he fears their rejection if they knew he was gay. Given that, he had avoided being tested and remains fairly uneducated about HIV prevention and treatment. When confronted with his HIV diagnosis and treatment options, Anton begs the staff to not tell his family and is unwilling to discuss starting ARVs. Upon discharge, he never follows up with his doctor, and is hospitalized again within 2 months. During this second admittance, he is also diagnosed with lymphoma. Upon hearing about the cancer, Anton is relieved, feeling that he finally has a legitimate reason to give his family for his continued poor health. His family holds vigils around his bedside and are extremely supportive and attentive to his needs around having cancer. He still refuses to share his HIV status or sexual orientation with them, and dies from his lymphoma 3 months later.

The psychosocial meaning around having HIV, for Anton, is complete and utter rejection by his family unit. So fearful is he of their reaction that he steadfastly avoids potentially life saving treatment. At 22, Anton's normal life cycle stage would be to develop independence and accept responsibility for himself,[38] and yet his first dabbles with differentiation (separation) from his family and development of intimate peer relationships leave him with a disease that he fears would be completely unacceptable to his family, and ultimately contributes to his death. In contrast, he receives his cancer diagnosis very differently—with ironic relief, as it provides him with an acceptable reason—one in which he can maintain blamelessness, to be sick to his family. The cancer diagnosis unites his family, calls upon their collective resources for support, and provides a socially acceptable reason for Anton to be ill and to die.

In describing how certain diseases evoke powerful societal metaphors, Susan Sontag stated, "societies need to have one illness that becomes identified with evil, and attaches blame to its 'victims.'"[33] Before the first case of AIDS, cancer was such a disease, a deep societal metaphor centering on lack of control and certain death. To protect against the fears this elicits, blame was often assigned to its victims for behaviors which may have contributed to their plight. Over the past two decades, HIV/AIDS has become an even more powerful metaphor—the impact of this metaphor is clearly depicted in situations like the aforementioned case, in which the family belief system around what it means to have HIV serves as a barrier from benefiting from medical advances. In doing so, the psychosocial typology of HIV/AIDS harkens back to the pre-HAART era with a fatal outcome and severe incapacitation.

CASE #3

"Sam" is a 55-year-old African American openly gay male, who considers himself a "longtime survivor" after living with the HIV virus for the past 20 years. He has lived through seeing many of his friends and lovers die, through hopes for new treatments, and ups and downs in his own health. In the early days of the epidemic, he steadfastly avoided "AZT" (azidothymidine, the first approved ARVs), watching his friends and lovers suffer serious side effects. He conquered a serious cocaine addiction, and relishes the fact that his years of homelessness and addiction are long behind him. Now at 55, he is more stable than ever—he works as a peer educator, using his story to give the message of HIV prevention to younger generations. His virus is well controlled with his ARV regimen, and he lives with his longtime partner who is also HIV positive. After receiving a diagnosis of prostate cancer, he finds himself depressed and deeply angry. He feels it is unfair that after all he is survived through, he is struck by yet another hurdle to overcome.

Unlike the first two cases, the psychosocial meaning of having HIV is quite different for Sam: he has a community of social support, and many models for coping with the tremendous stress of having HIV. He has, in a sense, aged with the epidemic and, in so doing; the history of HIV and his life story have become intricately linked. In his personal narrative around having HIV, he has overcome his addictions, engaged in fuller self-care and contributed to future generations through education and advocacy. At 55, he has lived longer than he expected, and while he still fears the toll HIV is taking on his body, HIV has become a known entity, and thus is less frightening. He has a long-term partner and a community whose illness belief model empowers and helps him in his healing. A new diagnosis of cancer is a very different story. At 55, a diagnosis of prostrate cancer is more timely, as he enters a phase in his life where chronic illness is to be more expected. Yet for Sam, he has no cognitive model for what to expect in having cancer. Further, in his life narrative, he has already struggled with a deadly disease and to be struck with a second one feels unjust and reactivates fears about his own mortality.

As of 2003, the CDC reported that more than 60,000 people in the United States were estimated to be over 50 with AIDS. Older adults also represent a substantial share of new diagnoses[39] with the number of new diagnoses in people aged 65 and older having grown 10-fold between 1994 and 2004 (from 1008 to 10,002); this number is expected to keep growing.[39-41] As people with HIV grow older and live longer, and as older adults increase among numbers of the newly infected, diagnoses of non-ADMs are becoming more common.[39-41]

The risk of one such non-ADM, prostate cancer, appears to be higher and more virulent among HIV-infected men; and African-American men, who are also disproportionately affected by the HIV epidemic, have a higher incidence of, and mortality, due to prostate cancer.[31] Thus, it is particularly problematic for HIV positive, gay, African-American men who experience being "triply biased" by their race, sexual orientation, and HIV status. Further, many such men find that disclosing a prostate cancer diagnosis is yet another "coming out" reactivating past anxieties around coming out as a gay man and coming out as being HIV positive.[30] Treatment for prostate cancer can cause ejaculation problems and erectile dysfunction[28];

impacting sexuality which furthers feelings of stigmatization. Finally, within the gay community, many HIV-positive men have found HIV specializing physicians who are more sensitive and knowledgeable about the health issues of gay men. Finding urologists who are sensitive to issues faced by gay HIV-positive men can be far more challenging.[30]

PALLIATIVE CARE AND END OF LIFE ISSUES

The availability of HIV-specific therapies has altered the way in which palliative care is viewed for patients with HIV. In the first decade of the epidemic, death swiftly followed an HIV diagnosis, usually within months, and HIV care was almost fully understood in the context of palliative care.[42] Yet as protease inhibitors became available in the mid-1990s, and mortality rates began to decline, the view of HIV care shifted to a chronic disease model, and thus interest in HIV palliative care was replaced by optimism for "curative" therapies. Despite this, HIV/AIDS continues to cause considerable morbidity and mortality.[43]

While the death rate due to HIV/AIDS dropped sharply following the advent of HAART, that decline has since plateaued; currently there are approximately 15,000 deaths per year due to HIV/AIDS. The reduction in morbidity and mortality has not universally affected all demographic groups: HIV-infected Whites have experienced improved outcomes while this has been less so for African Americans and Latinos with HIV. HIV/AIDS continues to be the leading cause of death for young African-American and Latino men and women aged 20–50.[42] Ability to access or adhere to treatment regimens has been problematic for patients with psychiatric illness, substance abuse, or other severe psychosocial stressors. Even patients who have the social and emotional resources to access and adhere to HAART can still experience progressive viral resistance despite therapy.[43] Finally, mortality rates among HIV patients have been steadily increasing from co-occurring diseases such as both ADMs and non-ADMs, as well as Hepatitis B. Analyses of causes of death among AIDS patients consistently found between 19% and 28% were due to malignancies.[44–46] Thus, palliative care remains a focal point in HIV care.

As HIV-infected patients live longer and develop more symptoms related to opportunistic infections and medication neurotoxicity, a more integrated palliative care model is required, one which allows for the continuation of potential "curative therapies" with symptom-specific treatments.[47] In the HAART era, HIV palliative care issues include diagnosis, management, and treatment of pain; management of medical and mental health symptoms; attention to drug–drug interactions; prognosis and advance care planning; and decisions around when is the right time to withdraw disease-specific therapies.[42] Major challenges currently exist to incorporate the science of palliative care with the hopefulness of life-sustaining treatments, especially in the context of co-developing malignancies and other significant morbidities.

REFERENCES

1. Joint United Nations Programme on HIV/AIDS. *Overview of the global AIDS epidemic. 2006 Report on the global AIDS epidemic.* Geneva: UNAIDS; 2006.
2. Centers for Disease Control and Prevention. Cases of HIV infection and AIDS in the United States and dependent areas. *HIV/AIDS Surveillance Report.* 2006;18.
3. Berretta M, Cinelli R, Martellotta F, Spina M, Vaccher E, Tirelli U. Therapeutic approaches to AIDS-related malignancies. *Oncogene.* 2003;22(42):6646–6659.
4. Holtgrave DR, Curran JW. What works, and what remains to be done, in HIV prevention in the United States. *Annu Rev Public Health.* 2006;27:261–275.
5. Scadden DT. AIDS-related malignancies. *Annu Rev Med.* 2003;54:285–303.
6. Bower M, Palmieri C, Dhillon T. AIDS-related malignancies: changing epidemiology and the impact of highly active antiretroviral therapy. *Curr Opin Infect Dis.* 2006;19(1):14–19.
7. Cheung MC, Pantanowitz L, Dezube BJ. AIDS-related malignancies: emerging challenges in the era of highly active antiretroviral therapy. *Oncologist.* 2005;10(6):412–426.
8. Powles T, Nelson M, Bower M. HIV-related lung cancer—a growing concern? *Int J STD AIDS.* 2003;14(10):647–651.
9. Santos J, Palacios R, Ruiz J, Gonzalez M, Marquez M. Unusual malignant tumours in patients with HIV infection. *Int J STD AIDS.* 2002;13(10):674–676.
10. Santos J, Palacios R. Another reason to stop smoking. *Int J STD AIDS.* 2004;15(7):497.
11. Chu C, Selwyn PA. Current health disparities in HIV/AIDS. *AIDS Read.* 2008;18(3):144–148, C3.
12. Tiamson ML. Challenges in the management of the HIV patient in the third decade of AIDS. *Psychiatr Q.* 2002;73(1):51–58.
13. Wells K, Klap R, Koike A, Sherbourne C. Ethnic disparities in unmet need for alcoholism, drug abuse, and mental health care. *Am J Psychiatry.* 2001;158(12):2027–2032.
14. Schnittker J. Misgivings of medicine?: African Americans' skepticism of psychiatric medication. *J Health Soc Behav.* 2003;44(4):506–524.
15. Snowden LR. Bias in mental health assessment and intervention: theory and evidence. *Am J Public Health.* 2003;93(2):239–243.
16. Remien RH, Stirratt MJ, Dolezal C, et al. Couple-focused support to improve HIV medication adherence: a randomized controlled trial. *AIDS.* 2005;19(8):807–814.
17. Tegger MK, Crane HM, Tapia KA, Uldall KK, Holte SE, Kitahata MM. The effect of mental illness, substance use, and treatment for depression on the initiation of highly active antiretroviral therapy among HIV-infected individuals. *AIDS Patient Care STDS.* 2008;22(3):233–243.
18. Bing EG, Burnam MA, Longshore D, et al. Psychiatric disorders and drug use among human immunodeficiency virus-infected adults in the United States. *Arch Gen Psychiatry.* 2001;58(8):721–728.
19. Israelski DM, Prentiss DE, Lubega S, et al. Psychiatric co-morbidity in vulnerable populations receiving primary care for HIV/AIDS. *AIDS Care.* 2007;19(2):220–225.
20. Baillargeon JG, Paar DP, Wu H, et al. Psychiatric disorders, HIV infection and HIV/hepatitis co-infection in the correctional setting. *AIDS Care.* 2008;20(1):124–129.
21. Hays RD, Cunningham WE, Sherbourne CD, et al. Health-related quality of life in patients with human immunodeficiency virus infection in the United States: results from the HIV Cost and Services Utilization Study. *Am J Med.* 2000;108(9):714–722.
22. Heckman TG. The chronic illness quality of life (CIQOL) model: explaining life satisfaction in people living with HIV disease. *Health Psychol.* 2003;22(2):140–147.
23. Lee K, Solts B, Burns J. Investigating the psychosocial impact of anti-HIV combination therapies. *AIDS Care.* 2002;14(6):851–857.
24. Remien RH, Hirky AE, Johnson MO, Weinhardt LS, Whittier D, Le GM. Adherence to medication treatment: a qualitative study of facilitators and barriers among a diverse sample of HIV+ men and women in four US cities. *AIDS Behav.* 2003;7(1):61–72.
25. Bedino R, Chen RY, Accortt NA, et al. Trends in AIDS-defining and non-AIDS-defining malignancies among HIV-infected patients: 1989–2002. *Clin Infect Dis.* 2004;39(9):1380–1384.
26. Palefsky JM, Holly EA, Efirdc JT, et al. Anal intraepithelial neoplasia in the highly active antiretroviral therapy era among HIV-positive men who have sex with men. *AIDS.* 2005;19(13):1407–1414.
27. Palefsky JM. Anal squamous intraepithelial lesions in human immunodeficiency virus-positive men and women. *Semin Oncol.* 2000;27(4):471–479.
28. Mitteldorf D. Psychotherapy with gay prostate cancer patients. *J Gay Lesbian Psychother.* 2005;9(1/2):57–67.
29. Jackson L. Surviving yet another challenge. *J Gay Lesbian Psychother.* 2005;9(1/2):101–107.
30. Perlman G. Prostate cancer, the group, and me. *J Gay Lesbian Psychother.* 2005;9(1/2):69–90.
31. Santillo V, Lowe FC. Prostate cancer and the gay male. *J Gay Lesbian Psychother.* 2005;9(1/2):9–27.
32. Fife BL, Wright ER. The dimensionality of stigma: a comparison of its impact on the self of persons with HIV/AIDS and cancer. *J Health Soc Behav.* 2000;41(1):50–67.
33. Rolland JS. *Families, illness, & disability.* New York: Basic Books; 1994.
34. Frye V, Latka MH, Wu Y, et al. Intimate partner violence perpetration against main female partners among HIV-positive male injection drug users. *J Acquir Immune Defic Syndr.* 2007;46(Suppl 2):S101–S109.
35. El-Bassel N, Gilbert L, Wu E, et al. Intimate partner violence prevalence and HIV risks among women receiving care in emergency departments: implications for IPV and HIV screening. *Emerg Med J.* 2007;24(4):255–259.
36. Gilbert L, El-Bassel N, Wu E, Chang M. Intimate partner violence and HIV risks: a longitudinal study of men on methadone. *J Urban Health.* 2007;84(5):667–680.
37. Gielen AC, Ghandour RM, Burke JG, Mahoney P, McDonnell KA, O'Campo P. HIV/AIDS and intimate partner violence: intersecting women's health issues in the United States. *Trauma Violence Abuse.* 2007;8(2):178–198.
38. Carter EA, McGoldrick M. *The changing family life cycle: A framework for family therapy.* 2nd ed. Boston, MO: Alleyn & Bacon; 1989:15.
39. Mack KA, Ory MG. AIDS and older Americans at the end of the twentieth century. *J Acquir Immune Defic Syndr.* 2003;33(Suppl 2):S68–S75.

40. Stoff DM, Khalsa JH, Monjan A, Portegies P. Introduction: HIV/AIDS and aging. *AIDS.* 2004;18(Suppl 1):S1–S2.

41. Stoff DM. Mental health research in HIV/AIDS and aging: problems and prospects. *AIDS.* 2004;18(Suppl 1):S3–S10.

42. Selwyn PA. Palliative care for patient with human immunodeficiency virus/acquired immune deficiency syndrome. *J Palliat Med.* 2005;8(6):1248–1268.

43. Selwyn PA, Rivard M. Palliative care for AIDS: challenges and opportunities in the era of highly active anti-retroviral therapy. *J Palliat Med.* 2003;6(3):475–487.

44. Bonnet F, Lewden C, May T, et al. Malignancy-related causes of death in human immunodeficiency virus-infected patients in the era of highly active anti-retroviral therapy. *Cancer.* 2004;101(2):317–324.

45. Lewden C, Salmon D, Morlat P, et al. Causes of death among human immunodeficiency virus (HIV)-infected adults in the era of potent antiretroviral therapy: emerging role of hepatitis and cancers, persistent role of AIDS. *Int J Epidemiol.* 2005;34(1):121–130.

46. Krentz HB, Kliewer G, Gill MJ. Changing mortality rates and causes of death for HIV-infected individuals living in Southern Alberta, Canada from 1984 to 2003. *HIV Med.* 2005;6(2):99–106.

47. Selwyn PA, Forstein M. Overcoming the false dichotomy of curative vs palliative care for late-stage HIV/AIDS: "let me live the way I want to live, until I can't". *JAMA.* 2003;290(6):806–814.

CHAPTER 28

Tumor of Unknown Primary Site

Leonard B. Saltz, Steven D. Passik, and Tatiana D. Starr

INTRODUCTION

The term "cancer of unknown primary" (CUP) represents a diverse group of diseases which present complex challenges in diagnosis and therapy. Unknown primary cancer represents approximately 2% of current cancer diagnoses. Older series report the incidence to be as high as 7.8%[1]; however, many of these cases would be unlikely to remain of unknown origin with current diagnostic imaging techniques. In general, CUP implies a poor prognosis; older literature indicates extremely limited therapeutic options and an overall median survival of 4–10 months.[2-5] More recent trials have suggested a somewhat better outcome; however, these trials have been more selective of favorable performance status patients, which may account in total or in part for the better outcomes than some historical comparators.[6,7] Favorable clinical outcomes are typically limited to those patients in more treatable subgroups of CUP or to instances where a more favorable histological diagnosis can be identified.[6,8-11] Oncologic management of CUP consists of: (1) reasonable attempts to establish the CUP diagnosis; (2) a search for alternative diagnoses with better prognoses, and (3) attempts to identify factors which would establish the patient as a member of one of the more treatable subgroups of unknown primary cancer. In this chapter, we provide background medical information that serves to highlight some of the more salient psychological and psychosocial issues that arise within this patient population. Psycho-oncologists need to acknowledge that patients with CUP contend with even higher than typical levels of uncertainty than most cancer patients' face. Also, due to the fact that an unknown primary cancer is by definition metastatic, and therefore advanced, at the time of initial diagnosis, issues reflective of the advanced stage of disease must be confronted quite early in the patient's adjustment to the illness.

Definition of CUP. The term "cancer of unknown primary" (CUP) lacks a strict, universally accepted definition and is frequently also referred to as carcinoma of unknown primary, adenocarcinoma of unknown primary, occult primary cancer, or anaplastic tumor of unknown primary.[12] The lack of strictly defined criteria makes interpretation of the literature regarding unknown primary cancers difficult. In light of the more advanced techniques presently available, many tumors included in previously published series would quite likely be categorized as other diagnoses. It is therefore difficult to ascertain how this inaccuracy has affected the interpretability of survival data and other pertinent information. Reasonable criteria for establishing the diagnosis includes a thorough medical history; physical examination; and a chest, abdomen, and pelvic computed tomography (CT) scan. Some have advocated use of positron emission tomography (PET) scans,[13] however, the evidence that this is truly useful in identifying a primary is debatable. A biopsy of tumor, metastatic site or otherwise, is necessary to confirm a cancer diagnosis. The biopsy will also permit immunohistochemical evaluation, although the utility of this in definitively identifying a primary site is minimal.[14,15]

In a large number of CUP patients, the primary site of the tumor will never be found. Even in autopsy series, 15%–27% of patients will not have a discernible origin of their disease,[2,4,5,16] possibly attributed either to the extensive carcinomatosis that obscures the primary or to the immunological destruction of the original primary tumor. Primary sites of lung, pancreas, and colon have been most commonly identified during postmortem investigation, while primary sites of the liver, ovary, prostate, kidney, and bile duct account for the primary to a lesser extent.[17]

The diagnostic evaluation of CUP. As mentioned above, the evaluation of the patient with CUP begins with a detailed medical history and physical examination. Laboratory evaluation includes a complete blood count and biochemical screening profile to assess hepatic and renal function.

The use of CT scanning in unknown primary patients has become relatively routine; however, there remains a relative lack of truly useful information that would be likely to be obtained that would substantially influence the effectiveness of treatment.[14,15] In the absence of symptoms or signs suggesting a gastrointestinal primary (e.g., blood in the stool, microcytic anemia, abdominal pain, etc.), an evaluation of the gastrointestinal tract is not routinely indicated in the workup of unknown primary cancers. That having been said, such endoscopic workups are commonly performed.[18] Such workups rarely identify the primary. Furthermore, the treatment of metastatic digestive tract cancers is generally unsuccessful. The rediagnosis from metastatic CUP to metastatic gastric, pancreatic, or colorectal cancer does not improve the patient's prognosis or the efficacy of treatment. An exception would be in a patient with potentially resectable metastatic disease confined only to the liver (i.e., no nodal, mesenteric, or extraabdominal disease). In such a patient, identification of a colon primary could open up a possible surgical treatment option with the potential for cure.

Pathologic evaluation. Following the initial clinical diagnosis of CUP, expert histological evaluation is required to ensure that the tumor is indeed a carcinoma and does not represent a more treatable form of malignancy. Adenocarcinoma of the moderately- or well-differentiated variety represents a majority of cases reviewed. If indicated, the pathologist may employ specific-immunohistochemical stains to confirm this diagnosis. Further pathological characterization is rarely of substantial benefit should the pathologic evaluation reveal a moderately- to well-differentiated adenocarcinoma, although some investigators have attempted to utilize immunohistochemical characterization for further analysis.[19] However, further study is warranted should the tumor display a poorly differentiated or anaplastic appearance. Specific-immunohistochemical studies may be employed to confirm or exclude a lymphoma, a far more treatable malignancy with a significantly more favorable prognosis.[20] Although not specific, the leukocyte common antigen (LCA) is a highly sensitive marker for lymphoma and is frequently employed in this type of evaluation. A diagnosis of lymphoma is essentially excluded in the presence of a negative LCA and a positive cytokeratins, the hallmark of carcinomas. Within the cytokeratin-positives carcinomas, a thyroglobulin stain should be sought to rule out a thyroid primary. Markers for neuroendocrine differentiation, such as chromogranin, synaptophytin, or a Gremilius stain is used to rule out the presence of neuroendocrine tumor of unknown primary.[21]

Cytogenetics. Cytogenetic evaluation has recently been employed to facilitate the identification of the origin of poorly differentiated tumors. A study at Memorial Sloan-Kettering Cancer Center examined 40 patients who presented with a poorly differentiated carcinoma.[22] Using a southern blot analysis and florescence in situ hybridization for the identification of an isochromosome 12p abnormality in a midline tumor distribution, which is a chromosomal aberration associated with germ cell tumors, a specific diagnosis of germ cell tumor was suggested in 30% of patients. This group of patients achieved a 75% response rate to cisplatin therapy as compared to a response rate of 18% in the larger group of patients who presented with a carcinoma. Cytogenetics can also be used to identify mutations suggestive of Ewing sarcoma, or lymphomas, both of which have specific and effective chemotherapeutic treatment options.

Tumor markers. In contrast to patients with moderately- to well-differentiated cancers, the evaluation of germ cell tumor markers is indicated when evaluating a male patient with a poorly differentiated unknown primary cancer. An elevated prostate-specific antigen (PSA) may open the option for hormonal therapy and should be obtained in appropriate older male patients. A serum thyroglobulin can be used to rule out a thyroid primary. Other serum tumor markers are of less usefulness. Markers such as carcinoembryonic antigen (CEA), CA-125 and CA 19–9 are not specific enough for any particular tumor to be used for diagnostic purposes. Considering the high cost of these markers and the lack of useful information provided to the management of the patient, they are not appropriate for the workup of an unknown primary cancer.

Treatable types of carcinoma. Except in cases where the primary being sought is responsive to available treatments or will otherwise change the patient's clinical management, costly radiographic studies, and invasive diagnostic procedures do not benefit the patient and may heighten anxiety. Therefore, the workup should be geared toward ruling in or out identifiable primaries or histologies that will convey either a specific therapy or a more favorable prognosis. In men, germ cell cancers, either extragonadal or gonadal, are highly curable with chemotherapy and should not be overlooked. Thus, testicular ultrasound is performed and serum levels of tumor markers alpha fetal protein (AFP) and beta human choriogonadotropin (βHCG) are drawn in male patients with a histology of either consistent with a germ cell tumor or with poorly differentiated carcinoma. Similarly, a diagnosis of prostate carcinoma would result in specific therapy. Many prostate cancers are hormonally sensitive and respond well initially to androgen-ablative therapy. Therefore, a serum PSA is drawn in male patients, especially in the presence of bone metastases.

In women, breast carcinomas are frequently hormonally responsive and amenable to systemic chemotherapy. Thus, a careful breast examination and mammography is performed in female patients with unknown primary cancers. Ovarian cancer, especially when confined to the abdomen, carries a more favorable prognosis and also responds to specific therapy. A gynecologic evaluation of this possibility through a careful pelvic examination (with transvaginal ultrasound if indicated) is performed. Because the ovary is frequently the site of metastasis from other tumors, the presence of an ovarian mass does not necessarily identify that mass as the primary.

Finally, thyroid carcinomas may be treatable with radioactive iodine and should, therefore, be taken into diagnostic consideration in CUP patients as well. A serum thyroglobulin level or stain of the tumor tissue for thyroglobulin may be helpful.

The identification of treatable subgroups within the CUP population. In cases where the workup outlined above fails to redefine the diagnosis beyond that of unknown primary, the oncologist is then obligated to look for specific subgroups within this diagnostic category that may carry a more favorable prognosis. Several such subgroups have been identified.

Male patients, typically under the age of 50, who have a poorly differentiated histology and a tumor distribution more or less symmetrical about the midline (i.e., retroperitoneal or mediastinal adenopathy, bilateral multiple lung masses, cervical adenopathy, etc.) are felt to potentially have an unrecognized extragonadal germ cell tumor and represent one such subgroup. Careful testicular examination and testicular ultrasound is obtained, but cisplatin-based therapy along the lines of a testicular regimen is indicated even in the absence of an identified primary. One study of 71 such patients demonstrated a partial response rate of 54%, complete response rate of 22%, and a 5-year disease-free survival rate of 13%.[23]

Solitary site of disease. Several small series and anecdotes have suggested that patients with a solitary site of disease inconsistent with a primary site (i.e., carcinoma in a lymph node or cluster of lymph nodes) carry a superior prognosis compared to patients with multiple sites of disease. Definitive local management including surgical resection, localized radiation therapy, or a combination of the two, has resulted in prolonged disease-free survival and some apparent cures. These data cannot be extrapolated to patients with more than one site of disease. Surgical debulking of unknown primary cancers and the administration of adjuvant postoperative chemotherapy should not be routinely undertaken.

Axillary mass. The presentation of an isolated lymph node containing carcinoma in an axilla of a female patient represents a specific and prognostically favorable subgroup of CUP. Such patients are considered to have stage II breast cancer until/unless proven otherwise. Mammography and careful examination of the ipsilateral breast may reveal the primary and remove the patient from the category of unknown primary. Even if this workup is negative, evidence suggests that a primary tumor of the breast will be identified in greater than 50% of mastectomy specimens in patients who undergo this procedure. Modified radical mastectomy with axillary dissection has been recommended as initial management for otherwise healthy patients.[24,25] The option of axillary dissection and whole breast radiotherapy has also been advocated.[26] While at least short-term follow-up appears favorable, there is potential concern regarding the risk of local recurrence in the breast, since the exact site in the breast is unknown, and localized excision or "lumpectomy" with a radiation cone-down or "boost" to the primary site is not possible.

Since the disease has been clinically defined as stage II, adjuvant chemotherapy routinely used for stage II breast cancer would be appropriate. An investigation for estrogen and progesterone receptors of the tumor in patients with an axillary mass/unknown primary, with subsequent hormonal therapy for receptor-positive tumors, is also indicated.

Neuroendocrine differentiation. Investigations have shown that poorly differentiated tumors of unknown primary that demonstrate immunohistochemical evidence of neuroendocrine differentiation have a high clinical response rate to cisplatin-based chemotherapy. In a study of 29 such patients, 24% had a partial response and 48% achieved a complete response, with 13% alive and disease-free at 2 years.[27] Chromogranin, synaptophytin, or Gremelius stains should be utilized to investigate for neuroendocrine differentiation.

Oncologic therapy of unknown primary cancers. The therapy for more favorable prognostic subgroups of unknown primary cancers has been outlined above. Such therapies frequently involve aggressive treatments such as high-dose cisplatin-based chemotherapy, surgery, or combined modality approaches. Patients with unknown primary cancers who do not fall into one of these specific favorable subgroups have, in general, a poor prognosis, and available data do not suggest that systemic chemotherapy or other aggressive measures are capable of conferring a survival advantage to treated patients. Therefore, any therapy undertaken in these patients should be regarded as strictly palliative. For this reason, patients who are relatively asymptomatic may achieve no discernible benefit from palliative chemotherapy, and expectant observation and supportive care are often the most appropriate initial treatment options for these patients. The oncologist must remain cognizant that there are, both, limited benefits and potential toxicity involved with chemotherapeutic treatments in this group of patients with CUP.

A trial of systemic chemotherapy may be justified in patients who have or develop symptoms attributable to his/her malignant disease if there is reason to believe that a decrease in tumor size or bulk will result in the improvement of such symptoms. Patients with rapidly progressing disease under observation may also be appropriate candidates for treatment, since such patients could be expected to imminently develop symptoms.

The choice of chemotherapy for unknown primary cancers, other than in patients with better prognostic subgroups, has not been well defined. In the absence of demonstrated efficacious therapy, enrollment in a clinical trial of investigational agents may be appropriately considered. In the absence of a clinical trial, treatments have frequently been recommended on the basis of predominant tumor location site. Tumors predominantly above the diaphragm are often treated with a relatively well-tolerated lung cancer regimen such as mitomycin plus vinblastine. Tumors predominantly below the diaphragm are presumed to be more likely of gastrointestinal origin. Fluorouracil, either alone or modulated with leucovorin, is the typical chemotherapeutic agent employed. Whether combined use of cytotoxic agents is more efficacious than single agents in the CUP population is unclear at this time. Outside of a clinical trial, one must be cautiously aware of the increased toxicity associated with such combinations.

Several trials have reported the use of various chemotherapy regimens for unknown primary cancer patients. It is important to remember that to enter these trials; patients were required to have sufficient renal, hepatic, and bone marrow function, as well as high enough performance status to meet the study's eligibility criteria. Performance status (a measure of the patients overall energy level and state of well-being) is a strong prognostic indicator. Patients with a good performance status, who are up and about most of the day and who are not actively losing weight, have a much higher response rate and lower toxicity rate for chemotherapies than do more debilitated patients. Thus, results of clinical trials may not be generalizable to more debilitated patients. Also, appreciation of the importance of performance status has increased in recent years, and eligibility criteria for trials have gotten stricter. Thus more recent trial may well represent a better prognosis group of patients than older ones. Regardless of these study artifact issues, a patient who is not fully ambulatory, or is otherwise severely debilitated with multiple medical co-morbidities and who has an unknown primary cancer is therefore usually a poorer candidate for aggressive cytotoxic therapy. In these patients supportive care should be strongly considered as the primary mode of treatment.

PSYCHIATRIC AND PSYCHOSOCIAL ASPECTS OF CUP SITES

Unlike in cases of cancers of known primary sites, such as prostrate or breast cancer, the CUP diagnosis implies to the patient and their family a general lack of information among oncologists about their disease and higher than typical levels of uncertainty.[28] Patients generally need and desire an understanding of most or all aspects of their disease. Patients who are better educated about the various aspects of their illness generally have an increased sense of mastery and control, and thus adjust more successfully.[29] Because of the uncertainty that is engendered by a diagnosis of CUP, clinical experience suggests that this patient population is at elevated risk for problems of adjustment and the development of psychiatric symptoms. They are a diverse patient population and are poorly studied group from the vantage point of quality of life and psychosocial adjustment.

Psychological adjustment to CUP. In contrast to the somewhat more homogeneous populations of patients with cancer of common sites and the homogeneity of some of the accompanying psychosocial issues that correspond to these illnesses, patients with CUP comprise a population somewhat more highly diverse in age and gender and lack some of the important commonalities that other groups of patients share.[30] The most salient psychosocial aspects that this unfortunate group of patients share are: (1) the guarded to poor prognosis that results from the diagnosis of metastatic disease at initial presentation[31]; (2) the liability to psychological problems that is associated with the inability to traverse a process of adjustment to illness that accompanies the initial diagnosis being made in advanced stages of disease; (3) the uncertainty that is conveyed by the inability to locate a primary site of disease and thus, limited disease-related information; and (4) the psychological difficulties associated with expectant observation as a primary therapeutic approach and the failure to understand the oncology team's lack of aggressiveness toward further diagnostic evaluation and treatment. Research that identifies and better describes the psychiatric and quality of life issues in the CUP population is greatly needed. Given the grim prognosis and presence of advanced illness, psychosocial interventions for these patients are generally brief, supportive and psychoeducational in nature and focused upon issues common to patients with advanced illness (see Chapter 37).

A diagnosis of CUP often represents the presence of advanced, metastatic disease.[32] Unlike patients with localized disease and a more favorable prognosis, CUP patients are denied the opportunity to acclimate to the reality of having cancer before being confronted with issues of advanced, sometimes terminal illness. The oncologist and psycho-oncologist share the formidable task of engaging the patient in open and frank discussions regarding what, if any, treatment approaches are available and reaffirm their commitment to the total care for the patient. Clinical experience has shown that the typical levels of denial and disbelief common to the initial stages of adjustment to all cancer crises are sometimes more pronounced in CUP patients. These reactions often "crystallize" in the patient's failure to understand the futility of seeking out the primary cancer and the desire to initiate "psychological" chemotherapy (i.e., chemotherapy that is unlikely to benefit them other than to provide a sense of "doing something"). The recommendation of expectant observation to the asymptomatic patient that has metastatic cancer can be a difficult one for the patient to accept. Offering the patient emotional support and mobilizing them to utilize support groups and make positive changes in lifestyle (smoking cessation, healthful diet, stress management, exercise, if possible) will permit the patient to retain a sense of control, hope, and optimism.[28,33,34] When this disbelief gives way patient's generally need assistance with anticipatory grief.[35] The overwhelmingly mysterious nature of CUP may contribute to the patient's poor emotional adjustment to illness. Certain levels of depression and anxiety are to be expected in newly diagnosed CUP patients; however, prolonged symptoms of anxiety and depression can unnecessarily diminish the patient's quality of life and should be the focus of care.[36] Clinicians must take into consideration issues common to patients with advanced disease, such as communication with family and contemplation of one's mortality.[37] Psychiatric consultation should be utilized to evaluate and treat psychiatric co-morbidity. The use of brief psychotherapy that reinforces positive coping skills is beneficial in helping patients face advanced stages of illness.[28] Pharmacological interventions may be utilized to treat distressing symptoms such as fatigue, sleep disturbances, and more formal psychiatric syndromes, much as they are in other patients with advanced cancer. It is important to recognize the significant role of psychiatric treatment in the palliative care of CUP patients as untreated psychiatric conditions, such as depression, mistakenly viewed as normal consequences of such difficult situations, may be quite debilitating and worsen problems of patient and family adjustment.

Quality of life issues and the continuation of treatment. A diagnosis of CUP presents a multitude of complex issues to the patient, family and staff. Decision-making about treatment can be highly emotional and draining and a source of family disagreement. Patients diagnosed with CUP frequently believe that further diagnostic evaluation will increase the likelihood of identifying the primary tumor and improve their prognosis. Unfortunately, this is generally not the case and may unnecessarily contribute to anxiety and psychological distress on the part of the patient. Once the more treatable subtypes of unknown primary cancer are ruled out, identification of the primary is often not an important. Other possible diagnoses carry an equally poor prognosis and limited number of therapeutic options. Therefore, it is crucial for the oncologist and other physicians involved to carefully communicate to the patient and family the insignificance of identification of the primary tumor. Futile attempts by, both, the oncologist and the patient to locate the primary tumor will subject the patient to an exhaustive and costly series of diagnostic tests that will ultimately increase the risk of complications and psychological distress.

Consultation by psycho-oncologists may assist the CUP patient in evaluating impact of continuing diagnostic workups to locate the primary tumor and subsequent treatment options on their quality of life. The patient's age, family and social structure, religious beliefs, and value system should be taken into consideration when evaluating the patient with CUP who is considering various treatment options as the two vignettes below illustrate: A 35-year-old married father of two young children and a 75-year-old male, also married with two adult children both with CUP are given the opportunity to participate in a experimental protocol involving the administration of a combination chemotherapy modality. Both patients are informed by researchers of the potential for serious toxicity and the limited benefits to be expected from this treatment. A psycho-oncologist is requested for consultation with both patients. During consultation, the 35-year old CUP patient insists upon receiving the experimental chemotherapy regimen, regardless of the poor prognosis and high toxicity. The patient states to the clinician that the decision to not participate in the protocol would represent his "giving up" and subsequent "abandonment" of his family. He notes that even if he dies, he would have gone to his grave "knowing that (he) fought for (his) kids." In contrast, the older patient decides that, given the low likelihood of receiving benefits from the experimental chemotherapy, he would rather "be in my own home and spend the time I have left with my family."

The above situation represents how similar cases can greatly differ when issues regarding quality of life are taken into consideration. Psycho-oncologists can be instrumental in helping the CUP patient evaluate the continuation of treatment and the subsequent effects on their quality of life and fit the options to their value system. Even if the continuation of treatment is thought to be somewhat futile, the role of the clinician is not to outright discourage further treatment. Instead, the psycho-oncologist should assist the patient in evaluating the impact of further treatment on their quality of life. Discussion of issues regarding quality of life should proceed in a nonjudgmental and empathetic manner and respect the patient's wishes. Should the patient agree, family members should be included in all discussion of treatment options and quality of life to minimize the chance for miscommunication and allow for open exploration of differences of opinion amongst family members.

Dealing with anticipatory grief. The diagnosis of advanced cancer, such as CUP, is overwhelming and emotionally exhausting for both patient and family. Frequently, patients are aware of the seriousness of their disease, but are hesitant to discuss their approaching death with their family either because they do not wish to upset the family or appear to be "giving up the fight" against their cancer.[35] Family members may try to protect the patient from the burden of their fears and take the same approach when talking with the patient. Unfortunately, this approach may lead to isolation of the patient. The psycho-oncologist can be instrumental in facilitating open communication between the patient and family. After meeting with the family and patient separately, the clinician may feel it appropriate to hold a group discussion with the patient and family together to discuss the emotional issues of anticipatory grief. Such an approach may significantly improve the patient's quality of life in the terminal stage of illness and subsequently contribute to a healthier period of bereavement for family members.

Alternative therapies. Because of the limited therapeutic options available to treat CUP, clinicians should not be surprised to learn that the patient has begun to experiment with different alternative therapies. Alternative therapies are any treatments that have not either undergone clinical evaluation and/or been shown to demonstrate any medicinal value. The use of alternative approaches to therapy may reflect the patient's loss of hope and/or disillusionment with conventional medicine or simply the desire to mobilize all options for a sense of control over the unknown. Patients who utilize alternative therapies are frequently thought of as having psychological problems. However, they are typically well-adjusted, educated, and desire a sense of control over stressful situations. Psycho-oncologists can be helpful in conveying to the medical staff the patient's motives for taking an alternative approach to treatment. In addition, staff should be permitted to discuss their interpretations and feelings toward the patient actions in an attempt to minimize any resentment that may be present. The clinician should also confer with the patient and family about the use of alternative therapies in a nonjudgmental and empathetic manner, recognizing its psychological significance, while trying to dissuade patients from the use of dangerous alternatives and possibly very costly ones. Patients should be advised that the continued use of alternative therapies may negatively interact with medications they are receiving and could interfere with medical treatment.

CONCLUSION

Cancer of unknown primary constitutes a heterogeneous group of metastatic cancers. With a few notable exceptions, these patients carry a poor prognosis, and therapy is strictly palliative. Proper clinical management includes a careful evaluation to rule out the more treatable possible primaries and histologies, and to rule out those specific subgroups of unknown primary carcinoma patients in whom specific aggressive therapies have been shown to be efficacious. If the clinical and pathological evaluation fails to identify a favorable prognostic histology or subgroup, then the team has an obligation to try and protect the patient from unwarranted exhaustive searches for the primary, and to communicate effectively to the patient the lack of utility of such searches. The potential for toxicities that may be encountered from chemotherapy must be carefully weighed against the limited possibility of clinical benefit in this patient population when deciding upon the appropriateness of therapy.

Psycho-oncologists must be cognizant of the patient's perception and the potential psychological impact of the term "unknown" on CUP patients and their families. Patients may experience many negative emotions (i.e., anger, frustration, anxiety, depression) that are both a part of and can interfere with normal adjustment. Given the uncertainty that constitutes CUP, the psycho-oncologist should act to improve communication between the patient and physician regarding the insignificance of locating an unknown primary when other subtypes have been excluded, and its prognosis, and treatment. Research is needed to further identify psychosocial issues, including the prevalence of psychiatric disorders, and the development of interventions designed specifically for patients with CUP. CUP presents a difficult challenge to the psycho-oncologist and medical staff in helping both the patient and family adjust to this frightening group of diseases.

REFERENCES

1. Greco FA, Hainsworth JD. Cancer of unknown primary site. In: DeVita VT Jr, Lawrence T, Rosenberg SA, (eds). *Cancer: Principles and practice of oncology, eighth edition.* 7th ed. Philadelphia, PA: Lippincott Williams & Wilkins; 2008:2363–2387.

2. Jordan WE III, Shildt RA. Adenocarcinoma of unknown primary site. The brooke army medical center experience. *Cancer.* 1985;55(4):857–860.

3. Moertel DG, Reitemeier RJ, Schutt AJ, Hahn RG. Treatment of the patient with adenocarcinoma of unknown origin. *Cancer.* 1972;30(6):1469–1473.

4. Nystrom JS, Weiner JM, Heffelfinger-Juttner J, Irwin LE, Bateman JR, Wolf RM. Metastatic and histologic presentations in unknown primary cancer. *Semin Oncol.* 1977;4:53–58.

5. Schildt RA, Lennedy PS, Chen TT, Athens JW, O'Bryan RM, Blacerzak SP. Management of patients with metastatic carcinoma of unknown origin: a Southwest Oncology Group study. *Cancer Treat Rep.* 1983;67:77–79.

6. Greco FA, Burris HA III, Litchy S, et al. Gemcitabine, Carboplatin, and Paclitaxel for patients with carcinoma of unknown primary site: a Minnie Pearl Cancer Research Network Study. *J Clin Oncol.* 2002 Mar 15;20(6):1651–1656.

7. Greco FA, Rodriguez GI, Shaffer DW, et al. Carcinoma of unknown primary site: sequential treatment with Paclitaxel/Carboplatin/Etoposide and Gemcitabine/Irinotecan: A Minnie Pearl Cancer Research Network Phase II Trial. *Oncologist.* 2004 Nov 1;9(6):644–652.

8. Greco FA, Hainsworth JD. The management of patients with adenocarcinoma and poorly differentiated carcinoma of unknown primary site. *Semin Oncol.* 1989;16(Suppl 6):116–122.

9. Greco FA, Hainsworth JD. Cancer of unknown primary site. In: DeVita VT, Hellman S, Rosenberg SA, (eds). *Cancer : Principles & practice of oncology : Pancreatic cancer.* 4th ed. Philadelphia: Lippincott Williams & Wilkins; 1993:2072–2092.

10. Raber MN. Cancers of unknown primary origin. In: MacDonald JS HD, Mayer RJ, (eds). *Manual of oncologic therapeutics.* 3rd ed. Philadelphia, PA: JB Lippincott; 1995:308–311.

11. Sporn JR, Greenberg BR. Empiric chemotherapy in patients with carcinoma of unknown primary site. *Am J Med.* 1990;88(1):49–55.

12. Pavlidis N, Briasoulis E, Hainsworth J, Greco FA. Diagnostic and therapeutic management of cancer of an unknown primary. *Eur J Cancer.* 2003 Sep;39(14):1990–2005.

13. Seve P, Billotey C, Broussolle C, Dumontet C, Mackey JR. The role of 2-deoxy-2-[F-18]fluoro-D-glucose positron emission tomography in disseminated carcinoma of unknown primary site. *Cancer.* 2007 Jan 15;109(2):292–299.

14. Abbruzzese JL, Abbruzzese MC, Lenzi R, Hess KR, Raber MN. Analysis of a diagnostic strategy for patients with suspected tumors of unknown origin. *J Clin Oncol.* 1995 Aug;13(8):2094–2103.

15. Frost P, Raber MN, Abbruzzese JL. Unknown primary tumors as a unique clinical and biologic entity: a hypothesis. *Cancer Bull.* 1989;41:139–141.

16. Didolkar MS, Fanous N, Elias EG, Moore RH. Metastatic carcinomas from occult primary tumors. A study of 254 patients. *Ann Surg.* 1977 Nov;186(5):625–630.

17. Greco FA. Therapy of adenocarcinoma of unknown primary: are we making progress? *J Natl Compr Canc Netw.* 2008 Nov;6(10):1061–1067.

18. Casciato DA, Tabbarah HJ. Metastases on unknown origin. In: Haskell CM, (ed). *Cancer treatment.* 3rd ed. Philadelphia: WB Saunders; 1990.

19. van de Wouw AJ, Jansen RL, Griffioen AW, Hillen HF. Clinical and immunohistochemical analysis of patients with unknown primary tumour. A search for prognostic factors in UPT. *Anticancer Res.* 2004 Jan-Feb;24(1):297–301.

20. Horning SJ, Carrier EK, Rouse RV, Warnke RA, Michie SA. Lymphomas presenting as histologically unclassified neoplasms: characteristics and response to treatment. *J Clin Oncol.* 1989 Sep;7(9):1281–1287.

21. Mackay B, Ordonez NG. Pathological evaluation of neoplasms with unknown primary tumor site. *Semin Oncol.* 1993 Jun;20(3):206–228.

22. Ilson DH, Motzer RJ, Rodriguez E, Chaganti RS, Bosl GJ. Genetic analysis in the diagnosis of neoplasms of unknown primary tumor site. *Semin Oncol.* 1993 Jun;20(3):229–237.

23. Greco FA, Vaughn WK, Hainsworth JD. Advanced poorly differentiated carcinoma of unknown primary site: recognition of a treatable syndrome. *Ann Intern Med.* 1986 Apr;104(4):547–553.

24. Ashikari R, Rosen PP, Urban JA, Senoo T. Breast cancer presenting as an axillary mass. *Ann Surg.* 1976 Apr;183(4):415–417.

25. Patel J, Nemoto T, Rosner D, Dao TL, Pickren JW. Axillary lymph node metastasis from an occult breast cancer. *Cancer.* 1981 Jun 15;47(12):2923–2927.

26. Ellerbroek N, Holmes F, Singletary E, Evans H, Oswald M, McNeese M. Treatment of patients with isolated axillary nodal metastases from an occult primary carcinoma consistent with breast origin. *Cancer.* 1990 Oct 1;66(7):1461–1467.

27. Hainsworth JD, Johnson DH, Greco FA. Poorly differentiated neuroendocrine carcinoma of unknown primary site. A newly recognized clinicopathologic entity. *Ann Intern Med.* 1988 Sep 1;109(5):364–371.

28. Loscalzo M, Brintzenhofeszoc K. Brief crisis counseling. In: Holland JC, Breitbart W, Jacobsen PB, et al., (eds). *Psychooncology.* New York, NY: Oxford University Press; 1998:662–675.

29. Merluzzi TV, Nairn RC, Hegde K, Martinez Sanchez MA, Dunn L. Self-efficacy for coping with cancer: revision of the Cancer Behavior Inventory (version 2.0). *Psychooncology.* 2001 May-Jun;10(3):206–217.

30. Pavlidis N, Briasoulis E, Hainsworth J, Greco FA. Diagnostic and therapeutic management of cancer of an unknown primary. *Eur J Cancer.* 2003;39(14):1990–2005.

31. Neumann KH, Nystrom JS. Metastatic cancer of unknown origin: nonsquamous cell type. *Semin Oncol.* 1982;9(4):427–434.

32. Hainsworth JD, Greco FA. Treatment of patients with cancer of an unknown primary site. *N Engl J Med.* 1993 July 22;329(4):257–263.

33. Holland JC, Gooen-Piels J. Principles of psycho-oncology. In: Holland JC FE, (eds). *Cancer medicine,* Vol 5th ed. Hamilton, ON: B.C. Decker Inc; 2000:943–958.

34. Spencer SM, Carver CS, Price AA. Psychological and social factors in adaptation. In: Holland JC, Breitbart W, Jacobsen PB, et al., (eds). *Psycho-oncology.* New York, NY: Oxford University Press; 1998:211–222.

35. Casarett D, Kutner JS, Abrahm J, for the End-of-Life Care Consensus Panell. Life after death: a practical approach to grief and bereavement. *Ann Intern Med.* 2001 Feb 6;134(3):208–215.

36. Wilson KG, Chochinov HM, Graham Skirko M, et al. Depression and anxiety disorders in palliative cancer care. *J Pain Symptom Manage.* 2007;33(2):118–129.

37. National Comprehensive Cancer Network. NCCN practice guidelines for the management of psychosocial distress. *Oncology (Huntingt).* 1999;13(5A):113–147.

CHAPTER 29

Psychological Issues Related to Common Tumors in the Developing World

Twalib A. Ngoma and Diwani B. Msemo

INTRODUCTION

There is common understanding among clinicians treating cancer patients in the developing world that the suffering of the body as a result of growing tumors leads to the suffering of the mind. In spite of this, it is appalling that few clinicians in these countries translate this understanding into action in their practice. In most cases the psychological issues receive very little attention and most patients make their psychological cancer journeys alone. The diagnosis of cancer to patients in developing countries is in most instances equated to death. This evokes intense emotional crisis and loss of hope.

The loss of hope, a fundamental human experience manifesting as an energy which brings life and joy, influences the psychological state and behavior of patients. As patients continue on the cancer illness trajectory which is marked by increasing disability, pain and realization that cure or prolonged reprieve from death is impossible they experience multiple psychological problems. The diagnosis of cancer also brings out family issues such as—How will the children live without their father or mother? How will other dependants in the extended family live once the patient dies? A lot of questions remain unanswered and this leads to further psychological damage.

Most of these problems are left unresolved in developing countries because most clinicians do not have adequate skills to deal with them. The impact of this on the quality of life of the patients and their family members is immense.

This chapter highlights with case reports some psychological issues which have an impact on the quality of life of patients with common cancers in developing countries. The areas which are addressed include

- Myths about cancer
- Fear of Recurrence
- Sexual problems
- Pain perception
- Fatigue
- Guilty of delaying diagnosis
- Guilty for doing things that may have caused cancer
- Changes in physical appearance
- Depression
- Sleep difficulties
- Changes in what they are able to do after cancer treatment
- The burden the cancer may have on finances
- The burden the cancer may have on the loved ones
- Concerns about whether they will be able to father children or get pregnant

MYTHS ABOUT CANCER

Some cultures in developing countries, associate cancer with evil spirits sent by their ancestors because the ancestors are not happy with how the patients conduct their life. In this scenario, the patient feels guilty of misconduct and/or violation of cultural taboos. Furthermore the patient is made to strongly believe that disease can only be cured by appeasing the ancestors through traditional healers. No matter what is done in the hospital it is hard to make these patients find peace within themselves. In addition, majority of the patients believe that both radiotherapy and surgery are bad treatments which no one should try on them because they make the disease worse. There is belief in some developing countries

that surgery makes cancer spread and radiotherapy kills' patient and not the cancer. Although this is not true, since most patients present with very advanced disease and die as a result of it whenever radiotherapy or any form of surgery is performed most people associate the death with the treatment given.

FEAR OF CANCER RECURRENCE

Cancer recurrence is defined as return of cancer after treatment and after a period of time during which the cancer could not be detected. (The length of time is not clearly defined.) The same cancer may come back in the same place where it first started or in another place in the body. For example, breast cancer may return in the chest wall (even if the breast was removed).

CASE STUDY

Zuwena, 40-year-old lady, had a mastectomy for breast cancer, followed by chemotherapy and radiation to her chest wall. Following the treatment, her doctor told her that no cancer could be found in her body and although she would be given an appointment to be seen for follow-up every 4–6 months for the next 5 years, he feels like the worst was over. Zuwena responded by saying it was hard for her to trust that her cancer was gone and she wanted to know whether her cancer would come back after the 5 years. Specifically she wanted to know the odds of her cancer coming back. But what she really wanted was to feel sure that she would never have cancer again. She was in a "holding pattern." She felt like a cancer survivor, ready to put the experience behind her. On the other hand, she was afraid that she would be reliving it all again soon if the cancer does come back. In addition to this she still had issues and concerns. She had been seeing her doctor quite regularly; now, suddenly, she is told she doesn't have to visit for many months at a time. The thought of not seeing her doctor made her anxious and sad because she felt alone and lost without the support of her healthcare team who had become an important part of her life. She was also not sure whether she would be able to raise some money for the bus fare from her village to the hospital. When she came back for the first follow-up visit she reported that she found that going back to her family role was not as easy as she had thought it would be. Things that she did before the cancer were now being done by others. The mother-in-law was not willing to give the tasks back to her because she was of the opinion that she was not well completely. As a result of this the emotions that were put aside during cancer treatment came flooding back and she felt overwhelmed with sadness, anger, and fear. She felt emotionally exhausted and tired all the time. Although she wanted to believe it's over and put the cancer behind her she couldn't. She was all the time occupied with thoughts like,

> Will it come back?
> What are the chances it will come back?
> How will I know it has come back?
> What will I do if it comes back?
> When will it come back?

The fear gripped her; she had trouble sleeping, being close with her partner, and even had trouble making simple decisions. In short she says she was emotionally overwhelmed and has never been herself after the diagnosis of cancer.

SEXUALITY

In developing countries women with breast cancer feel less feminine than the rest of women because they have lost their breast. Those who are sexually active and have cancer of the cervix are more vulnerable since they cannot perform as they used to do and cannot bear children after radiotherapy. Owing to lack of awareness about cancer, its causes, and its treatment, some men and other family members tend to stigmatize cancer patients making their life miserable. Foul smelling discharge as it happens to most of them with locally advanced disease makes women unattractive to their spouses hence increasing the chance for separation. For those who get a fistulae, the situation becomes more complicated psychologically and the majority end up getting divorced by their spouses.

PAIN PERCEPTION

Cancer in developing countries is synonymous with pain. Most patients present with advanced disease with pain as the commonest symptom. It is therefore no wonder that the word cancer is associated with pain. Since pain control and palliative care services are nonexistent or less developed in most developing countries most patients endure agonizing pain to the end of their lives.

SOCIAL ECONOMIC ISSUES

Most people in developing countries are very poor, living with less than a dollar per day. This makes it very difficult for them to afford cancer treatment which is very expensive. Even in countries which offer free cancer treatment, the indirect costs such as fares to the hospital and food are too high for poor patients. In most cases the family has to raise funds by selling family assets only to be frustrated by the eventual outcome which is death. When death occurs in the hospital which in most cases is very far from the home of the patient, transporting the dead body back home is the expected norm. This is very expensive and a great source of stress to the family.

CANCER OF CERVIX

This is the most common cancer affecting women in developing countries. Initially the age group affected was mostly postmenopausal women who are sexually inactive. Recently there has been a significant shift toward young and sexually active women. Psychological impact of this disease is devastating in both morbidity and mortality. Further more human immunodeficiency virus/acquired immunodeficiency syndrome (HIV/AIDS) has complicated the problems especially when women are affected by both. This again happens in young productive and sexually reproductive women hence increasing family psychological burden. Late presentation is the main problem in these patients. Lack of awareness about cancer, ignorance, poverty, and strong cultural belief in traditional medicine are some of the contributing factors to these late presentations. This brings about tremendous psychological effects as seen in case report below.

CASE STUDY

Mwanamvua, 45 years old, presented to hospital with a history of frequent postcoital bleeding for the past 3 years. She says she could not share this problem with her husband for fear that her husband might think she had contracted sexually transmitted diseases. The husband would divorce her for being dishonest, although the truth is that she had never had any sexual affair outside her marriage during the 29 years of their marriage as the third wife. Her sex life became painful and unpleasant as days went. She felt uneasy when the night set in and the thought of being asked for sex crept into her conscious mind. She could not dare to reveal this to her husband and whenever the husband wanted sex she always accepted as she strongly believed that it is disrespect to deny sex to her husband. As time went on the condition worsened and she started getting unprovoked bleeding with foul smelling discharge. When she shared this information with her mother Nanzia who was 75 years old, Nanzia agreed that she should not share the information with her husband because it was very shameful. The mother advised her to consult a traditional healer Mr. Kokoto who is very famous and practicing in another part of the country. The next hurdle was how she would ask for permission from her husband to travel. She had no alternative but to lie that her relative had died and she felt duty bound to travel to extend their condolences. The journey to see the traditional healer took 1 week in very difficult road conditions. When Mr. Kokoto saw her he comforted her and gave her a lot of hopes. He told her that she had cancer of the womb and that he has drugs which could cure it completely as long as she doest not go for modern medicine particularly radiation therapy because it has adverse effect on his good medicine. She started taking the drugs but she never got cured let alone getting better. Three months later she started leaking stool per vagina together with urine. Her life became more miserable and when she asked Mr. Kokoto as to why she is getting worse, Mr. Kokoto who believes that his treatments never fail had two answers to give her. First was that patients get worse before they get better, secondly her faith is not strong enough so she may not benefit from the treatment. A month later she could no longer bear the false reassurance from Kokoto hence she went back to her home. Even though she still had some herbs with her she no longer believed that herbs will work. At this point she picked the courage to inform her husband that she was not well and she wanted to go to the hospital. She had unbearable severe pains and foul smelling discharge per vagina. The husband decided not to sit close to her because of the terrible smell. After 2 weeks of no communication the husband sent a messenger to Mwanamvua's home that he has divorced her and would not be responsible for her treatment. Mwanamvua was shocked, she cried for 7 consecutive days. A Nongovernmental organization (NGO) working in Mwanamvua's village got word of her predicament hence advised and assisted her to travel to Ocean Road Cancer Institute (ORCI) where she was diagnosed with advanced cervical cancer with both vesico and rectovagina fistula. She also had widespread bone and lung metastasis. She was very much depressed at the time of her arrival at ORCI. At ORCI she was referred to palliative care team for pain and other symptom control. The head of the team admits that although they successfully controlled her pain in addition to addressing other psychosocial issues, the case was the most challenging case they have ever encountered during their decade of palliative care practice.

KAPOSI SARCOMA

This is the most common cancer affecting men in Sub-Sahara Africa. Patients usually present with infected nodules and foul smelling discharges. Severe lymphoedema like elephantiasis is one of the complications. This obvious AIDS clinical presentation has a lot of psychological impact to patients because everybody can actually recognize that one is affected by AIDS. Stigmatization is often seen in this condition because relatives fear getting infected while others just feel embarrassed by such a situation.

CASE STUDY

Mr Nzaro, a 32-year-old businessman was admitted to a private hospital with HIV-related Kaposis Sarcoma. In addition to the typical generalized Kaposis Sarcoma lesions he had fever, fatigue, anorexia, vomiting, and weight loss. His CD4 count was only 25 cells/mm3. He had been separated from his wife and lived with his relatives.

Mr. Nzaro was started on highly active antiretroviral (HAART) regimen, Cotrimazole, azithromycin, and vincristine. After 6 weeks Mr. Nzaro improved and was discharged from hospital. He still had difficulty holding food down and ate small frequent meals. While at home, 1 month later Nzaro's condition took unexpected turn for the worse and within 24 hours he slipped into coma and died. In a letter found at his bedside, Mr Nzaro thanked the hospital staff for their unconditional care, he also said that he had forgiven his wife, who had abandoned him when he needed her the most. In this message the importance of unconditional love and caring presence were reinforced.

CANCER OF BREAST

This is the second most common cancer affecting women in developing countries. Despite the fact that breasts are anatomically located in easily accessible part of the body the majority of the patients in developing countries present with advanced disease. Owing to late-stage presentation conservative treatment is in most cases not possible and mastectomy becomes the only option. This form of treatment has great psychological impact on the patients. Removal of the breast for whatever reasons is not well accepted in most cultures and some people would rather die of their disease than have their organ removed. Unlike in the past when most of these cancers were happening to older women, now majority of affected people are young and productive as well as reproductive. Since it is a well known fact that breast cancer can be inherited, the diagnosis leads to psychological effects to the female relative of the patients. When death from breast cancer occurs, family members become apprehensive and repeatedly ask whether they will be the next person to suffer and die like their sister.

CASE STUDY

Mrs Senzota, a 40-yrear-old housewife and mother of five children was referred for oncology consultation following simple mastectomy for Stage IV breast cancer with 16 positive nodes and bone metastases on her right hip. On being told that she required both radiotherapy and chemotherapy, she refused, saying "It is hopeless—why bother." The oncologist persuaded her to discuss her decision with the nurse counselor and she reluctantly agreed. She was anxious, depressed, and withdrawn. During the counseling session she wrung her hands throughout the interview, reporting intrusive thoughts of death that kept her from sleeping at night and stated that she preferred her husband remembering her as she was and early death would be preferable to loss of hair and the lingering debilitation she believed would be associated with chemotherapy. On further review she described being 15 years old when her mother was diagnosed with breast cancer and that she had since then feared that it would happen to her. Her mother's mastectomy had been followed by painful bone metastases despite chemotherapy. Mrs Senzota had distressing memories of her mother's suffering and had taken precautions to have regular self and clinician breast examination to ensure that if breast cancer were to develop it would be diagnosed at an early stage. She now had anger that something that she had attempted to prevent for so long had happened. The anger and hopelessness together were overwhelming and she could not focus on anything else.

OESOPHAGEAL CANCER

In Africa, this is the second most common cancer in males after Kaposi sarcoma. Unlike other cancers for which various effective modalities of palliation and prolongation of life can be offered, cancer of esophagus has a poor outcome due to limited options. Its psychological impact to the patient and family is great. Family members on seeing their loved one being wasted away slowly find it hard to comprehend. They would always come and ask what they can do to pass a glass of milk

through the patient's throat. The patient will always say that they are hungry but few of them would accept a feeding gastrostomy or nasogastric tube for the reason that it is no longer food but feed. Some even say that it is psychologically torturing to get down food which you do not feel the taste of. In that situation they feel that they are as good as dead yet a feeding tube is one of the palliative modality recognized for cancer of esophagus globally. Very few can be motivated to accept this procedure. After the patient dies essentially of starvation, it leaves very bad memories to those left behind whenever they remember how he/she was to the last minute and this makes bereavement period more complicated.

NASOPHARYNGEAL CARCINOMA

Nasopharyngeal carcinoma (NPC) arises from the mucosal *epithelium* of the *nasopharynx*, most often within the lateral nasopharyngeal recess or fossa of Rosenmüller. There are three *microscopic* subtypes of NPC: a well-differentiated *keratinizing* type, a moderately-differentiated nonkeratinizing type, and an undifferentiated type, which typically contains large numbers of noncancerous lymphocytes (chronic inflammatory cells), thus giving rise to the name *lymphoepithelioma*. The undifferentiated form is most common, and is most strongly associated with *Epstein-Barr virus* (EBV) infection of the cancerous cells.

Symptoms and signs. Nasopharyngeal carcinoma produces few symptoms early in its course, with the result that most cases are quite advanced when detected. Once the tumor has expanded from its site of origin in the lateral wall of the nasopharynx, it may obstruct the nasal passages and cause *nasal discharge* or nosebleed. Obstruction of the *auditory tubes* may cause chronic *ear infections*, and patients may experience *referred* pain to the *ear*. *Metastasis* of cancer to the *lymph nodes* of the *neck* may also be the first noticeable sign of the disease.

Numerous studies have linked common subtypes of NPC to infection with the EBV, which has also been implicated in the development of other cancers such as Hodgkin disease, Burkitt lymphoma (BL), and HIV-associated lymphomas. There is some evidence that genetic factors, such as HLA type may play a role in the susceptibility of certain ethnic groups to NPC. Finally, dietary risk factors, such as the consumption of salt-cured fish high in nitrosamines, may play a role in the Asian endemic regions. Well-differentiated NPC, with a microscopic appearance most similar to other squamous cell cancers of the head and neck may be more closely associated with the standard risk factors for that disease, such as cigarette smoking.

Treatment. Since NPC occurs in an anatomical site which is poorly accessible to surgeons, and is often advanced at presentation, the most effective means of treatment is generally radiation therapy, either with or without concurrent chemotherapy. While the undifferentiated subtype of NPC is highly radiosensitive, this is less true of the more differentiated subtypes.

CASE STUDY

Mwajuma is an albino woman of 23 years who looks older than her years. She presented with NCP and huge ulcerated super infected neck nodes. The nasopharyngeal tumor and ulcerated neck nodes emanated a very offensive smell. During the consultation, the attending doctor's reaction was to accept the unpleasant situation and avoid to offend the patient, for whom he had wanted to give great respect although she had a very offensive smell. On realizing that the situation is very unbearable, the doctor decided to ask one of the nurses to open all the windows in an attempt to suppress the smell. This trick did not work. Before the doctor could think of what else he could do, the smell triggered some vomiting in one of the student nurses. Then there were some murmurs from other nurses that the smell was so intolerable to the extent that it would be impossible to continue working without addressing the smell problem. At this juncture, the doctor asked for an air freshener. The answer was that the last time it was available and used was 4 years ago. Because there was no air freshener in the hospital the doctor decided to buy an air freshener from his pocket but this also did not help matters very much. At this point the patient felt very embarrassed and started crying in spite of all the assurances that her problem with the offensive smell would be sorted out very soon. As a long-term solution to her problem of offensive smell the doctor resolved to start her on a combination of oral metronidazole 400 mg tabs, three times a day for 7 days and amoxycillin 500 mg four times a day for 7 days and prescribed local treatment, which included wound dressing with metronidazole cream after cleansing with 3% solution of boric acid and external beam radiotherapy. This treatment was very effective and in 5 days time the patient was thankful for the prescribed treatment, which provided relief for her pain and eliminated the smell completely. She looked and behaved like a different person.

BURKITT LYMPHOMA

Burkitt lymphoma (BL) was first recognized in Africa as a tumor of the jaw occurring in high frequency in children. Although it is believed that BL has existed in Africa for thousands of years, the earliest documentation of this tumor, apart from in carvings from Lorenco Marques, in Mozambique, was at the beginning of the twentieth century when its unusual and prominent features were observed and recorded by European missionary doctors. Hospital records from Mulago Hospital in Uganda analyzed in the late 1950s revealed a high frequency of tumors of the jaw and orbit in children and analysis of these records strongly suggested that over 50% of the cases of childhood cancer were what we would now call BL. During the 1950s and 1960s, in-depth clinical and pathological descriptions of the features of this tumor were made by Dennis Burkitt, Greg O'Conor, Dennis Wright, and others. An important epidemiological observation was the delineation of the geographical distribution of this tumor in Africa. The findings of an extensive survey in Africa suggested that this disease had a high incidence in an area that is approximately 15 degrees north and south of the equator with a prolongation southward in the eastern side of the African continent. This was shown to be a consequence of climatic factors and led to the hypothesis, likely, but still unproven, that malaria predisposes to BL. It also led to the discovery of EBV in cell lines derived from tumors, a search stimulated by the earlier hypothesis that the disease might be caused by a virus vectored by a mosquito.

Shortly after the descriptions of the African lymphoma were published, pathologists recognized that some childhood lymphomas occurring in the United States and Europe at low incidence (sporadically) were histologically identical to African BL, whose incidence was considered high enough for the disease to be referred to as endemic. In equatorial African countries, the average annual incidence is four to ten per 100,000 children less than the age of 16 years whereas, in western countries, it accounts for a few percent of all childhood cancers and has an annual incidence rate of 0.2 per 100,000.

CASE STUDY

Jacqueline is a 9-year-old girl who developed a jaw swelling in April 1994. This was initially attributed, by her parents, to a recent tooth extraction. The swelling progressively increased in size. When the parents noticed that their daughter was sitting on the sand by herself and looked extremely tired while all the other children were playing in the playground, they developed an unsettled feeling which made them to take her to the nearby district hospital right away.

After examining the patient, the doctor—a medical assistant at the district hospital—suspected that the patient might have BL but had no facilities to perform tests to confirm the diagnosis. The clinical diagnosis was conveyed to the parents. When the word cancer was mentioned, the parents were overcome with shock, fear, and denial. The doctor recommended that the patient be referred to the Consultant Hospital in Dar es Salaam, which is 1000 km from the district hospital. Since at that time it was the rainy season and most of the roads were not easily passable, it took about 10 days for the family to arrive at the Consultant Hospital.

THE DIAGNOSIS. The patient and her parents had a horrible trip to Dar es Salaam. She developed malaria on the way. The deterioration in her health only emphasized the seriousness of the situation. The parents were physically and financially exhausted and could only watch in utter despair as the staff at the casualty department of the Consultant Hospital whisked their daughter off to the pediatric ward for supportive care and work-up to establish the diagnosis. The investigations included a full blood count, chest x ray, ultrasound of the abdomen and pelvis, spinal fluid examination, touch imprint, and tissue biopsy. The diagnosis of BL was confirmed in the third week of her stay at the Consultant Hospital. During the weekly Tumor Board meeting in her fourth week at the consultant Hospital, the Tumor Board recommended that the patient be transferred to the ORCI where she was to receive her chemotherapy.

THE TREATMENT. Burkitt lymphoma is a very aggressive cancer but it is also exquisitely sensitive to chemotherapy. This patient's prognosis was extremely good. At the ORCI the expected cure rate for a patient with her stage of disease is 85%. Although cytotoxic drugs are usually not affordable to most Tanzanians due to their high costs, at the ORCI we have a policy of supporting all pediatric oncology patients with free chemotherapy treatment. Therefore the patient was assured of receiving the ORCI recommended combination chemotherapy despite the fact that her family could not afford to pay for the treatment.

THE VICTORY. In July 1994 the patient was started on cyclophosphamide 30 mg/kg IV bolus, vincristine 1.4 mg/m2, methotrexate 15 mg/m2, and allopurinol 100 mg three times a day—repeated at two weekly intervals. After four cycles the tumor had melted away. Throughout the grueling ordeal the patient gained weight and her general condition improved. We advised the patient to continue with chemotherapy for another two cycles to ensure that the cancer did not come back. In October 1994 the patient was finally free—free from intravenous fluid administration, free from the raid of cytotoxic drugs on her body, and free from disease. The mother was ecstatic. As for the patient, all she could really think about was school, home, and her friends.

THE PATIENT IN 2008. The patient is well and attending high school. When asked what she plans to do with her life—a life she so nearly lost—she says that she intends to become a doctor.

CONCLUSION

Psychological problems are a part of cancer patient's experience of living and dying with cancer in developing countries. Unfortunately these problems are not addressed adequately. Clinicians and nurses should strive to play an important role in helping patients cope with these problems by providing expert physical, psychosocial, and spiritual care. There is evidence that sensitive, skillful attention to psychological issues can enhance quality of life and contribute significantly to "good death" as defined by the patient and family. In summary, addressing psychological issues adequately is an important means by which healthcare providers accompany patients and families through the cancer illness trajectory that may be marked by increasing disability and uncontrolled pains.

SUGGESTED READING

Holland J, Lewis S. *The human side of cancer: living with hope, coping with uncertainity.* New York:Quill; 2000.

Sepkwotz A. AIDS—the first 20 years. *N Engl J Med.* 2001;344:1764–1772.

Fraser J. Sharing the challenge: intergration of cancer and AIDS. *J. Palliat Care.* 1995;11:23–25.

Walsh TD. An overview of palliative care in cancer and AIDS. *Oncology.* 1991;6:7–11.

Holland J, Massie MJ, Straker N. Pyschotherapeutic interventions. In Holland TC, Rowlands JH, (eds). *Handbook of pyschooncology: Pyschological care of patient with cancer.* New York: Oxford University Press; 1989:455–469.

Ferrel BR, Coyle N. (eds). *Textbook of palliative care nursing.* New York: Oxford University Press; 2001.

Back AL, Arnold RM, Quill TE. Hope for the best, and prepare for the worst. *Ann Intetrn Med.* 2003;138:439–443.

Schwartz M. (ed). *Letting go: Morrie's reflections on living while dying.* New York: Delta; 1997.

PART VI

Management of Specific Symptoms

William S. Breitbart, ED

CHAPTER 30

Pain

William S. Breitbart, Jessica Park, and Aviva M. Katz

INTRODUCTION

Pain is perhaps among the most prevalent and distressing symptoms encountered in patients with cancer. Psychiatric and psychological consultation in the psycho-oncology setting must take into account the important relationships between pain and psychological and psychiatric morbidity. Uncontrolled pain can mimic psychiatric disorders, so mental health clinicians must be knowledgeable about pain and its appropriate management to recognize cancer-related pain when it is present. In addition, psychiatrists and psychologists can play a vital role in the multidisciplinary approach to managing cancer pain at all stages of disease. This chapter reviews the prevalence of pain in cancer, pain syndromes, and pain assessment issues, as well as pharmacologic and nonpharmacologic interventions for cancer-related pain. Psychiatric and psychological interventions in the treatment of cancer pain have now become an integral part of a comprehensive approach to pain management, and these are highlighted in this chapter.

PREVALENCE OF PAIN

Pain is a common problem for cancer patients, with approximately 70% of patients experiencing severe pain at some time in the course of their illness.[1] It has been suggested that nearly 75% of patients with advanced cancers have pain,[2] and that 50% of terminally ill patients are in moderate to severe pain.[3] It is also estimated that 25% of cancer patients die in severe pain.[4] There is considerable variability in the prevalence of pain among different types of cancer. For example, approximately 5% of leukemia patients experience pain during the course of their illness, compared to 50%–75% of patients with tumors of the lung, gastrointestinal (GI) tract, or genitourinary system. Patients with cancers of the bone or cervix have been found to have the highest prevalence of pain, with as many as 85% of patients experiencing significant pain during the course of their illness.[5] Despite the high prevalence of pain, however, studies have shown that it is frequently underdiagnosed and inadequately treated.[4] It is important to remember that pain is frequently only one of several symptoms that occur as part of a "cluster" of physical and psychological symptoms.[6] With disease progression, the number of distressing physical and psychological symptoms increases so that patients with advance disease report an average of 11 symptoms. A global evaluation of the symptom burden allows for a more complex understanding of the impact of pain.[7]

PAIN TYPES AND SYNDROMES IN CANCER

The International Association of Pain has defined pain as "an unpleasant sensory and emotional experience associated with actual or potential tissue damage or described in terms of such damage."[8] This definition of pain has disconnected the concept of pain intensity being directly proportional to the objectively observable tissue damage, emphasizing the subjective nature of the pain experience. In cancer pain patients however, there is typically dramatic evidence of tissue damage that is etiologically related to the pain complaint. This definition, particularly the component which emphasizes pain as an emotional experience as well as a sensory one, clearly demonstrates the need for psychosocial involvement in pain assessment and management.

Pain is often characterized by type on the basis of temporal factors as well as pathophysiology. Pain is often subtyped as acute pain or chronic pain based on temporal characteristics. A well-defined temporal pattern of

Table 30–1. Classification of pain

Nociceptive pain

Results from stimulation of intact "nociceptors" (pain receptors)

Includes somatic pain (involving skin, soft tissue, muscle, bone); visceral pain (involving internal organs, hollow viscera)

Responds to opioid and nonopioid analgesics

Neuropathic pain

Results from stimulation of damaged or compromised nerve tissue

Responds to opioid and nonopioid analgesics AND adjuvant medications

---

onset and termination characterizes acute pain. Generally, it is associated with subjective and objective physical or behavioral signs (e.g., grimacing, guarding, restlessness) and evidence of hyperactivity of the autonomic nervous system (e.g., rapid pulse, sweating). In contrast, chronic pain is pain that is experienced for longer than 3–6 months, or pain that persists beyond evidence of tissue damage healing. Patients with chronic pain often do not "look as if they are in pain" because adaptation of the autonomic nervous system occurs, and acute pain behaviors become replaced by depression, disability, and dysfunction. Chronic cancer pain can lead to significant changes in mood, personality, quality of life, relational problems, and functional ability.[1] As such, this type of pain requires an approach that includes treatment of the cause of the pain as well as treatment of its psychological and social consequences.[9]

Pain can be further classified into two major categories based on pathophysiology: *nociceptive* and *neuropathic* pain (Table 30–1).[10] Nociceptive pain derives from the stimulation of intact "nociceptors" or pain receptors in afferent nerves and is further subdivided into *somatic pain* (involving skin, soft tissue, muscle, and bone) and *visceral pain* (involving internal organs and hollow viscera). Nociceptive pain may be well-localized (common in somatic pain) or more diffuse (common in visceral pain), and may be sharp, dull, aching, gnawing, throbbing, constant, or spasmodic, with varying intensity. Neuropathic pain involves stimulation of damaged or compromised nerve tissue, and may be burning, tingling, stabbing, shooting, with a sensation of electric shock, or allodynia (the sensation of pain or discomfort produced by a minimal stimulus such as light touch to the skin). The differentiation of pain into one of these subtypes (particularly nociceptive vs. neuropathic) can help in determining appropriate therapy, as discussed below.

Foley[1] has categorized cancer pain syndromes based on temporal, etiologic, and contextual factors (Table 30–2). This approach to understanding cancer pain syndromes provides clinicians with a useful classification when considering therapeutic approaches.

MULTIDIMENSIONAL CONCEPT OF PAIN IN TERMINAL ILLNESS

Pain, and especially pain in cancer, is not a purely nociceptive or physical experience but involves complex aspects of human functioning, including personality, affect, cognition, behavior, and social relations.[11] It is important to note that the use of analgesic drugs alone does not

Table 30–2. Types of patients with pain from cancer

1. Patients with acute cancer-related pain
   Associated with the diagnosis of cancer
   Associated with cancer therapy (surgery, chemotherapy, or radiation)
2. Patients with chronic cancer-related pain
   Associated with cancer progression
   Associated with cancer therapy (surgery, chemotherapy, or radiation)
3. Patients with preexisting chronic pain and cancer-related pain
4. Patients with a history of drug addiction and cancer-related pain
   Actively involved in illicit drug use
   In methadone maintenance programs
   With a history of drug use
5. Dying patients with cancer-related pain

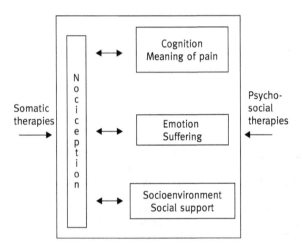

Fig. 30–1. The multidimensional nature of pain in cancer.

always lead to pain relief and that the psychological factors play a modest but important role in pain intensity.[12] The interaction of cognitive, emotional, socio-environmental, and nociceptive aspects of pain shown in Fig. 30–1 illustrates the multidimensional nature of pain in terminal illness and suggests a model for multimodal intervention.[13] The challenge of untangling and addressing both the physical and the psychological issues involved in pain is essential in developing rational and effective management strategies. Psychosocial therapies directed primarily at psychological variables have profound impacts on nociception, while somatic therapies have beneficial effects on the psychological aspects of nociceptive pain. Ideally, such somatic and psychosocial therapies are used simultaneously in a multidisciplinary approach to pain management in the cancer patient.[14]

PSYCHOLOGICAL FACTORS IN THE CANCER PAIN EXPERIENCE

Among the many stressors faced by patients with cancer are dependency, disability, and fear of painful death. Such fears are universal; however, the level of psychological distress is variable and depends on medical factors, social support, coping capacities, and personality.

Cancer pain and distress. Cancer-related pain has profound effects on psychological distress; and psychological factors such as anxiety, depression, and the meaning of pain for the patient can intensify the cancer pain experience. Daut and Cleeland[15] demonstrated that cancer patients who attribute a new pain to an unrelated benign cause report less interference with their activity and quality of life than patients who believe their pain represents progression of disease. Spiegel and Bloom[9]

found that women with metastatic breast cancer experience more intense pain if they believe their pain represents spread of their cancer and if they are depressed. Belief about the meaning of pain and the presence of a mood disturbance were better predictors of pain level than number or site of metastases.

Cancer pain and quality of life. In an attempt to define the potential relationships between cancer pain and psychosocial variables, Padilla et al.[16] found that there were pain-related quality-of-life variables in three domains: physical well-being; psychological well-being (consisting of affective factors, cognitive factors, spiritual factors, communication skills, coping skills, and meaning attribute to pain or cancer); and interpersonal well-being (focusing on social support or role functioning). The perception of marked impairment in activities of daily living has been shown to be associated with increased pain intensity.[17] Measures of emotional disturbance have been reported to be predictors of pain in the late stages of cancer, and cancer patients with less anxiety and depression are less likely to report pain.[18] In a prospective study of cancer patients, it was found that maladaptive coping strategies, lower levels of self-efficacy, and distress specific to treatment or disease progression were modest but significant predictors of reports of pain intensity.[12]

Psychological variables, such as the amount of control people believe they have over pain, emotional associations and memories of pain, fear of death, depression, anxiety, and hopelessness, contribute to the experience of pain and can increase suffering. Singer and colleagues[19] reported an association among the frequency of multiple pains, increased disability, and higher levels of depression. All too frequently, psychological variables are proposed to explain continued pain or lack of response to therapy when in fact medical factors have not been adequately appreciated. Often, the psychiatrist is the last physician to consult on a cancer patient with pain. In that role, one must be vigilant that an accurate pain diagnosis is made and must be able to assess the adequacy of the medical analgesic management provided. Personality factors may be quite distorted by the presence of pain, and relief of pain often results in the disappearance of a perceived psychiatric disorder.[20]

CANCER PAIN AND PSYCHIATRIC DISORDERS

There is an increased frequency of psychiatric disorders in cancer patients with pain. In the Psychosocial Collaborative Oncology Group Study[21] on the prevalence of psychiatric disorders in cancer patients, 39% of the patients who received a psychiatric diagnosis (Table 30–3) reported significant pain, whereas only 19% of patients without a psychiatric diagnosis had significant pain. The psychiatric disorders in cancer patients with pain primarily included adjustment disorder with depressed or anxious mood (69%) and major depression (15%). This finding of increased frequency of psychiatric disturbance in cancer pain patients also has been reported by other investigators.[22] The incidence and patterns of psychiatric disorders may vary systematically in subgroups of patients. For example, Steifel et al.[23] described the psychiatric complications seen in cancer patients undergoing treatment for epidural spinal cord compression (ESCC), which may include high-dose dexamethasone (as much as 96 mg/day for up to a week, followed by a tapering course for up to 3 or 4 weeks). Twenty-two percent of patients with ESCC had a major depressive syndrome diagnosed as compared to 4% in the comparison group. Also, delirium was much more common in the dexamethasone-treated patients with ESCC, with 24% diagnosed with delirium during the course of treatment as compared to only 10% in the comparison group.

Although there is limited information about patterns of disorders in other subpopulations, it is apparent that advanced disease itself, at least among patients with cancer, is associated with a relatively high prevalence of depression and delirium.[24] Approximately 25% of all cancer patients experience severe depressive symptoms, with the prevalence increasing to 77% in those with advanced illness. The prevalence of organic mental disorders (delirium) among cancer patients requiring psychiatric consultation has been found to range from 25% to 40%, and to be as high as 85% during the terminal stages of illness.[25] Opioid

Table 30–3. Rates of DSM-III psychiatric disorders and prevalence of pain observed in 215 cancer patients from three cancer centers

Diagnostic category	Number in diagnostic class	Percentage of psychiatric diagnoses	Number with significant pain[a]
Adjustment disorders	69	32	68
Major affective disorders	13	6	13
Organic mental disorders	8	4	8
Personality disorders	7	3	7
Anxiety disorders	4	2	4
Total with psychiatric diagnosis	101	47	39 (39%)
Total with no psychiatric diagnosis	114	53	21 (19%)
Total patient population	215	100	60 (28%)

[a] Score greater than 50 mm on a 100 mm VAS pain severity.
ABBREVIATION: VAS, visual analogue scale

analgesics and many other drugs can cause confusional states, particularly in the elderly and terminally ill.[6]

CANCER PAIN AND SUICIDE

Uncontrolled pain is a major factor in suicide and suicidal ideation in cancer patients.[26] The majority of suicides observed among patients with cancer had severe pain, which was often inadequately controlled or tolerated poorly.[27] Although relatively few cancer patients commit suicide, they are at increased risk. Pain is both a unique and synergistic contributor to suicide risk in cancer patients. For more details on suicide and desire for hastened death in cancer patients, please refer to Chapter 43.

CANCER PAIN ASSESSMENT

The initial step in cancer pain management is a comprehensive assessment of pain symptoms. An important element in assessment of pain is the concept that assessment is continuous and needs to be repeated over the course of pain treatment. There are essentially four aspects of pain experience in cancer that require ongoing evaluation, and they include pain intensity, pain relief, pain-related functional interference (e.g., mood state, general and specific activities), and monitoring of intervention effects (e.g., analgesic drug side effects, abuse).[28] Table 30–4 outlines the principles of pain assessment as described by Foley.[1] The Memorial Pain Assessment Card (MPAC)[29] is also a helpful clinical tool that allows patients to report their pain experience. The MPAC consists of visual analog scales that measure pain intensity, pain relief, and mood. Patients can complete the MPAC in less than 30 seconds. Patients' reports of pain intensity, pain relief, and present mood state provide the essential information required to help guide their pain management. The Brief Pain Inventory[30] is another pain assessment tool that has useful clinical and research applications.

Table 30–4. Principles of pain assessment

1. Believe the patient's complaint of pain
2. Take a detailed history
3. Assess the psychosocial status of the patient
4. Perform a careful medical and neurological examination
5. Order and personally review the appropriate diagnostic procedures
6. Evaluate the patient's extent of pain
7. Treat the pain to facilitate the diagnostic work-up
8. Consider the alternative methods of pain control during the initial evaluation
9. Reassess the pain complaint during the prescribed therapy

INADEQUATE CANCER PAIN MANAGEMENT

Inadequate management of cancer pain is often a result of the inability to properly assess pain in all its dimensions.[14] All too frequently, psychological variables are proposed to explain continued pain or lack of response to therapy, when in fact medical factors have not been adequately appreciated. Other causes of inadequate pain management include lack of knowledge of current pharmacotherapeutic or psychotherapeutic approaches; focus on prolonging life rather than alleviating suffering; lack of communication between doctor and patient; limited expectations of patients regarding pain relief; limited communication capacity in patients impaired by organic mental disorders; unavailability of opioids; doctors' fear of causing respiratory depression; and, most important, doctors' fear of amplifying addiction and substance abuse. In cancer, several additional factors have been noted to predict the undermanagement of pain, including a discrepancy between physician and patient in judging the severity of pain; the presence of pain that physicians do not attribute to cancer; better performance status; age of 70 years or more; and female sex.[31]

Fear of addiction and inadequate cancer pain management. Fear of addiction affects both patient compliance and physician management of narcotic analgesics, leading to undermedication of pain in cancer patients.[32] Studies of the patterns of chronic narcotic analgesic use in patients with cancer have demonstrated that, although tolerance and physical dependence commonly occur, addiction (psychological dependence) is rare and almost never occurs in individuals without a history of drug abuse before cancer illness.[32] Studies of the patterns of chronic narcotic analgesic use in patients with cancer have demonstrated that, although tolerance and physical dependence commonly occur, addiction (psychological dependence) is rare and almost never occurs in individuals without a history of drug abuse before cancer illness[33] reported on their experience in managing cancer pain in such a population. Of 468 inpatient cancer-pain consultations, only eight patients (1.7%) had a history of intravenous (IV) drug abuse, but none had been actively abusing drugs in the previous year. All eight of these patients had inadequate pain control, and more than half were intentionally undermedicated because of staff concern that drug abuse was active or would recur. Adequate pain control was ultimately achieved in these patients by using appropriate analgesic dosages and intensive staff education.

Concerns over respiratory depression and inadequate cancer pain management. The risk of inducing respiratory depression is too often overestimated and can limit appropriate use of narcotic analgesics for pain and symptom control. Bruera et al.[34] demonstrated that, in a population of terminally ill cancer patients with respiratory failure and dyspnea, the administration of subcutaneous morphine actually improved dyspnea without causing a significant deterioration in respiratory function.

Lack of concordance between patient and caregiver assessment of pain intensity. The adequacy of cancer pain management can be influenced by the lack of concordance between patient ratings or complaints of their pain and those made by caregivers. Persistent cancer pain is often ascribed to a psychological cause when it does not respond to treatment attempts. In our clinical experience, we have noted that patients who report their pain as severe are quite likely to be viewed as having a psychological contribution to their complaints. Staff members' ability to empathize with a patient's pain complaint may be limited by the intensity of the pain complaint. Grossman et al.[35] found that, while there is a high degree of concordance between patient and caregiver ratings of patient pain intensity at the low and moderate levels, this concordance breaks down at high levels. Thus, a clinician's ability to assess a patient's level of pain becomes unreliable once a patient's report of pain intensity rises above 7 on a visual analogue rating scale of 0–10. Physicians must be educated as to the limitations of their ability to objectively assess the severity of a subjective pain experience. In addition, patient education is often a useful intervention in such cases.

PSYCHIATRIC MANAGEMENT OF PAIN IN CANCER

Optimal treatment of pain associated with cancer may require a multimodal strategy, including pharmacological, psychotherapeutic, rehabilitative, and interventional approaches. Psychiatric participation in pain management involves the use of psychotherapeutic, cognitive-behavioral, and psychopharmacologic interventions, usually in combination.

PSYCHOTHERAPY AND CANCER PAIN

The goals of psychotherapy with cancer patients with pain are to provide support, knowledge, and skills (Table 30–5). Utilizing short-term supportive psychotherapy focused on the crisis created by the medical illness, the therapist provides emotional support, continuity, information, and assists in adaptation. The therapist has a role in emphasizing past strengths, supporting previously successful coping strategies, and teaching new coping skills, such as relaxation, cognitive coping, use of analgesics, self-observation, documentation, assertiveness, and communication skills. Communication skills are of paramount importance for both patient and family, particularly around pain and analgesic issues. The patient and family are the unit of concern, and need a more general, long-term, supportive relationship within the healthcare system in addition to specific psychological approaches dealing with pain and dying, which a psychiatrist, psychologist, social worker, chaplain, or nurse can provide.

Utilizing psychotherapy to diminish symptoms of anxiety and depression, factors that can intensify pain, empirically has beneficial effects on cancer pain experience. Spiegel and Bloom[36] demonstrated, in a controlled randomized prospective study, the effect of both supportive group therapy for metastatic breast cancer patients in general and, in particular, the effect of hypnotic pain control exercises. Their support group focused not on interpersonal processes or self-exploration, but rather on a series of themes related to the practical and existential problems of living with cancer. Patients were divided into two treatment groups and a control group.

The treatment patients experienced significantly less pain than the control patients. Those in the group that combined a self-hypnosis exercise group showed a slight increase, and the control group showed a large increase in pain.

Group interventions for individuals with cancer pain (even in advanced stages of disease) are a powerful means of sharing experiences and identifying successful coping strategies. The limitations of using group interventions for patients with advanced disease are primarily pragmatic. The patient must be physically comfortable enough to participate and have the cognitive capacity to be aware of group discussion. It is often helpful for family members to attend support groups during the terminal phases of the patient's illness. Interventions aimed at spouses and family members of cancer pain patients can also be beneficial (see section on Novel Psychosocial Interventions). Passik et al.[37] have worked with spouses of brain tumor patients in a psychoeducational group that has included spouses at all phases of the patient's diagnosis and treatment. They have demonstrated how bereavement issues are often a focus of such interventions from the time of diagnosis. The leaders have been impressed by the increased quality of patient care that can be given at home by the spouse (including pain management and all forms of nursing care) when the spouses engage in such support.

Psychotherapeutic interventions that have multiple foci may be most useful. On the basis of a prospective study of cancer pain, cognitive-behavioral and psychoeducational techniques based on increasing support, self-efficacy, and providing education may prove to be helpful in assisting patients in dealing with increased pain.[38] Results of an evaluation of patients with cancer pain indicate that psychological and social variables are significant predictors of pain. More specifically, distress specific to the illness, self-efficacy, and coping styles were predictors of increased pain.

Cognitive-behavioral techniques. Cognitive-behavioral techniques can be useful as adjuncts to the management of pain in cancer patients (Table 30–6). These techniques fall into two major categories: cognitive

Table 30–6. Cognitive-behavioral techniques used by pain patients with advanced disease

Psychoeducation
Preparatory information
Self-monitoring

Relaxation
Passive breathing
Progressive muscle relaxation

Distraction
Focusing
Controlled by mental imagery
Cognitive distraction
Behavioral distraction

Combined techniques (relaxation and distraction)
Passive/progressive relaxation with mental imagery
Systematic desensitization
Meditation
Hypnosis
Biofeedback
Music therapy

Cognitive therapies
Cognitive distortion
Cognitive restructuring

Behavioral therapies
Modeling
Graded task management
Contingency management
Behavioral rehearsal

Table 30–5. Goals and forms of psychotherapy for pain in patients with advanced disease

Goals	Form
Support—provide continuity	Individuals—supportive/crisis intervention
Knowledge—provide information	Family—patient and family are the unit of concern
Skills—relaxation cognitive coping use of analgesics communication	Group—share experiences identify successful coping strategies

Table 30–7. Cognitive-behavioral techniques: definitions and descriptions

Behavioral therapy	The clinical use of techniques derived from the experimental analysis of behavior, i.e. learning and conditioning for the evaluation, prevention, and treatment of physical disease or physiological dysfunction
Cognitive therapy	A focused intervention targeted at changing maladaptive beliefs and dysfunctional attitudes. The therapist engages the client in a process of collaborative empiricism, where these underlying beliefs are challenged and corrected
Operant pain	Pain behaviors resulting from operant learning or conditioning. Pain behavior is reinforced and continues because of secondary gain, i.e. increased attention and caring
Respondent pain	Pain behaviors resulting from respondent learning or conditioning. Stimuli associated with prior painful experiences can elicit increased pain and avoidance behavior
Cognitive restructuring	Redefinition of some or all aspects of the patient's interpretation of the noxious or threatening experience, resulting in decreased distress, anxiety, and hopelessness
Self-monitoring (pain diary)	Written or audiotaped chronicle that the patient maintains to describe specific agreed-upon characteristics associated with pain
Contingency management	Focusing of patient and family member responses that either reinforce or inhibit specific behaviors exhibited by the patient. Method involves reinforcing desired "well" behaviors
Grade task assignments	A hierarchy of tasks, i.e. physical, cognitive, and behavioral are compartmentalized and performed sequentially in manageable steps ultimately achieving an identified goal
Systematic desensitization	Relaxation and distraction exercises paired with a hierarchy of anxiety-arousing stimuli presented through mental imagery, or presented in vivo, resulting in control of fear

techniques and behavioral techniques. Both techniques comprise a range of techniques including passive relaxation with mental imagery, cognitive distraction or focusing, progressive muscle relaxation, biofeedback, hypnosis, and music therapy.[39] The goal of treatment is to guide the patient toward a sense of control over pain. Some techniques are primarily cognitive in nature, focusing on perceptual and thought processes, and others are directed at modifying patterns of behavior that help cancer patients cope with pain. Behavioral techniques for pain control seek to modify physiologic pain reactions, respondent pain behaviors, and operant pain behaviors (see Table 30–7 for definitions).

Relaxation techniques. Several techniques can be used to achieve a mental and physical state of relaxation. Muscular tension, autonomic arousal, and mental distress exacerbate pain.[40,41] Some specific relaxation techniques include (1) passive relaxation focusing attention on sensations of warmth and decreased tension in various parts of the body, (2) progressive muscle relaxation involving active tensing and relaxing of muscles, and (3) meditation.

Hypnosis. Hypnosis can be a useful adjunct in the management of cancer pain.[36,39,42–45] Hypnotherapy, usually involving the teaching of self-hypnotic techniques, can be used effectively in the management of pain associated with invasive procedures.[46] In a controlled trial comparing self-hypnosis with cognitive-behavioral therapy in relieving mucositis following a bone marrow transplant, patients utilizing self-hypnosis reported a significant reduction in pain compared to patients who used cognitive-behavioral techniques.[38] The hypnotic trance is essentially a state of heightened and focused concentration, and thus it can be used to manipulate the perception of pain.

Biofeedback. Fotopoulos et al.[47] noted significant pain relief in a group of cancer patients who were taught electromyographic (EMG) and electroencephalographic (EEG) biofeedback-assisted relaxation. Only 2 out of 17 were able to maintain analgesia after the treatment ended. A lack of generalization of effect can be a problem with biofeedback techniques. Although physical condition may make a prolonged training period impossible, especially for the terminally ill, most cancer patients can often use EMG and temperature biofeedback techniques for learning relaxation-assisted pain control.[48]

Novel psychosocial interventions. It should be noted that nontraditional psychosocial interventions for cancer pain hold great promise. For example, Keefe et al.[49] tested the efficacy of a partner-guided cancer pain management protocol. The partner-guided pain management training protocol was a three-session intervention conducted in patients' homes that integrated educational information about cancer pain with systematic training of patients and partners in cognitive and behavioral pain coping skills. Data analyses revealed that the partner-guided pain management protocol produced significant increases in partners' ratings of their self-efficacy for helping the patient control pain and self-efficacy for controlling other symptoms.

AROMA THERAPY

Aromas have been shown to have innate relaxing and stimulating qualities. Our colleagues at Memorial Hospital have recently begun to explore the use of aroma therapy for the treatment of procedure-related anxiety (i.e., anxiety related to magnetic resonance imaging [MRI] scans). Utilizing the scent heliotropin, Manne et al.[50] reported that two-thirds of the patients in their study found the scent especially pleasant and reported feeling much less anxiety than those who were not exposed to the scent during MRI. As a general relaxation technique, aroma therapy may have an application for pain management, but this is as yet unstudied.

PHARMACOTHERAPIES FOR PAIN

Although the management of analgesic medications is more often undertaken by the oncologist or palliative care specialist, it is essential that the psycho-oncologist have a thorough understanding of the analgesic medications most often used in the management of cancer-related pain. The World Health Organization (WHO) has devised guidelines for analgesic management of cancer pain that the Agency for Health Care Policy and Research (AHCPR) has endorsed for the management of pain related to cancer.[51] These guidelines, also known widely as the WHO Analgesic Ladder (see Fig. 30–2), have been well validated.[52] This approach advocates selection of analgesics on the basis of severity of pain. For mild to moderately severe pain, nonopioid analgesics such as nonsteroidal antiinflammatory drugs (NSAIDs) and acetaminophen are recommended. For pain that is persistent and moderate to severe in intensity, opioid analgesics of increasing potency (such as morphine) should be used. Adjuvant agents, such as laxatives and psychostimulants, are useful in preventing as well as treating opioid side effects such as constipation or sedation, respectively. Adjuvant analgesic drugs, such as the

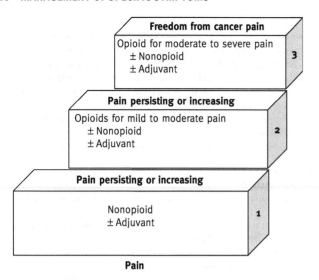

Fig. 30-2. WHO Analgesic Ladder.
SOURCE: Adapted from *Cancer pain relief, with a guide to opioid availability.* 2nd ed. Geneva: World Health Organization; 1996.

antidepressant analgesics, are suggested for considered use, along with opioids and NSAIDs, in all stages of the analgesic ladder (mild, moderate, or severe pain).

Portenoy[53] have described the indications for and the use of three classes of analgesic drugs that have applications in the management of cancer and acquired immunodeficiency syndrome (AIDS) patients with pain: nonopioid analgesics (such as acetaminophen, aspirin, and other NSAIDs), opioid analgesics (of which morphine is the standard), and adjuvant analgesics (such as antidepressants and anticonvulsants).

NONOPIOD ANALGESICS (NSAIDs)

The nonopioid analgesics (Table 30–8) are prescribed principally for mild to moderate pain or to augment the analgesic effects of opioid analgesics in the treatment of severe pain. The analgesic effects of the NSAIDs result from their inhibition of cyclooxygenase and the subsequent reduction of prostaglandins in the tissues. The concurrent use of NSAIDs or acetaminophen and opioids provides more analgesia than does either of the drug classes alone. In contrast to opioids, NSAIDs have a ceiling effect for analgesia, do not produce tolerance or dependence,

have antipyretic effects, and have a different spectrum of adverse side effects.[51]

The NSAIDs' mechanisms of action, pharmacokinetics, and pharmacodynamics influence the analgesic response. The selection of the NSAID should take into account the etiology and severity of the pain, concurrent medical conditions that may be relative contraindications (e.g., bleeding diathesis), associated symptoms, and favorable experience by the patient as well as the physician. From a practical point of view, an NSAID should be titrated to effect as well as to side effects. There is also variability in patient response to both relief and adverse reactions; if the results are not favorable, an alternative NSAID should be tried.

MAJOR ADVERSE EFFECTS OF NSAIDs

The major adverse effects associated with NSAIDs include gastric ulceration, renal failure, hepatic dysfunction, and bleeding. The use of NSAIDs has been associated with a variety of GI toxicities, including minor dyspepsia and heartburn, as well as major gastric erosion, peptic ulcer formation, and GI hemorrhage. The nonacetylated salicylates, such as salsalate, sodium salicylate, and choline magnesium salicylate, theoretically have fewer GI side effects and might be considered in cases where GI distress is an issue. Prophylaxis for NSAID-associated GI symptoms includes H2-antagonist drugs (cimetidine 300 mg tid-qid or ranitidine 150 mg bid); misoprostal 200 mg qid; omeprazole 20 mg qd; or an antacid. Patients should be informed of these symptoms, issued guaiac cards with reagent, and taught to check their stool weekly. NSAIDs affect kidney function and should be used with caution. Prostaglandins are involved in the autoregulation of renal blood flow, glomerular filtration, and the tubular transport of water and ions. NSAIDs can cause a decrease in glomerular filtration, acute and chronic renal failure, interstitial nephritis, papillary necrosis, and hyperkalemia.[54] In patients with renal impairment, NSAIDs should be used with caution, since many (i.e., ketoprofen, feroprofen, naproxen, and carpofen) are highly dependent on renal function for clearance. The risk of renal dysfunction is greatest in patients with advanced age, preexisting renal impairment, hypovolemia, concomitant therapy with nephrotoxic drugs, and heart failure. Prostaglandins modulate vascular tone, and their inhibition by the NSAIDs can cause hypertension as well as interference with the pharmacologic control of hypertension.[55] Caution should be used in patients receiving β-adrenergic antagonists, diuretics, or angiotensin-converting enzyme inhibitors. Several studies have suggested that there is substantial biliary excretion of several NSAIDs, including indomethacin and sulindac. In patients with hepatic dysfunction, these drugs should be used with caution. NSAIDs, with the exception of the nonacetylated salicylates (e.g., sodium salicylate, choline magnesium trisalicylate), produce inhibition of platelet aggregation (usually reversible, but irreversible with aspirin). NSAIDs should be used with extreme caution or avoided in patients who are thrombocytopenic or who have clotting impairment.

Table 30-8. Oral analgesics for mild to moderate pain in cancer

Analgesic (by class)	Starting dose (mg)	Plasma duration (hrs)	Half-life (hrs)	Comments
Nonsteroidal				
Aspirin	650	4–6	4–6	The standard for comparison among nonopioid analgesics
Ibuprofen	400–600	—	—	Like aspirin, can inhibit platelet function
Choline magnesium trisalicylate	700–1500	—	—	Essentially no hematologic or gastrointestinal side effects
Weaker opioids				
Codeine	32–65	3–4	—	Metabolized to morphine, often used to suppress cough in patients at risk of pulmonary bleed
Oxycodone	5–10	3–4	—	Available as a single agent and in combination with aspirin or acetaminophen
Proxyphene	65–13	4–6	—	Toxic metabolite norpropoxy accumulates with repeated usage

The use of NSAIDs in patients with cancer and AIDS must be accompanied by heightened awareness of toxicity and adverse effects. NSAIDs are highly protein bound, and the free fraction of available drug is increased in cancer patients who are cachectic, wasted, and hypoalbuminic, often resulting in toxicities and adverse effects. Patients with cancer are frequently hypovolemic and on concurrent nephrotoxic drugs and so are at increased risk for renal toxicity related to NSAIDs. Finally, the antipyretic effects of the NSAIDs may interfere with early detection of infection in patients with cancer.

COX-2 inhibitors have an analgesic action equal to that of conventional NSAIDs, but with fewer GI complications and have been widely used for rheumatic diseases.[56] COX-2 inhibitors are associated with an increased risk of adverse cardiovascular events, including infarction, stroke and new onset or worsening of preexisting hypertension, GI irritation, ulceration, bleeding and perforation, and are contraindicated for the treatment of perioperative pain in the setting of coronary artery bypass graft (CABG).

OPIOID ANALGESICS

Opioid analgesics are the mainstay of pharmacotherapy of moderate to severe intensity pain in the patient with cancer (see Table 30–9).

In choosing the appropriate opioid analgesic for cancer pain, Portenoy[57] highlights the following important considerations: opioid class, choice of "weak" versus "strong" opioids, pharmacokinetic characteristics, duration of analgesic effect, favorable prior response, and opioid side effects (Table 30–10).

Opioid classes. Opioid analgesics are divided into two classes: the agonists and the agonist-antagonists, on the basis of their affinity to opioid receptors. Pentazocine, butorphanol, and nalbuphine are examples of opioid analgesics with mixed agonist-antagonist properties. These drugs can reverse opioid effects and precipitate an opioid withdrawal syndrome in patients who are opioid tolerant or dependent. They are of limited use in the management of chronic pain in cancer and AIDS. Oxycodone (in combination with either aspirin or acetaminophen), hydrocodone, and codeine are the so-called weaker opioid analgesics and are indicated for use in step 2 of the WHO ladder for mild to moderate pain. More severe pain is best managed with morphine or another of the "stronger" opioid analgesics, such as hydromorphone, methadone, levorphanol, or fentanyl. Oxycodone, as a single agent without aspirin or acetaminophen, is available in immediate and sustained-release forms and is considered a stronger opioid in these forms. Oxymorphone, including Numorphan, Opana, and Opana ER, is a potent opioid analgesic. They act quickly when taken orally and have significantly longer half-lives than morphine. Rectal administration is an alternative for those patients unable to take oral medications. Equianalgesic dosages may be due to pharmacokinetic differences.

Pharmacokinetics. A basic understanding of the pharmacokinetics of the opioid analgesics[58] is important for the cancer and AIDS care provider. Opioid analgesics with long half-lives, such as methadone and levorphanol, require approximately 5 days to achieve a steady state. Despite their long half-lives, the duration of analgesia that they provide is considerably shorter (i.e., most patients require administration of the drug every 4–6 hours). As both methadone and levorphanol tend to accumulate with early initial dosing, delayed effects of toxicity can develop (primarily sedation and, more rarely, respiratory depression).

Duration of effects. The duration of analgesic effects of opioid analgesics varies considerably. Immediate-release preparations of morphine or oxycodone often provide only 3 hours of relief and must be prescribed on an every 3-hour, around-the-clock basis (not as needed). Methadone and levorphanol may provide up to 6 hours of analgesia. There is individual variation in the metabolism of opioid analgesics, and there can be significant differences between individuals in drug absorption and disposition. These differences lead to a need for alterations in dosing, route of administration, and scheduling for maximum analgesia in individual patients. While parenteral administration (IV, intramuscular, subcutaneous) yields a faster onset of pain relief, the duration of analgesia is shorter unless a continuous infusion of opioid is instituted. The use of continuous subcutaneous or IV infusions of opioids, with or without patient-controlled analgesia (PCA) devices, has become commonplace in caring for cancer patients with escalating pain and in hospice and home settings during late stages of disease.

Routes of administration. The oral route is often the preferred route of administration of opioid analgesics from the perspectives of convenience and cost. Immediate-release oral morphine or hydromorphone preparations require that the drug be taken every 3–4 hours. Longer-acting, sustained-release oral morphine preparations and oxycodone preparations are now available that provide up to 8–12 hours of analgesia (or longer), minimizing the number of daily doses required for the control of persistent pain. Rescue doses of immediate-release, short-acting opioid are often necessary to supplement the use of sustained-release morphine or oxycodone, particularly during periods of titration or pain escalation. The transdermal fentanyl patch system (Duragesic) also has applications in the management of severe pain in cancer. Each transdermal fentanyl patch contains a 48- to 72-hour supply of fentanyl, which is absorbed from a depot in the skin. Levels in the plasma rise slowly over 12–18 hours after patch placement, so, with the initial placement of a patch, alternative opioid analgesia (oral, rectal, or parenteral) must be provided until adequate levels of fentanyl are attained. The elimination half-life of this dosage form of fentanyl is long (21 hours), so it must be noted that significant levels of fentanyl remain in the plasma for approximately 24 hours after the removal of a transdermal patch. The transdermal system is not optimal for rapid dose titration of acutely exacerbated pain; however, a variety of dosage forms are available. As with sustained-release morphine preparations, all patients should be provided with oral or parenteral rapidly acting short-duration opioids to manage breakthrough pain. The transdermal system is convenient and eliminates the reminders of pain associated with repeated oral dosing of analgesics. In patients with cancer and AIDS, it should be noted that the absorption of transdermal fentanyl can be increased with fever, resulting in increased plasma levels and shorter duration of analgesia from the patch.

It is important to note that opioids can be administered through various routes: oral, rectal, transdermal, IV, subcutaneous, intraspinal, and even intraventricularly.[59] There are advantages and disadvantages, as well as indications, for the use of these various routes. Further discussion of such alternative delivery routes as the intraspinal route are beyond the scope of this chapter; however, interested readers are directed to the Agency for Health Care Policy and Research Clinical Practice Guideline: Management of Cancer Pain[51] available free of charge through 1-800-4 cancer.

Appropriate dosage. The adequate treatment of pain in cancer also requires consideration of the equianalgesic doses of opioid drugs, which are generally calculated using morphine as a standard. Cross-tolerance is not complete among these drugs. Therefore, one-half to two-thirds of the equianalgesic dose of the new drug should be given as the starting dose when switching from one opioid to another.[60] For example, if a patient receiving 20 mg of parenteral morphine is to be switched to hydromorphone, the equianalgesic dose of parenteral hydromorphone would be 3.0 mg. Thus, the starting dose of parenteral hydromorphone should be approximately 1.5 to 2 mg. There is also considerable variability in the parenteral-to-oral ratios among the opioid analgesics. Both levorphanol and methadone have 1:2 intramuscular/oral ratios, whereas morphine has a 1:6 and hydromorphone a 1:5 intramuscular/oral ratio. Failure to appreciate these dosage differences in route of administration can lead to inadequate pain control.

Standing dose scheduling. Regular ("standing") scheduling of the opioid analgesics is the foundation of adequate pain control. It is

Table 30–9. Opioid analgesics for moderate to severe pain in cancer patients

Analgesic	Equianalgesic route	Dose (mg)	Analgesic onset (hrs)	Duration (hrs)	Plasma half-life (hrs)	Comments
Morphine	PO IM, IV, SC	30–60*10	1–1½ ½–1	4–6 3–6	2–3	Standard of comparison for the narcotic analgesics. 30 mg for repeat around-the-clock dosing; 60 mg for single dose or intermittent dosing
Morphine	PO	90–120	1–1½	8–12	———	Now available in long-acting sustained-release forms
Oxycodone	PO PO	20–30 20–40	1 1	3–6 8–12	2–3 2–3	In combination with aspirin or acetaminophen it is considered a weaker opioid; as a single agent it is comparable to the strong opioids, like morphine Available in immediate-release and sustained-release preparation
Hydromorphone	PO IM, IV	7.5 1.5	½–1 ¼–½	3–4 3–4	2–3 2–3	Short half-life; ideal for elderly patients. Comes in suppository and injectable forms
Methadone	PO IM, IV	20 10	½–1 ½–1	4–8 ———	15–30 15–30	Long half-life; tends to accumulate with initial dosing, requires careful titration. Good oral potency
Levorphanol	PO IM	4 2	½–1½ ½–1	3–6 3–4	12–16 12–16	Long half-life; requires careful dose titration in first week. Note that analgesic duration is only 4 hrs
Meperidine	PO IM	300 75	½–1½ ½–1	3–6 3–4	3–4 3–4	Active toxic metabolite, ormeperidine, tends to accumulate (plasma half-life is 12–16 hrs), especially with renal impairment and in elderly patients, causing delirium, myoclonus, and seizures
Fentanyl Transdermal System	TD IV	0.1–01	12–18	48–72 ———	20–22 ———	Transdermal patch is convenient, bypassing GI analgesia until depot is formed. Not suitable for rapid titrationw
Oxymorphone	PO IV, IM, SC	10 mg	½–1	4–6	8	Long half-life but low oral bioavailability Rectal administration is an alternate route for patients unable to take oral medications. More frequent dosing may be required

ABBREVIATIONS: GI, gastrointestinal tract; PO, per oral; IM, intramuscular; IV, intravenous; SC, subcutaneous; TD, transdermal.

preferable to prevent the return of pain as opposed to treating pain as it reoccurs. "As needed" orders for chronic cancer pain often create a struggle among patient, family, and staff that is easily avoided by regular administration of opioid analgesics. The typical prescribing of methadone is a notable exception. It is often initially prescribed on an as-needed basis to determine the patient's total daily requirement and to minimize toxicity (due to its long half-life).

Opioid rotation is a useful strategy to improve pain management especially in long-term treatment. Accumulation of toxic metabolites can lead to the development of symptoms that include hallucinations,

Table 30–10. Principles of opioid analgesic use

1. Choose an appropriate drug
2. Start with lowest dose possible
3. Titrate dose
4. Use "as needed" doses selectively
5. Use an appropriate route of administration
6. Be aware of equivalent analgesic doses
7. Use a combination of opioid, nonopioid, and adjuvant drugs
8. Be aware of tolerance
9. Understand physical and psychological dependence

myoclonus, nausea and vomiting, and persisting pain. Several strategies of opioid rotation using equianalgesic doses have been reported to be useful in managing pain while decreasing the tolerance as well as the frequency and severity of opioid toxicity.[60]

Side effects. While the opioids are extremely effective analgesics, their side effects are common and can be minimized if anticipated in advance. Sedation is a common central nervous system (CNS) side effect, especially during the initiation of treatment. Sedation usually resolves after the patient has been maintained on a steady dosage. Persistent sedation can be alleviated with a psychostimulant, such as dextroamphetamine, pemoline, or methylphenidate. All are prescribed in divided doses in early morning and at noon. In addition, psychostimulants can improve depressed mood and enhance analgesia.[61] Delirium, of either an agitated or a somnolent variety, can also occur while the patient is on opioid analgesics and is usually accompanied by attentional deficits, disorientation, and perceptual disturbances (visual hallucinations and, more commonly, illusions). Myoclonus and asterixis are often early signs of neurotoxicity that accompany the course of opioid-induced delirium. Meperidine (Demerol), when administered chronically in patients with renal impairment, can lead to a delirium resulting from accumulation of the neuroexcitatory metabolite normeperidine.[62] Opioid-induced delirium can be alleviated through the implementation of three possible strategies: lowering the dose of the opioid drug presently in use, changing to a different opioid, or treating the delirium with low doses of high-potency neuroleptics, such as haloperidol. The third strategy is especially useful for agitation and clears the sensorium.[63] For agitated states, IV haloperidol in doses starting at between 1 and 2 mg is useful, with rapid escalation of dose if no effect is noted. Gastrointestinal side effects of opioid analgesics are common. The most prevalent are nausea, vomiting, and constipation.[64] Concomitant therapy with prochlorperazine for nausea is sometimes effective. Since all opioid analgesics are not tolerated in the same manner, switching to another narcotic can be helpful if an antiemetic regimen fails to control nausea. Constipation caused by narcotic effects on gut receptors is a problem frequently encountered, and it tends to be responsive to the regular use of senna derivatives. A careful review of medications is imperative, since anticholinergic drugs such as the tricyclic antidepressants (TCAs) can worsen opioid-induced constipation and can cause bowel obstruction. Respiratory depression is a worrisome but rare side effect of the opioid analgesics. Respiratory difficulties can almost always be avoided if two general principles are adhered to: start opioid analgesics in low doses in opioid-naive patients; and be cognizant of relative potencies when switching opioid analgesics, routes of administration, or both.

PSYCHOTROPIC ADJUVANT ANALGESICS

The patient with advanced disease and pain has much to gain from the appropriate and maximal utilization of psychotropic drugs. Psychotropic drugs, particularly the TCAs, are useful as adjuvant analgesics in the pharmacological management of cancer pain and neuropathic pain. Table 30-11 lists the various psychotropic medications with analgesic properties, their routes of administration, and their approximate daily doses. These medications are not only effective in managing symptoms of anxiety, depression, insomnia, or delirium that commonly complicate

Table 30–11. Psychotropic adjuvant analgesic drugs for pain in patients with advanced disease

Generic name	Approximate daily dosage range (mg)	Route
Tricyclic antidepressants		
Amitriptyline	10–150	PO, IM
Nortriptyline	10–150	PO
Imipramine	15.5–150	PO, IM
Desipramine	10–150	PO
Clomipramine	10–150	PO
Doxepin	12–150	PO, IM
Heterocyclic and noncyclic antidepressants		
Trazodone	125–300	PO
Maprotiline	50–300	PO
Serotonin-reuptake inhibitors		
Fluoxetine	20–80	PO
Paroxetine	10–60	PO
Sertraline	50–200	PO
Citalopram	10–40	PO
Escitalopram	10–20	PO
Newer agents		
Nefazodone	100–500	PO
Venlafaxine	75–300	PO
Duloxetine	20–90	PO
Mirtazapine	7.5–60	PO
Psychostimulants		
Methylphenidate	2.5–20 bid	PO
Dextroamphetamine	2.5–20 bid	PO
Pemoline	13.75–75 bid	PO
Modafinil	100–400	PO
Phenothiazines		
Fluphenazine	1–3	PO, IM
Methotrimeprazine	10–20 q6h	IM, IV
Butyrophenones		
Haloperidol	1–3	PO, IV
Pimozide	2–6 bid	PO
Antihistamines		
Hydroxyzine	50 q4h–q6h	PO
Anticonvulsants		
Carbamazepine	200 tid–400 tid	PO
Phenytoin	300–400	PO
Valproate	500 tid–1000 tid	PO
Gabapentin	300 tid–1000 tid	PO
Oxcarbazepine	300 bid–1800 daily	PO
Pregabalin	50 tid–150 bid	PO
Oral local anesthetics		
Mexiletine	600–900	PO
Corticosteroids		
Dexamethasone	4–16	PO, IV
Benzodiazepines		
Alprazolam	0.25–2.0 tid	PO
Clonazepam	0.5–4 bid	PO

ABBREVIATIONS: PO, per oral; IM, intramuscular; IV, intravenous; q6h, every 6 hrs; Bid, twice a day; tid, three times a day; qid, four times a day.

the course of advanced disease in patients who are in pain, but also potentiate the analgesic effects of the opioid drugs and have innate analgesic properties of their own.[61] A common use of adjuvant analgesics is to manage neuropathic pain. In this population, nonopioid adjuvant drugs that are neuroactive or neuromodulatory may be needed to complement opioid therapy. The primary adjuvant analgesics are anticonvulsant and antidepressant medications but a variety of other drugs are used.[65]

ANTIDEPRESSANTS

The current literature supports the use of antidepressants as adjuvant analgesic agents in the management of a wide variety of chronic pain syndromes, including cancer pain.[66]

Tricyclics. Amitriptyline is the TCA most studied, and proven effective as an analgesic, in a large number of clinical trials, addressing a wide variety of chronic pains.[67] Other TCAs that have been shown to have efficacy as analgesics include imipramine,[68] desipramine,[69] nortriptyline,[70] clomipramine,[71] doxepin,[72] and sertraline.[73] In a placebo-controlled double-blind study of imipramine in chronic cancer pain, Walsh[74] demonstrated that imipramine had analgesic effects independent of its mood effects, and was a potent co-analgesic when used along with morphine. Sertraline has been showed to reduce hot flashes in early stage breast cancer patients taking tamoxifen; however, compared to a placebo the reduction was not significant.[75] In general, the TCAs are used in cancer pain as adjuvant analgesics, potentiating the effects of opioid analgesics, and are rarely used as the primary analgesic.[76] Ventafridda et al.[76] reviewed a multicenter clinical experience with antidepressant agents (trazodone and amitriptyline) in the treatment of chronic cancer pain that included a deafferentation of neuropathic component. Almost all of these patients were already receiving weak or strong opioids and experienced improved pain control. A subsequent randomized double-blind study showed both amitriptyline and trazodone to have similar therapeutic analgesic efficacy.[76] Magni et al.[77] reviewed the use of antidepressants in Italian cancer centers and found that a wide range of antidepressants were used for a variety of cancer pain syndromes, with amitriptyline being the most commonly prescribed, for a variety of cancer pains. In nearly all cases, antidepressants were used in association with opioids. There is some evidence that there may be a subgroup of patients who respond differentially to tricyclics and therefore if amitriptyline fails to alleviate pain, another tricyclic should be tried. The TCAs are effective as adjuvants in cancer pain through a number of mechanisms that include (1) antidepressant activity, (2) potentiation or enhancement of opioid analgesia,[78] and (3) direct analgesic effects.[79]

The heterocyclic and noncyclic antidepressant drugs such as trazodone, mianserin, maprotiline, and the newer SSRIs, fluoxetine, and paroxetine may also be useful as adjuvant analgesics for cancer patients with pain; however, clinical trials of their efficacy as analgesics have been equivocal. There are several case reports that suggest that fluoxetine may be a useful adjuvant analgesic in the management of headache,[80] fibrositis,[81] and diabetic neuropathy.[82] In a recent clinical trial, fluoxetine was shown to be no better than placebo as an analgesic in painful diabetic neuropathy.

SSRIs. Paroxetine is the first SSRI shown to be a highly effective analgesic in the treatment of neuropathic pain,[83] and may be a useful addition to our armamentarium of adjuvant analgesics for cancer pain. Although it has not been tested on cancer pain, SSRI such as citalopram has also been shown to help with neuropathic pain.[84] Escitalopram, a newer SSRI, has advantages over other SSRIs; it has the highest selectivity in its class, no active metabolite, and does not significantly affect the CYP450 isoenzyme.[85] While Escitalopram has not been tested on cancer pain, it has been shown to lessen both depression and anxiety.[86] SSRIs may offer greater benefit to these patients as evidenced by greater improvements in quality-of-life measures.[87]

Newer antidepressants as analgesics. Newer antidepressants such as sertraline, venlafaxine, nefazodone, and duloxetine also appear to be clinically useful as adjuvant analgesics. Nefazodone, for instance, has

been demonstrated to potentiate opioid analgesics in an animal model[88]; and venlafaxine has been shown by Tasmuth et al.[89] to decrease the maximum pain intensity following treatment of breast cancer. Duloxetine, a dual reuptake inhibitor of serotonin and norepinephrine, has been shown to be an effective treatment for depression and for neuropathic pain[90]; however, there are no trials in cancer patients. At this point, it is clear that many antidepressants have analgesic properties. There is no definite indication that any one drug is more effective than the others, although the most experience has been accrued with amitriptyline, and most recently with duloxetine.

In a small sample, mirtazapine has been shown to improve, though not statistically significant, pain, nausea, appetite, insomnia, and anxiety. Gains were small, but one must consider that patients left untreated are likely to show decline in these symptoms, not improvement.[91] Freynhagen et al.[92] has shown that in a large sample of 594 patients, from baseline to endpoint (a 6-week period), mirtazapine significantly improves pain, sleep disturbances, irritability, and exhaustion.

Appropriate dosage of antidepressant adjuvant analgesics. In terms of appropriate dosage, there is evidence that the therapeutic analgesic effects of amitriptyline are correlated with serum levels just as the antidepressant effects are, and analgesic treatment failure is due to low serum levels.[93] A high-dose regimen of up to 150 mg of amitriptyline or higher is suggested.[94] As to the time course of onset of analgesia or with antidepressants, there appears to be a biphasic process that occurs with immediate or early analgesic effects that occur within hours or days[71] and later, longer analgesic effects that peak over a 4- to 6-week period.[67]

Treatment should be initiated with a small dose of amitriptyline; for instance, that is, 10–25 mg at bedtime especially in debilitated patients, and increased slowly by 10–25 mg every 2–4 days toward 150 mg with frequent assessment of pain and side effects until a beneficial effect is achieved. Maximal effect as an adjuvant analgesic may require continuation of drug for 2–6 weeks. Serum levels of antidepressant drug, when available, may also help in management to assure that therapeutic serum levels of drug are being achieved.

Both pain and depression in cancer patients often respond to lower doses (25–100 mg) of antidepressant than are usually required in the physically healthy (100–300 mg), most probably because of impaired metabolism of these drugs.

Choosing the appropriate antidepressant adjuvant analgesic drug. The choice of drug often depends on the side-effect profile, existing medical problems, the nature of depressive symptoms if present, and past response to specific antidepressants. Sedating drugs like amitriptyline are helpful when insomnia complicates the presence of pain and depression on a cancer patient. Anticholinergic properties of some of these drugs should also be kept in mind. Occasionally, in patients who have limited analgesic response to a tricyclic, potentiation of analgesia can be accomplished with the addition of lithium augmentation.[95]

Tricyclic antidepressants have been shown to be as effective as analgesics for mucositis when compared to opioids and for patients for whom opioids are contraindicated TCAs may be used.[96]

MONOAMINE OXIDASE INHIBITORS

Monoamine oxidase inhibitors (MAOIs) are less useful in the cancer setting because of dietary restriction and potentially dangerous interactions between MAOIs and narcotics such as meperidine. Amongst the MAOI drugs available, phenelzine has been shown to have adjuvant analgesic properties in patients with atypical facial pain and migraine.[97]

ANTICONVULSANTS

Selected anticonvulsant drugs appear to be analgesic for the lancinating dysesthesias that characterize diverse types of neuropathic pain.[64] Clinical experience also supports the use of these agents in patients with paroxysmal neuropathic pains that may not be lancinating and, to a far lesser extent, in those with neuropathic pains characterized solely by continuous dysesthesias. Although, in the past, practitioners used carbamazepine because of the good response rates observed in trigeminal neuralgia, it is, generally, not currently perceived as a first-line anticonvulsant analgesic. Carbamazepine must be used cautiously in patients with thrombocytopenia, those at risk for marrow failure, and those whose blood counts must be monitored to determine disease status. Several newer anticonvulsants are now commonly used in the treatment of neuropathic pain, particularly in cancer patients with chemotherapy-induced neuropathic pain syndromes. These drugs include gabapentin, pregabalin, oxcarbazepine, lamotrigine, and felbamate. Of these anticonvulsants, anecdotal experience has been most favorable with gabapentin, which is now being widely used by pain specialists to treat neuropathic pain of various types. Gabapentin has a relatively high degree of safety, including no known drug–drug interactions and a lack of hepatic metabolism.[64] Treatment with gabapentin is usually initiated at a dose of 300 mg per day and then gradually increased to a dose range of 900–3200 mg per day in three divided doses. Pregabalin is Food and Drug Administration (FDA)-approved for neuropathic pain associated with diabetic neuropathy as well as for postherpetic neuralgia. A randomized placebo-controlled trial reported by Dworkin et al.[98] demonstrated that pregabalin at doses of 300 mg or 600 mg daily, significantly reduced pain by 30% after 8-week treatment. Oxcarbazepine has shown in small clinical trials to be effective in the management of trigeminal neuralgia and diabetic neuropathy.[99]

PSYCHOSTIMULANTS

The psychostimulants dextroamphetamine and methylphenidate are useful antidepressant agents prescribed selectively for medically ill cancer patients with depression.[99] Psychostimulants are also useful in diminishing excessive sedation secondary to narcotic analgesics, and are potent adjuvant analgesics. Bruera et al[69] demonstrated that a regimen of 10 mg methylphenidate with breakfast and 5 mg with lunch significantly decreased sedation and potentiated the analgesic effect of narcotics in patients with cancer pain. Dextroamphetamine has also been reported to have additive analgesic effects when used with morphine in postoperative pain.[100]

In relatively low dose, psychostimulants stimulate appetite, promote a sense of well-being, and improve feelings of weakness and fatigue in cancer patients. Treatment with dextroamphetamine or methylphenidate usually begins with a dose of 2.5 mg at 8 a.m. and at noon. The dosage is slowly increased over several days until a desired effect is achieved or side effects (overstimulation, anxiety, insomnia, paranoia, confusion) intervene. Typically, a dose greater than 30 mg per day is not necessary although occasionally patients require up to 60 mg per day. Patients usually are maintained on methylphenidate for 1–2 months, and approximately two-thirds will be able to be withdrawn from methylphenidate without a recurrence of depressive symptoms. Those who do recur can be maintained on a psychostimulant for up to 1 year without significant abuse problems. Tolerance will develop and adjustment of dose may be necessary. A strategy we have found useful in treating cancer pain associated with depression is to start a psychostimulant (starting dose of 2.5 mg of methylphenidate at 8 a.m. and at noon) and then to add a TCA after several days to help prolong and potentiate the short effect of the stimulant.

Modafinil is a wakefulness agent, FDA approved for the treatment of excessive daytime sedation secondary to sleep disorders (e.g., narcolepsy, sleep apnea), but often used clinically in the palliative care setting as a mild psychostimulant.[101] A study by DeBattista et al.[102] tested modafinil on subjects with major depression and partial response to antidepressants, and found that adjunctive treatment with modafinil significantly improved fatigue and depressive symptoms. Furthermore, modafinil was found to increase attention, concentration, and cognitive functioning. Fatigue is a common symptom of cancer and cancer treatment, and modafinil has been shown to improve fatigue in patients with multiple sclerosis and in cancer populations.[103] Modafinil, in doses ranging from 50 to 400 mg, is used in the palliative care settings to treat fatigue as well as to counteract the sedation caused by opioids in the setting of pain management. Modafinil is not a sympathomimetic agent, and its

mechanism of action is distinct from classic psychostimulants, suggesting that issues of dependence, tolerance, and abuse may be significantly less of a concern with modafinil than with agents such as dextroamphetamine or methylphenidate.[104]

NEUROLEPTICS AND ANTIPSYCHOTIC AGENTS FOR CANCER PAIN

Methotrimeprazine is a phenothiazine that is equianalgesic to morphine, has none of the opioid effects on gut motility, and probably produces analgesia through α-adrenergic blockade.[105] In patients who are opioid tolerant, it provides an alternative approach in providing analgesia by a nonopioid mechanism. It is a dopamine blocker and so has antiemetic as well as anxiolytic effects. Methotrimeprazine can produce sedation and hypotension and should be given cautiously by slow IV infusion. Unfortunately, methotrimeprazine has limited availability (e.g., unavailable in the United States, but available in Canada). Other phenothiazines such as chlorpromazine and prochlorperazine (Compazine) are useful as antiemetics in cancer patients, but probably have limited use as analgesics.[106] Fluphenazine in combination with TCAs has been shown to be helpful in neuropathic pains.[107] Haloperidol is the drug of choice in the management of delirium or psychoses in cancer patients, and has clinical usefulness as a co-analgesic for cancer pain.[106] Pimozide (Orap), a butyrophenone, has been shown to be effective as an analgesic in the management of trigeminal neuralgia, at doses of 4–12 mg per day.[105]

Atypical antipsychotics, such as olanzapine, risperidone, quetiapine, apiprazole, and ziprasidone are primarily used to treat delirium in the palliative care setting. Boettger and Breitbart[106] suggest that olanzapine and risperidone are the atypical antipsychotics with the most demonstrated efficacy for managing the symptoms of delirium; however, smaller studies and case series reports suggest potential benefit for quetiapine,[108] ziprasidone,[109] and apiprazole.[110] Olanzapine[111] has been used to treat unmanaged pain in the context of anxiety and mild cognitive impairment. Patients received 2.5–7.5 mg of olanzapine daily. Daily pain scores decreased; anxiety and cognitive impairment resolved. Aripiprazole has been shown to be potentially beneficial in reducing bone pain.[112]

ANXIOLYTIC AGENTS AND CANCER PAIN

Hydroxyzine is a mild anxiolytic with sedating and analgesic properties that are useful in the anxious cancer patient with pain.[113] This antihistamine has antiemetic activity as well. One hundred milligrams of parenteral hydroxizine has analgesic activity approaching 8 mg of morphine, and has additive analgesic effects when combined with morphine. Benzodiazepines have not been felt to have direct analgesic properties, although they are potent anxiolytics and anticonvulsants.[114] Some authors have suggested that their anticonvulsant properties make certain benzodiazepine drugs useful in the management of neuropathic pain. Recently, Fernandez et al.[115] showed that alprazolam, a unique benzodiazepine with mild antidepressant properties, was a helpful adjuvant analgesic in cancer patients with phantom limb pain or deafferentation (neuropathic) pain. Clonazepam (Klonopin) may also be useful in the management of lancinating neuropathic pains in the cancer setting, and has been reported to be an effective analgesic for patients with trigeminal neuralgia, headache, and posttraumatic neuralgia.[116] With the use of midazolam by IV in a patient-controlled dosage, there was no reduction in the use of postoperative morphine requirements or in the patient's perception of pain.[117] Intrathecal midazolam in animal models, however, has been shown to potentiate morphine analgesia.[118]

CORTICOSTEROIDS

Corticosteroid drugs have analgesic potential in a variety of chronic pain syndromes, including neuropathic pains and pain syndromes resulting from inflammatory processes.[64] Like other adjuvant analgesics, corticosteroids are usually added to an opioid regimen. In patients with advanced disease, these drugs may also improve appetite, nausea, malaise, and overall quality of life. Adverse effects include neuropsychiatric syndromes, GI disturbances, and immunosuppression.

ORAL LOCAL ANESTHETICS

Local anesthetic drugs may be useful in the management of neuropathic pains characterized by either continuous or lancinating dysesthesias. Controlled trials have demonstrated the efficacy of tocainide and mexiletine, and there is clinical evidence that suggests similar effects from flecainide and subcutaneous lidocaine.[64] It is reasonable to undertake a trial with oral local anesthetic in patients with continuous dysesthesias who fail to respond adequately to, or who cannot tolerate, the TCAs and with patients with lancinating pains refractory to trials of anticonvulsant drugs and baclofen. Mexiletine is preferred in the United States.[18]

PLACEBO

A mention of the placebo response is important to highlight the misunderstandings and relative harm of this phenomenon. The placebo response is common, and analgesia is mediated through endogenous opioids. The deceptive use of placebo response to distinguish psychogenic pain from "real" pain should be avoided. Placebos are effective in a portion of patients for a short period of time only and are not indicated in the management of cancer pain.

REFERENCES

1. Foley KM. The treatment of cancer pain. *N Engl J Med.* 1985 Jul 11;313(2):84–95.
2. Fitzgibbon DR. Cancer pain: management. In: Loeser JD, Butler SH, Chapman CR, Turk DC (eds). *Bonica's management of pain.* Philadelphia, PA: Lippincott Williams & Wilkins; 2001:659–703.
3. Weiss SC, Emanuel LL, Fairclough DL, Emanuel EJ. Understanding the experience of pain in terminally ill patients.[see comment]. *Lancet.* 2001 Apr 28;357(9265):1311–1315.
4. Twycross RG, Lack SA. *Symptom control in far advanced cancer: Pain relief.* London: Pitman Brooks; 1983.
5. Foley KM. Pain syndromes in patients with cancer. In: Bonica JJ (ed). *Advances in pain research and therapy.* New York: Raven Press; 1975:59–75.
6. Grond S, Zech D, Diefenbach C, Bischoff A. Prevalence and pattern of symptoms in patients with cancer pain: a prospective evaluation of 1635 cancer patients referred to a pain clinic. *J Pain Symptom Manage.* 1994 Aug;9(6):372–382.
7. Achte KA, Vanhkonen ML. Cancer and the psych. *Omega.* 1971;2:46–56.
8. IASP Subcommittee. Taxonomy pain terms: a list with definitions and notes on usage. *Pain.* 1979;6:249–252.
9. Spiegel D, Bloom JR. Pain in metastatic breast cancer. *Cancer.* 1983;52:341–345.
10. Doyle D, Hanks GWC, MacDonald N. *Oxford textbook of palliative medicine.* 2nd ed. New York: Oxford University Press; 1998.
11. Breitbart W, Stiefel F, Kornblith A, Pannulo S. Neuropsychiatric disturbances in cancer patients with epidural spinal cord compression receiving high dose corticosteroids: a prospective comparison study. *Psychooncology.* 1993;2:233–245.
12. Syrjala K, Chapko M. Evidence for a biopsychosocial model of cancer treatment-related pain. *Pain.* 1995;61:69–79.
13. Breitbart W, Holland J. Psychiatric aspects of cancer pain. In: Foley KM (ed). *Advances in pain research and therapy.* Vol 16. New York: Raven Press; 1990:73–87.
14. Breitbart W. Psychiatric management of cancer pain. *Cancer.* 1989;63:2336–2342.
15. Daut RL, Cleeland CS. The prevalence and severity of pain in cancer. *Cancer.* 1982;50:1913–1918.
16. Padilla G, Ferrell B, Grant M, Rhiner M. Defining the content domain of quality of life for cancer patients with pain. *Cancer Nurs.* 1990;13:108–115.
17. Payne D, Jacobsen P, Breitbart W, Passik S, Rosenfeld B, McDonald M. Negative thoughts related to pain are associated with greater pain, distress, and disability in AIDS pain. Presented at: *American Pain Society;* 1994; Vol Miami, FL.
18. McKegney FP, Bailey LR, Yates JW. Prediction and management of pain in patients with advanced cancer. *Gen Hosp Psychiatry.* 1981;3(2):95–101.
19. Singer EJ, Zorilla C, Fahy-Chandon B, Chi S, Syndulko K, Tourtellotte WW. Painful symptoms reported by ambulatory HIV-infected men in a longitudinal study. *Pain.* 1993;54(1):15–19.
20. Cleeland CS, Tearnan BH. Behavioral control of cancer pain. In: Holzman D, Turk D (eds). *Pain mangement.* New York: Pergamon Press; 1986:93–212.
21. Derogatis LR, Morrow GR, Fetting J, et al. The prevalence of psychiatric disorders among cancer patients. *JAMA.* 1983 Feb 11;249(6):751–757.
22. Ahles TA, Blanchard EB, Ruckdeschel JC. The multi-dimensional nature of cancer related pain. *Pain.* 1983;17:277–288.
23. Stiefel FC, Breitbart W, Holland J. Cortico-steroids in cancer: neuropsychiatric complications. *Cancer Invest.* 1989;7:479–91.
24. Bukberg J, Penman D, Holland JC. Depression in hospitalized cancer patients. *Psychosom Med.* 1984 May-Jun;46(3):199–212.
25. Massie MJ, Holland JC, Glass E. Delirium in terminally ill cancer patients. *Am J Psychiatr.* 1983;140:1048–1050.
26. Breitbart W. Suicide in cancer patients. *Oncology.* 1987;1:49–53.
27. Bolund C. Suicide and cancer: II. Medical and care factors in suicide by cancer patients in Sweden, 1973–1976. *J Psychosoc Oncol.* 1985;3:17–30.
28. Elliot K, Foley KM. Pain syndromes in the cancer patient. *J Psychosoc Oncol.* 1990;8:11–45.
29. Fishman BB, Pasternak SS, Wallenstein SL, Houde RW, Holland JC, Foley KM. The Memorial Pain Assessment Card. A valid instrument for the evaluation of cancer pain. *Cancer.* 1987;60(5):1151–1158.
30. Daut RL, Cleeland CS, Flanery RC. Development of the Wisconsin Brief Pain Questionnaire to assess pain in cancer and other disease. *Pain.* 1983;17:197–210.
31. Cleeland CS, Gonin R, Hatfield AK, et al. Pain and its treatment in outpatients with metastatic cancer. *N Engl J Med.* 1994 Mar 3;330(9):592–596.
32. Kanner RM, Foley KM. Patterns of narcotic use in a cancer pain clinic. *Ann N Y Acad Sci.* 1981;362:161–172.
33. Macaluso C, Weinberg D, Foley KM. Opioid abuse and misuse in a cancer pain population (Abstract). *Second International Congress on Cancer Pain.* Vol.
34. Bruera E, MacMillan K, Pither J, MacDonald, RN. Effects of morphine on the dyspnea of terminal cancer patients. *J Pain Symptom Manage.* 1990;5:341–344.
35. Grossman SA, Sheidler VR, Sweden K, Mucenski J, Piantadosi S. Correlations of patient and caregiver ratings of cancer pain. *J Pain Symptom Manage.* 1991;6:53–57.
36. Spiegel D, Bloom JR. Group therapy and hypnosis reduce metastatic breast carcinoma pain. *Psychosom Med.* 1983;4:333–339.
37. Passik S, Horowitz S, Malkin M, Gargan R. A psychoeducational support program for spouses of brain tumor patients (Abstract). Presented at: Symposium on New Trends in the Psychological Support of the Cancer Patient, American Psychiatric Association Annual Meeting; 1991; New Orleans, LA.
38. Syrjala K, Cummings C, Donaldson G. Hypnosis or cognitive behavioral training for the reduction of pai and nausea during cancer treatment: a controlled trial. *Pain.* 1992;48:137–146.
39. Tan SY, Leucht CA. Cognitive-behavioral therapy for clinical pain control: a 15-year update and its relationship to hypnosis. *Int J Clin Exp Hypn.* 1997 Oct;45(4):396–416.
40. Cleeland CS. Nonpharmacologic management of cancer pain. *J Pain Symptom Manage.* 1987;2:523–528.
41. Loscalzo M, Jacobsen PB. Practical behavioral approaches to the effective management of pain and distress. *J Psychosoc Oncol.* 1990;8:139–169.
42. Douglas DB. Hypnosis: useful, neglected, available. *Am J Hosp Palliat Care.* 1999 Sep-Oct;16(5):665–670.
43. Levitan A. The use of hypnosis with cancer patients. *Psychiatr Med.* 1992;10:119–131.
44. Montgomery GH, DuHamel KN, Redd WH. A meta-analysis of hypnotically induced analgesia: how effective is hypnosis? *Int J Clin Exp Hypn.* 2000 Apr;48(2):138–153.
45. Rajasekaran M, Edmonds PM, Higginson IL. Systematic review of hypnotherapy for treating symptoms in terminally ill adult cancer patients. *Palliat Med.* 2005 Jul;19(5):418–426.
46. Montgomery GH, Weltz CR, Seltz M, Bovbjerg DH. Brief presurgery hypnosis reduces distress and pain in excisional breast biopsy patients. *Int J Clin Exp Hypn.* 2002;50(1):17–32.
47. Fotopoulos SS, Graham C, Cook MR. Psychophysiologic control of cancer pain. In: Ventafridda JJBaV (ed). *Advances in pain research and therapy.* Vol 2. New York: Raven Press; 1979:231–244.
48. Kazak AE, Penati B, Brophy P, Himelstein B. Pharmacologic and psychologic interventions for procedural pain. *Pediatrics.* 1998;102(1 pt 1):59–66.
49. Keefe FJ, Ahles TA, Sutton L, et al. Partner-guided cancer pain management at the end of life: a preliminary study. *J Pain Symptom Manage.* 2005 Mar;29(3):263–272.
50. Manne S, Redd W, Jacobsen P, Georgiades I. Aroma for treatment of anxiety during MRI scans. (Abstract) Presented at: Meeting APAA (ed). Symposium on new trends in the psychological support of the cancer patient; 1991 Vol New Orleans, LA.

51. Jacox A, Carr D, Payne R, Berde CB, Breitbart W (ed). Clinical Practice Guideline Number 9: Management of Cancer Pain. In: U.S. Department of Health and Human Services PHS, Agency for Health Care Policy and Research, ed. Publication No. 94–0592. AHCPR 1994:139–141.

52. Fotopoulos SS, Graham C, Cook MR. Psychophysiologic control of cancer pain. In: Bonica JJ, Ventafridda V (eds). *Advances in pain research and therapy.* Vol 2. New York: Raven Press; 1979:231–244.

53. Portenoy RK. Pharmacologic approaches to the control of cancer pain. *J Psychosoc Oncol.* 1990;8:75–107.

54. Murray MD, Brater DC. Adverse effects of nonsteroidal anti-inflammatory drugs on renal function. *Ann Intern Med.* 1990;112:559–560.

55. Radack K, Deck C. Do nonsteroidal anti-inflammatory drugs interfere with blood pressure control in hypertensive patients? *J Gen Intern Med.* 1987;2(2):108–112.

56. Bolten WW. Symptomatic therapy of rheumatic diseases. How they reduce pain and thereby save costs. *MMW Fortschr Med.* 2002 Aug 22;144(33–34):30–36.

57. Portenoy RK. Acute and chronic pain. In: Lowinson J, Ruiz P, Millman R (eds). *Comprehensive textbook of substance abuse.* Baltimore: William and Wilkins; 1992:691–721.

58. Bruera E, Chadwick S, Brennels C, Hanson J, MacDonald RN. Methylphenidate associated with narcotics for the treatment of cancer pain. *Cancer Treat Res.* 1987;71:67–70.

59. Lefkowitz M, Newshan G. An evaluation of the use of analgesics for chronic pain in patients with AIDS (Abstract #684). Preented at: Proceedings of the 16th annual scientific meeting of the American Pain Society; 1997:71.

60. Freye E, Anderson-Hillemacher A, Ritzdorf I, Levy JV. Opioid rotation from high-dose morphine to transdermal buprenorphine (Transtec) in chronic pain patients. *Pain Pract.* 2007 Jun;7(2):123–129.

61. Breitbart W. Psychotropic adjuvant analgesics for pain in cancer and AIDS. *Psychooncology.* 1998;7(4):333–345.

62. Kaiko RF, Foley KM, Grabinski PY, et al. Central nervous system excitatory effects of meperidine in cancer patients. *Ann Neurol.* 1983;13(2):180–185.

63. Breitbart W, Sparrow B. Management of delirium in the terminally ill. *Prog Pall Care.* 1998;6:107–113.

64. Portenoy RK. Adjuvant analgesics in pain management. In: Doyle D, Hanks GWC, MacDonald N (eds). *Oxford textbook of palliative medicine.* New York: Oxford University Press; 1993:187–203.

65. Farrar JT, Portenoy RK. Neuropathic cancer pain: the role of adjuvant analgesics. *Oncology.* 2001 Nov;15(11):1435–1442.

66. Onghena P, Van Houdenhove B. Antidepressant-induced analgesia in chronic non-malignant pain: a meta-analysis of 39 placebo-controlled studies. *Pain.* 1992;49(2):205–219.

67. Max MB, Culnane M, Schafer SC, et al. Amitriptyline relieves diabetic-neuropathy pain in patients with normal and depressed mood. *Neurology.* 1987;37:589–596.

68. Sindrup SH, Ejlertsen B, Frøland A, Sindrup EH, Brøsen K, Gram LF. Imipramine treatment in diabetic neuropathy: relief of subjective symptoms without changes in peripheral and autonomic nerve function. *Eur J Clin Pharmacol.* 1989;37(2):151–153.

69. Bruera E, Fainsinger R, MacEachern T, Hanson J. The use of methylphenidate in patients with incident cancer pain receiving regular opiates: a preliminary report. *Pain.* 1992;50:75–77.

70. Gomez-Perez FJ, Rull JA, Dies H, Rodriquez-Rivera JG, Gonzalez-Barranco J, Lozano-Castañeda O. Nortriptyline and fluphenazine in the symptomatic treatment of diabetic neuropathy. A double-blind cross-over study. *Pain.* 1985;23:395–400.

71. Tiegno M, Pagnoni B, Calmi A, Rigoli M, Braga PC, Panerai AE. Chlorimipramine compared to pentazocine as a unique treatment in post-operative pain. *Int J Clin Pharmacol Res.* 1987;7:141–143.

72. Hameroff SR, Cork RC, Scherer K, et al. Doxepin effects on chronic pain, depression and plasma opioids. *J Clin Psychiatry.* 1982;2:22–26.

73. Lee RA, West RM, Wilson JD. The response to sertraline in men with chronic pelvic pain syndrome. *Sex Transm Infect.* 2005;81(2):147–149.

74. Walsh TD. Controlled study of imipramine and morphine in chronic pain due to advanced cancer (Abstract). Presented at: ASCO; May 4–6, 1986; Los Angeles.

75. Kimmick GG, Lovato J, McQuellon R, Robinson E, Muss HB. Randomized, double-blind, placebo-controlled, crossover study of sertraline (Zoloft) for the treatment of hot flashes in women with early stage breast cancer taking tamoxifen. *Breast J.* 2006;12(2):114–122.

76. Ventafridda V, Bonezzi C, Caraceni A, et al. Antidepressants for cancer pain and other painful syndromes with deafferentation component: comparison of Amitriptyline and Trazodone. *Ital J Neurol Sci.* 1987;8:579–587.

77. Magni G, Arsie D, DeLeo D. Antidepressants in the treatment of cancer pain. A survey in Italy. *Pain.* 1987;29:347–353.

78. Ventafridda V, Bianchi M, Ripamonti C, et al. Studies on the effects of antidepressant drugs on the antinociceptive action of morphine and on plasma morphine in rat and man. *Pain.* 1990;43:155–162.

79. Spiegel K, Kalb R, Pasternak GW. Analgesic activity of tricyclic antidepressants. *Ann Neurol.* 1983;13:462–465.

80. Diamond S, Frietag FG. The use of fluoxetine in the treatment of headache. *Clin J Pain.* 1989;5:200–201.

81. Geller SA. Treatment of fibrositis with fluoxetine hydrochloride (Prozac). *Am J Med.* 1989;87:594–595.

82. Max MB, Lynch SA, Muir J, Shoaf SE, Smoller B, Dubner R. Effects of desipramine, amitriptyline, and fluoxetine on pain in diabetic neuropathy. *N Engl J Med.* 1992;326:1250–1256.

83. Sindrup SH, Gram LF, Brosen K, Eshoj O, Mogenson EF. The selective serotonin reuptake inhibitor paroxetine is effective in the treatment of diabetic neuropathy symptoms. *Pain.* 1990;42:135–144.

84. Sindrup SH, Bjerre U, Dejgaard A, Brosen K, Aaes-Jorgensen T, Gram LF. The selective serotonin reuptake inhibitor citalopram relieves the symptoms of diabetic neuropathy. *Clin Pharmacol Ther.* 1992 Nov;52(5):547–552.

85. Sidney H, Kennedy HFA, Lam RW. Efficacy of escitalopram in treatment of major depressive disorder compared with conventional selective serotonin reuptake inhibitors and venlafaxine XR: a meta-analysis. J *Psychiatry Neurosci.* 2006;31(2):122–131.

86. Thase ME. Managing depressive and anxiety disorders with escitalopram. *Expert Opin Pharmacother.* 2006;7(4):429–440.

87. Holland JC, Romano SJ, Heiligenstein JH, Tepner RG, Wilson MG. A controlled trial of fluoxetine and desipramine in depressed women with advanced cancer. *Psychooncology.* 1998 Jul-Aug;7(4):291–300.

88. Pick CG, Paul D, Eison MS, Pasternak G. Potentiation of opioid analgesia by the antidepressant nefazodone. *Eur J Pharmacol.* 1992;211:375–381.

89. Tasmuth T, Hartel B, Kalso E. Venlafaxine in neuropathic pain following treatment of breast cancer. *Eur J Pain.* 2002;6:17–24.

90. Goldstein DJ, Lu Y, Detke MJ, Wiltse C, Mallinckrodt C, Demitrack MA. Duloxetine in the treatment of depression: a double-blind placebo-controlled comparison with paroxetine. *J Clin Psychopharmacol.* 2004;24(4):389–399.

91. Theobald DE, Kirsh KL, Holtsclaw E, Donaghy K, Passik SD. An open-label, crossover trial of mirtazapine (15 and 30 mg) in cancer patients with pain and other distressing symptoms. *J Pain Symptom Manage.* 2002;23(5): 442–447.

92. Freynhagen R, Muth-Selbach U, Lipfert P, et al. The effect of mirtazapine in patients with chronic pain and concomitant depression. *Curr Med Res Opin.* 2006;22(2):257–264.

93. McQuay HJ, Carroll D, Glynn CJ. Dose-response for analgesic effect of amitriptyline in chronic pain. *Anaesthesia.* 1993 Apr;48(4):281–285.

94. Watson CP, Evans RJ. A comparative trial of amitriptyline and zimelidine in post-herpetic neuralgia. *Pain.* 1985 Dec;23(4):387–394.

95. Tyler MA. Treatment of the painful shoulder syndrome with amitrityline and lithium carbonate. *Can Med Assoc J.* 1974;111:137–140.

96. Ehrnrooth E, Grau C, Zachariae R, Andersen J. Randomized trial of opioids versus tricyclic antidepressants for radiation-induced mucositis pain in head and neck cancer. *Acta Oncol.* 2001;40(6):745–750.

97. Anthony M. MAO inhibition in the treatment of migraine. *Arch Neurol.* 1969;21:263.

98. Dworkin RH, Corbin AE, Young JP Jr, et al. Pregabalin for the treatment of postherpetic neuralgia: a randomized, placebo-controlled trial. *Neurology.* 2003 Apr 22;60(8):1274–1283.

99. Fernandez F, Adams F, Holmes VF, Levy JK, Neidhart M. Methylphenidate for depressive disorders in cancer patients. An alternative to standard antidepressants. *Psychosomatics.* 1987 Sep;28(9):455–461.

100. Forrest WH Jr, Brown BW Jr, Brown CR, et al. Dextroamphetamine with morphine for the treatment of post-operative pain. *N Engl J Med.* 1977;296:712–715.

101. Morrow GR, Shelke AR, Roscoe JA, Hickok JT, Mustian K. Management of cancer-related fatigue. *Cancer Invest.* 2005;23(3):229–239.

102. DeBattista C, Lembke A, Solvason HB, Ghebremichael R, Poirier J. A prospective trial of modafinil as an adjunctive treatment of major depression. *J Clin Psychopharmacol.* 2004;24(1):87–90.

103. Kingshott RN, Vennelle M, Coleman EL, Engleman HM, Mackay TW, Douglas NJ. Randomized, double-blind, placebo-controlled crossover trial of modafinil in the treatment of residual excessive daytime sleepiness in the sleep apnea/hypopnea syndrome. *Am J Respir Crit Care Med.* 2001;163(4): 918–923.

104. Maltbie AA, Cavenar JO Jr, Sullivan JL, Hammett EB, Zung WW. Analgesia and haloperidol: a hypothesis. *J Clin Psychiatry.* 1979;40:323–326.

105. Lechin F, van der Dijs B, Lechin ME, et al. Pimozide therapy for trigeminal neuralgia. *Arch Neurol.* 1989;9:960–964.

106. Boettger S, Breitbart W. Atypical antipsychotics in the management of delirium: a review of the empirical literature. *Palliat Support Care.* 2005;3(3):227–237.

107. Langohr HD, Stohr M, Petruch F. An open and double-blind crossover study on the efficacy of clomipramine (anafranil) in patients with painful mono- and polyneuropathies. *Eur Neurol.* 1982;21:309–315.

108. Sasaki Y, Matsuyama T, Inoue S, et al. A prospective, open-label, flexible-dose study of quetiapine in the treatment of delirium. *J Clin Psychiatry.* 2003;64(11):1316–1321.

109. Leso L, Schwartz TL. Ziprasidone treatment of delirium. *Psychosomatics.* 2002;43(1):61–62.

110. Alao AO, Soderberg M, Pohl EL, Koss M. Aripiprazole in the treatment of delirium. *Int J Psychiatry Med.* 2005;35(4):429–433.

111. Khojainova N, Santiago-Palma J, Kornick C, Breitbart W, Gonzales GR. Olanzapine in the management of cancer pain. *J Pain Symptom Manage.* 2002;23(4):346–350.

112. Wilson MS. Aripiprazole and bone pain. *Psychosomatics.* 2005;46(2):187.

113. Rumore MA. Clinical efficacy of antihistamines as analgesics. *Pain.* 1986;25:7–22.

114. Coda B, Mackie A, Hill H. Influence of alprazolam on opioid analgesia and side effects during steady-stage morphine infusions. *Pain.* 1992;50: 306–316.

115. Fernandez F, Adams F, Holmes VF. Analgesic effect of alprazolam in patients with chronic, organic pain of malignant origin. *J Clin Psychiatry.* 1987;3:167–169.

116. Swerdlow M, Cundill JG. Anticonvulsant drugs used in the treatment of lancinating pains: a comparison. *Anesthesia.* 1981;36:1129–1134.

117. Egan K, Ready L, Nessly M, Greer B. Self administration of midazolam for post-operative anxiety: a double blinded study. *Pain.* 1992;49:3–8.

118. Liao J. Quantitative assessment of antinociceptive effects of midazolam, amitriptyline, and carbamazepine alone and in combination with morphine in mice. *Anesthesiology.* 1990;73:A753.

Nausea and Vomiting

Kavitha Ramchandran and Jamie H. Von Roenn

INTRODUCTION

Nausea and vomiting are two of the symptoms most feared by patients with cancer.[1] Although the prevention and treatment of nausea and vomiting has improved over the past 20 years, it continues to negatively impact quality of life.[2]

Definition. Nausea is a subjective symptom. It is the sensation of impending vomiting, of feeling "sick to your stomach" or "queasy." Vomiting, an objective, readily measurable symptom has two phases: retching and expulsion. Other autonomic changes during this process include pallor, sweating, hypotension, and salivation.[3] Overall, available antiemetics are more effective for the control of vomiting than nausea.[4] This is particularly true in the setting of chemotherapy-induced nausea and vomiting. Each of these symptoms, nausea and vomiting, must be evaluated.

Evaluation of the patient. A thorough history and physical examination are the first steps in the elucidation of the cause of nausea and vomiting. The history should establish the pattern of nausea and vomiting (i.e., time of day, association with meals or other symptoms, frequency). When did the nausea begin? How often does it occur? Does it occur at the same time of day? For example, early morning vomiting without nausea is associated with increased intracranial pressure. The quantity and content (i.e., hematemesis, undigested food, or bilious) of the emesis helps define its etiology; that is, large infrequent emesis that relieves nausea may indicate an obstruction. Associated or exacerbating symptoms such as pain, constipation, anxiety, anorexia, early satiety, dyspepsia, cough, further define the cause of nausea and vomiting and suggest specific treatment approaches. Additionally, medical interventions such as procedures, surgery, and radiation therapy can induce nausea and vomiting.

The patient's complete list of current medications and supplements is reviewed with special attention to recent changes in medication's dose and schedule. For example, escalation of opioid dose or discontinuation of high dose steroids, may lead to nausea and vomiting.

Comorbid disease or its therapy may be contributing factors to nausea and vomiting. For example, adrenal insufficiency, thyroid, cardiac and gastroesophageal reflux disease may present with nausea. Alcohol or illicit drug use may impact the incidence of nausea. For example, cannabinoids decrease nausea while excessive alcohol use may cause nausea.

Additionally, the primary cancer or its metastases may present with nausea. Central nervous system (CNS) primary tumors, brain metastases, or leptomeningeal disease present with nausea secondary to increased intracranial pressure and/or meningeal irritation. A gastrointestinal primary, such as gastric cancer, can cause obstructive symptoms including nausea and vomiting. Peritoneal carcinomatosis and ascites can cause "squashed stomach" syndrome and nausea.[5] Excessive cough may produce nausea secondary to increased intraabdominal pressure with coughing.

The physical examination includes an assessment of volume status (dry mucous membranes, skin tenting, orthostatics) since dehydration may lead to nausea. Mouth lesions may point toward stomatitis or thrush. Abdominal examination will identify changes in or lack of bowel sounds, masses, organomegaly, or ascites. Rectal examination may show fecal impaction suggesting constipation-induced nausea. Neurological signs such as cranial nerve abnormalities, papilledema would indicate increased intracranial pressure (see Table 31–1).

The laboratory work-up seeks to identify metabolic causes of nausea and vomiting including uremia, hypercalcemia, hyponatremia, and liver disease. Thyroid function tests and fasting cortisol are useful if the patient's clinical presentation suggests a diagnosis of hypothyroidism or adrenal insufficiency.

The history, physical examination, and initial laboratory studies suggest appropriate imaging studies. For a patient with new neurological findings magnetic resonance imaging (MRI) of the brain and/or spinal cord and meninges are indicated. The patient with abdominal distension, pain, decreased bowel movements, and hypoactive bowel sounds needs an acute abdominal series to rule out obstruction.

Pathophysiology. There are four major pathways involved in the pathogenesis of nausea and vomiting. The area postrema, or "vomiting center," is located in the medulla. The vomiting center receives input from the chemoreceptor trigger zone, the cortex, peripheral input, and the vestibular system.[6,7] The chemoreceptor trigger zone, located in the floor of the fourth ventricle, outside of the blood-brain barrier, is exposed to toxins in the bloodstream and cerebral spinal fluid that may stimulate vomiting. The cortex incorporates input from the five senses, as well as from other factors, such as meningeal irritation or increased intracranial pressure, and supplies input to the vomiting center. Peripheral pathways include mechanoreceptors and chemoreceptors in the gastrointestinal tract which transmit input to the vomiting center from the vagus, splachnic, glossopharyngeal nerves, and sympathetic ganglia. Finally, motion triggers nausea and vomiting via labyrinthine input to the vomiting center from the vestibulocochlear nerve (Fig. 31–1).

Multiple neurotransmitters (and neuroreceptors) mediate the symptoms of nausea and vomiting. These pathways include serotonin (5-HT3), substance P (NK1), dopamine (D2), histamine (H1), acetylcholine (muscarinic),[8,9] and the cannabinoid receptor (CB1). The predominant site of activity of these neurotransmitters and receptors are displayed in Fig. 31–1.

COMMON ETIOLOGIES OF NAUSEA AND VOMITING IN CANCER

Chemotherapy-induced nausea and vomiting. The incidence of chemotherapy-induced nausea and vomiting is influenced by age, gender, prior experience with chemotherapy, patient expectations, and the emetogenic potential and dose of the antineoplastic agent. Younger patients and women experience nausea more often than men or older patients.[10-12] Patients with a history of prior chemotherapy-induced nausea and vomiting, motion sickness, or the expectation of nausea have an increased likelihood of chemotherapy-induced nausea and vomiting.[13] Interestingly, alcoholics and chemotherapy naïve patients experience less nausea than the overall population.[8,9]

Chemotherapy-related nausea and vomiting is related to the chemotherapy agent and its dose. These drugs are classified on the basis of their emetogenic potential. Level 1 drugs are associated with a risk of nausea and vomiting of less than 10%, while Level 4 drugs have an emetogenic potential of >90% (Table 31–2).[14,15] Combination regimens containing multiple Level 1 drugs do not change the emetogenicity of the

Table 31–1. Common symptoms and signs of nausea and vomiting in patients with cancer

Symptoms	Evaluation	Etiology
Gastrointestinal		
Mouth pain/sores	Oropharynx examination Endoscopy if indicated	Oropharyngeal infection (i.e., thrush/viral) esophagitis
Large high volume emesis	Abdominal examination Acute abdominal series	High level obstruction
Hematemesis	History Oropharyngeal examination Abdominal examination Endoscopy	Varices Perforated ulcer/mass
Excessive cough	History Pulmonary examination Chest x ray	Cough→ increased abdominal pressure and nausea Pulmonary process→ infection
Right sided abdominal pain Colic	Abdominal examination Abdominal imaging	Liver, gallbladder disease
Constipation/Obstipation	Abdominal examination Rectal examination	Constipation related emesis Gastroparesis
Poor oral intake, cachexia	History Physical examination	Anorexia
Increased abdominal girth, palpable masses, small volume emesis	Abdominal examination, Abdominal imaging	Squashed stomach syndrome from mass effect, ascites, small bowel obstruction
Metabolic		
Abdominal discomfort, confusion, kidney stones	Laboratory studies	Hypercalcemia
Decreased urine output, confusion	Laboratory studies	Renal failure
Labile blood pressure, syncopal episodes	Laboratory studies including cortisol	Adrenal insufficiency
Confusion, changes in volume status	Laboratory studies	Hyponatremia
Neurologic		
Headaches, diplopia, early morning emesis, cranial nerve abnormalities	Neurological examination CNS imaging Lumbar puncture	Increased intracranial pressure
Anxiety/nervousness	History	Anxiety induced nausea

ABBREVIATION: CNS, central nervous system.

combination. However, a combination of more than one Level 2 drug increases the emetogenicity of the therapy by one level. The addition of a Level 3 or a Level 4 agent to a combination regimen increases the emetogenic potential of the therapy by one level per agent.[16]

Chemotherapy-induced nausea and vomiting is defined by its timing in relationship to treatment. Anticipatory nausea and vomiting (ANV) occurs before the initiation of treatment. Its pathophysiology appears to be an example of classical conditioning. A conditioned stimuli (i.e., the voice of the nurse, smells of the clinic) trigger nausea and vomiting before the initiation of treatment.[17] Poor control of nausea and vomiting during prior treatment cycles increases the risk of developing it. Additionally, with increasing cycles of therapy the risk of ANV increases.[18] Acute nausea and vomiting occurs within 24 hours of treatment. Delayed nausea and vomiting occurs 24–72 hours after chemotherapy.

The mechanism of chemotherapy-induced nausea and vomiting is multifaceted. Chemotherapy is thought to release free radicals that cause exocytic release of 5-HT from enterochromaffin cells in the gut. This stimulates nausea and vomiting via the vagal and splanchnic nerves. Additionally, chemotherapy acts directly on the vomiting center via 5-HT3 and NK1 receptors. Furthermore chemotherapy-induced nausea and vomiting may be driven by anxiety, as is the case with anticipatory symptoms.[19,20]

The recommended treatment of chemotherapy-induced vomiting depends on the emetogenicity of the treatment regimen. Multiple guidelines for the treatment of chemotherapy-induced nausea and vomiting have been published (Table 31-3). In general, treatment is more effective for the control of vomiting than it is for nausea.

Opioid-induced nausea and vomiting. Opioids stimulate nausea in one-half to two-thirds of opioid naïve patients. Nausea and emesis can occur with initiation or escalation of an opioid and with rotation of one opioid to another. The mechanism (and receptors involved) of opioid-induced nausea is multifactorial. Opioids slow gastrointestinal tract (GI) motility leading to constipation (H1, muscarinic acetylcholine receptor), delay gastric emptying (D2 receptor), stimulate the chemoreceptor trigger zone (CTZ) (D2 receptor), and may sensitize the labyrinth (H1, muscarinic acetylcholine receptor).

Opioid-induced nausea and vomiting generally resolves within 2–3 days of initiation or escalation of the medication. Prophylactic antiemetics, such as D2 antagonists, around the clock during the first 2–3 days of the opioid usually prevent nausea. If nausea occurs in spite of treatment, titrating up the antiemetic, rotation to an alternative opioid, or reduction of the opioid (if pain control allows) is usually effective.[21,22] If these initial steps are ineffective agents to increase gastric motility (i.e., metoclopramide) may be helpful. Development of nausea a week after initiation of opioid therapy suggests an alternate etiology for the nausea. Examples include an electrolyte abnormality, another offending drug, or constipation (another common opioid side effect).

Intestinal obstruction. Intestinal obstruction from external compression or internal occlusion by tumor frequently presents with nausea and vomiting. The most common cancers associated with bowel obstruction are gastric, ovarian, and colon cancer. In addition to progressive tumor, bowel obstruction may result from adhesions or postradiation fibrosis. The receptors involved in the nausea and vomiting associated

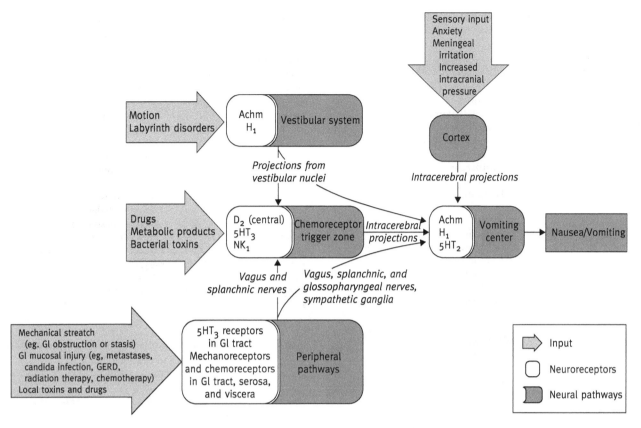

Fig. 31–1. Interrelationships between neural pathways that mediate nausea and vomiting.
ABBREVIATIONS: Achm, muscarinic acetylcholine receptor; D2, dopamine type 2 receptor; GERD, gastroesophageal reflux; GI, gastrointestinal; H1, histamine type 1 receptor; NK1, neurokinin type 1 receptor; 5HT2, 5-hydroxytryptamine type 2 receptor; 5-HT3, 5-hydroxytryptamine type 3 receptor.
SOURCE: Reprinted with permission from Wood G, et al., *J Am Med Ass.* 2007;298:1196–1207. Copyright © 2007 American Medical Association. All Rights reserved.

with bowel obstruction include peripheral receptors in the gut (H1, acetylcholine) as well as D2 receptors in the CTZ. The pathophysiology is multifactorial. Lumen occlusion prevents movement of intestinal contents from passing distally. The resultant accumulation of contents and nonabsorbed secretions produces distention and colic. The bowel also continues to contract in an uncoordinated fashion resulting in cramping and pain.

Symptoms of malignant obstruction differ based on the level of obstruction. With high level obstruction (i.e., stomach, duodenum, or jejunum) patients develop nausea early and usually have high volume emesis. Nausea usually persists even after an episode of emesis. Obstruction at lower levels present more classically with pain and colic rather than nausea and vomiting.

Nausea and vomiting associated with obstruction is usually relieved with insertion of a nasogastric tube as well as fluid and electrolyte replacement. This may be a bridging step to more definitive therapy such as surgery, a stent, or venting gastrostomy. Palliative surgery is an option in patients with good performance status, limited intra-abdominal tumor, minimal ascites, and a single site of obstruction.[23] For those patients who are not surgical candidates and who have a single site of obstruction stent placement may effectively relieve the obstruction. For patients with multiple sites of obstruction a venting gastrostomy may provide the best palliation of nausea, vomiting, and pain.

Pharmacologic therapy is an adjunct for the management of symptoms of nausea and vomiting from malignant bowel obstruction and is primary therapy for patients who cannot undergo a more definitive intervention. Recommended drugs include steroids, octreotide, anticholinergics, and promotility agents such as metoclopramide (if the obstruction is partial). Steroids work by reducing peritumoral edema

and increase water and salt absorption. Octreotide inhibits secretion of gastric acid, pepsin, pancreatic enzymes thus decreasing overall fluid output, and decreases peristalsis. Anticholinergics also have antisecretory effects and decrease contractions and tone.[24]

Radiation-induced nausea and vomiting. Management of radiation-induced nausea and vomiting includes both prevention and treatment. The incidence and severity of radiation-induced nausea and vomiting depends on the radiation site, port size, and dose.

Total body irradiation is associated with the highest risk of radiation-induced nausea and vomiting. Radiation therapy, which excludes the abdominal cavity has a low risk of nausea and vomiting.[25] Radiation-induced nausea and vomiting results from both central and peripheral mechanisms. Serotonin (5-hydroxytryptamine, 5-HT) is released from enterochromaffin cells located in the GI mucosa in response to radiation. Serotonin interacts with 5-HT3 receptors peripherally on vagal afferent neurons and centrally in the nucleus tractus solitarius, eliciting the vomiting reflex.[26] Guidelines for the treatment of radiation-induced nausea and vomiting are shown in Table 31–4.

Increased intracranial pressure. Parenchymal brain tumors, whether primary or metastatic can increase intracranial pressure and can cause nausea and vomiting. Symptoms frequently associated with increased intracranial pressure include morning headaches, diplopia, and cranial nerve abnormalities.

Increased intracranial pressure leads to meningeal irritation which activates meningeal mechanoreceptors that stimulate the vomiting center. This is also the mechanism of the nausea and vomiting secondary to meningeal irritation. While the nausea and vomiting associated with parenchymal brain metastases generally responds to steroids, the

Table 31–2. Emetogenicity of parenteral chemotherapeutic drugs

Level	Frequency of emesis, percent	Chemotherapeutic drug and dose
High	>90	Cisplatin
		Mechlorethamine
		Streptozotocin
		Cyclophosphamide ≥1500 mg/m²
		Carmustine
		Dacarbazine
		Dactinomycin
Moderate	30–90	Oxaliplatin
		Cytarabine >1 g/m²
		Carboplatin
		Ifosfamide
		Cyclophosphamide <1500 mg/m²
		Doxorubicin
		Daunorubicin
		Epirubicin
		Idarubicin
		Irinotecan
		Ixabepilone
Low	10–30	Paclitaxel
		Docetaxel
		Mitoxantrone
		Topotecan
		Etoposide
		Pemetrexed
		Methotrexate[a]
		Mitomycin
		Gemcitabine
		Cytarabine <=1000 mg/m²
		Fluorouracil
		Bortezomib
		Cetuximab
		Trastuzumab
Minimal	<10	Bevacizumab
		Bleomycin
		Busulfan
		2-Chlorodeoxyadenosine
		Fludarabine
		Rituximab
		Vinblastine
		Vincristine
		Vinorelbine

[a]At doses >1 gm, methotrexate has at least moderate emetogenic potential.
SOURCE: Adapted with permission from *Journal of Clinical Oncology* 24 (18), 2006: 2932–2947. © 2008 American Society of Clinical Oncology. All rights reserved.

Table 31–3. Drug regimens for the prevention of chemotherapy-induced emesis by emetic risk category

Emetic risk category (incidence of emesis without antiemetics)	Antiemetic regimens and schedules
High (>90%)	5-HT3 serotonin receptor antagonist: day 1
	Dexamethasone: days 1–4
	Aprepitant: days 1, 2, 3
Moderate (30%–90%)	5-HT₃ serotonin receptor antagonist: day 1
	Dexamethasone: day 1 (2, 3)[a]
	Aprepitant: days 1, 2, 3[b]
Low (10%–30%)	Dexamethasone: day 1
Minimal (<10%)	Prescribe as needed

ABBREVIATION: 5-HT3, 5-hydroxytryptamine-3.
[a]May omit days 2 and 3 if aprepitant is given.
[b]For patients receiving a combination of an anthracycline and cyclophosphamide.
SOURCE: Adapted with permission from *J Clin Oncol.* 2006;24:2932.

Table 31–4. Emetic risk category related to area of the body receiving radiation and treatment guidelines

Emetic risk category	Area receiving radiation	Antiemetic guideline
High	Total body irradiation	Before each fraction: 5-HT3 receptor antagonist + dexamethasone
Moderate	Upper abdomen	Before each fraction: 5-HT3 receptor antagonist
Low	Lower thorax, pelvis, cranium (radiosurgery), craniospinal	As needed: 5-HT3 receptor antagonist
Minimal	Head and neck, extremities, cranium, breast	As needed: dopamine receptor antagonist or 5-HT3 receptor antagonist

ABBREVIATION: 5-HT3, 5-hydroxytryptamine-3.
SOURCE: Adapted with permission from *J Clin Oncol.* 2006;24:2932.

nausea and vomiting due to meningeal infiltration by tumor is often difficult to control. Steroids and radiation therapy remain the most frequently prescribed therapy.[27] A centrally acting antiemetic may also be useful.

TREATMENT

Pharmacologic. A pathogenesis based treatment approach manages nausea and vomiting most effectively. A systematic approach to treatment minimizes the potential for overmedication and polypharmacy. The major classes of antiemetics are D2 antagonists, 5-HT3 antagonists, selective NK1 antagonists, antihistamines, and anticholinergics.

Dopamine 2(D2) receptor antagonists are among the oldest antiemetics. There are five groups of dopamine receptors (D1–D5). D2 is classically implicated in the pathogenesis of nausea and vomiting. D2 antagonists block CTZ-mediated nausea. Recent animal studies support a role for D3 in the generation of nausea from a central mechanism.[28] D2 receptor antagonists are the agents of choice for acute chemotherapy-induced nausea and vomiting with low-risk emetogenic regimens, opioid-induced nausea and vomiting, and in the setting of gastrointestinal dysmotility. The choice of a particular D2 receptor antagonist is generally based on the symptoms associated with the nausea. For example, a patient with constipation, early satiety or dyspepsia would benefit from metoclopramide and its promotility effects, whereas a patient who is

Table 31–5. Common antiemetics, indications, adverse effects, dose, route

Drug	Indications	Adverse effects[a]	Dosing/route
D2 receptor antagonists			
Reglan	Gastroparesis Chemotherapy induced	Drowsiness EPS symptoms Anticholinergic effects	1–2 mg/kg IV or 0.5 mg/kg PO
Prochlorperazine	Opiate induced Chemotherapy induced	Hyperprolactinemia Neuroleptic malignant syndrome Dystonic reactions	5–10 mg q 6 hours PO/IV
Haldol	Opiate induced Chemotherapy induced	Esophageal spasm and colic in GI obstruction	0.2–3 mg IV/PO/SQ q8–12 hours
NK receptor antagonists			
Aprepitant/ Fosaprepitant	Delayed N and V HEC/MEC	Fatigue, dizziness, constipation, diarrhea	125 mg PO 115 mg IV (fosaprepitant) Repeat doses at 80 mg PO/IV
5-HT3 receptor antagonists			
Ondansetron	MEC/HEC	Headache Diarrhea	4–8 mg PO/IV q 8–12 hours (up to 24 mg on day 1 of HEC)
Granisetron		Constipation Fatigue Transient transaminitis	1 mg PO BID (2 mg PO before day 1 of MEC or HEC)
Dolasetron			100 mg PO/IV daily
Tropisetron			3–5 mg PO/IV daily
Palonosetron			0.25 mg x1 on day 1
Corticosteroids			
Dexamethasone	MEC/HEC	Suppression of the hypothalamic pituitary axis Cushing syndrome Myopathy Osteoporosis Peptic ulcers/GERD/dyspepsia	Day 1 w/aprepitant 12 mg IV/PO w/o aprepitant—20 mg for HEC IV or PO, 8 mg for MEC IV or PO Day 2–3 8 mg days 2–4 for HEC 8 mg days 2–3 for MEC
CB1 receptor agonists			
Nabilone	Mild chemotherapy-induced N and V	Sympathomimetic activity Labile effects on mood/cognition/appetite/ perception	1–2 mg PO q 12 hours as needed
Dronabinol	Mild chemotherapy-induced N and V	Seizures	5mg/m2 q 2–4 hours PO

[a]Adverse effects reflects common reactions and is not inclusive of all possible adverse reactions.
ABBREVIATIONS: CB1, cannabinoid receptor; D2, dopamine; EPS, extrapyramidal side effects; GERD, gastroesophageal reflux; GI, gastrointestinal; HEC, high emetogenic chemotherapy; IV, intravenous; MEC, moderate emetogenic chemotherapy; NK, substance P; PO, per os, or orally.

anxious, agitated, or confused and has nausea would benefit most from haloperidol.

More than seven 5-HT receptors have been identified. The first 5-HT3 receptor antagonists were introduced in the 1990s and dramatically changed the management of nausea and vomiting. 5-HT3 is the receptor with the highest frequency in the gut and in the nucleus of the tractus solitarius. It is the primary target for 5-HT3 receptor antagonists. These agents are used to prevent radiation-induced nausea and vomiting and to prevent acute nausea and vomiting associated with moderately to highly emetogenic chemotherapy. The newest generation of drug in this class is palonosetron. It has a longer half-life and greater affinity for the 5-HT3 receptor than other 5-HT3 receptor antagonists. However, the specific indications for palonosetron over the older generation of 5-HT3 antagonists are not defined.

Tachykinins, such as substance P, exert their antiemetic effect centrally at NK receptor antagonists that cross the blood-brain barrier and decrease, both, acute and delayed chemotherapy-induced emesis. These agents have their greatest impact on delayed nausea and vomiting from chemotherapy (see Table 31–2).

Corticosteroids have been used as antiemetics for several decades. Their mechanism of action is poorly understood, but there are several proposed hypotheses. Steroids may produce their antiemetic effect by decreasing 5-HT release or antagonizing the 5-HT3 receptor. In addition they may activate the glucocorticoid receptor in the medulla and possibly increase drug levels of other antiemetics.[29] Steroids are the treatment of choice for nausea and vomiting secondary to increased intracranial pressure and are useful adjunctive therapy for the treatment of a malignant bowel obstruction.

Cannabinoids exert antiemetic effects by agonism of the CB1s. Dronabinol and nabilone are the two commercially available agents in the United States. They are approved for the treatment of nausea refractory to standard antiemetics though their efficacy appear about equal to that of prochlorperazine.[30] These drugs are reportedly more effective in patients previously exposed to cannabinoids.[31] Impaired psychomotor function and the psychoactive effects (dizziness, dysphoria, hallucinations) of cannabinoids limit their usefulness, particularly in older patients. See Table 31–5 for a list of commonly used antiemetics.

NONPHARMACOLOGIC TREATMENT OF NAUSEA AND VOMITING

Nonpharmacologic approaches to control nausea and vomiting include, but are not limited to, acupuncture, behavioral treatment, and nutritional interventions.

Acupuncture. A 1997 National Institutes of Health (NIH) consensus statement on acupuncture recognized the efficacy of needle acupuncture for adult postoperative and chemotherapy-induced nausea and vomiting.[32] This set the stage for additional research in this area. A recent Cochrane review of eleven acupuncture trials (N = 1247) reported that acupuncture point stimulation of all methods (needles, acupuncture trials, electrical stimulation, magnets, or acupressure) reduces the incidence of acute vomiting, but not nausea severity. However, when evaluated by modality, self- administered acupressure had a protective affect on the first day of nausea. Electroacupuncture (acupuncture supplied with electricity) reduced the incidence of acute vomiting while manual acupuncture did not. All of these trials, except the electroacupuncture trials, prescribed state-of-the-art antiemetics.[33]

Acupuncture techniques have not yet been evaluated for the treatment of nausea and vomiting induced by radiation therapy, opioids, or bowel obstruction.

Behavioral treatment. Behavioral therapies have a role in the treatment and prevention of nausea and vomiting. Examples of behavioral interventions include progressive muscle relaxation training (PMRT), systematic desensitization, hypnosis, and cognitive distraction. PMRT instructs patients to progressively stretch and relax specific muscle groups in combination with guided imagery. This appears to have its greatest benefit after chemotherapy is administered. It is less effective for anticipatory symptoms. Systematic desensitization, a method commonly used to train patients to overcome phobias, is helpful for control of ANV. Patients are taught to recreate the situation that causes the nausea (i.e., the infusion center) in their mind, while they are in a state of complete relaxation. This teaches patients to recondition themselves to be relaxed, instead of nauseated, in response to that stimuli. Hypnosis effectively prevents ANV in children but is less useful for adults. This may be because children are more easily hypnotized. Finally, cognitive distraction (i.e., video games) appears to be a cost-effective way to reduce ANV.[34]

Nutrition. Nutritional interventions have also been explored for their impact on nausea and vomiting. One trial randomized patients to receive a normal diet versus a diet high in protein (protein powder) and ginger (powdered ginger root). Patients who received the high protein/ginger diet experienced less nausea and used fewer antiemetics than the control group. Delayed nausea and vomiting was also reduced in the treatment group.[35] A phase I/II randomized controlled trial evaluating ginger for the control of postchemotherapy nausea is underway.[36]

CONCLUSIONS

Nausea and vomiting, distressing symptoms for patients with cancer, occur across the trajectory of disease, from diagnosis, through treatment, to end-of-life care. Careful evaluation of the patient, and awareness of the pathophysiology of nausea and vomiting, allows the development of a systematic, targeted approach to treatment and the most effective relief of symptoms.

REFERENCES

1. Coates A, Abraham S, Kaye SB, Sowerbutts T, Frewin C Fox, Tattersall MH. On the receiving end: patient perception of the side effects of cancer chemotherapy. *Eur J Cancer Clin Oncol.* 1983;19:203–208.

2. Carelle N, Piotto E, Bellanger A, Germanaud J, Thuillier A, Khayat D. Changing patient perceptions of the side effects of cancer chemotherapy. *Cancer.* 2002;95:155–163.

3. Pleuvry B. Physiology and pharmacology of nausea and vomiting. *Anaesth Intensive Care Med.* 2006;7(12):473–477.

4. Grunberg SM. Chemotherapy-induced nausea and vomiting: prevention, detection, and treatment—how are we doing? *J Support Oncol.* 2004;2(1, Suppl 1):1–10.

5. Regnard C, Comiskey M. Nausea and vomiting in advanced cancer: a flow diagram. *Palliat Med.* 1992;6:146–151.

6. Hornby PF. Central neurocircuitry associated with emesis. *Am J Med.* 2001;111(Suppl 8A):106S–112S.

7. Miller AD, Grelot S. Neural control of respiratory muscle activation during vomiting. In: Miller AD, Bianchi AL, Bishop BO, (eds). *Neural control of the respiratory muscles.* Boca Raton, FL: CRC Press; 1997:239–248.

8. Flake ZA, Scalley RD, Bailey AG. Practical selection of antiemetics. *Am Fam Physician.* 2004;69:1169–1174, 1176.

9. Wood G, Von Roenn JH, Lynch B. Management of intractable nausea and vomiting in patients at the end of life: "I was feeling nauseous all of the time...nothing was working." *JAMA.* 2007;298:1196–1207.

10. Pollera CF, Giannarelli D. Prognostic factors influencing cisplatin-induced emesis: definition and validation of a predictive logistic model. *Cancer.* 1989;64:1117–1122.

11. du Bois A, Meerpohl HG, Vach W, Kommoss FG, Fenzl E, Pfleiderer A. Course, patterns, and risk factors for chemotherapy-induced emesis in cisplatin-pretreated patients: a study with ondansetron. *Eur J Cancer.* 1992;28:450–457.

12. Osoba D, Zee B, Pater J, Warr D, Latreille J, Kaizer L. Determinants of postchemotherapy nausea and vomiting in patients with cancer. *J Clin Oncol.* 1997;15:116–123.

13. Roscoe JA, Bushunow P, Morrow GT, et al. Patient experience is a strong predictor of severe nausea after hemotherapy: a University of Rochester Community Clinical Oncology Program study of patients with breast carcinoma. *Cancer.* 2004;101:2701–2708.

14. Roila F, Hesketh PJ, Herrstedt J, Herrstedt J. Prevention of chemotherapy- and radiotherapy-induced emesis: results of the 2004 Perugia International Antiemetic Consensus Conference. *Ann Oncol.* 2006;17:20–28.

15. Hesketh PJ, Kris MG, Grunberg SM, et al. Proposal for classifying the acute emetogenicity of cancer chemotherapy. *J Clin Oncol.* 1997;15:103–109.

16. Hesketh P, Kris M, Grunberg SM, et al. Proposal for classifying the acute emetogenicity of cancer chemotherapy. *J Clin Oncol.* 1997;15:103.

17. Stockhorst U. Pavlovian conditioning of nausea and vomiting. *Auton Neurosci.* 2006;129:50–57.

18. Watson M. Psychological factors predicting nausea and vomiting in breast cancer patients on chemotherapy. *Eur J Cancer.* 1998;34:831–837.

19. Berger A, Clark-Snow R. Chemotherapy-related nausea and vomiting. In: Berger A, Schuster J, Von Roenn J, (eds). *Principles and practice of palliative care and supportive oncology,* 3rd ed. Philadelphia, PA: Lippincott Williams & Wilkins; 2007:139–149.

20. Warr DG. Chemotherapy- and cancer-related nausea and vomiting. *Curr Oncol.* 2008;15(Suppl 1):S4–S9.

21. Narabayashi M, Saijo Y, Takenoshita S, et al. Advisory Committee for Oxycodone Study. Opioid rotation from oral morphine to oral oxycodone in cancer patients with intolerable adverse effects: an open-label trial. *J Clin Oncol.* 2008;38:296–304.

22. Abrahm J. *Physician's guide to pain and symptom management in cancer patients.* The Johns Hopkins University Press; 2000, 2005.

23. Jong P, Sturgeon J, Jamieson CG. Benefit of palliative surgery for bowel obstruction in advanced ovarian cancer. *Can J Surg.* 1995;38:454–457.

24. Schwartzentruber DJ, Lublin M, Hostetter RB. Bowel obstruction. In: Berger A, Schuster J, Von Roenn J, (eds). *Principles and practice of palliative care and supportive oncology,* 3rd ed. Philadelphia, PA: Lippincott Williams & Wilkins; 2007:177–184.

25. The Italian Group for Antiemetic Research in Radiotherapy. Radiation-induced emesis: a prospective observational multicenter Italian trial. *Int J Radiat Oncol Biol Phys.* 1999;44:619–625.

26. Lindley C, Blower P. Oral serotonin type 3-receptor antagonists for prevention of chemotherapy-induced emesis. *Am J Health Syst Pharm.* 2000;57:1685–1697.

27. Mannix K. Palliation of nausea and vomiting in malignancy. *Clin Med.* 2006;6:144–147.

28. Yoshida N, Yoshikawa T, Kosoki K. A dopamine D3 receptor agonist, 7-OH-DPAT, causes vomiting in the dog. *Life Sci.* 1995;PL347–PL350.

29. Grunberg SM. Antiemetic activity of corticosteroids in patients receiving cancer chemotherapy: dosing, efficacy, and tolerability analysis. *Ann Oncol.* 2007;18:233–240.

30. Tramer MR, Carroll D, Campbell F, Reynolds D, Moore R, McQuay H. Cannabinoids for control of chemotherapy induced nausea and vomiting: quantitative systematic review. *BMJ.* 2001;323:16–21.

31. Slatkin NE. Cannabinoids in the treatment of chemotherapy-induced nausea and vomiting: beyond prevention of acute emesis. *J Support Oncol.* 2007; 5(5, Suppl 3):1–9.

32. NIH Consensus Statement. *Acupuncture.* 1997;15(5).

33. Ezzo JM, Richardson MA, Vickers A, Allen C, Dibble SL, Issell BF. Acupuncture-point stimulation for chemotherapy-induced nausea or vomiting. *Cochrane Database of Systemic Reviews* 2006, Issue 2, Art. No.: CD002285. DOI: 10.1002/14651858.CD002285.pub2.

34. Figueroa-Moseley C, Jean Pierre P, Roscoe J. Behavioral interventions in treating anticipatory nausea and vomiting. *J Natl Compr Canc Netw.* 2007;5:44–50.

35. Levine ME, Gillis MG, Koch SY, Voss AC, Stern RM, Koch KL. Protein and ginger for the treatment of chemotherapy-induced delayed nausea. *J Altern Complement Med.* 2008;14:454–551.

36. Hickok JT, Roscoe JA, Morrow GR, Ryan JL. A phase II/III randomized, placebo-controlled, double-blind clinical trial of ginger (zingiber officinale) for nausea caused by chemotherapy for cancer: a currently accruing URCC CCOP Cancer Control Study. *Support Cancer Ther.* 2007;4:247–250.

CHAPTER 32

Fatigue

William S. Breitbart and Yesne Alici

INTRODUCTION

Fatigue is a highly prevalent and distressing symptom of cancer, associated with decreased quality of life, as well as significant psychological and functional morbidity.[1-6] Fatigue in cancer patients has been significantly associated with depression, hopelessness, and overall psychological distress.[7] Fatigue has been shown to predict desire for hastened death among cancer patients.[8] Patients with cancer perceive fatigue as the most distressing symptom associated with cancer and its treatment, more distressing than pain, nausea, and vomiting.[3] As outlined in the National Comprehensive Cancer Network (NCCN) Practice Guidelines for Cancer-Related Fatigue,[9,10] "fatigue most commonly occurs with other symptoms, such as pain, distress, anemia, and sleep disturbances," thus cancer patients presenting with fatigue should be screened for all these symptoms.[9-11] Despite its impact on patients and their caregivers, cancer-related fatigue is underreported, underdiagnosed, and undertreated.[9,10] As growing attention is given to symptom management and quality of life in cancer patients, clinicians treating such patients should be familiar with major issues in assessment and management of fatigue. This chapter reviews the definition, prevalence, and assessment of cancer-related fatigue, as well as evidence-based strategies for treatment.

DEFINING CANCER-RELATED FATIGUE

Fatigue is a poorly defined symptom that may involve physical, mental, and motivational components. Cancer-related fatigue is defined by the NCCN[9,10] practice guidelines as "a distressing, persistent, subjective sense of physical, emotional, and cognitive tiredness or exhaustion related to cancer or cancer treatment that is not proportional to recent activity and interferes with usual functioning." Cancer-related fatigue is more severe and more distressing than fatigue experienced by healthy individuals and is less likely to be relieved by rest.[9,10] Recognizing the need for a standardized definition of fatigue, a group of expert clinicians[4] proposed a set of diagnostic criteria, which are included in the 10th edition of *International classification of diseases (ICD-10)* (Table 32–1). A standardized interview guide has been designed and validated for use in identifying patients with cancer-related fatigue.[12]

PREVALENCE OF FATIGUE

The reported prevalence of cancer-related fatigue ranges from 4% to 100%, depending on the specific cancer population studied and the methods of assessment.[13,14] Fatigue is present at the time of diagnosis in approximately 50% of patients with cancer. In a study of 179 cancer patients, 23.5% of patients reported "severe fatigue" at the time of diagnosis, before the start of therapy.[15]

Fatigue occurs in up to 75% of patients with bone metastases, and approximately 60%–96% of patients undergoing treatment for cancer report fatigue.[16] A national survey of 197 oncologists, 200 caregivers, and 419 cancer patients with various cancers, at various stages of illness, and treatment noted that more than 78% of patients experienced fatigue during the course of their disease and treatment. Thirty-two percent of patients experienced fatigue daily and 32% felt that fatigue significantly affected their daily routines. Sixty-one percent of patients said fatigue affected everyday life more than pain. Among the oncologists, 80% believed that fatigue was undertreated and that fatigue was infrequently discussed between patients and oncologists.[3] Chemotherapy, radiation therapy, and biologic and hormonal therapies have been shown to exacerbate fatigue.[9] Women with early-stage breast cancer before chemotherapy have reported a 4% rate of fatigue, which increased to 28% after four cycles of chemotherapy.[11] Fatigue was estimated to be a distressing symptom in up to 67% of hospitalized and ambulatory prostate cancer patients.[17] A study in men with localized prostate cancer showed that the fatigue rates increased from 4% to 25% after radiation treatment.[18] In a cross-sectional survey of 814 cancer patients receiving chemotherapy and/or radiotherapy, 80% of patients reported fatigue as a side-effect of cancer treatment. Female patients, younger and unemployed patients, and those with higher levels of depression and fatigue experienced more fatigue.[19]

Fatigue is a disruptive symptom months or even years after completion of cancer treatment, which ranges from 17% to 53% in different prevalence studies depending on the diagnostic criteria used to define fatigue.[10,13,20,21] A systematic review of fatigue among breast cancer survivors concluded that survivors experienced significant fatigue up to 5 years after completion of adjuvant chemotherapy.[22]

Fatigue is most common among cancer patients in palliative care settings reported by 84%–100% of patients in palliative care units.[23,24]

As evidenced by the prevalence studies, fatigue is a common symptom in cancer patients and survivors of cancer, from diagnosis through all stages of treatment and beyond.

PATHOPHYSIOLOGY OF FATIGUE

The exact mechanisms involved in the cancer-related fatigue are unknown. Studies have focused on understanding factors that contribute to fatigue, including the cancer itself, cancer-related treatments, and a variety of physical and psychological co-morbidities (e.g., anemia, pain, depression, anxiety, cachexia, sleep disturbances, and immobility).[9,10] Production of cytokines, abnormal accumulation of muscle metabolites, changes in neuromuscular function, abnormalities in adenosine triphosphate synthesis, serotonin dysregulation, disruption of the hypothalamic-pituitary-adrenal axis, modulation of the circadian rhythm, and vagal nerve activation have been proposed as possible mechanisms in the development of fatigue.[25-27] The role of cytokines in fatigue[25] has led researchers to consider cytokine-antagonist drugs, such as tumor necrosis factor (TNF) receptor etanercept, TNF-α antagonist thalidomide, to improve tolerability of chemotherapy regimens and potentially to treat fatigue and cachexia in cancer patients.[28-30] Genetic variables have also been implicated to play a role in the development of fatigue among cancer patients. Advanced colorectal cancer patients with two variant forms of the *DPYD* gene were significantly less likely than those patients with a form of the gene known as *DPYD*5 to report fatigue following treatment with a chemotherapy regimen of 5-fluorouracil, irinotecan, and oxaliplatin.[31]

The pathogenesis of fatigue among cancer survivors is unclear and most likely multifactorial.[10,27] A study comparing breast cancer survivors with and without fatigue (n = 20 in each group) has found significantly higher levels of interleukin-1 receptor antagonist, soluble TNF type II, and higher numbers of T lymphocytes among breast cancer survivors with fatigue suggesting a chronic inflammatory process involving the T-cell compartment in this group of patients.[32]

Table 32–1. ICD-10 criteria for cancer-related fatigue

A. Six (or more) of the following symptoms have been present every day or nearly every day during the same 2-week period in the past month, and at least one of the symptoms is (A1) significant fatigue:
   A1. Significant fatigue, diminished energy, or increased need to rest, disproportionate to any recent change in activity level
   A2. Complaints of generalized weakness or limb heaviness
   A3. Diminished concentration or attention
   A4. Decreased motivation or interest to engage in usual activities
   A5. Insomnia or hypersomnia
   A6. Experience of sleep as unrefreshing or nonrestorative
   A7. Perceived need to struggle to overcome inactivity
   A8. Marked emotional reactivity (eg, sadness, frustration, or irritability) to feeling fatigued
   A9. Difficulty completing daily tasks attributed to feeling fatigued
   A10. Perceived problems with short-term memory
   A11. Postexertional malaise lasting several hours
B. The symptoms cause clinically significant distress or impairment in social, occupational, or other important areas of functioning.
C. There is evidence from the history, physical examination, or laboratory findings that the symptoms are a consequence of cancer or cancer therapy.
D. The symptoms are not primarily a consequence of co-morbid psychiatric disorders, such as major depression, somatization disorder, somatoform disorder, or delirium.

SOURCE: Adapted from[4] Cella D, Peterman A, Passik S, Jacobsen P, Breitbart W. Progress toward guidelines for the management of fatigue. *Oncology (Williston Park)*. 1998;12:369–377.

ASSESSMENT OF FATIGUE

All cancer patients should be screened for fatigue at their initial visit, at regular intervals during and following cancer treatment, and as clinically indicated.[9,10] The NCCN practice guidelines on cancer-related fatigue recommend the use of numerical self-report scales or verbal scales to assess the severity of fatigue. As fatigue is a symptom that is perceived by the patient, like pain, it is most accurately described by self-report. If the severity is measured as moderate or severe (a score of 4 or more on a scale of 0 to 10 with higher numbers indicating increased severity) a focused history and physical examination; evaluation of the pattern, onset, and duration of fatigue; associated symptoms; and interference with normal functioning is recommended.[9,10] Description of patient behavior by family members and other caregivers is an important part of assessment among children and elderly patients. Precipitating factors, such as acute physical and psychological stresses should be identified, as should perpetuating factors such as physical inactivity and ongoing psychological or social stresses. Age specifications have been included in the NCCN practice guidelines for screening fatigue and assessing the severity of it highlighting the importance and variability of fatigue across the lifespan.[9,10]

Assessment of etiologies. The etiologies of fatigue are complex and varied, including tumor by-products, opioids or other drugs (such as antidepressants, β-blockers, benzodiazepines, antihistamines), hypogonadism, hypothyroidism, cachexia, anemia, malnutrition, pain, myopathy, nausea, hormonal therapy, chemotherapy, radiation therapy, bone marrow transplantation, and treatment with biological response modifiers (Table 32–2).[2,7,9,10,33] Potentially reversible causes of fatigue (such as pain, emotional distress, sleep disturbance, anemia, hypothyroidism) should be identified and treated, and nonessential centrally acting drugs (including prescription drugs, over-the-counter medications, and supplements) should be eliminated.[9,10] Clinicians should consider the possibility of depression due to its high prevalence in patients with cancer and provide treatment.[9,10] If anemia is the main cause of fatigue, the physician should determine the necessity of a transfusion in severely symptomatic patients. Clinical trials have shown that patients with anemia have improved energy and less fatigue after erythropoietin treatment.[34] Co-morbid conditions such as cardiac, pulmonary, renal, hepatic, endocrine, and neurologic dysfunction, and infections should be ruled out as potential causes of fatigue. Several chemotherapy agents and radiation therapy have been associated with endocrine abnormalities, including hypothyroidism and hypogonadism.[35,36] Assessment of nutrition (weight, caloric intake, fluid-electrolyte imbalances) and activity level are also

Table 32–2. Etiologies of cancer-related fatigue

Preexisting conditions
   –Congestive heart failure, chronic obstructive pulmonary disease

Direct effects of cancer, "tumor burden"

Effects of cancer treatment
   –Surgery, radiation therapy, chemotherapy, biological therapies

Psychological factors
   –Depression, anxiety

Immobility

Sleep disturbances (insomnia, excessive daytime sedation with or without narcolepsy, restless leg syndrome, obstructive sleep apnea)

Cancer-related symptoms
   –Pain, nausea

Conditions related to cancer or its treatment
   –Anemia, dehydration, malnutrition, infections, electrolyte abnormalities, cytokine production, myopathy

Medications and drugs
   –Opioid analgesics, psychotropic agents, β-blockers, alcohol

important elements of assessment.[9,10] Anemia, polypharmacy, cognitive impairment, malnutrition, and cachexia are the most likely etiologies of fatigue in palliative care settings.[37]

Assessment instruments. Fatigue is not only difficult to define but also difficult to assess and quantify. Nonetheless, reliable and valid tools for assessment are crucial for improved management and research progress. Various standardized self-report scales exist, developed mostly in the context of cancer.[38,39] Different scales may measure fundamentally different aspects or even potentially distinct conceptions of fatigue.

The oldest scales assessing fatigue are dichotomous. These include Pearson-Byers Fatigue Checklist, Profile of Mood States, Fatigue and Vigor Subscale, the Fatigue Severity Scale, and the European Organization for Research and Treatment of Cancer Quality of Life Questionnaire Fatigue Subscale.[38,39] Other scales have taken a unidimensional approach, namely the Visual Analogue Scale for Fatigue (VAS-F)[40] and the Karnofsky Performance Status.[41] VAS-F is organized into energy and fatigue dimensions and has good psychometric properties. The Karnofsky Performance Status probes mainly fatigue consequences. The limitations of such unidimensional scales include the presence of confounding factors such as pain.

Multidimensional fatigue instruments have been developed to assess a wide range of symptom domains that fatigue may present with.[39] Multidimensional scales include the Fatigue Symptom Inventory,[42] the Brief Fatigue Inventory,[43] The Piper Fatigue Scale (PFS),[44] and the Multidimensional Assessment of Fatigue (MAF).[45] PFS,[44] is comprised of affective, cognitive, sensory, and severity subscales. Its major shortcomings include the fact that it takes a long time to complete and is often difficult for patients to understand. The MAF[45] scale is a revision of the PFS developed for use in patients with rheumatoid arthritis.

The Patient-Reported Outcomes Management Information System (PROMIS) is a databank of survey questions, currently under development, designed to measure common symptoms in clinical trials.[46,47] The PROMIS includes 72 questions on fatigue that have been validated in cancer patients. A 1-minute short-version, cancer-specific fatigue short form, containing seven questions has recently been validated.[46,47]

Given the multifactorial nature of fatigue, accessory scales (e.g., depression scales) and measurements of certain biological parameters should be used in addition to fatigue assessment tools to evaluate a patient's fatigue comprehensively.[9,10,39] In particular, the complex interrelationship between fatigue and psychiatric disturbances such as depression and anxiety merit special attention.

Fatigue and depression. Depression is commonly co-morbid in patients with cancer-related fatigue. It is necessary to clarify the relationship between depression and fatigue to effectively evaluate and treat cancer-related fatigue. There is considerable overlap of symptoms in these two conditions, such as decreased energy and motivation, sleep disturbances, diminished concentration, attention, and memory. Depressive symptoms caused by fatigue are typically less severe and patients tend to attribute such symptoms to the consequences of fatigue. Depression, on the other hand, is more likely present with hopelessness, feelings of worthlessness and/or guilt, suicidal ideation, and a family history of depression.[9,10,39] It is also important to note that fatigue and depression may coexist in the same patient. In a study of chronic fatigue syndrome in primary care settings, a temporal relationship was found between depression and fatigue.[27,48] The nature of any causal relationship between cancer-related fatigue and depression remains unclear. In a study with 987 lung cancer patients, 33% were found to have depression; fatigue was identified as an independent predictor of depression.[49] In another study of 201 cancer patients, fatigue was found to be the most common symptom, with 25% of these patients experiencing depression.[50] A possible bidirectional relationship between fatigue and depression exists, with fatigue occurring as a symptom of depression or with depression occurring because of fatigue, due to interference with mood, work, and leisure activities.[9,10,20,51]

Fatigue and pain. Two most commonly reported symptoms among cancer patients, fatigue and pain, share several common features. Both symptoms are complex and multidimensional, largely based on subjective patient report, and require clear communication between patients and clinicians for timely recognition and treatment of these symptoms. Coexistence of pain and fatigue has been shown to worsen the overall symptom experience among elderly cancer patients, suggesting a synergistic effect between these two symptoms.[52]

MANAGEMENT OF FATIGUE

Given the multidimensional nature of fatigue, a biopsychosocial approach is recommended for treatment of fatigue. Interdisciplinary teams addressing needs of individual patients while implementing the treatment guidelines are critical to management of cancer-related fatigue.[9,10] Interventions can be tailored based on the stage of illness (e.g., active treatment phase, survivorship, and end-of-life). A three-stage hierarchy for the management of fatigue was proposed, namely to identify and treat any underlying causes of fatigue; to treat

fatigue directly; and finally to address and manage the consequences of fatigue.[4]

General strategies for management of fatigue. Self-monitoring of fatigue levels; energy conserving strategies such as setting priorities, scheduling activities at times of peak energy, postponing nonessential activities, structuring daily routine, attending to one activity at a time, and limiting naps to 45 minutes or less to minimize interference with nighttime sleep quality; and using distraction have been recommended by the NCCN practice guidelines for management of cancer-related fatigue.[9,10]

Nonpharmacologic interventions. Nonpharmacological approaches have been recommended by the NCCN guidelines for the treatment of cancer-related fatigue.[9,10] Increased physical activity and psychosocial interventions (i.e., education, support groups, cognitive-behavioral therapy, individual counseling, stress management training) in the treatment of fatigue have been well-supported by research.[9,10,53–56] There is also evidence supporting dietary management, attention-restoring therapy, and sleep therapy (e.g., sleep restriction, sleep hygiene, and stimulus control) in the treatment of fatigue.[9,10,55,56] Alternative therapies such as massage therapy, yoga, muscle relaxation, and mindfulness-based therapies have been evaluated pilot studies with results suggesting benefit in lowering fatigue in cancer patients.[9,10]

Pharmacologic interventions. A number of studies examined the efficacy and tolerability of different classes of pharmacologic agents for cancer-related fatigue, primarily psychostimulants and antidepressants. A recent meta-analysis of pharmacological treatment options for cancer-related fatigue has concluded that methylphenidate (a psychostimulant) might be effective for treating fatigue. There was also evidence that treatment with hematopoietic agents relieved fatigue due to chemotherapy-induced anemia.[57] Following is a review of pharmacologic interventions used in the treatment of cancer-related fatigue. Table 32–3 provides a list of commonly used psychostimulants and antidepressants in the treatment of cancer-related fatigue.

Psychostimulants. Psychostimulants are drugs that increase alertness and/or motivation and include methylphenidate, dextroamphetamine, and pemoline (withdrawn from the U.S. market). Methylphenidate and dextroamphetamine are sympathomimetic drugs. They stimulate adrenergic receptors directly as agonists and indirectly cause the release of dopamine and norepinephrine from presynaptic terminals. Dexmethylphenidate is the d-isomer of methylphenidate, has a longer duration of action (approximately 6 hours) than methylphenidate. Psychostimulants are scheduled as controlled drugs because of their rapid onset of action, immediate behavioral effects, and development of tolerance, which leads to an increased risk of abuse and dependence in vulnerable individuals. Existing neuropharmacologic data suggest that methylphenidate has pharmacokinetic properties that reduce its abuse potential as compared with stimulant drugs of abuse, such as cocaine.[58]

Agitation and insomnia are the most common side effects associated with the use of psychostimulants. Reducing the dosage and taking the medication early in the day may help. Rare side effects include hypertension, palpitations, arrhythmias, confusion, psychosis, tremor, and headache.[28] Methylphenidate and dextroamphetamine are contraindicated for patients with uncontrolled hypertension, underlying coronary artery disease, and tachyarrhythmias.

Psychostimulants show great promise in the treatment of medically induced fatigue in patients with cancer, multiple sclerosis, Parkinson's disease, opioid-induced sedation, and human immunodeficiency virus (HIV).[59–64] Breitbart and colleagues[59] conducted the first randomized, double-blind, placebo-controlled trial of two psychostimulants for the treatment of fatigue in ambulatory patients with HIV disease. They found that both methylphenidate and pemoline (no longer available) were equally effective and significantly superior to placebo in decreasing fatigue severity with minimal side effects. Psychostimulants also have been used in the treatment of fatigue-related conditions, such as pain, depression, opioid-related sedation, and cognitive impairment.[64,65] Table 32–4 is a summary of the psychotropic medication trials for the

Table 32–3. Psychotropic medications used in the treatment of cancer-related fatigue

Medication	Starting dose	Dose range	Comments
Psychostimulants			
Methylphenidate	2.5–5 mg daily or twice daily	5–30 mg/day, usually divided as twice daily	Longer-acting forms are available Capsule forms can be sprinkled on food
Dextroamphetamine	2.5–5 mg daily or twice daily	5–30 mg/day, usually divided as twice daily	Longer-acting formulations are available Capsule forms can be sprinkled on food
Wakefulness-promoting agents			
Modafinil	50–100 mg daily	50–400 mg daily, may be divided as twice daily	Favorable side-effect profile
Antidepressants			
Selective serotonin reuptake inhibitors			Well-tolerated Citalopram, escitalopram, and sertraline have the least drug-drug interactions
Fluoxetine[a]	10–20 mg/day	10–60 mg/day	
Paroxetine	10–20 mg/day	10–40 mg/day	
Citalopram[a]	10–20 mg/day	10–40 mg/day	
Escitalopram[a]	5–10 mg/day	5–20 mg/day	
Sertraline[a]	25–50 mg/day	25–200 mg/day	
Serotonin-norepinephrine reuptake inhibitors			Well-tolerated Monitor blood pressure regularly
Venlafaxine	37.5–75 mg/day	37.5–225 mg/day	
Duloxetine	20–30 mg/day	20–60 mg/day	
Norpinephrine-dopamine reuptake inhibitor			Doses higher than 300 mg a day should be administered twice daily to minimize the risk of seizures
Bupropion	75 mg/day	75–450 mg/day	
α-2 antagonist/5-HT2/5HT3 antagonist			Most helpful in patients with insomnia and anorexia
Mirtazapine	7.5–15 mg/day	7.5–45 mg/day	

ABBREVIATION: 5HT, 5-hydroxytryptamine.
[a]Available in liquid formulations.

Table 32–4. Psychotropic medication trials for the treatment of cancer-related fatigue

	Sample	Intervention	Results	Comments
Methylphenidate				
Sarhill et al. 2001[64]	Patients with advanced cancer Prospective, open-label design (n = 11)	Methylphenidate 10 mg twice daily	Decreased fatigue in 9 out of 11 patients, with sedation and pain improving in some patients	More than half of the patients experienced side effects, such as insomnia, agitation, anorexia, nausea, vomiting, and dry mouth
Sugawara et al. 2002[66]	Patients with advanced cancer Prospective, open-label study (n = 16)	Methylphenidate 5–30 mg/day, mean duration of treatment 8 days	Decreased fatigue scores ($p = 0.01$)	Two patients dropped out due to insomnia Visual analog scale was used for assessment of fatigue
Schwartz et al. 2002[67]	Patients with melanoma receiving interferon Prospective, open-label study (n = 12)	Exercise and methylphenidate 20 mg/day	Decreased fatigue scores	Unclear whether the positive effect was due to exercise or methylphenidate or both
Bruera et al. 2003[68]	Patients with advanced cancer. Prospective open-label (n = 30)	Patient-controlled methylphenidate 5 mg every 2 hours with a maximum of 4 caps in a day	Decrease in fatigue, depression, and overall well-being	None of the patients discontinued the medication

(Continued)

Table 32-4. Continued

	Sample	Intervention	Results	Comments
Hanna et al. 2006[69]	Patients with breast cancer, who were cancer free longer than 6 months but less than 5 years. Open-label, phase II study (n = 37)	Methylphenidate 5 mg twice daily for 6 weeks	54% of the patients responded with a decrease in BFI score of more than 2 points	16% of the patients withdrew from the study due to minor side effects
Bruera et al. 2006[70]	Patients with advanced cancer (n = 52 in medication arm, n = 53 in placebo arm). Randomized, double-blind, placebo-controlled trial	Patient-controlled methylphenidate (5 mg every 2 hours up to 4 caps a day) versus placebo for a total of 7 days	Fatigue scores improved both in placebo and medication arm on day 8	Open-label phase of the study following the randomized trial showed continued improvement in fatigue
Roth et al. 2006[71]	Ambulatory patients with prostate cancer Randomized, placebo-controlled, phase III trial (n = 15 in the placebo arm, n = 14 in the medication arm)	Methylphenidate versus placebo	13 patients taking placebo and 8 patients taking methylphenidate completed the study 73% of the patients in the methylphenidate arm, 23% of the patients in the placebo arm showed improvement in fatigue scores	Remarkable placebo effect was observed in the preliminary analysis of the study 43% of the patients dropped out due to cardiac side effects
D-methylphenidate				
Lower et al. 2005[72]	Adult patients with cancer, 2 months after chemotherapy Randomized, placebo-controlled, phase III trial (n = 75 placebo, n = 77 medication arm)	D-methylphenidate 10–50 mg/d for more than 2 weeks	Medication was found to be more effective compared to placebo in improving fatigue	Final data analysis has not been published yet
Butler et al. 2007[73]	Adult patients with primary or metastatic brain tumors on radiation therapy Double-blind, randomized, placebo-controlled trial (n=34 in each arm)	D-threo-methylphenidate 15 mg twice daily for 4–12 weeks	Prophylactic use of d-threo-methylphenidate did not result in improvement of fatigue scores or quality of life	Researchers concluded that therapeutic rather than prophylactic d-methylphenidate was recommended for patients undergoing brain RT who develop fatigue or cognitive dysfunction
Mar Fan et al. 2008[74]	Women with breast cancer undergoing adjuvant chemotherapy Randomized, double-blind, placebo-controlled trial (n = 29 on medication, n = 28 on placebo)	D-methylphenidate up to 10 twice daily for 20–140 days	There were no significant differences between the FACT-F scores of the randomized groups	Greater number of patients discontinued study drug in the d-MPH arm than the placebo arm, on the other hand equal numbers in each group required dose reduction for presumed d-MPH toxicity
Modafinil				
Morrow et al. 2005[79]	Women with breast cancer, 2 years after treatment Prospective, open-label study (n = 51)	Modafinil 200 mg/day for a month	86% reported improvement in fatigue	Final data analysis has not been published yet
Kaleita et al. 2006[80]	Adult patients with brain tumor. Phase III, open-label trial (n = 30)	Modafinil, mean dose 225 mg/day at week 8, 258 mg/day at week 12	Well-tolerated; mean fatigue score change at week 8 and 12 was significantly higher in the intervention arm	Only results from the open-label extension phase were reported in this abstract. Final data analysis has not been published yet

	Sample	Intervention	Results	Comments
Paroxetine				
Capuron et al. 2002[81]	Patients with malignant melanoma Double-randomized controlled trial (n = 40)	Paroxetine versus placebo 2 weeks before the start of interferon therapy	Paroxetine did not have an effect on the prevention of fatigue	Risk of depression was significantly reduced in the paroxetine arm
Morrow et al. 2003[82]	Patients with breast cancer receiving chemotherapy Randomized, double-blind, placebo-controlled trial (n = 479)	Paroxetine 20 mg/day versus placebo for 8 weeks	No significant difference was detected in fatigue improvement between placebo and paroxetine arms	There was a significant difference between groups in the mean level of depression
Roscoe et al. 2005[51]	Patients with breast cancer undergoing chemotherapy. Randomized, double-blind, placebo-controlled trial (n = 94)	Paroxetine 20 mg/day versus placebo	No significant difference was observed in fatigue scores between the placebo and paroxetine arms	Paroxetine was effective in treating depression, but not cancer-related fatigue
Sertraline				
Stockler et al. 2007[83]	Patients with advanced stage cancer (n = 189) without major depressive disorder Randomized, double-blind, placebo-controlled trial	Sertaline 50 mg/day (n = 95) versus placebo (n = 94)	No significant difference was observed in depression, anxiety, fatigue, and overall well-being	Sertraline was kept at the starting dose throughout the study duration of 8 weeks
Bupropion				
Cullum et al. 2004[84]	Adult patients with cancer Open-label, prospective design (n = 15).	Bupropion sustained release 100–150 mg/day	13 patients reported improvement in fatigue	Small sample size, open-label design
Moss et al. 2006[85]	Adult patients with cancer Prospective, case series (n = 21)	Bupropion sustained release 100–300 mg/day	Well-tolerated; both depressed and nondepressed patients reported improvement in their fatigue	Small sample size. Placebo-controlled studies are needed to confirm the results
Donepezil				
Bruera et al. 2003[90]	Adult patients with cancer Open-label trial (n=27)	Donepezil 5mg/day for 7 days	All of the 20 patients who completed the trial showed significant improvement in fatigue	7 patients dropped out. Open-label design limits the significance of positive results
Shaw et al. 2006[91]	Adult patients with brain tumor Open-label, phase II trial (n = 34).	Donepezil 5 mg/day for 24 weeks	Fatigue subscale of the Profile of Mood States scale showed improvement short of statistical significance, "trend toward significance" as noted by the researchers	Improvement in cognitive functioning and health-related quality of life were observed
Bruera et al. 2007[92]	Adult patients with advanced cancer Randomized, double-blind, placebo-controlled trial with donepezil (n = 47) versus placebo (n = 56)	Donepezil 5 mg/day for 7 days	There was no significant difference in fatigue scores between the donepezil and placebo groups	Improvement in sedation observed both in the placebo and donepezil arms Open-label phase of the study with donepezil showed sustained improvement in fatigue scores

ABBREVIATIONS: BFI, brief fatigue inventory; d-MPH, dexmethylphenidate hydrochloride; FACT-F, Functional Assessment of Cancer Therapy-Fatigue; RT, radiation therapy.

treatment of cancer-related fatigue. While open-label studies with psychostimulants have shown improvements in cancer-related fatigue, placebo-controlled randomized trials have found a remarkable placebo effect among cancer patients as well as improved fatigue scores with psychostimulants.[28]

The Food and Drug Administration (FDA) approved the use of wakefulness-promoting agent modafinil in adult patients with excessive sleepiness associated with narcolepsy, obstructive sleep apnea, and shift work sleep disorder.[75] It has been used to augment antidepressants in major depressive disorder, and as an adjunct treatment for bipolar depression.[76,77] Compared to the psychostimulants, modafinil has a novel mechanism of action and less abuse potential. It is well-tolerated and has a good safety profile. The mechanism of action is largely unknown. It presumably enhances activity in the hypothalamic wakefulness center (i.e., tuberomammillary nucleus), activates tuberomammillary nucleus neurons that release histamine, and activates other hypothalamic neurons that release orexin/hypocretin.

Modafinil is commonly used for the treatment of severe fatigue in multiple sclerosis[78] and has been studied as a treatment option for cancer-related fatigue with improvement of fatigue in open-label trials.[79,80] Well-designed, randomized, controlled clinical trials are necessary to further clarify the role of modafinil in the treatment of cancer-related fatigue.

Antidepressants. The phenomenological similarities and the possibility of a bidirectional relationship between fatigue and depression have led clinicians to consider antidepressants in the treatment of cancer-related fatigue.

The benefits of antidepressant use are not clear in patients with cancer-related fatigue in the absence of a depressive mood disorder. Research has suggested a common pathophysiological mechanism, such as serotonin insufficiency, in the development of both fatigue and depression.

Studies have examined the role of paroxetine,[51,81,82] sertraline,[83] and bupropion[84,85] in the treatment of cancer-related fatigue. Paroxetine[51,81,82] and sertraline[83] were effective in improving fatigue among cancer patients with co-morbid depressive symptoms. Bupropion was found to be effective and well-tolerated in both depressed and nondepressed cancer patients in open-label trials.[84,85] However controlled studies are required to determine whether the effect of bupropion on fatigue is independent of its antidepressant effects.

Underlying depression treated with selective serotonin-reuptake inhibitors (SSRIs) is generally better tolerated than tricyclic antidepressants in patients with cancer. Medications should be initiated at lower doses and drug-drug interactions should be carefully monitored among patients with cancer-related fatigue.[28]

Corticosteroids. Corticosteroids have been used in the treatment of cancer-related fatigue. In a survey among Swedish palliative care physicians, 40% of the clinicians reported using corticosteroids to treat fatigue, and 80% reported "very "or "some effect" of corticosteroids on fatigue.[86] Bruera and colleagues in their prospective, randomized, double-blind study observed that 40 palliative care patients who received a 2-week treatment with methylprednisolone demonstrated an increase in activity that became nonsignificant after 4 weeks of treatment.[87] This study suggests that the positive effects of corticosteroids in the treatment of fatigue may be transient. It is important to note that corticosteroids may have detrimental side effects such as muscle wasting with long-term use.

Megestrol acetate. Megestrol acetate, a progestational agent, which has been found to improve appetite in cancer-related cachexia, may have a role in the treatment of cancer-related fatigue. A double-blind crossover study comparing megestrol acetate (160 mg 3 times daily for 10 days) to placebo in the treatment of cachexia among patients with advanced cancer (n = 84, total number of patients) has shown significant improvement in overall fatigue scores measured by the PFS.[88] The effects of megestrol acetate on fatigue are not clear but probably involve anticytokine and corticosteroid-type effects.[88]

L-carnitine. L-carnitine is a cofactor that binds free long-chain fatty acids to transport them across mitochondrial membrane for fatty acid oxidation. Patients with advanced cancer are at risk for carnitine deficiency because of decreased intake and increased renal loss. L-carnitine supplements improved fatigue and depression in a group of patients with cancer with L-carnitine deficiency.[89] Although the use of L-carnitine in cancer-related fatigue is preliminary, carnitine supplementation shows some promise for management of fatigue.

Donepezil. Donepezil is a reversible cholinesterase inhibitor used in the treatment of Alzheimer's dementia. Studies have explored the role of donepezil in the treatment of cancer-related fatigue.[90-92] A double-blind randomized controlled trial has failed to show any difference between donepezil and placebo in improving fatigue among cancer patients.[92]

Other medications. Amantadine, an antiinfluenza agent with dopaminergic effects, used in Parkinson's disease and as an adjunct to interferon-based therapies for chronic hepatitis C. Amantadine has been utilized in the treatment of fatigue associated with multiple sclerosis, however it has not been studied in cancer-related fatigue.[93,94] Nonsteroidal antiinflammatory drugs, selective cyclooxygenase 2 inhibitors (e.g., celecoxib), monoclonal antibodies (e.g., infliximab), cytokine antagonists, and bradykinin antagonists have been considered as potential treatments for cancer-related fatigue through their direct and indirect cytokine antagonistic effects.[30,95]

CONCLUSIONS

Fatigue is highly prevalent among patients with cancer, and is associated with decreased quality of life. Fatigue should be recognized, assessed, monitored, and treated promptly for all age groups, at all stages of cancer, before, during, and following treatment as outlined by the NCCN Practice Guidelines on cancer-related fatigue.[9,10] Several nonpharmacologic and pharmacologic treatment options are available for management of fatigue. Increased physical activity, various types of psychosocial interventions, dietary management, and sleep hygiene are well-supported by research in the treatment of fatigue. Psychostimulants and antidepressants have been studied the most in the treatment of cancer-related fatigue. Psychostimulants are well-tolerated and appear to have a role in the improvement of fatigue despite a large placebo effect. Antidepressants are most effective in patients with underlying depression. Activating antidepressants such as bupropion may be more effective in the treatment of fatigue symptoms. However, it is important to emphasize that more research is needed to evaluate the efficacy of pharmacologic interventions, as current evidence falls short of providing sufficient evidence to recommend medications for treating cancer-related fatigue.

REFERENCES

1. Curt GA, Breitbart W, Cella D, et al. Impact of cancer-related fatigue on the lives of patients: new findings from the Fatigue Coalition. *Oncologist.* 2000;5:353–360.

2. Hwang SS, Chang VT, Rue M, Kasimis B. Multidimensional independent predictors of cancer-related fatigue. *J Pain Symptom Manage.* 2003;26:604–614.

3. Vogelzang NJ, Breitbart W, Cella D, et al. Patient, caregiver and oncologist perceptions of cancer-related fatigue: results of a tripart assessment survey. *Semin Hematol.* 1997;3:4–12.

4. Cella D, Peterman A, Passik S, Jacobsen P, Breitbart W. Progress toward guidelines for the management of fatigue. *Oncology (Williston Park).* 1998;12:369–377.

5. Beijer S, Kempen GI, Pijls-Johannesma MC, de Graeff A, Dagnelie PC. Determinants of overall quality of life in preterminal cancer patients. *Int J Cancer.* 2008 Jul 1;123(1):232–235.

6. Luciani A, Jacobsen PB, Extermann M, et al. Fatigue and functional dependence in older cancer patients. *Am J Clin Oncol.* 2008 Oct;31(5):424–430.

7. Kunkel EJ, Bakker JMR, Myers RE, Oyesanmi O, Gomella LG. Biopsychosocial aspects of prostate cancer. *Psychosomatics.* 2000;41:85–94.

8. Mystakidou K, Parpa E, Katsouda E, Galanos A, Vlahos L. The role of physical and psychological symptoms in desire for death: a study of terminally ill cancer patients. *Psychooncology.* 2006 Apr;15(4):355–360.

9. Mock V, Atkinson A, Barsevick A, et al. NCCN Practice Guidelines for Cancer-Related Fatigue. *Oncology (Williston Park).* 2000;14:151–161.

10. NCCN Cancer-Related Fatigue Panel Members. *National Comprehensive Cancer Network (v.1.2008) Cancer-Related Fatigue.* NCCN Practice Guidelines in Oncology. Available at: http://www.nccn.org/professionals/physician_gls/PDF/fatigue.pdf. Accessed August 12, 2009.

11. Jacobsen PB, Hann DM, Azzarello LM, Horton J, Balducci L, Lyman GH. Fatigue in women receiving adjuvant chemotherapy for breast cancer: characteristics, course, and correlates. *J Pain Symptom Manage.* 1999 Oct;18(4):233–242.

12. Sadler IJ, Jacobsen PB, Booth-Jones M, Belanger H, Weitzner MA, Fields KK. Preliminary evaluation of a clinical syndrome approach to assessing cancer-related fatigue. *J Pain Symptom Manage.* 2003;23:406–416.

13. Lawrence DP, Kupelnick B, Miller K, Devine D, Lau J. Evidence report on the occurrence, assessment, and treatment of fatigue in cancer patients. *J Natl Cancer Inst Monogr.* 2004;32:40–50.

14. Hofman M, Ryan JL, Figueroa-Moseley CD, Jean-Pierre P, Morrow GR. Cancer-related fatigue: the scale of the problem. *Oncologist*. 2007;12(Suppl 1): 4–10.

15. Goedendorp MM, Gielissen MF, Verhagen CA, Peters ME, Bleijenberg G. Severe fatigue and related factors in cancer patients before the initiation of treatment. *Br J Cancer*. 2008 Nov 4;99(9):1408–1414.

16. Flechtner H, Bottomley A. Fatigue and quality of life: lessons from the real world. *Oncologist*. 2003;(Suppl 8):5–9.

17. Portenoy R. The Memorial Symptom Assessment Scale: an instrument for the evaluation of symptom prevalence, characteristics and distress. *Eur J Cardiol*. 1994;30A.9:1326–1336.

18. Monga U, Kerrigan AJ, Thornby J, Monga TN. Prospective study of fatigue in localized prostate patients with cancer undergoing radiotherapy. *Radiat Oncol Invest*. 1999;7:178–185.

19. Henry DH, Viswanathan HN, Elkin EP, Traina S, Wade S, Cella D. Symptoms and treatment burden associated with cancer treatment: results from a cross-sectional national survey in the U.S. *Support Care Cancer*. 2008 Jul;16(7):791–801.

20. Bower JE, Ganz PA, Desmond KA, Rowland JH, Meyerowitz BE, Belin TR. Fatigue in breast cancer survivors: occurrence, correlates, and impact on quality of life. *J Clin Oncol*. 2000;18:743–753.

21. Cella D, Davis K, Breitbart W, Curt G, Fatigue Coalition. Cancer-related fatigue: prevalence of proposed diagnostic criteria in a United States sample of cancer survivors. *J Clin Oncol*. 2001;19:3385–3391.

22. Minton O, Stone P. How common is fatigue in disease-free breast cancer survivors? A systematic review of the literature. *Breast Cancer Res Treat*. 2008 Nov;112(1):5–13.

23. Lundh Hagelin C, Seiger A, Furst CJ. Quality of life in terminal care—with special reference to age, gender and marital status. *Support Care Cancer*. 2006 Apr;14(4):320–328.

24. Peters L, Sellick K. Quality of life of cancer patients receiving inpatient and home-based palliative care. *J Adv Nurs*. 2006 Mar;53(5):524–533.

25. Kurzrock R. The role of cytokines in cancer-related fatigue. *Cancer*. 2001;92(Suppl 6):1684–1688.

26. Ryan JL, Carroll JK, Ryan EP, Mustian KM, Fiscella K, Morrow GR. Mechanisms of cancer-related fatigue. *Oncologist*. 2007;12(Suppl 1):22–34.

27. Wang XS. Pathophysiology of cancer-related fatigue. *Clin J Oncol Nurs*. 2008 Oct;12(Suppl 5):11–20.

28. Breitbart W, Alici Y. Pharmacologic treatment options for cancer-related fatigue: current state of clinical research. *Clin J Oncol Nurs*. 2008; 12(Suppl 5):27–36.

29. Monk JP, Phillips G, Waite R, et al. Assessment of tumor necrosis factor alpha blockade as an intervention to improve tolerability of dose-intensive chemotherapy in cancer patients. *J Clin Oncol*. 2001;24:1852–1859.

30. Hussein MA. Research on thalidomide in solid tumors, hematologic malignancies, and supportive care. *Oncology (Williston Park)*. 2001;4(11, Suppl 12):9–15.

31. Sloan JA, Zhao CX. Genetics and quality of life. *Curr Probl Cancer*. 2006;30(6):255–60.

32. Bower JE, Ganz PA, Aziz N, Fahey JL, Cole SW. T-cell homeostasis in breast cancer survivors with persistent fatigue. *J Natl Cancer Inst*. 2003 Aug 6; 95(15):1165–1168.

33. Ahlberg K, Ekman T, Gaston-Johansson F, Mock, V. Assessment and management of cancer-related fatigue in adults. *Lancet*. 2003;362:640–650.

34. Savonije JH, van Groeningen CJ, Wormhoudt LW, Giaccone G. Early intervention with epoetin alfa during platinum-based chemotherapy: an analysis of the results of a multicenter, randomized, controlled trial based on initial hemoglobin level. *Oncologist*. 2006;11:206–216.

35. Canaris GJ, Manowitz NR, Mayor G, Ridgway EC. The Colorado thyroid disease prevalence study. *Arch Intern Med*. 2000 Feb 28;160(4):526–534.

36. Strasser F, Palmer JL, Schover LR, et al. The impact of hypogonadism and autonomic dysfunction on fatigue, emotional function, and sexual desire in male patients with advanced cancer: a pilot study. *Cancer*. 2006 Dec 15;107(12):2949–2957.

37. Yennurajalingam S, Bruera E. Palliative management of fatigue at the close of life: "it feels like my body is just worn out." *JAMA*. 2007 Jan 17;297(3): 295–304.

38. Piper BF, Borneman T, Sun VC, et al. Cancer-related fatigue: role of oncology nurses in translating national comprehensive cancer network assessment guidelines into practice. *Clin J Oncol Nurs*. 2008 Oct;12(Suppl 5):37–47.

39. Breitbart W, Dickerman AL. Fatigue and HIV. In: Cohen M, Gorman J, (eds). *Comprehensive textbook of AIDS psychiatry*. Oxford University Press; 2008:173–188.

40. Lee KA, Hicks G, Nino-Murcia G. Validity and reliability of a scale to assess fatigue. *Psychiatry Research*. 1991;36:291–298.

41. Schag CC, Heinrich RL, Ganz PA. Karnofsky performance status revisited: reliability, validity, and guidelines. *J Clin Oncol*. 1984;2:187–193.

42. Hann DM, Jacobsen PB, Azzarello LM, et al. Measurement of fatigue in cancer patients: development and validation of the Fatigue Symptom Inventory. *Qual Life Res*. 1998;7:301–310.

43. Mendoza TR, Wang XS, Cleeland CS, et al. The rapid assessment of fatigue severity in cancer patients: use of the Brief Fatigue Inventory. *Cancer*. 1999;85:1186–1196.

44. Piper B, Lindsey A, Dodd M, et al. Development of an instrument to measure the subjective dimension of fatigue. In: Funk SG, Turnquist EM, Campagne MT, et al. (eds). *Key aspects of comfort: Management of pain, fatigue and nausea*. New York, NY: Springer; 1998:199–208.

45. Belza BL. Comparison of self-reported fatigue in rheumatoid arthritis and controls. *J Rheumatol*. 1995;22:639–643.

46. McNeil C. No rest for fatigue researchers. *J Natl Cancer Inst*. 2008 Aug 20;100(16):1129–1131.

47. McNeil C. Quality of life researchers have new tool and new focus on measurement. *J Natl Cancer Inst*. 2008 Feb 20;100(4):234–236.

48. Skapinakis P, Lewis G, Mavreas V. Temporal relations between unexplained fatigue and depression: longitudinal data from an international study in primary care. *Psychosom Med*. 2004 May-Jun;66(3):330–335.

49. Hopwood P, Stephens RJ. Depression in patients with lung cancer: prevalence and risk factors derived from quality-of-life data. *J Clin Oncol*. 2000 Feb;18(4):893–903.

50. Newell S, Sanson-Fisher RW, Girgis A, Ackland S. The physical and psycho-social experiences of patients attending an outpatient medical oncology department: a cross-sectional study. *Eur J Cancer Care (Engl)*. 1999 Jun; 8(2):73–82.

51. Roscoe JA, Morrow GR, Hickok JT, et al. Effect of paroxetine hydrochloride on fatigue and depression in breast cancer patients receiving chemotherapy. *Breast Cancer Res Treat*, 2005;89:243–249.

52. Given B, Given C, Azzouz F, Stommel M. Physical functioning of elderly cancer patients prior to diagnosis and following initial treatment. *Nurs Res*. 2001 Jul-Aug;50(4):222–232.

53. Barsevick AM, Newhall T, Brown S. Management of cancer-related fatigue. *Clin J Oncol Nurs*. 2008 Oct;12(Suppl 5):21–25.

54. Kangas M, Bovbjerg DH, Montgomery GH. Cancer-related fatigue: a systematic and meta-analytic review of non-pharmacological therapies for cancer patients. *Psychol Bull*. 2008 Sep;134(5):700–741.

55. Mock V. Evidence-based treatment for cancer-related fatigue. *J Natl Cancer Inst Monogr*. 2004;32:112–118.

56. Mitchell SA, Beck SL, Hood LE, Moore K, Tanner ER. Putting evidence into practice: evidence-based interventions for fatigue during and following cancer and its treatment. *Clin J Oncol Nurs*,2007;11:99–113.

57. Minton O, Richardson A, Sharpe M, Hotopf M, Stone P. A systematic review and meta-analysis of the pharmacological treatment of cancer-related fatigue. *J Natl Cancer Inst*. 2008 Aug 20;100(16):1155–1166.

58. Kollins SH. Comparing the abuse potential of methylphenidate versus other stimulants: a review of available evidence and relevance to the ADHD patient. *J Clin Psychiatry*. 2003;64(Suppl 11):14–18.

59. Breitbart W, Rosenfeld B, Kaim M, Funesti-Esch J. A randomized, double-blind, placebo-controlled trial of psychostimulants for the treatment of fatigue in ambulatory patients with human immunodeficiency virus disease. *Arch Intern Med*. 2001;61:411–420.

60. Holmes VF, Fernandez F, Levy JK. Psychostimulant response in AIDS-related complex patients. *J Clin Psychiatry*. 1989;50:5–8.

61. Wagner GJ, Rabkin R. Effects of dextroamphetamine on depression and fatigue in men with HIV: a double-blind, placebo-controlled trial. *J Clin Psychiatry*. 2001;61:436–440.

62. Bruera E, Brenneis C, Paterson AH, MacDonald RN. Use of methylphenidate as an adjuvant to narcotic analgesics in patients with advanced cancer. *J Pain Symptom Manage*. 1989;4:3–6.

63. Mendonca DA, Menezes K, Joq MS. Methylphenidate improves fatigue scores in Parkinson disease: a randomized controlled trial. *Mov Disord*. 2007;22:2070–2076.

64. Sarhill N, Walsh D, Nelson KA, Homsi J, LeGrand S, Davis MP. Methylphenidate for fatigue in advanced cancer: a prospective open-label pilot study. *Am J Hosp Palliat Care*. 2001;18:187–192.

65. Homsi J, Walsh D, Nelson KA. Psychostimulants in supportive care. *Support Care Cancer*. 2000;8:385–397.

66. Sugawara Y, Akechi T, Shima Y, et al. Efficacy of methylphenidate for fatigue in advanced cancer patients: a preliminary study. *Palliat Med*. 2002;16:261–263.

67. Schwartz AL, Thompson JA, Masood N. Interferon-induced fatigue in patients with melanoma: a pilot study of exercise and methylphenidate. *Oncol Nurs Forum*. 2001;29:E85–E90.

68. Bruera E, Driver L, Barnes EA, et al. Patient-controlled methylphenidate for the management of fatigue in patients with advanced cancer: a preliminary report. *J Clin Oncol.* 2003;21:4439–4443.

69. Hanna A, Sledge G, Mayer ML, et al. A phase II study of methylphenidate for the treatment of fatigue. *Support Care Cancer.* 2006;4:210–215.

70. Bruera E, Valero V, Driver L, et al. Patient-controlled methylphenidate for cancer fatigue: a double-blind, randomized, placebo-controlled trial. *J Clin Oncol.* 2006;24:2073–2078.

71. Roth AJ, Nelson CJ, Rosenfeld B, et al. Randomized controlled trial testing methylphenidate as treatment for fatigue in men with prostate cancer [Abstract]. Proceedings of the 42nd Annual Meeting of the American Society of Clinical Oncology, 2009 (Abstract No. 275).

72. Lower E, Fleishman S, Cooper A, Zeldis J, Faleck H, Manning D. A phase III, randomized placebo-controlled trial of the safety and efficacy of d-MPH as new treatment of fatigue and "chemobrain" in adult cancer patients [Abstract]. Proceedings of the 41st Annual Meeting of the American Society of Clinical Oncology, 2005;23 (Abstract No. 8000).

73. Butler JM Jr, Case LD, Atkins J, et al. A phase III, double-blind, placebo-controlled prospective randomized clinical trial of d-threo-methylphenidate HCl in brain tumor patients receiving radiation therapy. *Int J Radiat Oncol Biol Phys.* 2007 Dec 1;69(5):1496–1501.

74. Mar Fan HG, Clemons M, Xu W, et al. A randomised, placebo-controlled, double-blind trial of the effects of d-methylphenidate on fatigue and cognitive dysfunction in women undergoing adjuvant chemotherapy for breast cancer. *Support Care Cancer.* 2008 Jun;16(6):577–583.

75. Prommer E. Modafinil: is it ready for prime time? *J Opioid Manag.* 2006;2:130–136.

76. Thase ME, Fava M, DeBattista C, Arora S, Hughes RJ. Modafinil augmentation of SSRI therapy in patients with major depressive disorder and excessive sleepiness and fatigue: a 12-week, open-label, extension study. *CNS Spectr.* 2006;11:93–102.

77. Frye MA, Grunze H, Suppes T, et al. A placebo-controlled evaluation of adjunctive modafinil in the treatment of bipolar depression. *Am J Psychiatry.* 2007;164:1242–1249.

78. MacAllister WS, Krupp LB. Multiple sclerosis-related fatigue. *Phys Med Rehabil Clin N Am.* 2005;16:483–502.

79. Morrow GR, Gillies LJ, Hickok JT, Roscoe JA, Padamanaban D, Griggs JJ. The positive effect of the psychostimulant modafinil on fatigue from cancer that persists after treatment is completed [Abstract]. Proceedings of the 41st Annual Meeting of the American Society of Clinical Oncology, 2005:23 (Abstract 8012).

80. Kaleita TA, Wellisch DK, Graham CA, et al. Pilot study of modafinil for treatment of neurobehavioral dysfunction and fatigue in adult patients with brain tumors [Abstract]. Proceedings of the 42nd Annual Meeting of the American Society of Clinical Oncology, 2006;24 (Abstract 1503).

81. Capuron L, Gumnick JF, Musselman DL, et al. Neurobehavioral effects of interferon alpha in cancer patients: phenomenology and paroxetine responsiveness of symptom dimensions. *Neuropsychopharmacology.* 2002;26:643–652.

82. Morrow GR, Hickok JT, Roscoe JA, et al. Differential effects of paroxetine on fatigue and depression: a randomized, double-blind trial from the University of Rochester Cancer Center Community Clinical Oncology Program. *J Clin Oncol.* 2003;21:4635–4641.

83. Stockler MR, O'Connell R, Nowak AK, et al. Effect of sertraline on symptoms and survival in patients with advanced cancer, but without major depression: a placebo-controlled double-blind randomised trial. *Lancet Oncol.* 2007;8:603–612.

84. Cullum JL, Wojciechowski AE, Pelletier G, Simpson JS. Bupropion sustained release treatment reduces fatigue in patients with cancer. *Can J Psychiatry.* 2004;49:139–144.

85. Moss EL, Simpson JS, Pelletier G, Forsyth P. An open-label study of the effects of bupropion SR on fatigue, depression and quality of life of mixed-site patients with cancer and their partners. *Psychooncology.* 2006;15:259–267.

86. Lundstrom SH, Furst CJ. The use of corticosteroids in Swedish palliative care. *Acta Oncol.* 2006;45(4):430–437.

87. Bruera E, Roca E, Cedaro L, Carraro S, Chacon R. Action of oral methylprednisolone in terminal patients with cancer: a prospective randomized double-blind study. *Cancer Treat Rep.* 2005;69:751–754.

88. Bruera E, Ernst S, Hagen N, et al. Effectiveness of megestrol acetate in patients with advanced cancer: a randomized, double-blind, crossover study. *Cancer Prev Control.* 1998;2:74–78.

89. Cruciani RA, Dvorkin E, Homel P, et al. Safety, tolerability and symptom outcomes associated with L-carnitine supplementation in patients with cancer, fatigue, and carnitine deficiency: a phase I/II study. *J Pain Symptom Manage.* 2006;32:551–559.

90. Bruera E, Strasser F, Shen L, et al. The effect of donepezil on sedation and other symptoms in patients receiving opioids for cancer pain: a pilot study. *J Pain Symptom Manage.* 2003;26:1049–1054.

91. Shaw EG, Rosdhal R, D'Agostino RB Jr, et al. Phase II study of donepezil in irradiated brain tumor patients: Effect on cognitive function, mood, and quality of life. *J Clin Oncol.* 2006;24:1415–1420.

92. Bruera E, El Osta B, Valero V, et al. Donepezil for cancer fatigue: a double-blind, randomized, placebo-controlled trial. *J Clin Oncol.* 2007;25(23):3475–3481.

93. Pucci E, Branãs P, D'Amico R, Giuliani G, Solari A, Taus C. Amantadine for fatigue in multiple sclerosis. *Cochrane Database Syst Rev.* 2007. Retrieved December 29 2008, from http://mrw.interscience.wiley.com/cochrane/clsysrev/articles/CD002818/frame.html. Accessed August 12, 2009.

94. Kronenberger B, Berg T, Herrmann E, et al. Efficacy of amantadine on quality of life in patients with chronic hepatitis C treated with interferon-alpha and ribavirin: results from a randomized, placebo-controlled, double-blind trial. *Eur J Gastroenterol Hepatol.* 2007;19:639–646.

95. Burks TF. New agents for the treatment of cancer-related fatigue. *Cancer.* 2001;92(Suppl 6):1714–1718.

CHAPTER 33

Sexuality after Cancer

Andrew J. Roth, Jeanne Carter, and Christian J. Nelson

INTRODUCTION

The Office of Cancer Survivorship now estimates cancer survivor to number over ten million. Many of these cancer patients will be challenged with changes in sexual function during the acute phase of treatment and/or in the aftermath of cancer survivorship. Intimacy can be an important part of quality of life (QOL) that is disrupted and altered in the setting of a cancer diagnosis and treatment, with estimates ranging in the literature from 30%–90%.[1-3] The most common changes in sexual function for cancer survivors include decreased libido or sexual interest, pain with penetration (dyspareunia) in women, or erectile dysfunction in men.[4] Despite these significant changes, solutions do exist to assist with sexual rehabilitation.

RISK FACTORS FOR SEXUAL DIFFICULTIES

Many factors can be associated with increased risk of sexual difficulties following cancer treatment, such as site and extent of disease, recommended treatment, and age of the patient. The effect of treatment (i.e., chemotherapy or radiation therapy) on ovarian and erectile functioning, as well as underlying psychological symptoms of depression or anxiety can also have a negative impact on sexuality. During or following treatment, issues of pain, energy level, and hormonal status can influence sexuality. The degree, frequency, and quality of sexual activity before the cancer is an additional factor that should be noted within the context of sexual difficulties after cancer.

EFFECTS OF DIFFERENT CANCER TREATMENTS ON SEXUAL FUNCTIONING

Surgical treatment. Various surgical procedures can directly affect sexual functioning,[5] depending on the anatomy involved. For women diagnosed with gynecological cancer, surgery could involve the removal of some or all of the reproductive organs and genitalia including the ovaries, uterus, cervix, vulva or vagina. Surgical procedures may lead to damage to nerves as well as the possibility of scarring or adhesions in the pelvic area as part of the healing process. When the ovaries are removed, hormonal deprivation can occur causing abrupt premature menopause for many women. Research on surgical treatment and sexual function demonstrates that hysterectomy for benign conditions does not appear to impair sexual function.[6] Recent studies investigating sexual function after treatment for cervical cancer noted changes in lubrication, vaginal elasticity, pain or arousal difficulties much of which resolves by 1 year.[7-9] However, vaginal dryness and decreased sexual satisfaction and interest have been shown to persist up to 2 years or longer after surgery.[8,9] Impairment can also be worsened if other treatments such as radiation therapy are used in conjunction with surgical treatment.[10] This issue has raised methodological concerns about the existing literature evaluating the impact of hysterectomy on sexual function. Many of these studies included patients who received chemotherapy and/or radiation therapy in addition to the surgical treatment of hysterectomy. As a result, it is difficult to discern the direct impact of surgical treatment alone on the sexual functioning of cancer survivors.[11] With the field expanding to explore the benefits of nerve sparing surgery for women being treated for gynecologic cancer, further research is warranted.

Surgical treatment also includes the constant reminder or reality of surgical scar(s) and loss of body parts. For example, women undergoing mastectomy for breast cancer not only deal with the loss of a sexual organ but also experience loss of sensation in the surgical area, and altered body image even in the setting of breast reconstruction.[12] Individuals receiving treatment for bladder, colon, and rectal cancer often require the placement of temporary or permanent ostomy(s) for urine or stool. Management of these appliances requires practice and practical advice from medical specialists and often from other veteran patients, in addition to the adjustment to one's body image.[13]

Men faced with prostatectomy or cystectomy for prostate or bladder cancer are at risk of erectile dysfunction. Following surgery, erectile dysfunction may improve for up to 18–24 months afterwards , however up to 85% of men may experience erectile dysfunction after they fully heal 24 months after surgery.[14] This percentage may be accurate for both nerve sparing and nonnerve sparing surgery.[15,16] During the healing process, medications that might otherwise assist with erections may not work as well. There is much variability in the clinical outcome of different urologists as well as important factors such as age and presurgical erectile function which may determine expected results. Men are also likely to experience urinary incontinence for at least a few months after prostatectomy. Fear of urine leakage during sex or at orgasm can be a deterrent to even getting started. Younger men who have an orchiectomy for testicular cancer face the challenge of adjusting to the changes in the look and feel of their testicles, even with surgical implants. In addition, the men who have had retro-peritoneal lymph node dissection may have retrograde ejaculation (semen that ejaculates into the bladder) which can be uncomfortable and awkward.

Radiation treatment. For men, radiation therapy to the pelvis can cause fibrosis over time and interfere with the nerves and blood vessels necessary for erections.[17] The rates of erectile dysfunction after radiation therapy increases with time for cancer survivors. It has been found that men who have undergone radiation therapy have equivalent rates of erectile dysfunction (ED) (although the onset is delayed) to those undergoing nerve sparing surgery at 5 year medical follow-up.[17] Urinary incontinence can also result from radiation therapy causing concern about leakage during sexual activity. In addition, disruption of the bowel from radiation scatter can result in diarrhea or rectal bleeding. Another side effect of radiation that may preclude romance is fatigue, which can become prominent during therapy and remain for weeks or months afterward.

The current literature notes radiation therapy to be more problematic for female cancer survivors. Radiation therapy has been shown to have direct adverse affects on sexual functioning. Inflammation to mucosal surfaces of the vagina can make intercourse uncomfortable. Issues of dyspareunia, vaginal stenosis, scaring, and fibrosis can emerge, in addition to the ramifications of these painful conditions on the sexual response.[18,19] Some authors have also noted that chronic fibrotic changes to the pelvis may worsen vaginal atrophy over time, thus creating chronic difficulties up to 5 or more years postradiation treatment.[10] Furthermore, radiation treatment that includes or focuses on the pelvis, as is the case with total body irradiation before bone marrow transplant or treatment for pelvic cancers (i.e., gynecologic, urologic, colorectal), presents the additional challenge of premature menopause and /or the loss of fertility for many young women. This situation creates a complex emotional and physical adjustment for female cancer survivorship.[13]

Chemotherapy. Multiple obstacles can influence sexual functioning during and following chemotherapy treatment. Symptoms of fatigue, changes in mucosal lining, side-effects of nausea, vomiting, and diarrhea can be a struggle in the acute phase of treatment[4,20]; and negatively impact the desire to be sexual or the ability to achieve adequate arousal. Some chemotherapy treatments can result in hair loss or thinning contributing to feelings of sexual unattractiveness or self-consciousness. Changes in hormonal levels, such as induction of premature menopause, and vaginal atrophy which can interfere with the sexual response can be a long term, late effect of chemotherapy treatment.

Psychological. Feelings of anxiety and depression, changes in relationships, concern about the loss of physical well-being, as well as the difficulty in coping with changes to the body secondary to cancer treatment all can have a bearing on sexual function.[12,21,22]

When a cancer diagnosis directly impacts sexual organs, as is the case with breast cancer, gynecological cancer, prostate cancer, or testicular cancer, choices of sexuality and QOL may be a secondary priority to issues of longevity and survival. If increased anxiety and procrastination in the decision-making process occurs, it can be helpful to provide a supportive setting so that questions can be asked and discussed, preferably with a multidisciplinary team consisting of medical and mental health professionals.

Most often when we think of sexual functioning as it relates to people with cancer we think about married, heterosexual couples. Sexual functioning is no less important nor less problematic for gay and lesbian patients and their partners, as well as the single patient dealing with a cancer diagnosis and treatment. Sexual issues that intrude on a long-term relationship or potentially on a future relationship are frightening. Though talking about sexuality is often uncomfortable, it may seem more acceptable in the setting of a long-term committed relationship. Needless to say, it is also paramount for the single patient coping with the uncertainty of future partners. Practical questions about "when do I talk about my cancer," "how do I discuss my scars" or "what if I have difficulty getting aroused" specific to concerns about erections or vaginal dryness are common in survivorship. Vulnerability and fears can also emerge, "Will anyone want to go out with me if I can't have sex anymore" or "What will happen if I tell them I can't have children?" Sexual and reproductive changes can cause feelings of shame and embarrassment as well as injury to one's self-esteem and sense of identity. These issues are not easy to talk about with others. Therefore it is important for medical professionals to raise the issue and inquire about the sexual and emotional well-being of their patients. Broaching the topic not only allows for the opportunity to educate patients, but also gives permission for the topic to be discussed either now or at a later date. Initiation of a conversation on this topic also provides the opportunity for referrals to be made for those patients who are struggling, and who may benefit from additional support or/therapy.

Other factors. There are a number of medications, both related and unrelated to the cancer treatment that can change sexual functioning. Some of the medicines that have been implicated as negatively affecting sexuality are antiemetics, such as prochlorperazine (Compazine) and metoclopramide (Reglan), antihypertensives, and narcotics for pain relief, such as morphine, hydromorphone, methadone, and Percocet.

Many men and women will utilize psychotropic medication to help them cope with the emotional toll of their cancer experience. Antidepressants, in particular the serotonin-specific reuptake inhibitors (SSRIs) and serotonin-norepinephrine reuptake inhibitors (SNRI's) are excellent medications for mood and anxiety but also have the potential to adversely affect sexual desire, ability to achieve orgasm in both genders, and ejaculation in men. Nevertheless, these medications can also be an excellent nonhormonal method to assist women struggling with menopausal symptoms, in particular hot flashes.[23–25] Anti-anxiety medicines such as Valium (diazepam), Xanax (alprazolam) and Ativan (lorazepam) are minor tranquilizers that can take the edge off of worrying too much or panic symptoms. They work in the same place in the brain as alcohol. But just like alcohol, they can have deleterious effect on sexual functioning. In addition, if used regularly they can cause physical dependence and tolerance. Similarly, sedative medications that induce sleep such as Ambien (zolpidem) or Restoril (temazepam) can also interfere with love-making.

Hormonal treatments may also be part of the prescribed treatment plan which can influence sexual function. In men with prostate cancer, hormones are used to lower testosterone levels. Adverse effects can include impaired sexual interest, as well as the inability to achieve an erection.[26,27] Hormone treatments also cause fatigue which secondarily affects interest in sex. One patient reported, "Since I've been on hormones, I have had no interest in sex and my wife is upset that I am not more intimate." Conversely, another patient receiving hormonal therapy said, "Since I found Viagra and the penile injections, I'm interested in having sex again, but…my wife doesn't want to be bothered so much." Adjuvant endocrine therapy (i.e., tamoxifen or aromatase inhibitors) is often part of the treatment for female breast cancer patients.[28] Vasomotor symptoms such as hot flashes are the most common side effect associated with these medications, negatively impacting intimacy and QOL. Other side-effects of vaginal discharge, vaginal dryness, and dyspareunia have also been noted.[29,30]

Other medical disorders such as diabetes, cardiovascular disease, and hypertension as well as medicines required to treat these conditions, such as antihypertensives, can negatively impact sexual functioning. It is important to consider the effect of alcohol and illicit drugs on sex. Though small amounts of alcohol may enhance the romantic feeling, too much can act as a depressant and sedative; this can derail sexual excitement for both men and women, as well as impede erections in men.

COMMUNICATION AND FEAR

Sexual compromise after a cancer diagnosis and treatment can lead to a number of fears and concerns. First, there is the fear of change: "If our sex life was so good before, how can it mean anything now if I/we can't do it the same way." In nonsupportive relationships these deficits can be brought out in angry and hurtful ways. However, supportive partners are often concerned about not wanting to hurt or embarrass their partner with vaginal changes, or with an erection insufficient for penetration. Discussing sexual issues may be avoided with the good intention of trying to protect a partner. But sometimes even good intentions have unintended negative consequences, so it is important to have open communication in survivorship.

Attitudes and behaviors can be shaped by other fears. Some women may worry that their husbands will not want to stay with them after mastectomy or hysterectomy because of the change in their bodies. They may feel as though their femininity is being challenged and question their own sexual attractiveness. Body image conflicts and insecurities may lead to individuals isolating themselves from others. Albeit, some healthy spouses, who fear the consequences of cancer and do not want to cope with it, may flee relationships. However, it may not be clear to what extent there were problems in the relationship before the cancer that were not identified or dealt with. Ideally, couples in crisis should be identified early for possible intervention. Couple's counseling can be helpful in expanding communication skills, dispelling unfounded fears and myths, and supporting patients and partners during the cancer experience.

Some patients feel guilty when they develop a genitally-related cancer because of past sexual experience or other activity—they feel as though they are being punished for those behaviors. These past behaviors may include sexual traumas, past sexual activity (i.e., multiple partners, sex before marriage, affairs) or even normal sexual activity like masturbation. Sexual practices are strongly influenced by an individual upbringing, culture, or religion. Guilt can cause patients to feel self-conscious about sexual activity or intimacy with a partner following a cancer diagnosis. Other myths include the fear that the cancer can be transmitted during sex via bodily fluids, such as semen (in the case of men with prostate, testicular, or bladder cancer) or vaginal lubrication (in the case of women with ovarian, vaginal, or uterine cancer). Cancers are not transmitted by semen or vaginal fluid. The issue of human papillomavirus (HPV) has heightened concerns about cervical cancer and sexual activity. Certain strains of this virus are considered high risk for development of cervical dysplasia or precancerous cells which could develop into cancer.[31] Recent vaccines have been developed to target high-risk HPV, but many misconceptions exist about HPV and cancer in the general population. Some men with prostate cancer and their partners, knowing that testosterone is needed both for tumor growth and for sexual performance, may fear that the tumor will grow if they have sex. This is not true. Patients who are receiving radiation therapy to their pelvic regions may worry that radiation will be transmitted to their partners during sexual intercourse. This is only true for brachytherapy while the seeds are implanted and for a brief period afterward. Therefore, it is important for patients to communicate these concerns to their physicians.

SOLUTIONS

For women. Women experiencing changes in sexual functioning following a cancer diagnosis and treatment will usually have difficulties with pain with intercourse (dyspareunia) and vaginal health issues of vaginal dryness, decreased lubrication, and/or atrophy. The first step in restoring vaginal health should address using water-based vaginal lubricants, nonhormonal vaginal moisturizers, and pelvic floor exercises. These simple strategies have been found to be helpful in several studies with breast cancer survivors,[32,33] and have been incorporated into a formal sexual health program at a National Cancer Institute (NCI) cancer center.[34]

For women with persistent vaginal dryness interfering with QOL, a low-dose vaginal estrogen may be considered for a short time period after thoughtful discussion with their oncologist. Many questions exist about the idea of hormone replacement in the setting of cancer survivorship. Low-dose vaginal estrogens may initially show a temporary increase in serum hormone levels which creates a complex and controversial issue for patients and the medical professionals caring for them in cancer survivorship[35]; however, these levels return to the normal postmenopausal range. This is not the case for systemic absorption of oral or transdermal administration of estrogen.[36,37] Clearly, more safety data is needed in cancer populations.

Most recently, the question of androgen therapy for treatment of loss of desire in women was explored. In December 2004, the Food and Drug Administration (FDA) reviewed data regarding the submission of a female testosterone patch for the treatment of hypoactive desire disorder. The FDA declined approval of the testosterone patch and requested more safety studies.[38] In the setting of cancer survivorship the topic becomes a point of debate. In a critical review of the literature on androgen therapy, it was concluded that testosterone supplementation should not be prescribed to women for treatment of low desire due to concerns of increased breast cancer risk, based on epidemiologic findings of higher endogenous serum androgen levels being associated with increased risk of breast cancer.[39] Long-term safety studies are crucial in deciphering the complexity between hormonal supplementation and cancer.

For treatment of dyspareunia, vaginal dilators can be beneficial in treating vaginal stenosis and adhesions.[40] Dilator therapy has been recommended as the only modality meeting reasonable standards for evidence-based medicine in the treatment of pelvic radiation-induced sexual dysfunction, by a recent Cochrane report.[41] The theory behind vaginal dilator therapy, is that it mechanically stretches the vaginal tissues allowing for breakdown of fibrotic tissue, thus improving elasticity.[41] However, some authors question whether stimulation of the vaginal walls improves blood flow to the affected area.[37] More research is needed, but our clinical experience has been to combine dilator therapy with pelvic floor exercises to get both potential benefits. However, embarrassment and fear have been shown to decrease compliance with dilator therapy. In most cases, education and support can enhance compliance with sexual rehabilitative techniques. Robinson and colleague demonstrated that brief psychoeducational interventions were helpful, resulting in increased compliance with dilator therapy and decreased fear of painful sexual activity in participants.[42,43]

For men. For men who have erectile difficulty, medications such as Viagra (sildenafil), Cialis (tadalafil), or Levitra (vardenafil) may help. These medicines block an enzyme called phosphodiesterase-5 (they are therefore known as PDE-5 inhibitors), and relax penile smooth musculature. Studies have shown that giving the muscles and tissue enough time to heal may allow these medications to work better. For instance, those men who have had a prostatectomy and have given up trying these medications just a few months after surgery may have been unknowingly shortchanging themselves. Had they tried the medication again after 12 or 18 months, after more postoperative healing could take place, they may have had better success. Ultimately the nerves need to be healthy for the pills to work. Men can try using the pills every month after recovery to observe when they become effective. Some men will use penile injections during the recovery period to try to assure penile blood flow.

Success after prostate cancer treatment does not necessarily mean achieving the same caliber erection as when a man was 20 years old. Success may now be considered the ability to have an erection that is firm enough for penetration to allow for intercourse. Many men can achieve orgasm even without attaining an erection. Some men discontinue the use of these medications prematurely because they are not being used correctly or are not dosed sufficiently. For instance, Viagra is best taken on an empty stomach a couple of hours before one is planning to have sex. Cialis, which has a very long half-life and therefore can maintain its effectiveness for up to 36 hours, may help relieve some of the awkwardness of breaking up the romantic moment over the course of a weekend. These medicines also require some degree of manual or psychological stimulation to work for some men. It is usually best to avoid alcohol when taking these medicines, as alcohol can also inhibit erectile activity. More urologists and radiation oncologists are recommending the prophylactic use of these medications before the prostate cancer treatment with continued use during treatment (for radiation) and soon after prostatectomy. This allows the muscles to maintain their architecture and blood flow integrity. The adage "If you don't use it, you'll lose it," appears to be true here. Experimentation with different positions during sex, with different degrees of foreplay or different romantic settings may be helpful. Erectile difficulty after prostatectomy is worse for those who have had erectile difficulty before their treatment. Though it is difficult to believe, there is potential for a more satisfactory sex life if one can accept some change in sexual activity when compared to life before the cancer.

There are a number of mechanical means of helping men achieve erections; however, most men are not comfortable hearing about these methods, let alone trying them. For instance, one of the most reliable ways to achieve an erection after treatment for prostate cancer is with a penile injection of a medication such as alprostadil, or a mixture of papavarine, phentolamine, and alprostadil (Trimix) which dilate the blood vessels in the penis. The injection is usually described as similar to a mosquito bite, in a place that most men associate with pleasure and manhood. Those men willing to try can improve their sexual functioning; however, it is helpful to have a supportive partner who can understand and accept interruptions and adaptations in "the romantic moment." This can feel much less like a disruption if the couple can work the mechanical aid into their sexual routine, much the same way other couples allow for placement of condoms or birth control devices such as diaphragms. Penile injection therapy is not free of problems; however, with proper training these can be minimized.

Some men prefer to use a vacuum erection device. This is a more cumbersome device; when placed over the penile shaft and pumped up, it helps men achieve an erection. The resulting erections are rigid but may not look or feel normal. Again, with a supportive partner and inclusion into the romantic routine, it can be seen as the aid that it is, not natural and romantic, but necessary and sufficient to allow a sexually intimate liaison to occur. Suppositories are available that fit inside the opening of the penis to allow delivery of a medication similar to that in the injection, that will cause dilation of the penile blood vessels and erections. The suppository eliminates the painful injections; however, the medicine itself can cause burning and pain. There are inconsistent results, and like the other mechanical methods, can significantly interfere with the romantic moment.

Because each of the above mechanical methods has to be used anew every time a man wants to have sex, some men opt for a penile implant or prosthesis which, with either a quick unfolding or a pumping action, will quickly lead to an erection. With an implant or prosthesis, the choice to have assistance with attaining an erection is made only once. Implants require a separate surgical procedure. The erection and ultimate intercourse does not always feel the same to a man as before prostate cancer treatment. Hopefully though, it falls into the "good enough" category to facilitate sexual intimacy. Just trying an aid for obtaining an erection may not be sufficient. Fifty-six percent of penile injection users stopped treatment in the first year.[44] In samples of cancer patients[45] only 38% of men felt that treatment for their sexual problem was at least "somewhat" helpful. Satisfaction with these treatments appears to be low because patients do not get very good training or instructions in how to use the pills or other devices. Many are not taking pills correctly, are getting an improper dosage, or they are giving up too early. Many of those who have tried penile injections are not injecting in the correct area of the penis or are getting an improper dose. A number of patients complain about the loss of spontaneity.[46] It is important to remind patients and partners that these alterations require changes in sexual practices that may take some trial and error and therefore time, practice, and patience to lead to success.

For the couple. At a time when a couple's communication needs to be at its best, it is often compromised because of the stress of the cancer experience. Some men tend to be uncomfortable sharing their emotions. They often have the experience of being the protector and provider for the family, however, incompatible this is with the new reality of their physical compromise. Even when communication has been open, honest, and productive between partners who have been together for many years, the introduction of a life-threatening illness like cancer can impede useful discussions about difficult issues. It is helpful if a couple can learn to discuss some of the physical and psychological changes in a supportive atmosphere. Understanding how vaginal lubrication is impaired and causes pain with intercourse, either because of older age or cancer treatments, can help reduce feelings of rejection or failure when a woman shies away from sex because she does not want to experience pain. An ability to discuss the benefits a partner gets from nonintercourse sexual activity can take the pressure off of a man who has difficulty getting an erection after a prostatectomy or a woman experiencing pain with penetration.

Again, it is important to note that any sexual rehabilitative method needs a motivated patient, and this process can be enhanced with a supportive and understanding partner. Therefore, it is important not only to understand a patient's level of precancer sexual functioning, but also to know how sexuality was dealt with and discussed among the couple before the cancer diagnosis. Were they comfortable discussing sexually intimate issues? Was sexual activity solely related to intercourse or were they comfortable with other forms of sexual intimacy? How often did they have sex? Or how satisfied was each partner beforehand? Who initiated sexual activity? For those patients who have experienced clear losses or changes physically due to their cancer or treatment, there is a need for the individual as well as their partner to recognize and acknowledge this loss. Often each may grieve for not only what was lost from life before cancer, but also the hopes, dreams, and expectations of the future as well.

When a couple finds that there are too many barriers to figuring out how to overcome their sexual problems on their own, they should seek professional help. If these barriers are more related to the couple's relationship, and existed before the cancer diagnosis, it may be more prudent to begin with a general couple's therapy. There are likely other areas of the relationship in which problems exist, but are most noticeable in the bedroom. When this distinction is not obvious, it may make sense to begin with the sex therapist. It will soon become clear whether the difficulties are related more to the sexual problems or larger relationship issues. It is also essential for the cancer survivor to have a comprehensive medical evaluation with a gynecologist and/or urologist as part of the sexual rehabilitative process to identify any underlying physiological issues while addressing the emotional adjustments.

SEXUAL REHABILITATION

Sex therapy provides information, support, and guidance. The issues discussed include practical strategies for communication, integrating therapeutic suggestions and treatments into the sexual relationship, and identification of different positions to decrease pain during sexual activity. Most patients are seen for one or two sessions[13] and most patients report improvements in sexual problems. In general, most patients can benefit from brief psychosexual interventions including education, counseling/support and symptom management. Effective and feasible interventions have been shown to increase compliance with vaginal dilation recommendations through provision of information, and support Robinson et al., 1998[47]; another example of a brief sexual intervention to address symptom management was reported by Ganz and colleagues.[32] This intervention focused on providing information, support and symptom management to breast cancer patients. Significant improvement in menopausal symptoms, including hot flashes and vaginal dryness, in addition to improved sexual function were achieved with this intervention.

Overall, it is helpful for the therapist to have some experience with working with cancer patients and perhaps specific familiarity with the couple's particular cancer-related sexual problem. A sex therapist will provide information about the sexual response cycle and anatomy, provide information about the effects of cancer treatment on sexuality, and provide information that normalizes the experience so the individual (or couple) does not feel alone or that this is only happening to them. In the therapy, the opportunity to learn techniques to discover nonsexual touch and intimacy, to expand the sexual repertoire and intimacy, and to assist in identifying other erotic zones will be reviewed. Positive affirmations, modification of negative cognitions, issues of body image, changes to one's body after treatment, and fears of intimacy are important themes to be addressed within the therapeutic process. Throughout, the sex therapist will help the individual (or couple) identify barriers and significant frustration while discussing methods to cope, adjust, and enhance intimacy after cancer, specific to a current or future relationship.

It is important when instituting any sexual treatment plan to recall the adage of start low and go slowly, but go. Reviewing some basic principles with couples may be helpful: (1) It is important to teach patients (men in particular) about the competitive aspects between pleasure and performance. Most men focus on performance as it relates to getting an erection and holding it as long as possible during intercourse. If they perform well, then they have been successful. This is a form of intimacy, but avoids the type of intimacy that many women are looking for in terms of their satisfaction. (2) Encourage the couple to create a safe space and time to discuss these issues and then to follow through on them. Though the couple may not have "dated" for many years, now is a good time to restart that type of physical and relationship intimacy. Often over time, couples lose some romance, and get in the rut of focusing just on having intercourse. (3) Of all the options that are presented by the therapist, the couple should remember to be specific and try to choose only one or two ideas at a time to work on. It is helpful to try to focus on the positive, to be aware of and try to use nonverbal sexual communication, to avoid arguments, to discuss fears, and to take the time to listen to their partner.

Sensate focus is a widely used sexual therapy technique developed to enhance sexual contact without the primary focus on genital contact, allowing for more relation in the setting of intimacy. This technique has been adapted by Leslie Schover and other sex therapists working with cancer patients. The goal is to try to remove the anxiety and distress that come about by focusing on the goal of sexual performance (i.e., orgasm or erection). Sensate focus teaches a couple how to take the emphasis off of goal-oriented sex and helps the couple discover more sensual contact and expand in the sexual repertoire.

RESOURCES

Unfortunately, sexual assessment and counseling are not routinely provided in the oncology setting. There are a number of different reasons for this, including time constraints and the need to prioritize critical and complex treatment issues, practitioner discomfort in initiating a conversation regarding sexual functioning, and patient discomfort or embarrassment with this subject.[48] Mismatched expectations between providers and patients have been found specific to communication about sexuality and intimacy after cancer. Cancer patients indicated a desire for open communication about intimacy and sexuality, however, medical professionals prefer to focus on topics related to combating the disease.[49] In addition the "medical environment" can also pose challenges to communication on this topic. In a study exploring sexual functioning after gynecologic cancer treatment it was found that 78% of the women wanted to have a discussion about sexual matters, but did not ask questions due to fear of rejection or inappropriate setting.[50] This finding indicates that discussion about sexual functioning would be welcomed by patients if done in a sensitive and appropriate manner. Basic questions regarding sexual functioning should be part of any complete medical history and part of the treatment plan discussion, in particular if the prescribed treatment has the potential to alter sexual function. Resources are needed to help medical professionals feel more comfortable in addressing this important topic with their patients. Urological and gynecological professionals can also be helpful in sharing information meaningfully and supportively with patients and their partners. Even so, it is still very important for all oncology professionals and staff to encourage open discussion in addition to making appropriate referrals, as needed.

Finding help for sexual problems can be difficult.[51] Ninety-five percent of patients are willing to meet with a health professional about sexual difficulty, even though 43% of the partners had encouraged treatment. Unfortunately, the available help is not always easily accessible. For many hospitals and office settings, it is not feasible or practical to have a sexual health program or professionals on staff. Therefore, it is important to identify a referral network of local professionals with experience in treating sexual difficulties which may include mental health professionals with training in sexual therapy or working with cancer survivors, as well as gynecologists and urologists who have expertise in treating patients with changes in sexual function (i.e., menopause and erectile dysfunction) related to medical illness. Educational resources are also available and can provide further information and support to help patients achieve greater comfort with these issues. Local and national support organizations, such as The Office of Cancer Survivorship (http://cancercontrol. cancer.gov/ocs/index.html); The American Cancer Society (www.cancer. org); The American Association for Sex Education, Counseling and Treatment (http://www.aasect.org/); The Lance Armstrong Foundation (http://www.livestrong.org); The Association of Reproductive Health Professionals (www.arhp.org) and North American Menopause Society (http://www.menopause.org/) have excellent informational resources both available in written form and via websites.

CONCLUSIONS

It is not uncommon for sexual function to be altered after cancer treatment. This is especially true depending on the particular cancer and the treatment offered. It is important for all members of the oncology treatment team to acknowledge sexuality as an important QOL variable for all cancer patients and to be prepared to initiate discussion on sexual issues as early in the diagnostic and treatment process as possible. Communication amongst a couple is a very important component in optimizing sexual functioning and intimacy after treatment. When communication breaks down, the possibilities of fixing the sexual problem are diminished considerably. The primary mode of assisting couples with sexual problems after cancer is to help them change expectations and to find alternative ways to bring relief and pleasure, which can be facilitated by sex and/or couples therapy.

REFERENCES

1. Andersen BL. Sexual functioning morbidity among cancer survivors. Current status and future research directions. *Cancer*. 1985;55(8):1835–1842.

2. Andersen BL, Anderson B, deProsse C. Controlled prospective longitudinal study of women with cancer: II. Psychological outcomes. *J Consult Clin Psychol*. 1989;57(6):692–697.

3. Matulonis UA, Kornblith A, Lee H, et al. Long-term adjustment of early-stage ovarian cancer survivors. *Int J Gynecol Cancer*. 2008 Nov-Dec;18(6):1183–1193.

4. Schover LR. Sexuality and fertility after cancer. *Hematology Am Soc Hematol Educ Program*. 2005:523–527.

5. Flay LD, Matthews JH. The effects of radiotherapy and surgery on the sexual function of women treated for cervical cancer. *Int J Radiat Oncol Biol Phys*. 1995;31(2):399–404.

6. Thakar R, Ayers S, Clarkson P, Stanton S, Manyonda I. Outcomes after total versus subtotal abdominal hysterectomy. *N Engl J Med*. 2002;347(17):1318–1325.

7. Grumann M, Robertson R, Hacker NF, Sommer G. Sexual functioning in patients following radical hysterectomy for stage IB cancer of the cervix. *Int J Gynecol Cancer*. 2001;11(5):372–380.

8. Jensen PT, Groenvold M, Klee MC, Thranov I, Petersen MA, Machin D. Early-stage cervical carcinoma, radical hysterectomy, and sexual function. A longitudinal study. *Cancer*. 2004;100(1):97–106.

9. Pieterse QD, Maas CP, ter Kuile MM, et al. An observational longitudinal study to evaluate miction, defecation, and sexual function after radical hysterectomy with pelvic lymphadenectomy for early-stage cervical cancer. *Int J Gynecol Cancer*. 2006;16(3):1119–1129.

10. Frumovitz M, Sun CC, Schover LR et al. Quality of life and sexual functioning in cervical cancer survivors. *J Clin Oncol*. 2005;23(30):7428–7436.

11. Downes M, Sonoda Y. A Review of hysterectomy and its effects on female sexual function. *Curr Sex Health Rep*. 2008;5:102–107.

12. Ganz PA. Psychological and social aspects of breast cancer. *Oncology (Williston Park)*. 2008;22(6):642–646, 650; Discussion 650, 653.

13. Schover LR. The impact of breast cancer on sexuality, body image and intimate relationships. *CA Cancer J Clin*. 1999;41:112–120.

14. Schover LR, Fouladi RT, Warneke CL, et al. The use of treatments for erectile dysfunction among survivors of prostate carcinoma. *Cancer*. 2002;95(11):2397–2407.

15. Potosky AL, McLerran D, Feng Z, et al. 5-year urinary and sexual outcomes after radical prostatectomy: results from the prostate cancer outcomes study. *J Urol*. 2005;173(5):1701–1705.

16. Potosky AL, Mori M, Hsieh YC, et al. Treatment of erectile dysfunction following therapy for clinically localized prostate cancer: patient reported use and outcomes from the Surveillance, Epidemiology, and End Results Prostate Cancer Outcomes Study. *J Urol*. 2005;174(2):646–650; Discussion 650.

17. Potosky AL, Davis WW, Hoffman RM, et al. Five-year outcomes after prostatectomy or radiotherapy for prostate cancer: the prostate cancer outcomes study. *J Natl Cancer Inst*. 2004;96(18):1358–1367.

18. Bergmark K, Avall-Lundqvist E, Dickman PW, et al. Vaginal changes and sexuality in women with a history of cervical cancer. *NEJM*. 1999;340:1383–1389.

19. Jensen PT, Groenvold M, Klee MC, Thranov I, Petersen MA, Machin D. Longitudinal study of sexual function and vaginal changes after radiotherapy for cervical cancer. *Int J Radiat Oncol Biol Phys*. 2003;56(4):937–949.

20. Krychman ML, Carter J, Aghajanian CA, Dizon DS, Castiel M. Chemotherapy-induced dyspareunia: a case study of vaginal mucositis and pegylated liposomal doxorubicin injection in advanced stage ovarian carcinoma. *Gynecol Oncol*. 2004;93(2):561–563.

21. McKee AL Jr, Schover LR. Sexuality rehabilitation. *Cancer*. 2001;92(Suppl 4): 1008–1012.

22. Wilmoth MC, Botchway P. Psychosexual implications of breast and gynecologic cancer. *Cancer Invest*. 1999;17(8):631–636.

23. Loprinzi L, Barton DL, Sloan JA, et al. Pilot evaluation of gabapentin for treating hot flashes. *Mayo Clin Proc*, 2002;77(11):1159–1163.

24. Loprinzi CL, Sloan JA, Perez EA, et al. Phase III evaluation of fluoxetine for treatment of hot flashes. *J Clin Oncol*. 2002;20(6):1578–1583.

25. Weitzer MA, Moncello J, Jacobsen PB, Minton S. *A Pilot trial of paroxetinefor the treatment of hot flashes and associated symptoms in women with breast cancer*. Psychosocial and Palliative Care Program, H. Lee Moffitt Cancer Center, Tampa FL 33612–9497, USA.

26. Crenshaw TL, Goldberg JP, Stern WC. Pharmacologic modification of psychosexual dysfunction. *J Sex Marital Therapy*. 1987;13(4):239–252.

27. Basaria S, Lieb J 2nd, Tang AM, et al. Long-term effects of androgen deprivation therapy in prostate cancer patients. *Clin Endocrinol (Oxf)*. 2002;56(6):779–786.

28. Cella D, Fallowfield LJ. Recognition and management of treatment-related side effects for breast cancer patients receiving adjuvant endocrine therapy. *Breast Cancer Res Treat*. 2008;107(2):167–180.

29. Ganz PA, Greendale GA, Petersen L, Kahn B, Bower JE. Breast cancer in younger women: reproductive and late health effects of treatment. *J Clin Oncol*. 2003;21(22):4184–4193.

30. Howell A, Cuzick J, Baum M, et al. Results of the ATAC (Arimidex, Tamoxifen, Alone or in Combination) trial after completion of 5 years' adjuvant treatment for breast cancer. *Lancet*. 2005;365(9453):60–62.

31. Al-Daraji WI, Smith JHF. Infection and cervical neoplasia: facts and fiction. *Int J Clin Exp Pathology.* 2009;2:48–64.

32. Ganz PA. Quality of life across the continuum of breast cancer care. *Breast J.* 2000;6(5):324–330.

33. Schover LR, Schover LR, Partridge AH, et al. American Society of Clinical Oncology recommendations on fertility preservation in cancer patients. *J Clin Oncol.* 2006;24(18):2917–2931.

34. Krychman ML, Pereira L, Carter J, Amsterdam A. Sexual oncology: Sexual health issues in women with cancer. *Oncology.* 2006;71(1–2):18–25.

35. Kendall A, Martinb L-A, Kendalla A, Dowsett M. The relationship between factors affecting endogenous oestradiol levels in postmenopausal women and breast cancer. *J Steroid Biochem Mol Biol.* 2006;102(1–5):250–255.

36. Cardozo L, Bachmann G, McClish D, Fonda D, Birgerson L. Meta-analysis of estrogen therapy in the management of urogenital atrophy in postmenopausal women: second report of the Hormones and Urogenital Therapy Committee. *Obstet Gynecol.* 1998;92(4, pt 2):722–727.

37. Schover LR, Jenkins R, Sui D, Adams JH, Marion MS, Jackson KE. Randomized trial of peer counseling on reproductive health in African American breast cancer survivors. *J Clin Oncol.* 2006;24(10):1620–1626.

38. Sparks RF. Intrinsa fails to impress FDA advisory panel. *Int J Impot Res.* 2005;17:283–284.

39. Schover LR. Androgen therapy for loss of desire in women: is the benefit worth the breast cancer risk? *Fertil Steril.* 2008;90(1):129–140.

40. Juraskova I, Butow P, Robertson R, Sharpe L, McLeod C, Hacker N. Post-treatment sexual adjustment following cervical and endometrial cancer: a qualitative insight. *Psychooncology.* 2003;12(3):267–279.

41. Denton AS, Maher EJ. Interventions for the physical aspects of sexual dysfunction in women following pelvic radiotherapy. *Cochrane Database Syst Rev.* 2003(1):CD003750.

42. Robinson JW, Faris PD, Scott CB. Psychoeducational group increases vaginal dilation for younger women and reduces sexual fears for women of all ages with gynecological carcinoma treated with radiotherapy. *Int J Radiat Oncol Biol Phys.* 1999;44:497–506.

43. Jeffries SA, Robinson JW, Craighead PS, Keats MR. An effective group psychoeducational intervention for improving compliance with vaginal dilation: a randomized controlled trial. *Int J Radiat Oncol Biol Phys.* 2006;65(2):404–411.

44. Sundaram CP, Thomas W, Pryor L, Ami Sidi A, Billups K, Pryor J. Long-term follow-up of patients receiving injection therapy for erectile dysfunction. *Urology.* 1997;49(6):932–935.

45. Schover LR, Fouladi RT, Warneke CL, et al. Defining sexual outcomes after treatment for localized prostate carcinoma. *Cancer.* 2002;95(8):1773–1785.

46. Sexton WJ, Benedict JF, Jarow JP. Comparison of long-term outcomes of penile prostheses and intracavernosal injection therapy. *J Urol.* 1998;159(3):811–815.

47. Robinson JW. Sexuality and cancer. Breaking the silence. *Aust Fam Physician.* 1998;27:45–47

48. Schover LR. Counseling cancer patients about changes in sexual function. *Oncology (Williston Park).* 1999;13(11):1585–1591; Discussion 1591–1592, 1595–1596.

49. Hordern AJ, Street AF. Communicating about patient sexuality and intimacy after cancer: mismatched expectations and unmet needs. *MJA.* 2007; 186:5.

50. Lancaster J. Women's experiences of gynecologic cancer treated with radiation. *Curationis.* 1993;16(1):37–42.

51. Neese LE, Schover LR, Klein EA. Finding help for sexual problems after prostate cancer treatment: a phone survey of men's and women's perpectives. *Psychooncology.* 2003;12(5):463–473.

CHAPTER 34

Neuropsychological Impact of Cancer and Cancer Treatments

Tim A. Ahles and Denise D. Correa

INTRODUCTION

Increasing research has focused on cognitive changes associated with cancer and cancer treatments. Although cognitive problems associated with cancer of the central nervous system (CNS) have been recognized for many years,[1,2] more recent research has been focused on cognitive side effects of non-CNS tumors.[3] The current chapter will review the most studied examples of each type: brain tumors and early stage breast cancer. However, emerging areas of neurocognitive research are focusing on cognitive changes associated with androgen ablation for the treatment of prostate cancer,[4] chemotherapy for the treatment of colon, ovarian, and testicular cancers,[5] and high-dose chemotherapy and bone marrow transplantation.[6]

COGNITIVE FUNCTIONS IN PATIENTS WITH PRIMARY BRAIN TUMORS

Primary brain tumors are classified by their predominant histologic appearance and location. Gliomas are the most common tumors accounting for 40% of all CNS neoplasms and include low-grade astrocytomas (grades I, II) and high-grade or anaplastic astrocytomas and glioblastoma multiforme (grades III, IV). Other less frequent tumors include primary central nervous system lymphoma (PCNSL), oligodendrogliomas, ependymomas, meningiomas, and medulloblastomas.[7]

Cognitive dysfunction is common in brain tumor patients, and can be related to both the disease and its treatment including surgery, radiotherapy (RT) and chemotherapy. The side effects of medications such as corticosteroids and antiepileptics often contribute to or exacerbate their cognitive difficulties. Clinical trials in neuro-oncology have focused primarily on survival and time to disease progression, and cognitive outcome was often based on performance status and mental state examinations. These methods have low sensitivity to detect cognitive impairment in this population,[8-10] and as a result, the incidence of cognitive dysfunction was most likely underestimated in several studies. As effective treatment interventions have increased survival, there has been greater awareness that many brain tumor patients experience cognitive dysfunction despite adequate disease control.[11] The relevance of including cognitive and quality of life (QOL) evaluations as outcome variables in neuro-oncology research has been recognized by many professionals in the field,[12] and the National Cancer Institute (NCI) Brain Tumor Progress Review Group Report has recommended that routine cognitive and QOL assessment become the standard care for patients with brain tumors.[13]

DISEASE AND TREATMENT EFFECTS ON COGNITION

Seizures, headaches, increased intracranial pressure, focal neurological signs, and cognitive impairment are among the most common presenting symptoms in patients with brain tumors. The specific effects of tumor on cognitive abilities have not been systematically investigated as most of the research evaluated cognitive functions subsequent to treatment intervention. Nevertheless, recent studies documented cognitive impairment at diagnosis and before RT or chemotherapy in patients with high-grade gliomas,[14] low-grade gliomas,[15] and PCNSLs.[16] Cognitive difficulties present at the time of diagnosis are often related to the location and side of the tumor,[14] but a diffuse pattern of deficits has also been reported.[17] Rate of tumor growth is a predictor of cognitive impairment, as slow tumor growth is often associated with less severe cognitive dysfunction than rapid tumor growth.[18,19]

Surgical resection can be associated with neurological and cognitive deficits due to damage to tumor surrounding tissue, but these have been reported to be mild and transient in most cases.[20,21] However, studies including both pre- and postsurgery cognitive evaluations are few suggesting that the incidence and extent of cognitive dysfunction specifically related to surgical intervention is unknown. In addition, the contribution of corticosteroids, frequently given to many brain tumor patients subsequent to diagnosis, has not been assessed systematically. Although steroids may improve cognitive deficits due to resolution of edema,[14] they have also been associated with mood disturbance and cognitive difficulties,[22-24] and may contribute to cognitive changes in some brain tumor patients.

Treatment-related neurotoxicity

Whole-brain and conformal RT. The late-delayed effects of RT become apparent a few months to many years after treatment, and often produce irreversible and progressive damage to the CNS through vascular injury causing ischemia of surrounding tissue, and demyelination of the white matter and necrosis.[25] Suggested mechanisms include depletion of glial progenitor cells and perpetuation of oxidative stress induced by radiation.[26] Radiation may diminish the reproductive capacity of the O-2A progenitors of oligodendrocytes, disrupting the normal turnover of myelin.[27] This progressive demyelination may take months to cause symptoms, contributing to the latency in onset of neurotoxicity and its progressive nature. In addition, recent animal and human studies have documented that RT, as well as chemotherapy can disrupt hippocampal neurogenesis.[28-30] Risk factors for developing delayed RT-induced brain injury include greater volume of radiated tissue, higher total dose of RT, >2Gy dose per fraction, concomitant administration of chemotherapy, age greater than 60 years, and presence of co-morbid vascular risk factors.[31]

A substantial number of brain tumor patients treated with RT develop cognitive dysfunction that vary from mild to severe, and it is currently considered the most frequent complication among long-term survivors.[32] The peak of neurocognitive abnormalities resulting from RT occurs approximately 6 months to 2 years after treatment completion, and its incidence is proportional to the percentage of patients with disease-free survival.[33] The variability in the documented frequency of RT-induced cognitive deficits may be partially associated with the insensitivity of the methods of assessment used, duration of follow-up, retrospective nature of many studies, inclusion of patients treated with different regimens, and population discrepancies. In addition, the high incidence of tumor recurrence and short-term survival in patients with high-grade malignancies have often been considered confounding variables that hampered the ability to quantify the frequency, onset, and course of the delayed cognitive effects of RT.[34] Overall, the literature suggests that the pattern of neuropsychological impairments associated with the delayed effects of whole-brain RT is diffuse and relatively independent of tumor location.[35] The cognitive deficits are consistent with frontal-subcortical dysfunction,

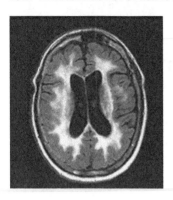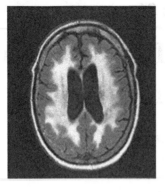

Fig. 34–1. Periventricular white matter disease on MRI images of a 60-year-old PCNSL patient 5 years after treatment with high-dose chemotherapy and whole-brain radiotherapy.

ABBREVIATIONS: MRI, magnetic resonance imaging; PCNSL, primary central nervous system lymphoma.

SOURCE: Reproduced from Correa, DD. Primary central nervous system lymphoma. In Meyers CA, Perry JR, (eds). *Cognition and cancer.* New York: Cambridge University Press; 2008:187–197.

and domains suggested to be particularly sensitive to treatment-induced cognitive dysfunction include attention, executive functions, learning and retrieval of new information, and psychomotor speed.[10,24,34,36–39]

In recent years, conformal RT that includes the area of the tumor and a variable surrounding margin, has supplanted whole-brain RT in the treatment of gliomas due to equivalent efficacy and reduced neurotoxicity.[40] Most studies examining the effects of partial RT have been retrospective and revealed variable outcomes ranging from no morbidity to marked cognitive deficits.[41–45] Several studies that documented cognitive dysfunction in low-grade glioma patients found that the tumor itself rather than RT was the primary contributing factor,[45–47] but other studies reported that conformal RT and antiepileptic treatment contributed to mild cognitive dysfunction.[48–50] In patients who had cognitive dysfunction, psychomotor speed, and verbal and nonverbal memory were the domains most likely to be affected.[51]

Chemotherapy alone or combined with RT. Neurotoxicity has been reported after high-dose regimens with procarbazine, lomustine, and vincristine (PCV) chemotherapy,[52] and after high-dose methotrexate (HD-MTX) and high-dose cytarabine often used in the treatment of PCNSL, particularly if RT is administered before or during chemotherapy[53] (Fig. 34–1). Chemotherapy administered intrathecally is more likely to cause CNS toxicity than when it is applied systemically. Combined treatment with RT and chemotherapy may have a synergistic effect,[54] as chemotherapy agents may interfere with the same cellular structures as radiation and may act as a radiosensitizer. Radiation may alter the distribution kinetics of chemotherapeutic agents in the CNS by increasing the permeability of the blood-brain barrier (BBB), affecting the ability of arachnoid granulations or choroid plexus to clear the drug, or interrupting the ependymal barrier to allow drugs in the cerebrospinal fluid to enter the white matter. Finally, RT-induced cellular changes may allow greater amounts of the drug to enter nontumor cells or less drug to exit. The interactions between RT and HD-MTX are the most clearly demonstrated.[54] Other chemotherapy agents that may produce CNS damage when combined with RT are nitrosoureas, cytosine arabinoside, and vincristine[53]; however, the injury mechanisms are not as well understood.

Patients with PCNSL have a favorable response to HD-MTX-based chemotherapy alone or in combination with whole-brain RT.[33,55] A literature review of cognitive outcome in PCNSL[51] reported that in patients treated with whole-brain RT and HD-MTX-based chemotherapy, or with whole-brain RT and chemotherapy with BBB disruption, there was evidence of significant cognitive impairment. The pattern of cognitive deficits was diffuse and the domains most commonly disrupted included attention and executive functions, psychomotor speed, and learning and retrieval of new information.[56–59] However, the retrospective nature of

these studies limited the ability to examine the specific contributions of tumor and the delayed effects of treatment. In PCNSL patients treated with high-dose chemotherapy alone or with BBB disruption chemotherapy there was evidence of diffuse cognitive impairment before treatment. Posttreatment follow-ups were variable across studies, but several reported either stable or improved cognitive performance[60–64]; however, methodological problems such as small number patients in each study, inclusion of patients with partial response to therapy or tumor recurrence, and incomplete reporting of cognitive test results limited the conclusions regarding the chemotherapy effects.

BREAST CANCER

For many years, breast cancer survivors have been reporting changes in multiple areas of cognitive functioning including attention and concentration, short-term memory, and the ability to multi-task. Reports of the potential cognitive effects of chemotherapy can be found in the scientific literature dating back to the 1970s[65]; however, concerted scientific attention to this area began only in the 1990s. Starting in the mid-1990s several posttreatment, cross-sectional studies were reported that supported the hypothesis that chemotherapy can negatively impact cognitive functioning in a subgroup of breast cancer survivors who were 6 months to 10 years posttreatment,[66–72] although negative studies were reported.[73,74] In importance, cognitive functioning was found to be independent of mood or fatigue. Interestingly, many of the initial cross-sectional studies evaluated cancer survivors who had been treated before the routine use of endocrine therapies; however, latter studies suggested that treatment with chemotherapy and tamoxifen produced greater impact on cognitive functioning than chemotherapy alone.[75]

Although these studies were informative, the interpretation of these results was limited by the lack of pretreatment evaluations of neuropsychological functioning. Consequently, as recommended by the International Cognition and Cancer Task Force, investigators began a series of longitudinal studies.[5,76] Longitudinal studies (Table 34–1) to date have reported that chemotherapy[77–80] or the combination of chemotherapy and endocrine therapy[81,82] can negatively impact cognitive functioning. However, the findings have not been completely consistent. For example, Schagen et al.[83] reported that patients treated with high-dose chemotherapy, but not patients treated with standard-dose chemotherapy, were significantly more likely to experience posttreatment cognitive changes as compared to matched healthy controls. Further, Jenkins et al.[84] reported no group differences in posttreatment cognitive functioning in a study comparing breast cancer patients exposed to chemotherapy, endocrine therapy and/radiation therapy, and healthy controls. Several factors may have contributed to the variability in the results across studies: (1) type of chemotherapy regimen, (2) timing of cognitive assessment and length of follow-up, (3) study design, (4) small number of patients studied, (5) type of comparison control group (healthy vs. patient controls, published normative data), (6) sensitivity/ reliability of neuropsychological measures, (7) and definition of cognitive impairment.[2]

An unexpected finding from the initial prospective studies was the identification of 20%–30% of patients who demonstrated lower than expected performance (based on age and education) before beginning adjuvant treatment.[5,85] Cognitive performance in this subgroup could not be explained by factors such as anxiety, depression, or fatigue, suggesting that there may be aspects of the biology of breast cancer that influence cognitive functioning and/or shared risk factors for the development of cancer and mild cognitive changes.[85] Further, preliminary analyses from the Dartmouth longitudinal study demonstrated that lower than expected pretreatment cognitive performance was predictive of posttreatment decline in the processing speed domain.[86] This stands in contrast to general improvement in patients with normal pretreatment performance and healthy controls who generally demonstrated an improvement over time in all domains, consistent with a practice effect.[5] This pattern of results could be interpreted as indicating that patients with lower cognitive reserve are more vulnerable to cognitive side effects of adjuvant treatments for breast cancer.

Finally, the impact of endocrine therapy alone on cognitive functioning is beginning to be studied but remains an open question.[87] Further,

Table 34-1. Longitudinal studies of cognitive effects of adjuvant therapy in women with breast cancer

Authors	Participants	Assessment schedule	Cognitive domains	Outcomes
Bender et al. (2006)	Pre- and perimenopausal patients n = 46; mean age 42.57 years; divided in 3 groups: Group 1—Stage I or II, receptor negative, receiving only chemotherapy Group 2—Stage I or II, receptor positive, receiving chemotherapy and tamoxifen Group 3—ductal carcinoma in situ (DCIS), receiving no chemotherapy or tamoxifen	T_1—postsurgery, but before starting adjuvant therapy for Groups 1 and 2 T_2—within 2 weeks of completing chemotherapy for Groups 1 and 2; a similar time period for Group 3 T_3—one year after T2	Attention; learning; memory; psychomotor speed; mental flexibility; executive function; visuoconstructional ability; and general intelligence	Women who received chemotherapy plus tamoxifen declined in visual memory and verbal working memory; women who received chemotherapy alone showed decline in verbal working memory only
Collins et al. (2008)	Postmenopausal patients divided in 2 groups: Group 1—Stage I–III, receiving chemotherapy n = 53; mean age 57.9 years Group 2—Stage I–III, receiving only hormone therapy n = 40; mean age 57.6 years	T_1—postsurgery, but before starting chemotherapy for Group 1 T_2—within 1 month of completing chemotherapy or 5–6 months following baseline T_3—one year after T_2	Executive function; language function; motor; processing speed; verbal learning and memory; visual learning and memory; visuospatial function; and working memory	Women who received chemotherapy plus hormone therapy performed more poorly on measures of processing speed and verbal memory at T_3
Hurria et al. (2006)	Patients over 65 years of age, Stages I–II, n = 31; mean age 71 years	Before and after chemotherapy	Attention; verbal memory; visual memory; and verbal, spatial, psychomotor, and executive functions	Women who received cyclophospamide, methotrexate, and 5-fluorouracil (CMF; 91%) declined in visual memory, spatial function, attention and psychomotor function
Jenkins et al. (2006)	Patients divided into 2 groups; healthy control group: Scheduled to receive chemotherapy n = 85; mean age 51.49 years Scheduled to receive endocrine therapy and/or radiotherapy n = 43; mean age 58.93 years Healthy control subjects n = 49; mean age 51.90 years	T1—baseline T2—postchemotherapy or 6 months postbaseline T3—18 months postbaseline	Intelligence; verbal memory; visual memory; working memory; executive function; and processing speed and vigilance	Treatment regimens were not found to affect cognitive performance at group or individual levels
Quesnel et al. (2007)	Group 1—Patients receiving chemotherapy and radiotherapy n = 41; mean age 50.3 years Group 2—Patients receiving only radiotherapy n = 40; mean age 57.7 years Group 3—Healthy controls matched to those patients receiving chemotherapy and radiotherapy n = 23; mean age 47.9 years	Group 1—before and after chemotherapy, and 3 months posttreatment Group 2—before and after radiotherapy, and 3 months posttreatment Groups 3 and 4—baseline only	Verbal and visual memory; attention; concentration; executive functions; speed of information; and verbal fluency	At baseline, patients showed lower performance on attention measures in comparison to healthy controls; both patient groups declined in verbal memory; patients receiving chemotherapy also declined in verbal fluency

(Continued)

Table 34–1. Continued

Authors	Participants	Assessment schedule	Cognitive domains	Outcomes
	Group 4—Healthy controls matched to those patients receiving only radiotherapy n = 22; mean age 55.0 years			
Shagen et al. (2006)	Group 1—Patients who received high-dose chemotherapy with cyclophosphamide, thiotepa, and carboplatin (CTC) n = 28; mean age 45.5 years	Groups 1 and 2—before and 6 months after completion of chemotherapy (12-month interval)	Attention; working, verbal, and visual memory; processing speed; executive function; and verbal and motor function	Patients who received CTC chemotherapy declined in cognitive performance
	Group 2—Patients who received standard-dose chemotherapy with 5-fluorouracil, epirubicin, and cyclophosphamide (FEC) n = 39; mean age 45.2 years	Group 3—baseline and 12 month interval to mirror Groups 1 and 2		
	Group 3—Stage I patients who did not receive chemotherapy n = 57; mean age 50.5 years	Group 4—baseline and 6-month interval		
	Group 4—Healthy controls n = 60; mean age 48.8 years			
Shilling et al. (2004)	Group 1—Patients to receive chemotherapy and patients receiving radiotherapy and/or endocrine therapy n = 50; mean age 51.1 years	Baseline; 4 weeks after completion of chemotherapy (6 months for controls); and 18 months	Intelligence; verbal memory; visual memory; working memory; executive function; and processing speed and vigilance	Chemotherapy patients declined in cognitive performance in comparison to controls
	Group 2—Healthy controls n = 43; mean age 52.3 years			
Wefel et al. (2004)	Patients receiving chemotherapy n = 18; mean age 45.4 years	Baseline; 3 weeks postchemotherapy; and 1 year postchemotherapy	Attention; processing speed; learning; memory; executive function; visuospatial function; and motor skills	Women who received chemotherapy declined in attention, learning and processing speed

although menopausal status has not been predictive of posttreatment cognitive changes in the longitudinal studies reviewed,[83] the role of chemotherapy-induced menopause and associated abrupt changes in estrogen levels has not been carefully evaluated.

NEUROIMAGING STUDIES

Recent studies have reported structural brain abnormalities in patients treated with chemotherapy. Saykin and colleagues[88] used magnetic resonance imaging (MRI) to assess structural brain changes associated with chemotherapy in long-term survivors (>5 years after diagnosis) of breast cancer and lymphoma (n = 12) and healthy controls (n = 12). Using voxel-based morphometry, the authors documented a bilateral reduction of gray matter, and cortical and subcortical white matter in patients treated with chemotherapy. Inagaki and colleagues[89] used voxel-based morphometry to assess regional brain volume in breast cancer patients who received either chemotherapy or no adjuvant therapy. Patients treated with chemotherapy (n = 51) had reductions in the gray matter (i.e., right prefrontal and parahippocampal gyrus), and in the white matter (i.e., bilateral middle frontal gyrus, left parahippocampal gyrus, left precuneus, and right cingulate gyrus) at the 1-year MRI study in comparison

to the no chemotherapy group (n = 54) and healthy controls (n = 55); these regional volumes were significantly correlated with performance on cognitive tests of attention and visual memory. No volume differences between patients and controls were observed in the 3-year study, although data for this analysis represented a different cohort from the 1-year analyses. Abraham and colleagues[90] used diffusion tensor imaging (DTI) to assess the integrity of white matter tracts in 10 breast cancer patients treated with chemotherapy who reported cognitive change as compared to 9 age- and education-matched healthy controls. Patients had decreased white matter integrity (fractional anisotropy) in the genu of the corpus callosum and this was correlated with reduced graphomotor speed.

Saykin and colleagues[91] used functional MRI to study patterns of regional brain activation associated with the performance of an auditory verbal working memory test in breast cancer patients before receiving either chemotherapy or local radiation, and 1 month after treatment; healthy controls were evaluated at similar intervals. Patients not exposed to chemotherapy and healthy controls showed greater activation in the bilateral anterior frontal regions at the 1-month follow-up compared to patients exposed to chemotherapy. Patients treated with chemotherapy showed increased activation in more posterior frontal and parietal regions. Decreased frontal activation in the chemotherapy group was interpreted as indicative of dysfunction in areas involved in working memory, whereas increased activation was interpreted as compensatory activation since the groups did not differ in task performance. Ferguson and colleagues[92] studied one set of monozygotic twins who were discordant for breast cancer and chemotherapy. Although there were no significant differences on tests of memory and executive functions, the twin treated with chemotherapy had substantially more cognitive complaints, greater white matter lesion volumes on MRI, and a broader spatial extent of activation in typical working memory circuitry (bifrontal and biparietal regions) on functional MRI. Silverman and colleagues[93] used [O-15] water positron emission tomography (PET) to study cerebral blood flow during a task requiring short-term word recall. They studied 16 breast cancer survivors who had chemotherapy 5–10 years before enrollment, 8 controls with a history of breast cancer but no exposure to chemotherapy; 11 patients who received chemotherapy also had tamoxifen. Modulation of cerebral blood flow was altered in the inferior frontal cortex during performance of the memory task in the chemotherapy-treated group, suggesting that greater recruitment of frontal cortical regions was necessary to perform the task. The investigators also compared resting metabolism of the chemotherapy-treated patients to 10 healthy controls using [F-18] fluorodeoxyglucose (FDG) PET. The results showed decreased glucose metabolism in the left inferior frontal gyrus and in the contralateral cerebellum in the chemotherapy group relative to controls. In addition, metabolism in the basal ganglia was significantly decreased in patients treated with both chemotherapy and tamoxifen.

Overall, the neuroimaging studies suggest that chemotherapy is associated with changes in brain structure and function. The addition of endocrine therapy may contribute to these changes as suggested by the Silverman et al. study.[93] Several of the imaging studies have suggested that there is compensatory activation of alternate brain structures during performance of cognitive tasks during fMRI and fPET evaluations. These data suggest that cancer survivors are able to maintain normal performance during cognitive testing by compensatory activation of brain structures not typically utilized to accomplish the task. This may explain why breast cancer survivors who report cognitive changes frequently score within the normal range of neuropsychological tests and suggests that some of the traditional neuropsychological measures may not test the limits of cognitive capacity in patients with relatively subtle cognitive changes associated with adjuvant treatments for breast cancer.

Candidate mechanisms. The mechanisms of chemotherapy-induced cognitive change are not well understood. Investigators have assumed that most commonly used cytotoxic agents do not readily cross the BBB; however, recent animal studies suggest that higher levels of chemotherapy may reach the brain than previously assumed and that even very low doses of chemotherapy can increase cell death and decrease cell division in the hippocampus and corpus callosum[28,94] Further, a recent animal study demonstrated that 5-fluorouracil (5-FU), an agent that does cross the BBB, caused both acute and progressive, delayed damage to myelinated tracts.[95] Therefore, a direct effect of chemotherapy on the brain cannot be ruled out. Additional candidate mechanisms (Fig. 34–2) include chemotherapy-induced oxidative stress and DNA damage, immune dysregulation and/or stimulation of neurotoxic cytokines, and blood clotting in small CNS vessels.[96] Endocrine therapies presumably impact cognitive function through alteration of estrogen levels, although they also decrease antioxidant capacity, thereby, increasing DNA damage.[96]

Further, variation in genetic polymorphisms may also increase vulnerability to cognitive changes associated with cancer treatments. Long-term survivors of breast cancer and lymphoma who carried the E4 allele of apolipoprotein E (APOE) and received chemotherapy had poorer performance in several domains of neuropsychological functioning compared to survivors with other forms of the APOE allele.[97] Genetic polymorphisms related to the efficiency of the BBB (e.g., differential expression of MDR-1) and the functioning of cytokines (e.g., polymorphisms of interleukin-6), neurotransmitters (e.g., COMT), and DNA repair mechanism (e.g., XRCC1) may also be important.[5]

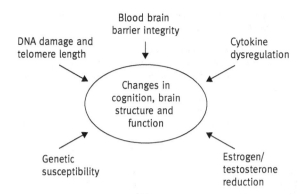

Fig. 34–2. Candidate mechanisms for chemotherapy-induced cognitive change.

INTERVENTIONS

Medication approaches that have been studied include the use of erythropoietin and methylphenidate; however, the results suggested moderate to no improvement in cognitive functioning.[98] Medications that have been proposed or that are currently under investigation include nonsteroidal antiinflammatory medications, aspirin, cholinesterase inhibitors, alpha-tocopherol (vitamin E), ascorbic acid (vitamin C), and gingko biloba.[98]

Ferguson et al.[99] developed a cognitive rehabilitation intervention for women with breast cancer who are experiencing postchemotherapy cognitive changes. The intervention, Memory/Attention Adaptation Training (MAAT), focused on arousal reduction through relaxation training and the use of tailored compensatory strategies such as memory and scheduling aids and establishment of routines. Preliminary results from a Phase I/feasibility trial were very positive and a randomized wait list control evaluation of the MAAT intervention is currently underway.[99]

SUMMARY/CONCLUSIONS

Brain tumor patients experience cognitive changes associated with their disease and a variety of aspects of their treatment, particularly RT and chemotherapy. Initially, cognitive changes for breast cancer patients were assumed to be primarily secondary to chemotherapy. However, increasing evidence suggests that there may be disease-related and treatment-related reasons for cognitive changes and that chemotherapy may only be one factor contributing to treatment-related cognitive changes. Future research in both populations is required to understand the impact of cognitive changes on functional capacity and quality of life. Further, the mechanism(s) for cognitive changes remain to be defined and targeted interventions designed to prevent or reduce the negative impact of cancer and cancer treatments remain to be developed. Finally, cognitive changes associated with other cancer diagnoses (e.g., colon, prostate, lung, ovarian) and treatment modalities (high-dose chemotherapy, biological response modifiers, hormone ablation therapy) require additional research attention.

REFERENCES

1. Taphoorn MJB, Klein M. Cognitive deficits in adult patients with brain tumours. *Lancet.* 2004;3:1–18.

2. Correa DD. Cognitive functions in brain tumor patients. *Hematol Oncol Clin North Am.* 2006;20:1363–1376.

3. Ahles TA, Correa DD. Neurocognitive changes in cancer survivors. *Cancer J: J Princ Prac Oncol. Cancer J* 2008;14:396–400.

4. Nelson CJ, Lee JS, Gamboa MC, Roth AJ. Cognitive effects of hormone therapy in men with prostate cancer. *Cancer.* 2008;113:1097–1106.

5. Vardy J, Wefel JS, Ahles TA, Tannock IF, Schagen SB. Cancer and cancer—therapy related cognitive dysfunction: an international perspective from the Venice cognitive workshop. *Ann Oncol.* 2007;19:623–629.

6. Syrjala KL, Dikmen S, Langer SL, Roth-Roemer S, Abrams JR. Neuropsychologic changes from before transplantation to 1 year in patients receiving myeloablative allogeneic hematopoietic cell transplant. *Blood.* 2004;104:3386–3392.

7. Bondy ML, El-Zein R, Wrench M. Epidemiology of brain cancer. In: Schiff D, O'Neill BP, (eds). *Principles of Neuro-Oncology*. New York: McGraw-Hill; 2005:3–16.

8. Bosma I, Vos MJ, Heimans JJ, et al. The course of neurocognitive functioning in high grade glioma patients. *Neuro Oncol*. 2007;9:53–62.

9. Meyers CA, Wefel JS. The use of the mini-mental state examination to assess cognitive functioning in cancer trials: no ifs, ands, buts, or sensitivity. *J Clin Oncol*. 2003;21:3557–3558.

10. Weitzner MA, Meyers CA. Cognitive functioning and quality of life in malignant glioma patients: a review of the literature. *Psychooncologyl*. 1997;6:169–177.

11. Poortmans PMP, Kluin-Nelemans HC, Haaxma-Reiche H, et al. High-dose methotrexate-based chemotherapy followed by consolidating radiotherapy in non-AIDS-related primary central nervous system lymphoma: European Organization for Research and Treatment of Cancer Lymphoma Group phase II Trial 20962. *J Clin Oncol*. 2003;21:4483–4488.

12. Meyers CA, Brown PD. Role and relevance of neurocognitive assessment in clinical trials of patients with CNS tumors. *J Clin Oncol*. 2006;24:1305–1309.

13. BTPRG. *Report of the Brain Tumor Progress Review Group (BTPRG)*. Baltimore, MD: National Institutes of Health; 2000.

14. Klein M, Taphoorn MJB, Heimans JJ, et al. Neurobehavioral status and health-related quality of life in newly diagnosed high-grade glioma patients. *J Clin Oncol*. 2001;19:4037–4047.

15. Klein M, Helmans JJ, Aaronson NK, et al. Effect of radiotherapy and other treatment-related factors on mid-term to long-term cognitive sequelae in low-grade gliomas: a comparative study. *Lancet*. 2002;360:1361–1368.

16. Correa DD, Anderson ND, Glass A, Mason WP, DeAngelis LM, Abrey LE. Cognitive functions in primary central nervous system lymphoma patients treated with chemotherapy and stem cell transplantation: preliminary findings. *Clin Adv Hematol Oncol*. 2003;1:490.

17. Crossen JR, Goldman DL, Dahlborg SA, Neuwelt EA. Neuropsychological asssessment outcomes of nonacquired immunodeficiency syndrome patients with primary central nervous system lymphoma before and after blood-brain barrier disruption chemotherapy. *Neurosurgery*. 1992;30:23–29.

18. Anderson SW, Damasio H, Tranel D. Neuropsychological impairments associated with lesions caused by tumor or stroke. *Arch Neurol*. 1990;47: 397–405.

19. Hom J, Reitan RM. Neuropsychological correlates of rapidly vs. slowly growing intrinsic cerebral neoplasms. *J Clin Neuropsychol*. 1984;6:309–324.

20. Duffau H. Lessons from brain mapping in surgery for low-grade glioma: insights into association between tumour and brain plasticity. *Lancet*. 2005;4:476–486.

21. Bosma I, Vos MJ, Heimans JJ, et al. The course of neurocognitive functioning in high grade glioma patients. *Neuro Oncol*. 2007;9:53–62.

22. Lupien SJ, Gillin CJ, Hauger RL. Working memory is more sensitive than declarative memory to the acute effects of corticosteroids: a dose-response study in humans. *Behav Neurosci*. 1999;113:420–430.

23. Young AH, Sahakian BJ, Robbins TW, Cowen PJ. The effects of chronic administration of hydrocortisone on cognitive function in normal male volunteers. *Psychopharmacol*. 1999;145:260–266.

24. Wefel JS, Kayl AE, Meyers CA. Neuropsychological dysfunction associated with cancer and cancer therapies: a conceptual review of an emerging target. *Br J Cancer*. 2004;90:1691–1696.

25. Sheline G, Wara WM, Smith V. Therapeutic irradiation and brain injury. *Int J Radiat Oncol Biol Phys*. 1980;6:1215–1228.

26. Tofilon PJ, Fike JR. The radioresponse of the central nervous system: a dynamic process. *Radiat Res*. 2000;153:357–370.

27. van der Maazen RW, Kleiboer BJ, Verhagen I, van der Kogel AJ. Repair capacity of adult rat glial progenitor cells determined by an in vitro clonogenic assay after in vitro or in vivo fractionated irradiation. *Int J Radiat Biol*. 1993;63:661–666.

28. Dietrich J, Han R, Yang Y, Mayer-Pröschel M, Noble M. CNS progenitor cells and oligodendrocytes are targets of chemotherapeutic agents in vitro and vivo. *J Biol*. 2006;5:1–23.

29. Monje ML, Palmer T. Radiation injury and neurogenesis. *Curr Opin Neurol*. 2003;16:129–134.

30. Santarelli L, Saxe M, Gross C, et al. Requirment of hippocampal neurogenesis for the behavioral effects of antidepressants. *Science*. 2003;301:805–809.

31. Constine LS, Konski A, Ekholm S, McDonald S, Rubin Pl. Adverse effects of brain irradiation correlated with MR and CT imaging. *Int J Radiat Oncol Biol Phys*. 1988;15:319–330.

32. Behin A, Delattre, J-Y. Neurologic sequelae of radiotherapy on the nervous system. In: Schiff D, Wen PY, (eds). *Cancer neurology in clinical practice*. Totowa, NJ: Humana Press Inc.; 2003:173–191.

33. DeAngelis, LM, Yahalom J, Thaler HT, Kher U. Combined modality therapy for primary CNS lymphoma. *J Clin Oncol*. 1992;10:635–643.

34. Crossen, JR, Garwood D, Glatstein E, Neuwelt EA. Neurobehavioral sequelae of cranial irradiation in adults: a review of radiation-induced encephalopathy. *J Clin Oncol*. 1994;12:627–642.

35. Duffey P, Chari G., Cartlidge NEF, Shaw PJ. Progressive deterioration of intellect and motor function occurring several decades after cranial irradiation. *Arch Neurol*. 1996;53:814–818.

36. Archibald YM, Lunn D, Ruttan LA, et al. Cognitive functioning in long-term survivors of high-grade glioma. *J Neurosurg*. 1994;80:247–253.

37. Salander P, Karlsson T, Bergenheim T, Henrikson R. Long-term memory deficits in patients with malignant gliomas. *J Neurooncol*. 1995;25:227–238.

38. Scheibel RS, Meyers CA, Levin VA. Cognitive dysfunction following surgery for intracerebral glioma: influence of histopathology, lesion location, and treatment. *J Neurooncol*. 1996;30:61–69.

39. Taphoorn MJB, Klein M. Cognitive deficits in adult patients with brain tumours. *Lancet*. 2004;3:1–18.

40. De Groot JF, Aldape KD, Colman H. High-grade astrocytomas. In: Schiff D, O'Neill BP, (eds). *Principles of neuro-oncology*. New York: McGraw-Hill; 2005:259–288.

41. Armstrong CL, Corn BW, Ruffer JE, Pruitt AA, Mollman JE, Phillips PC. Radiotherapeutic effects on brain function: double dissociation of memory systems. *Neuropsychiatr Neuropsychol Behav Neurol*. 2000;13:101–111.

42. Armstrong CL, Hunter JV, Ledakis GE, et al. Late cognitive and radiographic changes related to radiotherapy. *Neurology*. 2002;59:40–48.

43. Postma TJ, Klein M, Verstappen CCP, et al. Radiotherapy-induced cerebral abnormalities in patients with low-grade glioma. *Neurology*. 2002;59:121–123.

44. Surma-aho O, Niemela M, Vikki J, et al. Adverse long-term effects of brain radiotherapy in adult low-grade glioma patients. *Neurology*. 2001;56:1285–1290.

45. Taphoorn, MJB, Schiphorst, AK, Snoek, FJ, Lindeboom J, Karim AB. Cognitive functions and quality of life in patients with low-grade gliomas: the impact of radiotherapy. *Ann Neurol*. 1994;36:48–54.

46. Laack NN, Brown PD, Furth A, et al. Neurocognitive function after radiotherapy (RT) for supratentorial low-grade gliomas (LGG): results of a north central cancer treatment group (NCCTG) prospective study. *Int J Radiat Oncol Biol Phys*. 2003;57:S134.

47. Torres IJ, Mundt AJ, Sweeney PJ, et al. A longitudinal neuropsychological study of partial brain radiation in adults with brain tumors. *Neurology*. 2003;60:1113–1118.

48. . Correa DD, DeAngelis LM, Shi W, Thaler HT, Lin M, Abrey LE. Cognitive functions in low-grade-gliomas: disease and treatment effects. *J Neurooncol*. 2007;81:175–184.

49. Correa DD, Shi W, Thaler HT, Cheung AM, DeAngelis LM, Abrey LE. Longitudinal cognitive follow-up in low-grade gliomas. *J Neurooncol*. 2008;86:321–327.

50. Klein M, Postma TJ, Taphoorn MJB, et al. The prognostic value of cognitive functioning in the survival of patients with high-grade glioma. *Neurology*. 2003;61:1796–1798.

51. Correa DD, Maron L, Harder H, et al. Cognitive functions in primary central nervous system lymphoma: literature review and assessment guidelines. *Ann Oncol*. 2007;18:1145–1151.

52. Postma TJ, van Groeningen CJ, Witjies RJ, et al. Neurotoxicity of combination chemotherapy with procarbazine, CCNU and vincristine (PCV) for recurrent glioma. *J Neuro Oncol*. 1998;38:69–75.

53. DeAngelis LM, Shapiro WR. Drug/radiation interactions and central nervous system injury. In: Gutin PH, Leibel SA, Sheline GE, (eds). *Radiation injury to the nervous system*. New York: Raven Press; 1991:361–382.

54. Keime-Guibert F, Napolitano M, Delattre J-Y. Neurological complications of radiotherapy and chemotherapy. *J Neurol*. 1998;245:695–708.

55. Abrey LE, DeAngelis LM, Yahalom J. Long-term survival in primary CNS lymphoma. *J Clin Oncol*. 1998;16:859–863.

56. Correa DD, DeAngelis LM, Shi W, et al. Cognitive functions in survivors of primary central nervous system lymphoma. *Neurology*. 2004;62:548–555.

57. Harder H, Holtel H, Bromberg JEC, et al. Cognitive status and quality of life after treatment for primary CNS lymphoma. *Neurology*. 2004;62:544–547.

58. Neuwelt EA, Goldamn DA, Dahlborg SA, et al. Primary CNS lymphoma treated with osmotic blood-brain barrier disruption: prolonged survival and preservation of cognitive function. *J Clin Oncol*. 1991;9:1580–1590.

59. Pels H, Deckert-Schulter M, Glasmacher A, et al. Primary central nervous system lymphoma: a clinicopathological study of 28 cases. *Hematol Oncol*. 2000;18:21–32.

60. Fliessbach K, Urbach H, Helmstaedter C, et al. Cognitive performance and magnetic resonance imaging findings after high-dose systemic and intraventricular chemotherapy for primary central nervous system lymphoma. *Arch Neurol*. 2003;60:563–568.

61. Fliessbach K, Helmstaedter C, Urbach H, et al. Neuropsychological outcome after chemotherapy for primary CNS lymphoma: a prospective study. *Neurology*. 2005;64:1184–1188.

62. McAllister LD, Doolittle ND, Guastadisegni PE, et al. Cognitive outcomes and long-term follow-up results after enhanced chemotherapy delivery for primary central nervous system lymphoma. *Neurosurgery*. 2000;46:51–61.

63. Pels H, Schmidt-Wolf IGH, Glasmacher A, et al. Primary central nervous system lymphoma: results of a pilot study and phase II study of systemic and intraventricular chemotherapy with deferred radiotherapy. *J Clin Oncol*. 2003;21:4489–4495.

64. Schlegel U, Pels H, Glasmacher A, et al. Combined systemic and intraventricular chemotherapy in primary CNS lymphoma: a pilot study. *J Neurol Neurosurg Psychiatry*. 2001;71:118–122.

65. Silberfarb PM. Chemotherapy and cognitive defects in cancer patients. *Ann Rev Med*. 1983;34:35–46.

66. Wieneke MH, Dienst ER. Neuropsychological assessment of cognitive functioning following chemotherapy for breast cancer. *Psychooncology*. 1995;4:61–66.

67. van Dam FS, Schagen SB, Muller MJ, et al. Impairment of cognitive function in women receiving adjuvant treatment for high-risk breast cancer: high-dose versus standard-dose chemotherapy. [Comment]. *J Natl Cancer Inst*. 1998;90(3):210–218.

68. Schagen SB, van Dam FS, Muller MJ, Boogerd W, Lindeboom J, Bruning PF. Cognitive deficits after postoperative adjuvant chemotherapy for breast carcinoma. *Cancer*. 1999;85:640–650.

69. Schagen SB, Muller MJ, Boogerd W, et al. Late effects of adjuvant chemotherapy on cognitive function: a follow-up study in breast cancer patients. *Ann Oncol*. 2002;13:1387–1397.

70. Brezden CB, Phillips KA, Abdolell M, Bunston T, Tannock IF. Cognitive function in breast cancer patients receiving adjuvant chemotherapy. *J Clin Oncol*. 2000;18:2695–2701.

71. Ahles TA, Saykin AJ, Furstenberg CT, et al. Neuropsychological impact of standard-dose chemotherapy in long-term survivors of breast cancer and lymphoma. *J Clin Oncol*. 2002;20:485–493.

72. Tchen M, Juffs HG, Downie FP, et al. Cognitive function, fatigue, and menopausal symptoms in women receiving adjuvant chemotherapy for breast cancer. *J Clin Oncol*. 2003;21:4175–4183.

73. Donovan KA, Small BJ, Andrykowski MA, Schmitt FA, Munster P, Jacobsen PB. Cognitive functioning after adjuvant chemotherapy and/or radiotherapy for early stage breast carcinoma. *Cancer*. 2005;104:2499–2507.

74. Scherwath A, Mehnert A, Schleimer B, et al. Neuropsychological function in high risk breast cancer survivors after stem-cell supported high-dose therapy versus standard-dose chemotherapy: evaluation of long-term effects. *Ann Oncol*. 2006;17:415–423.

75. Castellon SA, Ganz PA, Bower JE, Petersen L, Abraham L, Greendale GA. Neurocognitive performance in breast cancer survivors exposed to adjuvant chemotherapy and tamoxifen. *J Clin Exp Neuropsychol*. 2004;26:955–969.

76. Tannock IF, Ahles TA, Ganz PA, van Dam FS. Cognitive impairment associated with chemotherapy for cancer: report of a workshop. *J Clin Oncol*. 2004;22:2233–2239.

77. Wefel JS, Lenzi R, Theriault RL, Davis RN, Meyers CA. The cognitive sequelae of standard-dose adjuvant chemotherapy in women with breast carcinoma: results of a prospective, randomized, longitudinal trial. *Cancer*. 2004;100:2292–2299.

78. Schilling V, Jenkins V, Morris R, Deutsch G, Bloomfield D. The effects of adjuvant chemotherapy on cognition in women with breast cancer-preliminary results of an observational study. *Breast*. 2005;14:142–150.

79. Hurria A, Rosen C, Hudis C, et al. Cognitive function of older patients receiving adjuvant chemotherapy for breast cancer: a pilot prospective longitudinal study. *J Am Geriatr Soc*. 2006;54:925–931.

80. Quesnel C, Savard J, Ivers H. Cognitive impairments associated with breast cancer treatments: results from a longitudinal study. *Breast Cancer Res Treat*. 2009;116:113–123.

81. Bender CM, Sereika SM, Berga SL, et al. Cognitive impairment associated with adjuvant therapy in breast cancer. *Psychooncology*. 2006;15:422–430.

82. Collins B, Mackenzie J, Stewart A, Bielajew C, Verma S. Cognitive effects of chemotherapy in post-menopausal breast cancer patients 1 year after treatment. *Psychooncology*. 2009;18:134–143.

83. Schagen SB, Muller MJ, Boogerd W, Mellenbergh GJ, van Dam FS. Change in cognitive function after chemotherapy: a prospective longitudinal study in breast cancer patients. *J Natl Cancer Inst*. 2006;98:1742–1745.

84. Jenkins V, Shilling V, Deutsch G, et al. A 3-year prospective study of the effects of adjuvant treatments on cognition in women with early stage breast cancer. *Br J Cancer*. 2006;94:828–834.

85. Ahles TA, Saykin AJ, McDonald BC, et al. Cognitive function in breast cancer patients prior to adjuvant treatment. *Breast Cancer Res Treat*. 2008;110:143–152.

86. Ahles TA. Assessing and managing cognitive dysfunction in an elderly population. *ASCO Educational Book*. 2007;283–286.

87. Schilder CMT, Schagen SB. Effects of hormonal therapy on cognitive functioning in breast cancer patients: review of the literature. *Minerva Ginecologica*. 2007;59:387–401.

88. Saykin AJ, Ahles TA, McDonald BC. Mechanisms of chemotherapy-induced cognitive disorders: neuropsychological, pathophysiological and neuroimaging perspectives. *Semin Clin Neuropsychiatry*. 2003;8:201–216.

89. Inagaki M, Yoshikawa E, Matsuoka Y, et al. Smaller regional volumes of brain gray and white matter demonstrated in breast cancer survivors exposed to adjuvant chemotherapy. *Cancer*. 2007;109:146–156.

90. Abraham J, Haut MW, Moran MT, Filburn S, Lemiuex S, Kuwabara H. Adjuvant chemotherapy for breast cancer: effects on cerebral white matter seen in diffusion tensor imaging. *Clin Breast Cancer*. 2008;8:88–91.

91. Saykin AJ, McDonald BC, Ahles TA, et al. *Altered brain activation following systemic chemotherapy for breast cancer: Interim analysis from a prospective study*. Presented at the 34th Annual Meeting of the International Neuropsychological Society, Boston, MA, February 3, 2006.

92. Ferguson RJ, McDonald BC, Saykin AJ, Ahles T. Brain structure and function differences in monozygotic twins: possible effects of breast cancer chemotherapy. *J Clin Oncol*. 2007;25:3866–3870.

93. Silverman DHS, Dy CJ, Castellon SA, et al. Altered frontocortical, cerebellar, and basal ganglia activity in adjuvant-treated breast cancer survivors 5–10 years after chemotherapy. *Breast Cancer Res Treat*. 2006;103:303–311.

94. Reiriz AB, Reolon GK, Preissler T, et al. Cancer chemotherapy and cognitive function in rodent models: memory impairment induced by cyclophosphamide in mice. *Clin Cancer Res*. 2006;12:5000.

95. Han R, Yang YM, Dietrich J, Luebke A, Mayer-Proschel M, Noble M. Systemic 5-fluorouracil treatment causes a syndrome of delayed myelin destruction in the central nervous system. *J Biol*. 2008;7:12.

96. Ahles TA, Saykin AJ. Candidate mechanisms for chemotherapy-induced cognitive changes. *Nat Rev Cancer*. 2007;7:192–201.

97. Ahles TA, Saykin AJ, Noll WW, et al. The relationship of APOE genotype to neuropsychological performance in long-term cancer survivors treated with standard dose chemotherapy. *Psychooncology*. 2003;12:612–619.

98. Barton D, Loprinzi C. Novel approaches to preventing chemotherapy-induced cognitive dysfunction in breast cancer: the art of the possible. *Clin Breast Cancer*. 2002;3(Suppl 3):S121–S127.

99. Ferguson RJ, Ahles TA, Saykin AJ, et al. Cognitive-behavioral management of chemotherapy-related cognitive changes. *Psychooncology*. 2007;16:772–777.

CHAPTER 35

Sleep and Cancer

Herbert J. Yue and Joel E. Dimsdale

INTRODUCTION

Part of the burden of cancer is its associated sleep disruption. That disrupted sleep, when superimposed upon all of the other burdens that cancer patients face, casts an enormous shadow on their well-being. This chapter reviews the literature on sleep disruption in cancer patients. The prevalence of various types of sleep disruption will be discussed, as well as current ideas about the proposed causes of interrupted sleep. Finally, we will review the pharmacologic and nonpharmacologic treatments currently being utilized.

There has been an enormous increase in research in this area. Fig. 35–1 plots the growth of scientific literature published in the past decade. However, as this chapter will hopefully make clear, there are major gaps in our knowledge which pose a challenge, both, for researchers and clinicians in their efforts to provide outstanding care for cancer patients.

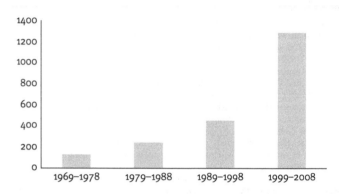

Fig. 35–1. Number of pubmed articles examining sleep disruption in cancer patients.

PREVALENCE OF SLEEP DISORDERS IN CANCER PATIENTS

Insomnia. Insomnia is a condition characterized by insufficient duration or poor quality of sleep. Patients typically report symptoms of difficulty falling asleep (sleep onset insomnia), staying asleep (middle or maintenance insomnia), or nonrestorative sleep.[1,2] The reported incidence of insomnia in the general population is approximately 10%, with higher rates seen in the elderly.[3,4] Insomnia is typically reported up to 25% of the time in patients in their 60s and 33% in patients in their 70s.[5]

There are numerous classification schemes for insomnia[6]:

i. The American Sleep Disorders Classification differentiates between acute insomnia less than 3 weeks) and chronic insomnia (greater than 3 weeks)[7]

ii. The National Institute of Mental Health Consensus Conference recognizes 3 types of insomnia transient (less than 1 week), short-term (1–3 weeks), and chronic (greater than 3 weeks)[8]

iii. The *Diagnostic and statistical manual of mental disorders*, fourth edition (DSM-IV) differentiates between primary insomnia, insomnia related to a psychiatric condition, insomnia related to a general medical condition, and insomnia related to substance abuse. All of these various insomnias require a duration greater than a month)[9]

iv. The international classification of sleep disorders (ICSD) lists >30 different categories with a significant insomnia component.[10] The large numbers of categories relates to an increased emphasis on etiologic factors (ranging from causes such as idiopathic etiologies to things such as food allergy associated sleep disruption and altitude insomnia.

Insomnia is typically the most common sleep disturbance experienced by patients with cancer. There are consistent reports suggesting elevated rates of insomnia in cancer patients, as compared with the rates experienced by the general population. Studies examining a heterogeneous population of malignancies have reported incidence rates of insomnia ranging from 23% to 60% of patients.[11-22] For instance, in a large community cohort of 772 patients, patients with cancer were more likely to complain of chronic insomnia than those without cancer (adjusted odds ratio of 2.50 after controlling for depression, anxiety, and other sleep disorders).[20] Symptoms of insomnia have been described in cancer patients throughout the course of their treatment, ranging from shortly after diagnosis to years after treatment has been completed. In a study of 300 patients with recently diagnosed breast cancer, patients who reported development of insomnia symptoms after their cancer diagnosis had a median duration of sleep difficulties of approximately 48 months.[21] In another study of 573 patients with newly diagnosed glioblastoma, approximately 30% of patients reported symptoms of insomnia that persisted for at least 1 year after the initial diagnosis.[23]

The impact of this insomnia on cancer patients is not well understood. Longitudinal outcome studies of cancer patients with insomnia are currently lacking. In the general population, sleep deprivation has been linked with deficits in cognitive function and quality of life, and, in both human and animal models, with altered immune function.[24-29] There have been few studies looking directly at quality of life outcomes in cancer patients with insomnia and many of these studies are difficult to interpret because of their cross sectional design. A few studies, however, have suggested that sleep deprivation in patients with cancer is associated with both decrements in quality of life as well as increased mortality. In a study of 29 patients with recently diagnosed lung cancer, participants had significant global disruptions in sleep (including insomnia) that were associated with lower levels of quality of life and decreased levels of daytime activity (as measured with daytime actigraphy).[15] Another study of 434 patients with a mixed population of cancers found that symptom distress (as measured with combined group of cancer-related symptoms which included insomnia) was predictive of decreased survival in the subset of lung cancer patients.[30] Unfortunately, the authors did not specifically analyze for the contribution of insomnia alone to cancer mortality and instead analyzed mortality changes in the context of a combined group of somatic complaints. As such, the effect of sleep disruption (particularly insomnia) on cancer mortality remains unclear.

Significant fatigue is also an exceptionally common complaint of patients with insomnia and cancer. Upwards of 70% of patients with cancer experience significant fatigue, either related to the malignancy itself or treatment.[31] Fatigue is associated with significant morbidity; for instance, cancer patients typically report that fatigue is their most troubling symptom.[32] Patients often experience cancer-related fatigue and insomnia simultaneously; approximately 30% of patients with recently diagnosed lung cancer were found to have significant concurrent fatigue and insomnia.[33] The specific nature of the relationship, however, is not clear. The literature suggests positive correlations between fatigue and sleep disruption in cancer patients but it is unclear which comes first.[34-36] Both fatigue and insomnia are now being examined in the context of a "symptom cluster" of multiple concurrent symptoms that are interrelated.[37] For instance, in a study of 69 patients with breast and prostate cancer, a symptom cluster of fatigue, insomnia, and depression showed significant interrelationships between all three symptoms.[38] The use of symptom clusters to help guide treatment of patients with cancer-associated co-morbidities has led to the hope for improved outcomes, although no studies to date have demonstrated such benefit.

Excessive daytime sleepiness. Not much is known about the prevalence of excessive daytime sleepiness (EDS) in patients with a cancer diagnosis. Much of the available literature involves subjective reports of sleepiness, typically measured with the Epworth Sleepiness Scale or the Stanford Sleepiness Scale. In a group of 93 women with metastatic breast cancer, approximately 25% of participants reported having problems with EDS.[39] When the authors looked for psychosocial factors that contributed significantly to daytime sleepiness, they found that baseline levels of depression and interval increases in depression scores over the follow-up period were associated with EDS. In another study of ~1000 patients with a mixed group of oncologic diagnoses, 37% of patients diagnosed reported EDS.[17] The incidence of sleepiness was associated with the time of treatment; patients generally reported more daytime sleepiness if they had been treated recently. This daytime sleepiness can persist for years, even after successful treatment of the cancer. In a large study of over 2500 survivors of childhood malignancies with at least a 5-year survival from the time of diagnosis, 14% of participants reported continued daytime sleepiness.[40] When compared to a sibling comparison group, those in the cancer cohort had significantly higher Epworth Sleepiness Scale scores. Depression and obesity contributed significantly to the increased risk of daytime sleepiness. More work with objective measures (such as multiple sleep latency or maintenance of wakefulness testing) is needed to better understand the incidence and impact of EDS in these patients.

Restless leg syndrome. Restless leg syndrome (RLS) is a condition characterized by symptoms of involuntary, intrusive leg movements, sometimes associated with paresthesias. Symptoms may occur during sleep in a periodic fashion and are referred to as periodic limb movement syndrome (PLMS). The two conditions are distinct entities, but can often co-exist in the same patient with up to 80% of patients with RLS demonstrating PLMS on overnight polysomnograms.[41] The symptoms can be particularly bothersome to patients and adversely affect subjective sleep quality.[42] The overall incidence of RLS and PLMS in the general population is approximately 10% for each condition.[43,44] RLS is characterized as primary or secondary to a number of general medical conditions. Iron deficiency anemia is the most relevant medical condition present in those with cancer and is a predisposing factor in the development of RLS and PLMS symptoms.

Little is known, however, about the incidence of either RLS or PLMS in cancer patients. A study of approximately 1000 patients with a mixed group of cancers noted that leg restlessness was the second most common sleep complaint of patients.[17] Of note, the authors did not formally diagnose RLS or PLMS in patients, and the leg restlessness was patient-reported on a brief sleep questionnaire. Given iron deficiency anemia is relatively common finding in cancer patients (particularly with gastrointestinal malignancies), there is a growing interest in RLS/PLMS as potentially important disruptors of sleep in cancer patients. There has been one study looking at a cohort of 500 patients with a mixed group of cancer diagnoses; the authors found 12% of men and 22% of women reported significant RLS symptoms, twice that expected for the general population.[45] Unfortunately, most of the available literature examining RLS and PLMS in cancer patients consists of case reports documenting RLS in iron deficient cancer patients or RLS as the presenting symptom in colon cancer.[46,47] Larger studies, particularly those using formal diagnostic criteria for RLS and PLMS, are needed to further understanding the potential sleep disruption in cancer patients.

Obstructive sleep apnea. The presence of obstructive sleep apnea (OSA) in the general oncologic population has not been frequently described, with the exception of the subset of patients with head and neck cancer. OSA (characterized by collapse of the upper airway during sleep, causing apneas and hypopneas) is typically associated with extrinsic soft tissue compression of the airway or diminished neural output to upper airway muscles. In comparison, OSA in head and neck cancer patients is often caused by intraluminal decreases in airway caliber by tumor or extrinsic compression of the airway by malignant invasion or growth. A study of 17 patients with either oral or oropharyngeal cancer found that >75% of patients had significant evidence of OSA (diagnosed with overnight polysomnograms) when compared to an age and body mass index matched control group.[48] Interestingly, this finding was independent of the size of the primary tumor. These patients also had a high rate of postoperative complications when compared to the non-OSA group (67% vs. 25% postoperative complication rate). There are case reports of improvement in OSA rates after treatment of the malignancy, although some have described worsening of the sleep apnea even after successful treatment of the malignancy. A study of 24 patients who had completed treatment for head and neck cancer examined the rates of OSA and found >90% of patients met criteria for OSA (on the basis of a respiratory disturbance index >15).[49] The authors suggest that despite successful treatment of a head and neck cancer, patients often are left with a partially obstructed upper airway that loses patency during sleep. More well-controlled studies are needed in patients with head and neck cancer to further evaluate the prevalence of OSA both before and after treatment.

OSA is a common disorder, with prevalence in the general population ranging from 5% to 20%, depending upon the sample frame.[50] Given its frequent occurrence and its debilitating effect on sleep and daytime functioning, it may be a "silent partner" with cancer; that is, while OSA may not be related to cancer or its treatment, it is an eminently treatable sleep disorder which may well be present in a high percentage of cancer patients.

Miscellaneous sleep disorders. Other sleep disorders, such as parasomnias and dysomnias, have been reported in patients with a cancer diagnosis, usually as single patient case reports. Night terrors, a parasomnia typically seen in childhood and adolescence, are associated with abrupt awakening from slow wave sleep followed by extreme terror. Night terrors were described in a 48-year-old patient who was found to have a low grade tumor of the thalamus.[51] Narcolepsy, a dysomnia characterized by severe EDS, has been reported in children who have central nervous system tumors, particularly those that affect the hypothalamus. Marcus et al. report on a group of three children with suprasellar tumors presenting with disabling EDS. Polysomnograms confirmed narcolepsy in all three children, who subsequently responded well to stimulants.[52]

SLEEP MEASURES

Sleep can be measured with various techniques. Actigraphy measures physical activity by means of a wrist-watch sized device which patients typically wear for multiple days. Actigraphy employs a portable accelerometer to measure movement over time and is used to differentiate sleep and wake cycles, as well as circadian rhythms. It has been validated with electroencephalogram (EEG) measures of sleep and arousals in, both, men and women and in, both, normal and disrupted sleep.[53,54] This apparatus is readily tolerated by patients, as actigraphs are designed to be minimally invasive. Their only limitation is that they should not be worn during swimming or bathing.

Polysomnography (PSG) is a technique that measures a number of modalities during sleep, including EEG waveforms, ocular movements, muscle activity, respiratory effort, and airflows. It provides the most amount of information regarding sleep quality, especially sleep architecture, and is required for diagnosis of a number of sleep-related disorders (such as PLMS). The main disadvantage of PSG is the need for expertise in setup for testing; often patients need to be examined overnight in a sleep laboratory (although devices now exist that allow home measurement of virtually all the same modalities as measured by inpatient polysomnograms). Traditional PSG requires a daunting electrical apparatus. However, the size of that apparatus has diminished greatly. The PSG hook-up is time consuming, requiring 30–60 minutes to place leads at meticulously determined sites. In addition, there is slight discomfort in attaching leads and the patient's mobility itself is obviously decreased with all of the monitoring equipment in place. In recent years, abbreviated PSGs have been used widely in epidemiological studies; such devices typically monitor somewhat fewer channels of data than a traditional PSG. Finally, sleep can be assessed through self-report questionnaires. Somewhat surprisingly, the correlation between self-report and PSG is not particularly strong.[55,56]

Sleep can be characterized in multiple ways. A number of variables are measured via actigraphy or PSG, including total time in bed, total sleep time, and wake time after sleep onset. Other variables, such as sleep efficiency, are calculated measures. PSG has the added ability to measure times in different stages of sleep, including light sleep (stages 1 and 2), deep sleep (stages 3 and 4), and rapid eye movement (REM sleep). Microarousals from sleep can also be seen, as well as periodic limb movements, episodes of desaturation, and episodes of decreased or absent airflow (hypopneas and apneas). Actigraphy has the advantage of being able to be worn continuously and is helpful in examining sleep-wake cycles by measuring physical activity at different times of the day.

Actigraphy and disturbed sleep in cancer patients. Despite a growing body of evidence demonstrating sleep disruption in cancer patients, much of the early work has relied on primarily subjective reports of sleep by patients. Given the heterogeneity of the instruments and differing criteria used to measure sleep quality, there has been a growing interest in measuring sleep quality through objective methods. Actigraphy has been employed in a number of cancer studies. The convenience of the device as well as the ability to take sleep measurements at home has made it an attractive modality to measure sleep quality.

The literature regarding actigraphy and sleep quality consistently demonstrates significant sleep disruption in patients with cancer, even before onset of treatment. Findings have included increased numbers of nighttime sleep interruptions and decreased overall sleep efficiency (percentage of sleep span actually spent sleeping). Two separate studies of approximately 30 patients each with recently diagnosed lung cancer found a significant increase in the numbers of nighttime arousals from sleep and overall duration of wakefulness from sleep, as well as significant decreases in sleep efficiency.[15,57] In a study of breast cancer in 85 women with varying stages of disease, increased nocturnal awakenings were noted, as well as decreased overall sleep time, sleep efficiency, and an increased wake after sleep onset time.[58] Similar findings were found in another study of 130 patients with breast cancer, although total sleep time and sleep efficiency were normal.[59]

Little is known about what happens to objective measures of sleep quality after cancer treatment. A number of studies have examined patients who were either undergoing or had completed treatment for their malignancy (either chemotherapy or radiation therapy) and again found disrupted sleep (i.e., increased arousals, decreased sleep time and efficiency).[60,61] Unfortunately, no comparisons were made with pretreatment actigraphy results in most studies. One study that examined 21 patients who had just completed the first cycle of chemotherapy found an increased number and duration of night awakenings, with otherwise normal sleep parameters.[61] Another study, however, examined changes in sleep actigraphy in 11 women over 4 cycles of adjuvant chemotherapy. The latter study specifically examined changes across days of an individual cycle and across each of 2 cycles in the study (specifically across cycle 1 and 4). The investigators found decreased amount of total sleep time on night 2 compared to night 1 of the first cycle of chemotherapy, but found no other significant objective sleep changes across any combination of day or cycle.[62]

PSG and disturbed sleep in cancer patients. Despite the growing interest and use of actigraphy as an objective measure of sleep quality in cancer patients, PSG remains the gold standard.

A few studies have looked at sleep quality in cancer patients with PSG, although the results have been somewhat inconsistent. One study examined sleep polysomnograms of 14 patients with different cancer diagnoses, half with subjective reports of poor sleep and half with subjectively normal sleep, and found no significant differences in the sleep architecture of either group, with the exception of a mean difference of 4 minutes of delta (i.e., deep) sleep between the two groups.[63] Another study examined 32 patients (half with breast cancer and half with lung cancer) with overnight polysomnograms and compared them to a group of normals and a group of patients with chronic insomnia. That study found that cancer patients had lower sleep efficiency and higher amounts of stage 1 sleep as compared to normals.[64] No other differences in terms of awakenings or sleep stages were seen. Of note, when subgroup analyses of the cancer patients were performed, lung cancer patients slept much more poorly than the breast cancer patients and had sleep efficiencies comparable to the insomniac group. Finally, a study of 114 patients with advanced stage malignancies underwent continuous ambulatory PSG over a period of two nights and one day. These patients manifested decreased sleep efficiency, increased REM latency, and increased number of nocturnal awakenings.[65] No significant changes in total sleep time or sleep stages were observed when compared to a reference population.

Self-report measures and disturbed sleep in cancer patients. Most of the literature examining sleep disruption has used either validated questionnaires, instruments specifically designed for a study, or patient self-report. This heterogeneity has led to a large variety of measures, each defined differently and potentially measuring different things. For instance, many studies have considered insomnia as a symptom, a condition, or both.[66] These are important distinctions, as more stringent criteria are used to define an insomnia syndrome, as opposed to a simple symptom. Fortner et al. have reviewed studies of sleep and quality of life; in their examination of 36 studies, approximately 18 different measures of sleep quality were used, ranging from the Pittsburgh Sleep Quality Index (PSQI) to chart reviews and sedative-use records.[67]

Of these self-report measures, the PSQI and Epworth Sleepiness Scale are among the best validated and widely used. The PSQI is a 24-item questionnaire with 19 items self-rated and 5 questions answered by a bed partner. Scores are generated across 7 scales, including sleep quality, sleep efficiency, sleep disturbances, and daytime function.[68] It has been validated in a number of different populations, including insomniacs and cancer patients.[69,70] The Epworth Sleepiness scale is an 8-item questionnaire designed to measure daytime sleepiness and asks participants about their chances of dozing off in a variety of situations.[71] It has been primarily validated for use in patients with suspected OSA, although it has also been used in other populations to measure EDS.[72]

ETIOLOGIES OF SLEEP DISTURBANCE IN CANCER

Much of the work examining etiology of sleep disruption has centered on insomnia, as it is the most commonly reported sleep disturbance in cancer patients. A review by Savard et al. provides a framework for evaluation of the etiology of insomnia, based on Spielman's three factor model.[73] Although this framework was developed primarily for insomnia, many of the etiologic factors described are applicable to other sleep disorders. The framework is divided into three main categories and is summarized in Table 35–1[66]:

i. Predisposing factors: Preincident or enduring traits that increase the vulnerability of developing insomnia.
ii. Precipitating factors: Factors or conditions that incite the development of insomnia.
iii. Perpetuating factors: Factors contributing to the maintenance of insomnia over time.

These factors are associated with insomnia in normal patients as well. We will consider some of the pertinent etiologic factors uniquely applicable to cancer patients.

Predisposing factors of insomnia. Many of the basic predisposing factors towards the development of insomnia in cancer patients are identical to those in the general population, including age, prior history

Table 35-1. Potential etiologic factors of insomnia in cancer patients

Predisposing factors	Precipitating factors	Perpetuating factors
Hyperarousability Female gender Age Familial or personal history of insomnia Psychiatric disorder, such as depression or anxiety	Surgery Hospitalization Radiation therapy Chemotherapy as well as chemotherapy-related side effects; side effects from medications used to palliate chemotherapy symptoms Pain Delirium	Maladaptive sleep behaviors such as excessive time in bed, napping, poor sleep hygiene Circadian rhythm disruption Faulty beliefs and attitudes about sleep such as misattributions of daytime impairments, unrealistic sleep expectation, inaccurate appraisals of sleep difficulties

of insomnia, or gender. However, two conditions deserve special note in a cancer population, specifically depression and anxiety disorders.

Depression. The relationship between depression and sleep disruption is complex. While insomnia is an important symptom of depression, it is not clear if depression itself worsens insomnia or if insomnia worsens depressive symptoms. For instance, longitudinal studies in the general population have suggested that persistent insomnia can lead to the development of depression.[74,75] In groups of women with insomnia and breast cancer, successful treatment of their sleep disruption was associated with decreased reports of depression and anxiety.[76,77] A large study of approximately 400 patients with, both, depression and insomnia found that concurrent treatment with, both, sedative hypnotics and antidepressants resulted in faster improvements in depressive symptoms and a greater magnitude of antidepressant benefit when compared to antidepressants alone.[78]

Depression rates approaching as high as 50% have been described in a variety of cancer diagnoses and stages, although there is some variability in how depression is defined and diagnosed.[79–82] Strong associations between depressive symptoms and insomnia have been frequently reported. A study of >2600 women less than 4 years out from treatment for breast cancer examined specific risk factors that were associated with insomnia. The investigators found that depressive symptoms were the most important individual risk factor that significantly contributed to insomnia scores.[16] In another study of 327 patients undergoing radical prostatectomy for prostate cancer, depressive symptoms were the strongest risk factor associated with the development of an insomnia syndrome.[22] Interpretation across studies is difficult, however, because of disparities in definition of depression.

Despite the significant amount of evidence demonstrating correlations between depressive symptoms and insomnia, there are contrary reports. Several studies have found no significant increase in depression diagnoses in cancer patients and longitudinal studies found no increase in depressive symptoms years after cancer treatment, suggesting that insomnia cannot be caused by depression alone.[83,84] Indeed, in some studies, insomnia persists despite the resolution or absence of depressive symptoms. Further work is needed to examine the role of depression in the development of insomnia, particularly via the concept of a symptoms cluster (i.e., depression, fatigue, and insomnia as a cluster of symptoms that influence quality of life in an interrelated fashion).

Anxiety disorders. Less work has been done on anxiety disorders as a predisposing factor in the development of insomnia in cancer. Anxiety disorder rates have been estimated to be in the 10% range for a mixed group of patients with cancer. Positive associations with sleep disruption have been described, albeit with less frequency.[85] In prostate cancer patients, anxiety symptoms were the greatest risk factor for the development of nonspecific sleep difficulties, but not insomnia.[22] Palesh et al. looked at a group of 93 women with metastatic breast cancer and

examined psychosocial factors predictive of sleep disturbance. They did not measure anxiety but measured life stress (using a 37-item questionnaire developed by Horowitz et al.) and found that levels of stress were strongly associated with difficulties falling asleep and EDS.[39,86] Similar findings were observed in two studies of patients enrolled in a symptom control clinic or palliative care unit; anxiety levels were most closely associated with difficulties falling asleep, EDS, and nightmares.[18,87]

Precipitating factors of insomnia. The factors that precipitate disruption of sleep in cancer patients are typically significant stressors, either emotional or physiologic. The diagnosis of cancer itself can represent a tremendous emotional burden on patients, whereas treatment can impose direct derangements on normal physiologic sleep or can act by virtue of side effects. A number of important cancer- and treatment-associated effects on sleep will be briefly considered.

Pain. Pain is one of the most common symptoms reported by patients with cancer. In a study of ~1300 outpatients with metastatic cancer, over 60% of patients reported having significant cancer related pain.[88] Another study of over 3000 patients with a diagnosis of cancer who were subsequently admitted to a nursing home found that at least 30% of the patients had significant levels of pain that required treatment.[89] Chronic pain is a known disruptor of sleep; in a group of nearly 300 patients with chronic pain issues (but no cancer diagnosis), at least 90% of participants had at least one symptom of sleep disruption.[90] Similar findings are noted in the cancer literature; in analyses of correlates of sleep disruption (particularly insomnia), pain is often a significant finding.[17,21] This is a consistent finding across a variety of cancer diagnoses and stages, with insomnia being reported as the most common symptom associated with pain.[16,91] How pain symptoms specifically disrupt sleep in cancer patients is not entirely understood, although some studies have noted that pain may interfere with mechanisms of sleep initiation and maintenance.[92,93] The path between pain and sleep is bidirectional, as decreased sleep is associated with a decreased threshold for pain.[94–96] More needs to be known about specific effects of adequate pain control on sleep. For instance, Wirz et al. noted that insomnia rates improved with rotation of pain medications to hydromorphone in a group of 50 patients with suspected tolerance to their current pain regimen.[97] There has been some thought that with improved pain control in cancer patients that improvements in insomnia rates would be seen, although the empirical literature supporting that idea is sparse. Pain medications themselves have side effect profiles that potentially disrupt sleep. Opioids are among the most commonly prescribed medications for pain relief in cancer patients, as such patients often have intractable symptoms that are unresponsive to other classes of agents. While opioids have a known effect of sedation, studies have also suggested that they also can disrupt sleep architecture. Several studies of either methadone or heroin have shown significant decreases in REM and slow wave sleep, with some increase in nocturnal awakenings.[98–100] The clinical significance of these findings is unclear; the studies are limited by their sample size and the lack of

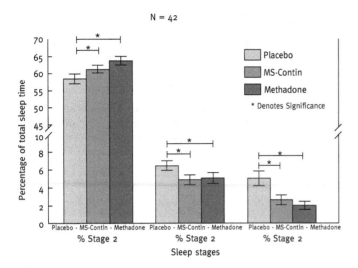

Fig. 35–2. Effects of opioids on sleep architecture.
SOURCE: Reprinted from Dimsdale JE, Norman D, DeJardin D, Wallace MS. The effect of opioids on sleep architecture. *J Clin Sleep Med.* 2007 Feb 15;3(1):33–36. With permission from the American Academy of Sleep Medicine.

measures of subjective sleep quality, but they do suggest more work is needed to examine the role of opioids in sleep disruption. One recent study employed multiple cross-overs between placebo, MS-Contin, and methadone and found that in healthy normals, both opioids decimated slow wave sleep (see Fig. 35–2).[101]

Chemotherapy. Despite chemotherapy's role in treatment in many cancer patients, not much is known about the potential sleep disruption caused by these agents. Studies examining subjective reports of sleep in breast cancer patients have noted increased sleep disruption in those undergoing chemotherapy compared to those who did not undergo treatment. A majority of patients associated their chemotherapy as an aggravating or etiologic factor in their sleep problems.[21,67] Studies looking at objective measure of sleep have been inconsistent. A study examining sleep actigraphy in women who had just completed the first cycle of chemotherapy observed an increased number of nocturnal awakenings; however, another study of 11 women examining changes over 4 cycles of chemotherapy found only decreased sleep time on the second night of the first cycle of chemotherapy and no other significant differences.[61,62] There is a great deal of heterogeneity across different chemotherapy regimens, with some containing medications that are potentially much more disruptive to sleep than others. Without attempting to control for different chemotherapy regimens given to women, it would be difficult to interpret the literature with adequate clarity.

Side effects associated with chemotherapy are other important factors in the disrupted sleep of treated cancer patients. A closely studied group has been breast cancer survivors who have vasomotor symptoms related to treatment-associated menopause. Cytotoxic chemotherapy regimens can cause premature ovarian failure leading to menopausal symptoms while other medications given to reduce the risk of recurrent disease (such as tamoxifen) are also associated with hot flashes.[102–104] Symptoms can include sensations of sudden flushing, palpitations, irritability, and headaches. Menopausal symptoms are a common problem in patients treated for breast cancer. Breast cancer patients commonly complain of significant vasomotor symptoms.[105,106] Symptoms that occur at night can be particularly bothersome and can also interfere with sleep; upwards of 70% of patients in a breast cancer study reported nocturnal hot flashes with symptoms more frequent and severe when compared to a control group.[107] Several studies have observed vasomotor symptoms strongly associated with subjective sleep disruption; in a large study of 2600

women with breast cancer, menopausal symptoms were the strongest factor associated with insomnia.[16,106,108] Savard et al. reported fragmented sleep with increased arousals from sleep associated with measured hot flashes and increased amount of wake time and REM latency.[109]

Radiotherapy. Radiation therapy is commonly a first line treatment in patients with cancer; it is commonly utilized in a variety of malignancies including breast, lung, prostate, and lymphoma. There have been some studies looking at the effect of radiation on sleep in cancer patients, although many of the studies did not control for other factors that may contribute to sleep disruption (such as concurrent chemotherapy/tamoxifen, surgical status, or postmenopausal state). Wengstrom et al. evaluated a group of 134 women undergoing radiation therapy for breast cancer and noted increasing rates of insomnia peaking at 5 weeks into the treatment course.[110] Similar findings were noted in a study of 30 women with early stage cancer undergoing radiation treatment, with approximately 60% of participants reporting significant sleep problems 3 weeks into the study. Neither study, however, controlled for the presence of other sleep disrupting treatments and there were no statistical analyses reported for either study. Increased rates of symptoms such as daytime sleepiness have been reported in patients who had received cranial radiation for brain tumors as well as head and neck cancer.[12,111]

Surgery. Little literature is available looking at the effect of surgery on sleep in cancer patients. Some authors have suggested that more disfiguring surgeries such as total mastectomies may increase psychological distress with subsequent sleep disruption, although there are no current data to support this hypothesis.[66] In a study of 99 women who underwent either breast conserving therapy or total mastectomy, no significant differences in sleep disruption were found either between group or after either type of surgery.[112] Another study of quality of life study in patients who underwent colorectal cancer surgery noted some increases in reported insomnia 1 month after surgery, but with a subsequent return to the presurgery baseline within 3 months.[113]

Perpetuating factors of insomnia. Factors in this category have been suggested to propagate sleep disruption; they include items such as some aspects of poor sleep hygiene, misconceptions about the causes of sleep disruption, and maladaptive responses to disturbed sleep. One condition in the group of perpetuating factors is circadian rhythm disruption, which deserves some special consideration.

Circadian rhythms refer to the manner by which a number of basic biologic functions are arranged along a ~ 24-hour cycle. Processes such as metabolism, cellular propagation, and sleep are governed by such periodicity; animal models have shown a genetic component to these rhythms with specific gene disruption (such as the *clock* gene in mice) associated with disordered sleep-wake cycles.[114] Similar genes have been discovered in human cell lines, suggesting that genetic control of circadian rhythms is a ubiquitous component of life. Anatomically, the suprachiasmatic nucleus in the hypothalamus is directly responsible for regulation of circadian rhythms. The rest-activity cycle in humans has been demonstrated to be an accurate marker of the innate circadian clock and has been used in a number of studies examining the role of circadian rhythm disruption in patient outcomes.

There has been a growing interest in examining circadian rhythms in cancer patients, as there is a suggestion that disruption of such cycles may be linked with poorer outcomes. In normal humans, there is commonly a sharp contrast between rest and awake cycles, with significant actigraphic activity during awake (day periods) times and minimal movement during sleep (night periods). Fig. 35–3 shows an actigraph of a breast cancer patient before treatment.

In cancer patients, a number of investigators have noted dampening of this contrast between daytime and nighttime activity. For instance, Chevalier et al. investigated a group of 10 patients with metastatic colon cancer using actigraphy; they noted a significant loss of contrast between awake and sleep times, with considerable amounts of activity noted throughout night periods and increased periods of sleep during the day.[115]

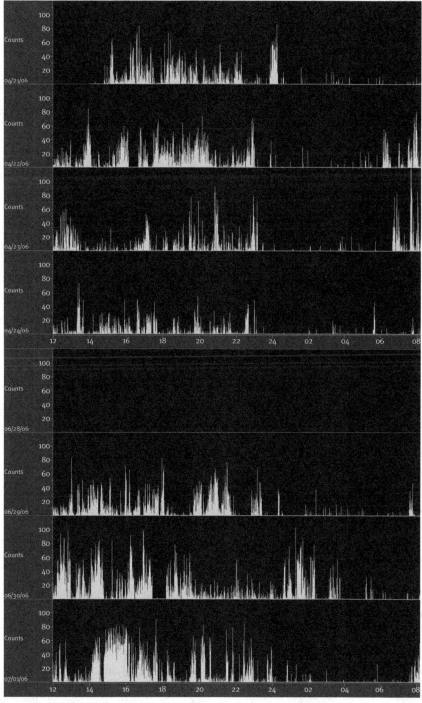

Fig. 35–3. Actigraph of breast cancer patient before and after treatment. Each row represents a separate day. The numbers at the bottom are the time of the day. Each row represents a separate day. The numbers at the top are the time of the day. Each black mark represents activity, with white representing rest periods. The two blocks represent actigraphs taken of the same patient before and after treatment.

Similar findings have been noted for breast and lung cancer patients as well.[15,57,65] These disrupted circadian rhythms in cancer patients have been linked with factors such as fatigue, daytime sleepiness, and overall quality of life. In three separate studies of patients with cancer, the investigators noted significant dampening of circadian rhythms that was associated with decreased subjective report of quality of life and ability to complete activities of daily living.[15,57,58] Another study in patients with colon cancer found that patients with a preserved circadian rhythm had significantly less subjective report of fatigue.[116] Some early studies have even suggested a connection between circadian rhythms and chemotherapy response

and mortality. A pilot study of 13 patients with metastatic breast cancer noted correlations between circadian rhythms and the number of sites of metastasis and performance status.[117] Finally, Mormont et al. examined 200 patients with colorectal cancer and found that those with a disrupted circadian rhythm had a poorer response to chemotherapy and significantly decreased overall survival at 2 years after diagnosis.[118]

Work is starting to focus on the possible underlying biological basis for these differences in outcomes in these cancer patients. Studies in both animal and human tumor cell lines have demonstrated that cancer cells have an inherent circadian rhythm as well.[114] This rhythm is

Table 35-2. Response rates of cancer patients receiving chronotherapy chemotherapy versus those receiving constant-rate infusions

	Number of Patients	
Endpoint	Constant-rate infusion (n = 93)	Chronotherapy (n = 93)
Objective response		
Partial	24 (26%)	42 (45%)
Complete	3 (3%)	5 (5%)
All	27 (29%)	47 (51%)
Success rate* (95% CI)	29% (19.6–38.4)	51% (40.0–61.0)
Surgery		
Secondary surgery	17 (18%)	23 (25%)
Complete response after surgery	11 (12%)	16 (17%)
All complete responses	13 (14%)	20 (22%)
3-year survival	22%	21%

*$p = 0.003$.

The left column represents constant-rate infusion patients and the right column represents patients who received chronotherapy. As noted, there was an increase in the number of patients with a partial response with a statistically significant increase in the overall success rate.

SOURCE: Reprinted with permission from Levi F, Zidani R, Misset JL. Randomised multicentre trial of chronotherapy with oxaliplatin, fluorouracil, and folinic acid in metastatic colorectal cancer. International Organization for Cancer Chronotherapy. *Lancet.* 1997 Sep 6;350(9079):681–686. With permission from Elsevier.

associated with cell growth and division, two particularly important therapeutic targets in cancer cells. This has led to an interest in chronotherapy of chemotherapeutic agents, in the hope that by adjusting the time when chemotherapy is administered, it might be possible to maximize antitumor efficacy and minimize toxicity. Time-adjusted chemotherapy was first studied in colorectal cancer. A study of 180 patients who received their chemotherapy at the standard time or else at times selected according to cell division activity observed significantly higher response rates in the group of patients who had time-adjusted infusions.[119] The authors also noted significantly less mucositis and neuropathy in the rhythm-adjusted group compared to controls (Table 35–2) (Figs. 35–4 and 35–5).

Tumor effects on sleep disruption. There has been a growing interest in the role of inflammation on behavior in cancer patients. Studies in animals have demonstrated links between inflammatory cytokines and the development of sickness behaviors, including fatigue, anorexia, pain, depression, and sleep disturbance. These cytokines act through activation of inflammatory pathways in the central nervous system to produce nonspecific symptoms associated with infection.[120,121] For instance, mice injected with interleukin (IL)-1β and interferon-α demonstrated significant alterations in their behavior, including changes in appetite and cognitive ability.[122,123] In a recent large meta-analysis of the available literature on fatigue and cytokines, the authors noted some positive associations with IL-1 and IL-6, although they also found a significant number of studies without any significant associations as well.[124] In studies of patients with cancer, investigators have demonstrated that increased levels of IL-1 and IL-6 were associated with higher levels of fatigue and depression, although the literature is inconsistent on this matter.[120] Patients with chronic insomnia and OSA also have increased levels of IL-6 and tumor necrosis factor (TNF)-α that are thought to have a potentially etiologic role in the pathogenesis of the disease.[125–127]

Despite the growing literature examining cytokines and various components of sickness behavior, little is known about the relationship between sleep disturbance and inflammation in cancer patients. Much of the cytokine-sleep literature involves patients without a cancer diagnosis, making interpretation of the findings difficult. One study of approximately 30 patients with breast cancer undergoing cognitive-behavioral therapy (CBT) for insomnia found increased levels of

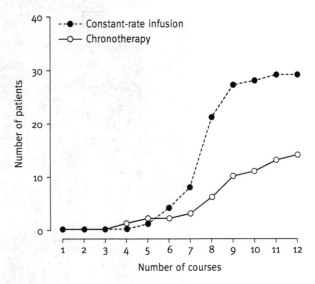

Fig. 35-4. Occurrence of peripheral neuropathy in patients receiving chronotherapy chemotherapy versus those receiving constant-rate infusions. The above two lines represent the number of patients who reported significant symptoms of peripheral neuropathy in either the constant-rate infusion group versus those that received chronotherapy. As noted above, by the 7th course of treatment, patients receiving chronotherapy had significantly less peripheral neuropathy than the standard treatment group.

SOURCE: Reprinted from Levi F, Zidani R, Misset JL. Randomised multicentre trial of chronotherapy with oxaliplatin, fluorouracil, and folinic acid in metastatic colorectal cancer. International Organization for Cancer Chronotherapy. *Lancet.* 1997 Sep 6;350(9079):681–686. With permission from Elsevier.

IFN-γ and IL-1β after completion of the program; cytokine levels were strongly associated with decreased subjective reports of insomnia from patients.[128] Rich et al. evaluated a group of colon cancer patients with either disrupted or normal circadian rhythms and measured cytokines

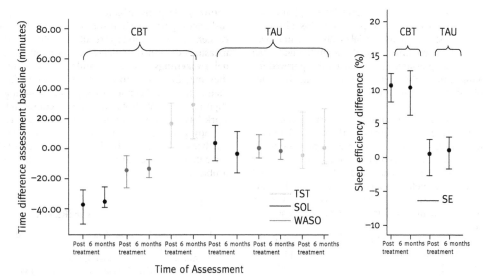

Fig. 35–5. Comparison of cognitive-behavioral therapy to therapy as usual in cancer patients with persistent insomnia. Each pair of points represents a different sleep parameter immediately post treatment and 6 months later.

ABBREVIATIONS: CBT, cognitive-behavioral therapy; SE, sleep efficiency; SOL, sleep onset latency; TAU, therapy as usual; TST, total sleep time; WASO, wake after sleep onset.

SOURCE: Reprinted with permission from Espie CA, Fleming L, Cassidy J, et al. Randomized controlled clinical effectiveness trial of cognitive behavior therapy compared with treatment as usual for persistent insomnia in patients with cancer. *J Clin Oncol.* 2008 Jun 30. © 2008 American Society of Clinical Oncology. All rights reserved.

before and after chemotherapy treatment. They found that patients with abnormal circadian rhythms (as well as disrupted sleep) had higher pretreatment levels of tumor growth factor (TGF)-α, TNF-α, and IL-6; increased levels of IL-6 were correlated with poor outcomes.[129] Much more work is needed in this area; more consistency across measured cytokines and an evaluation of cancer treatment effects on cytokines would facilitate progress.

TREATMENT OF SLEEP DISORDERS IN CANCER PATIENTS

Pharmacotherapy. As insomnia is a prevalent problem among patients with a cancer diagnosis, a significant proportion of patients are treated symptomatically with medications. An estimated 40%–50% of patients with cancer are estimated to have used a hypnotic at least once a month.[130] We will review the most commonly used medications for insomnia and examine the evidence for their efficacy.

Barbiturates. These medications act at the gamma-aminobutyric acid (GABA)$_A$ receptor, an inhibitory neuroreceptor in the central nervous system. Barbiturates were first synthesized in the 1860s and were among the first medications prescribed for insomnia. Members of this class include medications such as secobarbital (Seconal) and pentobarbital (Nembutal). Barbiturates are associated with a high risk of dependency and toxicity and have been largely replaced by benzodiazepine receptor agonists for the treatment of insomnia.

Antihistamines. Antihistamines are occasionally used for mild cases of insomnia and are a significant component of many over the counter hypnotic agents. Prototypes of this class include diphenhydramine and hydroxyzine; both work as antagonists of the H1 histamine receptor, resulting in drowsiness and sedation. There have been a number of placebo controlled trials examining the efficacy of antihistamines, with some demonstrated benefits on subjective sleep onset latency and duration of sleep.[131,132] However, antihistamines have anticholinergic properties as well and have been associated with symptoms such as excessive next day sleepiness, malaise, and even delirium in some older patients.[131] Chronic use of antihistamines is also associated with tolerance.

Benzodiazepine hypnotics. This class of medications includes members marketed specifically as hypnotics (such as flurazepam, estazolam, quazepam, temazepam, and triazolam), although other benzodiazepines used for anxiolysis (such as lorazepam and diazepam) are often prescribed as well.[133] These medications act through binding to the benzodiazepine receptor-GABA$_A$ complex and act in an inhibitory fashion, much like barbiturates.[134] They have been shown to decrease sleep latency and wake time after sleep onset, although the actual effects are modest (decreases in sleep latency average 3 minutes).[135,136] Some studies have suggested high use of benzodiazepines in cancer patients.[17,137] Their use can be associated with symptoms of excessive next day sleepiness and cognitive impairment, as well as increased risk of falls and hip fractures.[138,139] Rebound insomnia (recurrence or worsening of insomnia after discontinuation of the medication) is also a significant adverse reaction associated with chronic benzodiazepine use.[133] In the cancer population, benzodiazepine use has been linked with poorer subjective quality of life and paradoxically, increased rates of insomnia.[140] The majority of the members of this class have only been approved for short-term treatment of insomnia, as tolerance and dependence can develop.

Nonbenzodiazepine hypnotics. These medications represent the next generation of benzodiazepine receptor agonists. They work in a similar fashion, with less reported next day somnolence and adverse drug reactions. Members of this class include zolpidem, zaleplon, and eszoplicone. Similar effects on sleep architecture are seen, with improvement in sleep onset latency and wake after sleep onset time comparable to those seen in benzodiazepines.[141–143] Tolerance is not typically seen and rebound insomnia has only been reported with zolpidem.[133]

Antidepressants. Occasionally, antidepressants with sedating qualities are used for the treatment of insomnia. Commonly used members of this class include trazodone, amitriptyline, and doxepin. They can sometimes be helpful in the treatment of insomnia in depressed patients, although studies to support such an observation are scant. A comparison study examining trazadone with zolpidem and placebo noted some improvements in sleep latency and total sleep time, although these improvements were short lived.[144] Some studies have examined amitriptyline, but found no significant changes in sleep onset or total sleep times.[145] Doxepin, a tricyclic antidepressant, has been studied in a few trials with some improvements in sleep latency and total sleep time, although the studies had small sample sizes.[146,147] Of note, antidepressants are not currently approved for use for the treatment of insomnia in the United States and some have significant side-effect profiles that limit their usage.

Other medications. Melatonin is a naturally occurring hormone that is implicated in the regulation of the circadian rhythms in humans. It has some sleep-inducing qualities and has been used to regulate circadian rhythms. Some studies have evaluated melatonin as treatment for primary insomnia with mixed results. A small study of 10 patients noted no significant benefit whereas a meta-analysis observed some benefits for sleep efficiency and sleep latency.[148,149] Melatonin is sold over the counter as a nutritional supplement; appropriate dosing regimens have not yet been well validated.

Some of the newer generation antipsychotics (such as quetiapine and olanzapine) have been used in some patients to help with symptoms of insomnia, although patients typically had concurrent schizophrenia.[150] These drugs are not commonly used in the general population or in those with cancer and have significant adverse drug reaction profiles.

Nonpharmacologic treatments. Given the side-effect profiles of many of the medications used to treat insomnia and the high prevalence of co-morbid symptoms of depression and anxiety in cancer patients, there has been a growing interest in nonpharmacologic treatments. CBT has been the best studied of these interventions. CBT focuses on the impact of patients' cognitions on how patients feel or act. CBT changes distorted views, with the hope of improving a variety of symptoms. When used as a treatment for sleep disturbances (particularly insomnia), CBT is often linked with an educational component that emphasizes aspects of good sleep hygiene.

There have been a large number of studies demonstrating the efficacy of CBT on insomnia. Three meta-analyses (spanning over 60 studies in the last decade) looking at outcomes of CBT for chronic insomnia have observed improvements in sleep architecture measurements such as time to sleep onset, time awake after sleep onset, and duration of awakenings at night.[151–153] Participants also reported subjective improvements in their sleep with benefits lasting for at least 6 months after completion of therapy. While these studies were performed in patients without a cancer diagnosis, similar findings have been reported for patients with malignancy as well. One study examined a group of 12 cancer survivors who completed a 6 week course of CBT and found subjective improvements in the number of nighttime awakening, sleep efficiency, and global sleep quality.[154] These improvements in sleep architecture have been confirmed with objective measurements, albeit with some inconsistency. Sleep efficiency, total awake time, and sleep onset latency were improved after CBT in two separate studies using either actigraphy or PSG, whereas another study of 27 patients noted only equivocal changes on the polysomnogram after completion of CBT.[76,77,155] Finally, a recent study in cancer patients with persistent insomnia compared treatment with CBT versus conventional treatment; the authors found significant improvements in insomnia and nighttime wakefulness that persisted for at least 6 months.[156]

Other nonpharmacologic modalities being investigated include relaxation treatment, muscle relaxation and imagery training, individualized sleep promotion plans, and exercise programs.[61,157–159] These studies have generally reported some improvements in sleep onset latency and global sleep quality, although objective evaluation of sleep quality was not examined.

CONCLUSION

We started this chapter by pointing to the recent and substantial growth in interest in sleep and cancer. We have tried to summarize the sorts of directions that are being pursued in studying this important area and have emphasized (perhaps tediously) that despite the recent publications, much more work needs to be done to understand the complex nature of sleep disturbances found in cancer patients. These sleep disturbances, particularly insomnia, are very distressing to patients with cancer. Patients often report subjectively poor sleep, and objective sleep measures demonstrate decreased sleep efficiency and frequent nocturnal awakenings. There are multiple causes of sleep interruption and they may be related to the effects of the malignancy itself or to treatment. There has been a growing understanding of the role of circadian rhythms in the quality of life and outcomes in these patients, and some work has begun to examine if chronotropic administration of chemotherapy may enhance treatment response and minimize side effects. Further work needs to be done in all aspects of sleep disruption in cancer patients, as we currently have only a limited understanding of the problem.

REFERENCES

1. Fiorentino L, Ancoli-Israel S. Insomnia and its treatment in women with breast cancer. *Sleep Med Rev.* 2006 Dec;10(6):419–429.
2. Aldrich M. Cardinal manifestations of sleep disorders. In: Kryger M, Roth T, Dement WC, (eds). *Principles and practice of sleep medicine.* Philadelphia, PA: WB Saunders; 1994:418.
3. Ford DE, Kamerow DB. Epidemiologic study of sleep disturbances and psychiatric disorders. An opportunity for prevention? *JAMA.* 1989 Sep 15;262(11):1479–1484.
4. Morphy H, Dunn KM, Lewis M, Boardman HF, Croft PR. Epidemiology of insomnia: a longitudinal study in a UK population. *Sleep.* 2007 Mar 1;30(3):274–280.
5. Foley DJ, Monjan A, Simonsick EM, Wallace RB, Blazer DG. Incidence and remission of insomnia among elderly adults: an epidemiologic study of 6,800 persons over three years. *Sleep.* 1999 May 1;22(Suppl 2):S366–S372.
6. Epidemiology and causes of insomnia. Available at: http://www.uptodate.com/online/content/topic.do?topicKey=sleepdis/12754&selectedTitle=1~150. Accessed July 1, 2008.
7. Diagnostic classification of sleep and arousal disorders. 1979 first edition. Association of Sleep Disorders Centers and the Association for the Psychophysiological Study of Sleep. *Sleep.* 1979;2:1.
8. Drugs and insomnia. *NIH consensus development conference. Consensus development conference summary.* Vol 4, No 10. Bethesda, MD: National Institutes of Health; 1984:1.
9. American Psychiatric Association. *Diagnostic and statistical manual of mental disorders,* 4th ed, DSM-IV. Washington, DC: American Psychiatric Association; 1994.
10. Diagnostic Classification Steering Committee. The International Classification of Sleep Disorders, Revised: Diagnostic and Coding Manual. Rochester, MN: American Sleep Disorders Association; 1997.
11. Couzi RJ, Helzlsouer KJ, Fetting JH. Prevalence of menopausal symptoms among women with a history of breast cancer and attitudes toward estrogen replacement therapy. *J Clin Oncol.* 1995 Nov;13(11):2737–2744.
12. Harrison LB, Zelefsky MJ, Pfister DG, et al. Detailed quality of life assessment in patients treated with primary radiotherapy for squamous cell cancer of the base of the tongue. *Head Neck.* 1997 May;19(3):169–175.
13. Lindley C, Vasa S, Sawyer WT, Winer EP. Quality of life and preferences for treatment following systemic adjuvant therapy for early-stage breast cancer. *J Clin Oncol.* 1998 Apr;16(4):1380–1387.
14. Portenoy RK, Thaler HT, Kornblith AB, et al. Symptom prevalence, characteristics and distress in a cancer population. *Qual Life Res.* 1994 Jun;3(3):183–189.
15. Le Guen Y, Gagnadoux F, Hureaux J, et al. Sleep disturbances and impaired daytime functioning in outpatients with newly diagnosed lung cancer. *Lung Cancer.* 2007 Oct;58(1):139–143.
16. Bardwell WA, Profant J, Casden DR, et al. The relative importance of specific risk factors for insomnia in women treated for early-stage breast cancer. *Psychooncology.* 2008 Jan;17(1):9–18.
17. Davidson JR, MacLean AW, Brundage MD, Schulze K. Sleep disturbance in cancer patients. *Soc Sci Med.* 2002 May;54(9):1309–1321.
18. Sela RA, Watanabe S, Nekolaichuk CL. Sleep disturbances in palliative cancer patients attending a pain and symptom control clinic. *Palliat Support Care.* 2005 Mar;3(1):23–31.
19. Skaug K, Eide GE, Gulsvik A. Prevalence and predictors of symptoms in the terminal stage of lung cancer: a community study. *Chest.* 2007 Feb;131(2):389–394.
20. Taylor DJ, Mallory LJ, Lichstein KL, Durrence HH, Riedel BW, Bush AJ. Comorbidity of chronic insomnia with medical problems. *Sleep.* 2007 Feb 1;30(2):213–218.

21. Savard J, Simard S, Blanchet J, Ivers H, Morin CM. Prevalence, clinical characteristics, and risk factors for insomnia in the context of breast cancer. *Sleep*. 2001 Aug 1;24(5):583–590.

22. Savard J, Simard S, Hervouet S, Ivers H, Lacombe L, Fradet Y. Insomnia in men treated with radical prostatectomy for prostate cancer. *Psychooncology*. 2005 Feb;14(2):147–156.

23. Taphoorn MJ, Stupp R, Coens C, et al. Health-related quality of life in patients with glioblastoma: a randomised controlled trial. *Lancet Oncol*. 2005 Dec;6(12):937–944.

24. Killgore WD, Killgore DB, Day LM, Li C, Kamimori GH, Balkin TJ. The effects of 53 hours of sleep deprivation on moral judgment. *Sleep*. 2007 Mar 1;30(3):345–352.

25. Broughton R, Ghanem Q, Hishikawa Y, Sugita Y, Nevsimalova S, Roth B. Life effects of narcolepsy in 180 patients from North America, Asia and Europe compared to matched controls. *Can J Neurol Sci*. 1981 Nov;8(4):299–304.

26. Everson CA. Sustained sleep deprivation impairs host defense. *Am J Physiol*. 1993 Nov;265(5, pt 2):R1148–R1154.

27. Irwin MR, Wang M, Campomayor CO, Collado-Hidalgo A, Cole S. Sleep deprivation and activation of morning levels of cellular and genomic markers of inflammation. *Arch Intern Med*. 2006 Sep 18;166(16):1756–1762.

28. Redwine L, Dang J, Irwin M. Cellular adhesion molecule expression, nocturnal sleep, and partial night sleep deprivation. *Brain Behav Immun*. 2004 Jul;18(4):333–340.

29. Shearer WT, Reuben JM, Mullington JM, et al. Soluble TNF-alpha receptor 1 and IL-6 plasma levels in humans subjected to the sleep deprivation model of spaceflight. *J Allergy Clin Immunol*. 2001 Jan;107(1):165–170.

30. Degner LF, Sloan JA. Symptom distress in newly diagnosed ambulatory cancer patients and as a predictor of survival in lung cancer. *J Pain Symptom Manage*. 1995 Aug;10(6):423–431.

31. Ahlberg K, Ekman T, Gaston-Johansson F, Mock V. Assessment and management of cancer-related fatigue in adults. *Lancet*. 2003 Aug 23;362(9384): 640–650.

32. Vogelzang NJ, Breitbart W, Cella D, et al. Patient, caregiver, and oncologist perceptions of cancer-related fatigue: results of a tripart assessment survey. The fatigue coalition. *Semin Hematol*. 1997 Jul;34(3, Suppl 2):4–12.

33. Sarna L. Correlates of symptom distress in women with lung cancer. *Cancer Pract*. 1993 May-Jun;1(1):21–28.

34. Roscoe JA, Kaufman ME, Matteson-Rusby SE, et al. Cancer-related fatigue and sleep disorders. *Oncologist*. 2007;1(Suppl 12):35–42.

35. Broeckel JA, Jacobsen PB, Horton J, Balducci L, Lyman GH. Characteristics and correlates of fatigue after adjuvant chemotherapy for breast cancer. *J Clin Oncol*. 1998 May;16(5):1689–1696.

36. Reyes-Gibby CC, Aday LA, Anderson KO, Mendoza TR, Cleeland CS. Pain, depression, and fatigue in community-dwelling adults with and without a history of cancer. *J Pain Symptom Manage*. 2006 Aug;32(2):118–128.

37. Dodd MJ, Miaskowski C, Paul SM. Symptom clusters and their effect on the functional status of patients with cancer. *Oncol Nurs Forum*. 2001 Apr;28(3):465–470.

38. Stone P, Richards M, A'Hern R, Hardy J. Fatigue in patients with cancers of the breast or prostate undergoing radical radiotherapy. *J Pain Symptom Manage*. 2001 Dec;22(6):1007–1015.

39. Palesh OG, Collie K, Batiuchok D, et al. A longitudinal study of depression, pain, and stress as predictors of sleep disturbance among women with metastatic breast cancer. *Biol Psychol*. 2007 Apr;75(1):37–44.

40. Mulrooney DA, Ness KK, Neglia JP, et al. Fatigue and sleep disturbance in adult survivors of childhood cancer: a report from the childhood cancer survivor study (CCSS). *Sleep*. 2008 Feb 1;31(2):271–281.

41. Montplaisir J, Boucher S, Poirier G, Lavigne G, Lapierre O, Lesperance P. Clinical, polysomnographic, and genetic characteristics of restless legs syndrome: a study of 133 patients diagnosed with new standard criteria. *Mov Disord*. 1997 Jan;12(1):61–65.

42. Carrier J, Frenette S, Montplaisir J, Paquet J, Drapeau C, Morettini J. Effects of periodic leg movements during sleep in middle-aged subjects without sleep complaints. *Mov Disord*. 2005 Sep;20(9):1127–1132.

43. Allen RP, Walters AS, Montplaisir J, et al. Restless legs syndrome prevalence and impact: REST general population study. *Arch Intern Med*. 2005 Jun 13;165(11):1286–1292.

44. Hornyak M, Feige B, Riemann D, Voderholzer U. Periodic leg movements in sleep and periodic limb movement disorder: prevalence, clinical significance and treatment. *Sleep Med Rev*. 2006 Jun;10(3):169–177.

45. Saini A, Ostacoli L, Sguazzotti E, et al. High prevalence of restless legs syndrome in cancer patients undergoing chemotherapy: relationship with anxiety, depression and quality of life perception. *JCO ASCO Annual Meeting Proceedings Part I*. 2007;25(18S).

46. Parish JM. "I can't sleep at night" an unusual case of insomnia. *J Clin Sleep Med*. 2005 Jul 15;1(3):305–308.

47. Brocklehurst J. Restless legs syndrome as a presenting symptom in malignant disease. *Age Ageing*. 2003 Mar;32(2):234.

48. Payne RJ, Hier MP, Kost KM, et al. High prevalence of obstructive sleep apnea among patients with head and neck cancer. *J Otolaryngol*. 2005 Oct;34(5):304–311.

49. Friedman M, Landsberg R, Pryor S, Syed Z, Ibrahim H, Caldarelli DD. The occurrence of sleep-disordered breathing among patients with head and neck cancer. *Laryngoscope*. 2001 Nov;111(11, pt 1):1917–1919.

50. Hiestand DM, Britz P, Goldman M, Phillips B. Prevalence of symptoms and risk of sleep apnea in the US population: results from the national sleep foundation sleep in America 2005 poll. *Chest*. 2006 Sep;130(3):780–786.

51. Di Gennaro G, Autret A, Mascia A, Onorati P, Sebastiano F, Paolo Quarato P. Night terrors associated with thalamic lesion. *Clin Neurophysiol*. 2004 Nov;115(11):2489–2492.

52. Marcus CL, Trescher WH, Halbower AC, Lutz J. Secondary narcolepsy in children with brain tumors. *Sleep*. 2002 Jun 15;25(4):435–439.

53. Ancoli-Israel S, Cole R, Alessi C, Chambers M, Moorcroft W, Pollak CP. The role of actigraphy in the study of sleep and circadian rhythms. *Sleep*. 2003 May 1;26(3):342–392.

54. Sadeh A, Hauri PJ, Kripke DF, Lavie P. The role of actigraphy in the evaluation of sleep disorders. *Sleep*. 1995 May;18(4):288–302.

55. Weaver EM, Kapur V, Yueh B. Polysomnography vs self-reported measures in patients with sleep apnea. *Arch Otolaryngol Head Neck Surg*. 2004 Apr;130(4):453–458.

56. Kapur VK, Baldwin CM, Resnick HE, Gottlieb DJ, Nieto FJ. Sleepiness in patients with moderate to severe sleep-disordered breathing. *Sleep*. 2005 Apr 1;28(4):472–477.

57. Levin RD, Daehler MA, Grutsch JF, et al. Circadian function in patients with advanced non-small-cell lung cancer. *Br J Cancer*. 2005 Nov 28;93(11): 1202–1208.

58. Ancoli-Israel S, Liu L, Marler MR, et al. Fatigue, sleep, and circadian rhythms prior to chemotherapy for breast cancer. *Support Care Cancer*. 2006 Mar;14(3):201–209.

59. Berger AM, Farr LA, Kuhn BR, Fischer P, Agrawal S. Values of sleep/wake, activity/rest, circadian rhythms, and fatigue prior to adjuvant breast cancer chemotherapy. *J Pain Symptom Manage*. 2007 Apr;33(4):398–409.

60. Berger AM. Patterns of fatigue and activity and rest during adjuvant breast cancer chemotherapy. *Oncol Nurs Forum*. 1998 Jan-Feb;25(1):51–62.

61. Berger AM, VonEssen S, Kuhn BR, et al. Adherence, sleep, and fatigue outcomes after adjuvant breast cancer chemotherapy: results of a feasibility intervention study. *Oncol Nurs Forum*. 2003 May-Jun;30(3):513–522.

62. Payne J, Piper B, Rabinowitz I, Zimmerman B. Biomarkers, fatigue, sleep, and depressive symptoms in women with breast cancer: a pilot study. *Oncol Nurs Forum*. 2006 Jul;33(4):775–783.

63. Silberfarb PM, Hauri PJ, Oxman TE, Lash S. Insomnia in cancer patients. *Soc Sci Med*. 1985;20(8):849–850.

64. Silberfarb PM, Hauri PJ, Oxman TE, Schnurr P. Assessment of sleep in patients with lung cancer and breast cancer. *J Clin Oncol*. 1993 May;11(5): 997–1004.

65. Parker KP, Bliwise DL, Ribeiro M, et al. Sleep/Wake patterns of individuals with advanced cancer measured by ambulatory polysomnography. *J Clin Oncol*. 2008 May 20;26(15):2464–2472.

66. Savard J, Morin CM. Insomnia in the context of cancer: a review of a neglected problem. *J Clin Oncol*. 2001 Feb 1;19(3):895–908.

67. Fortner BV, Stepanski EJ, Wang SC, Kasprowicz S, Durrence HH. Sleep and quality of life in breast cancer patients. *J Pain Symptom Manage*. 2002 Nov;24(5):471–480.

68. Buysse DJ, Reynolds CF, 3rd, Monk TH, Berman SR, Kupfer DJ. The Pittsburgh Sleep Quality Index: a new instrument for psychiatric practice and research. *Psychiatry Res*. 1989 May;28(2):193–213.

69. Beck SL, Schwartz AL, Towsley G, Dudley W, Barsevick A. Psychometric evaluation of the Pittsburgh Sleep Quality Index in cancer patients. *J Pain Symptom Manage*. 2004 Feb;27(2):140–148.

70. Backhaus J, Junghanns K, Broocks A, Riemann D, Hohagen F. Test-retest reliability and validity of the Pittsburgh Sleep Quality Index in primary insomnia. *J Psychosom Res*. 2002 Sep;53(3):737–740.

71. Johns MW. A new method for measuring daytime sleepiness: the Epworth sleepiness scale. *Sleep*. 1991 Dec;14(6):540–545.

72. Gander PH, Marshall NS, Harris R, Reid P. The Epworth Sleepiness Scale: influence of age, ethnicity, and socioeconomic deprivation. Epworth Sleepiness scores of adults in New Zealand. *Sleep*. 2005 Feb 1;28(2):249–253.

73. Spielman AJ, Caruso LS, Glovinsky PB. A behavioral perspective on insomnia treatment. *Psychiatr Clin North Am*. 1987 Dec;10(4):541–553.

74. Breslau N, Roth T, Rosenthal L, Andreski P. Sleep disturbance and psychiatric disorders: a longitudinal epidemiological study of young adults. *Biol Psychiatry*. 1996 Mar 15;39(6):411–418.

75. Gillin JC. Are sleep disturbances risk factors for anxiety, depressive and addictive disorders? *Acta Psychiatr Scand Suppl*. 1998;393:39–43.

76. Savard J, Simard S, Ivers H, Morin CM. Randomized study on the efficacy of cognitive-behavioral therapy for insomnia secondary to breast cancer, part I: Sleep and psychological effects. *J Clin Oncol*. 2005 Sep 1;23(25):6083–6096.

77. Quesnel C, Savard J, Simard S, Ivers H, Morin CM. Efficacy of cognitive-behavioral therapy for insomnia in women treated for nonmetastatic breast cancer. *J Consult Clin Psychol*. 2003 Feb;71(1):189–200.

78. Fava M, McCall WV, Krystal A, et al. Eszopiclone co-administered with fluoxetine in patients with insomnia coexisting with major depressive disorder. *Biol Psychiatry*. 2006 Jun 1;59(11):1052–1060.

79. Fann JR, Thomas-Rich AM, Katon WJ, et al. Major depression after breast cancer: a review of epidemiology and treatment. *Gen Hosp Psychiatry*. 2008 Mar-Apr;30(2):112–126.

80. Lydiatt WM, Denman D, McNeilly DP, Puumula SE, Burke WJ. A randomized, placebo-controlled trial of citalopram for the prevention of major depression during treatment for head and neck cancer. *Arch Otolaryngol Head Neck Surg*. 2008 May;134(5):528–535.

81. Massie MJ. Prevalence of depression in patients with cancer. *J Natl Cancer Inst Monogr*. 2004(32):57–71.

82. van't Spijker A, Trijsburg RW, Duivenvoorden HJ. Psychological sequelae of cancer diagnosis: a meta-analytical review of 58 studies after 1980. *Psychosom Med*. 1997 May-Jun;59(3):280–293.

83. Ginsburg ML, Quirt C, Ginsburg AD, MacKillop WJ. Psychiatric illness and psychosocial concerns of patients with newly diagnosed lung cancer. *CMAJ*. 1995 Mar 1;152(5):701–708.

84. Ganz PA, Desmond KA, Leedham B, Rowland JH, Meyerowitz BE, Belin TR. Quality of life in long-term, disease-free survivors of breast cancer: a follow-up study. *J Natl Cancer Inst*. 2002 Jan 2;94(1):39–49.

85. Teunissen SC, de Graeff A, Voest EE, de Haes JC. Are anxiety and depressed mood related to physical symptom burden? A study in hospitalized advanced cancer patients. *Palliat Med*. 2007 Jun;21(4):341–346.

86. Horowitz M, Schaefer C, Hiroto D, Wilner N, Levin B. Life event questionnaires for measuring presumptive stress. *Psychosom Med*. 1977 Nov-Dec;39(6):413–431.

87. Mercadante S, Girelli D, Casuccio A. Sleep disorders in advanced cancer patients: prevalence and factors associated. *Support Care Cancer*. 2004 May;12(5):355–359.

88. Cleeland CS, Gonin R, Hatfield AK, et al. Pain and its treatment in outpatients with metastatic cancer. *N Engl J Med*. 1994 Mar 3;330(9):592–596.

89. Teunissen SC, Wesker W, Kruitwagen C, de Haes HC, Voest EE, de Graeff A. Symptom prevalence in patients with incurable cancer: a systematic review. *J Pain Symptom Manage*. 2007 Jul;34(1):94–104.

90. McCracken LM, Iverson GL. Disrupted sleep patterns and daily functioning in patients with chronic pain. *Pain Res Manag*. 2002 Summer;7(2):75–79.

91. Grond S, Zech D, Diefenbach C, Bischoff A. Prevalence and pattern of symptoms in patients with cancer pain: a prospective evaluation of 1635 cancer patients referred to a pain clinic. *J Pain Symptom Manage*. 1994 Aug;9(6):372–382.

92. Strang P. Emotional and social aspects of cancer pain. *Acta Oncol*. 1992;31(3):323–326.

93. Dorrepaal KL, Aaronson NK, van Dam FS. Pain experience and pain management among hospitalized cancer patients. A clinical study. *Cancer*. 1989 Feb 1;63(3):593–598.

94. Kundermann B, Spernal J, Huber MT, Krieg JC, Lautenbacher S. Sleep deprivation affects thermal pain thresholds but not somatosensory thresholds in healthy volunteers. *Psychosom Med*. 2004 Nov-Dec;66(6):932–937.

95. Moldofsky H, Scarisbrick P. Induction of neurasthenic musculoskeletal pain syndrome by selective sleep stage deprivation. *Psychosom Med*. 1976 Jan-Feb;38(1):35–44.

96. Onen SH, Alloui A, Gross A, Eschallier A, Dubray C. The effects of total sleep deprivation, selective sleep interruption and sleep recovery on pain tolerance thresholds in healthy subjects. *J Sleep Res*. 2001 Mar;10(1):35–42.

97. Wirz S, Wartenberg HC, Elsen C, Wittmann M, Diederichs M, Nadstawek J. Managing cancer pain and symptoms of outpatients by rotation to sustained-release hydromorphone: a prospective clinical trial. *Clin J Pain*. 2006 Nov-Dec;22(9):770–775.

98. Kay DC. Human sleep during chronic morphine intoxication. *Psychopharmacologia*. 1975 Oct 31;44(2):117–124.

99. Kay DC, Pickworth WB, Neidert GL, Falcone D, Fishman PM, Othmer E. Opioid effects on computer-derived sleep and EEG parameters in nondependent human addicts. *Sleep*. 1979;2(2):175–191.

100. Lewis SA, Oswald I, Evans JI, Akindele MO. Heroin and human sleep. *Electroencephalogr Clin Neurophysiol*. 1970 Apr;28(4):429.

101. Dimsdale JE, Norman D, DeJardin D, Wallace MS. The effect of opioids on sleep architecture. *J Clin Sleep Med*. 2007 Feb 15;3(1):33–36.

102. Knobf MT. Reproductive and hormonal sequelae of chemotherapy in women. Premature menopause and impaired fertility can result, effects that are especially disturbing to young women. *Am J Nurs*. 2006 Mar;106(Supp 3):60–65.

103. Shapiro CL, Recht A. Side effects of adjuvant treatment of breast cancer. *N Engl J Med*. 2001 Jun 28;344(26):1997–2008.

104. Love RR, Cameron L, Connell BL, Leventhal H. Symptoms associated with tamoxifen treatment in postmenopausal women. *Arch Intern Med*. 1991 Sep;151(9):1842–1847.

105. Harris PF, Remington PL, Trentham-Dietz A, Allen CI, Newcomb PA. Prevalence and treatment of menopausal symptoms among breast cancer survivors. *J Pain Symptom Manage*. 2002 Jun;23(6):501–509.

106. Carpenter JS, Johnson D, Wagner L, Andrykowski M. Hot flashes and related outcomes in breast cancer survivors and matched comparison women. *Oncol Nurs Forum*. 2002 Apr;29(3):E16–25.

107. Carpenter JS, Elam JL, Ridner SH, Carney PH, Cherry GJ, Cucullu HL. Sleep, fatigue, and depressive symptoms in breast cancer survivors and matched healthy women experiencing hot flashes. *Oncol Nurs Forum*. 2004 May;31(3):591–5598.

108. Stein KD, Jacobsen PB, Hann DM, Greenberg H, Lyman G. Impact of hot flashes on quality of life among postmenopausal women being treated for breast cancer. *J Pain Symptom Manage*. 2000 Jun;19(6):436–445.

109. Savard J, Davidson JR, Ivers H, et al. The association between nocturnal hot flashes and sleep in breast cancer survivors. *J Pain Symptom Manage*. 2004 Jun;27(6):513–522.

110. Wengstrom Y, Haggmark C, Strander H, Forsberg C. Perceived symptoms and quality of life in women with breast cancer receiving radiation therapy. *Eur J Oncol Nurs*. 2000 Jun;4(2):78–88; discussion 89–90.

111. Van Someren EJ, Swart-Heikens J, Endert E, et al. Long-term effects of cranial irradiation for childhood malignancy on sleep in adulthood. *Eur J Endocrinol*. 2004 Apr;150(4):503–510.

112. Omne-Ponten M, Holmberg L, Burns T, Adami HO, Bergstrom R. Determinants of the psycho-social outcome after operation for breast cancer. Results of a prospective comparative interview study following mastectomy and breast conservation. *Eur J Cancer*. 1992;28A(6–7):1062–1067.

113. Tsunoda A, Nakao K, Hiratsuka K, Tsunoda Y, Kusano M. Prospective analysis of quality of life in the first year after colorectal cancer surgery. *Acta Oncol*. 2007;46(1):77–82.

114. Mormont MC, Levi F. Cancer chronotherapy: principles, applications, and perspectives. *Cancer*. 2003 Jan 1;97(1):155–169.

115. Chevalier V, Mormont MC, Cure H, Chollet P. Assessment of circadian rhythms by actimetry in healthy subjects and patients with advanced colorectal cancer. *Oncol Rep*. 2003 May-Jun;10(3):733–737.

116. Mormont MC, Waterhouse J. Contribution of the rest-activity circadian rhythm to quality of life in cancer patients. *Chronobiol Int*. 2002 Jan;19(1):313–323.

117. Touitou Y, Levi F, Bogdan A, Benavides M, Bailleul F, Misset JL. Rhythm alteration in patients with metastatic breast cancer and poor prognostic factors. *J Cancer Res Clin Oncol*. 1995;121(3):181–188.

118. Mormont MC, Waterhouse J, Bleuzen P, et al. Marked 24-h rest/activity rhythms are associated with better quality of life, better response, and longer survival in patients with metastatic colorectal cancer and good performance status. *Clin Cancer Res*. 2000 Aug;6(8):3038–3045.

119. Levi F, Zidani R, Misset JL. Randomised multicentre trial of chronotherapy with oxaliplatin, fluorouracil, and folinic acid in metastatic colorectal cancer. International Organization for Cancer Chronotherapy. *Lancet*. 1997 Sep 6;350(9079):681–686.

120. Miller AH, Ancoli-Israel S, Bower JE, Capuron L, Irwin MR. Neuroendocrine-immune mechanisms of behavioral comorbidities in patients with cancer. *J Clin Oncol*. 2008 Feb 20;26(6):971–982.

121. Kelley KW, Bluthe RM, Dantzer R, et al. Cytokine-induced sickness behavior. *Brain Behav Immun*. 2003 Feb;17(Suppl 1):S112–S118.

122. Spadaro F, Dunn AJ. Intracerebroventricular administration of interleukin-1 to mice alters investigation of stimuli in a novel environment. *Brain Behav Immun*. 1990 Dec;4(4):308–322.

123. Segall MA, Crnic LS. An animal model for the behavioral effects of interferon. *Behav Neurosci*. 1990 Aug;104(4):612–618.

124. Schubert C, Hong S, Natarajan L, Mills PJ, Dimsdale JE. The association between fatigue and inflammatory marker levels in cancer patients: a quantitative review. *Brain Behav Immun*. 2007 May;21(4):413–427.

125. Alberti A, Sarchielli P, Gallinella E, Floridi A, Mazzotta G, Gallai V. Plasma cytokine levels in patients with obstructive sleep apnea syndrome: a preliminary study. *J Sleep Res*. 2003 Dec;12(4):305–311.

126. Minoguchi K, Tazaki T, Yokoe T, et al. Elevated production of tumor necrosis factor-alpha by monocytes in patients with obstructive sleep apnea syndrome. *Chest*. 2004 Nov;126(5):1473–1479.

127. Vgontzas AN, Zoumakis M, Papanicolaou DA, et al. Chronic insomnia is associated with a shift of interleukin-6 and tumor necrosis factor secretion from nighttime to daytime. *Metabolism.* 2002 Jul;51(7):887–892.

128. Savard J, Simard S, Ivers H, Morin CM. Randomized study on the efficacy of cognitive-behavioral therapy for insomnia secondary to breast cancer, part II: immunologic effects. *J Clin Oncol.* 2005 Sep 1;23(25):6097–6106.

129. Rich T, Innominato PF, Boerner J, et al. Elevated serum cytokines correlated with altered behavior, serum cortisol rhythm, and dampened 24-hour rest-activity patterns in patients with metastatic colorectal cancer. *Clin Cancer Res.* 2005 Mar 1;11(5):1757–1764.

130. Kripke DF, Klauber MR, Wingard DL, Fell RL, Assmus JD, Garfinkel L. Mortality hazard associated with prescription hypnotics. *Biol Psychiatry.* 1998 May 1;43(9):687–693.

131. Kudo Y, Kurihara M. Clinical evaluation of diphenhydramine hydrochloride for the treatment of insomnia in psychiatric patients: a double-blind study. *J Clin Pharmacol.* 1990 Nov;30(11):1041–1048.

132. Rickels K, Morris RJ, Newman H, Rosenfeld H, Schiller H, Weinstock R. Diphenhydramine in insomniac family practice patients: a double-blind study. *J Clin Pharmacol.* 1983 May-Jun;23(5–6):234–242.

133. Bhat A, Shafi F, El Solh AA. Pharmacotherapy of insomnia. *Expert Opin Pharmacother.* 2008 Feb;9(3):351–362.

134. Mohler H, Fritschy JM, Vogt K, Crestani F, Rudolph U. Pathophysiology and pharmacology of GABA(A) receptors. *Hand Exp Pharmacol.* 2005(169):225–247.

135. Nowell PD, Mazumdar S, Buysse DJ, Dew MA, Reynolds CF, 3rd, Kupfer DJ. Benzodiazepines and zolpidem for chronic insomnia: a meta-analysis of treatment efficacy. *JAMA.* 1997 Dec 24–31;278(24):2170–2177.

136. Holbrook AM, Crowther R, Lotter A, Cheng C, King D. Meta-analysis of benzodiazepine use in the treatment of insomnia. *CMAJ.* 2000 Jan 25;162(2):225–233.

137. King SA, Strain JJ. Benzodiazepines and chronic pain. *Pain.* 1990 Apr; 41(1):3–4.

138. Roth T, Roehrs TA. A review of the safety profiles of benzodiazepine hypnotics. *J Clin Psychiatry.* 1991 Sep;52 Suppl:38–41.

139. Nurmi-Luthje I, Kaukonen JP, Luthje P, et al. Use of benzodiazepines and benzodiazepine-related drugs among 223 patients with an acute hip fracture in Finland: comparison of benzodiazepine findings in medical records and laboratory assays. *Drugs Aging.* 2006;23(1):27–37.

140. Paltiel O, Marzec-Boguslawska A, Soskolne V, et al. Use of tranquilizers and sleeping pills among cancer patients is associated with a poorer quality of life. *Qual Life Res.* 2004 Dec;13(10):1699–1706.

141. Scharf MB, Roth T, Vogel GW, Walsh JK. A multicenter, placebo-controlled study evaluating zolpidem in the treatment of chronic insomnia. *J Clin Psychiatry.* 1994 May;55(5):192–199.

142. Zammit GK, Corser B, Doghramji K, et al. Sleep and residual sedation after administration of zaleplon, zolpidem, and placebo during experimental iddle-of-the-night awakening. *J Clin Sleep Med.* 2006 Oct 15;2(4): 417–423.

143. Krystal AD, Walsh JK, Laska E, et al. Sustained efficacy of eszopiclone over 6 months of nightly treatment: results of a randomized, double-blind, placebo-controlled study in adults with chronic insomnia. *Sleep.* 2003 Nov 1;26(7): 793–799.

144. Mendelson WB, Roth T, Cassella J, et al. The treatment of chronic insomnia: drug indications, chronic use and abuse liability. Summary of a 2001 New Clinical Drug Evaluation Unit meeting symposium. *Sleep Med Rev.* 2004 Feb;8(1):7–17.

145. Wilson S, Argyropoulos S. Antidepressants and sleep: a qualitative review of the literature. *Drugs.* 2005;65(7):927–947.

146. Rodenbeck A, Cohrs S, Jordan W, Huether G, Ruther E, Hajak G. The sleep-improving effects of doxepin are paralleled by a normalized plasma cortisol secretion in primary insomnia. A placebo-controlled, double-blind, randomized, cross-over study followed by an open treatment over 3 weeks. *Psychopharmacology (Berl).* 2003 Dec;170(4):423–428.

147. Hajak G, Rodenbeck A, Voderholzer U, et al. Doxepin in the treatment of primary insomnia: a placebo-controlled, double-blind, polysomnographic study. *J Clin Psychiatry.* 2001 Jun;62(6):453–463.

148. Almeida Montes LG, Ontiveros Uribe MP, Cortes Sotres J, Heinze Martin G. Treatment of primary insomnia with melatonin: a double-blind, placebo-controlled, crossover study. *J Psychiatry Neurosci.* 2003 May;28(3):191–196.

149. Brzezinski A, Vangel MG, Wurtman RJ, et al. Effects of exogenous melatonin on sleep: a meta-analysis. *Sleep Med Rev.* 2005 Feb;9(1):41–50.

150. Salin-Pascual RJ, Herrera-Estrella M, Galicia-Polo L, Laurrabaquio MR. Olanzapine acute administration in schizophrenic patients increases delta sleep and sleep efficiency. *Biol Psychiatry.* 1999 Jul 1;46(1):141–143.

151. Murtagh DR, Greenwood KM. Identifying effective psychological treatments for insomnia: a meta-analysis. *J Consult Clin Psychol.* 1995 Feb;63(1):79–89.

152. Morin CM, Culbert JP, Schwartz SM. Nonpharmacological interventions for insomnia: a meta-analysis of treatment efficacy. *Am J Psychiatry.* 1994 Aug;151(8):1172–1180.

153. Montgomery P, Dennis J. Cognitive behavioural interventions for sleep problems in adults aged 60+. *Cochrane Database Syst Rev.* 2003(1):CD003161.

154. Davidson JR, Waisberg JL, Brundage MD, MacLean AW. Non-pharmacologic group treatment of insomnia: a preliminary study with cancer survivors. *Psychooncology.* 2001 Sep-Oct;10(5):389–397.

155. Epstein DR, Dirksen SR. Randomized trial of a cognitive-behavioral intervention for insomnia in breast cancer survivors. *Oncol Nurs Forum.* 2007 Sep;34(5):E51–E59.

156. Espie CA, Fleming L, Cassidy J, et al. Randomized controlled clinical effectiveness trial of cognitive behavior therapy compared with treatment as usual for persistent insomnia in patients with cancer. *J Clin Oncol.* 2008 Jun 30;26(28):4651–4658.

157. Cannici J, Malcolm R, Peek LA. Treatment of insomnia in cancer patients using muscle relaxation training. *J Behav Ther Exp Psychiatry.* 1983 Sep;14(3):251–256.

158. Stam HJ, Bultz BD. The treatment of severe insomnia in a cancer patient. *J Behav Ther Exp Psychiatry.* 1986 Mar;17(1):33–37.

159. Coleman EA, Coon S, Hall-Barrow J, Richards K, Gaylor D, Stewart B. Feasibility of exercise during treatment for multiple myeloma. *Cancer Nurs.* 2003 Oct;26(5):410–419.

CHAPTER 36

Weight and Appetite Loss in Cancer

Stewart B. Fleishman and Juskaran S. Chadha

INTRODUCTION

Weight loss from cancer is a multidetermined sign that includes each of the domains affecting patients, their families and caregivers, as well as the whole oncology treatment team. Weight loss affects one's ability to survive cancer and its treatment, and greatly impacts on quality of life. Unintended weight loss is often the presenting feature drawing a patient to seek medical attention, and the diagnostic work-up that leads to the initial cancer diagnosis. During treatment, weight loss despite reasonable nutritional intake is perceived as a serious warning signal to the oncology treatment team, patients, families, and the prudent layperson alike. Before corroboration through imaging studies, tumor markers or clinical examination, weight loss is often a *herald* sign of recurrence or relapse with its associated expectable fears and distress of progressive disease or death.

Cancer cachexia is a major morbidity of cancer. The goal of cancer-specific nutritional intervention is to provide the calories and protein together with a metabolically active nutritional substrate, to provide safe and effective tools to help prevent weight loss, and to promote gain in lean body mass and ultimately improve outcomes and quality of life in patients with cancer-induced weight loss. As pharmacological intervention can increase appetite, retention of calories and weight, its timing needs to be proactive. Early intervention can prevent cancer-associated weight loss.

IMPORTANCE OF WEIGHT MAINTENANCE

Weight loss is experienced by 80% of patients presenting with any cancer, excluding the superficial skin cancers. It may be the root cause of mortality in up to 20%[1] of patients with cancer, with an estimated 10 million deaths projected for 2010.[2-4] The prevalence of this problem highlights the importance of a variety of nutritional factors that should be evaluated for symptom management and support of patients throughout their life after a diagnosis of cancer.

Most religious and legal belief systems contend that nutrition and hydration are essential individual rights, and virtually every culture sees the provision of food as a basic entitlement. Optimal nutrition during initial treatment or with progressive disease is yet to be defined, but basic clinical principles and research have yielded useful techniques for the present generation of patients. As the nutritional needs associated with different forms of cancer at various stages are better understood by those who treat cancer, there will be further guidance on the requirements for "optimal nutrition."

The modern understanding of weight loss in cancer has advanced with the better understanding of the biology of cancer itself. More is known about and yet more needs to be identified in the pathogenesis of weight loss in cancer. Formerly ascribed to a patient "giving up" or being "depressed," the intrinsic and extrinsic factors responsible in large part for weight loss align with the inflammatory underpinnings of cancer and its systemic effects. Understanding the contributions of these biological processes expands our knowledge about weight loss so that patients and families do not believe it is their fault that weight loss occurs, or that the cancer itself or its recurrence is solely due to faulty nutrition. Such knowledge can relieve a great burden, but likewise leave a patient and family with little else they believe they can control in their environment.

Cachexia versus anorexia. *Cachexia*, a term from the Greek meaning "a bad condition," is a severe depletion of muscle (lean body mass), and, to a lesser extent, fat, directly or indirectly from cancer and its treatment. *Cachexia* is a more accurate descriptor than *anorexia,* whose unfortunate association with *anorexia nervosa* may bring the clinician, patient, or family member to the *erroneous* conclusion that the condition is mainly psychologically based. *Anorexia* usually refers only to a loss of appetite, which is part of—but not the principal driver of—weight loss in cancer.

Cachexia in noncancer illness. *Cachexia* is seen with a variety of other acute diseases (such as sepsis, trauma, burns) and chronic diseases (such as human immunodeficiency virus/acquired immunodeficiency syndrome [HIV/AIDS], chronic pulmonary disease, liver or renal failure). In the acute diseases, the onset of *cachexia* is often sudden in a patient who is inherently healthy and close to, or exceeds his or her ideal body weight, so the immediate reduction in caloric intake is blunted by the physiologic cushion of a robust state. For acute noncancer patients, parenteral nutrition (central or peripheral hyperalimentation) would be the logical treatment to maintain adequate caloric intake. However, for patients with progressive cancer, parenteral nutrition is burdensome, risks infection, and often has no clear clinical benefit. Other chronic illnesses each provide a somewhat differing set of nutritional challenges. Some of the advances in the treatment of cancer *cachexia* are owed to innovations in the treatment of HIV/AIDS-related wasting.

THE IMPORTANT ROLE OF BEHAVIORAL HEALTH SPECIALISTS

Traditionally, regardless of culture or tradition, food symbolizes basic sustenance, respect, celebration, socialization and/or diversion. Woven into the fabric of daily life and ritual, when food is connected to medical treatment, decision making takes on additional layers of complexity. For example, in the health professions we know that withholding food evolves into a moral, ethical, and religious issue that overarches society and medicine. The emblematic significance of food as succor—for patients as well as their caregivers—cannot be disregarded or taken lightly. Consider the poignant scene often played out at home or in a tertiary care cancer center: A well-meaning and frightened family member bends over at a loved-one's bedside, slowly feeding scant milliliters of soup or dairy product right after the patient's episode of vomiting or as the patient is at end-of-life. This all-too-frequent, tender gesture represents the belief that maintaining nutrition maintains the patient's life force. With so much of modern cancer treatment a passive experience for a patient and family, feeding translates into an opportunity to "do something" active and participatory. Such noble efforts must, of course, be weighed against the risk of aspiration in the seriously ill who may actually crave the taste and texture of a familiar food as well as appreciate the human kindness and interaction. Unfortunately, such feedings add too few calories to change the course of the weight loss itself, despite its secondary benefits. The psychosocial dimension of the caretaker's behavior can be seen as an *anticipatory bereavement* and is best identified by a counselor who can help the treatment team as a whole to recognize the changing goals of care.

With the loss of weight and/or appetite a hallmark sign and symptom of major depression, behavioral health specialists in cancer must be able to ascribe them to cancer itself, its treatment or major depression.

Although it is yet to be shown as psychometrically valid, looking at the cause of the symptom can help make a differential diagnosis between *cachexia* and depression. A differentiation is often made: the *lack of motivation to eat* though able is often associated with *depression*; and the *lack of the ability to eat sufficiently* is more associated with the *cancer itself* or its treatment. Patients with significant weight loss can often smile and show a sparkle in their eyes when asked about their "favorite foods," a practical question when distinguishing between weight loss secondary to cancer *cachexia* or major depression.

CANCER-INDUCED VERSUS CANCER-ASSOCIATED WEIGHT LOSS

Cancer-associated weight loss encompasses the extrinsic mechanical and practical factors that affect caloric supply. **Cancer-induced** weight loss refers to the specific metabolic abnormalities, mediated by inflammatory cytokines, and their effect on energy retention and calories expended.

Eating well is time-consuming and requires much energy for the related tasks: shopping, cooking, chewing, swallowing, digesting, cleaning up, and evacuating waste products from the bowel and bladder. Cancer itself and its treatment, both, affect the sense of smell and taste which are so important to good nutrition, chewing with adequate salivary function, and swallowing. Both, chemotherapy and radiation therapy can induce varying degrees of nausea—with or without vomiting—as well as gastritis. Bowel function is often compromised by anticholinergic effects of opiate analgesics or some antiemetics. Resulting constipation or urinary changes may lead to proctitis or hemorrhoids, making evacuation painful. Opiates or other anticholinergic medications used in cancer may also contribute to urinary hesitancy or retention. These practical, mechanical, and extrinsic factors are *associated* with weight loss in patients with cancer and reduce the adequate caloric supply. To compensate for the poor oral intake, alternative routes may help circumvent total reliance on the oral or *po* intake with percutaneous enteral gastrostomies (PEG) or percutaneous enteral jejunostomies (PEJ). Limitations exist on the volume of supplements that can be given by alternative route when patients rely on oral liquid or parenteral feedings for their total nutritional intake. The quality of the calories, relying on the optimal mixture of proteins and complex carbohydrates, remains important to weight maintenance. Pharmacologic intervention to increase *appetite* provides limited but meaningful help.

The mechanisms of *cancer-induced* weight loss underscore the interference of cell-mediated inflammatory cytokines in the maintenance of weight during treatment for cancer. Cachectin (tumor necrosis factor alpha [TNF-α]), interleukins-1 and 6, and C-reactive protein have an imputed role in the inability to retain protein stored as lean body mass for energy and well-being. The circulating cytokines enter the cell and encourage metabolic activity of cancer cells, raising the energy requirements even more. Glucose serves as an energy supply for only a few hours after it is consumed and digested. Extra calories are stored as glycogen, providing another few hours of energy supply. After these initial glycogen stores are depleted, extraction of energy from fat cells uses up too many calories, so proteins stored as lean body mass are accessed. An additional cytokine, proteolysis-inducing factor (PIF), further fuels the use of lean body mass for energy, depleting muscles and worsening fatigue, and *cachexia* even more. Support of the resting energy expenditure, the amount of energy the body needs for minimal sustenance, is mediated through the same cytokines which use further calories as tissues demand energy. These processes are schematically presented in Figs. 36–1 and 36–2.

THE ECONOMIC MODEL OF CACHEXIA: SUPPLY, RETENTION, AND DEMAND

A realistic *economic model* helps understand the causes of weight loss in cancer as well as its remedies. This model breaks weight loss into components of: *inadequate supply*, *inability to retain calories*, and *increased energy demand*. With oral routes rendered ineffective by obstructive lesions, mucositis and stomatitis, caloric intake is reduced, lowering the nutritional *supply*. Proinflammatory cytokines (TNF-α, interleukin-6, χ interferon, PIF) access energy stores in muscles and vital organs after glycogen stores are depleted, affecting energy *retention*, and an increase in the resting energy expenditure increases *demand*. Such a situation results in a "downward spiral" of weight: a patient is less hungry, eats less which induces fatigue, and that fatigue leads to more weight loss in a continuous descending progression.

The optimal *anticachexia* agent has not yet been discovered. Ideally, such an agent would maintain the skeletal muscle mass so that lean body tissues would *not* be digested as a source of energy. One such drug, with a socially charged history, thalidomide, has been shown to reduce

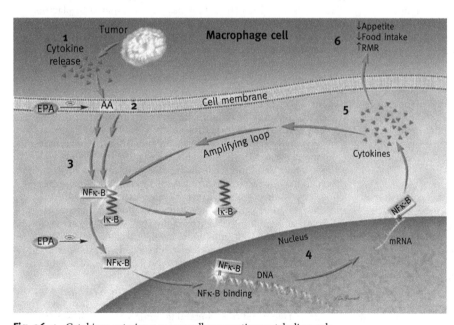

Fig. 36–1. Cytokines entering a cancer cell augmenting metabolic needs.
ABBREVIATIONS: AA, arachidonic acid; EPA, eicosapentanoic acid; mRNA, messenger ribonucleic acid; NF-Kb, *nuclear factor-kappaB*; PIF, proteolysis-inducing factor; RMR, resting metabolic rate.
SOURCE: Reprinted with the permission of © Abbott Laboratories.

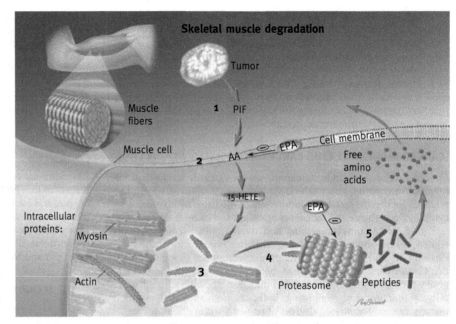

Fig. 36–2. Cytokine proteolysis-inducing factor (PIF) entering skeletal muscle cell facilitating its degradation for energy.
ABBREVIATIONS: AA, arachidonic acid; EPA, eicosapentanoic acid; HETE,.
SOURCE: Reprinted with the permission of © Abbott Laboratories.

cytokines, particularly TNF-α, enhancing weight gain. Other cytokines, such as *nuclear factor-kappaB* (NF-kB) may also block muscle atrophy.[5]

Supply. Interventions to overcome weight loss in cancer also address the three components of supply, energy, and demand. Provision of adequate proteins, high-quality complex carbohydrates and lipids are the cornerstone to overcome *supply* deficits. Nutritional counseling and the use of fortified, specially prepared foods that can be swallowed or administered via PEG or PEJ are tailor-made to an individual's co-morbidities, including diabetes or protein intolerance, such as sprue. Commercially made food supplements can be used orally or parenterally, though some trial and error may be necessary to find a brand or product easily tolerated. Insurance reimbursement identifying preferred products based on contractual agreements may also dictate which supplement is used. Small regular feeds through a plunger or overnight feeds via pump allow for the adequate caloric intake.

The dietary patterns in patients with advanced cancer are not well known. In a study on 151 patients a wide variation in the intake of energy and protein was observed.[6] Even the subjects with highest intake had a recent history of weight loss, suggesting that diets of even those people were consistently inadequate for weight maintenance. Cluster analysis found three dietary patterns that differed in food choice and caloric intake: (1) the milk and soup pattern; (2) the fruit and white bread pattern; and (3) the meat and potato pattern of intake. Low intakes and high risk of weight loss were associated with decreased frequency of eating, and the subjects' dietary profiles included little variety and had unusually high proportions of liquids. It was postulated that a doubling or even tripling of dietary intake would be necessary to maintain weight. This is an unrealistic goal when patients are suffering from *cachexia*.

Retention. Pharmacologic stimulation of appetite by corticosteroids, megesterol acetate, or dronabinol (cannabis congeners) can each encourage maintenance or additional intake (see Table 36–1.). It has been shown that that one of the possible mechanisms that antagonize the progression of *cachexia-anorexia* is the endocannabinoid system. Cannabinoid type 1 receptor activation is shown to stimulate appetite promoting lipogenesis and energy storage.[7] Further development of safe cannabinoids may help reduce cancer patient's cachectic state. Cyproheptadine, a seratonergic antihistamine has been used despite its sedative properties. Prokinetic agents such as metoclopramide may help with feelings of early satiety or when PEG feedings leave one feeling "full" even though small quantities have been instilled. Omega-3 fatty acids containing eicosapentanoic acid (EPA) and docosahexenoic acid (DHA) are thought to down-regulate the cytokines to help maintain lean body

mass and minimize the use of proteins as an energy source to augment energy retention. As a food supplement rather than a prescription drug item, omega-3s have been overlooked as a mainstay in the treatment of cancer *cachexia*. It has been tested alone and in conjunction with high protein and carbohydrate food supplements, and is currently marketed outside the United States for cancer *cachexia*. Studies in pancreatic cancer, head and neck cancer and lung cancer have shown merit in omega-3s' effectiveness in the retention of lean body mass, and the optimal component of weight gain at approximately 2000 mg/day. Although omega-3 fatty acid esters are Food and Drug Administration (FDA)-approved as a prescription drug for hypertriglyceridemia (Lovaza®; formerly Omacor®) they can be recommended as an *off-label* indication in the United States.[8] The purported mechanism of EPA and DHA is illustrated in Fig. 36–1. EPA is shown binding to AA, arachiadonic acid in the cell wall, blocking the passage of the destructive cytokines into the cell, reducing the inflated caloric needs and preserving weight.

In the Bruera 2003 trial,[9] EPA has been compared to placebo. The patients were randomized to receive capsules of 180 mg EPA, 120 DHA, and 1 mg Vitamin E or placebo. In this trial, the patients were not able to tolerate 18 capsules per day. The comparison of results showed a slight weight gain with EPA, DHA, and Vitamin E. Another study compared different doses of EPA alone and megestrol acetate alone to combinations of EPA and megestrol acetate.[10] The combination of EPA with megestrol acetate resulted in a worse outcome versus megestrol acetate alone. The benefits of weight gain showed no significant difference between EPA alone and megestrol alone.

Antilypolytic treatment is shown to prevent *cachexia* progression. Lundholm[11] evaluated whether daily, long-acting insulin attenuates the progression of weight loss in cancer patients without any harmful side effects. Criteria used for measuring results were: nutritional assessment, blood tests, indirect calorimetry, maximum exercise test, quality of life, and daily physical activity. The results showed body fat in the trunk and legs was significantly higher among the patients receiving insulin compared to controls. Insulin improved the metabolic efficiency during exercise, ultimately leading to the conclusion that insulin is a significant metabolic treatment in the multimodal palliation of weight loss in cancer patients.

Essential amino acids such as arginine, glutamine, and *hydroxy*methylbutyric acid (HMB) further inhibit PIF to maintain lean body mass. Commercial preparations containing amino-acid rich supplements (Juven® and others) have also been used for the frail elderly without cancer to promote wound healing. These essential amino acids are also marketed separately as food supplements.[12,13] An early attempt to prove the efficacy of another supplement, hydrazine sulfate, failed to show it as

Table 36–1. Pharmacologic stimulation of appetite or weight gain

Class of agent	Name	Effects	Side effects
Glucocorticoids	Methylprednisone (Prednisone®) Dexamethasone (Decadron®)	↓nausea, antiemetic Transient ↑ appetite No effect on lean body mass	Jittery → agitation; Insomnia, mood swings Gastritis, reflux Weaken proximal muscles (to stand from prone or seated position); avascular necrosis of the hips (protracted course)
Progestational Agents	Megestrol acetate (Megace®)	Increase appetite No effect on lean body mass	Risk of blood clots (thrombosis) surprising lack of feminizing side effects
Cannaboids	Dronabinaol (Marinol®)	↓ nausea, antiemetic "munchies"	"stoned," "high"
Antisertonergic Antihistamine	Cyproheptadine (Periactin®)	Minimal weight gain	Drowsiness, sedation
Neuroleptics	Olanzipine (Zyprexa®)	Increased weight	Relative hyperglycemia? Responsible for weight Can lead to type II diabetes
Omega-3 fatty acids	Omega-3 esters Lovaza® (Omacor®)	Increased lean body mass	Underutilized due to stigma as a nonprescription Food supplement
Thalidomide	Thalomid®	Decreased weight loss	Some sedation; must use effective barrier contraception to avoid teratogenic effects

an effective substance in cancer *cachexia* in patients with advanced lung or colorectal cancer.[14]

Studies looking at ghrelin-like compounds are underway and have received a "fast-track" designation by the U.S. FDDA.[15–17] Ghrelin is a circulating peptide hormone, principally produced in stomach cells, which has various physiological actions, including appetite stimulation and muscle-building (anabolic) effects which oppose leptin. Where leptin is thought to decrease appetite, Ghrelin can increase food intake.

Thalidomide can help in calorie retention. When using thalidomide, the need for barrier contraceptive protection and the drug's associated fatigue often make the burden outweigh the benefit. However, in a study of 50 patients with advanced pancreatic cancer did find it well-tolerated and demonstrated reduced weight loss in the experimental group.[18]

Protection of skeletal muscle from use as an energy source both helps retain weight and allows maintenance of functioning in the most efficient way, helping both retention and demand. The same proposed mechanism that prevents the entry of cytokines into cancer cells is also understood to prevent PIF from entering and degrading the skeletal muscle cell. EPA binds the AA in the cell wall, it is understood to prevent the destructive cytokines from entering the cell that access muscle protein for energy (see Fig. 36–2.).

Demand. Moderating the amount of calories a patient uses—*demand*—can help maintain weight when caloric *supply* and *retention* are maximized. A certain amount of energy, resting energy potential, is used by the individual to maintain basic metabolic function. "Budgeting" activities by prioritizing how and what one can and will do is an often difficult accommodation to cancer illness. Restorative sleep and naps may help further make the most out of preserved energy. The role of exercise in preserving function for both basic metabolic processes and necessary and enjoyable activities has encouraged a number of clinical trials of exercise to improve quality of life during and after cancer treatment.

These practical solutions may be enhanced by optimal energy *supply* and *retention*, demonstrating how these areas are interrelated. The *resting energy potential* or the energy required to maintain functioning has been enhanced with EPA in one pancreatic cancer study.[19]

MODEL OF EARLY NUTRITIONAL INTERVENTION AS PART OF COMPREHENSIVE SYMPTOM MANAGEMENT

Nutritional intervention and support is a cornerstone of early, comprehensive symptom management in cancer. It can easily be implemented in outpatient ambulatory and inpatient practices, and requires clinician, patient, and family participation. Nutritional intervention should be incorporated as part of routine care along with the other core services provided by the physician, nurse, nutritionist, and oncology social worker. Physical, occupational therapists, speech and swallowing therapists, psychologists, and pastoral care counselors can each bring their expertise to help patients and families receive *early* in treatment.

TEAM APPROACH

Because of the importance placed on maintaining the patient's state of nourishment, a multidimensional approach is warranted. After initial contact with the oncologist and oncology nurse in the inpatient or ambulatory setting, patients should be referred to the other disciplines for screening and initial evaluation. Patients are sometimes seen by the inpatient hospital dietician, who may provide initial information and reinforce the importance of proper nutrition. Since most cancer treatment continues on an ambulatory basis, patients undergoing radiotherapy or chemotherapy are regularly seen and evaluated by the multidisciplinary oncology team. As a patient requires assistance with food choices, better defining quantities to eat, or specific instruction regarding oral supplements, PEGs, enteral supplies or the optimal use of vitamins, antioxidants, or over-the-counter supplements, the oncology nutritionist serves a vital role in the continuity of care and education.

IMPORTANCE OF PSYCHOSOCIAL INTERVENTION WITH WEIGHT LOSS

Clarification of information reinforces contact with the other team members and often creates the bridge for a patient and family to access psychosocial care. Instead of being an "add-on" service or selected by only the most distressed patients and or families, good psychosocial support provides multiple benefits. Ameliorating any of distress within the dimensions of cancer treatment, including the nutritional needs, can offer a solid entry point for patients and families who may initially refuse meeting the social worker or pastoral counselor for fear of stigma or weakness. Practical issues involved in nutritional management, such as accessing insurance or entitlements for oral or enteral supplements or opening doors to community-based agencies, easily segue into an opportunity to assess the patient and family's coping styles.

BEYOND THE INITIAL TREATMENT PERIOD

The treatment team must monitor patients during treatment and then through the recovery process. This is especially important during the transitions onto and then off enteral tube feeding, where there is a particular need to provide in-depth counseling for patients with altered taste and special food texture requirements. Creating this structure gives patients and families the optimal information and guidance, and limits their acting on untested information from well-meaning friends or internet sites. The treatment team benefits as well, emphasizing multidisciplinary input and cohesion while improving patient satisfaction with care, outcomes, and quality of life.

Too often, concerned patients and families hope "If he would only eat just a little more...," would reverse the complexities of cancer-associated and cancer-induced weight and appetite loss. Sadly, such a uni-dimensional approach will not reverse the intricate phenomena that so greatly diminish physical and psychic energy. With the efforts of the multidisciplinary team, the effects of weight and appetite loss can be blunted or forestalled resulting in improving the patient's and family's quality of life.

REFERENCES

1. Muscurtoli M, Bossola M, Aversa Z, Bellantone R, Fanelli FR Prevention and treatment of cancer cachexia: new insights into an old problem. *Eur J Ca.* 2006 Nov;42:31–41.

2. Kondrup J, Johansen N, Plum L, et al. Incidence of nutritional risk and causes of inadequate nutritional care in hospitals. *Clin Nutr.* 2002 Dec;21(6):461–468.

3. DeWys WD, Begg C, Lavin PT, et al. Prognostic effect of weight-loss prior to chemotherapy in cancer patients. *Am J Med.* 1980;69:491–497.

4. Andreyev HJ, Norman AR, Oates J, Cunningham D. Why do patients with weight loss have a worse outcome when undergoing chemotherapy for gastrointestinal malignancies? *Eur J Cancer.* 1998;34(4):503–509.

5. Boddaert MS, Gerritsen WR, Pinedo HM. On our way to targeted therapy for cachexia in cancer? *Curr Opin Oncol.* 2006;18(4):335–340.

6. Hutton JL, Martin L, Field CJ, et al. Dietary patterns in patients with advanced cancer: implications for anorexia-cachexia therapy. *Am J Clin Nutr.* 2006;84(5):1163–1170.

7. Osei-Hyiaman D. Endocannabinoid system in cancer cachexia. *Curr Opin Clin Nutr Metab Care.* 2007;10(4):443–448.

8. Dewey A, Baughan C, Dean T, et al. Eicosapentaenoic acid (EPA, an omega-3 fatty acid from fish oils) for the treatment of cancer cachexia. *Cochrane Database Syst Rev.* 2007;(1):CD004597.

9. Bruera E, Strasser F, Palmer JL, et al. Effect of fish oil on appetite and other symptoms in patients with advanced cancer and anorexia/cachexia: a double blind, placebo controlled study. *J Clin Oncol.* 2003;21(1):129–134.

10. Jatoi A, Rowland K, Loprinzi CL, et al. An eicosapentaenoic acid supplement versus megestrol acetate versus both for patients with cancer-associated wasting: a north central cancer treatment group and national cancer institute of Canada collaborative effort. *J Clin Oncol.* 2004;22(12):2469–2476.

11. Lundholm K, Körner U, Gunnebo L, et al. Insulin treatment in cancer cachexia: effects on survival, metabolism, and physical functioning. *Clin Cancer Res.* 2007;13(9):2699–2706.

12. Nissen SL, Abumrod NN. Nutritional role of leucine metabolite β-hydroxymethylbutyrate. *J Nutr Biochem.* 1997;8:300–311.

13. May, PE, Barber A, D'Olimpio J. Reversal of cancer-related wasting using oral supplementation with a combination of β-hyroxymethyl butyrate, arginine and glutamine. *Am J Surg.* 2002;183:471–479.

14. Kosty MP, Fleishman SB, Herndon JE, et al. Cisplatin, Vinblastine and Hydrazine Sulfate (NSC 150014) in advanced non-small cell lung cancer (NSCLC): a Randomized Placebo Controlled Double-Blind Phase III Study. A Trial of the Cancer and Leukemia Group B (CALGB 8931). *J Clin Oncol.* 1994;13:1113–1120.

15. DeBoer MD, Zhu XX, Levasseur P, et al. Ghrelin treatment causes increased food intake and retention of lean body mass in a rat model of cancer cachexia. *Endocrinology.* 2007;148(6):3004–3012.

16. Bossola M, Pacelli F, Tortorelli A, Doglietto GB . Cancer cachexia: it's time for more clinical trials. *Ann Surg Oncol.* 2007;14(2):276–285.

17. Business News Rejuvenon's RC-1291 Ghrelin Mimetic Receives Fast Track January 11, 2005. Available at: http://www.ergogenics.org/rc1291.html. Accessed August 31, 2008.

18. Gordon JM, Trebble TM, Ellis RD, Duncan HD, Johns T, Goggin PM Thalidomide in the treatment of cancer cachexia: a randomized controlled trial. *Gut.* 2005;54:540–545.

19. Barber MD, McMillan DC, Preston T, et al. Metabolic response to feeding in weight-losing pancreatic cancer patients and its modulation by a fish-oil-enriched nutritional supplement. *Clin Sci.* 2000;98:389–399.

PART VII

Palliative and Terminal Care

William S. Breitbart, ED

CHAPTER 37

The Role of Palliative Care in Cancer Care Transitions

Scott A. Irwin and Charles F. von Gunten

INTRODUCTION

Transitions are difficult for everyone. In the course of cancer care, many transitions occur for patients, families, and the care teams. The "transition" to palliative care is perceived to be one of the more difficult, but it need not be. Psycho-oncologists are well positioned to support patient, family, and oncologist while they navigate changes in goals of care throughout an illness course.

Palliative care is an approach to the relief of suffering. It grew out of, and includes, hospice care for the terminally ill. It is now clear that it applies to the entire course of illness—from diagnosis to death.[1] As in the situation for Phase I studies of new cancer agents studied first in the terminally ill, palliative care was first demonstrated effective for those near the end of life. However, just as with new anticancer agents, it may be even more effective when it is used earlier in the course of an illness.

Suffering from cancer is substantial. Suffering can have physical, psychological, social, and spiritual components.[2] Of the more than one-third of Americans who will be diagnosed with some type of malignancy during their lifetime, all will suffer in some respects,[1] often beginning with the diagnosis. Attention to the suffering caused by cancer and its treatment is fairly recent, despite the myriad reports describing its manifestations and significance.[3-7] Of all patients with cancer, only 50% will be cured, meaning the cancer is gone and will never come back. Even those that find cure will often continue to suffer in some respect. Despite the many advances in cancer care, the proportion cured has not increased over the past 40 years.[8-10] Over the same period, there has been an increased interest in the field of psycho-oncology. Recently, there have been calls for the seamless integration of palliative care with anticancer care that mirror the calls for integration of psycho-oncology.[11]

It is the purpose of this chapter to describe a model of palliative care that can be woven into oncologic care from diagnosis. When palliative care is seen as extending throughout the course of illness and overall goals of care determine the treatment plan, then transitions can be straightforward and transparent. First, palliative care will be defined. Then, several conceptual frameworks for its role in the comprehensive care of patients with cancer will be presented. Finally, an approach to structuring the conversation for setting goals of care and making transitions when goals of care change will be described. All of these issues are well within the realm of the oncologist and psycho-oncologist in support of the entire cancer care team.

PALLIATIVE CARE

Since the time of Hippocrates there have been two overall goals of medical care: relief of suffering and cure of disease.[12] These goals are shared by the patient as well as healthcare providers. The relative emphasis on cure versus relief of suffering is best determined by, both, the underlying illness and the overall goals of the person who has the illness, within the context of his or her family and culture.

The term "palliate" originated with the Latin term *pallium* which means "cloak" or "cover."[13] While at one time the term palliative care was used as a pejorative for "covering up" the real problem; it is now a superlative; "covering up" the suffering and letting the patient experience the best quality of life possible. The field of palliative care encompasses a wide range of therapeutic interventions that aim to prevent and relieve suffering caused by the multiple issues that patients, families, and caregivers face at any stage during an acute or chronic life-threatening illness. In providing whole-person care to relieve suffering, palliative care attends to all domains of the human experience of illness that may be involved: physical, psychological, social, and spiritual.[14] Quality of life rather than quantity of life is most often the chief aim of those engaged in the delivery of palliative care. Since suffering is experienced by persons, its existence, character, and criteria for relief are best defined by the patient rather than by the physician.[12-14] As persons do not exist in isolation, the relief of suffering requires attention to the care of patients within their framework of beliefs, culture, and loved ones. Suffering is caused by many factors that are rarely limited to the physical domain. As such, tending to the relief of suffering in these domains cannot possibly be accomplished by a single medical discipline—a team approach is required.

Palliative care can be delivered at primary (generalist), secondary (specialist), or tertiary (academic) levels.[15] At the primary level, all physicians, nurses, and other health professionals need basic skills in relieving suffering. In this sense, the palliative care skills one would expect of every medical, radiation, surgical, or pediatric oncologist qualify as primary palliative care. One might expect oncology professionals to even have exemplary skills in this area. Secondary levels refer to specialist physicians and services. Palliative Medicine is the term coined to denote the physician subspecialty concerned with the relief of suffering within the larger interdisciplinary model of palliative care.

Palliative medicine is now a recognized specialty. The Royal College of Physicians in Great Britain recognized palliative medicine as a physician specialty in 1987.[16] This recognition came only after it had been demonstrated that there was an established body of medical knowledge that uniquely pertained to a distinct patient population. Later, the Royal College of Physicians and Surgeons in Australia recognized the specialty. The Royal College of Physicians and Surgeons and the College of Family Physicians of Canada established 1-year postgraduate training programs in the field in 1999. Similar recognition as a subspecialty followed in the United States in 2006.[17]

CONCEPTUAL FRAMEWORK

The mental model of the cancer professional treating patients with cancer is of critical importance. Treating cancer is not equivalent to treating a person with cancer. Failure to recognize this has led, in some circumstances, to cause increased suffering while administering anticancer treatment. An exclusively "cure-oriented" approach to cancer can be conceptualized in the following diagram where the time course and goals of such treatment are illustrated (Fig. 37–1).

A patient is first evaluated for some constellation of symptoms for which a diagnosis of cancer is made. Evaluation and treatment is directed toward the eradication, reversal, or substantial control of the disease. Symptoms help elucidate the diagnosis and course of treatment. This model of treatment can be characterized as disease-oriented and pathophysiologically based. Clinicians are engaged in a "war on cancer" and the patient dies in spite of "doing everything" and maintaining a "fighting spirit" to the end. The death is often viewed as a "casualty" in the war on the cancer.

Unfortunately this model leaves many patients and the doctors feeling as if they have failed if the cancer "wins" and the patient dies. Following the logic of this model may actually cause suffering. Working within this

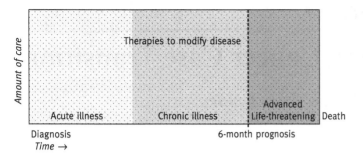

Fig. 37–1. Model of cancer care where only therapies directed at the disease are considered as part of standard care.

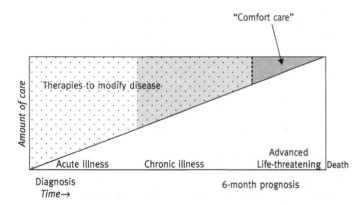

Fig. 37–2. Model of cancer care where anti–disease therapy diminishes over time as it becomes less and less effective.

framework, well-meaning clinicians may administer anticancer or other therapies of which there is no evidence of benefit as a way to demonstrate their character as "fighters" and demonstrating rejection of the possibility that they are "quitters" often with substantial adverse effects.

For oncologists who try to modify the approach diagrammed in Fig. 37–1 to include only medical care for which there is evidence of efficacy for the stage of disease and the likely outcomes of treatment, the patient and family may perceive the care to be more like that shown in Fig. 37–2.[18] In recognition of the situation when the disease is progressive and treatment modalities are no longer effective, "comfort care" measures may be instituted. This last period, if it occurs at all, is often of short duration (sometimes hours to days) and may consist only of analgesics, sedatives, and a private room. Quite often, this model does not include explicit consideration of nonphysical aspects of a person's illness experience or that of the person's family. Further, once "comfort care" has been recommended, there can be a perception that the oncologists are no longer engaged in the care of the patient. That is to say, the patient and family often feel that the oncologist shows diminished attention to the patient over time. Unfortunately, in many instances, this is true, as the oncologist struggles with feelings of failure and discomfort with the death and dying.[19]

This can lead to a major cause for patient and family dissatisfaction with the healthcare system—a feeling of abandonment. Although the severity of illness may be increasing, within this framework the attention of the oncologist and other healthcare providers often diminishes when the evidence shows there is "nothing more to do" for the disease.

In addition, the implication of abandonment may lead to strident demands from patients and families to "do more, do everything." In the absence of a better treatment framework that addresses these issues, the oncologist may give in to patient demands and revert to the model in Fig. 37–1, offering treatment that is of no medical benefit in the service of patient autonomy. Such treatment results in increased suffering for the patient and family independent of adverse events, as important issues that surround death and dying are ignored.

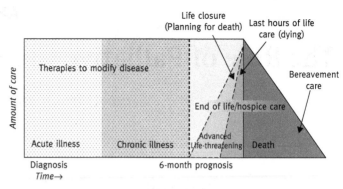

Fig. 37–3. Model of cancer care where palliative care begins after efforts directed at the cancer end.

In appreciation that the models of care diagrammed in Figs. 37–1 and 37–2 do not adequately address issues of patient suffering, Dr. Cicely Saunders in England introduced the hospice model of palliative care.[14] Working primarily with cancer patients, she recognized that suffering might be produced not only from the cancer, but also by medical efforts to control the disease. She also recognized that the physical, psychological, social, and spiritual aspects of suffering were inadequately addressed. Dr. Saunders founded St. Christopher's Hospice in 1967 to pilot a new model of inpatient care for patients for whom curative therapy was not available or was no longer desired. It is useful to note that she tried to advance these ideas in standard hospitals and hospices at the time. However, because she was unable to influence contemporary patterns of care for these patients, she developed her own facility where she could test her ideas. She demonstrated that an interdisciplinary team approach to the care of the patient and family that continues into a bereavement period after the patient's death is effective for the relief of suffering. The hospice concept has been widely adopted because of its demonstrated benefits for patients and families.

Sadly, this model leaves a sharp demarcation between disease-oriented therapy and hospice care. Fig. 37–3 shows the most common position of hospice care in the overall scheme of cancer patient care introduced in Fig. 37–1. This model suggests that the goal of medical care is *first* cure of cancer, *then* relieve suffering. Although hospice care aims to address aspects of patient suffering not usually addressed during "standard medical treatment," the period of hospice care espoused in Fig. 37–3 is often short and comes at the end of a long care process. The median length of hospice care for 1.3 million patients in the United States in 2006 was 20.6 days with about one-third of patients receiving hospice care for 7 days or less.[20] Only approximately one-third of eligible patients received hospice care in the United States that year. With this model there is a sharp discontinuity between the previous cancer care and hospice care, which can leave patients feeling abandoned by their oncologists. Another problem with this model is it suggests a dichotomy between curative/life-prolonging care and palliative care. Yet, good sense dictates that the two goals are not mutually exclusive and can be pursued simultaneously. Integrating curative or life-prolonging treatments with the relief of suffering should be the goal. Palliative treatments are not adjuncts or complementary to "conventional" cancer care, but are an essential part of good cancer care. In fact, when oncologists integrate palliative care in their practice, the role of the palliative care specialist is only to help with the difficult cases. When considered carefully, no care provider would suggest waiting to introduce measures for alleviating suffering and improving quality of life until either all attempts at cure have been exhausted or the patient and family plead for such efforts to stop.

Many palliative care approaches to illness can and should precede the point at which referral to a hospice program is appropriate. For example, aggressive control of pain and other bothersome symptoms, setting goals of care, and addressing the psychosocial effects of a cancer diagnosis should co-dominate the very *beginning* of contemporary cancer care.[1,21–24] Where the oncologist feels uncertain with addressing these symptoms, a palliative care specialist can be helpful as a consultant or in a co-management role. Palliative care specialists can be especially helpful when it comes to setting goals of care, both for curative

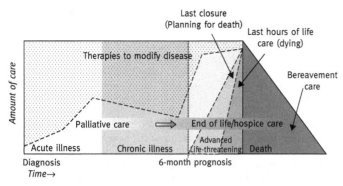

Fig. 37-4. Model of cancer care where palliative care begins at diagnosis and is integrated throughout the course of cancer care.

treatment and symptom relief, though the whole illness experience. A psycho-oncologist can facilitate these discussions as well. In addition to their disease status, a patient's goals and priorities should determine which treatment approaches will be most valuable to them. A treatment plan that is directed by those goals should be provided and adhered to by the care team.[25] These goals and treatment plans will usually evolve as the illness changes and should be reevaluated often. This care scheme is shown in Fig. 37-4.

In this model, palliative care is given simultaneously with curative care, and hospice care represents the completion of comprehensive cancer care, not an alternative to, or an abrupt change from, the preceding care plan.[26] Thus abrupt transitions are avoided and the best of all types of care are provided throughout the illness.

NEGOTIATING TRANSITIONS AND GOALS OF CARE

Clearly, negotiating goals of care throughout an illness process is the important clinical skill rather than conceptualizing care as abrupt transitions. In other words, an abrupt transition from curative care to palliative care suggests earlier communication and conceptualizing were omitted or were incomplete.

Along the trajectory of cancer care, several trigger situations invite the patient and healthcare provider to reflect upon and discuss goals of care. These include general advance care planning[27,28] (1) at the time of diagnosis, (2) at first and subsequent episodes of progression or relapse, and (3) when initiation of hospice care is recommended.

Evidence shows that patients are open to such discussions. Studies done in North America and Europe show that between 85% and 95% of patients want to have honest discussions with their healthcare providers regarding life-threatening diseases.[29,30] Evidence also suggests that oncologists struggle with and often avoid such discussions.[31,32] Some studies suggest that oncologists generally fail to adequately address their patients' emotional concerns and often are deficient in the skills necessary to handle the emotional component of discourse with patients. Fortunately, research shows oncologists and others can learn these skills.[33-36]

A six-step approach to structuring such conversations can be used for any situation during the disease trajectory such as advance care planning, discussing treatment options, or when introducing hospice care. This protocol has been adapted from a widely used communication model for the delivery of bad news.[35,36] Specific examples for the discussion of resuscitation orders or when introducing hospice care have been described elsewhere.[37,38]

The protocol uses the general principle of shared decision making. Shared decision making as a process puts great emphasis on patient autonomy while acknowledging the physician's responsibility to make treatment recommendations that are based both on the patient's stated overall goals of care as well as the physician's medical expertise and evidence-based medicine. Psycho-oncologists and palliative medicine specialists are well poised to facilitate such conversations.

This approach for determining goals of care discussions reflects common communication patterns in North America. Studies of healthcare decision making in other parts of the world show that different cultures prioritize these values differently. The most common variation is to place less emphasis on autonomy in favor of family-centered decision making (examples of beneficence and nonmalefeasance). For example, more than 90% of U.S. oncologists share a new diagnosis of cancer with their patients.[39] In contrast, only 44% of hospital-based and 25% of outpatient oncologists in Great Britain have been shown to do so.[40,41] A study of European physicians showed that, in northern and western parts of Europe, they generally feel that a new cancer diagnosis should be shared with patients whereas their colleagues in southern and eastern parts of Europe considered withholding information regarding the diagnosis of a life-threatening condition as part of their duty to protect their patients, even if patients expressed a wish to be informed. A study from China indicates that patients there are only rarely informed of a new diagnosis of cancer.[42] In African countries such as Nigeria, Egypt, or South Africa, the type and amount of information shared seems to depend on patient factors such as level of education or socioeconomic status. Only 18% of South American oncologists think their patients would want to know a diagnosis of cancer.[43-45]

Asking patients and families what they want to know before giving information can be helpful in guiding further discussion while staying within cultural norms and the wishes of the patient.[46-48] In some cases, patients quite happily prefer their families to hear the news and to make decisions for them. Even in North America, there is nothing to prevent a patient from giving his or her autonomy to others.

USING GOALS OF CARE TO NEGOTIATE TRANSITIONS

Eliciting patient preferences is at the center of goals-of-care discussions. Empathic listening, a highly underestimated skill in medical practice, is required to negotiate goals of care. Therefore, it is imperative to start the conversation with an open-ended question followed by active listening. This allows the patient to focus on his or her major concerns and sets the stage for patient-centered care. Active or empathic listening then includes nonverbal communication skills that show full attention such as good eye contact and leaning toward the patient as well as verbal empathic listening techniques such as reflection, paraphrasing, and validation.[49]

Psychooncolgists and palliative medicine specialists can be of great help in these discussions, as there exists evidence that oncologists struggle with these discussions. For example, it has been shown that oncologists, on average, interrupt their patients only 20 seconds after they begin to speak. It has also been shown that oncologists often miss empathic opportunities[50] and tend to use close-ended questions in an attempt to retrieve information as fast as possible. This risks that patients never get to address their major concerns. Unfortunately, under these circumstances, the majority of patients leave the office without ever having their concerns addressed or with a feeling that they have been "heard."[51]

It is helpful to give medical information in short phrases using words that the patient can understand, with frequent pauses to check for patient response and understanding. The higher the emotional impact of the given information, the less likely the patient is to hear what is being said. It might therefore be necessary to repeat the information at a later time and more than once. Not only can psycho-oncologists and palliative medicine specialists facilitate these discussions, they might also be able to reflect back to their oncologist colleagues these facts in the service of educating and improving oncologist skill and sense of competence in having these discussions.[52-55]

6 STEPS TO SETTING GOALS

A step-wise approach to goals-of-care discussions helps to remind the clinician to include all major components of the discussion. This is particularly true for those who are inexperienced or early in their training where this skill has generally not yet been learned.[48] The six steps include (1) preparing and establishing an appropriate setting for the discussion, (2) asking the patient and family what they understand about the patient's health situation, (3) finding out what they expect will happen in the future and what they want to know, (4) discussing overall goals and treatment options, (5) responding to emotions, and (6) establishing and implementing a plan.[56]

Prepare and establish an appropriate setting for the discussion. Preparation for a goal-setting conversation by knowledge of the clinical facts of the case and the evidence-based outcomes regarding stage specific prognosis, chemotherapy, radiation, surgery, and cardiopulmonary resuscitation is a must. In general, patients are more interested in concrete descriptions of abilities ("Life is not worth living if I won't be able to speak.") than in the details of interventions ("That means that we would have to put a tube down your throat that is about as thick as your finger."), where often functional consequences are omitted.

Reflection upon the expected emotional responses and possible identity issues that might arise for the patient or the physician before entering the discussion is helpful. The phrase, "I'm a fighter" or "I always fight for my patients" are expressions of patient identity, not expressions of desire for a specific plan of cancer care.

The meeting should occur in a private and comfortable place when those who need to be present can be present. The atmosphere should be unhurried and undisturbed, with the clinician sitting at eye level. After general introductions, the purpose of the meeting should be made clear. Examples of introductory phrases are

- I'd like to talk to you about your overall goals of cancer care.
- I'd like to review where we are with your cancer and make plans for the future.
- I'd like to discuss aspects of your cancer care today that I discuss with all my patients.

Before continuing, asking if anyone else should be present for this discussion can avoid serious pitfalls. If others need to be present, the meeting can be postponed accordingly.

Ask the patient and family what they understand. Starting with an open-ended question to elicit what the patient understands about his or her current health situation is the best approach. This is an important question, and one that many clinicians skip as their nervousness drives them to speak first. If the physician is doing all the talking, the rest of the conversation is unlikely to go well. Example phrases are

- What do you understand about the cancer?
- Tell me about how you see things are going.
- What do you understand from what I and the other doctors have told you about your cancer?

Open-ended questions have been shown to establish trust and set the tone for patient-centered decision making. Structured this way, the answers help the care team assess and address misconceptions or conflicting or missing information. They also allow a quick glimpse into the patient's emotional response to his or her current health state, such as fear, anger, or acceptance. More time might need to be spent to clarify the current situation before the patient is able to address future medical decisions.

Find out what they expect will happen. For the patient who has a good understanding of the status of their disease, the third step is to ask the patient to consider their future. Examples of how to start are

- What do you expect in the future?
- Have you ever thought about how you want things to be if you were much more ill?
- What are you hoping for?

This step allows the care provider to listen while the patient contemplates and verbalizes his/her goals, hopes, and fears. This step creates an opportunity to clarify what is likely or unlikely to happen. Follow-up questions might be needed to better understand the patient's vision of the future, as well as his or her values and priorities. If there is a significant discrepancy between what the physician expects and what the patient expects from the future, this is the time to discover it.

Some cancer care teams find they are speaking for the first time with a patient and family late in the course of treatment. Consequently, this should be acknowledged, and often, before proceeding, it is wise to ask how much the patient wants to know about his/her condition. This provides a protection against giving unwanted information to a patient whose culture or personal preferences are either not to know or not to take the decision-making role. Examples include

- Some patients like all the information, others like me to speak with someone else in the family. I wonder what is true for you.
- Tell me how you like to receive medical information.
- Some people are detail oriented, some want just the big picture, which do you prefer?

Discuss overall goals and specific options. Now that the stage has been set with a mutual understanding of the patient's present and anticipated future, a discussion of overall goals of care and specific options can ensue. Allowing the patient to reflect upon goals that might still be realistic despite reduced functional abilities and a limited life expectancy can be a very effective tool to maintain hope.[36,49] Insight into the patient's values and priorities will help structure the conversation of medical options and guide expert opinion. Using language that the patient can understand and giving information in short phrases is best. In general, patients prefer a focus on treatment outcomes rather than the details of medical interventions. Stopping frequently to check for emotional reactions, to ask for clarifications, and to clarify misunderstandings will improve the communication between patient and care team.

As an introduction to specific treatment options, summarize the patient's stated overall goals and priorities. In following the principle of shared decision making, clarify that recommendations are based, both, on the patient's stated overall goals of care as well as medical expert opinion. For example

- You have told me your goal is to try for a cure while staying pain free.
- I understand your goal is to feel like you are a fighter and not a quitter. You also said you understand that you can both hope for the best, but plan for the worst.
- You have told me that being at home with your family is your number one priority and that the frequent trips to the hospital have become very bothersome for you.
- If I heard you correctly, your first priority is to live to participate in your granddaughter's wedding in June.
- I heard you say that your goal is not to be a burden to your wife and children.

Beginning the discussion of treatment options from the patient's perspective and evaluating treatment options according to their potential to achieve the patient's overall goals can be a great help in building trust between the patient and healthcare provider. Working to achieve realistic goals is inherently hopeful. The goals may change over time, but the hopeful attitude about achieving them can be sustained.

Respond to emotions. Patients, families, and healthcare providers may experience profound emotions in response to an exploration of goals of care. It shouldn't be surprising that patients, when confronting evidence that initial therapy didn't work or that the end of their life is sooner than they thought, might cry, become angry, or myriad other responses. Parents of children with life-threatening diseases are especially likely to be emotional and will need extra support from the healthcare team. In contrast to common worries in the healthcare community though, emotional responses tend to be brief and therapeutic. Psycho-oncologists should be well versed in providing this type of support and can help both the oncologist and patient to deal with the emotional response.

Responses should be sympathetic. The most profound initial response a physician can make might be silence and the offering of a facial tissue. Consider using phrases such as

- I can see this makes you sad.
- Tell me more about how you are feeling.
- People in your situation often get angry. I wonder what you are feeling right now.
- I notice you are silent. Will you tell me what you are thinking?
- Many people experience strong emotions. I wonder if that is true for you.

A common barrier to this step is the physician's fear to precipitate overwhelming emotional outbursts that they might not be able to handle. As such, conversations between physicians and their patients often remain in the cognitive realm where emotions are not addressed. The best way to overcome this barrier is to learn how to sympathetically respond to patient emotions and to learn to be comfortable with silence. The majority of patients are embarrassed by being emotional and keep their expressions brief. This is because most patients have adequate coping skills and appreciate the presence of a doctor while they work through the experience and their emotions. As with most aspects of being a physician, a sense of competence and confidence imparted to the patient leads to a willingness to engage in the challenge on the part of both parties.

Establish and implement the plan. Establishing and implementing a plan that will meet the agreed upon goals, aids in coping, sets goals and expectations, and lays out the tasks at hand. The plan should be clear and roles and responsibilities should be understood by everyone involved. Consider using language like the following:

- You said that it is most important for you to continue to live independently for as long as possible. Since you are doing so well right now and need your current breathing machine only at night, we will continue what we are doing. However, when your breathing becomes worse, you do not want to be placed on a continuous breathing machine. We will then focus on keeping you comfortable with medicines to making sure that you do not feel short of breath.
- The different regimens we have used to fight your cancer are not working. There is no other anticancer therapy that I think will be effective. We discussed your options at this point including getting a second opinion from one of my oncology colleagues or asking a hospice program to get involved in your care. In light of what you told me about your worries about being a burden to your family, you thought that hospice care might be the best option at this point because you would get extra help at home from the hospice team members that come to see you at your house. I am going to call the hospice team today and arrange for them to call you in the morning so they can see you and explain more about what they offer. We can talk more after you see them.
- We'll start combination chemotherapy and radiotherapy next week. We won't know whether it's working for about 2 months when we repeat your scans. If it is not working at that time, we will have exhausted all of our anticancer therapy options. I'll ask the palliative care team to see you after you're admitted so they can help me with your symptoms and to give you and your family some support. They can continue to see you when you follow-up with me as an outpatient.
- I'll ask our social worker to help you finish those advance directive forms I gave you at your next office visit. She can then make copies and get them into the medical record.
- From what you've said, I think getting hospice care involved at home seems to be the option that best helps you to realize your goals.
- Let's try this third-line chemotherapy and treat your nausea with a different drug regimen. We'll repeat the scans after the second cycle. If the cancer is smaller or the same size, we'll continue. If it's bigger, we'll stop chemotherapy and get the hospice program involved.
- You don't feel you need the help, but the hospice team can help your family cope through the support from the nurse, chaplain, and social worker. In addition, the bereavement team will look out for them after you are gone.
- It is clear you want to try all options to extend your life as long as possible, even if there is a small chance they will work. So, we'll start fifth-line chemotherapy. If you develop an infection that is serious, we will care for you in an intensive care setting with maximal support. However, if you are unable to communicate, and there is no reasonable chance of recovery, you want life support to be stopped and for us to let you die comfortably.

It is often helpful to ask the patient or family member to summarize the plan and underlying reasoning in their own words to ensure understanding. Especially for the emotionally overwhelmed patient, it is important that there is good continuity of care. Ensuring this continuity, for example, by arranging for follow-up appointments, speaking to the referring clinician, or writing the appropriate orders, is part of the oncologist's and care team's responsibility.

COMMON PITFALLS IN GOALS-OF-CARE DISCUSSIONS

There are a number of common pitfalls that fall into several categories. These are outlined below.

Inadequate preparation

- **Having an agenda:** If a physician enters a room with a predetermined agenda (e.g., to "get the DNR" or to "stop this futile treatment") trouble may ensue.[53] By trying to understand patient values and priorities first, the care team can make appropriate medical recommendations which are most likely to achieve the patient's goals. An awareness of possible agendas of all parties involved in a goals-of-care discussion such as the physicians, patients and families, consultants, or even hospital administrators assists in understanding the different perspectives and can help prevent adversarial outcomes.
- **Stakeholders not identified:** A picture-perfect goals-of-care discussion might have occurred and everyone seemed to have agreed upon a reasonable plan, but then the "cousin from out of town" flew in and threw out the whole plan. Before starting a goals-of-care discussion, make sure that all stakeholders are either physically present, included over the phone, or otherwise represented to the extent possible. Stakeholders also include other healthcare providers involved in the patient's care.
- **Homework not done:** Be prepared to answer questions regarding the outcomes and evidence of discussed interventions, such as resuscitation survival data, prognosis, and the risks and benefits of various of treatment interventions. Just as in any other informed consent discussion, patients need accurate information to make good decisions.

Inadequate discussion of overall goals and specific options

- **Inadequate information giving:** Each person handles information differently. While some patients want to understand the numerical probability of success or failure of specific interventions, most people do not comprehend statistical information. Many clinicians share an excessive amount of medical details (because its familiar or interesting to themselves) using language that the patient cannot understand. The actual information given should be tailored to the patient's needs and learning style. It might be helpful to ask the patient to repeat the information back using his own words.

Improper shared decision making, informed consenting, and decision-making capacity assessment

- **The person either does not have, or is inappropriately denied, decision-making capacity:** Before asking someone to make a decision regarding goals of care, assess if that person has decision-making capacity. This is usually the case if a person can summarize the decision in his or her own words, including weighing the risks and benefits and demonstrating appropriate underlying reasoning. Patients with delirium, dementia, depression, or other mental health problems may be able to demonstrate decision-making capacity. Since decision-making capacity is specific for each decision and at a specific point in time, patients might very well be able to make consistent decisions regarding their care. This right should not be taken away from them inappropriately. Nor should a choice that was stable while the person had decision-making capacity be reversed if they lose that capacity but other stakeholders have different opinions on that decision. Furthermore, simple "yes" or "no" answers do not imply understanding, and decision-making capacity should never be assumed.

- **"Restaurant-menu medicine"**: The process of shared decision making strongly values patient autonomy but also recognizes the duty of the healthcare provider to make recommendations, based on his or her medical expertise, that are most likely to achieve the patient's stated goals. Many physicians skip the step of giving an expert opinion, often leaving themselves frustrated as the "waiter," offering a wide array of all possible medical options, as if they were items on a restaurant menu for the patient to choose. This can leave the patient feeling lost and overwhelmed as well. Physicians are under no obligation to offer any single therapy, especially if there is no belief of benefit to the patient and possible risk of harm. Only those options with potential benefit and within the patients goals of care should be offered.

PEARLS REGARDING THE DISCUSSION OF GOALS OF CARE

- **Start with the "big picture"**: Many healthcare providers skip steps 2 and 3 (finding out what the patient understands and expects to happen) and lunge straight into detailed descriptions of medical interventions. These two simple steps help set the stage. They show that the clinician is interested in the patient and his/her experience and wants to support them to achieve their goals. Starting from the patient's perspective not only establishes trust and a feeling of safety for the patient, it also makes giving recommendations much easier later on. When the "big picture" goals are clearly understood, the discussion of specific medical interventions most commonly fall quickly into place.
- **Pay attention to nonverbal language**: Approximately 50% of communication between people happens nonverbally. Sitting down, maintaining eye contact, leaning forward, and a nod of the head in response to a patient talking all communicate interest and concern.[57] Similar behaviors in the patient or family member suggest they are listening. Standing, pacing, breaking eye contact, scowling, or whispering to other family members suggest there may be a problem.
- **Deferring autonomy is an act of autonomy**: Concerned family member sometimes ask that healthcare information not be disclosed to the identified patient. This can make clinicians feel very uneasy, as it interferes with their understanding of patient autonomy. Less skilled oncologists tell the truth over the objections of patient or family in a misplaced sense of duty. More skilled oncologists verbalize understanding for the family members concerns and then convey a need to check with the patient if this is how he/she would like to proceed (if the care team hasn't done that already). When the patient is seen alone, he/she can be asked how they would like to handle medical information and decision making. Questions such as: "Some people want to know all medical information as we find it and discuss all options with the doctor. Others would rather have their children make decisions and do not want to have to deal with the medical information. Where do you stand?" can be helpful.
- **Cultural competence**: In multicultural societies, such as the United States, physicians are apt to care for patients and families from many different backgrounds. The term culture is used here in the broad sense and includes ethnic, religious, and social. Each culture has its own values and language. Sensitivity to differences in cultural background helps to facilitate communication and understanding. When inquiring about cultural backgrounds sentences such as: "People from different backgrounds handle medical decision making very differently. Is there anything that we should be aware of regarding your care?" might be appropriate. It can also be very helpful to be sensitive to the "culture" of the facilities or other medical specialties involved in the patients' care to help avoid conflicts or misunderstandings.
- **Validate "unrealistic" or conflicting goals**: Physicians are sometimes frustrated by their patients' "unrealistic" goals. "They just don't get it." is a common reason for palliative care consultation requests. Many people have some hopes that might not be very realistic ("I wish I could win the lottery."), but still valid. The great difference lies in how these hopes are handled: are people leading a life counting on what seems an unrealistic hope? An often cited example of this is a terminally ill parent who is unable to make the necessary arrangements for his/her minor children. A useful strategy is to support hope, but at the same time assist in making appropriate plans for future needs with a "Plan B" approach: "While we hope for plan A, lets also prepare for plan B, just in case." Another useful way to validate the patient's hope is the "I wish" statement, for example: "I wish that were possible. Whatever happens we will be there for you."[58] It is often similarly distressing to healthcare providers when patients verbalize conflicting goals over time. "I want to be aggressive but I don't want to keep coming to the hospital" is an example. Acknowledge that conflicting goals are common, for example, "I wish I could eat ice cream three times a day and still be as slim as I was when I was 20." In end-of-life care especially, intermittent denial of terminal prognoses verbalized as unrealistic hopes can be an effective way of coping. As long as patients are not making decisions that will harm them or others, it can be accepted and worked with as a coping mechanism.
- **Pay attention to emotions and identity issues**: Promoting understanding, comfort, trust, and thereby successful discussion and decision making is of the upmost importance. Emotional awareness is at core of empathic healthcare and allows for a true, authentic, and ultimately successful relationship between clinician and patient.[59]

SUMMARY

The mental model of the relationship between palliative care and anticancer care is important to negotiating transitions in care. For most patients with cancer, transitions can be predicted at four times: (1) diagnosis of cancer, (2) recurrence of cancer, (3) worsening cancer despite therapy, and (4) lack of efficacy of cancer treatment. A model of integrated anticancer and palliative care can help smooth these transitions. Preparing for and addressing goals of care periodically over the course of a patient's illness is an important part of patient-centered care and has been shown to increase patient satisfaction and decrease patient stress and anxiety. Simple steps can be taken to ensure good goals of care discussions. Psycho-oncologists are well poised to assist oncologists with these discussions and educate physicians about improving such interactions. Goal-oriented care sustains hopefulness for both patient and clinician.

REFERENCES

1. World Health Organization. *Palliative care*. Geneva; 2007. Available at: http://www.who.int/cancer/palliative/definition/en/. Accessed September 30, 2008.

2. National Consensus Project for Quality Palliative Care. Clinical practice guidelines for quality palliative care, executive summary. *J Palliat Med*. 2004;7:611–627.

3. The SUPPORT Principal Investigators. A controlled trial to improve care for seriously ill hospitalized patients. *JAMA*. 1995;274:1591–1598.

4. Vachon ML, Kristjanson L, Higginson I. Psychosocial issues in palliative care. *J Pain Symptom Manage*. 1995;10:142–50.

5. Field MJ, Cassel, CK. Approaching death: improving care at the end of life. Committee on care at the end of life, Division of Health Care Services, Institute of Medicine, National Academy of Sciences; 1997.

6. Foley K, Gelband H, (eds). *Improving palliative care for cancer*. National Cancer Policy Board, National Research Council, National Academy of Sciences; 2001.

7. National Institutes of Health. State-of-the-Science Conference Statement on Improving End-of-Life Care, NIH Consensus Development Program, December 6–8, 2004.

8. Surveillance Epidemiology and End Results (SEER). National Cancer Institute. Available at: http://seer.cancer.gov/faststats. Accessed September 30, 2008.

9. Bailar JC III, Gornick HC. Cancer undefeated. *N Engl J Med*. 1997;336:1569–1574.

10. Bailar JC III, Smtih EM. Progress against cancer? *N Engl J Med*. 1986;314:1226–1232.

11. Ferris FD, Bruera D, Cherny N, et al. Palliative cancer care a decade later: accomplishments, the need, next steps—from the American Society of Clinical Oncology. *J Clin Oncol*. 2009;27:3052–3058.

12. Cassel EJ. *The nature of suffering and the goals of medicine.* New York: Oxford University Press; 1991.

13. Doyle, D, Hanks GWC, MacDonald N. Introduction. In: Doyle D, Hanks GWC, MacDonald N, (eds). *Oxford textbook of palliative medicine*, 2nd ed. New York: Oxford University Press; 1998.

14. Saunders C. Introduction-history and challenge. In: Saunders C, Sykes N, (eds). *The management of terminal malignant disease.* Boston: Edward Arnold; 1993.

15. von Gunten CF. Secondary and tertiary palliative care in US hospitals. *JAMA.* 2002;287:875–881.

16. Doyle D. Palliative medicine: a UK specialty. *J Palliat Care.* 1994;10:8–9.

17. Von Gunten CF. Bedazzled by a home run. *J Palliat Med.* 2006;9:1036.

18. Mitchell WM, von Gunten CF. The role of palliative medicine in cancer patient care. In: Angelos P, (ed). *Ethical issues in cancer patient care.* 2nd ed. New York City: Springer; 2008.

19. Jackson VA, Mack J, Matsuyama R, et al. A qualitative study of oncologists' approaches to end of life care. *J Palliat Med.* 2008;11:893–906.

20. NHPCO Facts and Figures: Hospice Care in America. November 2007. Available at: http://www.nhpco.org/files/public/Statistics_Research/NHPCO_facts-and-figures_Nov2007.pdf. Accessed September 30, 2008.

21. Task Force on Cancer Care at the End of Life. Cancer care during the last phase of life. *J Clin Oncol.* 1998;1986–1996.

22. National Comprehensive Cancer Network. Clinical Practice Guidelines in Oncology, National Comprehensive Cancer Network, 2005. Available at: www.nccn.org. Accessed August 12, 2009.

23. Gillick M. Rethinking the central dogma of palliative care. *J Palliat Med.* 2005;909–913.

24. MacDonald N. The interface between oncology and palliative medicine. In: Doyle D, Hanks GWC, MacDonald N, (eds). *Oxford textbook of palliative medicine*, 2nd ed. New York: Oxford University Press; 1998.

25. Vollrath A, von Gunten CF. Negotiating goals of care along the illness trajectory. In: Emanuel L, Librach 1, (eds). *Palliative care: Core skills and clinical competencies.* Philadelphia, PA: WB Saunders; 2007:70–82.

26. Levy MH, Back A, Bazargan S, et al. Palliative care. Clinical practice guidelines in oncology. *J Natl Compr Canc Netw.* 2006 Sep;4(8):776–818.

27. Emanuel LL, von Gunten CF, Ferris FD. Advance care planning. *Arch Fam Med.* 2000;9(10):1181–1187.

28. Hickman SE, Hammes BJ, Moss AH, Tolle SW. Hope for the future: achieving the original intent of advance directives. *Hastings Cent Rep.* 2005 Nov-Dec;S26–S30.

29. Meredith C, Symonds P, Webster L, et al. Informational needs of cancer patients in West Scotland: cross sectional survey of patients' views. *BMJ.* 1996;313:724–726.

30. Parker PA, Baile WF, de Moor C, Lenzi R, Kudelka AP, Cohen L. Breaking bad news about cancer: patients' preferences for communication. *J Clin Oncol.* 2001;19:2049–2056.

31. Back AL, Arnold RM, Baile WF, Tulsky JA, Fryer-Edwards K. Approaching difficult communication tasks in oncology. *CA Cancer J Clin.* 2005;55:164–177.

32. Maguire P. Improving communication with cancer patients. *Eur J Cancer.* 1999;35:2058–2065.

33. Lenzi R, Baile WF, Berek J, et al. Design conduct and evaluation of a communication course for oncology fellows. *J Cancer Educ.* 2005;20:143–149.

34. Back AL, Arnold RM, Tulsky JA, et al. Teaching communication skills to medical oncology fellows. *J Clin Oncol,* 2003;21:2433–2436.

35. von Gunten CF, Ferris FD, Emanuel L. Ensuring competency in end-of-life care: communication and relational skills. *JAMA.* 2000;284(23):3051–3057.

36. Von Roenn J, von Gunten CF. Setting goals to maintain hope. *J Clin Oncol.* 2003;21:570–574.

37. von Gunten CF. Discussing do-not-resuscitate status. *J Clin Oncol.* 2001;19:1576–1581.

38. von Gunten CF. Discussing hospice care. *J Clin Oncol.* 2002;20:1419–1424.

39. Novack, DH, Plumer R, Smith RL, Ochitill H, Morrow GR, Benett JM. Changes in physicians attitudes toward telling the cancer patient. *JAMA.* 1979;241:897–900.

40. Wilkes E. Rethinking established dogma. Is good general practice possible? *BMJ.* 1984;289:85–86.

41. Thomsen OO, Wulff HR, Martin A, Singer PA. What do gastroenterologists in Europe tell cancer patients? *Lancet.* 1993;341:473–478.

42. Li S, Chou JL. Communication with the cancer patient in China. *Ann N Y Acad Sci.* 1997;809:243–248.

43. Solanke, T. Communication with the cancer patient in Nigeria: information and truth. In Surbone A, Zwitter M, (eds). *Communication with the cancer patient.* New York: New York Academy of Sciences; 1997:109–118.

44. El Ghazali S. Is it wise to tell the truth, the whole truth, and nothing but the truth to a cancer patient? *Ann NY Acad Sci.* 1997;20:809:97–108.

45. Bezwoda WR, Colvin H, Lehoka J. Transcultural and language problems in communicating with cancer patients in southern Africa. *Ann N Y Acad Sci.* 1997 Feb 20;809:119–132.

46. Bruera E, Neumann CM, Mazzocato C, Stiefel F, Sala R. Attitudes and beliefs of palliative care physicians regarding communication with terminally ill cancer patients. *Palliat Med.* 2000 Jul;14(4):287–298.

47. Beckman HB, Frankel RM. The effect of physician behavior on the collection of data. *Ann Intern Med.* 1984 Nov;101(5):692–696.

48. Back AL, Arnold RM, Baile WF, et al. Efficacy of communication skills training for giving bad news and discussing transitions to palliative care. *Arch Intern Med.* 2007 Mar 12;167(5):453–460.

49. Curtis JR, Engelberg R, Young JP, et al. An approach to understanding the interaction of hope and desire for explicit prognostic information among individuals with severe chronic obstructive pulmonary disease or advanced cancer. *J Palliat Med.* 2008 May;11(4):610–620.

50. Sell L, Devlin B, Bourke SJ, Munro NC, Corris PA, Gibson GJ. Communicating the diagnosis of lung cancer. *Respir Med.* 1993 Jan;87(1):61–63.

51. Levinson W, Gorawara-Bhat R, Lamb J. A study of patient clues and physician responses in primary care and surgical settings. *JAMA.* 2000 Aug 23–30;284(8):1021–1027.

52. Eden OB, Black I, MacKinlay GA, Emery AE. Communication with parents of children with cancer. *Palliat Med.* 1994;8(2):105–114.

53. Tulsky JA, Chesney MA, Lo B. See one, do one, teach one? House staff experience discussing do-not-resuscitate orders. *Arch Intern Med.* 1996 Jun 24;156(12):1285–1289.

54. Pfeifer MP, Sidorov JE, Smith AC, Boero JF, Evans AT, Settle MB. The discussion of end-of-life medical care by primary care patients and physicians: a multicenter study using structured qualitative interviews. The EOL Study Group. *J Gen Intern Med.* 1994 Feb;9(2):82–88.

55. Frankl D, Oye RK, Bellamy PE. Attitudes of hospitalized patients toward life support: a survey of 200 medical inpatients. *Am J Med.* 1989 Jun;86(6):645–648.

56. Baile WF, Buckman R, Lenzi R, Glober G, Beale EA, Kudelka AP. SPIKES-A six-step protocol for delivering bad news: application to the patient with cancer. *Oncologist.* 2000;5:302–311.

57. Bruera E, Palmer JL, Pace E, et al. A randomized, controlled trial of physician postures when breaking bad news to cancer patients. *Palliat Med.* 2007 Sep;21(6):501–505.

58. Back AL, Arnold RM, Quill TE. Hope for the best, and prepare for the worst. *Ann Intern Med.* 2003 Mar 4;138(5):439–443.

59. Tierney WM, Dexter PR, Gramelspacher GP, Perkins AJ, Zhou XH, Wolinsky FD. The effect of discussions about advance directives on patients' satisfaction with primary care. *J Gen Intern Med.* 2001 Jan;16(1):32–40.

CHAPTER 38

Hospice and Home Care

Stephen R. Connor

Hospice care continues to be viewed in many countries as an inpatient setting for the care of those at life's end. Increasingly, hospice care is now viewed as palliative care provided to people in the place they call home. Home can be the house one has lived in for a long time, or it can be an assisted living setting where one has moved, or the nursing facility one has to live in to meet basic needs. It could also be the street, the city park, the village, the homeless shelter, or even the prison.

Unlike hospice development in the United Kingdom, which was centered primarily in inpatient facilities, in the United States hospice grew primarily as a home-care program. In 2007 there were over 4700 unique hospice programs operated by 3700 different companies or organizations. There has been enormous growth in the number of hospices in the United States in recent years (see Fig. 38–1). All these programs provide home care. Hospice care in the United States is measured by days of care. In 2007 over 96% of patient days were provided at the routine or continuous home-care level, while only approximately 4% were at the general inpatient or inpatient respite levels (see Fig. 38–2).

What little we know about where people say they want to spend their last days comes from public opinion surveys that probe what people believe they would do if facing a life limiting illness or condition. In the United States over 90% of people say when asked if they would prefer to die at home or in a hospital that they would prefer to be at home. The reality is that approximately 50% of American's die in acute care facilities. Hospice patients predominantly die in the place they call home (see Table 38–1). In 2007, over 70% of hospice patients died in personal residences, assisted living facilities, or nursing homes. Only 10.5% of hospice patients died in acute care hospitals in units that are not run by the hospice program. An increasing number of hospice patients are dying in freestanding hospices (12.5%) or in hospice run units (6.7%).[1]

HOME CARE AND PALLIATIVE HOME CARE

Home care in general can be provided to many people with health conditions that do not require hospitalization. To qualify for home care, patients usually have to have a condition that requires skilled intervention that cannot be done by the patient or family alone. The objective in home health care is to help the patient to return to a level of functioning that allows for self-care. This can include postsurgical patients requiring wound care, new diabetics needing help with insulin, patients recovering from an episode of congestive heart failure, postinjury patients requiring rehabilitative physical therapy, and so forth.

Home health care can also be provided to patients with a life-limiting prognosis, especially if their prognosis is uncertain or likely to be greater than 6–12 months. Palliative or hospice home care is a specialized form of home care that brings to bear specialized skills and interdisciplinary team care delivery. What distinguishes palliative home care from general home care is that the focus of care is not on rehabilitation or achieving a higher level of functioning, but on helping patients and families to achieve a preferred level of quality of life while completing their lives. Hospice home care focuses on the relief of suffering and preparation for death in a manner consistent with the goals and values of the individual patient in a family system.

Palliative home care utilizes a broad array of different disciplines to achieve these goals. While general home care is mainly nursing and the rehabilitative therapies, hospice home care adds more emphasis on psychosocial and spiritual-care providers, especially social workers and chaplains. There is also a considerable emphasis on the use of volunteers to expand care and to provide practical and emotional support.

Hospice home care uses an interdisciplinary approach to care delivery. In multidisciplinary teams, care is provided by a variety of different professionals; however, each discipline provides its own service and there is not as much emphasis on collaboration. In interdisciplinary care there is interaction among the disciplines. Each adds to the picture of the whole patient. An interdisciplinary team values the input of all members. There are boundaries as to what each member is expected to do and focus on, but there is some blurring of boundaries. The nurse pays attention to psychosocial concerns, and the social worker attends to how symptoms may be affecting the person's ability to meet emotional needs. The home health aide may be the one the patient wants to pray with and the chaplain may hear about the family's financial concerns.[2]

HOME-BASED CARE AROUND THE WORLD

In many parts of the developing world the majority of people may not see a nontraditional healthcare professional from the time they are born until the time they die. Increasingly, health care is delivered by home-based care workers. Many of these paraprofessionals lack appropriate support and supervision from competent medical and psychosocial professionals. In Africa, a significant portion of health care is delivered by faith-based organizations that have created not only networks of congregations but healthcare delivery systems.

In Tanzania, the Evangelical Lutheran Church operates a network of 18 hospitals and one medical college that serve about 20% of the country's healthcare needs. Using their network of congregations, voluntary healthcare workers are recruited to help care for those in villages with healthcare needs. Many of those with HIV/AIDS are cared for. With funding from the United States Agency for International Development (USAID), through the President's Emergency Plan for AIDS Relief (PEPFAR) program, an effort is underway to expand this home-based care system to include training and support in home-based palliative care. Home-based care teams anchored at the system's hospitals and treatment centers include physicians and nurses trained in palliative care to back up home-based care workers.

In Kerala, India, the Neighborhood Network in Palliative Care (NNPC) Program[3] has developed an effective model engaging large numbers of volunteers to care for those in their immediate neighborhoods. In one region, 7 physicians and 200 nurses support over 4000 volunteers in caring for the chronically ill and dying. The NNPC is an attempt to develop a sustainable "community led" service capable of offering comprehensive long-term care and palliative care to the needy in the developing world. In this program, volunteers from the local community are trained to identify problems of the chronically ill in their area and to intervene effectively with active support from a network of trained professionals. NNPC aims at empowering local communities to look after the chronically ill and dying patients in that community using a primary healthcare model.

These and other programs developed to meet the needs of communities provide learning laboratories for how health care can be redesigned and delivered to meet the needs of an increasingly aged and chronically ill population, whether it is in the developed or developing world.

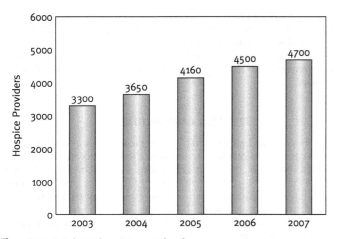

Fig. 38-1. Total U.S. hospice providers by year.

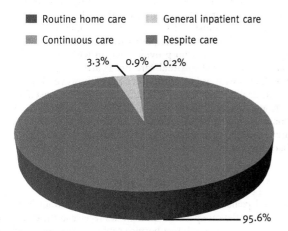

Fig. 38-2. Days of care by level of care—2007.

Table 38-1. Location of death

	2007 (%)	2006 (%)
Patient's place of residence	70.3	74.1
Private residence	42.0	47.1
Nursing facility	22.8	22.5
Residential facility	5.5	4.6
Hospice inpatient facility	19.2	17.0
Acute care hospital	10.5	8.8

PSYCHOSOCIAL CARE IN HOSPICE AND PALLIATIVE HOME CARE

Psychosocial care is underdeveloped in home care generally. Some social work services are available and there are some home-based mental health programs, but unless there is a major mental health issue interfering with care, not much attention is paid to the provision of mental health services. Hospice home care puts increased emphasis on psychosocial support for both patient and family with a focus on family dynamics and life closure issues. However, even in hospice care, the provision of services beyond some social work intervention is limited.

There is a lot of provision of emotional support, which is a rather nonspecific intervention consisting primarily of active listening. Depending on the clinical skills of the social worker there may be quite competent team intervention but many social workers lack graduate training and competency in the provision of psychosocial interventions aligned with the specific issues patients and families present with. If you consider that few competent therapists could work effectively in the home setting by themselves when dealing with a family in crisis with often multiple dysfunctional behaviors, it is no wonder that services are limited.

When working with patients and families in their residential settings, it is important to focus on the immediate needs that when dealt with help support the ability to meet the patients needs. Trying to resolve long-standing emotional conflicts and dynamics is usually unrealistic in these situations. The focus must be on achieving closure and support for whatever adaptive coping mechanisms can be drawn upon. Sometimes family members need care to provide care. An overwhelmed caregiver or spouse may need individualized attention to stress and self-care and may need help in mobilizing social and emotional resources to help instead of trying to meet all the patient's needs alone.

The International Work Group on Death Dying and Bereavement (IWG) has published a set of Assumptions and Principles for Psychosocial Care of Dying Persons and Their Families[4] that address some of the major concerns faced by patients, families, and caregivers at the end of life and provide guidance in dealing with these concerns. These assumptions are summarized here.

Assumptions and Principles. The dying and their families face numerous psychosocial issues as death approaches. In writing the following assumptions and principles concerning these issues, we hope to counteract the tendency to focus too much on physical and technical care, to stimulate readers to test the following assumptions against their own experience, and to incorporate them into their work.

By psychosocial we mean the emotional, intellectual, spiritual, interpersonal, social, cultural, and economic dimensions of the human experience. Assumptions and principles for spiritual care have been developed by other work groups of the IWG.

By family we mean those individuals who are part of the dying person's most immediate attachment network, regardless of blood or matrimonial ties. The family, which includes the dying person, is the unit of care. By caregivers we mean those professionals and volunteers who provide care to dying persons and their families. We have separated the dying person, the family, and caregivers for the purpose of discussion only. Many of these assumptions and principles apply equally to dying persons and their families. They may not apply to all cultures and belief systems.

Issues for dying persons

Assumptions

1. Dying persons may choose to acknowledge or not acknowledge their impending death.
2. Dying persons can communicate about their impending death in different cultural ways, encompassing verbal, nonverbal, or symbolic ways of communicating.
3. Dying persons have the right to information on their changing physical status, and the right to choose whether to be told they are dying.
4. Dying persons may be preoccupied with dying, death itself, or with what happens after death.
5. Dying persons can have a deep-seated fear of abandonment. They may therefore continue treatment for the sake of the family or physician rather than in the belief that it will be of personal benefit.
6. Many dying persons experience multiple physical and psychological losses before their death.
7. Dying persons exhibit a variety of coping strategies in facing death.
8. Dying persons generally need to express feelings.
9. Dying persons communicate when they feel safe and secure.
10. Dying persons may find it helpful to communicate with others who are terminally ill.

11. A dying person's communication of concern about death may be inhibited by a number of psychosocial and culturally determined expectations.
12. Dying persons have a right to be acknowledged as living human beings until their death.
13. Dying persons' psychological suffering may be greater than their physical pain or discomfort.
14. Dying persons may have difficulty in dealing with the different or conflicting needs of family members.

Issues for families

Assumptions

1. Families have fundamental needs to care and be cared for.
2. The need to care and the need to be cared for sometimes conflict.
3. People vary in their coping abilities and personal resources. Moreover, competing priorities may hamper the amount and quality of care people are able to give.
4. The approach of death may disrupt the structure and functioning of the family.
5. Families need to have information about a dying person's condition, although in cases of conflict his or her desire for confidentiality must be respected.
6. Families often need to be involved with the dying person in decision making.
7. Families have a right to know that their affairs will be shared only with those that have a need to know.
8. Family members need to maintain self-esteem and self-respect.
9. Sexual needs may continue up to the point of death.
10. Families coping with terminal illness frequently have financial concerns.
11. Faced with death, the family may imagine that changes will be greater than they are.
12. Families have a need and a right to express grief for the multiple losses associated with illness and for impending death.

Issues for caregivers

Assumptions

1. Caregivers need education and experience in addressing the psychosocial needs of dying persons and their families.
2. Caregivers need to be aware of the dying person's and family's psychosocial frame of reference in acknowledging and coping with impending death.
3. Caregivers bring their own values, attitudes, feelings, and fears into the dying person's setting.
4. Caregivers are exposed to repeated intense emotional experiences, loss, and confrontation with their own death in their work with dying persons.
5. Caregivers dealing with family groups sometimes experience conflicting needs and requests for information and confidentiality.
6. Caregivers may sometimes not communicate with each other about their own needs and feelings.

Many of these psychosocial principles apply as well to those living with chronic illness who are not yet at the point of being identified as a dying person. Nonhospice palliative home care is not that well developed at this point in the United States. A significant number of hospice programs have added palliative home care for patients who cannot qualify for hospice benefits or who chose not to enroll in hospice. The services are similar to hospice home care and hospices provide these programs as a kind of bridge to hospice; however, experience has shown that the majority of these patients never transition to hospice care.

In the United Kingdom there is a system of public health community nursing and a specialized group of home-care nurses for cancer patients referred to as Macmillan nurses. Many of these nurses provide basic palliative care and may try to help the patient to get hospice care when needed. Ideally, in any healthcare system, all professionals should have a basic competency in the principles of palliative care. There will likely continue to be a need for specialist palliative care in health care because not everyone will be good at or want to meet the complex and challenging needs of patients with life-limiting illnesses.

SPIRITUAL CARE IN HOME CARE

Even more limited are spiritual-care services in home care. Although home-care staff is certainly sensitive to the existence of spiritual and religious concerns, there is practically no mechanism for chaplaincy service outside the acute hospital except for hospice care. Many hospitals have a multidenominational roster of clergy who visit hospitalized patients and community clergy do try to visit seriously ill members of their congregations at home or in nursing facilities; however, there is usually no organized program for the delivery of spiritual-care services outside hospice and even those services vary quite a bit.

In 2007 only 3.4% of full time equivalent hospice staff were identified as chaplains or spiritual-care providers. There are also hospice volunteers with a ministerial background who may provide services, and for the hospice with no chaplains there must be a staff member, usually a social worker, who provides liaison with community clergy to make sure identified spiritual-care needs are being addressed. One of the problems with use of community clergy, however, is their lack of training in dealing with issues of death and dying. We usually assume that fears and concerns about dying are the province of the clergy; however, many clergy express inadequacy in dealing with these issues as they are not taught in seminaries or other schools for priests, ministers, rabbi's, or imams.

CONCLUSION

Hospice and palliative care delivered in residential settings is becoming more and more the care patients and families receive at the end of life; in spite of the continuing myth that hospice care is a place you go when terminally ill. Increasingly, residential settings are not just personal residences but assisted living facilities, nursing facilities, group care homes, and other alternative living arrangements especially for an increasingly elder population.

Home hospice care is growing rapidly in the United States and is being embraced by health systems wishing to avoid the large health-care costs associated with inpatient facility care. In the developing world, home-based care workers are the primary deliverers of palliative care with back up from interdisciplinary healthcare professionals.

The need for palliative care worldwide is enormous. Less than 8% of those dying each year worldwide are accessing palliative care. While palliative care is increasingly available in the developed world it is rarely available in the developing world. Some innovative models of home-based palliative care are developing around the world but major barriers including lack of education, lack of access to essential palliative medications, and lack of supportive governmental policies continue to limit availability.[5]

Home-based hospice and palliative care is distinguished by a focus not only on the physical and medical needs of patients but a rich understanding of the psychosocial and spiritual or transcendent dimensions of care. Patients and their families as well as those who provide care face many challenges triggered by some degree of knowledge of impending death and need specialized intervention that should be guided by the patient's goals, needs, and desire to explore or not explore sensitive psychological, interpersonal, and transcendent concerns.

We hopefully will see home-based hospice and palliative care continue to grow in the coming years to meet the increasing demand for competent decent care[6] for those nearing the end of life. No healthcare system can claim to be comprehensive without the inclusion of palliative care for those in need.

REFERENCES

1. National Hospice and Palliative Care Organization. NHPCO Facts and Figures: Hospice Care in America. 2008. Available at: www/nhpco.org/research. Accessed 10/2/08.

2. Connor S, Egan K, Kwilosz D, Larson D, Reese D. Interdisciplinary approaches to assisting with end-of-life care and decision making. *Am Behav Sci.* 2002;46(3):340–356.

3. Kumar S, Numpeli M. Neighborhood network in palliative care. *Indian J Palliat Care.* 2005;11:6–9.

4. International Work Group on Death, Dying & Bereavement. International Work Group on Death, Dying & Bereavement: Assumptions and principles for psychosocial care of dying patients and their families. *J Palliat Care.* 1993;9(3):29–32. (Assumptions reprinted with permission.)

5. Mwangi-Powell F. Palliative care and public health. A perspective from the African Palliative Care Association. *J Public Health Policy.* 2007;28: 59–61.

6. Karpf T, Ferguson T, Swift R, Lazarus, JV. (Ed.). *Restoring hope: Decent care in the midst of HIV/AIDS.* London: Blackwell Publishing; 2008.

International Aspects of Palliative Care

Liliana De Lima

INTRODUCTION

The World Health Organization (WHO) estimates that 58 million deaths occur annually around the world. Approximately 76% of these deaths occur in developing countries, where over three-fourths of the people in the world live. According to the data, the main causes of the total mortality are noncommunicable conditions, including cancers and cardiovascular diseases, and communicable diseases, including acquired immunodeficiency syndrome (AIDS), maternal and perinatal conditions, and nutritional deficiencies (over 58% and 32%, respectively).[1]

Cancer is among the major noncommunicable causes of death worldwide and accounted for 12.6% of the total deaths in 2001.[1] The International Agency for Research on Cancer (IARC), projects that global cancer rates will increase by 50% from 10 million new cases worldwide in 2000, to 15 million new cases in 2020, primarily due to the ageing of population and increases in smoking. Fifty percent of the world's new cancer cases and deaths occur in developing nations and approximately 80% of these cancer patients are already incurable at the time of diagnosis. Regarding communicable diseases, approximately 8% of the adult population is infected with the human immunodeficiency virus (HIV) virus in sub-Saharan African, and global AIDS deaths are approximately 3 million per year.[2] The vast majority of these patients diagnosed with advanced cancer or in advanced stages of HIV/AIDS would benefit from palliative care. However, availability of and access to palliative care services, including medications, is none or very limited to most of the population in need in the world.

PALLIATIVE CARE

Palliative care is defined by the WHO as an approach that improves the quality of life of patients and their families facing the problem associated with life-threatening illness, through the prevention and relief of suffering by means of early identification and impeccable assessment and treatment of pain and the physical, psychosocial and spiritual problems.[3]

The WHO definition expands the following about palliative care

- provides relief from pain and other distressing symptoms;
- affirms life and regards dying as a normal process;
- intends neither hastening nor postponing death;
- integrates the psychological and spiritual aspects of patient care;
- offers a support system to help patients live as actively as possible until death;
- offers a support system to help the family cope during the patient's illness and in their own bereavement;
- uses a team approach to address the needs of patients and their families, including bereavement counseling, if indicated;
- enhances quality of life, and may also positively influence the course of illness.

According to WHO, 60% of the people who die each year have a prolonged advanced illness and would benefit from palliative care. Palliative care is applicable early in the course of illness, in conjunction with other therapies that are intended to prolong life, such as chemotherapy, radiation therapy, Highly Active AntiRetroviral Therapy (HAART), and includes those investigations needed to better understand and manage distressing clinical complications.

Access to palliative care. Access to palliative care services is often limited, even in developed countries, due to several reasons, some of which include lack of political will, insufficient information and education, and excessive regulation of opioids. For several years, the International Observatory in End of Life Care (IOELC) at the University of Lancaster in England has been documenting and reporting on the progress in the development of palliative care around the world. For this task, the IOELC identified a set of criteria to measure the rate of development of a country which include capacity for service provision, availability of morphine, appropriate policies, a national association, and others. On the basis of these criteria, countries are placed in one of four categories of development: (1) no known activity; (2) capacity building; (3) localized provision, and (4) approaching integration. Table 39–1 includes the typology and criteria used by the IOELC.[4] Using this typology, the IOELC constructed a "world map" of palliative care service development which has served as a comparative tool among countries and also one which will be extremely useful in the future to compare progress within countries throughout the years.[5] Table 39–2 includes the list of the countries and their corresponding categories of development at the time of the study. According to the IOELC study, about half of the 234 countries included in the review have established one or more hospice-palliative care services. Of those, only 15% countries have achieved a measure of integration with wider mainstream service providers, while in about one-third of the countries, no palliative care activity was identified. An important finding of this study was that the researchers found a strong association between palliative care and the human development index (HDI). The majority of the countries in Group 4 have a high level HDI, while 54% of the countries in Group 1 have no HDI.[4]

A recent study on advanced-cancer care in Latin America demonstrated that most of the care given to persons with advanced cancer occurs in hospitals as compared to other facilities or at home, whereas the majority of cancer deaths take place at home. The study also identified the following barriers to cancer pain management as reported by the respondents: (1) inadequate staff knowledge of pain management; (2) patients' inability to pay for services or analgesics; (3) inadequate pain assessment; and (4) excessive state/legal regulations of prescribing opiates.[6]

Even if the availability and access to curative therapies may be limited in developing countries, the balance and integration of disease-specific and palliative therapies must be constantly sought for. The existence of global and within-country variations in resources and health services should never lead to a system which endorses curative therapy for those with resources and palliative care for the poor. In any setting, policy and health advocacy must seek to obtain the best available curative treatments in whatever manner is feasible, at the same time as seeking to obtain accessible and effective palliative care services for all those who may need them.

ACCESS TO MEDICATIONS

According to data from the WHO, in spite of recent progress, about one-third of the world's population still has little or no access to essential and often life-saving medicines. This results in enormous suffering and loss of life, particularly among the poor, and massive damage to national economies. The problem is particularly severe in the poorest parts of Africa and Asia.[7] The WHO Essential Medicines concept has over a

Table 39-1. Typology of hospice-palliative care service development[4]

No known activity	Capacity building	Localized provision	Approaching integration
	Presence of sensitized personnel	A range of capacity building activities, but also:	Capacity building and localized activities, but also:
	Expressions of interest with key external organizations	Critical mass of activists in one or more locations.	Critical mass of activists countrywide
	Links established (international) with service providers	Service established often linked to home care	Range of providers and service types
	Conference participation	Local awareness/support	Broad awareness of palliative care
	Visits to hospice and palliative care organizations	Sources of funding established, though may be heavily donor dependent and relatively isolated from one another, with little impact on wider health policy	Measure of integration with mainstream service providers
	Education and training (visiting teams)		Impact on policy
	External training courses undertaken		Established education centers
			Academic links
	Preparation of a strategy for service development	Morphine available	Research undertaken
	Lobbying of policymakers/health ministries	Some training undertaken by hospice organization	National association in existence

Reprinted from Journal of Pain and Symptom Management, Vol. 33 No. 5, Clark D, Wright M, The International Observatory on End of Life Care: A Global View of Palliative Care Development, pg 542–546, Copyright (2007), with permission from Elsevier.

Table 39-2. Categorization of palliative care development (countries by group)[4]

Group 4 Approaching integration (n ¼ 35)	Argentina, Australia, Austria, Belgium, Canada, Chile, Costa Rica, Denmark, Finland, France, Germany, Hong Kong, Hungary, Iceland, Ireland, Israel, Italy, Japan, Kenya, Malaysia, Mongolia, New Zealand, Netherlands, Norway, Poland, Romania, Singapore, Slovenia, South Africa, Spain, Sweden, Switzerland, Uganda, United Kingdom, United States of America
Group 3 Localized provision (n ¼ 80)	Aland Islands, Albania, Armenia, Azerbaijan, Bangladesh, Barbados, Belarus, Bermuda, Bosnia and Herzegovina, Botswana, Brazil, Bulgaria, Cameroon, Cayman Islands, China, Colombia, Congo, Croatia, Cuba, Cyprus, Czech Republic, Dominican Republic, Ecuador, Egypt, El Salvador, Estonia, Georgia, Gibraltar, Greece, Guadeloupe, Guatemala, Guernsey, Guyana, Honduras, India, Indonesia, Iraq, Isle of Man, Jamaica, Jersey, Jordan, Kazakhstan, Korea (South), Kyrgyzstan, Latvia, Lithuania, Luxembourg, Macau, Macedonia, Malawi, Malta, Mexico, Moldova, Morocco, Myanmar, Nepal, Nigeria, Pakistan, Panama, Peru, Philippines, Portugal, Russia, Saudi Arabia, Serbia, Sierra Leone, Slovakia, Sri Lanka, Swaziland, Tanzania, Thailand, The Gambia, Trinidad and Tobago, Ukraine, Uruguay, United Arab Emirates, Venezuela, Vietnam, Zambia, Zimbabwe
Group 2 Capacity building (n ¼ 41)	Algeria, Bahrain, Belize, Bolivia, British Virgin Islands, Brunei, Cambodia, Democratic Republic of Congo, Cote d'Ivoire, Dominica, Ethiopia, Fiji, Ghana, Haiti, Holy See (Vatican), Iran, Kuwait, Lebanon, Lesotho, Madagascar, Mauritius, Mozambique, Namibia, Nicaragua, Oman, Palestinian Authority, Papua New Guinea, Paraguay, Qatar, Reunion, Rwanda, Saint Lucia, Seychelles, Sudan, Suriname, Tajikistan, The Bahamas, Tunisia, Turkey, Uzbekistan, Puerto Rico
Group 1 No known activity(n ¼ 78)	Afghanistan, American Samoa, Andorra, Angola, Anguilla, Antigua and Barbuda, Aruba, Benin, Bhutan, Burkina Faso, Burundi, Cape Verdi, Central African Republic, Chad, Comoros, Cook Islands, Djibouti, Equatorial Guinea, Eritrea, Falkland Islands, French Guiana, French Polynesia, Gabon, Greenland, Grenada, Guam, Guinea, Guinea-Bissau, Kiribati, Korea (DPR), Laos, Liberia, Libya, Liechtenstein, Maldives, Mali, Marshall Islands, Martinique, Mauritania, Mayotte, Micronesia, Monaco, Montenegro, Montserrat, Nauru, Netherlands Antilles, New Caledonia, Niger, Niue, Norfolk Island, Northern Mariana Islands, Palau, Pitcairn, Saint Helena, Saint Kits and Nevis, Saint Pierre and Miquelon, Saint Vincent and the Grenadines, Samoa, San Marino, Sao Tome and Principe, Senegal, Solomon Islands, Somalia, Svalbard, Syria, Timor-Leste, Togo, Tokelau, Tonga, Turkmenistan, Turks and Caicos Islands, Tuvalu, US Virgin Islands, Vanuatu, Wallis and Fortuna, Western Sahara, Yemen

Reprinted from Journal of Pain and Symptom Management, Vol. 33 No. 5, Clark D, Wright M, The International Observatory on End of Life Care: A Global View of Palliative Care Development, pg 542–546, Copyright (2007), with permission from Elsevier.

period of nearly more than 30 years laid the basis for numerous national Essential Medicines programs in which countries developed their own lists based on the needs of the local populations. This has resulted in better access to care and treatment.

In regards to medications for palliative care, the International Association for Hospice and Palliative Care (IAHPC), in collaboration with several organizations, recently developed a consensus based List of Essential Medicines in Palliative Care. The list includes 33 medications to treat the most common symptoms in palliative care resulting from cancer, HIV/AIDS, renal failure, cardiovascular diseases, and others.[8]

A significant problem is the lack of access to analgesics for the treatment of pain. The *Three Step Analgesic Ladder* developed in the 1980s by the WHO and its Expert Committee on Cancer relies on the availability of a number of analgesics, including oral morphine and codeine.[9] Both morphine (short-acting oral and long-acting oral and injectable ampoules) and codeine (oral) are included in the current WHO Model List of Essential Medicines.[10] In addition, the IAHPC List of Essential Medicines for Palliative Care[8] includes morphine as well as oral methadone, oral oxycodone, and transdermal fentanyl as analgesics for the third step of the *WHO Ladder*. The inclusion of several opioids and different formulations in the IAHPC List is based on the premise that short-acting morphine should always be available.

In spite of this recognition, it is estimated that 80% of patients in pain do not have access to pain relieving medications.[11] Patients in the developing world suffer much more than those in the developed world: A review done by the Pain and Policy Studies Group (PPSG) a WHO Collaborating Center for Policy and Communications in Cancer Care of the University of Wisconsin, of the 2006 International Narcotics Control Board (INCB) morphine data reported by governments revealed that 7 high-income countries (United States, France, Canada, United Kingdom, Germany, Austria, and Australia) accounted for nearly 84% of medical morphine consumed in the world. These seven countries comprise less than 12% of the world's population.[12] These reports and figures point to the large and continuing disparity in morphine consumption among countries, and provide further evidence of the inadequate global treatment of pain, especially in low- and middle-income countries.

Some of the reasons why opioids are unavailable in developing countries are misconceptions and attitudes on opioids; insufficient knowledge on how to asses and treat pain; economic and procurement impediments; and regulatory impediments.[11]

Recently the WHO launched a special program called Access to Controlled Medications Program, to address the main causes for impaired access to controlled medications, including opioids for pain relief. These causes are essentially an imbalance between the prevention of abuse of controlled substances and their use for legitimate medical purposes. The program as proposed, will address regulatory barriers, the functioning of the estimate system for importing/exporting by the countries and education of healthcare professionals and others involved.[13]

In addition to the WHO, the INCB has also asked governments to ensure availability and accessibility of opioid medications to satisfy the needs of the population.[14]

POLICY ISSUES

Palliative care public health policy. In the majority of cases, the development of palliative care has been a "bottom up" approach in which individuals and groups have started programs or initiatives that eventually are incorporated into academic programs and generate enough demand and awareness to motivate changes in health policy. The limitation to this system is that it lacks official recognition and therefore reimbursement issues, budget, and resource allocation are unavailable, making these very fragile programs with no viability over time.

For public health strategies to be effective, they must be incorporated by governments into all levels of their healthcare systems. In 1990, the WHO pioneered a public health strategy to integrate palliative care into existing healthcare systems which included advice and guidelines to governments on priorities and how to implement national palliative care programs.[15] On the basis of this a Public Health Model was developed and has now evolved, which includes four components: (1) appropriate policies,

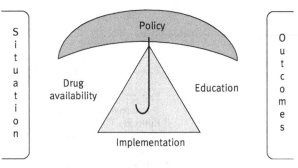

Fig. 39–1. WHO public health model.
SOURCE: Reprinted from Stjernsward J, Foley KM, Ferris FD. The public health strategy for palliative care. *J Pain Symptom Manage.* 2007;33(5):486–493. With permission from Elsevier.

(2) adequate availability of medications, (3) education of healthcare workers and the public, and (4) implementation of palliative care services at all levels throughout the society. This model is depicted in Fig. 39–1.[16]

GLOBAL ADVOCACY CAMPAIGNS

Several organizations and associations designed advocacy campaigns which have been successful at increasing awareness of palliative care, underscoring the importance of ensuring access to pain treatment and the need to implement changes in policy and practice. Some of these campaigns are aimed at governments, others at the general public and others at caregivers and providers. All these recognize the critical role played by the civil society and the community in helping move forward the palliative care agenda. Two examples of successful campaigns are described below.

World hospice and palliative care day. World Hospice and Palliative Care Day[17] is a unified day of action to celebrate and support hospice and palliative care around the world. It takes place on the second Saturday of October, every year. The day is a Worldwide Palliative Care Alliance (WPCA) activity.

The aims of the World Hospice and Palliative Care Day are to

- share our vision to increase the availability of hospice and palliative care throughout the world;
- create opportunities to speak out about the issues which affect provision of hospice and palliative care around the world, to influence opinion formers including healthcare funders and policy makers;
- raise awareness and understanding of the needs—medical, social, practical, and spiritual—of people living with a life-limiting illness and their families. To explain how hospice and palliative care can transform people's lives and to show how it can help to meet those needs;
- raise funds to support and develop hospice and palliative care services around the world.

The World Day calls for:

- individuals worldwide to participate in World Day to demand their right to palliative care;
- all countries to include palliative care in their national healthcare programs and to make it available throughout existing healthcare infrastructures;
- greater and more secure funding to support hospice and palliative care services worldwide;
- essential low-cost opioid analgesics for pain and symptom control to be made available, particularly in resource-limited countries;
- adequate care to be provided to people affected by a wide variety of life-limiting illnesses, including HIV and cancer;
- increased availability of palliative care for people in developing countries—particularly in rural areas. Also, to reach marginalized groups throughout the world, such as prisoners, the homeless, and those with special needs such as learning difficulties;
- the integration of hospice and palliative care into all healthcare professionals' education programs, both undergraduate and postgraduate;

- palliative care to be provided not as a last resort but concurrently with disease treatment such as antiretrovirals (ARVs) or cancer treatment.

The World Day has been successful in creating awareness of hospice and palliative care throughout the world, by involving members of the civil society in the celebration and activities.

Palliative care and pain treatment as human rights. The Joint Declaration and Statement of Commitment for the recognition of palliative care and pain treatment as human rights[18] was developed by the IAHPC and the WPCA, and signed by representatives of several international and regional organizations from Africa, Latin America, Eastern Europe, Western Europe, Asia, and North America. The Declaration identifies the international covenants and treaties which are unmet whenever patients are denied access to palliative care and pain treatment and calls for individuals and representatives of organizations to sign the Declaration through an online signature page.

The Declaration also lists seven goals which are to be met to make this recognition possible:

1. Identify, develop, and implement strategies for the recognition of palliative care and pain treatment as fundamental human rights.
2. Work with governments and policy makers to adopt the necessary changes in legislation to ensure appropriate care of patients with life-limiting conditions.
3. Work with policy makers and regulators to identify and eliminate regulatory and legal barriers that interfere with the rational use of controlled medications.
4. Advocate for improvements in access to and availability of opioids and other medications required for the effective treatment of pain and other symptoms common in palliative care, including special formulations and appropriate medications for children.
5. Advocate for adequate resources to be made available to support the implementation of palliative care and pain treatment services and providers where needed.
6. Advocate for academic institutions, teaching hospital and universities to adopt the necessary practices and changes needed to ensure that palliative care and pain positions, resources, personnel, infrastructures, review boards, and systems are created and sustained.
7. Encourage and enlist other international and national palliative care, pain treatment, related organizations, associations, federations, and interested parties to join this global campaign for the recognition of palliative care and pain treatment as human rights.

The Declaration is intended to be used by nongovernmental organizations, professional organizations, federations, alliances, and civic-minded individuals to bring palliative care and pain treatment to the attention of policy makers, regulators, governments and organizations to improve the care of patients with life-limiting conditions, and to provide support to their families and loved ones.

This Declaration is an unprecedented collective effort by representatives from healthcare and patient advocacy organizations from around the world working together to achieve seven specific goals in palliative care and pain management. To date, more than 4500 individuals and more than 400 organizations representing different sectors of the civil society have signed the Declaration. The Declaration and signature page are available in http://www.hospicecare.com/resources/pain_pallcare_hr/

REGIONAL ORGANIZATIONS

A significant indicator of improvement has been the development of regional organizations in palliative care. Most of the regions of the world have an organization, with the exception of the Middle East and North America. In the case of North America, this may be due to the limited number of countries making up the Region—both the United States and Canada have strong national associations and professional organizations, and Mexico is usually included in Latin America and the Caribbean. A Regional organization of two countries would be an unnecessary use of resources. Some regions have more than one organization: one usually encompasses the whole region while the other includes a subgroup of countries sharing similar characteristics such as geographical location, language, ethnical or religious beliefs. This section will only describe the major regional organizations, while recognizing that subregional organizations have also had a strong influence in the development of palliative care in the countries under their influence.

African palliative care association. The African Palliative Care Association (APCA) was founded in 2003, to help support and promote the development of palliative care and palliative care professionals throughout Africa. Members include professionals, individuals with a special interest in the promotion of palliative care, and national and local palliative care associations/programs. APCA held its inaugural conference in Arusha, Tanzania where also a new journal was created.[19]

Objectives

- To promote the availability of palliative care for all in need.
- To encourage governments in sub-Saharan Africa to support affordable and appropriate palliative care which is incorporated into the whole spectrum of healthcare services.
- To promote the availability of palliative care drugs for all in need.
- To encourage the establishment of national palliative care associations in all African countries.
- To promote palliative care training programs suitable for sub-Saharan African countries.
- To develop standard guidelines for training and care at different levels of health professional and care providers.

APCA Web site: http://www.apca.co.ug/

Asia Pacific hospice and palliative care network. The Asia Pacific Hospice and Palliative Care Network (APHN) has been established to link all those who are interested in developing hospice and palliative programs in Asia and the Pacific. There are now more than 700 members. Sixteen percent of these are organizations that have joined as Organizational Members; the rest are individuals who are working with some of the 500 hospices and palliative care services in the Asia Pacific region.[20] The APHN evolved over a series of meetings from March 1995 until March 2001 when the organization was registered in Singapore. Although the Secretariat has been established in Singapore, the APHN is a regional organization with fourteen founding sectors.

Objectives[21]

- To facilitate the development of hospice and palliative care programs.
- To promote professional and public education in palliative care.
- To enhance communication and dissemination of information among members.
- To foster research and collaborative activities.
- To encourage co-operation with other relevant professional and public organizations.

APHN Web site: http://www.aphn.org/

European association for palliative care. The European Association for Palliative Care (EAPC) was established on December 1988, with 42 founding members after an important initiative by Professor Vittorio Ventafridda and the Floriani Foundation. The aim of the EAPC is to promote palliative care in Europe and to act as a focus for all of those who work, or have an interest, in the field of palliative care at the scientific, clinical, and social levels.[22] Since 1990 the Head Office of EAPC has been based at the Division of Rehabilitation and Palliative Care in the National Cancer Institute in Milan (Italy). The EAPC includes individual and collective members from 30 National Associations in 20 European countries, representing a movement of some 50,000 healthcare workers and volunteers working or interested in palliative care.

Aims of EAPC

- Promote the implementation of existing knowledge; train those who at any level are involved with the care of patients and families affected by incurable and advanced disease; and promote study and research.
- Bring together those who study and practice the disciplines involved in the care of patients and families affected by advanced disease (doctors, nurses, social workers, psychologists, and volunteers).
- Promote and sponsor publications or periodicals concerning palliative care.
- Unify national palliative care organizations and establish an international network for the exchange of information and expertise.
- Address the ethical problems associated with the care of terminally ill patients

EAPC Web site: http://www.eapcnet.org/index.html

Latin American association for palliative care (*Asociación Latinoamericana de Cuidados Paliativos*). The Asociación Latinoamericana de Cuidados Paliativos (ALCP) was incorporated as a legal entity in 2002, but for more than 14 years, Latin American palliative care workers have been meeting every 2 years to discuss problems, review recent developments and establish networks of support. For some years, the participants voiced their interest in establishing a formal organization to represent the needs and goals of the Region.

The mission of the ALCP is to promote the development of palliative care in Latin America and the Caribbean by integrating all those interested in helping improve the quality of life of patients with incurable progressive diseases as well as their families.[23]

The Association recognizes palliative care as "the active total care of patients and their families by a multi-professional team when the patients' disease is no longer responsive to the curative treatment. Control of pain, of other symptoms, and of psychological, social and spiritual problems is paramount."

Objectives

- To associate all those who are interested in caring for patients with incurable diseases and their families.
- To promote regional information exchange of experiences to strengthen the existing programs and help in the development of new programs.
- To promote the implementation of existing available knowledge, study, and research.
- To develop a basic system to be adapted and applied in every country for the accreditation of institutions and the certification of health personnel of different disciplines.
- To collaborate with its members in:
  - their relationships with the community and the sanitary authorities;
  - the identification and planning of the best healthcare model for their country or region;
  - the development of systems of economic retribution applicable to their country;
  - the development of norms of quality applicable to their country;
  - the procurement of resources;
  - training of healthcare personnel;
  - obtaining regional information to identify needs and collaborate in the design of strategic plans based on this information;
  - publishing guidelines and papers in Spanish and Portuguese;
  - providing information on educational activities for healthcare professionals, patients, legislators, and the general public;
  - supporting initiatives for changes in public health policies which seek to endorse and ensure adequate palliative care;
  - Promoting the necessary changes in policies and regulations to ensure that the necessary drugs for pain relief and other symptoms are available in all countries, in rural and urban regions

ALCP Web site: www.cuidadospaliativos.org

CHALLENGES

There are several challenges to the provision of palliative care in the world, especially in developing countries. Some of the most critical include the following:

Weak health systems. Many donor led strategies and programs from multilateral organizations have focused on the prevention, treatment, and care of specific diseases and conditions. This vertical approach has led in many developing countries, to a disparity in the availability of treatment options for patients who are diagnosed with conditions other than those for which the funding is available. It is important to develop tools to improve systems and not approaches to ones particular disease by focusing on horizontal integrations and strengthening the healthcare systems. Palliative care is applicable in almost all life-limiting conditions and diseases and it should be a component of care for all, not just cancer, HIV, and others.

Political, social, and economic instability. In addition to the limited resources, many developing countries also face political instability and conditions which lead to economic constraints such as shortages in food, water, and medications. In some countries, there are also internal wars among factions, groups, or guerrillas while others face conflicts with their neighbors. In addition to the usual challenges of implementing and developing palliative care programs, many workers have to face additional ones, including risking their personal safety. Bringing relief to the suffering of patients with life-limiting conditions and at their end of their lives in these regions is an extraordinary example of human solidarity.

Misconceptions about palliative care and pain treatment. There are still many misconceptions about palliative care—in some countries caregivers think palliative care is the same as euthanasia and others believe palliative care will provide second class medical care. In the same way, there are many misconceptions about pain treatment and opioids. Many fear that the use of opioids for pain treatment will lead to addiction, while some care providers and health workers have prejudices, believing that people who have not been exposed to analgesics do not feel pain as intensely as those in developed countries.

CONCLUSION

The development of palliative care in the world has been an increasing trend in the last few decades. This has been largely the result of the commitment of extraordinary individuals and the financial support provided by generous donors and organizations. Organizations such as the ones described in this chapter have done an enormous effort and have had a large impact in the development of palliative care globally.

Many patients are now benefiting of hospice and palliative care services in developed countries, but services in developing countries are scarce and very fragile and more is needed to guarantee their permanence and survival.

Education needs to be incorporated in the underground medical and nursing curricula to guarantee the provision of services by a large body of healthcare providers, especially in developing countries. Services and medications need to be subsidized for those who are unable to pay and should be incorporated in the public healthcare systems and reimbursement plans for providers.

More studies are needed on the status of palliative and hospice care services in the world and should be the focus of future research projects.

USEFUL WEB SITES

Pain and Policy Studies Group: http://www.painpolicy.wisc.edu/
The International Association for Hospice and Palliative Care (IAHPC): www.hospicecare.com
The International Observatory in End of Life Care (IOELC): http://www.eolc-observatory.net/
Worldwide Palliative Care Alliance (WPCA): www.wwpca.net

REFERENCES

1. The World Health Report 2002. *Reducing risks, promoting healthy life.* Geneva: WHO; 2002.

2. UNAIDS/WHO. *AIDS epidemic update, December 2004.* Geneva: UNAIDS/WHO; 2004.

3. World Health Organization. *Cancer control program: Policies and managerial guidelines.* Geneva: WHO; 2002.

4. Clark D, Wright M. The international observatory on end of life care: a global view of palliative care development. *J Pain Symptom Manage.* 2007;33(5):542–546.

5. Wright M, Wood J, Lynch T, Clark D. Mapping levels of palliative care development: a global view. International observatory on end of life care. UK: Lancaster University; 2006 November.

6. Torres-Vigil I, Aday LA, Reyes-Gibby C, et al. Health care providers' assessments of the quality of advanced-cancer care in Latin American medical institutions: a comparison of predictors in five countries: Argentina, Brazil, Cuba, Mexico, and Peru. *J Pain Palliat Care Pharmacother.* 2008;22(1):7–20.

7. World Health Organization. *Essential drugs and medicines policy. The essential drug strategy.* Geneva: WHO; 2000.

8. De Lima L, Krakauer EL, Lorenz K, Praill D, MacDonald N, Doyle D. Ensuring palliative medicines availability: The development of the IAHPC list of essential medicines for palliative care. *J Pain Symptom Manage.* 2007;33(5):521–526.

9. World Health Organization. *Cancer pain relief and palliative care.* Report of a WHO Expert Committee, World Health Organization Technical Report Series No 804; Geneva: WHO; 1990.

10. World Health Organization. *WHO model list of essential medicines,* 15th ed. WHO; 2007.

11. World Health Organization. *Access to controlled medications programme.* Geneva: WHO; 2007. Available at: http://www.who.int/medicines/areas/quality_safety/access_to_controlled_medications_brnote_english.pdf. Accessed August 12, 2009.

12. Pain and Policy Studies Group. *Global, regional and national consumption statistics for 2006.* Madison: PPSG; 2008. Available at: http://www.painpolicy.wisc.edu/news/international.htm#041508. Accessed August 12, 2009.

13. World Health Organization Briefing Note. *Access to controlled medications programme.* WHO: Geneva; March 2007.

14. International Narcotics Board. UN Drug Control Body concerned over inadequate medical supply of narcotic drugs to relieve pain and suffering. Press Release, Vienna: INCB, February 23, 2000.

15. World Health Organization. *National cancer control programs: Policies and managerial guidelines.* Geneva: World Health Organization CAN/92.1; 1993, 1995.

16. Stjernsward J, Foley KM, Ferris FD. The public health strategy for palliative care. *J Pain Symptom Manage.* 2007;33(5):486–493.

17. World Hospice and Palliative Care Day. Available at: http://www.worldday.org/. Accessed December 12, 2008.

18. IAHPC and WPCA. Joint declaration and statement of commitment on palliative care and pain treatment as human rights. Retrieved December 15, 2008. Available at: http://www.hospicecare.com/resources/pain_pallcare_hr/. Accessed August 12, 2009.

19. African Palliative Care Association. Available at: http://www.apca.co.ug/. Accessed September 12, 2009.

20. Goh CR. The Asia Pacific hospice palliative care network: a network for individuals and organizations. *J Pain Symptom Manage.* 2002;24(2):128–133.

21. APHN. Information retrieved from the WWW on September 23, 2004. Available at: http://www.aphn.org/. Accessed August 12, 2009.

22. Blumhuber H, Kaasa S, De Conno F. The European association for palliative care. *J Pain Symptom Manage.* 2002;24(2):124–127.

23. Asociación Latinoamericana de Cuidados Paliativos. Mission and objectives. Retrieved December 3, 2008. Available at: http://www.cuidadospaliativos.org/quienes-somos/mision-y-objetivos#Mission. Accessed August 12, 2009.

PART VIII

Psychiatric Disorders

William S. Breitbart, ED

CHAPTER 40

Psychiatric Emergencies

Andrew J. Roth and Talia R. Weiss

INTRODUCTION

A psychiatric emergency is an unforeseen combination of medical and/or psychiatric problems that calls for immediate action to insure safety of the patient or others.[1] These emergencies result from dangerous behaviors or altered mental states, such as thought or mood changes. The first priority is the safety of the patient and anyone else in danger (e.g., family members and staff). Psychiatric emergencies in the medical setting share a number of characteristics with general psychiatric emergencies; however, the setting, the experience, and the availability of trained staff to handle these emergencies and medical co-morbidities all add significant challenges to successful outcomes. Psychiatric emergencies in the oncology setting have their own unique aspects that oncology staff and mental health providers need to be aware of.[2]

Patients often exhibit *intense behaviors or emotions* such as aggression, violence, impulsivity, and agitation[3] before or during a psychiatric emergency. Identifying these behaviors in the earliest phases can assist in the safest management of the patient and the situation. Common manifestations include pulling out tubes or intravenous lines, pacing, becoming demanding or threatening, restlessness, destructiveness, impulsivity, violence, acting on psychotic symptoms, suicidal behavior, or threatening potential harm to self or others (Table 40–1). Some *psychiatric symptoms* constitute an emergency, such as, acute psychosis including paranoid ideation, manic agitation or menacing behavior, irritability and extreme anger, panic attacks, suicidal ideation or hysterical or dramatic behavioral exhibitions. Psychiatric emergencies in the cancer setting may be related to patients in regard to their cancer diagnosis or cancer treatment, or to family members or friends and their reactions to the events and situations of their loved ones and include acute grief reactions after a loved one dies.

This chapter provides a set of strategies to handle a psychiatric emergency which can be implemented by the oncologist or the primary care team initially, with eventual access to a psychiatric consultant. The goals of this chapter are threefold: (1) to teach what types of behaviors, diagnoses, and symptoms lead to emergency psychiatric consultation in the cancer setting; (2) to inform the reader about how to manage psychiatric emergencies in patients with agitation related to delirium, and cognitive impairment disorders, anxiety disorders, depression, and suicidal ideation and behavior in the cancer setting; (3) to convey the indications and suggestions for using physical restraints in the cancer setting; and (4) to discuss how to deal with assessment for capacity and refusal of treatment in the oncology setting.

Common psychiatric emergencies. The most common psychiatric emergencies in medical settings are related to drug or alcohol intoxication or withdrawal syndromes,[4] delirium (due to opioids, steroids, or central nervous system (CNS) disease), suicidality (due to depression; akathisia; suffering related to pain and debilitation, disinhibition, or confusion), panic attacks, manic syndromes (usually due to medications), or patients attempting to leave the hospital against medical advice or refusing treatment. Without comparable prevalence data available, anecdotal experience suggests that these are the most common psychiatric emergencies in the oncology setting as well. Psychiatric emergencies in older patients can be secondary to numerous factors: depression and suicide ideation and attempts, behavioral disturbance secondary to underlying organic conditions, substance abuse, elder abuse, and medication-induced adverse events[5] and can be life threatening.[6]

Risk factors leading to different types of psychiatric emergencies. There are six main risk factors for emergent psychiatric complications in oncology settings (Table 40–2): *advanced stage of disease, unresolved physical symptoms, disease-related factors, treatment-related factors, psychiatric premorbidity, and social factors*.[7] Pain, depression, and delirium all increase in patients with advancing disease.[7-9] Physical symptom burden such as severe, uncontrolled pain, nausea, fatigue, and functional limitations are more likely to lead to acute psychological distress. Disease or medically related factors such as CNS spread, brain cancer, or metabolic abnormalities are more likely to result in delirium or cognitive disorders such as dementia. Treatment-related factors such as recent use of corticosteroids,[10,11] chemotherapeutic agents (vincristine, vinblastine, asparaginase, intrathecal methotrexate, interferon, interleukin, amphotericin),[12] and whole brain irradiation[13] have all been associated with the development of agitation, panic symptoms, depression, delirium, or dementia. In addition finding out about progression of disease or the failure of a treatment regimen can sometimes lead to strong emotional reactions. Advanced cancer patients experience major psychiatric disorders at a rate similar to the general population, but affected individuals have a low utilization of mental health services.[14] Treatment for severe pain with high-dose opioid infusions or drugs such as meperidine can be associated with acute confusional states (delirium), particularly in the elderly and terminally ill. Psychiatric premorbidity, a past history of major depressive disorder or bipolar disorder, a history of substance abuse or major psychotic illness increases the risk of psychologic distress during treatment. In addition, patients with preexisting anxiety disorders, panic disorder, or phobias are likely to experience exacerbations during cancer treatment. Social factors such as prior experience with cancer illness in family members as well as existing social supports influence the experience of a patient with cancer.[15] Recent bereavement and past experiences of loss of a family member with cancer, as well as other recent losses, are important considerations. The role of social support in vulnerability to developing frank psychiatric disorders in cancer is unclear, but certainly it has been shown to serve as a buffer for the degree of psychologic distress and hopelessness experienced by cancer patients, risk for suicide, as well as aiding in the amelioration of these symptoms.[16,17]

AGITATION

Causes. Perhaps the most frightening situation for patients, staff, and family is to see a patient who is out of control and not consolable. A chief assessment goal during a psychiatric emergency is to evaluate for risk and safety.[18] It is useful to assume a medical cause of agitation or confusion in the oncology setting until proven otherwise, since this is considerably more common than functional causes. The following problems often present first with psychological symptoms, but if not recognized and addressed quickly, may become medical emergencies with behavioral changes: progression of disease; CNS involvement or brain metastases; pulmonary emboli; uncontrolled pain; intraabdominal malignancies; metabolic abnormalities (i.e., hyperthyroidism, hypoglycemia, hypocalcemia); medications and other cancer treatments (i.e., opioids, corticosteroids; antiemetics causing akathisia, chemotherapeutic agents, whole brain irradiation); and substances of abuse (i.e., alcohol intoxication or withdrawal, delirium tremens, cocaine use).

Table 40–1. Common behaviors or situations that may constitute psychiatric emergencies

Violence or threatening harm to others
Suicidal ideation or attempts
Restlessness, agitation, or pacing
Threatening or demanding behavior
Pulling out IV or other medical or surgical tubes
Manic behavior
Refusal of urgent treatment or questions of capacity to make medical decisions

Table 40–2. Risk factors for psychiatric emergencies

Advanced stage of disease
Unresolved physical symptoms
Disease or medically related factors
Treatment-related factors
Psychiatric premorbidity
Social factors

Management of the agitated patient. There is usually safety and success in numbers with appropriate staff members.[1] Security, nursing, oncology, and psychiatric staff will be most advantageous in handling a psychiatric emergency. The following guidelines will help in the management of psychiatric emergencies (Table 40–3) and calm agitated patients (Table 40–4).

Ideally, the oncologist treating the patient should be present since s/he knows the medical details best and is known to the patient as a familiar face and voice. In managing an agitated patient, try talking to the patient to decrease agitation and calm excited behavior. The environment can play a key role in exacerbating or reducing the agitation a patient is experiencing. When a patient has been agitated, threatening, expressing suicidality, or violent in the hospital, it is important to have security or nursing staff search the patient's room to remove any dangerous or sharp objects, as well as search for substances of abuse; security or other staff should be available for constant observation until the situation is clearly safe. This may mean having security or nursing staff in or near the patient's room and available to observe visits from family or friends. When agitation or suicidal behavior is a concern in an outpatient clinic, similar guidelines must be in place. If you are responding to a call from family managing the patient at home similar suggestions for constant observation and access to 911 may be recommended. The goal is to reduce the tumult of the situation. This can be accomplished in several ways: isolating the patient from other patients; escorting the patient to a quiet environment, with security, if needed; clearing out a lounge area for the patient, to allow for fewer distractions; and putting the patient in a single room to decrease distractions and danger to others. Assessment of the patient's mental status, the timeline of changes in behavior, the medical status of the patient, past or current psychiatric history including drug and alcohol use, or history of agitation, violence, or suicidality in the past are crucial to optimal management of the emergent situation. Consider whether familiar family or friends are helping to calm the patient or hindering by inadvertently agitating the patient. Consider who/which staff member the patient trusts (e.g., male, female, older, younger, trusted before, speaks the same language) and also, ask staff members toward whom the patient is suspicious or paranoid about not to participate temporarily, if feasible.

Once you have decided on the least invasive management plan to safely calm the patient, explain the plan to the patient with other staff present. If s/he resists, offer the patient the "non-choice choice": one of two or three acceptable modes of action described in a progression of options that suggests a spectrum of more to less freedom to the patient. For instance, "Because you have been so agitated and are in danger of

Table 40–3. Guidelines for managing psychiatric emergencies

In hospital: Call security and support staff for 1:1 observation if needed
At home: have family bring patient to the Emergency Room or call 911
Gather information about the nature of the emergent behavior:
Assess mental status of patient

- Assess timeline of change of behavior
- Assess medical status of patient
- Assess past or current psychiatric history including alcohol or substance use
- Assess whether the patient has been agitated, confused, suicidal, or violent in past?

Develop a working differential diagnosis as early as possible
Assume a medical cause of agitation or confusion until proven otherwise
Identify one staff person who can direct management of the emergency
A calm demeanor is critical to safety for the patient, family, staff, and others
Enlist the help of family, friends or staff members the patient trusts to reassure the patient
Give clear and concise instructions to all staff involved

Table 40–4. How to calm an agitated patient

- Talk to the patient to calm excited behavior
- Isolate the patient away from other patients and visitors
- Escort the patient to a quite room, with security, if needed
- Determine whether family or friends are helping to calm the patient or agitating further
- Identify a staff member the patient trusts to help and ask those who are the target of paranoia not to participate temporarily
- Offer the nonchoice choice: Tell the patient s/he may choose what to do from a couple of options: that is, "You can take the haloperidol liquid, a calming medication, by mouth or we can give you an injection of that medication, either in a muscle or by the IV. Which would you rather have?" With each request, offer a less or more invasive or coercive choice. The more rational the patient's thinking, the more likely s/he will choose the less intrusive option.

Calm, concise explanations help the patient cooperate. Allow the patient to express concerns or frustrations to reduce fears and lack of cooperation

hurting yourself or someone else, you will need to take this calming medicine, haloperidol. You can take the liquid medication, haloperidol, by mouth, or the security guards will have to restrain you so we can give you an injection of the medication. Which would you rather have?"; or "We can walk to your room so you can lie down and calm down, or the security guards will have to restrain you/escort you to your room." Each time, you offer less and more invasive or coercive choices; the more rational the patient's thinking, the more likely s/he will choose the less intrusive option. Allow the patient to express concerns or frustrations to reduce fears and lack of cooperation. Breitbart et al.[19] found that not only is delirium distressing for the patient and family, but also for the oncology staff. It may be even more so when the patient is agitated and in danger of hurting themselves or others. Explaining to family what is happening can be reassuring for them. Reviewing the events with the staff afterward can be helpful and can be a good learning and team building experience.

Use of restraints in psychiatric emergencies. There are many types of physical restraints in the oncology setting. Medical immobilization devices as well as postural and adaptive supports that do not require physician's orders are used to prevent and protect against injuries (i.e., using a belt to keep a patient secured to a surgical table; using a limb board to secure an IV placement). Physical restraints for control of agitated behaviors are usually used as either 2 point (arms) or 4 point (arms and legs) restraining devices. In some institutions, soft padded hand mitts are used to prevent a patient from pulling out tubes and lines or scratching themselves. Four point restraints usually require a physician's (or other licensed medical professional) order that must be renewed every 4 hours. Though the initial order may come by telephone, it, as well as subsequent orders, must be signed in the order sheet or electronic order form. Familiarize yourself with your institution's legal policies about this. Follow the guidelines for how often vital signs need to be checked and restraint sites rotated to decrease the likelihood of injury to the patient. Four point restraints require checking the patient's extremities every 15 minutes; these restraints should remain on as briefly as possible. Changing to a less restrictive form when safe is desirable. The patient should remain under 1:1 constant observation status while 4 point restraints are in use.

Medication—"Chemical Sedation." Psychotropic medications should not be used as chemical restraints just to keep patients quiet. Sometimes an emergency team must use physical restraint, by holding the patient down, to give medication to control agitated behavior. Care should be given in the oncology setting to aspects of the patient's medical condition that may compromise safety if the patient is restrained: platelet count, bone density, frailty. If the patient needs to be physically restrained and it is considered safe to do so, having a sufficient number of well-trained staff to secure each limb is imperative; thus four security guards or strong staff members might be needed to escort the patient and then hold each limb while a medication is given by injection by a nurse, or while the patient is put into restraints. Periodic practice of "psychiatric codes" help a multidisciplinary team become more comfortable with the procedure, and with each other, and may allow for a smoother, safer outcome when chaos presents itself.

Documentation. It is important to document the details of the medical and psychiatric situation, the reason for emergent intervention as well as the date and time on all chart notes. Make sure to include

- patient's medications
- pertinent lab results
- psychiatric history including alcohol and drug abuse
- history of self-destructive or violent behavior
- likelihood of the patient causing harm to himself or others
- whether there is a need, or not, for constant observation
- pertinent mental status examination findings
- whether restraints were required and why

It is always helpful in an emergency to be prepared. Have useful phone numbers on hand so you do not need to search for them in chaotic situations. It is important to have a psychiatrist available for immediate call who is familiar with the common as well as unusual presentations and management of agitation, withdrawal states, and suicidality in cancer patients, and who can work with you and the team. Other useful telephone numbers to have on hand are Hospital Security; Medical Records; Legal Affairs; Patient Representatives or Hospital Administration; Social Work; Emergency Room or Urgent Care Center; Outside Emergency Telephone Numbers; Central Intake for Psychiatric Admissions; and Chaplaincy. For outpatients in clinic or office settings, resources may be limited, but security should be available and a call to 911 for assistance is always available for local police and ambulance resources.

Psychopharmacological management of the agitated patient. There are many pharmacologic options available for treating agitated patients.[1-3] The following course of action has been found to be helpful. Haloperidol, a neuroleptic agent that is a potent dopamine blocker, is the drug of choice for agitated medically ill patients. If possible, check vital signs and obtain an electrocardiogram (EKG) to monitor QTc intervals.

Haloperidol in low doses (start with 0.5–2 mg IV, and double the dose every 30–60 minutes until agitation is decreased) is usually effective in targeting agitation, paranoia, and fear that have physiological causes. Parenteral doses are approximately twice as potent as oral doses. A common strategy is to add parenteral lorazepam (0.5–2 mg IV) to a regimen of haloperidol, which may help in rapidly sedating the agitated delirious patient. Lorazepam given alone is not a good choice when given for agitation caused by delirium.[20] It is important to realize that intravenous use of haloperidol has warnings about cardiac side effects; therefore documentation of why this method of treatment is being used (i.e., other means are not indicated, not available or ineffective) should be clearly stated in the chart. Risperidone, a less sedating atypical antipsychotic, may also be used with lorazepam, but is not available in intravenous form and also has the potential of causing extrapyramidal side effects (EPS).

Other atypical neuroleptic drugs with sedating qualities such as olanzapine and quetiapine show promise because of improved side-effect profiles, in particular, fewer EPS and cardiovascular problems than the high-potency haloperidol and risperidone and fewer cardiovascular side effects than chlorpromazine. Olanzapine and risperidone may be given in orally disintegrating tablets; ziprasidone, another atypical antipsychotic, may be given intramuscularly, however, none of the atypical antipsychotics are available in intravenous (IV) form. Elderly or frail patients require lower doses of these medications; there are warnings about using atypical antipsychotic medications in older patients with dementia because of the risk of cerebrovascular accidents.

When the combination of haloperidol and lorazepam or a sedating atypical neuroleptic is ineffective for calming an agitated or combative patient, consider using chlorpromazine intravenously. Be aware that this medicine may have hypotensive and anticholinergic side effects. Again, documentation in the chart is important when using medications for off label purposes or in nonofficially sanctioned formulations (e.g., intravenously) when other more standard trials have not been effective. Table 40–5 outlines an algorithm for medicating agitation, including the routes available for administration, and side effects to watch for.

After successfully calming the agitated patient, try to expedite any needed medical work-up that may explain the agitation or delirium (i.e., brain magnetic resonance imaging (MRI), computed tomography (CT) scans, lumbar puncture, other blood tests, x-rays, urinalysis); use the least amount of medication needed to keep the patient from harming self or others. A common approach to management of confusion caused by opioid therapy is to lower the dose of the opioid if the patient's pain is controlled, or to rotate to another opioid regimen that may be better tolerated, if there is still pain coincident with the confusion. Continue to monitor the patient closely to see whether more antipsychotic medication is needed to keep the patient and staff safe and to assure that the patient is not having side effects from the medications. Continue the neuroleptic regimen until symptoms improve and the etiology of the agitation is reversed; then taper off the medication (see Chapter 45).

ANXIETY-RELATED EMERGENCIES

Causes. Early recognition and treatment of severe anxiety is essential for optimal care and to hopefully prevent an emergent situation. Understanding the source of the many possible causes of anxiety is important in choosing an appropriate treatment as there are many causes of apprehension and worry in this population. Situations that lead to emergencies are often based on receiving unexpected bad news or anticipation of frightening situations. Patients may experience panic symptoms (i.e., pacing, heart palpitations, feeling the need to escape, shortness of breath, or a sense of impending doom). In addition, emergencies comprising anxiety and restlessness are frequently associated with medical problems such as uncontrolled pain, abnormal metabolic states, endocrine abnormalities, medications that produce anxiety, and withdrawal states.[2] Symptom control can significantly impact quality of life and a patient's sense of control over his/her situation, thus reducing anxiety, uncertainty, and potential danger.

Table 40–5. Algorithm for medicating agitation

Medication:	Haloperidol	OR SWITCH TO→	Chlorpromazine	OR USE/SWITCH TO↔	Olanzapine
Approximate Daily Dose (mg):	0.5–10 Q 2–12 hr		25–50 mg IV Q 4–12 hr if increased sedation desired OR if haloperidol or olanzapine regimen is not tolerated		2.5–5 mg BID if EPS is a concern OR if increased sedation is desired OR if haloperidol or Chloropamazine regimen is not tolerated
Route:	IV, IM, PO		IV, IM, PO		PO or Zydis wafer
Need to watch for:	Extrapyramidal symptoms (EPS), EKG		EKG, BP, Liver Function Tests, anticholinergic side effects		Increased glucose; anticholinergic side effects EKG-QTC
	If EPS is present, add benztropine 0.5–1 mg (po TID) If increased sedation desired, add lorazepam 0.5–2 mg q 4 hr EKG-QTC				
Alternative	Risperidone				Quetiapine

ABBREVIATIONS: BP, blood pressure; EKG, electrocardiogram; IM, intramuscular; IV, intravenous; PO, per oral; TID, *ter in die* (Latin). All neuroleptics may lower seizure threshold.

Patients with severe anxiety who are extremely fearful, unable to absorb information or cooperate with procedures require psychological support, medication, and/or behavioral interventions to reduce symptoms to a manageable level. It is important to note the duration and intensity of symptoms, the level of impairment of normal function, and the ability to comply with treatment.

Management. The initial management of an anxiety emergency requires that adequate information be given to patients in a supportive manner.[2] An attitude of ridicule or impatience makes their distress worse. Cognitive-behaviorally oriented techniques as well as crisis intervention principles are useful. Again, requesting the presence of supportive family or others familiar to the patient may help reduce tension and worry.

Psychopharmacological management. A benzodiazepine is often needed in combination with psychological support for severe anxiety.[1] The choice of medication depends on the severity of anxiety, desired duration of drug action and rapidity of onset needed, route of administration available, presence or absence of active metabolites, and metabolic problems that must be considered (see Chapter 44). Often fast acting benzodiazepines that can be given through a parenteral route, such as lorazepam, may be helpful in emergent situations. If a benzodiazepine cannot be used or tolerated because of sedation, confusion or respiratory depression, neuroleptics may bring the patient calm relatively quickly. In particular, the sedating atypical neuroleptics, olanzapine, and quetiapine have prominent antianxiety effects and help patients sleep better at night.

EMERGENCIES RELATED TO DEPRESSION

Causes. It is not normal or acceptable for a patient's mood to be severely depressed, accompanied by hopelessness, despondency, guilt, and suicidal thoughts; s/he likely has a major depression if symptoms have continued unabated for more than 2 weeks. Although sadness about illness is normally expected with any cancer, a major depressive episode is not. Depressive disorders lead to emergent situations when suicidality or self-harm is a possibility. Studies have found an increased suicide rate among patients with cancer.[21] A recent study found increased risk of suicidal ideation in middle-aged patients more so than older patients,[15] though the stigma of this symptom often makes it difficult to study this entity with precision. Suicidal risk must be assessed before an emergency is imminent. Physical symptoms must be carefully evaluated to determine whether uncontrolled pain, fatigue, immobility, insomnia, or nausea is so severe that they are leading to depression and thoughts of suicide. These symptoms often lead to hopeless, isolative, desperate feelings, and a sense that life is intolerable unless the symptoms are relieved. Patients interpret a new or increasingly severe symptom as a sign that the cancer has progressed, resulting in greater depression and hopelessness. Suicide is a real risk in these patients, especially if they do not believe that efforts are being made to control the symptom or that relief is possible. Suicidal ideation and depressive symptoms often abate when symptoms are controlled. A major depression likely needs to be treated with an antidepressant. It is important to remind all staff and family that *asking about suicide does not "put thoughts into patients' heads" or increase the risk of suicide attempts.* The thoughts are often present beforehand and asking about them can bring relief in knowing that the patient can now talk with someone about very upsetting thoughts.

Suicidal ideation as emergencies. Many cancer patients have thoughts about dying and, at times, that it might be better or easier if they were not alive. Some try to deal with the uncertainty of an unhappy, debilitated future by taking control with their thoughts, such as "if it gets bad enough I will kill myself." In reality, many of these people do not want to die or hurt themselves, but want to share their frustration and perhaps fears about not being able to have the kind of health or life that they wanted or expected. Suicidal ideation is frightening for the patient, family, and the medical staff. However, it is not always easy to make a distinction between passive thoughts of dying with no intent of self-harm and when someone is in acute danger of self-destructive behavior (see Chapter 41 and Chapter 43). Suicidal behavior can be seen in patients with depression or severe anxiety or panic symptoms[15] as well as fear of pain, disfigurement, and loss of function early in the patients' courses.[21] Desire for hastened death among terminally ill patients is often fueled by depression and hopelessness.[22] The seriousness of all expressions of suicidality, passive or active, should be explored with the patient.

Table 40–6. Questions to assess suicidal risk

- Do you feel hopeless about ever feeling better?
- What would you like to see happen for yourself?
- Have you had thoughts of not wanting to live?
- Have you had thoughts of doing something to hurt yourself if things get bad enough?
- Do you have any strong social supports?
- Do you have a problem with alcohol or drugs?
- Have you recently stopped either abruptly?
- Do you have pain or other debilitating symptoms that are not being relieved or addressed?
- Have you ever made a suicide attempt?
- Has anyone in your family made a suicide attempt?
- Do you have a plan in mind? In the last week?
- Do you have pills or other means of ending your life at home?
- Do you own or have access to a weapon?

Examples of less emergent expressions, that should still be addressed include

- "I've dealt with this illness for so many years; I don't think I can go through another procedure—I'd rather die."
- "This may be a new diagnosis, but it is Cancer. If the disease spreads and the pain ever gets bad enough, I may kill myself."

More emergent expressions of suicidality might include

- "This pain is unbearable. There's no way I can go on living like this." The patient has a gun at home.
- A nurse finds a number of pills under a patient's pillow when redoing bedding, a few days after he heard his disease had progressed. The patient was heard to mutter that everyone would be better off without him.

It is important to ask if the patient has made a definite plan to hurt him or herself. It bears repeating that asking the patient about suicide does not increase the risk of suicide! When assessing the risk of suicide it is important to acknowledge commonality, assess the presence of a plan and intent, assess their access to lethal methods of killing themselves, attain the patient's prior psychiatric history including substance abuse or prior self-destructive behavior, find out if the patient has recently lost a loved one, and if he/she has adequate social support.[2] Table 40–6 outlines questions to ask patients or family in the assessment of suicidal risk.

Medical predictors of enhanced suicidal risk are poorly controlled pain, fatigue, advanced stage of disease with debilitation, mild delirium with poor impulse control, psychiatric morbidity, and hopelessness or helplessness (loss of control) especially in the context of depression or anxiety.

Management of the suicidal patient. When you have determined that the patient is at risk for suicidal behavior it is important to inform family members of the risk, so they can assist in taking away weapons or other means of self-harm. Though it is unclear how beneficial a behavior contract is in preventing suicide,[23] it may be helpful in giving a patient the opportunity to think through other options when they may otherwise be too distressed to consider them, such as calling specific friends, family members or physicians. Symptoms such as pain, nausea, insomnia, anxiety, and depression should be treated as soon as possible. Engaging in symptom control can significantly impact quality of life and a patient's sense of control over his/her situation. For inpatients, room searches should be carried out to make sure there are no means available for self-destructive behavior. Patients should be under 1:1 constant observation from the time they express their active suicidal thoughts, though this too is not a foolproof deterrent to suicide. For severely suicidal outpatients whose suicidality is not acutely caused by their medical condition or medication, psychiatric hospitalization may be warranted, either by voluntary or involuntary means. A psychiatrist or social worker can assist in making these arrangements. Mobilizing the patient's support system is important. A close family member or friend should be involved to support the patient, provide information, and assist in treatment planning.

If a major depressive episode has been identified, and the patient is in a safe, protected environment, antidepressant therapy is initiated, recognizing that effectiveness will not be evident for a number of weeks. Additionally there are now warnings about the potential for antidepressants to cause suicidal ideation. Though rare, all patients started on antidepressants should be monitored closely, in particular for agitation and energizing effects of the medication that arise before the antidepressant effects have fully taken affect.

Psychostimulants are useful in low doses for patients who are suffering from depressed mood, apathy, decreased energy, poor concentration, and weakness. They promote a sense of well-being, decreased fatigue, and increased appetite. They are helpful in countering the sedating effects of opioids, and they produce a rapid effect in comparison with the other antidepressants. In fact they are often started along with antidepressants and can be discontinued when the antidepressant effects are likely to have begun in 4–8 weeks. Because of their rapid effect, psychostimulants are particularly useful in patients in the terminal phases of life. Side effects include insomnia, euphoria, and mood lability; suicidal patients should be monitored closely in the early, energizing period of treatment.

MANAGEMENT OF EMERGENCIES: SPECIAL CONSIDERATIONS

Capacity to make medical decisions, refusal of treatment or demands to leave the hospital. Another frequent reason to see a cancer patient emergently is to assess their capacity to make medical decisions, to refuse medical recommendations or to leave the hospital against medical advice. Emergent consults, interestingly, are usually not requested when the patient is agreeable to a treatment plan, even if they appear somewhat confused.[24] But when they refuse medical or surgical procedures (i.e., lumbar punctures, placement of central catheters), that are deemed to be medically appropriate, emergent consults are often requested. Discussions regarding appropriate levels of intervention based on issues such as patient wishes regarding advanced directives, clearly defined healthcare proxies, proper documentation of those wishes, location of care, cognitive status, and extent of clinical decline are useful to have before crisis situations.[25] Though the oncologist may evaluate the patient's capacity to make medical decisions, it may be advisable to ask for a psychiatric consultation. It is important to find people whom the patient knows and trusts (family, friends) to give information about cognitive and mental functioning before the current situation, and to help the patient feel calmer; this is especially true for patients whose first language is not English. Problems in staff-patient communication are often the cause of misunderstandings. In these situations, attaining adequate understanding and communication between doctor and patient about the medical situation may obviate the need for a definitive capacity examination. The issue of insight and judgment should turn on the question in hand, for example, regarding a specific procedure or situation. For instance, "Does the patient have the capacity to make a decision about refusing this MRI scan, (or lumbar puncture)?" The patient may be able to understand the issues related to some decisions and not to others, even if they have psychotic or depressive symptoms.

In general, the life-threatening nature or potential positive outcome of a medical decision will guide the needed depth of a patient's understanding of their illness, treatment recommendation and consequences of refusing those recommendations. For example: a patient's refusal of a well-accepted first line chemotherapy regimen with few side effects that has a good likelihood of curing a newly diagnosed cancer, would require more understanding about the benefits and consequences of this decision, than perhaps a terminally ill patient's refusal of a 4th line chemotherapy regimen that has little chance of cure and might cause severe side effects that severely diminish quality of life. Getting assistance from colleagues and hospital ethics committees may be helpful. Guidelines for assessing decision-making capacity and treatment refusal are listed in Table 40–7.

Table 40–7. Guidelines to assess decision-making capacity and refusal of medical and surgical treatment

- The patient may be detained until cognition and judgment are assessed
- Find out what the patient understands about the current medical situation
- Do a mental status examination and determine if cognition is compromised, including judgment and insight about the specific medical decision
- The patient may be able to understand issues related to some decisions and not to others
- Try to obtain corroborating information from family or friends about the patient's baseline mental status and end of life directives
- The seriousness of the decision to refuse treatment, as well as the life-threatening nature or potential benefit of a decision, guides the evaluation of the depth of a patient's understanding of the illness, treatment recommendations and consequences of refusing those recommendations.

In complex situations, a psychiatric consultation or an ethics committee review may be helpful

CONCLUSION

In summary, psychiatric emergencies can be amongst the most frightening and dangerous situations in the cancer setting. Of utmost importance is maintaining the safety of patients, staff, and family. Quick, efficient assessment of the possible etiology of the emergency as well as awareness of strategies for diffusing the distress and allowing either medical work-up or treatment to continue are primary goals of the oncology and psychiatry staff. Suggestions are presented in this chapter for preparing for and handling various psychiatric emergencies in the cancer setting. Discussions and planning among multidisciplinary groups about how to deal with these emergencies before they occur can help a staff deal with these situations more appropriately, efficiently, and safely.

ACKNOWLEDGMENTS

The authors wish to acknowledge the contribution of Jon Levenson to a chapter on a similar subject for the IPOS Quick Reference for Oncology Clinicians: The Psychiatric and Psychological Dimensions of Cancer Symptom Management that was the foundation for the current chapter. In addition, we want to acknowledge the important role of Michelle Ramsunder for her administrative and organizing skills in completing this and other chapters in this bible of Psycho-Oncology.

REFERENCES

1. Roth A, Levenson JA. *Psychiatric emergencies, in quick reference for oncology clinicians: the psychiatric and psychological dimensions of cancer symptom management.* Charlottesville, VA: IPOS Press; 2006.

2. Roth A, Breitbart W. Psychiatric emergencies in terminally ill cancer patients. *Hematol Oncol Clin North Am.* 1996;10:235–259.

3. Onyike C, Lyketsos CG. Aggression and violence. In: Levenson JL, (ed). *Textbook of psychiatric medicine.* Washington DC: American Psychiatric Publishing Inc; 2005:171–191.

4. Shakya D, Shyangw PM, Shakya R. Psychiatric emergencies in a tertiary care hospital. *JNMA J Nepal Med Assoc.* 2008;47:28–33.

5. Borja B, Borja CS, Gade S. Psychiatric emergencies in the geriatric population. *Clin Geriatr Med.* 2007;23:391–400.

6. Tueth M, Zuberi P. Life-threatening psychiatric emergencies in the elderly: overview. *J Geriatr Psychiatry Neurol.* 1999;12:60–66.

7. Bukberg J, Penman D, Holland JC. Depression in hospitalized cancer patients. *Psychosomatic Med.* 1984;46:199–212.

8. Foley K. The Treatment of cancer pain. *N Engl J Med.* 19985;313:84–95.

9. Massie M, Holland JC, Glass E. Delirium in terminally ill cancer patients. *Am J Psychiatry.* 1983;140:1048–1050.

10. Breitbart W, Stiefel F, Pannulo S, et al. Neuropsychiatric cancer patients with epidural spinal cord compression receiving high dose corticosteroids: a prospective comparison study. *Psychooncology.* 1993;2:233–245.

11. Stiefel F, Breitbart WS, Holland JC. Corticosteroids in cancer: neuropsychiatric complications. *Cancer Invest.* 1989;7:479–491.

12. Weddington W. Delirium and depression associated with amphotericin B. *Psychosomatics.* 1982;23:1076–1078.

13. DeAngelis L, Delattre J, Toma T. Radiation-induced dementia in patients cured of brain metastases. *Neurology.* 1989;39:789–796.

14. Kadan-Lottick N, Vanderwerker LC, Block SD, Zhang B, Prigerson HG. Psychiatric disorders and mental health service use in patients with advanced cancer: a report from the coping with cancer study. *Cancer.* 2005; 104:2872–2881.

15. Rasic D, Belik SL, Bolton JM, et al. Cancer, mental disorders, suicidal ideation and attempts in a large community sample. *Psychooncology.* 2008;17: 660–667.

16. Breitbart W. Suicide in the cancer patient. *Oncology.* 1987;1:49–54.

17. Goldberg J, Cullen LO. Factors important to psychological adjustment to cancer: a review of the evidence. *Soc Sci Med.* 1985;20:803–807.

18. Lee T, Renaud EF, Hills OF. An emergency treatment hub-and-spoke model for psychiatric emergency services. *Psychiatr Serv.* 2003;54: 1590–1594.

19. Breitbart W, Gibson C, Tremblay A. The delirium experience: delirium recall and delirium-related distress in hospitalized patients with cancer, their spouses/caregivers, and their nurses. *Psychosomatics.* 2002;43: 183–194.

20. Breitbart W, Marotta R, Platt MM, et al. A double-blinded trial of haloperidol, chlorpromazine, and lorazepam in the treatment of delirium in hospitalized AIDS patients *Am J Psychiatry.* 1996;152(2):231–237.

21. Bostwick J, Levenson, JL. Suicidality. In: Levenson JL, (ed). *Textbook of psychiatric medicine.* Washington DC: American Psychiatric Publishing Inc.; 2005:219–234.

22. Breitbart W, Rosenfeld, B, Pessin, H, et al. Depression, hopelessness, and desire for hastened death in terminally ill patients with cancer. *JAMA.* 2000;284:2907–2911.

23. Lewis L. No-harm contracts: a review of what we know. *Suicide Life Threat Behav.* 2007;37:50–57.

24. Stowell C, Barnhill J, Ferrando S. *Characteristics of patients with impaired decision-making capacity.* Paper presented at: Academy of Psychosomatic Medicine Annual Meeting; 2007.

25. Wrede-Seaman L. Management of emergent conditions in palliative care. *Prim Care.* 2001;28:317–328.

Adjustment Disorders

Madeline Li, Sarah Hales, and Gary Rodin

Adjustment disorder refers to a condition in which there is distress in excess of what would normally be expected or significant functional impairment following exposure to an identifiable stressor.[1] It is the most commonly reported psychiatric diagnosis in patients with cancer[2,3] but the most problematic in terms of its conceptualization and evidence base.[4,5] Although the diagnosis, treatment and recovery from cancer is universally associated with multiple, unavoidable, internal, chronic, or recurrent cancer-related stressors and perceived trauma, the normative response to these stressors is not well established. Consequently, the diagnostic thresholds for adjustment disorder are uncertain and the reliability and validity of this diagnosis have been questioned. Although the adjustment disorder category has undoubted descriptive value, whether it should be regarded as a psychiatric disorder has been the subject of debate.

It is a commonplace observation that psychological distress follows traumatic life events and the more severe manifestations of this phenomenon have been included in most diagnostic classifications of psychiatric disorders. The adjustment disorder diagnosis first appeared in the *Diagnostic and Statistical Manual of Mental Disorders*, Second Edition (DSM-II) in 1968 to replace the category of transient situational disturbance and it was subsequently included in the *International Statistical Classification of Diseases and Related Health Problems*, Ninth Edition (ICD-9) in 1978.[4] Adjustment disorder was included in these diagnostic systems, in part, to compensate for the elimination of the category of reactive depression[4] and to provide a category that would allow third party reimbursement for psychiatric care of patients whose psychological disturbance did not otherwise meet the criteria for a major mental disorder.[5] The categorization of discrete distress syndromes, such as adjustment disorder, may also satisfy certain research and publication requirements, although there is a growing consensus that dimensional assessments of distress may actually have better reliability and construct validity.[6]

Adjustment disorder lies in a transitional zone on the continuum of distress between normative adaptation and psychopathology. Although it is regarded as an Axis I disorder in the DSM, Strain[7] has proposed a hierarchical classification in which it is located between V codes or problem-level diagnoses and subthreshold psychiatric disorders. This approach has some heuristic value, although the distinction between adjustment disorder and subthreshold depression may be arbitrary. The diagnosis of adjustment disorder may be of clinical value when used to capture prodromal or transient states of distress that are amenable to preventive or early interventions. Such interventions are justified given that psychological distress is associated with decreased satisfaction and participation in medical treatment,[8,9] the desire for hastened death, requests for physician-assisted suicide and/or euthanasia,[10,11] reduced quality of life,[12-14] and distress in family caregivers.[15]

This chapter will focus on adjustment disorders in patients with cancer. The validity and utility of the current diagnostic criteria for adjustment disorders and potential new directions for the diagnostic classification of such disturbances in patients with cancer will be discussed. Evidence regarding epidemiology, pathogenesis, and potential interventions for adjustment disorders will be reviewed.

CURRENT DIAGNOSTIC CRITERIA

The diagnosis of adjustment disorder, according to the *Diagnostic and Statistical Manual of Mental Disorders*, Fourth Edition, Text Revision

(DSM-IV-TR) (see Table 41-1), requires that a clinically significant psychological response to an identifiable stressor develop within 3 months of its onset (Criterion A). The DSM-IV-TR specifies that this response must be characterized either by marked distress, in excess of what would be expected with the specific stressor, or by significant impairment in social or occupational functioning (Criterion B). The latter criterion allows for a normal or expectable level of distress in response to a stressor if it is severe enough to cause significant impairment. This specification circumvents the uncertainty about what is a normative response to major life stress, although it contains the contradiction that a "normal" emotional response can simultaneously be considered to be psychopathological.

DSM-IV-TR excludes co-morbidity with other Axis I or Axis II disorders and bereavement (Criterion C and D) if the other disorder accounts for the pattern of symptoms observed in response to the stressor. Finally, the symptoms must not persist more than 6 months after the termination of the stressor (Criterion E), although there is a chronic specifier for stressors or their consequences that have a prolonged course. Subtypes of adjustment disorder are coded according to the predominant symptom: "with depressed mood" for symptoms of depression, tearfulness, or hopelessness; "anxiety" for nervousness, worry, jitteriness, or fears of separation from attachment figures (in children); and "disturbance of conduct" for violation of the rights of others or of major age-appropriate societal norms and rules. Mixed subtypes can also be specified with "mixed anxiety and depressed mood," and "mixed disturbance of emotions and conduct." There is also an "unspecified" subtype for maladaptive reactions not otherwise classified (i.e., physical complaints, social withdrawal, work, or academic inhibition).

The diagnostic criteria for adjustment disorder depart from the general conceptual and operational principles of the DSM-IV-TR in two important respects. First, unlike the criteria listed for virtually all other major psychiatric disorders, there is a lack of specificity that is provided for other diagnoses by symptom checklists, quantifiable attributes, or diagnostic algorithms. Secondly, whereas it is purported that most DSM-IV-TR diagnoses are atheoretical (i.e., based on phenomenologic symptomatology and not linked to any specific pathogenesis or etiology), adjustment disorder is linked to a specific triggering event, as is the case with posttraumatic stress disorder (PTSD) and acute stress disorder (ASD).

There are a number of differences in the categorization of adjustment disorder in the DSM-IV-TR and the *International Statistical Classification of Diseases and Related Health Problems*, Tenth Edition (ICD-10), a diagnostic system developed by the World Health Organization[16] and commonly used in Europe and other parts of the world. In contrast to the DSM-IV-TR, adjustment disorder in the ICD-10 is classified within the anxiety disorders category, must have an onset within 1 month of the stressful event and is subtyped into brief depressive reaction and prolonged depressive reaction. The ICD-10 specifies that in children adjustment disorder may be characterized by regressive behaviors, and has no chronic specifier, although the prolonged depressive reaction subtype may extend up to 2 years (Table 41-2).

The nature of what is captured in the category of adjustment disorder may be best illustrated by case examples, such as those described below.

Table 41-1. DSM-IV diagnostic criteria for adjustment disorders

A. The development of emotional or behavioral symptoms in response to an identifiable stressor(s) occurring within 3 months of the onset of the stressor(s).
B. These symptoms or behaviors are clinically significant as evidenced by either of the following:
  1. marked distress that is in excess of what would be expected from exposure to the stressor
  2. significant impairment in social or occupational (academic) functioning
C. The stress-related disturbance does not meet the criteria for another specific Axis I disorder and is not merely an exacerbation of a preexisting Axis I or Axis II disorder.
D. The symptoms do not represent bereavement.
E. Once the stressor (or its consequences) has terminated, the symptoms do not persist for more than an additional 6 months.

Specify:
Acute: if the disturbance lasts less than 6 months.
Chronic: if the disturbance lasts for 6 months or longer.
Adjustment disorders are coded based on the subtype, which is selected according to the predominant symptoms. The specific stressor(s) can be specified on Axis IV.
  With depressed mood
  With anxiety
  With mixed anxiety and depressed mood
  With disturbance of conduct
  With mixed disturbance of emotions and conduct
  Unspecified

SOURCE: Reprinted with permission from Association AP. Diagnostic and statistical manual of mental disorders, text revision. 4th ed. Washington, DC: American Psychiatric Association Press; 2000.

Table 41-2. ICD-10 diagnostic criteria for adjustment disorders

A. Onset of symptoms must occur within 1 month of exposure to an identifiable psychosocial stressor, not of an unusual or catastrophic type.
B. The individual manifests symptoms or behavior disturbance of the types found in any of the affective disorders (except for delusions and hallucinations), any disorder in neurotic, stress-related, and somatoform disorders, and conduct disorders, but the criteria for an individual disorder are not fulfilled. Symptoms may be variable in both form and severity.

The predominant feature of the symptoms may be further specified.
Brief depressive reaction
A transient mild depressive state of a duration not exceeding 1 month.
Prolonged depressive reaction
A mild depressive state occurring in response to a prolonged exposure to a stressful situation but of a duration not exceeding 2 years.
Mixed anxiety and depressive reaction
Both anxiety and depressive symptoms are prominent, but at levels no greater than those specified for mixed anxiety and depressive disorder or other mixed anxiety disorders.
With predominant disturbance of other emotions
The symptoms are usually of several types of emotions, such as anxiety, depression, worry, tensions, and anger. Symptoms of anxiety and depression may meet the criteria for mixed anxiety and depressive disorder or for other mixed anxiety disorders, but they are not so predominant that other more specific depressive or anxiety disorders can be diagnosed. This category should also be used for reactions in children in whom regressive behavior such as bed-wetting or thumb-sucking is also present.

With predominant disturbance of conduct
The main disturbance is one involving conduct, for example, an adolescent grief reaction resulting in aggressive or dissocial behavior.
With mixed disturbance of emotions and conduct
Both emotional symptoms and disturbances of conduct are prominent features.
With other specified predominant symptoms
Except in prolonged depressive reaction, the symptoms do not persist for more than 6 months after the cessation of the stress or its consequences. However, this should not prevent a provisional diagnosis being made if this criterion is not yet fulfilled.

C. Except in prolonged depressive reaction, the symptoms do not persist for more than 6 months after the cessation of the stress or its consequences. However, this should not prevent a provisional diagnosis being made if this criterion is not yet fulfilled.

SOURCE: Reprinted with permission from Organization WH. International classification of diseases. 10th ed. Geneva: World Heath Organization; 1995.

CASE STUDY 1: ADJUSTMENT DISORDER WITH DEPRESSED MOOD

Mr. L was a 37-year-old divorced male of Italian descent, with no children, living with his parents and working in construction when he was diagnosed with a locally advanced laryngeal cancer. He was referred for psychiatric assessment by his oncology team, who said that he had "run away" before he was scheduled to begin his first cycle of induction chemotherapy. His family reported that he had "gone missing" the day before his first chemotherapy appointment and returned home without explanation 4 days later, telling them that he had decided not to have chemotherapy.

When interviewed, Mr. L was downcast but did not demonstrate psychomotor retardation. He expressed a belief that treatment with chemotherapy was futile—that it would only prolong the burden on his family and prevent him from enjoying the limited time remaining in his life. The expected period of disability from work and the enforced dependence on his family was highly distressing to him. He endorsed significant dysphoria, with frequent episodes of tearfulness, which he found intolerable, feelings of guilt about the burden on his family, and hopelessness about his future and about a favorable response to treatment. He denied anhedonia, neurovegetative symptoms or suicidal ideation and revealed that he spent the 4 days in which he was "missing" enjoying a fishing trip which had distracted him from his dilemma.

Mr. L agreed to accept individual psychological support, initially undertaken to determine his capacity to refuse treatment. The treatment focused both on his negative cognitions about the futility of treatment and on his attachment insecurity in the context of an increased dependency on others. Over the following 3 weeks, he was able to reframe his negative beliefs about the futility of treatment and to consider other potential outcomes. He developed insight into his difficulty accepting help and became more able to tolerate receiving support from his family. He eventually agreed to chemotherapy, and adopted a "fighting spirit" toward his cancer. He completed a course of combined chemoradiation treatment, requiring only intermittent subsequent sessions for psychological support.

CASE STUDY 2: ADJUSTMENT DISORDER WITH MIXED ANXIETY AND DEPRESSED MOOD

Mrs. F was a 47-year-old married woman with three children who had been diagnosed 3 years earlier with a rare T-cell leukemia. Her treatment was marked by numerous medical complications and a relapse within 2 months of completing her initial chemotherapy. She understood that her disease was incurable at the time of diagnosis, but had managed to avoid dwelling on such thoughts. She maintained a positive, hopeful attitude, accepting disease complications as they arose and focusing on enjoying her life. However, this adaptive approach was undermined by the complications of a stem-cell transplant that included viral nephritis and severe pedal edema that impaired her ability to walk.

Mrs. F was referred for psychiatric assessment following a 5-day history of uncontrollable crying and anxiety which were highly unusual for her. She reported intense and persistent feelings of terror, with intrusive thoughts about her current medical complications which she believed marked "the beginning of the end." She was afraid to spend any time alone but was distressed that her husband took a leave of absence from his work to be at her side. She endorsed significant anhedonia and impaired concentration, and reported that she had completely stopped her usual comfort strategies of meditation, reading, and singing. She felt hopeless about regaining the ability to walk or to garden and indicated that she did not wish to live if her current emotional state could not be alleviated.

Mrs. F's anxiety responded to a low dose of clonazepam which enabled her to engage in supportive-expressive therapy, reflecting on the feelings of grief and the existential concerns that had been activated by the progression of her disease. With support, she was more able to tolerate disturbing feelings and she began to engage in end-of-life preparations, including developing legacy projects for her children. Over the next few weeks, the clonazepam was gradually reduced in dosage and then discontinued without recurrence of her anxiety. As her medical condition improved, she began to reengage in and to enjoy meditation and reading.

LIMITATIONS OF THE ADJUSTMENT DIAGNOSIS IN CANCER

A major short-coming of the adjustment disorder category is the lack of operational criteria for its diagnosis. Indeed, all of the core diagnostic criteria for adjustment disorder lack specificity, particularly in the context of cancer. With respect to Criterion A, it may be difficult to identify a discrete stressor with a temporal relationship to the onset of symptoms. Distress in patients with cancer most often fluctuates across the course of illness and the multitude of stressors frequently obfuscates temporal relationships. Changes in bodily appearance and functioning, significant physical symptoms, impairment of occupational and family role functioning, perceived alterations in life trajectory, uncertainty about the future, and the threat of mortality all may contribute to distress at various time-points in the cancer trajectory. The impact of these stressors may vary considerably depending on individual differences in social support, personal strengths and vulnerabilities, past experience, age, gender, culture, and the personal meaning assigned to the stressor. As a result of the cumulative impact of multiple and repetitive stressors, a relatively minor subsequent stressor may precipitate symptoms that cross the threshold from normal adaptation to disorder. In some cases, distress emerges after the 3-month-time restriction in the DSM-IV-TR criteria for adjustment disorder. This may occur in the months following completion of all active cancer treatment, often due to a process of reflection that had been derailed or delayed due to a prolonged state of crisis and narrowed attention. In other cases, the precise timing and duration of specific stressors may be difficult to establish.

With respect to Criterion B, it can be difficult to determine whether significant impairment in social or occupational functioning is related to the psychological disturbance associated with cancer or to medical morbidity. Physical symptoms, such as pain, nausea, and fatigue, may require patients to take leave from work and may limit pleasure in social activities and the ability to continue social engagements. In addition, there are no standards by which to determine what constitutes "distress in excess of what would be expected" in the context of the multiple, chronic, or recurrent biological, psychological, and social stressors of cancer. While there are clear DSM criteria for determining when psychological disturbances cross the threshold into a full syndrome disorder such as major depression, there is no such guidance provided to determine when

distress should be considered to have crossed the threshold of severity from "normality" to minor disorders.[17,18]

The diagnosis, treatment, and recovery from cancer are inevitably experienced as stressful and traumatic, and can be expected universally to elicit at least transient feelings of anxiety and sadness. The psychological response may meet criteria for an anxiety or depressive disorder, although many[18,19] have cautioned against the pathologizing of such sadness. Horwitz and Wakefield argue against the atheoretical approach of the DSM and emphasize the need to assess symptoms within their etiological context. Their suggested approach for demarking the boundaries of psychopathology follows an assumption of a linear model of stress-disorder interaction, in which there is assumed to be a direct correlation between the severity of an identifiable stressor and the magnitude of the psychological response.[20] The adjustment disorder category is consistent with this assumption, the diagnosis being made when there is a response to a stressor that is considered to be disproportionate. It should be noted, however, that the degrees of distress following exposure to trauma is related not only to the severity of the stressor but also to other social and developmental factors.[21,22]

Criterion D for the diagnosis of adjustment disorder, according to the DSM-IV-TR, specifically excludes distress related to bereavement, although grief reactions are common in response to the multiple and profound losses associated with cancer. Cancer-related losses include those related to body image and identity, sexuality, employment and financial status, social and family relationships, and anticipated future accomplishments and events. Grief and prolonged or unresolved mourning related to all of these losses may be associated with persistent distress in cancer patients.

Finally, Criterion E states that once the stressor or consequences have terminated, the symptoms do not continue for more than 6 months. This does not account for the complicated situation of prolonged medical illness which may be associated with persistent, repeated, or sequential stressors. A chronic course specifier was added to the DSM-IV-TR, to allow for symptoms continuing beyond 6 months when a stressor is ongoing or has enduring consequences. This expanded the category of adjustment disorder, a diagnosis that was originally constructed to describe transient distress, to include the persistent distress that may occur throughout the course of cancer and cancer survivorship.

RECONCEPTUALIZATIONS OF PSYCHOLOGICAL RESPONSE TO MEDICAL ILLNESS

Several authors have proposed alternate classification schemes in response to questions that have been raised regarding the clinical utility of the adjustment disorder diagnosis in medical populations.[4,23–26] Some have suggested placing adjustment disorder in the stress response spectrum, along with PTSD, ASD, and complicated bereavement.[27] In that regard, Ronson[23] has proposed completely eliminating the diagnosis of adjustment disorder and considering the psychological response to cancer entirely in terms of traumatic distress. From this perspective, initial cancer-related distress is viewed on the continuum of full or subthreshold ASD, or PTSD after 4 weeks, with depressive syndromes considered as a secondary response.[28] Ronson has further proposed a category of disorders of extreme stress not otherwise specified (DESNOS), that would apply in some circumstances to cancer patients.[29] The DESNOS category includes six psychological disturbances that occur in response to trauma: dysregulation of affects and impulses, disorders of attention, disorders of consciousness and self-perception, distorted interpersonal relationships, distortion of systems of meaning, and somatisation.[30]

Considering adjustment disorder as a stress response syndrome has logical appeal and is consistent with the etiological linkage of symptoms to a stressor as outlined in DSM. In this vein, Maercker et al. operationalized new diagnostic criteria for adjustment disorders, categorizing them as stress response syndromes and demonstrating their internal and discriminant validity in both a medical sample and a geriatric community population.[24,31] Their model, based on the core posttraumatic symptoms of intrusion, avoidance and failure to adapt, permits co-morbidity with other Axis I disorders, and is congruent with Ronson's traumatic stress theory.[23] However, there are limitations to the applicability of trauma nosography to cancer, because of the nondiscrete nature of the trauma in cancer, the internality and unavoidable nature of the threat, and the future-oriented and anticipatory aspects of the threat.[21,29] As well, classification within the anxiety disorders spectrum would not account for the other commonly observed and problematic emotional and behavioral sequelae of cancer, such as depressed mood and disturbance of conduct.

Others have proposed entirely new taxonomies to characterize illness-related distress. Clarke et al.[25] used latent trait analysis to identify dimensions of distress, followed by cluster analysis to classify five common distress syndromes in medical patients. These syndromes—demoralization, anhedonic depression, demoralized grief, uncomplicated grief, and a nonspecific moderate distress—are distinguished from each other by the severity of distress, anhedonia, and grief.[25] Clarke has gone on to explore demoralization in medical patients, including its prevalence and distinction from depression.[32,33] Defined as the subjective experience of an inability to cope, helplessness, hopelessness, diminished personal esteem, and existential despair, demoralization has been equated by some to adjustment disorder.[34,35] However, the specific characteristics of demoralization may make it more suitable to be considered as a separate or at least a distinct category of disturbance.[33]

Demoralization is one of 12 psychological clusters derived from the Diagnostic Criteria for Psychosomatic Research (DCPR), a structured interview to characterize the psychosocial dimensions of patients with medical illness.[36] Along with other DCPR clusters, including alexithymia, thanatophobia, illness denial, Type A behavior, and irritable mood, demoralization may contribute to or be a manifestation of distress in cancer.[37] There is, in fact, an emerging call to reformulate the DSM-IV-TR category of psychological factors affecting a medical condition, by incorporating specific DCPR clusters to replace the classifications of somatoform disorders[38] and adjustment disorders.[26] Currently, the category of psychological factors affecting a medical condition is relegated to the diverse group of "other conditions that may be a focus of clinical attention." Recognizing psychological factors affecting a medical condition as a distinct diagnostic category may serve to emphasize the bidirectional relationship between medical illness and psychological distress, an important consideration in the conceptualization of adjustment disorders.

Despite the problematic aspects of the adjustment disorder category, there are also several arguments in favor of retaining this diagnosis. Its ill-defined boundaries may be valued by clinicians who wish to label distress in a way that is nonstigmatizing, and that provides an acceptable diagnosis that allows third party reimbursement of legitimate mental health care costs. Recent evidence also suggests that this frequently used diagnosis has correlates and a clinical course distinct from major psychiatric disorders in medical populations.[39,40] Research has shown that those diagnosed with adjustment disorders differ from those diagnosed with depressive disorders in the medical setting.[41] The former were found to be associated with higher ratings of stress and lower severity of illness while the latter were associated with older age, isolation, and less improvement in psychiatric condition.

EPIDEMIOLOGY

The ambiguity surrounding the adjustment disorder category has contributed to its relative neglect in psychiatric research.[4] Consequently, there is little data available regarding its epidemiology, pathogenesis, course, prevention, identification, and treatment. Research which has been conducted has been limited by the uncertain reliability and validity of the diagnosis and, in cancer in particular, by the difficulty identifying a singular etiological stressor and determining when it has stabilized or abated.[5]

Perhaps the greatest testament to the clinical utility of the diagnosis of adjustment disorder is the frequency with which it is used clinically. Despite the lack of attention and weight given to adjustment disorder in the healthcare and psychiatric research literature, it appears to be the most common psychiatric diagnosis made in cancer patients. Studies employing diagnostic interviews have found the prevalence of adjustment disorder in cancer patients to range from 16% to 42%.[2,14,42–45] These rates are far higher than those found either in the general population or in outpatient psychiatry settings. The first and the only large

community-based study examining prevalence of adjustment disorders, the European Outcome of Depression International Network (ODIN) study,[46] found the prevalence of adjustment disorder with depressed mood to be 0.5% in adults 18–64 years old.[47] However, the researchers in that study considered that methodological limitations may have led to overdiagnosis of depressive disorders and underdiagnosis of adjustment disorder.[48] In the general psychiatry outpatient treatment setting, adjustment disorder has been reported to be the principal diagnosis in 5%–20% of cases.[1]

It is unclear to what extent trends in psychiatry affected the usage of specific psychiatric diagnoses. In a 10-year longitudinal observational study of referrals to a consultation-liaison psychiatric service from 1988 to 1997, Diefenbacher and Strain[49] found that the diagnosis of adjustment disorder with depressed mood decreased by half (30%–14%), while the frequency of the diagnosis of depressive disorders more than doubled (6%–15%) during that same time period. This shift has been attributed to the increased emphasis on biological psychiatry and on psychiatric disorders with presumed biological bases.[4] As well, the advent of serotonin selective-reuptake inhibitors (SSRIs), regarded as safer in the medically ill, may have created a change in the "culture of prescription" and therefore a change in the "culture of diagnosis" of both disorders.[5]

Within the general population, adjustment disorders have been associated with specific sociodemographic variables, including younger age, female gender, and greater severity of the stressor.[50] Within the cancer population specifically, adjustment disorders have been associated with such disease-related factors as the stage of disease,[44] prognosis and disease burden,[51,52] earlier recurrence,[45] lower performance status,[42,51] and pain[2]; and social factors, including living alone,[44] concern about burdening others, and satisfaction with social support.[42] Further research is needed to investigate the impact of cultural factors on the occurrence of adjustment disorder. However, Akechi et al.[42] reported that certain characteristics of Japanese society (i.e., the low divorce rate and the low proportion of individuals living alone) may have contributed to the lower prevalence of distress in their research, compared to similar North American and European studies.

PATHOGENESIS

Most models of the pathogenesis of adjustment disorder are based on that of stress response symptoms, in which a stressor precipitates symptoms and maladaptation until the stressor is attenuated or a new state of adaptation occurs.[5] The severity and/or chronicity of the stressor may overwhelm the resources of the individual and preexisting vulnerabilities in the biological, psychological, social, and existential domains may increase the likelihood of symptom development. This is consistent with the view that depression and other manifestations of distress arise as a final common pathway in patients with cancer and other diseases.[53,54] The emergence of distress is conceptualized, from this perspective, as a consequence of multiple risk and protective factors (see Fig. 41–1).

In cancer, the stressors arising from the disease are both psychosocial and biological. The former include the psychological and social impact of illness-related events, such as diagnosis, recurrence, disease advancement, and disability. These events and their sequelae may be associated with attendant changes in role functioning, physical appearance, identity, and the sense of certainty and hope for the future. The biological effects of the disease and its treatment may be associated with profound and disturbing physical symptoms, neurobiological changes, and psychological distress. Emerging evidence suggests that stress-related alterations in neuroendocrine, neuroimmune, and neurotransmitter function may contribute to the development of distress in cancer, as part of a group of behavioral changes termed "sickness behaviour."[55–57] These behavioral changes, including anhedonia, anxiety, fatigue, cognitive disturbance, anorexia, sleep alterations, and hyperalgesia are thought to reflect temporary, adaptive psychobiological responses that may be pro-inflammatory in origin and may serve to promote healing. As such, they suggest a biological model in which prolonged illness and failure to regulate the neurobiological alterations contribute, along with the psychosocial factors, to the eventual development of full threshold psychiatric disorders such as adjustment disorder and depression.

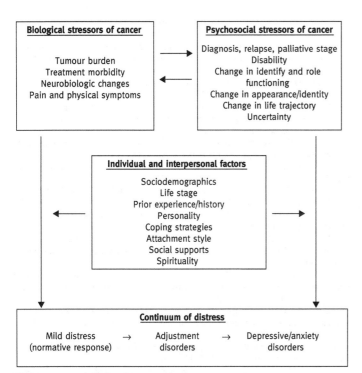

Fig. 41–1. Model of pathways to distress.

Individual and interpersonal factors likely moderate the relationship between cancer-related stressors and the development of distress. These include a broad range of variables such as age, gender, life stage, prior experiences, available social supports, personality, and coping strategies.[58] Individual factors such as self-esteem and spirituality[11,58] and the capacity to express affect[59,60] correlate with the severity of distress. An individual's expectations of support and their capacity to make use of social support, captured in the construct of attachment style, have also been shown to influence the emergence of distress in cancer.[58]

The model of distress as a final common pathway resulting from multiple psychological, social and biological factors draws attention to the diverse interventions that may be employed for prevention and early intervention, including those directed toward psychoeducation, spiritual well-being, family functioning, and the relief of pain and other physical symptoms. Recent research also suggests the potential for novel neurobiological treatments, some of which are already being evaluated in clinical trials, targeted toward corticotropin-releasing hormone (CRH) antagonists, cyclooxygenase (COX) inhibitors, cytokine antagonists, immunosuppressant, prostaglandin inhibitors, nitric oxide synthase (NOS) inhibitors and Substance P inhibitors.[61–67]

It remains unclear whether the symptoms of adjustment disorder represent an attenuated form of a mood or anxiety disorder or a clinical syndrome with unique determining factors and sequelae. A longitudinal positron emission tomography (PET) study in cancer patients has shown that effects in similar brain regions (e.g., decreased metabolism in the right medial frontal gyrus, and increased metabolism in the right posterior cingulate, right anterior cingulate, left subcallosal gyrus, and left caudate) associated with vulnerability to major depression also were associated with adjustment disorder.[68] It is possible that these are nonspecific brain changes linked to affective arousal and that they do not distinguish among diagnostic categories. More longitudinal research is needed to build upon the pathways to distress model, clarify the construct validity of the adjustment disorder category, and account for protection from distress and healthy adjustment in the cancer population.

COURSE

The DSM-IV-TR criteria for adjustment disorder specify that once the stressor or its consequences have terminated, the symptoms resolve within 6 months.[1] The lack of quantitative or qualitative specificity

regarding the definitions of "stressor" and "consequences" may obscure this endpoint. Nevertheless, research in the general psychiatry population suggests that those patients who have been given diagnoses of adjustment disorder have less long-term psychosocial morbidity than those with other psychiatric disorders. When compared to depression, patients with adjustment disorders require less treatment and have a more rapid return to work and less recurrence of psychological distress.[69,70]

The adjustment disorder diagnosis is often unstable, especially when it is made at the onset of investigation or treatment of the psychological disturbance. For example, in one study of psychiatric patients admitted to hospital with a diagnosis of adjustment disorder, 40% were discharged with a different diagnosis.[70] With regard to its clinical course, adjustment disorder may resolve, become chronic, or develop into a full-blown mood or anxiety disorder. Andreasen and Hoenk[71] followed patients diagnosed with adjustment disorder for 5 years and found that 21% developed major depression during this period. In an advanced cancer population, Akechi et al.[42] found that 83% of patients diagnosed with adjustment disorder had a change of diagnosis at follow-up (median 58 days after the time of diagnosis), with half of these diagnosed with major depression and half having no diagnosis at follow-up. In cancer patients, adjustment disorder may not be as likely to resolve given that the etiological stressor(s) may be ongoing, compounded, or worsen.

There is debate about whether psychological distress may impact on the course and prognosis of the cancer itself via changes in the hypothalamic-pituitary axis and immune function.[72] A recent review of prospective research determined there is no clear relationship between symptoms of anxiety or depression and cancer initiation or progression, although research continues to be conducted regarding the interactive effects of demographic, psychological, and medical variables.[73]

PREVENTION AND EARLY DETECTION

It is possible that early or proactive interventions could prevent or diminish distress in cancer patients, thereby reducing the prevalence of adjustment disorders and other manifestations of psychological distress. Unfortunately, however, the rates of detection of significant distress and the rates of referral for specialized psychosocial care remain low in cancer patients.[74–78] This may be due to physicians' lack of awareness or training in detecting significant distress and/or to the reluctance of patients to discuss emotional symptoms or adjustment difficulties with their physicians. This reluctance may be due to shame or embarrassment about emotional distress, beliefs about the lack of availability or interest of medical caregivers to hear about and respond to such symptoms, or a lack of awareness of other resources that might be mobilized to help them. As well, the prevailing myth that depressive and anxiety symptoms are "normal" in the context of cancer may prevent both physicians and patients from considering early intervention.

There may be less awareness in clinical settings of the category of adjustment disorders, compared to anxiety and depressive disorders, because current screening instruments have not been structured to detect adjustment disorders.[14,48] The Hospital Anxiety and Depression Scale,[79] One-Question Interview,[43] and Distress Thermometer[80] have been used in the detection of adjustment disorders in cancer, but do not reliably distinguish them from depressive disorders.[42,43] In a study of commonly used distress screening tools in patients undergoing bone marrow transplantation, it was concluded that currently available tools are not predictive of adjustment disorders.[14] This group went on to develop a specific measure to screen for adjustment disorders in cancer, the Coping Flexibility Scale for Cancer (C-Flex), which also proved to lack sensitivity and specificity for adjustment disorder, possibly related to the vague nature of the diagnostic criteria.[14]

TREATMENT

Psychotherapeutic interventions are generally the first line of treatment for adjustment disorders. The primary goals of most interventions are to reduce the severity of the stressor, enhance coping skills, and strengthen the available support system. In cancer patients, a wide range of interventions, including education, relaxation, guided-imagery, music therapy, individual (supportive, cognitive-behavioral, interpersonal, problem-solving, meaning-centered, dignity), couple, family, or group therapy have been shown to result in distress reduction, improved coping, and better functioning.[81,82] Many of these interventions must be delivered by highly experienced therapists but some can be delivered by nurses, social workers, occupational therapists, and peer counselors. No studies on the outcome of psychotherapeutic treatments specifically for adjustment disorder in cancer patients have been reported. In general psychiatry, modalities that have been shown to be effective in treating adjustment disorder include cognitive-behavioral therapy, interpersonal psychotherapy, ego enhancing therapy, eye movement desensitization and reprocessing (EMDR), and support groups.[5]

It has been suggested that medications may be indicated for patients with adjustment disorder who do not benefit from supportive measures or psychotherapy.[5] In cancer patients, the temporary use of medications for insomnia or anxiety and depressive symptoms may be helpful, particularly since these drugs have a dual benefit, potentially alleviating cancer-related physical symptoms such as fatigue (i.e., bupropion), nausea and loss of appetite (i.e., mirtazapine, olanzapine), pain (i.e., duloxetine), and hot-flashes (i.e., venlafaxine).[83] However, research evidence guiding pharmacotherapy for adjustment disorders is limited. There has been only one randomized controlled trial (RCT) of pharmacotherapy for adjustment disorders in cancer which showed that trazodone was more effective than clorazepate in treatment of anxious and depressed symptoms.[84] In general psychiatry, a retrospective review found that SSRIs were effective treatment for adjustment disorders in a general primary care sample with sustained response rates double that of major depression.[85] RCTs have supported the use of lorazepam and the nonbenzodiazepine etifoxine,[86] tianeptine, alprazolam, and mianserin in improving adjustment disorder with anxiety.[87] There is also RCT evidence supporting use of plant extracts including extracts of kava-kava and gingko biloba for adjustment disorder with anxiety.[88–90]

One concern that has been raised regarding adjustment disorders, as a category of psychiatric diagnosis, is the potential medicalization of distress and emphasis on pharmacological solutions to the stresses of everyday life that may result from the use of such lables.[17] In that regard, it has been questioned whether treatment for adjustment disorder is necessary at all.[4] However, proponents of the category point to the high rates of distress reported by cancer patients, their interest in and appreciation of psychological or psychiatric interventions that are offered, and the fact that both psychotherapeutic and pharmacotherapeutic treatments have been shown to decrease levels of distress in these patients.[82]

The goals and endpoint of treatment for adjustment disorders in cancer patients may be unclear, given the chronic, compounded, or worsening nature of many cancer-related stressors. Nevertheless, this diagnosis is compatible with an approach in which brief interventions are used to relieve distress in cancer patients. These patients may benefit from such interventions, in spite of the enormous challenges that they may face, because of the relative absence of psychiatric co-morbidity and the presence of supportive social and family environments.

CONCLUSION

Adjustment disorder is a psychiatric categorization of distress that captures symptoms that impair well-being and quality of life but which do not fulfill the criteria for another psychiatric condition. There has been debate about whether the category of adjustment disorder is valid, and whether it constitutes the medicalization of distress that will then be treated unnecessarily with psychopharmacological interventions. These are legitimate concerns that should be considered seriously. However, evidence suggests that categorization of distress as adjustment disorder may allow it to be prevented or treated by interventions which are primarily psychosocial. Further research may be needed to refine the criteria for the diagnosis of adjustment disorder and to evaluate treatment outcomes. In the meantime, this category may help to facilitate treatment for many cancer patients who are suffering unnecessarily from psychological distress.

REFERENCES

1. Association AP. *Diagnostic and statistical manual of mental disorders, text revision.* 4th ed. Washington, DC: American Psychiatric Association Press; 2000.
2. Derogatis LR, Morrow GR, Fetting J, et al. The prevalence of psychiatric disorders among cancer patients. *JAMA.* 1983;249(6):751–757.
3. Strain JJ, Smith GC, Hammer JS, et al. Adjustment disorder: a multisite study of its utilization and interventions in the consultation-liaison psychiatry setting. *Gen Hosp Psychiatry.* 1998;20(3):139–149.
4. Casey P, Dowrick C, Wilkinson G. Adjustment disorders: fault line in the psychiatric glossary. *Br J Psychiatry.* 2001;179:479–481.
5. Strain JJ, Diefenbacher A. The adjustment disorders: the conundrums of the diagnoses. *Compr Psychiatry.* 2008;49(2):121–130.
6. Cohen J. The cost of dichotomization. *App Psychol Meas.* 1983;7:249–253.
7. Strain J, Newcorn J, Cartagena-Rochas A. Adjustment disorders. In: Gelder M, Lopez-Ibor J, Andreasen N (eds). *New Oxford textbook of psychiatry.* Oxford, England: Oxford University Press; 2000:774–783.
8. Colleoni M, Mandala M, Peruzzotti G, Robertson C, Bredart A, Goldhirsch A. Depression and degree of acceptance of adjuvant cytotoxic drugs. *Lancet.* 2000;356(9238):1326–1327.
9. Bui QU, Ostir GV, Kuo YF, Freeman J, Goodwin JS. Relationship of depression to patient satisfaction: findings from the barriers to breast cancer study. *Breast Cancer Res Treat.* 2005;89(1):23–28.
10. Breitbart W, Rosenfeld B, Pessin H, et al. Depression, hopelessness, and desire for hastened death in terminally ill patients with cancer. *JAMA.* 2000;284(22):2907–2911.
11. Chochinov HM, Wilson KG, Enns M, et al. Desire for death in the terminally ill. *Am J Psychiatry.* 1995;152(8):1185–1191.
12. Stark D, Kiely M, Smith A, Velikova G, House A, Selby P. Anxiety disorders in cancer patients: their nature, associations, and relation to quality of life. *J Clin Oncol.* 2002;20(14):3137–3148.
13. Skarstein J, Aass N, Fossa SD, Skovlund E, Dahl AA. Anxiety and depression in cancer patients: relation between the Hospital Anxiety and Depression Scale and the European Organization for Research and Treatment of Cancer Core Quality of Life Questionnaire. *J Psychosom Res.* 2000;49(1): 27–34.
14. Kirsh KL, McGrew JH, Dugan M, Passik SD. Difficulties in screening for adjustment disorder, Part I: use of existing screening instruments in cancer patients undergoing bone marrow transplantation. *Palliat Support Care.* 2004;2(1):23–31.
15. Fang CY, Manne SL, Pape SJ. Functional impairment, marital quality, and patient psychological distress as predictors of psychological distress among cancer patients' spouses. *Health Psychol.* 2001;20(6):452–457.
16. Organization WH. *International classification of diseases.* 10th ed. Geneva: World Heath Organization; 1995.
17. Kleinman A. The normal, the pathological, and the existential. *Compr Psychiatry.* 2008;49(2):111–112.
18. Horwitz AV, Wakefield JC. *The loss of sadness: How psychiatry transformed normal sorrow into depressive disorder.* New York Oxford University Press; 2007.
19. Mulder RT. An epidemic of depression or the medicalization of distress? *Perspect Biol Med.* 2008;51(2):238–250.
20. Holmes TH. Life situations, emotions, and disease. *Psychosomatics.* 1978;19(12):747–754.
21. Gurevich M, Devins GM, Rodin GM. Stress response syndromes and cancer: conceptual and assessment issues. *Psychosomatics.* 2002;43(4):259–281.
22. Iversen AC, Fear NT, Ehlers A, et al. Risk factors for post-traumatic stress disorder among UK Armed Forces personnel. *Psychol Med.* 2008;38(4): 511–522.
23. Ronson A. Adjustment disorders in oncology: a conceptual framework to be refined. *Encephale.* 2005;31(2):118–126.
24. Maercker A, Forstmeier S, Enzler A, et al. Adjustment disorders, posttraumatic stress disorder, and depressive disorders in old age: findings from a community survey. *Compr Psychiatry.* 2008;49(2):113–120.
25. Clarke DM, Smith GC, Dowe DL, McKenzie DP. An empirically derived taxonomy of common distress syndromes in the medically ill. *J Psychosom Res.* 2003;54(4):323–330.
26. Grassi L, Mangelli L, Fava GA, et al. Psychosomatic characterization of adjustment disorders in the medical setting: some suggestions for DSM-V. *J Affect Disord.* 2007;101(1–3):251–254.
27. Horowitz M. *Stress response syndromes.* Northvale, NJ: Aronson; 1997.
28. Ronson A. Psychiatric disorders in oncology: recent therapeutic advances and new conceptual frameworks. *Curr Opin Oncol.* 2004;16(4):318–323.
29. Desaive P, Ronson A. Stress spectrum disorders in oncology. *Curr Opin Oncol.* 2008;20(4):378–385.
30. Wheeler K. Psychotherapeutic strategies for healing trauma. *Perspect Psychiatr Care.* 2007;43(3):132–141.

31. Maercker A, Einsle F, Kollner V. Adjustment disorders as stress response syndromes: a new diagnostic concept and its exploration in a medical sample. *Psychopathology.* 2007;40(3):135–146.

32. Clarke DM, Cook KE, Coleman KJ, Smith GC. A qualitative examination of the experience of 'depression' in hospitalized medically ill patients. *Psychopathology.* 2006;39(6):303–312.

33. Clarke DM, Kissane DW. Demoralization: its phenomenology and importance. *Aust N Z J Psychiatry.* 2002;36(6):733–742.

34. Angelino AF, Treisman GJ. Major depression and demoralization in cancer patients: diagnostic and treatment considerations. *Support Care Cancer.* 2001;9(5):344–349.

35. Slavney PR. Diagnosing demoralization in consultation psychiatry. *Psychosomatics.* 1999;40(4):325–329.

36. Fava GA, Freyberger HJ, Bech P, et al. Diagnostic criteria for use in psychosomatic research. *Psychother Psychosom.* 1995;63(1):1–8.

37. Grassi L, Biancosino B, Marmai L, Rossi E, Sabato S. Psychological factors affecting oncology conditions. *Adv Psychosom Med.* 2007;28:57–71.

38. Fabbri S, Fava GA, Sirri L, Wise TN. Development of a new assessment strategy in psychosomatic medicine: the diagnostic criteria for psychosomatic research. *Adv Psychosom Med.* 2007;28:1–20.

39. Kovacs M, Ho V, Pollock MH. Criterion and predictive validity of the diagnosis of adjustment disorder: a prospective study of youths with new-onset insulin-dependent diabetes mellitus. *Am J Psychiatry.* 1995;152(4):523–528.

40. Bronisch T, Hecht H. Validity of adjustment disorder, comparison with major depression. *J Affect Disord.* 1989;17(3):229–236.

41. Snyder S, Strain JJ, Wolf D. Differentiating major depression from adjustment disorder with depressed mood in the medical setting. *Gen Hosp Psychiatry.* 1990;12(3):159–165.

42. Akechi T, Okuyama T, Sugawara Y, Nakano T, Shima Y, Uchitomi Y. Major depression, adjustment disorders, and post-traumatic stress disorder in terminally ill cancer patients: associated and predictive factors. *J Clin Oncol.* 2004;22(10):1957–1965.

43. Akizuki N, Akechi T, Nakanishi T, et al. Development of a brief screening interview for adjustment disorders and major depression in patients with cancer. *Cancer.* 2003;97(10):2605–2613.

44. Kugaya A, Akechi T, Okuyama T, et al. Prevalence, predictive factors, and screening for psychologic distress in patients with newly diagnosed head and neck cancer. *Cancer.* 2000;88(12):2817–2823.

45. Okamura H, Watanabe T, Narabayashi M, et al. Psychological distress following first recurrence of disease in patients with breast cancer: prevalence and risk factors. *Breast Cancer Res Treat.* 2000;61(2):131–137.

46. Dowrick C, Casey P, Dalgard O, et al. Outcomes of Depression International Network (ODIN). Background, methods and field trials. ODIN Group. *Br J Psychiatry.* 1998;172:359–363.

47. Ayuso-Mateos JL, Vazquez-Barquero JL, Dowrick C, et al. Depressive disorders in Europe: prevalence figures from the ODIN study. *Br J Psychiatry.* 2001;179:308–316.

48. Casey P, Maracy M, Kelly BD, et al. Can adjustment disorder and depressive episode be distinguished? Results from ODIN. *J Affect Disord.* 2006;92(2–3):291–297.

49. Diefenbacher A, Strain J. Consultation-liaison psychiatry: stability and change over a 10-year-period. *Gen Hosp Psychiatry.* 2002;24:249–256.

50. Despland JN, Monod L, Ferrero F. Clinical relevance of adjustment disorder in DSM-III-4 and DSM-IV. *Compr Psychiatry.* 1995;36(6):454–460.

51. Dugan W, McDonald MV, Passik SD, Rosenfeld BD, Theobald D, Edgerton S. Use of the Zung Self-Rating Depression Scale in cancer patients: feasibility as a screening tool. *Psycho-oncology.* 1998;7(6):483–493.

52. Zabora J, BrintzenhofeSzoc K, Curbow B, Hooker C, Piantadosi S. The prevalence of psychological distress by cancer site. *Psychooncology.* 2001;10(1):19–28.

53. Rodin G, Zimmermann C, Rydall A, et al. The desire for hastened death in patients with metastatic cancer. *J Pain Symptom Manage.* 2007;33(6):661–675.

54. Lo C, Li M, Rodin G. The assessment and treatment of distress in cancer patients: overview and future directions. *Minerva Psichiatr.* 2008;49:129–143.

55. Dantzer R, O'Connor JC, Freund GG, Johnson RW, Kelley KW. From inflammation to sickness and depression: when the immune system subjugates the brain. *Nat Rev Neurosci.* 2008;9(1):46–56.

56. Miller AH, Capuron L, Raison CL. Immunologic influences on emotion regulation. *Clin Neurosci Res.* 2005 2005;4:325–333.

57. Raison CL, Capuron L, Miller AH. Cytokines sing the blues: inflammation and the pathogenesis of depression. *Trends Immunol.* 2006;27(1):24–31.

58. Rodin G, Walsh A, Zimmermann C, et al. The contribution of attachment security and social support to depressive symptoms in patients with metastatic cancer. *Psychooncology.* 2007;16(12):1080–1091.

59. Classen CC, Kraemer HC, Blasey C, et al. Supportive-expressive group therapy for primary breast cancer patients: a randomized prospective multicenter trial. *Psychooncology.* 2008;17(5):438–447.

60. Spiegel D, Morrow GR, Classen C, et al. Group psychotherapy for recently diagnosed breast cancer patients: a multicenter feasibility study. *Psychooncology.* 1999;8(6):482–493.

61. Cleeland CS, Bennett GJ, Dantzer R, et al. Are the symptoms of cancer and cancer treatment due to a shared biologic mechanism? A cytokine-immunologic model of cancer symptoms. *Cancer.* 2003;97(11):2919–2925.

62. Holmes A, Heilig M, Rupniak NM, Steckler T, Griebel G. Neuropeptide systems as novel therapeutic targets for depression and anxiety disorders. *Trends Pharmacol Sci.* 2003;24(11):580–588.

63. Keller M, Montgomery S, Ball W, et al. Lack of efficacy of the substance p (neurokinin1 receptor) antagonist aprepitant in the treatment of major depressive disorder. *Biol Psychiatry.* 2006;59(3):216–223.

64. Kramer MS, Winokur A, Kelsey J, et al. Demonstration of the efficacy and safety of a novel substance P (NK1) receptor antagonist in major depression. *Neuropsychopharmacology.* 2004;29(2):385–392.

65. Nielsen DM. Corticotropin-releasing factor type-1 receptor antagonists: the next class of antidepressants? *Life Sci.* 25 2006;78(9):909–919.

66. Zobel AW, Nickel T, Kunzel HE, et al. Effects of the high-affinity corticotropin-releasing hormone receptor 1 antagonist R121919 in major depression: the first 20 patients treated. *J Psychiatr Res.* 2000;34(2):171–181.

67. Tyring S, Gottlieb A, Papp K, et al. Etanercept and clinical outcomes, fatigue, and depression in psoriasis: double-blind placebo-controlled randomised phase III trial. *Lancet.* 2006;367(9504):29–35.

68. Kumano H, Ida I, Oshima A, et al. Brain metabolic changes associated with predisposition to onset of major depressive disorder and adjustment disorder in cancer patients—a preliminary PET study. *J Psychiatr Res.* 2007;41(7):591–599.

69. Bronish T. Adjustment reactions: a long-term prospective and retrospective follow-up of former patients in a crisis intervention ward. *Acta Psychiatr Scand.* 1991;84:86–93.

70. Greenberg WM, Rosenfeld DN, Ortega EA. Adjustment disorder as an admission diagnosis. *Am J Psychiatry.* 1995;152(3):459–461.

71. Andreasen NC, Hoenk PR. The predictive value of adjustment disorders: a follow-up study. *Am J Psychiatry.* 1982;139(5):584–590.

72. Spiegel D, Giese-Davis J. Depression and cancer: mechanisms and disease progression. *Biol Psychiatry.* 2003;54(3):269–282.

73. Garssen B. Psychological factors and cancer development: evidence after 30 years of research. *Clin Psychol Rev.* 2004;24(3):315–338.

74. Fallowfield L, Ratcliffe D, Jenkins V, Saul J. Psychiatric morbidity and its recognition by doctors in patients with cancer. *Br J Cancer.* 2001;84(8):1011–1015.

75. Keller M, Sommerfeldt S, Fischer C, et al. Recognition of distress and psychiatric morbidity in cancer patients: a multi-method approach. *Ann Oncol.* 2004;15(8):1243–1249.

76. Sharpe M, Strong V, Allen K, et al. Major depression in outpatients attending a regional cancer centre: screening and unmet treatment needs. *Br J Cancer.* 2004;90(2):314–320.

77. Sollner W, DeVries A, Steixner E, et al. How successful are oncologists in identifying patient distress, perceived social support, and need for psychosocial counselling? *Br J Cancer.* 2001;84(2):179–185.

78. Ellis J, Lin J, Walsh A, et al. Predictors of referral for specialized psychosocial oncology care in patients with metastatic cancer: the contributions of age, distress and marital status. *J Clin Oncol.* 2009;27(5):699–705.

79. Zigmond AS, Snaith RP. The hospital anxiety and depression scale. *Acta Psychiatr Scand.* 1983;67(6):361–370.

80. Roth AJ, Kornblith AB, Batel-Copel L, Peabody E, Scher HI, Holland JC. Rapid screening for psychologic distress in men with prostate carcinoma: a pilot study. *Cancer.* 1998;82(10):1904–1908.

81. Daniels J, Kissane DW. Psychosocial interventions for cancer patients. *Curr Opin Oncol.* 2008;20(4):367–371.

82. Newell SA, Sanson-Fisher RW, Savolainen NJ. Systematic review of psychological therapies for cancer patients: overview and recommendations for future research. *J Natl Cancer Inst.* 2002;94(8):558–584.

83. Rodin G, Lloyd N, Katz M, Green E, Mackay JA, Wong RK. The treatment of depression in cancer patients: a systematic review. *Support Care Cancer.* 2007;15(2):123–136.

84. Razavi D, Kormoss N, Collard A Farvacques C, Delvaux N. Comparative study of efficacy and safety of trazodone versus clorazepate in the treatment of adjustment disorders in cancer patients: a pilot study. *J Int Med Res.* 1999;27:264–272.

85. Hameed U, Schwartz TL, Malhotra K, West RL, Bertone F. Antidepressant treatment in the primary care office: outcomes for adjustment disorder versus major depression. *Ann Clin Psychiatry.* 2005;17(2):77–81.

86. Nguyen N, Fakra E, Pradel V, et al. Efficacy of etifoxine compared to lorazepam monotherapy in the treatment of patients with adjustment disorders with anxiety: a double-blind controlled study in general practice. *Hum Psychopharmacol.* 2006;21(3):139–149.

87. Ansseau M, Bataille M, Briole G, et al. Controlled comparison of tianeptine, alprazolam and mianserin in the treatment of adjustment disorders with anxiety and depression. *Hum Psychopharm Clin Experiment.* 1996;11:293–298.

88. Bourin M, Bougerol T, Guitton B, Broutin E. A combination of plant extracts in the treatment of outpatients with adjustment disorder with anxious mood: controlled study versus placebo. *Fundam Clin Pharmacol.* 1997;11(2):127–132.

89. Volz HP, Kieser M. Kava-kava extract WS 1490 versus placebo in anxiety disorders—a randomized placebo-controlled 25-week outpatient trial. *Pharmacopsychiatry.* 1997;30(1):1–5.

90. Woelk H, Arnoldt KH, Kieser M, Hoerr R. Ginkgo biloba special extract EGb 761 in generalized anxiety disorder and adjustment disorder with anxious mood: a randomized, double-blind, placebo-controlled trial. *J Psychiatr Res.* 2007;41(6):472–480.

CHAPTER 42

Depressive Disorders

Kimberley Miller and Mary Jane Massie

INTRODUCTION

Distress is common and can take many forms in a cancer patient who is burdened by multiple physical and psychological symptoms. Biological, psychological, and social factors all contribute to distress variability. Themes of uncertainty, loss of control, and increased dependency affect most cancer patients at some point. Many fear future suffering, including a painful death, as well as loss of relationships and roles through advancing illness. Although feelings of sadness, grief, and anxiety develop in most patients, they usually resolve spontaneously when supported by family, friends, and a physician who clarifies a treatment plan forward that offers hope and alleviation of suffering. Intolerable or prolonged distress that interferes with function requires evaluation and management. Developing major depression is not a normal or expected response, and is considered a significant complication that requires individualized assessment and treatment, given its propensity to worsen quality of life and functional status. Distress develops at different points throughout the illness trajectory, including at initial diagnosis, initiation or completion of treatment, recurrence, and during the transition to the palliative phase.

PREVALENCE OF DEPRESSION IN CANCER

The 12-month and lifetime-prevalence rates for major depressive disorder (MDD) in the general population are 6.6% and 16.6%,[1] respectively, with prevalence rates in cancer patients ranging from 0% to 38% for major depression, and 0%–58% for depression spectrum syndromes.[2] Most of this variance can be attributed to the lack of standardization of methodology and diagnostic criteria used. An evidence-based review of cancer patients found the prevalence rates of MDD to be between 10% and 25%, with similar rates for other depressive syndromes.[3] Such chronic medical illnesses like diabetes and cardiac disease show similar rates, while neurological diseases are slightly more prevalent.

An observational cohort study involving 222 early stage breast cancer patients revealed prevalence rates in depression and anxiety of 33% at diagnosis, 15% after 1 year and 45% after a recurrence was diagnosed.[4] In patients with advanced cancer depression has been reported to be as high as 26%.[2,5]

ASSESSMENT OF DEPRESSION

Screening. Physicians identify only one-third of patients who score highly on measures of distress, suggesting the need to develop better detection strategies.[6] However, despite attempts to increase awareness in distress screening, only 14% of oncologists used formal screening tools, instead relying on clinical judgment.[7] Additional barriers to universal screening include format and length of instrument used, administration time, and associated resources required for scoring and interpreting results, leading to the development of several ultrashort screening tools, including 1-or 2-item screening questions and computer touch screens. Table 42–1 reviews commonly administered screening measures in depressed cancer patients, the topic being more thoroughly reviewed elsewhere (see Chapter 52). Intended for the busy oncologist, Hoffman provides a succinct review of diagnosing depression in cancer patients.[11]

A Cochrane systematic review revealed that screening alone does not impact outcome of depression, emphasizing the need for coordinated and multidisciplinary interventions.[12] Many advocate for a two-stage screening process involving an initial self-report scale, followed by a diagnostic interview, which remains the gold standard for diagnosing depression.

Diagnosing depression in cancer patients. In the cancer setting, assessing depression often involves differentiating between an adjustment disorder with depressed mood, major depression, mood disorder due to cancer, and substance-induced mood disorder. Considering a patient's psychological and physical symptoms, placing them in their individual social and medical context, and having an understanding of the neuropsychiatric sequelae of chemotherapeutic and other biological cancer treatments, as well as psychosocial impacts of the disease, are essential in this process. An episode of major depression is diagnosed when a person experiences a 2-week history of either depressed mood or anhedonia, along with four of the following symptoms, nearly every day: increased or decreased appetite; insomnia or hypersomnia; psychomotor agitation or retardation; fatigue, guilt, or worthlessness; diminished concentration; or recurrent thoughts of death, including suicidal ideation. Many of the somatic symptoms caused by cancer or its treatment overlap with the diagnostic criteria for major depression, including disturbances in sleep, appetite, energy, psychomotor activity, and concentration. Controversy continues over how to weight the psychological (depressed mood, anhedonia, guilt, worthlessness, hopelessness, helplessness, and suicidal ideation) versus the aforementioned somatic symptoms in evaluating the depressed cancer patient, although most recommend the inclusive approach clinically. Just as the somatic symptoms may inaccurately be ascribed solely to the cancer or its treatment, the psychological symptoms may also be normalized as an expected consequence of dealing with a life-threatening illness. Pervasiveness, quantity, and severity of symptoms, as well as associated impact on functioning help to differentiate major depression from an adjustment disorder. Although not included as a diagnosis in the *Diagnostic and statistical manual of mental disorders* (DSM), demoralization syndrome has been described to include existential despair, hopelessness, helplessness, with loss of meaning and purpose for life, differing from depression by its lack of anhedonia.[13]

Mood disorder due to cancer is diagnosed when the direct physiologic effects of illness cause the depressive episode, such as in primary or secondary brain tumors. The potential role of proinflammatory cytokines contributing to depression might imply that any new onset of major depression, especially those with significant somatic symptoms, developing in the midst of acute cancer could be considered in this diagnostic category. Substance-induced depression may develop from cancer treatments, most commonly exogenous cytokines and corticosteroids. Discontinuation or dosage reduction of the causative agent may not always be possible, resulting in concomitantly prescribing an antidepressant. Hypoactive delirium may resemble depression, as patients may appear less engaged, less motivated to participate in their care, and may voice suicidal ideation. Disturbances in consciousness, impaired attention and cognition, as well as perceptual disturbances suggest a delirious process, which should always be ruled out when evaluating a cancer patient for depression, given the significant treatment differences between the two disorders. Although an underlying depression may be present, treating the delirium takes priority and reevaluation of mood symptoms follows resolution of the delirium.

A complex relationship exists between mood and physical symptoms, including pain and fatigue, in the depressed cancer patient. Patients in an

Table 42–1. Screening instruments for depression in cancer

Single item	Two item
Are you depressed?[8]	
Please grade your mood during the past week by assigning it a score from 0 to 100, with a score of 100 representing your usual relaxed mood. A score of 60 is considered a passing grade[9]	1. Have you often been bothered by feeling down, depressed, or hopeless?
	2. Have you often been bothered by having a lack of interest or pleasure in doing things?[10]

Beck depression inventory (BDI)
Beck depression inventory-short form (BDI-SF)
Brief symptom inventory (BSI)
Brief version, Zung self-rating depression scale (BZSDRS)
Center for epidemiologic studies depression scale (CES-D)
General health questionnaire (GHQ)
Hamilton rating scale for depression (Ham-D)
Hospital and anxiety depression scale (HADS)
Montgomery asberg depression rating scale (MADRS)
Profile of mood states (POMS)
Rotterdam symptom checklist (RSCL)
Zung self-rating depression scale (ZSRDS)

acute pain crisis may express depression, despair, and suicidal ideation, symptoms which can not be considered evidence of depression until the pain is adequately controlled. Fatigue is a common side effect of cancer and its treatment and can mimic depression through its impact on concentration, activity level, and sleep. Differentiating between the two has significant implications at the intervention level. For example, a systematic review of 27 trials involving 6746 patients showed that erythropoietin, darbopoetin (for anemic patients receiving chemotherapy) and psychostimulants, but not paroxetine or progestational steroids, improved cancer-related fatigue.[14]

Barriers to diagnosis. Several barriers to the diagnosis of depression in cancer patients exist.[15] In addition to the difficulty in evaluating the etiology of somatic symptoms in diagnosing depression, busy oncology clinics may also have uncertainty about the effectiveness of treatment for depression, impacting referrals for psychosocial interventions. Lack of access to psychosocial resources as well as a lack of patient awareness of supportive services are additional barriers. However, even depressed patients who are informed of services may not seek treatment, related to reluctance to report depression, focusing more on their physical treatments and need for aggressive cancer treatment, especially soon after diagnosis. Similar to the general population, cancer patients may fear psychotropic medication side effects, while others may have a discomfort with reporting psychological suffering, related to stigma of contact with psychosocial services. Many patients may have a strong need to maintain a "fighting spirit," believing this will positively impact their cancer course, inhibiting them from disclosing or acknowledging any distress or perceived "negativity." Cultural differences may impact the reporting of psychological symptoms. Asian patients focus more on their physical than psychological symptoms.[16] In 472 low-income ethnic minority women receiving cancer care, 24% reported moderate to severe major depression, yet only 12% of them had received medications for depression and 5% received any other form of psychosocial support, significantly less than that reported by higher income Caucasian populations.[17]

Risk factors for depression in cancer. Consistently, studies have found that younger age, low social supports, and advanced disease are risk factors for patients with cancer developing depression. Although major depression is more common in women in the general population, this gender difference is inconsistently found in the oncology population.[3,18,19] Strong found that female gender, being younger than 65 and having active disease predicted Hospital Anxiety and Depression Scale (HADS) >15 in 674/3071 mixed cancer patients.[18] Similarly another large Canadian study of 2276 mixed cancer patients examining distress using the Brief Symptom Inventory (BSI)-18 found that more men met case criteria for the subscale of somatization, whereas more women for the subscale of depression.[20] Differentiating these two large studies was the role of specific cancer diagnosis on distress. Strong et al. did not find cancer diagnosis to be a predictor for distress, whereas Carlson et al. found that patients with lung, pancreatic, head and neck, Hodgkin's disease, and brain cancer were most distressed, which is consistent with another large study examining distress by cancer site.[21] Rodin et al. examined the interaction of individual, social, and disease-related factors with the development of depressive symptoms in advanced cancer patients in Canada.[19] In 326 outpatients with metastatic gastrointestinal or lung cancer, they demonstrated a strong relationship between disease burden (especially pain and fatigue), perceived social support and insecure attachment style, both, of the anxious and avoidant type, and depression. In a large study of 2595 early stage breast cancer patients, stressful life events, less optimism, ambivalence overexpressing negative emotions, sleep disturbance, and poorer social functioning better predicted risk for elevated depressive symptoms than cancer-related variables.[22]

Certain cancer treatments, including corticosteroids, exogenous cytokines, hormonal treatments, and chemotherapeutic agents have been shown to contribute to depressive symptoms (see Table 42–2). A recent case control study followed 138 stage II/III breast cancer patients undergoing adjuvant chemotherapy, and subsequently, over a 5-year period. Controlling for poor physical functioning, patients who received taxanes had higher emotional distress and worse mental quality of life throughout adjuvant treatment, and took longer (2 years on average) to recover emotionally than patients in the no-taxane group (6–12 months).[23]

Biopsychosocial risk factors most commonly associated with depression in cancer are listed in Table 42–3.

Biological mechanism of depression. Much of the current interest and research in pathophysiology of depression in cancer focuses on psychoneuroimmunologic pathways. Low natural killer cell (NK) activity has been associated with depression. And within depressed patients, greater life stress, smoking status, symptoms of psychomotor retardation, and insomnia, and co-morbid anxiety and alcohol dependence contribute to even greater declines in NK activity, factors commonly seen in some cancer populations.[24] Twenty three depressed hepatobiliary cancer patients showed significantly lower NK cell numbers compared to 77 nondepressed patients.[25] Further suggesting an association, antidepressants and group therapy improve NK activity in depressed patients.[24] Activation of proinflammatory cytokines results in a "sickness syndrome," many of its symptoms overlapping with major depression, including anhedonia, fatigue, anorexia, weight loss, insomnia, cognitive

Table 42–2. Anticancer treatment associated with depression

Corticosteroids
Interferon-alpha
Interleukin 2
Tamoxifen
Cyproterone
Leuprolide
Vincristine
Vinblastine
Vinorelbine
Procarbazine
Asparaginase
Paclitaxel
Docetaxel

Table 42–3. Biopsychosocial risk factors associated with depression in cancer

Biological	Psychological	Social
Younger age	Relational	Low supports
Family history of depression	Perceived low supports	Poorer social functioning
Personal history of depression	Anxious or avoidant attachment	Recent loss
Cancer-related factors	Attitudinal	Stressful life events
Advanced disease	Less optimism	History of trauma/ abuse
Low PS	Ambivalence in expressing negative emotions	Substance use disorder
Physical burden		
Pain	Low self-esteem	
Fatigue		
Tumor sites		
Pancreas, head and neck, lung, brain, Hodgkin's		
Treatment		

ABBREVIATION: PS, performance status.

impairment, psychomotor retardation, and hyperalgesia.[26] Increased levels of cytokines, including interleukin (IL)-6, tumor necrosis factor ∝ (TNF), IL-1 and IL-12 have also been found in depressed patients. Cytokines may cause depression or "sickness behavior" by altering the metabolism of monoamines, tryptophan, or thyroid hormones, as well as by activating corticotropin-releasing factor (CRF), thereby stimulating the hypothalamic-pituitary-adrenal (HPA) axis.[26] Administering exogenous cytokines, including interferon-alpha, contributes to depression in patients with malignant melanoma.[27] However, a recent small Dutch study only found 2/43 patients with renal cell carcinoma and malignant melanoma developed depressive episodes, although more depression was seen when higher doses were used.[28] It has been suggested that novel treatments, including cytokine antagonists, which manipulate the psychoneuroimmunologic pathways, may target both depression and "sickness behavior."

Impact of depression in Cancer. Depressed cancer patients report a poorer quality of life, are less adherent to medical interventions and have longer hospital stays.[29] A meta-analysis of the effects of depression on adherence to general medical treatment reveals that depressed patients are three times more likely to be nonadherent than nondepressed patients.[30] In addition, depression may impair a patient's capacity to understand and process information about their prognosis.

Many have investigated the role depression and other psychological factors have in initiating or advancing cancer, and contributing to a poorer prognosis. One review in 2004 examined a series of 70 studies, and concluded that no psychological factor, including depression, convincingly influenced the initiation or progression of cancer, although suggested repression, helplessness, and chronic depression may be contributing factors.[31] The evidence associating depression with cancer incidence is weaker than that for cancer progression.[32] The literature regarding depression contributing to increased risk of mortality in cancer patients is less clear and mixed results have been reported, likely due to methodological problems, as well as different interpretations of the available data, suggesting the need for ongoing prospective studies on the topic. Most agree that a complex relationship exists between depression and mortality in cancer patients, involving multiple biologic (increases in proinflammatory cytokines, decreased NK cell numbers) and behavioral (treatment nonadherence, smoking, alcohol use, and suicide) mechanisms.[33] Thus although it remains unclear if treating a cancer patient's depression will prolong survival, there may be opportunity to improve treatment adherence and quality of life.

Suicide and desire for hastened death. Suicide accounts for a very low number of deaths in cancer patients, 0.2%, including in the terminally ill population, 0.03%.[34] In a recent study of a community dwelling population, cancer was only associated with suicidal ideation in the 55–74-year-old age group, but did not hold significance when other influences, such as social supports, mental disorders, and sociodemographic factors, were excluded.[35] Social supports are protective, resulting in cancer patients having an increased will to live[36] and less severe depression.[37]

Factors such as poor prognosis, delirium, uncontrolled pain, depression, and hopelessness often occur in a patient with advanced disease, increasing the risk of suicide. Hopelessness is an even stronger predictive factor than depression itself.[38] Studies exploring the desire for hastened death (DHD) have found that 1%–17% of terminally ill cancer patients wish to have their lives end naturally or by suicide, or euthanasia. A nonpalliative sample found that of 326 advanced gastrointestinal and lung cancer patients, only 2% expressed a desire for hastened death, suggesting resilience overall in this population.[34] This was found despite 20% reporting significant depression and hopelessness and 50% reporting pain and other physical symptoms. DHD was positively correlated with hopelessness, depression and physical distress, and negatively with physical functioning, spiritual well being, social support, and self esteem. In a patient expressing suicidal ideation, differentiating a depressive illness from a desire to have control over intolerable symptoms is vital, and has a clear impact on intervention. The management of the suicidal cancer patient involves a careful consideration of the context of the problem. Identifying and alleviating physical (e.g., pain, nausea, fatigue) and emotional (e.g., depression, anxiety, insomnia, confusion) suffering is paramount. Conveying the attitude that much can be done to improve the quality, if not the quantity, of life even if the prognosis is poor can reassure patients. Maintaining a supportive presence and availability to patients and their families can reduce fears of abandonment, and help at times of crisis.

When the need to hospitalize a suicidal patient is considered, evaluation of the risk factors, including the presence of a plan and its lethality, and associated intent ensues. If the suicidal patient does not have any clear physiologic cause contributing to their psychiatric presentation, admitting the patient to a psychiatric unit may be indicated. However, during the palliative phase, when patients are too ill to be psychiatrically hospitalized, they may be admitted to oncology wards, palliative care units, or hospice settings, where 24-hour companions can be provided to ensure safety.

Treatment. As in the general population, understanding a depressed cancer patient from a biopsychosocial perspective allows individual and personally relevant interventions to be implemented. Evaluating co-morbid physical symptoms, in addition to psychiatric symptoms, optimizes somatic treatments. A thoughtful exploration of patients' understanding of their illness and prognosis, previous personal experience with cancer, including cancer losses, concurrent stressors, and current level of supports helps to develop an individualized psychosocial intervention. Depressed cancer patients may receive psychopharmacologic and/or psychosocial treatments. Practice guidelines for the psychosocial care of cancer patients have been developed in several countries, aiding in treatment decision making, while highlighting the need for additional well-designed intervention studies for this population.[39,40] Both nonpharmacological and pharmacological studies are limited by small sample sizes, high withdrawal rates, contributing to selection bias, as well as the presence of significant confounding factors. As well, few studies have examined the effect of combined modalities, with Akechi et al. recently showing feasibility and promise with their multifaceted psychosocial intervention program in fifty breast cancer patients experiencing their first recurrence.[41]

PSYCHOLOGICAL

Meta-analyses have shown improvement in depression and depressive symptoms with psychosocial treatments, however, when systematic reviews examine depression per se, versus depressive symptoms alone, the quantity of available evidence diminishes significantly, including in the advanced incurable population.[42-44] Modalities found to be effective in depression include counseling/psychotherapy, counseling/relaxation, as well as various nurse-delivered interventions, components of which have included psychoeducation, problem solving, coordination of, both, oncological and psychiatric care, orientation to an oncology unit, and education about procedural issues at the clinic level.[42,43,45] In 227 metastatic breast cancer patients, Kissane et al. found that new cases of clinical depression were prevented in those women participating in supportive-expressive group therapy and relaxation therapy versus those in relaxation therapy alone.[46] Evidence for cognitive-behavior therapy (CBT), social, including web-based, support groups also reduce depressive symptoms. In the incurable population, a meta-analysis of six studies showed improvement in depressive symptoms, using supportive psychotherapy, CBT, and problem solving. However, the evidence does not support the effectiveness of psychotherapy in patients diagnosed with depression with advanced cancer.[44]

As some of the trials proven effective involve multiple components, a multi-modal individualized approach may be best. Data on impacting survival through psychosocial treatments is varied and covered in more detail elsewhere (see Chapter 52).

Psychotherapy may be delivered to the patient individually, in a group setting, or with their partner and/or family. Extrapolating from the general population, as well as clinical experience, suggests incorporating elements of other models of psychotherapy in treating depressed cancer patients, including interpersonal and psychodynamic. In the advanced or terminally ill cancer population, existential, life narrative, dignity conserving, and meaning-centered interventions may be more appropriate. Offering a supportive, validating, and nonjudgmental presence, providing realistic reassurance, and emphasizing prior strengths and coping are therapeutic. Living with uncertainty, as well as balancing hope and grief are difficult tasks for the depressed cancer patient, which can be managed with support and behavioral interventions.

PSYCHOPHARMACOLOGICAL

Choosing a medication to alleviate depressive symptoms requires careful consideration of a number of factors, including a patient's medical co-morbidities, potential drug interactions (Table 42-4), route of administration (as many cancer patients may be unable to take oral medications), onset of action required and associated estimate of patient prognosis, somatic symptom profile (e.g., pain, insomnia, agitation, hot flashes), and adverse effect profile of the intended psychotropic medication. Okamura et al have developed a treatment algorithm to help guide treatment decisions based on the above-mentioned factors.[49]

Although there is much clinical experience in using antidepressants in cancer patients, there are few randomized placebo-controlled trials in depressed cancer patients.[42,43] To date, seven placebo-controlled trials have shown a reduction in either caseness of depression or depressive symptoms, using the antidepressants, fluoxetine, paroxetine, or mianserin.[27,50-55] Another study found that fluoxetine did not improve depressive symptoms significantly over placebo,[56] and no significant differences in Ham-D and CGI-S scores were found in 35 patients with major depression randomized to paroxetine, desipramine or placebo.[57] Excluding patients with major depression, sertraline did not improve depression, anxiety, fatigue, well being or survival in patients with advanced cancer, leading the authors to recommend avoiding its use in patients without a clear proven indication.[58]

In studies comparing active treatments, Holland et al found alprazolam superior to progressive muscle relaxation in reducing depressive symptoms.[59] No between group differences were seen in two other studies; one compared paroxetine to amitriptyline,[60] the other compared fluoxetine to desipramine,[61] with all four active treatments improving depressive symptoms.

ANTIDEPRESSANTS

SSRIs and SNRIs. Selective serotonin reuptake inhibitors (SSRIs) and serotonin norepinephrine reuptake inhibitors (SNRIs) tend to be used first line due to their tolerability and safety profile. They are equally efficacious, with depressive symptoms improving after 2 to 4 weeks of an adequate dose (Table 42-5). In addition to relieving symptoms of depression and anxiety, many of the SSRIs and venlafaxine have also been shown to alleviate hot flashes by approximately 50% (37%-61%), depending on dosage and agent used, in breast cancer survivors.[62] Venlafaxine (37.5-150 mg daily), fluoxetine (20 mg daily), paroxetine (10-20 mg daily), and citalopram (10-20 mg daily) and sertraline (50 mg daily) have been shown to be effective.

Recent reports suggest that more potent inhibitors of the cytochrome P450 isoenzyme 2D6, such as paroxetine and fluoxetine, may reduce the level of one of the more active metabolites of tamoxifen, 4-hydroxy-N-desmethyl-tamoxifen (endoxifen), by inhibiting its metabolism.[63,64] Patients with decreased metabolism, through genetic variation and enzyme inhibition, have been found to have shorter time to recurrence and worse relapse-free survival, resulting in some recommending the use of a weaker 2D6 inhibitor, such as venlafaxine, in these patients until further information is known.[64,65] However, at this time no definitive recommendations regarding specific antidepressant use in this patient population can be made. All SSRIs share a similar side effect profile in that there is a risk of gastrointestinal disturbance, headache, fatigue or insomnia, sexual dysfunction and increased anxiety after initiation. However, there are some unique differences between each SSRI that may impact a physician's treatment decision making (Table 42-5). Owing to its long half life fluoxetine should be used with caution in patients whose chemotherapy regimens are anticipated to change, given its risk of interaction with anti cancer treatments metabolized through the cytochrome P450 system. The other SSRIs have a relatively short half life (approximately 24 hours), and their abrupt discontinuation (e.g., postoperatively, or due to acute bowel obstruction and inability to take oral medications) may result in psychiatric, gastrointestinal, neurologic, or flulike symptoms.

Antidepressant-related hyponatremia has been reported in case reports, retrospective chart reviews, case-control studies, and one prospective observational trial.[66] All of the SSRIs, venlafaxine and mirtazapine have been associated with hyponatremia. A review of 736 cases of hyponatremia and SIADH associated with SSRI use and found that the mean time to onset was 13 days (range 3-120 days), with normalization of the sodium values 2-28 days after the discontinuation of SSRIs.[67] Risk factors include advanced age, female gender, low baseline sodium levels, co-morbid medical conditions, including congestive heart failure, pneumonia, and small cell lung cancer, concomitant medications, including diuretics, and vincristine. Routine monitoring of electrolytes is advisable, especially in cancer patients with additional risk factors. Educating patients about the signs and symptoms of hyponatremia and the importance of seeking medical assessment if lethargy, delirium or nausea develop, is recommended. Risk of hemorrhage has also been widely reported with SSRIs, most commonly gastrointestinal (GI) bleeding, and to a lesser extent uterine bleeding.[68] The mechanism is believed to be related to SSRIs depleting platelet serotonin through its action on the serotonin transporter, which reduces coagulation and increases risk of bleeding in vulnerable patients, especially those taking acetylsalicylic acid (ASA) or nonsteroidal anti-inflammatory medications (NSAIDS). It is unknown if cancer patients, who often have chemotherapy or disease-related thrombocytopenia are at higher risk, but caution is advised.

Venlafaxine and duloxetine are serotonin norepinephrine reuptake inhibitors (SNRIs), with venlafaxine inhibiting serotonin reuptake at lower doses, thereby sharing some of the side effects with the SSRIs, while inhibiting norepinephrine reuptake at higher doses. Dose-dependent hypertension may occur in patients taking venlafaxine. Both duloxetine and venlafaxine have been shown to improve neuropathic pain.

Atypical and mixed antidepressants. Bupropion is a dual norepinephrine and dopamine reuptake inhibitor that has been shown to improve sexual function and fatigue in cancer patients.[69,70] Unlike the SSRIs and venlafaxine, a pilot study of bupropion did not improve hot flashes.[71] It tends to be weight neutral, or in some cases promotes weight

Table 42–4. Common cytochrome P450 interactions in psycho-oncology

Agents	1A2	2B6	2C9	2C19	2D6	3A4
Substrates	Doxepin Imipramine Mirtazapine Clozapine Olanzapine Ziprasidone Dacarbazine	Bupropion Cyclophosphamide Ifosfamide Tamoxifen Tramadol Aripiprazole	Paclitaxel Tamoxifen	Amitriptyline Clomipramine Imipramine Diazepam Clozapine Cannabinoids Tamoxifen Cyclophosphamide Ifosfamide	Sufentanil Amitriptyline Clomipramine Desipramine Doxepin Imipramine Nortriptyline Venlafaxine Duloxetine Fluoxetine Paroxetine Mirtazapine Trazodone Haloperidol Chlorpromazine Perphenazine Clozapine Olanzapine Risperidone Aripiprazole Oxycodone Hydrocodone ?Methadone Odansetron Tamoxifen Tramadol	Alprazolam Midazolam Triazolam Clonazepam Diazepam Buspirone Methadone Alfentanil Fentanyl Sufentanil Hydrocodone ?Oxycodone Tramadol Cyclosporine Prednisone Tacrolimus Cyclophosphamide Daunorubicin Dexamethasone Docetaxel Doxorubicin Etoposide Ifosfamide Paclitaxel Tamoxifen Vinblastine Vincristine Vinorelbine Amitriptyline Clomipramine Doxepin Imipramine Mirtazapine Trazodone Haloperidol Aripiprazole Clozapine Quetiapine Risperidone Ziprasidone Pimzide Zolpidem Zopiclone Modafinil
Inhibitors	Anastrozole Fluvoxamine	Paroxetine		Fluoxetine Fluvoxamine	Fluoxetine Paroxetine Sertraline Bupropion Chlorpromazine Haloperidol Metoclopramide Methadone Doxorubicin Vinblastine Ritonavir Lopinavir/ritonavir (Kaletra)	Nefazodone Fluoxetine Fluvoxamine Grapefruit juice HIV protease inhibitors Cyclosporine ?Fentanyl Methadone Anastrozole ?Doxorubicin ?Paclitaxel Tamoxifen
Inducers			Cyclophosphamide Ifosfamide	Corticosteroids		St John's wort Barbiturates Phenytoin Corticosteroids Rifampin Cisplatin Cyclophosphamide Ifosfamide

SOURCE: References 47,48.

Table 42–5. Medications used for depression in cancer patients

Drug	Starting Daily Dosage mg (po)	Therapeutic Daily Dosage mg (po)	Comments
SSRIs			
Fluoxetine	5–10	20–60	Stimulating, longest half life (5 weeks), no risk serotonin discontinuation syndrome
Sertraline	25–50	50–200	Relatively few drug interactions
Paroxetine	10	20–60	More anticholinergic effects, weight gain, more sedating
Escitalopram	5–10	10–20	Relatively few drug interactions
Citalopram	10	20–60	Relatively few drug interactions
Fluvoxamine	25	50–300	More sedating, more drug interactions
Mixed Action			
Trazodone	25–50	50–300	Sedating, orthostatic hypotension, priapism
Bupropion	75–100	150–450	Stimulating, seizure risk, minimal effect on weight and sexual functioning, useful for smoking cessation
Venlafaxine	37.5	75–300	Adjuvant for neuropathic pain, causes elevated diastolic BP at higher doses
Mirtazapine	7.5–15	15–45	Sedating, anxiolytic, antiemetic, appetite stimulating, available in orally disintegrating tablet
Duloxetine	30	30–60	Treats diabetic neuropathy, pain syndromes
TCAs			
Amitriptyline	10–25	50–150	Sedating
Imipramine	10–25	50–200	
Desipramine	10–25	50–150	Least sedating TCA
Nortriptyline	10–25	50–150	Least anticholinergic TCA, serum levels
Psychostimulants			
Methylphenidate	2.5 q am, 2.5 q noon	5–60	Insomnia, anxiety, tremor, achycardia, hypertension, confusion, delirium
Dextroamphetamine	same	same	same
Modafinil	50–100	100–400	Similar side effects as stimulants, but less frequent, more costly

ABBREVIATIONS: BP, blood pressure; SSRI, selective serotonin reuptake inhibitor; TCA, tricyclic antidepressant.
SOURCE: Adapted from "Drugs with Clinically Significant Cytochrome P450 Interactions" from the *American psychiatric publishing textbook of psychosomatic medicine.* © 2004 American Psychiatric Publishing, Inc.

loss, and thus may not be used first line in depressed cachectic cancer patients. Nausea has been reported to occur as frequently, 15%, as in the SSRIs, and other common adverse effects include dry mouth, constipation, headaches, agitation and insomnia. Daily doses exceeding 450 mg increase the seizure threshold tenfold, and its use is contraindicated in patients with seizure disorders, eating disorders or patients experiencing alcohol withdrawal. It has also been shown to prevent seasonal affective disorder and aid in smoking cessation.[72] Although rare, it may contribute to confusion or psychotic symptoms in vulnerable patients, due to its effect on dopamine.

Mirtazapine is a noradrenergic and specific serotonergic antidepressant. It has high affinity for H1 histaminic receptors and antagonizes 5HT2 and 5HT3 receptors. Through these mechanisms, anxiolysis, sedation, appetite stimulation and antiemesis occurs. Thus, in addition to alleviating depressive symptoms, it also improves cancer-related anorexia, cachexia, nausea and vomiting. Its structure is similar to mianserin, an antidepressant proven effective in depressed cancer patients. Side effects include constipation, drowsiness, and rarely reversible neutropenia. The side effect of weight gain may be advantageous in the cachectic cancer patient, and less so to those cancer patients who have gained weight from corticosteroids or chemotherapy. Another benefit of mirtazapine is its availability as a rapidly dissolving tablet, making it useful in patients who can not tolerate oral medications, and has also been shown to reduce hot flashes.[73]

Trazodone is a weak but specific inhibitor of serotonin and a post-synaptic serotonin receptor blocker which has been used to treat insomnia, usually at doses under 100 mg nightly. However, there is limited evidence showing its benefit in nondepressed patients with insomnia.[74] Its alpha blocking properties contribute to risks of priapism and orthostatic hypotension.

TCAs. Seldom used first line as antidepressants due to their side effect profile, the tricyclic antidepressants (TCAs) may be used in patients who have co-morbid neuropathic pain, usually at lower doses than are used for depression. Caution is used when prescribing TCAs to elderly patients, due to the anticholinergic activity that may contribute to confusion, as well as the alpha adrenergic blockade, which may contribute to orthostatic hypotension and increase risk of falls. Blocking muscarinic receptors may alter cardiac conduction, and thus caution is used in prescribing TCAs in patients with pre-existing arrythmias. H-1 histaminic blockade results in sedation, and possibly weight gain. Other anticholinergic side effects may result in constipation, urinary retention, dry mouth, and blurred vision.

Psychostimulants. Due to their rapid onset of action (days rather than weeks), the psychostimulants(methylphenidate and dextroamphetamine) are often used for their euphoric and energizing effects in depressed cancer patients, especially those with advanced or terminal disease. There have been five non placebo-controlled studies, as well as case series and reports, examining the effect of the psychostimulants in cancer patients, with four of the studies showing an improved mood in 73%–100% of patients.[75] Four of the studies used methylphenidate (doses ranging from 5 to 80 mg daily) and one used methylphenidate or dextroamphetamine (doses ranging from 2.5 to 20 mg daily). In addition to their impact on mood, the psychostimulants also reduce anorexia and fatigue, improve attention and concentration, counteract opiate-induced sedation and improve pain. The psychostimulants appear to be safe for long-term use with minimal risk for dependence, misuse, or tolerance in this population.[75] Despite the optimistic results of the studies done to date, these were open label trials and retrospective chart reviews; well-designed placebo-controlled studies are still needed. The most common adverse effects reported from the psychostimulants include insomnia and agitation. Due to their ability to stimulate the cardiovascular system, caution is advised when considering their use in patients with hypertension or arrhythmias. Rarely, psychosis can develop. Unlike the typical stimulant medications, Modafinil, a wakefulness promoting agent, does not effect the release of dopamine or noradrenaline, but instead, likely works through histamine release and agonism of noradrenaline receptors. There are no published trials of its use in the depressed cancer patient, however, extrapolating from other patient populations suggests that it is likely helpful and has less risk of dependency or side effects than the older stimulant medications.

CONCLUSION

As depression develops in approximately 25% of cancer patients, and has numerous negative consequences, its identification and management are important aspects of quality care. Individualizing interventions for the depressed cancer patient based on biopsychosocial needs, while using available evidence, including extrapolating from the general population, is recommended.

REFERENCES

1. Kessler RC, Chiu WT, Demler O, Walters EE. Prevalence, severity, and comorbidity of 12-month DSM-IV disorders in the National Comorbidity Survey Replication. *Arch Gen Psychiatry*. 2005;62:617–627.

2. Massie MJ. Prevalence of depression in patients with cancer. *J Natl Cancer Inst Monogr*. 2004;32:57.

3. Pirl WF. Evidence report on the occurrence, assessment, and treatment of depression in cancer patients. *J Natl Cancer Inst Monogr*. 2004;32:32–39.

4. Burgess C, Cornelius V, Love S, Graham J, Richards M, Ramirez A. Depression and anxiety in women with early breast cancer: five year observational cohort study. *BMJ*. 2005;330:702–707.

5. Hotopf M, Chidgey J, Addington-Hall J, Lan Ly K. Depression in advanced disease: a systemic review. *Palliat Med*. 2002;16:81–97.

6. Fallowfield L, Ratcliffe D, Jenkins V, Saul J. Psychiatric morbidity and its recognition by doctors in patients with cancer. *Br J Cancer*. 2001;84:1011–1015.

7. Pirl WF, Muriel A, Hwang V, et al. Screening for psychosocial distress: a national survey of oncologists. *J Supp Oncol*. 2007;5:499–504.

8. Chochinov H, Wilson K, Enns M, Lander S. 'Are you depressed?' Screening for depression in the terminally ill. *Am J Psychiatry*. 1997;154:674–676.

9. Akikuzi N, Akechi T, Nakanishi T, et al. Development of a brief screening interview for adjustment disorders and major depression in patients with cancer. *Cancer*. 2003;97:2005–2013.

10. Whooley M, Avins A, Mranda J, Browner W. Case-finding instruments for depression: two questions are as good as many. *J Gen Intern Med*. 1997;12:439–445.

11. Hoffman MA, Weiner JS. Is Mrs S depressed? Diagnosing depression in the cancer patient. *J Clin Oncol*. 2007;25:2853–2856.

12. Gilbody S, Sheldon T, House A. Screening and case-finding instruments for depression: a meta-analysis. *CMAJ*. 2008;178:997–1003.

13. Clarke DM, Kissane DW. Demoralization: its phenomenology and importance. *Aust N Z J Psychiatry*. 2002;36:733–742.

14. Minton O, Stone P, Richardson A, Sharpe M, Hotopf M. Drug therapy for the management of cancer related fatigue. *Cochrane Database Syst Rev*. 2008;1:CD006704.

15. Greenberg DB. Barriers to the treatment of depression in cancer. *J Natl Cancer Inst Monogr*. 2004;32:127–135.

16. Bailey RK, Geyen DJ, Scott-Gurnell K, Hipolito MMS, Bailey TA, Beal JM. Understanding and treating depression among cancer patients. *Int J Gynecol Cancer*. 2005;15:203–208.

17. Ell K, Sanchez K, Vourlekis B, et al. Depression, correlates of depression, and receipt of depression care among low-income women with breast or gynecologic cancer. *J Clin Oncol*. 2005;23:3052–3060.

18. Strong V, Waters R, Hibberd C, et al. Emotional distress in cancer patients: the Edinburgh cancer center symptom study. *Br J Cancer*. 2007;96:868–874.

19. Rodin 1 G, Walsh A, Zimmerman C, et al. The contribution of attachment security and social support to depressive symptoms in patients with metastatic cancer. *Psychooncology*. 2007;16:1–12.

20. Carlson LE, Angen M, Cullum J, et al. High levels of untreated distress and fatigue in cancer patients. *Br J Cancer*. 2004;90:2297–2304.

21. Zabora J, BrintzenhofeSzoc K, Curbow B, Hoker C, Piantadosi S. The prevalence of psychological distress by cancer site. *Psychooncology*. 2001;10:19–28.

22. Bardwell WA, Natarajan L, Dimsdale JE, et al. Objective cancer-related variables are not associated with depressive symptoms in women treated for early-stage breast cancer. *J Clin Oncol*. 2006;24:2420–2427.

23. Thornton LM, Carson WE, Shapiro CL, Farrar WB, Andersen BL. Delayed emotional recovery after taxane-based chemotherapy. *Cancer*. 2008;113:638–647.

24. Irwin MR, Miller AH. Depressive disorders and immunity: 20 years of progress and discovery. *Brain Behav Immun*. 2007;21:374–383.

25. Steel JL, Geller DA, Gamblin TC, Olek MC, Carr BI. Depression, immunity and survival in patients with hepatobiliary carcinoma. *J Clin Oncol*. 2007;25:2397–2405.

26. Raison CL, Miller AH. Depression in cancer: new developments regarding diagnosis and treatment. *Biol Psychiatry*. 2003;54:283–294.

27. Musselman DL, Lawson DH, Gumnick JF, et al. Paroxetine for the prevention of depression induced by high-dose interferon alpha. *N Engl J Med*. 2001;344:961–966.

28. Bannink M, Kruit WHJ, Van Gool AR, et al. Interferon-∝ in oncology patients: fewer psychiatric side effects than anticipated. *Psychosomatics*. 2008;49:56–63.

29. Newport DJ, Nemeroff CB. Assessment and treatment of depression in the cancer patient. *J Psychosom Res*. 1998;45:215–237.

30. DiMatteo MR, Lepper HS, Croghan TW. Depression is a risk factor for noncompliance with medical treatment: a meta-analysis of the effects of anxiety and depression on patient adherence. *Arch Int Med*. 2000;160:2101–2107.

31. Garssen B. Psychological factors and cancer development: evidence after 30 years of research. *Clin Psychol Rev*. 2004;24:315–338.

32. Spiegel D, Giese-Davis J. Depression and cancer: mechanisms and disease progression. *Biol Psychiatry*. 2003;54:269–282.

33. Irwin MR. Depression and risk of cancer progression: an elusive link. *J Clin Oncol*. 2007;25:2343–2344.

34. Rodin G, Zimmerman C, Rydall A, et al. The desire for hastened death in patients with metastatic cancer. *J Pain Symptom Manage*. 2007;33:661–675.

35. Rasic DT, Belik SL, Bolton JM, Chochinov HM, Sareen J. Cancer, mental disorders, suicidal ideation and attempts in a large community sample. *Psychooncology*. 2008;17:660–667.

36. Chochinov HM, Hack T, Hassard T, Kristjanson LJ, McClement S, Harlos M. Understanding the will to live in patients nearing death. *Psychosomatics*. 2005;46:7–10.

37. Hann D, Baker F, Denniston M, et al. The influence of social support on depressive symptoms in cancer patients: age and gender differences. *J Psychosom Res*. 2002;52:279–283.

38. Chochinov HM, Wilson KG, Enns M, Lander S. Depression, hopelessness, and suicidal ideation in the terminally ill. *Psychosomatics*. 1998;39:366–370.

39. Turner J, Zapart S, Pedersen K, Rankin N, Luxford K, Fletcher J. Clinical practice guidelines for the psychosocial care of adults with cancer. *Psychooncology*. 2005;14:159–173.

40. Rodin G, Katz M, Lloyd N, Green E, Mackay JA, Wong RKS, and the Supportive Care Guidelines Group of Cancer Care Ontario's Program in Evidence-Based Care. Treatment of depression in cancer patients. *Curr Oncol*. 2007;14:180–188.

41. Akechi T, Taniguchi K, Suzuki S, et al. Multifaceted psychosocial intervention program breast cancer patients after first recurrence: feasibility study. *Psychooncology*. 2007;16:517–524.

42. Rodin G, Lloyd N, Katz M, Green E, Mackay J, Wong R. The treatment of depression in cancer patients: a systematic review. *Support Care Cancer*. 2007;15:123–136.

43. Williams S, Dale J. The effectiveness of treatment for depression/depressive symptoms in adults with cancer: a systemic review. *Br J Cancer*. 2006;94:372–390.

44. Akechi T, Okuyama T, Onishi J, Morita T, Furukawa TA. Psychotherapy for depression among incurable cancer patients (review). *Cochrane Lib*. 2008;2:1–27.

45. Strong V, Waters R, Hibberd C, et al. Management of depression for people with cancer (SmaRT oncology 1): a randomized trial. *Lancet*. 2008;372:40–48.

46. Kissane DW, Grabsch B, Clarke DM, et al. Supportive-expressive group therapy for women with metastatic breast cancer: survival and psychosocial outcome from a randomized controlled trial. *Psychooncology*. 2007;16:277–286.

47. Cozza K, Armstrong S, Oesterheld JR. *Concise guide to drug interaction principles for medical practice: cytochrome p450s, ugts, p-glycoproteins*, 2nd ed. Washington, DC, American Psychiatric Publishing; 2003.

48. Robinson MJ, Owen JA. Psychopharmacology. In: Levenson JL, (ed). *Textbook of psychosomatic medicine.* Washington, DC: American Psychiatric Publishing, Inc; 2005:876–879.

49. Okamura M, Akizuki N, Nakano T, et al. Clinical experience of the use of a pharmacological treatment algorithm for major depressive disorder in patients with advanced cancer. *Psychooncology.* 2008;17:154–160.

50. Fisch MJ, Loehrer PJ, Kristeller J, et al. Fluoxetine versus placebo in advanced cancer outpatients: a double-blinded trial of the Hoosier Oncology Group. *J Clin Oncol.* 2003;21:1937–1943.

51. Navari RM, Brenner MC, Wilson MN. Treatment of depressive symptoms in patients with early stage breast cancer undergoing adjuvant therapy. *Breast Cancer Res Treat.* 2007 online publication

52. Roscoe JA, Morrow GR, Hickok JT, et al. Effect of paroxetine hydrochloride (Paxil) on fatigue and depression in breast cancer patients receiving chemotherapy. *Breast Cancer Res Treat.* 2005;89:243–249.

53. Morrow GR, Hickok JT, Roscoe JA, et al. Differential effects of paroxetine on fatigue and depression: a randomized double-blind trial from the University of Rochester Cancer Center Community Clinical Oncology Program. *J Clin Oncol.* 2003;21:4635–4641.

54. Van Heeringen K, Zivkov M. Pharmacological treatment of depression in cancer patients. A placebo-controlled study of mianserin. *Br J Psychiatry.* 1996;169:440–443.

55. Costa D, Mogos I, Toma T. Efficacy and safety of mianserin in the treatment of depression of women with cancer. *Acta Psychiatr Scand Suppl.* 1985;320:85–92.

56. Razavi D, Allilaire JF, Smith M, et al. The effect of fluoxetine on anxiety and depression in cancer patients. *Acta Psychiatr Scand.* 1996;94:205–210.

57. Musselman DL, Somerset WI, Guo Y, et al. A double-blind, multicenter, parallel-group study of paroxetine, desipramine, or placebo in breast cancer patients (stages I, II, III, and IV) with major depression. *J Clin Psychiatry.* 2006;67:288–296.

58. Stockler MR, O'ConnellR, Kowak AK, et al. Effect of sertraline on symptoms and survival in patients with advanced cancer, but without major depression: a placebo-controlled double-blind randomized trial. *Lancet.* 2007; 8:603–612.

59. Holland l JC, Morrow GR, Schmale A, et al. A randomized clinical trial of alprazolam versus progressive muscle relaxation in cancer patients with anxiety and depressive symptoms. *J Clin Oncol.* 1991;9:1004–1011.

60. Pezella G, Moslinger-Gehmayr R, Contu A. Treatment of depression in patients with breast cancer: a comparison between paroxetine and amitriptyline. *Breast Cancer Res Treat.* 2001;70:1–10.

61. Holland JC, Romano SJ, Heiligenstein JH, Tepner RG, Wilson MG. A controlled trial of fluoxetine and desipramine in depressed women with advanced cancer. *Psychooncology.* 1998;7:291–300.

62. Bordeleau L, Pritchard K, Goodwin P, Loprinzi C. Therapeutic options for the management of hot flashes in breast cancer survivors: an evidenced-based review. *Clin Ther.* 2007;29:230–241.

63. Stearns V, Johnson MD, Rae JM, et al. Active tamoxifen metabolite plasma concentrations after coadministration of tamoxifen and the selective serotonin reuptake inhibitor paroxetine. *J Natl Cancer Inst.* 2003;95:1758–1764.

64. Jin Y, Desta Z, Stearns V, et al. CYP2D6 genotype, antidepressant use, and tamoxifen metabolism during adjuvant breast cancer treatment. *J Natl Cancer Inst.* 2005;97:30–39.

65. Goetz MP, Knox SK, Suman VJ, et al. The impact of cytochrome P450 2D6 metabolism in women receiving adjuvant tamoxifen. *Breast Cancer Res Treat.* 2007;101:113–121.

66. Jacob S, Spinler SA. Hyponatremia associated with selective serotonin-reuptake inhibitors in older adults. *Ann Pharmacother.* 2006;40:1618–1622.

67. Liu BA, Mittman N, Knowles SR, Shear NH. Hyponatremia and the syndrome of inappropriate secretion of antidiuretic hormone associated with the use of selective serotonin re-uptake inhibitors: a review of spontaneous reports. *Can Med Assoc J.* 1996;155:519–527.

68. Looper K. Potential medical and surgical complications of serotonergic antidepressant medications. *Psychosomatics.* 2007;48:1–9.

69. Mathias C, Cardeal Mendes CM, et al. An open-label, fixed-dose study of bupropion effect on sexual function scores in women treated for breast cancer. *Ann Oncol.* 2006;17:1792–1796.

70. Moss EL, Simpson JSA, Pelletier G, Forsyth P. An open-label study of the effects of bupropion SR on fatigue, depression and quality of life of mixed-site cancer patients and their caregivers. *Psychooncology.* 2005;15:259–267.

71. Perez DG, Loprinzi CL, Sloan J, et al. Pilot evaluation of bupropion for the treatment of hot flashes. *J Palliat Med.* 2006;9:631–637.

72. Foley KF, DeSanty KP, Kast RE. Bupropion: pharmacology and therapeutic applications. *Expert Rev. Neurotherapeutics.* 2006;6:1249–1265.

73. Biglia N, Kubatzki F, Sgandurra P, et al. Mirtazapine for the treatment of hot flushes in breast cancer survivors: a prospective pilot trial. *Breast J.* 2007;13:490–495.

74. Mendelson WB. A review of the evidence for the efficacy and safety of trazodone in insomnia. *J Clin Psychiatry.* 2005;66:469–476.

75. Orr K, Taylor D. Psychostimulants in the treatment of depression: a review of the evidence. *CNS Drugs.* 2007;21:239–257.

Suicide

Haley Pessin, Lia Amakawa, and William S. Breitbart

Unfortunately, the assessment and identification of those individuals at risk for suicide continues to remain a vital topic for clinicians working with cancer patients, as individuals with cancer are at increased risk for suicidal ideation and behavior when compared to the general population[1] and other medically ill populations.[2,3] Suicidal thoughts and behaviors in cancer patients are associated with a number of psychosocial and physical risk factors. This chapter will describe suicidality in cancer, prevalence rates, risk factors, and will provide clinical guidelines for assessment and intervention.

KEY CONCEPTS AND DEFINITIONS

Suicidal ideation and behavior varies widely with regard to severity and risk. *Suicidal ideation* can, but does not necessarily, reflect an actual wish to harm oneself. In fact, less severe forms of suicidal ideation, such as a fleeting wish to die, are often normal in cancer patients at all stages of disease. When suicidal ideation occurs and becomes severe in patients who are survivors or those who have a good prognosis the likelihood of an underlying significant depression with suicidal potential should be considered. Suicidal ideation is of greatest concern when it persists or involves an actual *suicidal intent or plan,* where a desire to act on these feelings is expressed and a potential method is described. The term *desire for hastened death* is utilized when suicidal wishes occur in the context of advanced disease, such as terminal cancer. Desire for hastened death represents a person's wish to die sooner than might occur by natural disease progression. It may be manifested among patients with varying degrees of severity: (1) a passive wish (either fleeting or persistent) for death without an active plan; (2) a request for assistance in hastening death through withdrawal of essential aspects of medical care (e.g., feeding tube); or (3) an active desire and plan to commit suicide.[4] Finally, other terms closely related to suicidality in end-of-life care are *physician-assisted suicide* (PAS), which is used when a physician provides a prescription for medication to a patient to end his or her life, and *euthanasia,* which is the term used when a physician administers a fatal overdose of medication at the patient's request.[5]

SUICIDE RISK IN CANCER

While occasional thoughts of suicide are relatively common among cancer patients, research suggests that persistent suicidal ideation is far less frequent, existing mostly among patients with advanced disease, in hospital or palliative care settings, or experiencing severe pain or significant depression.[6,7] Although few cancer patients actually commit suicide compared to the number who report passive suicidal ideation and desire for hastened death, individuals with cancer have approximately twice the risk of suicide compared to the general population.[1,3] A recent study of completed suicide among the general population in the United States and Australia from 1999 though 2003 identified cancer as the only physical disease associated with significant suicide mortality.[3]

Despite the association between cancer and suicide, few studies have focused on the frequency of suicide in this population. A recent study using data from the Cancer Registry of Norway addresses this gap, reporting that males are 55% more likely and females are 35% more likely to die by suicide than the general population.[8] This study found the first months following diagnosis to be the period of greatest risk. There is also evidence that cancer patients more frequently commit suicide in the advanced stages of disease.[9-11] The preponderance of suicides in advanced cancer may be attributable to the increased likelihood of other risk factors for suicide such as depression, pain, delirium, and deficit symptoms.[12] However, the available data may actually underestimate the true prevalence of suicidal ideation in cancer, due to the limitations of research interviews and measures to elicit this information, and may also underestimate suicide rates, given the unknown frequency of unreported overdoses assisted by families or decisions to stop critical aspects of care such as nutrition and hydration.[6] Finally, patients at the end of life may be utilizing euthanasia and PAS far more frequently than the literature indicates as healthcare professionals may be reluctant to report euthanasia and PAS to avoid possible legal and political ramifications.[13]

SPECIFIC RISK FACTORS IN CANCER SUICIDE

Primary demographic, physical, and psychosocial risk factors for suicide in cancer patients have been identified in the literature and will be outlined below. Awareness of these risks factors should serve as red flags for further evaluation. Effective assessment and management of suicidal ideation and behavior in cancer requires a thorough understanding of the potential complications associated with these risk factors.

Demographic characteristics. Several studies have noted the effects of age on suicide in cancer patients, particularly among individuals in the sixth and seventh decades of life.[9,10,14] While men with cancer may have over twice the risk of suicide compared to the general population, the relative risk of suicide in women with cancer is less clear.[8-10] Furthermore, there may be an interaction between gender and type of cancer. For example, data from the Cancer Registry of Norway attributed the highest suicide risk to males with respiratory cancers.[8] This may relate to the presence of other risk factors such as the higher use of alcohol and tobacco, suggesting preexisting psychological problems.

Depression. The co-morbidity of suicide and major depression is common both in the general population and among cancer patients. Depression factors into 50% of all suicides. The incidence of depression is particularly high for individuals with cancer. Approximately 25% of all cancer patients endorse severe depressive symptoms with 6% meeting criteria for a major depression diagnosis.[15] Massie (2004) reviewed over 100 studies with prevalence rates for depression in cancer and reported a close association between cancer and depression regardless of stage and site of disease.[16] Chochinov and colleagues' (1995) study in advanced cancer patients found that 58% of patients reporting significant desire for hastened death also met criteria for major depression.[15] Moreover, depression emerged as the strongest predictor of desire for hastened death. The authors concluded that many individuals with cancer who express interest in a hastened death may suffer from an unrecognized depressive disorder.

Hopelessness. Once subsumed under depressive symptoms, hopelessness has emerged as a unique risk factor for suicidal ideation and behavior.[17] Past studies in a general population have linked hopelessness and suicidal ideation,[18,19] with a stronger association between hopelessness and suicidal intent than depression and suicidal intent.[20] Chochinov and colleagues (1998) found hopelessness to be a stronger predictor of suicidal ideation than severity of depression among individuals with terminal cancer.[17] More recently, hopelessness has been identified as the strongest predictor of desire for hastened death in advanced cancer.[21] However, the presence of both depression and hopelessness may be the strongest clinical marker for high desire for hastened death.[22]

Helplessness, control, and burden to others. Individuals with cancer who present with an excessive need to control all aspects of living or dying may be particularly vulnerable to suicide. In one study cancer patients who reportedly approached their medical care with acceptance and adaptability were less likely to commit suicide than those who did not.[23] Other personality factors such as concerns about loss of autonomy, dependency, and a strong need to control the circumstances of one's death are important predictors of desire for hastened death.[4] However, cancer-related events may elicit feelings of helplessness among any patient with cancer. Distressing physical impairment such as loss of mobility, paraplegia, amputation, sensory loss, and inability to eat or swallow can elicit helplessness. Patients may be most distraught by the sense that they have lost "control" of their minds, due to heavy sedation or episodes of delirium.[12] Feelings of excessive burden may accompany perceptions of helplessness and loss of control among cancer patients. Research highlights the association between concerns about burdening others and suicidal ideation and desire for hastened death.[22] A study of Oregonian patients who died by assisted suicide reported that 63% of patients felt that they had become a significant burden to family, friends, or other caregivers.[24] Kelly and colleagues (2003) found similar perceptions of burden to others to be significantly associated with a wish to hastened death among cancer patients receiving hospice care.[25]

Pain. Uncontrolled pain plays an important role in vulnerability to cancer suicide.[6,10,12,26] Physicians have reported that persistent or uncontrolled pain fuels the majority of cancer patients' requests for assisted suicide.[10] Studies have demonstrated that most cancer suicides were preceded by inadequately managed or poorly tolerated pain.[23–26] Mystakidou and colleagues (2005) found that severity of pain as well as the extent to which pain interfered with activity significantly predicted desire for death.[26] Moreover, for advanced cancer patients, the presence of pain increases the likelihood of the co-occurrence of several risk factors for suicide: depression, delirium, loss of control, and hopelessness.[6]

Physical symptoms. Physical symptoms other than pain also have a relationship with suicide and desire for hastened death, as they can induce psychological distress and escalate to suicidal thoughts or behaviors. Conversely, the presence of psychological disorders may heighten perceptions of pain and other physical symptoms and contribute to suicidal thoughts. Regardless of causality, studies have demonstrated a link between specific physical symptoms (i.e., shortness of breath) and frequency of suicidal ideation[27] and the number of physical symptoms, symptom distress, and a higher desire for hastened death.[22,28]

Cognitive dysfunction and delirium. Past studies have revealed a high prevalence of organic mental disorders, primarily delirium, among cancer patients receiving psychiatric consultation. These estimates range from 25% to 40%, reaching 85% during the terminal stages of disease.[29] Psychiatric consultation data at Memorial Sloan-Kettering Cancer Center showed that one-third of suicidal patients were simultaneously suffering from delirium.[30] Pessin and colleagues (2003) found a significant association between moderate cognitive impairment and desire for hastened death in other acutely medically ill populations.[31] Because delirium and cognitive impairment cloud a patient's reasoning ability, these factors may result in an inability to judge consequences of one's behavior and increase the risk of impulsive behavior. In fact, the majority of treatment delays or refusals in cancer patients occur in the context of psychoses, organic mental disorders, and/or depression.[32]

Social support. A growing body of research has demonstrated the important relationship between social support and suicide. Social and psychological factors (e.g., concern regarding a loss of dignity; fear of becoming a burden to others) comprised four of the five most frequently cited reasons for euthanasia requests.[33] Several studies have found a significant correlation between lower levels of social support and a higher desire for death in advanced cancer patients.[15,21–22]

Psychiatric history and personality factors. Preexisting psychiatric disturbance significantly increases the risk for desire for hastened death and suicidal ideation.[34] In fact, Holland (1982) argued that it is extremely rare for a cancer patient to actually commit suicide without some degree of premorbid psychopathology.[35] Psychiatric consultation data from Memorial Sloan-Kettering Cancer Center indicates that half of the suicidal cancer patients who were assessed had a diagnosable personality disorder. Furthermore, one-third of these patients were also diagnosed with a major depression and half were diagnosed with an adjustment disorder with both depressed and anxious features during the psychiatric consultation.[30] In addition, a history of past suicide attempts or a family history of suicide also increases suicide risk significantly.[6]

Spiritual and existential concerns. When faced with a cancer diagnosis, individuals often experience distress and despair, posing the critical question, "Why me?"[36] The newly diagnosed commonly dwell on issues of life and death for the first few months following diagnosis.[37] For cancer patients with terminal illness, existential issues become paramount as they consider loss of meaning, purpose, or dignity; awareness of incomplete life tasks; regret; and anxiety around what happens after death. These difficulties with existential issues has been tied to desire for hastened death.[36] Terminally ill cancer patients reporting low spiritual well-being were more likely to endorse desire for hastened death, hopelessness, and suicidal ideation.[38]

LEGAL AND ETHICAL ISSUES IN ASSISTED SUICIDE

Several important legal and ethical issues should be considered with regard to assisted suicide. First, this area continues to change and evolve both within the field of palliative care and the judicial system. Second, there is potential for emotionally charged ethical dilemmas, as demonstrated by high-profile media coverage of assisted suicide cases. Finally, the controversial nature of assisted suicide is likely to play a role in providers' assessment of and responses to patients' wishes to die, impacting subsequent treatment decisions.

Those opposing legalization have expressed concerns that requests for assisted suicide are often due to depression, distorted beliefs that one is a burden, or the other potentially treatable clinical correlates of desire for hastened death described above.[39] Others have argued that aspects of the quality of end-of-life care, including an increase in referrals to palliative care, have improved since assisted suicide was legalized.[40,41] Regardless of one's position on the issue of assisted suicide, comprehensive and detailed assessment of palliative care patients is critical to determine if conditions related to desire for hastened death can be modified to enhance patients' quality of life, ameliorate unnecessary suffering, and ensure that patients are not requesting assisted suicide impulsively or without a clear understanding of possible alternative solutions.

In spite of the heated debate, the practice of assisted suicide by providers is still relatively rare. The legalization of assisted suicide remains under the jurisdiction of each state in the United States. Currently, Oregon is the only state in the United States that has legalized physician-assisted suicide, permitting physicians to write prescriptions for lethal doses of medication for terminally ill residents who make this request. Legalization occurred in 1997 when the state legislature passed the Oregon Death with Dignity Act, which the U.S. Supreme Court upheld with the Gonzales *v.* Oregon decision in 2006.[42] Assisted suicide and euthanasia are also legal in the Netherlands, comprising approximately 1%–5% of all deaths and 7.4% of deaths among cancer patients, and these rates have remained stable over the past decade.[43]

PRACTICE GUIDELINES

Assessment. The careful assessment of suicide risk is the first step toward appropriate intervention. Early and comprehensive psychiatric involvement with high-risk cancer patients can often avert suicide.[44] However, healthcare professionals may remain wary of conducting suicide risk assessment or responding to desire to die statements because of fear of diminishing patients' hope or provoking emotional discussions.[45] There is no clinical research evidence to support the myth that asking about suicidal thoughts increases suicidal acts.[46] In fact, such reservations run counter to evidence that patients report a sense of relief and diminished suicidal urges once their distress and need for control over death have been acknowledged.[34] Furthermore, it is recommended that practitioners use the assessment as a therapeutic opportunity to ask patients about their concerns about the future, provide accurate information to allay unwarranted fears, and allow patients to express feelings that may be difficult to discuss with others.[47] Hudson, Schofield, and colleagues (2006) proposed guidelines for health professionals conducting suicide assessment[47] (see Table 43-1). Although developed for use among patients with advanced disease, these principles and strategies for therapeutic communication are applicable to cancer patients at all stages. Systematic reviews of randomized controlled trials have shown that this approach ameliorates distress and promotes psychological well-being.[46]

Among those who directly endorse desire for death, suicidal ideation, suicidal behaviors, or depression, clinicians should thoroughly evaluate extent of ideation, plan, and intent (see Table 43-2). Evaluations of the severity and intensity of suicidal ideation will inform appropriate intervention and treatment planning.

In addition, Rudd and Joiner (1999) have recommended evaluating the following factors to identify those individual who are at highest risk for suicidal behavior (see Table 43-3). These include predisposition to suicidal behavior (i.e., a history of suicidal behavior, psychiatric diagnosis, and demographic risk factors); precipitants or stressors; symptomatic presentation (i.e., depression, anger, and agitation); nature of suicidal thinking (frequency, intensity, duration, specificity of plans, availability of means, and explicitness of intent); hopelessness; previous suicidal behavior (frequency, method, lethality, and outcome); impulsivity and lack of protective factors (social support, problem-solving skills, and mental health treatment).[48] In addition, evaluation of palliative care patients requires careful assessment of somatic symptoms to determine whether their etiology is psychiatric or organic in nature.[49,50]

Table 43-1. General guidelines for the assessment suicide[46,47]

Be alert to your own responses	Be aware of how your responses influence discussions
	Monitor your attitude and responses
	Demonstrate positive regard for the patient
	Seek supervision
Be open to hearing concerns	Gently ask about emotional concerns
	Be alert to verbal and nonverbal distress cues
	Encourage expression of feelings
	Actively listen without interrupting
	Discuss desire for death using patient's words
	Permit sadness, silence, and tears
	Express empathy verbally and nonverbally
	Acknowledge differences in responses to illness
Assess contributing factors	Prior psychiatric history
	Prior suicide attempts
	History of alcohol or substance abuse
	Lack of social support
	Feelings of burden
	Family conflict
	Need for additional assistance
	Depression and anxiety
	Existential concerns, loss of meaning and dignity
	Cognitive impairment
	Physical symptoms, especially severe pain
Respond to specific issues	Acknowledge patient or family fears and concerns
	Address modifiable contributing factors
	Recommend interventions
	Develop plan to manage more complicated issues
Conclude discussion	Summarize and review important points
	Clarify patient perceptions
	Provide opportunity for questions
	Assist in facilitating discussion with others
	Provide appropriate referrals
After discussion	Document discussion in medical records
	Communicate with members of the treatment team

Table 43-2. Assessing severity of suicidal ideation[51]

Suicidal ideation	Many patients have passing thoughts of suicide, such as, "If my pain was bad enough, I might…" Have you had thoughts like that?
	Have you found yourself thinking that you do not want to live or that you would be better off dead?
Suicidal plan	Have you stopped or wanted to stop taking care of yourself?
	Have you thought about how you would end your life?
Suicidal intent	Do you plan or intend to hurt yourself? What would you do?
	Do you think you would carry out these plans?

Table 43-3. Questions to ask patients and family when assessing suicidal risk

Acknowledge that these are common thoughts that can be discussed	Most patients with cancer have passing thoughts about suicide, such as "I might do something if it gets bad enough." Have you ever had thoughts like that?
	Have you had any thoughts of not wanting to live?
	Have you had those thoughts in the past few days?
Assess level of risk	Do you have thoughts about wanting to end your life? How?
	Do you have a plan?
	Do you have any strong social supports?
	Do you have pills stockpiled at home?
	Do you own or have access to a weapon?
Obtain prior history	Have you ever had a psychiatric disorder, suffered from depression, or made a suicide attempt?
	Is there a family history of suicide?
Identify substance abuse	Have you had a problem with alcohol or drugs?
Identify bereavement	Have you lost anyone close to you recently?
Identify medical predictors of risk	Do you have pain that is not being relieved?
	How has the disease affected your life?
	How is your memory and concentration?
	Do you feel hopeless?
	What do you plan for the future?

SOURCE: Adapted from APOS. *Quick Reference for Oncology Clinicians: The Psychiatric and Psychological Dimensions of Cancer Symptom Management*; 2006.[52]

Intervention strategies. Thorough psychological assessment and competent intervention for suicide may provide cancer patients with great relief from distress and suffering and ultimately save lives. It is essential that all treatments targeting suicidality, regardless of technique and modality, are informed by careful attention to the risk factors for suicide. An appropriate therapeutic response to these discussions should include empathy, active listening, management of realistic expectations, permission to discuss psychological distress, and a referral to other professionals when appropriate.

Initial interventions should focus on determining imminent risk and making necessary plans and arrangements for patient safety (see Table 43–4). Appropriate interventions may include psychiatric hospitalization for severely suicidal patients, the use of suicide prevention resources, contracting with the patient for safety, limiting access to potential means such as pills or guns, and involvement of family or friends in monitoring the patient[52] However, it should be noted that psychiatric hospitalization may not be ideal or realistic for severely medically ill patients and other strategies may have to be utilized. In these cases, crisis intervention and the mobilization of support systems may act as external controls and strongly reduce the risk of suicide.[12]

Recognition of the prominent risk factors for suicide (see Table 43–1) should also inform targeted intervention strategies and treatment plans that may reduce suicidality, such as the aggressive management of pain, physical symptoms, delirium, and cognitive impairment.[34] Antidepressant medications in tandem with supportive psychotherapy, cognitive-behavioral techniques, and patient and family education are the most effective means of improving depressive symptoms, hopelessness, and suicidal ideation.[53,54] Pharmacological interventions should also include analgesics, anxiolytics, or narcoleptics to treat any accompanying symptoms of anxiety, agitation, psychosis, or pain.[50,4] Cognitive-behavioral techniques can be tailored to manage cancer patients' physical symptoms and challenge cognitive distortions driving suicidal ideation.[55–57] Both individual and group supportive psychotherapy for cancer patients can provide additional support by assuaging feelings of isolation, bolstering coping skills, and addressing existential concerns.[36,52,58]

Table 43–4. Interventions for the suicidal patient

For patient whose suicidal threat is seen as serious	Provide constant observation and further assessment.
	Dangerous objects like guns or intoxicants should be removed from the room or home.
	The risk for suicidal behavior should be communicated to family members.
For patient who is not acutely suicidal and is medically stable	Patient should agree to call when feeling overwhelmed, making a contract with the physician to talk about suicidal thoughts in the future rather than to act on them.
For inpatients	Room searches should be carried out to make sure there no means available for self-destructive behavior.
	The patient should be under constant observation from the time suicidal thoughts are expressed.
For severely suicidal outpatients whose suicidal thoughts are not acutely caused by their medical condition or medication	Psychiatric hospitalization is warranted, either by voluntary or by involuntary means.
	A psychiatrist can assist in making these arrangements. Document medical action and reasoning in the crisis.

SOURCE: Adapted from APOS. *Quick Reference for Oncology Clinicians: The Psychiatric and Psychological Dimensions of Cancer Symptom Management*; 2006.[52]

REFERENCES

1. Levi F, Bulliard JL, La Vecchia C. Suicide risk among incident cases of cancer in the Swiss Canton of Vaud. *Oncology*. 1990;48:44–47.

2. Mishara, BL. Synthesis of research and evidence on factors affecting the desire of terminally ill or seriously chronically ill persons to hasten death. *Omega (Westport)*. 1999;39:1–70.

3. Rockett IRH, Wang S, Lian Y, Stack S. Suicide-associated comorbidity among U.S. males and females: a multiple cause-of-death analysis. *Injury Prev.* 2007;13:311–315.

4. Hudson PL, Kristjanson LJ, Ashby M, et al. Desire for hastened death in patients with advanced disease and the evidence base of clinical guidelines: a systematic review. *Palliat Med.* 2006;20:693–701.

5. Cohen JS, Fihn SD, Boyko EJ, Jonsen AR, Wood RW. Attitudes toward assisted suicide and euthanasia among physicians in Washington state. *New Engl J Med.* 1994;89–94.

6. Breitbart W. Suicide risk and pain in cancer and AIDS patients. In: Chapman CR, Foley KM (eds). *Current and emerging issues in cancer pain: Research and practice.* New York: Raven Press; 1993:49–65.

7. Breitbart W, Levenson JA, Passik SD. Terminally ill cancer patients. In: Breitbart W, Holland JC (eds). *Psychiatric aspects of symptom management in cancer patients.* Washington, DC: American Psychiatric Press;1993:192–194.

8. Hem E, Loge JH, Haldorsen T, Ekeberg O. Suicide risk in cancer patients from 1960 to 1999. *J Clin Oncol.* 2004;22:4209–4216.

9. Bolund C. Suicide and cancer I. Demographic and social characteristics of cancer patients who committed suicide in Sweden, 1973–1976. *J Psychosoc Oncol.* 1985;3:17–30.

10. Bolund C. Suicide and cancer II. Medical and care factors in suicide by cancer patients in Sweden, 1973–1976. *J Psychosoc Oncol.* 1985;3:31–52.

11. Ransom S, Sacco WP, Weitzner MA, Azzarello LM, McMillan SC. Interpersonal factors predict increased desire for hastened death in late-stage cancer patients. *Ann Behav Med.* 2006;31:63–69.

12. Breitbart W, Gibson C, Abbey J, Iannarone N, Borenstein, R. Suicide in palliative care. In: Bruera E, Higginson IJ, Ripamonti, C, Von Guten C (eds). *Textbook of palliative medicine.* London: Hodder Arnold; 2006:860–868.

13. Rosenfeld B. Methodological issues in assisted suicide and euthanasia research. *Psychol Public Pol L.* 2000;6:559–574.

14. Hietanen P, Lönnqvist J, Henriksson M, Jallinoja P. Do cancer suicides differ from others? *Psychooncology.* 1994;3:189–195.

15. Chochinov HM, Wilson KG, Enns M, et al. Desire for death in the terminally ill. *Am J Psychiat.* 1995;152:1185–1191.

16. Massie MJ. Prevalence of depression in patients with cancer. *JNCI Monographs.* 2004;32:57–71.

17. Chochinov HM, Wilson KG, Enns M, Lander S. Depression, hopelessness, and suicidal ideation in the terminally ill. *Psychosomatics.* 1998;39:366–370.

18. Beck AT, Kovacs M, Weissman A. Hopelessness and suicidal behavior. An overview. *JAMA.* 1975;234:1146–1149.

19. Minkoff K, Bergman E, Beck AT, Beck RD. Hopelessness, depression, and attempted suicide. *Am J Psychiatry.* 1973;130:455–459.

20. Wetzel RD. Hopelessness, depression, and suicide intent. *Arch Gen Psychiatry.* 1976;33:1069–1073.

21. Rodin G, Zimmermann C, Rydall A, et al. The desire for hastened death in patients with metastatic cancer. *J Pain Symptom Manage.* 2007;33:661–675.

22. Breitbart W, Rosenfeld B, Pessin H, et al. Depression, hopelessness, and desire for hastened death in terminally ill patients with cancer. *JAMA.* 2000;284:2907–2911.

23. Farberow NL, Schneiderman ES, Leonard, CV. Suicide among general medical and surgical hospital patients with malignant neoplasms. *Med Bull.* 1963;9:1–11. Washington DC: U.S. Veterans Administration.

24. Sullivan AD, Hedberg K, Hopkins, MS. Legalized physician-assisted suicide in Oregon, 1998–2000. *New Engl J Med.* 2001;344:605–607.

25. Kelly B, Burnett, P, Pelusi D, Badger S, Varghese F, Robertson M. Factors associated with the wish to hasten death: a study of patients with terminal illness. *Psychol Med.* 2003;33:75–81.

26. Mystakidou K, Parpa E, Katsouda E, Galanos A, Vlahos L. Pain and desire for hastened death in terminally ill cancer patients. *Cancer Nurs.* 2005;28:318–324.

27. Suarez-Almazor ME, Newman C, Hanson J, Bruera E. Attitudes of terminally ill cancer patients about euthanasia and assisted suicide: predominance of psychosocial determinants and beliefs over symptoms distress and subsequent survival. *J Clin Oncol.* 2002;20:2134–2141.

28. Sullivan M, Rapp S, Fitzgibbon D, Chapman CR. Pain and the choice to hasten death in patients with painful metastatic cancers. *J Palliat Care.* 1997;13:18–28.

29. Massie MJ, Holland JC, Glass E. Delirium in terminally ill cancer patients. *Am J Psychiatry.* 1983;140:1048–1050.

30. Breitbart W. Suicide in cancer patients. *Oncology.* 1987;1:49–54.

31. Pessin H, Rosenfeld B, Burton L, Breitbart W. The role of cognitive impairment in desire for hastened death: a study of patients with advanced AIDS. *Gen Hosp Psychiatry.* 2003;25:194–199.

32. Filiberti A, Ripamonti C. Suicide and suicidal thoughts in cancer patients. *Tumori.* 2002;88:193–199.

33. van der Maas PJ, van der Wal G, Haverkate I, et al. Euthanasia, physician-assisted suicide, and other medical practices involving the end of life in the Netherlands, 1990–1995. *New Engl J Med.* 1996;335:1699–1705.

34. Pessin H, Evcimen YA, Apostolatos A, Breitbart W. Diagnosis, assessment, and treatment of depression in palliative care. In: Lloyd-Williams M (ed). *Psychosocial issues in palliative care.* New York: Oxford University Press; 2008:129–159.

35. Holland, JC. Psychological aspects of cancer. In: Holland, JF, Frei E III (eds). *Cancer medicine,* 2nd ed. Philadelphia, PA: Lea & Febiger; 1982:1175–1203.

36. Breitbart W. Spirituality and meaning in supportive care: spirituality- and meaning-centered group psychotherapy interventions in advanced cancer. *Support Care Cancer.* 2002;10:272–280.

37. Weisman A, Worden J. The existential plight in cancer: significance of the first 100 days. *Intl Psychiatry Med.* 1976–1977;7:1–15.

38. McClain CS, Rosenfeld B, Breitbart W. Effect of spiritual well-being on end-of-life despair in terminally-ill cancer patients. *Lancet.* 2003;361:1603–1607.

39. Okie S. Physician-assisted suicide—Oregon and beyond. *N Engl J Med.* 2005;352:1627–1630.

40. Ganzini L, Nelson HD, Lee MA, Kraemer DF, Schmidt TA, Delorit MA. Oregon physicians' attitudes about and experiences with end-of-life care since passage of the Oregon Death with Dignity Act. *JAMA.* 2001;285(18):2363–2369.

41. National Health and Medical Research Council, Australia. *Clinical practice guidelines for the psychosocial care of adults with cancer.* National Health and Medical Research Council, Australia; 2003.

42. Oregon Department of Health Services. *Death with dignity act annual report 2006—Year 9 summary.* Oregon Department of Health Services; 2007.

43. Onwuteaka-Philipsen BD, van der Heide A, Koper D, et al. Euthanasia and other end-of-life decisions in the Netherlands in 1990, 1995, 2001. *Lancet.* 2003;362:395–397.

44. Dubovsky SL. Averting suicide in terminally ill patients. *Psychosomatics.* 1978;19:113–115.

45. Schwarz JK. Understanding and responding to patients' requests for assistance in dying. *J Nurs Scholarsh.* 2003;35:377–384.

46. National Breast Cancer Centre and National Cancer Control Initiative. *Clinical practice guidelines for the psychosocial care of adults with cancer.* Camperdown, NSW: National Breast Cancer Centre; 2003.

47. Hudson PL, Schofield P, Kelly B, et al. Responding to desire to die statements from patients with advanced disease: recommendations for health professionals. *Palliat Med.* 2006;20:703–710.

48. Rudd M D, Joiner T. Assessment of suicidality in outpatient practice. In VandeCreek L, Jackson R (eds). *Innovation in clinical practice: A sourcebook.* Sarasota, FL: Professional Resource Press; 1999(17):101–117.

49. Pessin H, Olden M, McClain CS, Kosinski A. Clinical assessment of depression: a practical guide. *Palliat Support Care.* 2005;3:319–324.

50. Pessin H, Potash M, Breitbart W. Diagnosis, assessment, and treatment of depression in palliative care. In: Lloyd-Williams M (ed). *Psychosocial issues in palliative care.* Oxford: Oxford University Press; 2003:81–103.

51. Breitbart W. Cancer pain and suicide In: Foley K, Bonica JJ, Venafridda V (eds). *Advances in pain research and therapy.* New York: Raven Press; 1990(16):399–412.

52. American Psychosocial Oncology Society. *Quick reference for oncology clinicians: The psychiatric and psychological dimensions of cancer symptom management.* Charlottesville, VA: IPOS Press; 2006.

53. Maguire P, Hopwood P, Tarrier N, Howell T. Treatment of depression in cancer patients. *Acta Psychiatr Scand. Suppl.* 1985;320:81–84.

54. Block SD. Psychological issues in end-of-life care. *J Palliat Med.* 2006;9:751–772.

55. Moorey S, Greer S. *Cognitive behaviour therapy for people with cancer.* 2nd ed. New York: Oxford University Press; 2002.

56. Tatrow K, Montgomery GH. Cognitive behavioral techniques for distress and pain in breast cancer patients: a meta-analysis. *J Behav Med.* 2006; 29:17–27.

57. Massie MJ, Holland JC. Depression and the cancer patient. *J Clin Psychiatry.* 1990;51(Suppl):12–17. Discussion 18–9.

58. Spiegel D, Bloom JR, Yalom I. Group support for patients with metastatic cancer: a randomized outcome study. *Arch Gen Psychiatry.* 1981;38:527–533.

CHAPTER 44

Anxiety Disorders

Tomer T. Levin and Yesne Alici

INTRODUCTION

Anxiety is an unpleasant psychobiological emotion that forms part of the defensive structure. Mobilizing resources to reduce exposure to a perceived danger, it activates the primal fight, flight, freeze, and faint reaction. The cognitive appraisal, affective, behavioral, and physiological components of anxiety[1] are detailed in Table 44–1.

Anxiety, like pain and fever, is not of itself pathological, but rather a response to perceived threats. When adaptive, via accurate information processing, it motivates an individual to take steps to reduce or avoid the danger.

Anxiety is maladaptive when it is activated disproportionately, inappropriately, or independently of the actual danger. Maladaptive anxiety has a noxious intensity and chronicity that impairs functioning, wears out family and friends, and serves no end point, such as better problem solving. The danger sensor is conceptualized as having been set too sensitively, resulting in false alarms and needless anxiety.[1]

For example, an anxious patient who fears cancer recurrence may expend considerable effort on fruitless worry. Nonspecific physical sensations are cognitively amplified and misperceived as being a sign of cancer causing secondary worry and anxiety. A person who is overwhelmed by anxiety has a reduced sense of self-efficacy to problem-solve and therefore reduce the impact of potential threats. Avoidance lessens the chance of habituation to the perceived theat. The paradox is that hypervigilance is unlikely to produce better results than rational vigilance by empirically designed medical surveillance.

The term anxiety in this chapter is synonymous with the maladaptive variety. The following sections further explore anxiety subtypes and treatment issues.

PREVALENCE OF ANXIETY DISORDERS

The prevalence of cancer anxiety is in the 10%–30% range[2–7] but these data are limited by the use of varying instruments and criteria, small sample sizes, lack of prospective data, inclusion of anxiety due to a medical condition (e.g., steroid induced) within the anxiety category, heterogeneous cancer types, and cancer treatment confounders.

The prevalence of anxiety in cancer should be seen against the context of its ubiquity in the general population. It is usually higher in medical cohorts. For example, one study reported an 8% 12-month prevalence of generalized anxiety disorder (GAD) in primary care compared to 1.9%–5.1% in the general population.[8] Another epidemiological study showed that 12% of those with chronic medical problems had anxiety versus 6% of those without.[9]

Anxiety is commonly associated with other anxiety disorders.[10,11] It's covariance with depression is in the range of (0.45–0.75) in the general population[12] and 0.67–0.81 in cancer patients.[3,13–15]

Younger age, female sex, separated, divorced, widowed, and lower socio-economic status are associated with more anxiety in both general psychiatric populations and cancer cohorts.[3,16,17] Perhaps the reason for this is that with age comes experience and resilience and with improved socio-economic status come more resources to better cope with ill health.

Approaching death or worsening of the cancer is probably not associated with increased anxiety.[7,18]

The association between depression and suicide is well known. More recently, there has been an increasing awareness that anxiety is also a risk factor for suicide[19] and this likely applies to cancer patients too. The association is more likely to be complex rather than a direct anxiety-suicide relationship, largely because "anxiety" represents such a heterogeneous phenotype. For example, interactions between younger age, less social support, and specific anxiety subtypes (e.g., panic) might confer increased risk of suicidality.[16]

GENETIC AND ENVIRONMENTAL FACTORS INFLUENCING ANXIETY

Genetic factors are increasingly recognized as contributing to the risk for anxiety disorders. Studies in large cohorts of mono- and heterozygotic twins suggest that genetic influences on anxiety cluster around two groups, one shared by generalized anxiety, panic, and agoraphobia and the second by specific phobia.[20]

Moreover, genetic influences are dynamic rather than static over time. For example, a spider phobia may have more valence to a child as compared to a burly teenager.[21] This may offer a genetic hypothesis as to why anxiety in cancer patients decreases with age—older people are more likely to be able to modulate their environments in response to threats.

Childhood sexual abuse is associated with an increased risk for GAD and panic disorder (also major depression, substance abuse, and bulimia nervosa). This risk is doubled when the victim is subjected to sexual intercourse[22] highlighting the importance of considering sexual abuse when interviewing anxious cancer patients.

Thus, when considering how anxiety manifests in cancer patients, it is important to reflect on how genes and pre-illness environment interact with illness and treatment stressors.

SCREENING FOR ANXIETY

In psycho-oncology, anxiety can be assessed and diagnosed in three different ways:

1. **Single symptom assessment**: This categorical approach is common in busy practice where a clinician might ask, "Are you worried?" or observe nonverbal cues such as anxious facial expression. A variation on this is the distress thermometer, where patients are asked to rate their distress from 0 to 10.[23] The advantage of this approach is simplicity and lack of medical confounders such as fatigue or insomnia. The disadvantage of a single-item approach is a lack of reliability.
2. **Multiple symptom assessment**: Examples include screening measures such as the anxiety subscale of the Hospital Anxiety and Depression Questionnaire,[24] the State Trait Anxiety Inventory[25] and the anxiety subscale of the Brief Symptom Inventory.[26] More recently, the GAD-7 has shown proven utility in medical populations and has the advantage of matching DMS-IV criteria, with the exception of the time qualifier which is reduced to 2 weeks rather than 6 months.[27] The Primary Care Evaluation of Mental Disorders (PRIME MD) screens for panic disorder and somatization in medical populations.[28] Advantages of multisymptom measures are brevity, established reliability, and validity. All provide data on anxiety as a continuous variable with the exception of the GAD-7 that also has a categorical scoring system, reflecting anxiety severity thresholds.
3. **Clinical syndrome**: This describes a constellation of symptoms for example, GAD, panic disorder, social phobia disorder which comply to a classification system such as the *Diagnostic and statistical manual*

Table 44–1. Elements of the anxiety phenotype

Element	Manifestation
Cognitive	Evaluates the urgency of the threat and the people coping resources of dealing with the danger, focuses on threat to the exclusion of extraneous detail (tunnel vision)
Affective	Emotions such as nervous, edgy, scared, alarmed, terrified, worried
Behavioral	Avoidance, flight, fight, immobility, unable to speak
Physiological	Cardiovascular: palpitations, hypertension, faintness/fainting
	Respiratory: tachypnea, shortness of breath, shallow breathing, chest pain, choking, lump in throat
	Neuromuscular: startle reflex, twitching muscles, tremor, rigidity, wobbliness, restless
	Gastrointestinal: abdominal discomfort (butterflies), loss of appetite, nausea, diarrhea, vomiting
	Urinary: pressure and frequency
	Dermatological: flushed, pale, sweaty, itchy, hot, cold ashivers

Table 44–2. DSM-IV criteria for generalized anxiety disorder

A	Excessive anxiety and worry (apprehensive expectation), more days than not, ≥ 6 months
B	Difficulty controlling the worry
C	Associated with ≥ 3 of the following symptoms for more days than not:
	Restless, keyed-up, on edge
	Easily fatigued
	Difficulty concentrating my life will *never* be the same again, mind going blank
	Irritability
	Muscle tension
	Insomnia or unsatisfying, restless sleep
D	Other anxiety subtypes are excluded
E	Anxiety, worry, or physical symptoms cause clinically significant distress or impairment in social, occupational or other important areas of functioning
F	The following have been excluded: the physiological effects of a substance (drug, medication); a medical condition; and intercurrent mood, psychotic, or pervasive developmental disorder

SOURCE: Reproduced with permission from the American Psychiatric Association.

of mental disorders, 4th edition (DSM-IV).[29] This approach is clinically useful in aiding diagnosis and treatment. Disadvantages are all or nothing, categorical approach makes it difficult to measure change and that medical symptoms such as fatigue, insomnia, or somatic symptoms, such as muscle tension or pain, may act as confounders.[30] In research settings, a structured clinical interview is often used to identify eligibility criteria while continuous variables track symptom improvement. Clinical syndromes are discussed below.

ANXIETY SUBTYPES

GAD. Generalized anxiety disorder criteria are listed in Table 44–2. In psycho-oncology settings, the 6-month duration of symptoms is not tenable and a sensible clinical modification is a 2 week symptom duration.[27] This practical consideration does not detract from the fact that most GAD patients will have suffered from generalized anxiety, on and off, for many years previously. The average duration of symptoms before diagnosis is 5–10 years[31]; a careful past history is necessary as GAD rarely reaches psychiatric attention. In addition to chronicity, GAD sufferers have well documented impairment: they are greater users of primary and specialist medical care, have greater social impairment, less work productivity, and more absenteeism.[8] Another unsuitable DSM-IV criterion is an intercurrent mood disorder disqualifying the diagnosis of GAD because of the high frequency of covariance with mood disorders in the cancer setting, as discussed previously.

The cancer setting may uniquely color anxiety in GAD. Patients may worry about prognosis, uncertainty, or recurrence (described metaphorically as the sword of Damocles suspended above the patient's head), treatments, role changes, loss of income and status, transportation, and dependency.[32] "Markeritis," a tongue in cheek term, describes excessive worry about elevated cancer markers such as prostate-specific antigen (PSA) or carcinoembryonic antigen (CEA). Anxious patients may read more into fluctuations of these cancer markers than their physicians.

The power of positive thinking is a catch phrase of our times but it may also inadvertently feed into the worry cycle via the "tyranny of positive thinking." Here patients are told that they must think positively, the implication being that thinking negatively will adversely influence the oncology outcome. Because it is impossible to maintain a perpetually cheerful persona, even in the best of times, but especially when seriously ill, patients worry when pessimistic thoughts, quite understandably, cross their minds. Therefore, telling a cancer patient "not to think" negative is similar to saying, "don't think of a white elephant"—quite impossible.

If worry is an apprehensive expectation, meta-worry is worry about being worried. The conundrum is that worrying is seen as, both, useful

and uncontrollable and dangerous,[33] and in particular that excessive worry will worsen cancer outcomes.

Worry, in proportion, may have positive effects if it can motivate a person to change certain behaviors or minimize risk. For example, worry is associated with increased breast cancer screening via both self-examination and mammography (r = 0.12).[34]

Anxiety is moderated by a person's sense of self-efficacy or confidence in dealing with potential threats and this can be compromised by medical experiences. Loss of work or family roles, negative medical experiences such as misdiagnosis, physical weakness leading to a self-image of a weak or vulnerable person, can all erode confidence and increase anxiety.

Adjustment disorder with anxiety. The cardinal features of the adjustment disorder diagnostic category are a psychological response within 3 months of a stressor, clinically significant distress (in excess of what might be expected) or social impairment, the exclusion of other axis I or II diagnoses and bereavement. It should resolve within 6 months of termination of the stressful trigger. Subtypes are marked by either predominant anxiety or mixed anxiety and depressed mood. If symptoms last for less than 6 months, it is classified as acute; more than 6 months is considered chronic.[29]

Clinically, the symptoms of an adjustment disorder with anxiety are similar to generalized anxiety, with the caveat that, without the stressor, the patient would presumably not have anxiety or worry symptoms.

The advantages of this classification are that it is nonpejorative, semantically empathic, and conveys an expectation of recovery, rather than chronicity. One disadvantage is that it is hard to predict who will recover and who will have chronic symptoms. Secondly, in most cancer patients, even when cured or in remission, the cancer remains a long-term stressor with multilevel effects on the patient, family, employment, and finances. Therefore, it is somewhat simplistic to view the stressor as an on-off button. Thirdly, it invites the argument that excessive anxiety is to be expected in a cancer setting, raising doubts about the anxiety anchor qualifying the adjustment. Finally, there is a possibility that patients classified here may not be offered a trial of an evidence-based pharmacotherapy or psychotherapy. The DSM-IV does not actually classify adjustment disorders with anxiety under anxiety disorders, but rather, idiosyncratically, in a class of their own. Therefore, there is a real risk of minimizing the severity of the anxiety with this diagnostic classification.

Panic disorder with or without agoraphobia. The DSM describes panic attacks as discreet episodes of intense apprehension, fear, terror, or a sense of impending doom that peaks within 10 minutes, associated with physical symptoms such as chest pain, shortness of breath, choking, or smothering sensations and a fear of going crazy or losing control. Panic can be situational or out of the blue. Agoraphobia is anxiety about being in a place where escape might be difficult or embarrassing. When panic attacks become recurrent and unexpected, with persistent worry about additional attacks or worry about its implications (going crazy, heart attack) or there is a significant change in behavior because of the attacks, the threshold for panic disorder has been reached. Physiological and other psychiatric diagnoses are exclusion criteria.[29]

Panic in cancer patients may occur de novo or reflect an exacerbation of preexisting panic disorder. It may be underdiagnosed; one cancer center reported a fifth of referrals to its psycho-oncology service with panic symptoms.[35] Cognitively, panic is conceptualized as the misinterpretation of bodily symptoms, for example, a head and neck cancer patient who misinterprets postsurgery pain and discomfort catastrophically.[36] Not infrequently, panic disorder presents as a patient who has the urgent desire to leave the hospital against medical advice or suddenly refuses chemotherapy.[35]

Social anxiety disorder. This is characterized by a marked and persistent fear that social scrutiny will be humiliating or embarrassing. This provokes severe anxiety or a behavioral reaction such as avoidance or freezing that is recognized as being unreasonable or disproportionate. Anticipatory anxiety interferes with social and academic functioning. Since the disorder is largely a chronic condition that starts in teenage years, these patients are often underachievers in life.[29]

The cancer journeys of such painfully shy and inhibited patients are uncomfortable. They have difficulty negotiating the medical bureaucracy or advocating for themselves because, cognitively, their biggest fear is being the center of attention. Scars; radiations burns; or disfiguring surgery, such as radical neck dissection or mastectomy, can exacerbate social anxiety. Obtaining a second option may be an anxiety wrought experience, which is often avoided, to the patient's ultimate detriment. There is little psycho-oncology data on this subpopulation.

Specific phobia. Although these are common, seen in 3.5% of the general population,[37] they rarely come to the attention of psycho-oncologists. Blood-injection-injury phobias may result in fainting during medical procedures or perhaps, more importantly, avoidance of injections, blood tests, or dental care. Claustrophobia is very common in the setting of imaging (e.g., closed magnetic resonance imaging [MRI] scans) and head and neck radiation therapy. Self-injection is increasingly common; patients who have difficulty learning to self-inject may have a blood-injection-injury phobia.

Anticipatory anxiety and nausea. Anticipatory anxiety and nausea are classically conditioned responses (also called respondent or Pavlovian conditioning) to nausea induced by cancer treatment such as chemotherapy or radiation. The anxiety and nausea are generalized beyond the cancer treatment so that, for instance, all food cues result in anxiety and nausea. Subsequently, avoidance of food occurs. Preexisting trait anxiety, younger age, susceptibility to motion sickness, greater anxiety during treatment, more emetic chemotherapy, abnormal taste sensations during infusions, all predispose to anticipatory nausea and anxiety.[38]

Anxiety due to a general medical condition. Anxiety disorder due to a general medical condition is where symptoms are a direct physiological consequence of an underlying medical process. There is a temporal association between the onset and course of the medical condition and anxiety symptoms. Delirium is an exclusion criteria.[29]

This definition is not without limitations. The temporal association may be misleading because psychiatric symptoms may antedate the clinical recognition of the medical illness. Correction of the medical illness may also not result in elimination of anxiety.[39]

Anxiety in cancer is associated with a broad array of medical conditions (Table 44–3). Of note is the importance of processes associated with shortness of breath or tachypnea causing anxiety symptoms. Anxiety,

Table 44-3. Medical conditions and medications associated with anxiety

Metabolic	Hyperkalemia, porphyria, hypo- and hypercalcemia, hyperthermia, hypoglycemia, hyponatremia, vitamin deficiencies, hypovolemia, sepsis
Neurological Conditions	Pain, increased intracranial pressure, central nervous system neoplasms, postconcussion syndrome, seizure disorder, vertigo
Endocrine	Adrenal abnormalities, hyper-/hypothyroidism, parathyroid abnormalities, pituitary abnormalities, pheochromocytoma, carcinoid syndrome
Cardiovascular	Arrhythmia, congestive heart failure, coronary artery disease, anemia, valvular disease, cardiomyopathy
Pulmonary	Hypoxia, pulmonary embolism, asthma, chronic obstructive pulmonary disease, pneumothorax, pulmonary edema
Medications/toxic conditions	Corticosteroids, bronchodilators, antipsychotics, thyroid preparations, theophylline, sympathomimetic agents, levodopa, serotonergic agents, psychostimulants, antibiotics (cephalosporins, acyclovir, isoniazid), interferon, caffeine, cocaine, marijuana, withdrawal states (alcohol, opioid analgesics, benzodiazepines, caffeine)

conversely, may also worsen preexisting respiratory distress. Central nervous system tumors may also present with anxiety but often the psychiatric symptoms are not classical.[40,41] Symptom type is not indicative of localization[42,43] although there are reports of panic being associated with temporo-limbic lesions.[44] One study found that both state and trait anxiety did not worsen after brain surgery but trait anxiety was predictive of an increased risk of developing depression after surgery.[45]

Unrelieved pain is a common cause of anxiety in cancer patients.[46,47] Among cancer patients with a psychiatric diagnosis, 39% reported significant pain compared to 19% of those without a psychiatric diagnosis.[48] In a study among hospitalized cancer patients, the prevalence of pain was 96% for patients with anxiety as opposed to 80% for patients without anxiety.[49] Patients in severe pain appear diaphoretic, restless, and anxious. Anxiety assessment can only be completed after adequate pain relief. Anxiety often resolves after pain is treated.

Substance-induced anxiety disorder. Substance-induced anxiety is a direct physiological effect of a drug, medication, or toxin.[29] An extensive number of medications have been associated with anxiety.[50] Bronchodilators raise the pulse rate, compounding the anxiety caused by air hunger. Antiinflammatory cytokines such as interferons can cause anxiety and panic, perhaps via serotonergic and dopaminergic pathways,[51] although they may cause fewer psychiatric side effects than previously thought.[52,53] Psychiatric adverse effects of corticosteroids are common and include anxiety, emotional lability, insomnia, agitation, and restlessness.[54] Thyroxine, psychostimulants, sympathomimetic agents, serotonergic agents, anticholinergics, immunosuppressants, antihistamines, and certain antibiotics may produce symptoms of anxiety.

Akathisia, or motor restlessness, often misdiagnosed as anxiety, is commonly caused by antiemetics, prochlorperazine and metoclopramide.[55]

Anxiety due to substance withdrawal (alcohol, benzodiazepines, barbiturates, opioids) is common in the medical setting but often unrecognized. Abuse patterns are frequently underreported. Withdrawal may present with sudden, intense anxiety and agitation. Many patients stop smoking abruptly on receiving their diagnosis and may experience severe anxiety symptoms, sometimes associated with dissociative symptoms and bizarre behaviors.[56]

Acute and posttraumatic stress disorder (PTSD) are also classified as anxiety disorders and can occur in 3%–5% of cancer patient due to the arduous nature of the illness and treatment. These are discussed in Chapter 48.

ASSESSMENT AND DIFFERENTIAL DIAGNOSIS

At the heart of effective psycho-oncology treatment is an accurate evaluation. Any care pathway must be preceded by an evaluation by a competent psycho-oncology professional[57] and appropriate screening.[58]

Assessment of anxiety in cancer patients requires a comprehensive biopsychosocial evaluation. Consideration of the impact of biological factors on the anxiety phenotype is vital. A thorough medical history and physical examination should consider vital signs, cardiovascular, neurological, gastrointestinal, and respiratory systems. Diagnostic tests may include laboratory examination (such as electrolytes, thyroid function tests, liver function tests, albumin, blood urea nitrogen, creatinine), electrocardiogram, brain imaging studies to exclude structural CNS lesions, electroencephalogram when seizure activity is suspected and cerebrospinal fluid analysis (if CNS infection, subarachnoid hemorrhage, or leptomeningeal disease are suspected). Rating scales are also considered to be an integral part of the assessment process.[39]

An accurate multiaxial biopsychosocial formulation of the anxiety will enable the clinician to define potential treatment goals. These should be negotiated collaboratively with the patient and should have measurable outcomes. Here are some examples of treatment goals some of which are general and others uniquely tailored:

- A 50% reduction in the baseline GAD-7 score
- A 50% reduction in the fear of cancer recurrence as measured on a physician assessed Likert scale or a clinical global impression (CGI) scale
- Return to work
- Successful completion of the radiotherapy in a patient with treatment claustrophobia
- Reduction in the frequency of panic attacks.
- Resuming social activities (e.g., singing in the choir)

Where anxiety symptoms represent an exacerbation of a preexisting anxiety disorder, treatment of the underlying primary disorder may be the most expedient approach. Patients with comorbid psychiatric disorders may frequently experience anxiety and prioritizing the treatment of potential target symptoms is appropriate. For example, anxiety symptoms secondary to delirium mandate the treatment of the underlying delirium. In other instances where anxiety is the consequence of a medical condition, its treatment or substance induced, these underlying conditions should be corrected, if possible.

ANXIETY TREATMENTS

Evidence-based medicine suggests that effective treatments should be used ahead of treatments that have not been shown to be efficacious. One author suggests that psychosocial care that is ineffective is worse than no care at all,[30] highlighting the importance of trying to measure the impact of psycho-oncology care and skills on recipients, rather than relying on good intentions alone.

The following sections focus primarily on evidence-based treatments, where this data is available, for these have the largest probability of reproducible efficacy. Data supported by a systematic review of relevant randomized controlled trials (RCTs) is best but at least one well-designed RCT may be adequate.

Psychotherapy treatments

Psychoeducation. Psychoeducation interventions typically provide information which may be verbal, written, visual, or a combination such as an orientation to an oncology clinic. Acquisition of new knowledge is essential to help patients navigate the medical system and the treatment process as unfamiliarity increases anxiety and uncertainty. For example, one RCT which involved an orientation tour of the clinic, written

resources for coping (e.g., support groups) and a question and answer meeting with a counselor-reduced anxiety significantly at follow-up.[59] Devine's meta-analysis of 116 psychoeducational studies[60] reported a moderate effect size (ES) (d = .56, [95% CI = .42–.70) although another failed to show an effect.[61] A related concept is that of patient navigators, a barrier-focused intervention that helps patients complete a discrete episode of cancer-related care.[62] Anxiety has not yet been examined as an outcome for patient navigation but it contains elements that overlap with that of psychoeducation.

Cognitive therapy. Cognitive therapy is based on the principle that it is not a situation that results in an emotion but rather the preceding automatic thought.[63] A person's perception of a situation leads to the emotional or behavioral response. For example, one person undergoing a computed tomography (CT) scan may think, "I know that the pain is cancer," and feel anxious. Another may think, "I am glad that I will finally have an explanation for the pain," and feel relief.

Typical maladaptive cancer-related cognitions often associated with anxiety are listed in Table 44–4. These thoughts are characterized by an absolute quality and reflect cognitive thinking biases such as "all or nothing" thinking, overgeneralization, personalization, and "what if…" thinking. Therapy focuses on promoting self-regulation with more reasonable, realistic cognitions, and "de-catastrophizing."[1] Cognitive therapy uses behavioral techniques set up as empirical experiments. For example, anxiety levels are measured on a Likert scale before a diaphragmatic breathing exercise and then again afterward. This demonstrates the technique's efficacy and proves that control of anxiety is possible.

Regarding the efficacy of cognitive therapy for anxiety in cancer patients, Sheard reported a small ES of 0.42 [95% CI = .08–.74]. When a more robust subset of studies was examined and outliers removed, similar results were achieved (ES .39 [95% CI = .09%–.63%]). One limitation of these data is the inclusion of preventative studies, that is, subjects who are not necessarily anxious at baseline. The ES for anxiety reduction in cancer survivors in another meta-analysis was 1.99 [95% CI = 0.69–3.31].[61] A meta-analysis in advanced cancer patients did not support the efficacy of cognitive therapy in this challenging subpopulation.[64] In non-medical populations, data supporting the efficacy of cognitive therapy is

Table 44–4. Maladaptive cancer cognitions that are associated with anxiety

Cancer cognition	Consequence
I will die in my sleep	Insomnia, nocturnal anxiety, hypervigilance
Chemotherapy is like a poisonous chemical	Overgeneralization of *all* chemotherapy as toxic, minimization of the role for symptom management. May abandon treatment if perceived disadvantages are seen to outweigh advantages
Cancer rules my life; It's *all* luck	Underestimation of self-efficacy and over-estimation of cancer threat; "all or nothing" thinking. Anxiety increased
It's not fair!	Randomness of life and cancer are personalized
I *must* think positively!	The "tyranny of positive thinking" results in anxiety when invariably a realistic or pessimistic thought crosses the cancer patient's mind
What if the cancer *has* spread?	Worry and checking about potential signs of recurrence accompany "what if…" thinking.
Cancer *is* a death sentence	The term cancer is overgeneralized. In fact cancer is a heterogeneous, nonspecific term; 64% of cancer patients become survivors. This cognition often leads to paralysis and avoidance of problem solving

more robust and large ES's are reported for GAD, panic disorder with or without agoraphobia and social phobia.[65]

Problem-Solving therapy. Nezu developed this variant of cognitive therapy based on the hypothesis that the more efficient people are in solving or coping with their problems, the less distressed they will be. The standardized 90 minutes × 10 sessions program teaches patients to define the problem, brainstorm possible options, evaluate potential solutions, implement solutions, monitor their degree of success, and make adjustments to the solutions. The patient's significant other can also be incorporated as a coach, which is logical as most people solve problems collaboratively, especially in cancer care. A person's problem-solving attitudes are examined. For example, a person may erroneously believe that *all* of his problems are due to the cancer (the cancer is probably not to blame for every problem that he has), or that *only he* has trouble coping with cancer (every cancer patient has some difficulty coping), or that *no-one* can help (many patients are helped).[66] Problem solving was effective in reducing distress as measured by the Brief Symptom Inventory in a RCT although the specific anxiety subscale was not reported.[67]

Behavioral interventions: Distraction, systematic desensitization, hypnosis, relaxation training. Behavioral interventions are amongst the most widely used psychosocial services offered to cancer patients.[68] They constitute an array of interventions based on the theoretical foundation of Skinner, Pavlov, and Thorndike. These are particularly useful for managing the "here and now" distress associated with cancer treatment side effects. Four out of five RCT's of multimodal behavioral interventions summarized by Redd et al. showed a reduction in anxiety.[69] Luebbert estimated the ES for relaxation training as small, d = .45 [95% CI = .23–.67].[70] Behavioral interventions are additionally efficacious for anticipatory nausea.[38,69] The central behavioral techniques that are useful in reducing anxiety are summarized below:

Distraction. Attention is diverted away from the distressing stimulus, for example, wiggling toes during venipuncture, guided imagery, storytelling, and video games.[38]

Systematic desensitization. This involves gradual reexposure to a feared stimulus. It can be imaginal where relaxation is combined with gradual visualization of cues associated with the trigger or in vivo where the patient is gradually exposed to the actual stimulus in the context of relaxation or cognitive techniques. The end point is habituation to the feared stimulus so that the aversive reaction is contained. An example of this is an aversive reaction to eating after chemotherapy induced vomiting. The therapist does not have to be present during chemotherapy for this technique to be effective.[38]

Hypnosis. This is a behavioral technique where via relaxation techniques the patient learns to focus attention on thoughts and feelings unrelated to the source of distress, at which point the clinician can introduce suggestions, for example, for calm and wellbeing, and therefore anxiety can be reduced.

Relaxation training. A deep state of relaxation is induced by one or more of the following: progressive muscle relaxation, systematic tensing and releasing of muscle groups, deep breathing, narrative suggestion (audio-recorded or actual instructions from the therapist). Slowing down breathing is a key ingredient in relaxation training. This may come about indirectly through muscle relaxation or a meditative state. Slow breathing may be deliberately taught by techniques such as counting to seven on each inspiration and expiration or via diaphragmatic breathing where the patient places one hand on the anterior abdominal wall and learns to see it rise with each inspiration, rather than the panting, intercostal breathing seen in high anxiety states.

Some precautions should be noted. Relaxation type exercises may potentially make anxiety worse in people who have been traumatized or sexually abused for whom relaxation and letting down one's guard is perceived to be dangerous. Additionally, mastering behavioral techniques requires motivation and practice. If the groundwork is inadequate or the therapist's skills lacking, a failed behavioral exercise can leave a vulnerable patient with an even lower sense of self-esteem.

Behavioral interventions can also be self-administered, such as Jacobsen's stress management training for patients undergoing chemotherapy that uses print and audiovisual media to instruct patients in paced abdominal breathing, progressive muscle relaxation with guided imagery and coping-self statements, that are given to patients by a clinician in a 10 single minute encounter.[71]

Music therapy. Music therapy acts via multimodal pathways: behavioral activation, relaxation, regulation of breathing, distraction, cognitive and meaning-related pathways, and emotional expression. It can even be used in very ill patients, a territory that is more difficult to navigate with traditional psychotherapies.[72,73] There is preliminary evidence from several RCT's of its effectiveness in reducing short-term anxiety and distress.[73–75] One meta-analysis found a small ES (r = .34 [95% CI = −.06–.64], p=.09) for anxiety based on four studies which was not statistically significant.[76]

Support groups. Cancer support groups have a high degree of user satisfaction but heterogeneity in methodologies make it hard to compare their effects on anxiety.[77] More recently, online support groups such the Wellness Community (http://www.thewellnesscommunity.org/) have gained in popularity and represent an important future direction. Supportive-expressive group therapy may not be useful for anxiety symptoms in metastatic breast cancer patients, according to one study although they may be quite helpful for other symptoms such as depression or helplessness/hopelessness.[78,79]

Combination cognitive therapy and psychopharmacology. Psychopharmacology has been most widely studied in combination with cognitive-behavioral therapy. In meta-analyses, conducted on non-oncology patients, pharmacotherapy for anxiety is thought to work faster than psychotherapy but longer-term outcomes are more robust for psychotherapy.[80,81] Although combined cognitive and pharmacotherapy does not have a clear advantage in meta-analyses, these data are still considered to be early and not without controversy.[80,81] Side-effects of medications are a concern in combination therapy but, compared to medication alone, combined therapy patients suffer from fewer perceived side-effects of medications compared to those who receive the drug without psychotherapy.[82]

Whether benzodiazepines should be discontinued when a patient is being treated with cognitive therapy for panic disorder is a matter of controversy. Benzodiazepines may reinforce anxious avoidance because patients never learn to habituate to noxious levels of anxiety. On the other hand, there is, evidence that medications such as D-cycloserine, which facilitates glutaminergic transmission, may help extinguish the symptoms.[81] By extrapolation, therefore, similar antianxiety medications might help patients suffering from panic symptoms to break the anxious-avoidance vicious circle.

There are no comparable psycho-oncology data, however, in practice, combination therapy is common.[46,56,83] Psycho-oncology, due to the urgency of its context, also favors treatments that work faster; rapid symptom relief may facilitate more timely and definitive cancer treatment.

Psychopharmacological treatments

Benzodiazepines. Benzodiazepines are the most frequently used agents for anxiety and often considered the drugs of choice for anxiety in the terminally ill.[46,84–86] They can be administered in a variety of ways, which is an important consideration in medically settings where oral intake may be compromised (e.g., lorazepam: orally, intramuscularly; clonazepam: orally, orally disintegrating tablet). Longer-acting benzodiazepines, such as clonazepam or extended release alprazolam, may provide more persistent relief of anxiety symptoms.[83]

There are a few controlled trials of benzodiazepines for anxious cancer patients. For instance, one randomized trial of alprazolam versus progressive muscle relaxation found that both treatments resulted in a significant reduction in anxiety symptoms but alprazolam's effect was faster.[87]

The American College of Clinical Care Medicine and the Society of Critical Care Medicine guidelines for the management of anxiety in critically ill adult patients recommend use of lorazepam for prolonged (i.e., more than 24 hours) treatment of anxiety in critically ill patients.[88] Although a recent Cochrane review of pharmacotherapy for anxiety in palliative care concluded that there is lack of high level evidence on the role of antianxiety medications for reduction of anxiety in terminally ill patients,[86] they are widely used in this population.

Benzodiazepines are useful for anxiety, insomnia, nausea, vomiting, and panic attacks. Both lorazepam and alprazolam have been shown to reduce postchemotherapy nausea and vomiting, as well as anticipatory nausea and vomiting.[89,90] It is hypothesized that given before chemotherapy or a procedure, benzodiazepines may reduce conditioned aversion responses due to their amnesic properties.[46,89]

Sedation, drowsiness, and ataxia, the commonest side effects of benzodiazepines, increase falls risk in elderly patients. Memory difficulty, sexual dysfunction, and incontinence are encountered less frequently. Benzodiazepines predispose to delirium, especially in the elderly patients and in those with advanced disease. Impaired hepatic function and drugs that compete for liver enzymes that metabolize benzodiazepines (e.g., erythromycin, estrogen, isoniazid), may necessitate lower doses of benzodiazepines to minimize side effects. Lorazepam, oxazepam, and temazepam are preferred when hepatic function is impaired because they are metabolized by conjugation with glucuronic acid and have no active metabolites.[46,47]

Benzodiazepines have a dose-related effect on the respiratory center, however when their use is carefully monitored, they may reduce anxiety and improve the respiratory function amongst patients with anxiety due to dyspnea.[46]

Buspirone. Buspirone, a nonbenzodiazepine anxiolytic, lacks the sedative and cognitive side effects of benzodiazepines and may be considered in patients with high potential for benzodiazepine abuse. It is usually used for GAD. It cannot be used on an as needed basis, and its effects are not apparent for 1–2 weeks, often up to 4 weeks.[83]

Antipsychotics. Low-dose antipsychotics, such as haloperidol, olanzapine, risperidone, and quetiapine are commonly used to relieve anxiety symptoms among cancer patients, especially those who are both anxious and confused or at risk for delirium.[46,91] Antipsychotic medications are not, however, Food and Drug Administration (FDA) approved for the treatment of anxiety disorders. A few RCTs have investigated the role of atypical antipsychotics in as adjunctive treatment for anxiety disorders because of their broad neurochemical effects on postsynaptic 5-HT 2 receptors and the modulation of 5-HT1A.[92]

Clinicians should be familiar with several side effects and warnings associated with use of antipsychotic medications (e.g., extrapyramidal side effects, FDA warnings for increased risk of mortality and cerebrovascular disease in the elderly[93]). Olanzapine and risperidone have been suggested in the management of anxiety in patients with dementia and in patients with cancer-related pain, however, none of the antipsychotics have been systematically studied as treatment for anxiety among cancer patients.

Selective serotonin-reuptake inhibitors and serotonin-norepinephrine reuptake inhibitors. Selective serotonin-reuptake inhibitors (SSRIs), and serotonin-norepinephrine reuptake inhibitors (SNRIs) are considered first-line medications for the treatment of GAD, panic disorder, social anxiety disorder, and PTSD.[94–96] Blood pressure monitoring is recommended with the use of SNRIs especially with initiation of therapy and dose increases. SSRIs and SNRIs may alter the metabolism of drugs through inhibition of cytochrome P450 liver enzymes.[47,97] Initial worsening of anxiety or akathisia may occur with SSRIs. Gastrointestinal distress and nausea are transient side effects and

administration with food or a lower starting dose followed by gradual dose titration may help minimize these side effects.[56] As antidepressants may take 2–6 weeks to relieve anxiety, concomitant use of benzodiazepines initially may be helpful.[50]

Although older antidepressants such as tricyclic antidepressants (TCAs) and monoamine oxidase inhibitors (MAOIs) have been shown to be effective for anxiety disorders, SSRIs are commonly prescribed because of their favorable side-effect profile.[92] TCAs may potentially cause orthostatic hypotension, anticholinergic side effects, quinidine-like effects and are dangerous in overdose and MAOIs require a tyramine-free diet.[46]

Mirtazapine. Mirtazapine, an α-adrenoceptor antagonist and an antagonist at serotonin 5HT2A, 5HT2C, and 5HT3 receptors, is commonly used for anxiety in cancer patients with insomnia and anorexia as it is sedating and, in some patients, associated with weight gain.[47,56] It has no sexual side effects and has not been associated with serotonin syndrome.

Antihistamines. Antihistaminergic agents may be considered in anxious patients with severely compromised pulmonary function.[83] Antihistamines do not have anxiolytic properties; their sedative effects most likely result in a sense of anxiety relief.[98] The anticholinergic effects of these medications must be monitored carefully in patients at risk for delirium.[83]

Anticonvulsants. There is emerging evidence from RCTs for pregabalin in GAD and social anxiety disorder.[99,100] It is also FDA approved for partial seizures, diabetic peripheral neuropathy, postherpetic neuralgia and fibromyalgia. Pregabalin is an anticonvulsant that binds to the $\alpha 2\delta$ subunit of voltage-gated calcium channels, which reduces neurotransmitter release. The most common side effects are somnolence, dizziness, and weight gain. Pregabalin appears to be well tolerated in the elderly.[101] Evidence for the anticonvulsant tiagabine, a gamma-aminobutyric acid reuptake inhibitor, in GAD is limited.[92] Gabapentin, which is approved by the FDA for partial seizures, neuropathic pain, and postherpetic neuralgia, has been used "off-label" in anxiety disorders, although RCT data have shown only a modest benefit.[92] Evidence for use of other anticonvulsants in the treatment of anxiety disorders is lacking.

CONCLUSION

One challenge for psycho-oncology is detection of anxiety across the spectrum of cancer patients. This is difficult because of the variability in the anxiety phenotype—every anxious patient looks different. Furthermore, the detection of anxiety invariably must occur at a time of crisis when medical priorities are often seen to trump psychological. For these reasons screening and thorough evaluation by appropriately trained psycho-oncology professionals is essential.

Another challenge for psycho-oncology is delivering efficacious treatments for anxiety. Treatment should be evidence based and where this is not available, should be based on best practices. It should be tailored to the patient's and family's needs rather than assuming that one solution will fit all. Treatment of anxiety should take into account co-morbidity such as intercurrent depression, alcohol or nicotine dependence. It should also consider the risk of certain anxiety treatments triggering delirium symptoms. Treatment of anxiety should also be timely—the burden of anxiety can significantly add to the difficulties of negotiating cancer treatment, survivorship, or palliative care. Finally, anxiety needs to be considered from a systems perspective that spans the cancer trajectory from diagnosis, to treatment, to survivorship, and to palliative care. The diagnosis of anxiety should not come as a surprise. A considerable percentage of cancer patients will predictably have supra-threshold levels of anxiety and their needs should be anticipated.

Because anxiety is part of the defensive structure of all human beings, it cannot be eliminated entirely. The aim of treatment is to reduce its noxious intensity that serves no useful endpoint while capitalizing on the utility of mild anxiety to motivate more effective problem solving. Better managing anxiety symptoms and improving function is often a liberating process for the patient. For the psycho-oncologist, treating anxiety is often rewarding because of the dramatic, palpable, and sustained benefits to the patient.

REFERENCES

1. Beck AT, Emery G. *Anxiety disorders and phobias: A cognitive perspective.* New York: Basic Books; 1985.

2. Roy-Byrne PP, Davidson KW, Kessler RC, et al. Anxiety disorders and comorbid medical illness. *Gen Hosp Psychiatry.* 2008;30(3):208–225.

3. BrintzenhofeSzoc K, Levin TT, Li Y, Kissane DW, Zabora J. Mixed anxiety/depression symptoms in a large cancer cohort: prevalence by cancer type. *Psychosomatics.* 2009;50:383–391.

4. Watson M, Greer S, Rowden L, et al. Relationships between emotional control, adjustment to cancer and depression and anxiety in breast cancer patients. *Psychiatr Med.* 1991;21(1):51–57.

5. Carroll B, Kathol R, Noyes RJ, Wald TG, Clamon GH. Screening for depression and anxiety in cancer patients using the Hospital Anxiety and Depression Scale. *Gen Hosp Psychiatry.* 1993;15(2):69–74.

6. Roth A, Nelson CJ, Rosenfeld B, et al. Assessing anxiety in men with prostate cancer: further data on the reliability and validity of the Memorial Anxiety Scale for Prostate Cancer (MAX-PC). *Psychosomatics.* 2006;47(4):340–347.

7. Kissane DW, Grabsch B, Love A, Clarke DM, Bloch S, Smith GC. Psychiatric disorder in women with early stage and advanced breast cancer: a comparative analysis. *Aust N Z J Psychiatry.* 2004;38(5):320–326.

8. Wittchen H-U. Generalized anxiety disorder: prevalence, burden, and cost to society. *Depress Anxiety.* 2002;16(4):162–171.

9. Wells KB, Golding JM, Burnam MA. Chronic medical conditions in a sample of the general population with anxiety, affective, and substance use disorders. *Am J Psychiatry.* 1989;146(11):1440–1446.

10. Lenze EJ, Mulsant BH, Shear MK, et al. Comorbid anxiety disorders in depressed elderly patients. *Am J Psychiatry.* 2000;157(5):722–728.

11. Rush AJ, Zimmerman M, Wisniewski SR, et al. Comorbid psychiatric disorders in depressed outpatients: demographic and clinical features. *J Affect Disord.* 2005;87(1):43–55.

12. Clark LA, Watson D. Tripartite model of anxiety and depression: psychometric evidence and taxonometric implications. *J Abnorm Psychol.* 1991;100(3):316–336.

13. Cassileth B, Lusk E, Hutter R, Strouse TB, Brown LL. Concordance of depression and anxiety in patients with cancer. *Psychol Rep.* 1984;54(2):588–590.

14. Wilson KG, Chochinov HM, Skirko MG, et al. Depression and anxiety disorders in palliative cancer care. *J Pain Symptom Manage.* 2007;33(2):118–129.

15. Teunissen SC, de Graeff A, Voest EE, de Haes JC. Are anxiety and depressed mood related to physical symptom burden? A study in hospitalized advanced cancer patients. *Palliat Med.* 2007;21(4):341–346.

16. Rasic DT, Belik S-L, Bolton JM, Chochinov, HM, Sareen, J. Cancer, mental disorders, suicidal ideation and attempts in a large community sample. *Psychooncology.* 2008;17(7):660–667.

17. Grant B, Goldstein R, Chou S, et al. Sociodemographic and psychopathologic predictors of first incidence of DSM-IV substance use, mood and anxiety disorders: results from the Wave 2 National Epidemiologic Survey on Alcohol and Related Conditions. *Mol Psychiatry.* 2009 Nov;14(11)1051–1066.

18. Lichtenthal WG, Nilsson M, Zhang B, et al. Do rates of mental disorders and existential distress among advanced stage cancer patients increase as death approaches? *Psychooncology.* 2009 Jan;18(1):50–61.

19. Sareen J, Cox BJ, Afifi TO, et al. Anxiety disorders and risk for suicidal ideation and suicide attemps. *Arch Gen Psychiatry.* 2005;62:1249–1257.

20. Hettema JM, Prescott CA, Myers JM, Neale MC, Kendler KS. The structure of genetic and environmental risk factors for anxiety disorders in men and women. *Arch Gen Psychiatry.* 2005;62(2):182.

21. Kendler KS, Gardner CO, Annas P, Neale MC, Eaves LJ, Lichtenstein P. A longitudinal twin study of fears from middle childhood to early adulthood: evidence for a developmentally dynamic genome. *Arch Gen Psychiatry.* 2008;65(4):421–429.

22. Kendler KS, Bulik CM, Silberg J, Hettema JM, Myers J, Prescott CA. Childhood sexual abuse and adult psychiatric and substance use disorders in women: an epidemiological and cotwin control analysis. *Arch Gen Psychiatry.* 2000;57(10):953–959.

23. Roth AJ, Kornblith AB, Batel-Copel L, Peabody E, Scher HI, Holland JC. Rapid screening for psychologic distress in men with prostate carcinoma: a pilot study. *Cancer.* 1998;82(10):1904–1908.

24. Zigmond AS, Snaith RP. The hospital anxiety and depression scale. *Acta Psychiatr Scand.* 1983;67(6):361–370.

25. Speilberger CD. *Manual for the State-Trait Anxiety Inventory (Form Y).* Palo Alto: Consulting Psychologists Press; 1983.

26. Derogatis LR, Melisaratos N. The brief symptom inventory: an introductory report. *Psychiatr Med.* 1983;13(3):595–605.

27. Spitzer RL, Kroenke K, Williams JB, Williams JB, Löwe B. A brief measure for assessing generalized anxiety disorder: the GAD-7. *Arch Intern Med.* 2006;166(10):1092–1097.

28. Spitzer R, Kroenke K, Williams J. Validation and utility of a self-report version of PRIME-MD: the PHQ primary care study. Primary Care Evaluation of Mental Disorders. Patient Health Questionnaire. *JAMA.* 1999;282(18): 1737–1744.

29. *Diagnostic and statistical manual of mental disorders,* 4th ed, Text Revision. Washington DC: American Psychiatric Association; 2000.

30. Jacobsen PB, Jim HS. Psychosocial interventions for anxiety and depression in adult cancer patients: achievements and challenges. *CA.* 2008;58(4):214–230.

31. Kessler RC, Keller MB, Wittchen HU. The epidemiology of generalized anxiety disorder. *Psychiatr Clin North Am.* 2001;24(1):19–39.

32. Kornblith AB, Ligibel J. Psychosocial and sexual functioning of survivors of breast cancer. *Semin Oncol.* 2003;30(6):799–813.

33. Wells A. Preliminary tests of a cognitive model of generalized anxiety disorder. *Behav Res Ther.* 1999;37(6):585–594.

34. Hay JL, McCaul KD, Magnan RE. Does worry about breast cancer predict screening behaviors? A meta-analysis of the prospective evidence. *Prev Med.* 2006;42(6):401–408.

35. Slaughter JR, Jain A, Holmes S, Reid JC, Bobo W, Sherrod NB. Panic disorder in hospitalized cancer patients. *Psychooncology.* 2000;9(3):253–258.

36. Shimizu K, Kinoshita H, Akechi T, Uchitomi Y, Andoh M. First panic attack episodes in head and neck cancer patients who have undergone radical neck surgery. *J Pain Symptom Manage.* 2007;34(6):575–578.

37. Bienvenu OJ, Eaton WW. The epidemiology of blood-injection-injury phobia. *Psychol Med.* 1998;28(5):1129–1136.

38. Jacobsen PB, Redd WH. The development and management of chemotherapy-related anticipatory nausea and vomiting. *Cancer Invest.* 1988;6(3):329–336.

39. Colon EA, Popkin MK. Anxiety and panic. In: Rundell JR, Wise MG (eds). *The American psychiatric press textbook of consultation-liaison psychiatry.* Washington, DC: American Psychiatric Press; 1996:402–425.

40. Moise D, Madhusoodanan S. Psychiatric symptoms associated with brain tumors: a clinical enigma. *CNS Spectr.* 2006;11(1):28–31.

41. Bunevicius A, Deltuva VP, Deltuviene D, Tamasauskas A, Bunevicius R. Brain lesions manifesting as psychiatric disorders: eight cases. *CNS Spectr.* 2008;13(11):950–958.

42. Binder RL. Neurologically silent brain tumors in psychiatric hospital admissions: three cases and a review. *J Clin Psychiatry.* 1983;44(3):94–97.

43. Madhusoodanan S, Danan D, Moise D. Psychiatric manifestations of brain tumors: diagnostic implications. *Expert Rev Neurother.* 2007;7(4):343–349.

44. Filley CM, Kleinschmidt-DeMasters BK. Neurobehavioral presentations of brain neoplasms. *West J Med.* 1995;163(1):19–25.

45. D'Angelo C, Mirijello A, Leggio L, et al. State and trait anxiety and depression in patients with primary brain tumors before and after surgery: 1-year longitudinal study. *J Neurosurg.* 2008;108(2):281–286.

46. Noyes R, Holt CS, Massie MJ. Anxiety disorders. In: Holland JC, Breitbart W (eds). *Psychooncology.* New York: Oxford University Press; 1998:548–563.

47. Valentine AD. Anxiety Disorders. In: Holland JC, Greenberg DB, Hughes MK (eds). *Quick reference for oncology clinicians: The psychiatric and psychological dimensions of cancer symptom management.* Charlottesville, VA: The International Psycho-Oncology Society Press; 2006:39–44.

48. Derogatis LR, Morrow GR, Fetting J, et al. The prevalence of psychiatric disorders among cancer patients. *JAMA.* 1983;249(6):751–757.

49. Teunissen SC, de Graeff A, Voest EE, de Haes JC. Are anxiety and depressed mood related to physical symptom burden? A study in hospitalized advanced cancer patients. *Palliat Med.* 2007;21(4):341–346.

50. Epstein SA, Hicks D. Anxiety Disorders. In: Levenson JL (ed). *American psychiatric publishing textbook of psychosomatic medicine.* Washington, DC: American Psychiatric Publishing; 2004:251–270.

51. Miller AH. Mechanisms of cytokine-induced behavioral changes: psychoneuroimmunology at the translational interface. *Brain Behav Immun.* 2009 Feb;23(2):149–158.

52. Bannink M, Kruit WHJ, Van Gool AR, et al. Interferon-alpha in oncology patients: fewer psychiatric side effects than anticipated. *Psychosomatics.* 2008;49(1):56–63.

53. Quarantini LC, Bressan RA, Galvão A, Batista-Neves S, Paraná R, Miranda-Scippa A. Incidence of psychiatric side effects during pegylated interferon-alpha retreatment in nonresponder hepatitis C virus-infected patients. *Liver Int.* 2007;27(8):1098–1102.

54. Stiefel FC, Breitbart WS, Holland JC. Corticosteroids in cancer: neuropsychiatric complications. *Cancer Invest.* 1989;7(5):479–491.

55. Fleishman SB, Lavin MR, Sattler M, Szarka H. Antiemetic-induced akathisia in cancer patients receiving chemotherapy. *Am J Psychiatry.* 1994;151(5): 763–765.

56. Lederberg M. Psycho-oncology. In: Sadock BJ, Sadock VA (eds). *Kaplan and Sadock's comprehensive textbook of psychiatry*. Philadelphia, PA: Lippincott Williams & Wilkins; 2004:2196–2225.

57. NCCN practice guidelines for the management of psychosocial distress. National Comprehensive Cancer Network. *Oncology*. 1999;13(5A):113–147.

58. Holland JC, Reznik I. Pathways for psychosocial care of cancer survivors. *Cancer*. 2005;104(Suppl 11):2624–2637.

59. McQuellon RP, Wells M, Hoffman S, et al. Reducing distress in cancer patients with an orientation program. *Psychooncology*. 1998;7(3):207–217.

60. Devine EC, Westlake SK. The effects of psychoeducational care provided to adults with cancer: meta-analysis of 116 studies. *Oncol Nurs Forum*. 1995;22(9):1369–1381.

61. Osborn RL, Demoncada AC, Feuerstein M. Psychosocial interventions for depression, anxiety, and quality of life in cancer survivors: meta-analyses. *Int J Psychiatry Med*. 2006;36(1):13–34.

62. Wells KJ, Battaglia TA, Dudley DJ, et al. Patient navigation: state of the art or is it science? *Cancer*. 2008;113(8):1999–2010.

63. Beck AT, Rush AJ, Shaw BF, Emery, G. *Cognitive therapy of depression*. New York: Guilford Press; 1979.

64. Uitterhoeve RJ, Vernooy M, Litjens M, et al. Psychosocial interventions for patients with advanced cancer—a systematic review of the literature. *Br J Cancer*. 2004;91(6):1050–1062.

65. Butler AC, Chapman JE, Forman EM, Beck AT. The empirical status of cognitive-behavioral therapy: a review of meta-analyses. *Clin Psychol Rev*. 2006;26(1):17–31.

66. Nezu AM, Maguth Nezu C, Friedman SH, Faddis S, Houts PS. *Helping cancer patients cope. A problem solving approach*. Washington, DC: American Psychological Association; 1998.

67. Nezu AM, Nezu CM, Felgoise S, McClure KS, Houts PS. Project Genesis: assessing the efficacy of problem-solving therapy for distressed adult cancer patients. *J Consult Clin Psychol*. 2003;71(6):1036–1048.

68. Coluzzi PH, Grant M, Doroshow JH, Rhiner M, Ferrell B, Rivera L. Survey of the provision of supportive care services at National Cancer Institute-designated cancer centers. *J Clin Oncol*. 1995;13(3):756–764.

69. Redd WH, Montgomery GH, DuHamel KN. Behavioral intervention for cancer treatment side effects. *J Natl Cancer Inst*. 2001;93(11):810–823.

70. Luebbert K, Dahme B, Hasenbring M. The effectiveness of relaxation training in reducing treatment-related symptoms and improving emotional adjustment in acute non-surgical cancer treatment: a meta-analytical review. *Psychooncology*. 2001;10(6):490–502.

71. Jacobsen PB, Meade CD, Stein KD, Chirikos TN, Small BJ, Ruckdeschel JC. Efficacy and costs of two forms of stress management training for cancer patients undergoing chemotherapy. *J Clin Oncol*. 2002;20(12):2851–2862.

72. Magill L, Levin T, Spodek L. One-session music therapy and CBT for critically ill cancer patients. *Psychiatr Serv*. 2008;59(10):1216.

73. Cassileth BR, Vickers AJ, Magill LA. Music therapy for mood disturbance during hospitalization for autologous stem cell transplantation: a randomized controlled trial. *Cancer*. 2003;98(12):2723–2729.

74. Ferrer AJ. The effect of live music on decreasing anxiety in patients undergoing chemotherapy treatment. *J Music Ther*. 2007;44(3):242–255.

75. Newell SA, Sanson-Fisher RW, Savolainen NJ. Systematic review of psychological therapies for cancer patients: overview and recommendations for future research. *J Natl Cancer Inst*. 2002;94(8):558–584.

76. Dileo C. Effects of music and music therapy on medical patients: a meta-analysis of the research and implications for the future. *J Soc Integr Oncol*. 2006;4(2):67–70.

77. Gottlieb BH, Wachala ED. Cancer support groups: a critical review of empirical studies. *Psychooncology*. 2007;16(5):379–400.

78. Goodwin PJ, Leszcz M, Ennis M, et al. The effect of group psychosocial support on survival in metastatic breast cancer. *N Engl J Med*. 2001;345:1719–1726.

79. Kissane DW, Grabsch B, Clarke DM, et al. Supportive-expressive group therapy for women with metastatic breast cancer: survival and psychosocial outcome from a randomized controlled trial. *Psychooncology*. 2007;16(4):277–286.

80. Pull CB. Combined pharmacotherapy and cognitive-behavioural therapy for anxiety disorders. *Curr Opin Psychiatry*. 2007;20(1):30–35.

81. Zwanzger P, Diemer J, Jabs B. Comparison of combined psycho- and pharmacotherapy with monotherapy in anxiety disorders: controversial viewpoints and clinical perspectives. *J Neural Transm*. 2009;116(6):759–765.

82. Marcus SM, Gorman J, Shear MK, et al. A comparison of medications side effect reports by panic disorder patients with and without concomitant cognitve beahvior therapy. *Am J Psychiatry*. 2007;164(2):273–275.

83. Payne DK, Massie MJ. Anxiety in palliative care. In: Chochinov HM, Breitbart W (eds). *Handbook of psychiatry in palliative medicine*. New York: Oxford University Press; 2000.

84. Breitbart W, Jacobsen PB. Psychiatric symptom management in terminal care. *Clin Geriatr Med*. 1996;12(2):329–347.

85. Stiefel F, Razavi D. Common psychiatric disorders in cancer patients. II. Anxiety and acute confusional states. *Support Care Cancer*. 1994;2(4):233–237.

86. Jackson KC, Lipman AG. Drug therapy for anxiety in palliative care. *Cochrane Database Syst Rev*. 2004(1):CD004596.

87. Holland JC, Morrow GR, Schmale A, et al. A randomized clinical trial of alprazolam versus progressive muscle relaxation in cancer patients with anxiety and depressive symptoms. *J Clin Oncol*. 1991;9(6):1004–1011.

88. Shapiro BA, Warren J, Egol AB, et al. Practice parameters for intravenous analgesia and sedation for adult patients in the intensive care unit: an executive summary. Society of Critical Care Medicine. *Crit Care Med*. 1995;23(9):1596–1600.

89. Greenberg DB, Surman OS, Clarke J, Baer L. Alprazolam for phobic nausea and vomiting related to cancer chemotherapy. *Cancer Treat Rep*. 1987;71(5):549–550.

90. Triozzi PL, Goldstein D, Laszlo J. Contributions of benzodiazepines to cancer therapy. *Cancer Invest*. 1988;6(1):103–111.

91. Breitbart W, Marotta R, Platt MM, Weisman H, Derevenco M, Grau C. A double-blind trial of haloperidol, chlorpromazine, and lorazepam in the treatment of delirium in hospitalized AIDS patients. *Am J Psychiatry*. 1996;153(2):231–237.

92. Hoffman EJ, Mathew SJ. Anxiety disorders: a comprehensive review of pharmacotherapies. *Mt Sinai J Med*. 2008;75(3):248–262.

93. Schneider LS, Dagerman K, Insel PS. Efficacy and adverse effects of atypical antipsychotics for dementia: meta-analysis of randomized, placebo-controlled trials. *Am J Geriatr Psychiatry*. 2006;14(3):191–210.

94. Davidson JR. Pharmacotherapy of social anxiety disorder: what does the evidence tell us? *J Clin Psychiatry*. 2006;67(Suppl 12):20–26.

95. Stein DJ, Ipser JC, Seedat S. Pharmacotherapy for post traumatic stress disorder (PTSD). *Cochrane Database Syst Rev*. 2006(1):CD002795.

96. Katon WJ. Clinical practice. Panic disorder. *N Engl J Med*. 2006; 354(22):2360–2367.

97. de Jong JR, Vlaeyen JW, Onghena P, Goossens ME, Geilen M, Mulder H. Fear of movement/(re)injury in chronic low back pain: education or exposure in vivo as mediator to fear reduction? *Clin J Pain*. 2005;21(1):9–17.

98. Goldberg RJ, Posner DA. Anxiety in the medically ill. In: Stoudemire A, Fogel BS, Greenberg D (eds). *Psychiatric care of the medical patient*. New York: Oxford University Press; 2000:165–180.

99. Mula M, Pini S, Cassano GB. The role of anticonvulsant drugs in anxiety disorders: a critical review of the evidence. *J Clin Psychopharmacol*. 2007;27(3):263–272.

100. Pande AC, Feltner DE, Jefferson JW, et al. Efficacy of the novel anxiolytic pregabalin in social anxiety disorder: a placebo-controlled, multicenter study. *J Clin Psychopharmacol*. 2004;24(2):141–149.

101. Montgomery S, Chatamra K, Pauer L, Whalen E, Baldinetti F. Efficacy and safety of pregabalin in elderly people with generalised anxiety disorder. *Br J Psychiatry*. 2008;193(5):389–394.

CHAPTER 45

Delirium

William S. Breitbart and Yesne Alici

INTRODUCTION

Delirium is a common and often serious neuropsychiatric complication in the management of cancer patients, characterized by an abrupt onset of disturbances of consciousness, attention, cognition, and perception that fluctuate over the course of the day. Delirium is a medical emergency that needs to be prevented, identified, and treated vigorously. Delirium is associated with increased morbidity and mortality, increased length of hospitalization, causing distress in patients, family members, and staff.[1-4] Delirium is a sign of significant physiologic disturbance, usually involving multiple medical etiologies, including infection, organ failure, and medication adverse effects.[5-9] Delirium can interfere with the recognition and control of other physical and psychological symptoms, such as pain.[10-12] Unfortunately, delirium is often underrecognized or misdiagnosed and inappropriately treated or untreated in the medical setting. Clinicians who care for patients with cancer must be able to diagnose delirium accurately, undertake appropriate assessment of etiologies, and understand the benefits and the risks of the pharmacologic and nonpharmacologic interventions currently available for managing delirium.

EPIDEMIOLOGY

Delirium is one of the most prevalent neuropsychiatric disorders in inpatient settings. The reported prevalence and incidence of delirium varies widely in the medical literature. This is due to the diverse and complex nature of delirium and the heterogeneity of sample populations. Many predisposing factors influence the prevalence and incidence of delirium in the medically ill resulting in disparate estimates depending on the patients' characteristics, setting of care, and the assessment scale used.[4] The prevalence of delirium at hospital admission ranges from 14% to 24%, and the incidence of delirium during hospitalization ranges from 6% to 56% among general hospital populations.[4] Old age is a well-known risk factor for the development of delirium likely associated with increasing severity of medical illness, dementia, and physical frailty.[4] The community data from the Eastern Baltimore Mental Health survey suggested a low prevalence of delirium in younger populations with a significant increase associated with advancing age. The prevalence was 0.4% in patients over the age of 18, 1.1% in patients over the age of 55, and 13.6% in patients over the age of 85.[13] Postoperative patients, cancer and acquired immunodeficiency syndrome (AIDS) patients are also at greater risk for delirium.[14-16] Delirium occurs in up to 51% of postoperative patients.[4] Approximately 30%–40% of medically hospitalized AIDS patients develop delirium, and as many as 65%–80% develop some type of organic mental disorder.[4] Massie and coworkers found delirium in 25% of 334 hospitalized cancer patients evaluated in psychiatric consultation and in 85% of terminal cancer patients.[14] Advanced or severe illness involving multiorgan systems increases the risk of developing delirium. The highest prevalence and incidence of delirium is reported in hospices with terminally ill patients.[17] Pereira and coworkers found the prevalence of cognitive impairment among cancer inpatients to be 44%; the prevalence increased to 62.1% in the terminally ill.[15] Prospective studies conducted in inpatient palliative care units have found an occurrence rate of delirium ranging from 20% to 42% on admission,[9,16,18,19] and incident delirium developing during admission in 32%–45%.[6,18] In a cohort of cancer patients Lawlor et al. found that delirium was present for at least 6 hours before death in 88% of patients.[6]

PATHOPHYSIOLOGY

As reflected by its diverse phenomenology, delirium is a dysfunction of multiple regions of the brain, a global cerebral dysfunction characterized by concurrent disturbances of level of consciousness, attention, perception, cognition, psychomotor behavior, mood, and sleep-wake cycle. Fluctuations of these symptoms, as well as abrupt onset of such disturbances are other critical features of delirium.[20,21] Delirium is conceptualized as a reversible process as opposed to dementia.[20] Reversibility is often possible even in patients with advanced cancer; however, irreversible or persistent delirium have been described in the last days and among elderly patients.[6,8,22,23] Current literature on the pathophysiology of delirium is limited; however, study of the pathophysiology of delirium is vital to our understanding of the phenomenology, prognosis, treatment and prevention of delirium.

Delirium is a syndrome of generalized dysfunction in higher cortical cerebral processes.[24] Electroencephalogram (EEG) studies in delirious patients demonstrate diffuse slowing in the dominant posterior rhythm.[25] Functional brain imaging reveals general cortical hypofunction which normalizes with effective treatment of delirium.[26-28] At the subcortical level, both increased and decreased activity have been described for the thalamus, and basal ganglia structures.[29] Despite many different etiologies, symptoms of delirium are largely stereotypical, with a set of core symptoms. It appears that this diversity of physiological disturbances translates into a common clinical expression that may relate to dysfunction of a final common neuroanatomical and/or neurochemical pathway.[30] Investigators through brain imaging and lesion studies have postulated that the final common pathway involves the prefrontal cortex, posterior parietal cortex, temporo-occipital cortex, anteromedial thalamus, and right basal ganglia with an imbalance in the neurotransmitters acetylcholine and dopamine (DA).[26,30-35]

Many neurotransmitter systems including the serotonergic, noradrenergic, opiatergic, glutamatergic, and histaminergic systems, may contribute to delirium as a syndrome.[30-36] The most predominant evidence implies an underactivity of the cholinergic system as the final common pathway.[30-34,37] The cholinergic hypothesis is not separable from DA as these two neurotransmitters interact closely and usually reciprocally in the brain.[26] The acetylcholine-DA hypothesis explains the efficacy of DA antagonists in the treatment of delirium by regulating the imbalance between cholinergic and dopaminergic activity while the underlying etiology is being treated.[26] Increased serotonergic activity and decreased availability of the serotonin precursor tryptophan have both been associated with delirium.[26] The pathogenesis of delirium through serotonergic abnormalities may be related to the interaction of serotonergic, cholinergic, and dopaminergic systems,[26] resulting in an acetylcholine-DA imbalance. The association of delirium with abnormalities in noradrenergic transmission is less clear.[26] Glutamatergic hyperactivity can also contribute to delirium caused by hypoxia and quinolone antibiotics.[26] Gamma-amino butyric acid (GABA) dysregulation has been implicated in alcohol withdrawal delirium with decreased GABA activity.[26] Opioidergic transmission may cause delirium through interference at the anterior cingulate gyrus which has been implicated in the pathophysiology of delirium.[26,38] Cytokines (i.e., interleurkin-1, interleukin-2, interleukin-6, tumor necrosis factor alpha), chronic hypercortisolism, and high-dose interleukin therapy has been shown to be associated with delirium.[39,40]

CLINICAL FEATURES

The clinical features of delirium are numerous and include a variety of neuropsychiatric symptoms (Table 45-1).[17,21] Main features of delirium include prodromal symptoms (e.g., restlessness, anxiety, sleep disturbances, and irritability); rapidly fluctuating course; abrupt onset of symptoms; reduced attention (e.g., distractibility); altered level of arousal; increased or decreased psychomotor activity; disturbance of sleep-wake cycle; affective symptoms (e.g., emotional lability, depressed mood, anger, or euphoria); perceptual disturbances (e.g., misperceptions, illusions, and hallucinations); delusions; disorganized thinking and incoherent speech; disorientation; and memory impairment. Language disturbance may be evident as dysnomia (i.e., the impaired ability to name objects) or dysgraphia (i.e., the impaired ability to write). In some cases, speech is rambling and irrelevant, in others pressured and incoherent.[3,21] Neurologic abnormalities may include motor abnormalities such as tremor, asterixis, myoclonus, frontal release signs, and changes in muscle tone.[26]

Cognitive impairment was found to be the most common symptom noted in phenomenology studies with disorientation occurring in 78%–100%, attention deficits in 62%–100%, memory deficits in 62%–90%, and diffuse cognitive deficits in 77%.[41] Disturbance of consciousness was recorded in 65%–100% of patients with delirium. In addition, disorganized thinking was found in 95%, language abnormalities in 47%–93%, and sleep-wake cycle disturbances in 49%–96%.[41] A recent phenomenology study by Meagher and colleagues[42] has shown that sleep-wake cycle abnormalities (97%) and inattention (97%) were the most frequent symptoms, disorientation was found to be the least common symptom.

According to the latest edition of *Diagnostic and statistical manual of mental disorders*,[20] the essential features of delirium are as follows: disturbance of consciousness with reduced ability to focus, sustain, or shift attention; change in cognition that is not better accounted by a preexisting, established, or evolving dementia or development of a perceptual disturbance; development of the disturbance over a short period, usually hours to days, and fluctuation of symptoms during the course of the day; evidence from the history, physical examination, or laboratory tests that the delirium is a direct physiological consequence of a general medical condition, substance intoxication or withdrawal, use of a medication, or toxin exposure, or a combination of these factors. Abrupt onset and fluctuation of the symptoms is an integral part of the diagnostic criteria. The disturbance develops over a short period and tends to fluctuate during the course of the day. DSM-IV places less diagnostic emphasis on incoherent speech, disorganized thinking, disturbance of sleep-wake cycle, and disturbances in psychomotor activity.

On the basis of psychomotor behavior and arousal levels two subtypes of delirium were described by Lipowski.[43] The subtypes included the hyperactive (or agitated, or hyperalert) subtype and the hypoactive (or lethargic, hypoalert, or hypoaroused) subtype. A mixed subtype has since been proposed with alternating features of each.[21] The hypoactive subtype is characterized by psychomotor retardation, lethargy, sedation, and reduced awareness of surroundings.[9,16,42,44,45] Hypoactive delirium is often mistaken for depression, and is difficult to differentiate from sedation due to opioids, or obtundation in the last days of life.[46] The hyperactive subtype is commonly characterized by restlessness, agitation, hypervigilance, hallucinations, and delusions.[16,42,44,45] The hyperactive delirium is more easily recognized by clinicians and is more likely to be referred to psychiatrists compared to patients with other subtypes of delirium.[47]

A meta-analysis of delirium subtypes suggests that the mean prevalence of hypoactive delirium is 48% (ranging between 15% and 71%).[16] The prevalence of hyperactive delirium ranges from 13% to 46%.[16] A systematic review of delirium subtypes by de Rooij et al. has identified 10 studies[48] conducted in a variety of different settings, predominantly among older medically ill patients. Owing to lack of a standardized classification method, and different results obtained, it was difficult to draw any conclusions regarding the frequency of the three motoric subtypes of delirium, and their association with specific prognoses, etiologic factors, and therapeutic consequences. Peterson et al. studied delirium subtypes in patients admitted to a medical intensive care unit (ICU) and found that those aged 65 and older were almost twice as likely to have hypoactive delirium as younger patients.[49] In the palliative care setting, hypoactive delirium is most common. Spiller and Keen found a delirium prevalence of 29% in 100 acute admissions to a hospice centre, 86% of these had the hypoactive subtype.[9]

Both hypoactive and hyperactive subtypes of delirium have been shown to cause distress in patients, family members, clinicians, and staff.[1,2,50,51] In a study of 101 terminally ill cancer patients, Breitbart et al.[1] found that 54% of patients recalled their delirium experience after recovering from the episode. Patients with hypoactive delirium (i.e., with few outward manifestation of discomfort or distress) were just as distressed as patients with hyperactive delirium. Recent studies suggest that the experience of caring for a delirious family member or a patient is perhaps even more of a distressing experience than the experience of the patient.[1,51] In a study of delirium-related caregiver distress, Breitbart et al.[1] found that caregivers including spouses, family members, and staff experienced significant levels of distress. Predictors of spouse distress included the patients' Karnofsky Performance Status (the lower the Karnofsky, the worse the spouse distress), as well as the presence of hyperactive delirium, and delirium related to brain metastases.[1] Predictors of staff distress included delirium severity, the presence of perceptual disturbances, paranoid delusions, and sleep-wake cycle disturbance.

There is evidence suggesting that the subtypes of delirium may be related to different causes, and may have different treatment responses.[44–46,52,53] Hypoactive delirium has generally been found to occur due to hypoxia, metabolic disturbances, and hepatic encephalopathies.[16,45,46,52] Hyperactive delirium is correlated with alcohol and drug withdrawal, drug intoxication, or medication adverse effects.[16,45,46,52,53] A randomized controlled trial of haloperidol and chlorpromazine found that both medications were equally effective in hypoactive and hyperactive subtypes of delirium.[53] However, in an open-label trial, the hypoactive subtype was associated with poorer treatment response to olanzapine.[44] The hypoactive subtype of delirium is associated with higher mortality risk compared to hyperactive delirium.[23,52]

INTERFERENCE OF DELIRIUM WITH ASSESSMENT AND MANAGEMENT OF PAIN

It is well-recognized that success in the treatment of cancer pain is highly dependent on proper assessment.[54] However, the assessment of pain intensity becomes very difficult in patients with delirium. Delirium can interfere dramatically with the recognition and control of pain, and other physical and psychological symptoms in advanced cancer patients, particularly in the terminally ill.[10,11] Due to reversal of sleep-wake cycle, patients with delirium use a significantly greater number of "breakthrough" doses of opioids at nights compared to patients without delirium.[12] On the other hand, agitation may be misinterpreted as uncontrolled pain, resulting in inappropriate escalation of opioids,

Table 45–1. Common clinical features of delirium[26]

Disturbance in level of alertness (consciousness) and arousal
Attention disturbance
Rapidly fluctuating course and abrupt onset of symptoms
Increased or decreased psychomotor activity
Disturbance of sleep-wake cycle
Mood symptoms
Perceptual disturbances
Disorganized thinking
Incoherent speech
Disorientation and memory impairment
Other cognitive impairments (e.g., dysgraphia, constructional apraxia, dysnomia)
Asterixis, myoclonus, tremor, frontal release signs, changes in muscle tone

potentially exacerbating delirium.[11] Accurate pain reporting depends on the ability to perceive the pain normally and to communicate the experience appropriately. Delirium may, both, impair the ability to perceive and report pain accurately. A study of terminally ill hospice patients[55] found that their ability to communicate was frequently impaired, with the degree of impairment related, both, to delirium and to opioid dosage. Efforts have been made to improve assessment of pain in nonverbal palliative care patients.[56]

DIFFERENTIAL DIAGNOSIS

Many of the clinical features of delirium can be also be associated with other psychiatric disorders, such as depression, mania, psychosis, and dementia. When delirium presents with mood symptoms such as depression, apathy, euphoria, or irritability, these symptoms are not uncommonly attributed to depression or mania, especially in patients with a past psychiatric or family history of these conditions.[3,21] The hypoactive subtype of delirium is commonly misdiagnosed as depression.[17,48,57] Symptoms of major depression, including decreased psychomotor activity, insomnia, reduced ability to concentrate, depressed mood, and even suicidal ideation, can overlap with symptoms of delirium. In distinguishing delirium from depression, particularly in the context of advanced cancer, an evaluation of the onset and the temporal sequencing of depressive and cognitive symptoms is particularly helpful. It is important to note that the degree of cognitive impairment is much more pronounced in delirium than in depression, with a more abrupt onset. Also, in delirium the characteristic disturbance in level of arousal is present, while it is usually not a feature of depression. Similarly, a manic episode may share some features of delirium, particularly a hyperactive or mixed subtype of delirium. Again, the temporal onset and course of symptoms, the presence of a disturbance of level of arousal as well as cognition, and the identification of a presumed medical etiology for delirium are helpful in differentiating these disorders. Symptoms such as severe anxiety and autonomic hyperactivity can lead the clinician to an erroneous diagnosis of panic disorder. Delirium that is characterized by vivid hallucinations and delusions must be distinguished from a variety of psychotic disorders such as schizophrenia. Delusions in delirium tend to be poorly organized and of abrupt onset, and hallucinations are predominantly visual or tactile, rather than auditory, as is typical of schizophrenia. Acute onset, fluctuating course, disturbances of cognition, and consciousness, in the presence of one or more etiologic causes, are characteristic in the diagnosis of delirium.[21]

The most challenging differential diagnostic issue is whether the patient has delirium, dementia, or a delirium superimposed on a preexisting dementia. Both delirium and dementia are disorders of cognition and share common clinical features, such as disorientation, memory impairment, aphasia, apraxia, agnosia, and executive dysfunction.[21] Impairments in judgment, abstract thinking, and disturbances in thought process are seen in both disorders. Delusions and hallucinations can be central features of certain types of dementia (e.g., Lewy body dementia). It is the abrupt onset, fluctuating course, and disturbances of consciousness or arousal that differentiates delirium from dementia.[21] The temporal onset of symptoms in dementia is more subacute and chronically progressive. In delirium superimposed on an underlying dementia, such as in the case of an elderly patient, an AIDS patient, or a patient with a paraneoplastic syndrome, differential diagnosis becomes even more challenging. Delirium, unlike dementia, is by definition reversible, although as noted previously, in terminally ill patients, delirium may be irreversible.[3,21]

ASSESSMENT OF DELIRIUM

Clinically, the diagnostic gold standard for delirium is the clinician's assessment utilizing the DSM-IV-TR criteria[20] as outlined above. Several delirium screening and evaluation tools have been developed to maximize diagnostic precision for clinical and research purposes and to assess delirium severity.[58] A detailed review of these assessment tools is available elsewhere.[58] Several examples of delirium assessment tools currently used in cancer patients and in palliative care settings include the Memorial Delirium Assessment Scale (MDAS),[59,60] the Delirium-Rating Scale-Revised 98 (DRS-R-98),[61] and the Confusion Assessment Method (CAM).[62] Each of these scales has good reliability and validity.

The MDAS is designed to be administered repeatedly within the same day, to allow for objective measurement of changes in delirium severity in response to medical changes or clinical interventions. The MDAS is a 10-item, 4-point clinician-rated scale (possible range: 0–30) designed to quantify the severity of delirium, validated among hospitalized patients with advanced cancer and AIDS.[59] Items included in the MDAS reflect the diagnostic criteria for delirium in the DSM-IV, as well as symptoms of delirium from earlier or alternative classification systems (e.g., DSM-III, DSM-III-R, ICD-9). The MDAS is, both, a good delirium diagnostic screening tool as well as a reliable tool for assessing delirium severity among patients with advanced disease. Scale items assess disturbances in arousal and level of consciousness, as well as in several areas of cognitive functioning (memory, attention, orientation, disturbances in thinking) and psychomotor activity.[59] A cut off score of 13 is diagnostic of delirium. The MDAS has been revalidated among advanced cancer patients in inpatient palliative care settings with a sensitivity of 98% and a specificity of 96% at a cut off score of 7.[60]

The Delirium-Rating Scale (DRS)[63] is a numerical rating scale that specifically integrates DSM-III-R diagnostic criteria for delirium. DRS-R-98 is the revised version of the DRS.[61] The DRS-R-98 is a valid, sensitive, and reliable instrument for rating delirium severity.[61]

The CAM is a nine-item delirium diagnostic scale based on the DSM-III-R criteria for delirium.[62] A unique and helpful feature of the CAM is that it has been simplified into a diagnostic algorithm that includes only 4 items of the CAM designed for rapid identification of delirium by nonpsychiatrists. The 4 item algorithm requires the presence of: (1) acute onset and fluctuating course, (2) inattention, and either (3) disorganized thinking or (4) altered level of consciousness. CAM has recently been validated in palliative care settings with a sensitivity of 88% and a specificity of 100% when administered by well-trained clinicians.[64]

ETIOLOGIES AND REVERSIBILITY OF DELIRIUM

Delirium can have multiple potential etiologies. (Table 45–2) In patients with cancer, delirium can result either from the direct effects of cancer on the central nervous system (CNS) or from the indirect CNS effects of the disease or treatments (e.g., medications, electrolyte imbalance, dehydration, major organ failure, infection, vascular complications, paraneoplastic syndromes).[5,6,8,9,21,48,65] The diagnostic work-up of delirium should include an assessment of potentially reversible causes of delirium. The clinician should obtain a detailed history from family and staff of the patient's baseline mental status and verify the current fluctuating mental status. It is important to inquire about alcohol or other substance use disorders in hospitalized cancer patients to be able to recognize and treat alcohol or other substance-induced withdrawal delirium appropriately.[21] A full physical examination should assess for evidence of sepsis, dehydration, or major organic failure (renal, hepatic, pulmonary).[22,66] Medications that could contribute to delirium should be reviewed.

Table 45–2. Etiologies of delirium in cancer patients

Direct effects of cancer on the CNS
Primary CNS tumors
Metastatic brain tumors
Leptomeningeal carcinomatosis

Indirect CNS effects of cancer or treatments
Major organ failure (e.g., pulmonary, renal, hepatic)
Electrolyte imbalance
Medications (including chemotherapeutic agents)
Infection
Hematologic abnormalities
Paraneoplastic syndromes

ABBREVIATION: CNS, central nervous system.

Opioid analgesics, benzodiazepines, and anticholinergic drugs are common causes of delirium, particularly in the elderly and the terminally ill.[21,65-67] The challenge of assessing the opioid contribution to an episode of delirium is often compounded by the presence of many other potential contributors to cognitive impairment such as infection, metabolic disturbance, dehydration, or other medication effects. Reducing the dose of opioids or switching to another opioid have been demonstrated to reverse delirium due to opioids.[26] Chemotherapeutic agents known to cause delirium include methotrexate, fluorouracil, vincristine, vinblastine, bleomycin, bis-chloronitrosourea (BCNU), cis-platinum, ifosfamide, asparaginase, procarbazine, and gluco-corticosteroids.[3]

A screen of laboratory parameters will allow assessment of the possible role of metabolic abnormalities, such as hypercalcemia, and other problems, such as hypoxia or disseminated intravascular coagulation. In some instances, an EEG (to rule out seizures), brain imaging studies (to rule out brain metastases, intracranial bleeding, or ischemia), and lumbar puncture (to rule out leptomeningeal carcinomatosis or meningitis) may be appropriate.[17,21,66]

When assessing etiologies of delirium, an important challenge is the clinical differentiation of delirium as either a reversible complication of cancer or an integral element of the dying process in terminally ill patients. The potential utility of a thorough diagnostic assessment has been demonstrated in patients with advanced cancer. When diagnostic information points to a likely etiology, specific therapy may be able to reverse delirium. There is an ongoing debate as to the appropriate extent of diagnostic evaluation that should be pursued in a terminally ill patient with delirium.[65,68] When confronted with delirium in the terminally ill patients, the clinician must take a more individualized and judicious approach, consistent with the goals of care.[3]

Bruera et al. reported that an etiology was discovered in 43% of terminally ill patients with delirium, and one-third of the patients with delirium improved with treatment of the specific etiologies.[69] Lawlor and colleagues explored the etiologic precipitants and potential reversibility of delirium in advanced cancer patients admitted to a palliative care unit for symptom control and found an overall reversibility rate of 49%.[6] No difference was found in reversibility rates for delirium present on admission and that which developed subsequently. However, a significant difference existed in the reversibility of initial (56%) compared to repeated episodes (6%). The median number of precipitating factors for both reversible and irreversible delirium was 3 (range 1–6). The application of standardized criteria resulted in a classification of etiologic factors in 78% of episodes of reversible delirium and 59% of irreversible cases. Reversibility of delirium was significantly associated with opioids, other psychoactive medications, and dehydration. In contrast, irreversibility of delirium was significantly associated with hypoxic encephalopathy and metabolic factors related to major organ failure, including hepatic and renal insufficiency, and refractory hypercalcemia.[6] Ljubisavljevic and Kelly prospectively assessed the development of delirium in oncology patients, and found a delirium occurrence rate of 18% (26 out of 145 patients) and a reversal rate of 84.6% (22 out of 26 patients).[7] Morita examined factors associated with reversibility of delirium in another population of advanced cancer patients admitted to hospice.[8] This study's overall delirium reversibility rate was 20%, lower than that reported in prior studies. Patients with delirium had a 30-day mortality rate of 83% and a 50-day mortality rate of 91%. While reversibility of delirium was significantly associated with medications (37%) or hypercalcemia (38%), irreversibility was associated with infections (12%), hepatic failure, hypoxia, disseminated intravascular coagulation, and dehydration (<10%).

Leonard and colleagues[23] found a 27% recovery rate from delirium among patients in palliative care settings. Patients with irreversible delirium experienced greater disturbances of sleep and cognition. Mean time until death was 39.7 (SD, 69.8) days in patients with reversible delirium (n = 33) versus 16.8 (SD, 10.0) days in patients with irreversible delirium (n = 88).[23]

In light of the several studies on reversibility of delirium, the prognosis of patients who develop delirium is defined by the interaction of the patient's baseline physiologic susceptibility to delirium (e.g., predisposing factors), the precipitating etiologies, and any response to treatment.

If a patient's susceptibility or resilience is modifiable, then targeted interventions may reduce the risk of delirium upon exposure to a precipitant and enhance the capacity to respond to treatment.[3] Conversely, if a patient's vulnerability is high and resistant to modification, then exposure to precipitants enhances the likelihood of developing delirium and may diminish the probability of a complete restoration of cognitive function.[3]

MANAGEMENT OF DELIRIUM IN CANCER PATIENTS

The standard approach to managing delirium in cancer patients, even in those with advanced disease, includes a search for underlying causes, correction of those factors, and management of the symptoms of delirium.[21] Treatment of the symptoms of delirium should be initiated before, or in concert with, a diagnostic assessment of the etiologies to minimize distress to patients, staff, and family members. The desired and often achievable outcome is a patient who is awake, alert, calm, comfortable, cognitively intact, and communicating coherently with family and staff. In the terminally ill patient who develops delirium in the last days of life, the management of delirium is unique, presenting a number of dilemmas, and the desired clinical outcome may be significantly altered by the dying process.[17] The goal of care in the terminally ill may shift to providing comfort through the judicious use of sedatives, even at the expense of alertness.[66]

Nonpharmacological interventions. Nonpharmacologic and supportive therapies play an essential role in the treatment of cancer patients with delirium, especially in patients with terminal delirium.[66]

There is evidence that nonpharmacologic interventions in nonpalliative care settings result in faster improvement of delirium and slower deterioration in cognition. However, these interventions were not found to have any beneficial effects on mortality or health-related quality of life when compared with usual care.[70-72] Nonpharmacologic interventions used in these studies include oxygen delivery, fluid and electrolyte administration, ensuring bowel and bladder function, nutrition, mobilization, pain treatment, frequent orientation, use of visual and hearing aids, and environmental modifications (e.g., quiet, well-lit room with familiar objects, a visible clock or calendar) to enhance a sense of familiarity.[17,66,70-72] One-to-one nursing may be necessary for observation. Physical restraints should be avoided, when possible.[66,70] The use of physical restraints has been identified as an independent risk factor for delirium persistence at the time of hospital discharge.[70] Restraints should be used only when a patient represents a clear risk of harm to self and others and no less restrictive alternative is available. Restraint orders should be time-limited, and the patient's condition should be monitored closely.

Pharmacological interventions. Nonpharmacologic interventions and supportive measures alone are often not effective in controlling the symptoms of delirium. Symptomatic treatment with psychotropic medications is often essential to control the symptoms of delirium, although no medications have been approved by Food and Drug Administration (FDA) for treatment of delirium.

Antipsychotic medications. American Psychiatric Association (APA) practice guidelines provide directions for the use of antipsychotics in the treatment of delirium[21] and growing evidence supports their use (Table 45–3).[44,53,73-80]

Haloperidol (a "typical" antipsychotic) is often the gold-standard medication for treatment of delirium among cancer patients, due to its efficacy and safety (e.g., few anticholinergic effects, lack of active metabolites, and availability in different routes of administration).[21] Approximately 0.5%–2% of hospitalized cancer patients receive haloperidol for symptoms of delirium,[81] and only 17% of terminally ill patients receive any antipsychotic drugs for agitation or delirium.[81] Haloperidol in low doses (1–3 mg per day) is usually effective in targeting agitation and psychotic symptoms.[21] In general, doses of haloperidol need not exceed 20 mg in a 24-hour period; however, some clinicians advocate higher doses in selected cases.[21] In severe agitation related to delirium,

Table 45–3. Antipsychotic medications in the treatment of delirium in cancer patients

Medication	Dose range	Routes of administration	Side effects	Comments
Typical antipsychotics				
Haloperidol	0.5–2 mg every 2–12 hr	PO, IV, IM, SC	Extrapyramidal adverse effects can occur at higher doses Monitor QT interval on EKG	Remains the gold-standard therapy for delirium May add lorazepam (0.5–1 mg every 2–4 hr) for agitated patients
Chlorpromazine	12.5–50 mg every 4–6 hr	PO, IV, IM, SC, PR	More sedating and anti-cholinergic compared with haloperidol Monitor blood pressure for hypotension	May be preferred in agitated patients due to its sedative effect
Atypical antipsychotics				
Olanzapine	2.5–5 mg every 12–24 hr	PO,[a] IM	Sedation is the main dose-limiting adverse effect in short-term use	Older age, preexisting dementia, and hypoactive subtype of delirium have been associated with poor response
Risperidone	0.25–1 mg every 12–24 hr	PO[a]	Extrapyramidal adverse effects can occur with doses >6 mg/day Orthostatic hypotension	Clinical experience suggests better results in patients with hypoactive delirium
Quetiapine	12.5–100 mg every 12–24 hr	PO	Sedation, orthostatic hypotension	Sedating effects may be helpful in patients with sleep-wake cycle disturbance
Ziprasidone	10–40 mg every 12–24 hr	PO, IM	Monitor QT interval on EKG	Evidence is limited to case reports
Aripiprazole	5–30 mg every 24 hr	PO,[a] IM	Monitor for akathisia	Evidence is limited to case reports and case series

[a] Risperidone, olanzapine, and aripiprazole are available in orally disintegrating tablets.
ABBREVIATIONS: EKG, electrocardiogram; IM, intramuscular; IV, intravenous; PO, per oral; PR, per rectum; SC, subcutaneous.

clinicians may add lorazepam to haloperidol. This combination may be more effective in rapidly sedating patients and may help minimize any extrapyramidal adverse effects of haloperidol.[21]

Oral or intravenous (IV) chlorpromazine is considered to be an effective alternative to haloperidol (with or without lorazepam) when increased sedation is required, especially in the ICU setting where close blood pressure monitoring is feasible, and for severe agitation in terminally ill patients to decrease distress for the patient, family, and staff. It is important to monitor chlorpromazine's anticholinergic and hypotensive side effects, particularly in elderly patients.[17,21]

In a double-blind, randomized comparison trial (n = 30) of haloperidol, chlorpromazine, and lorazepam, Breitbart and colleagues[53] demonstrated that lorazepam alone, in doses up to 8 mg in a 12-hour period, was ineffective in the treatment of delirium, and in fact sometimes worsened it. Both haloperidol and chlorpromazine, in low doses (approximately 2 mg of haloperidol equivalent per 24 hours) were effective in controlling the symptoms of delirium and in improving cognitive function in the first 24 hours of treatment.[53] Both, hyperactive as well as hypoactive subtypes of delirium were equally responsive to treatment with haloperidol or chlorpromazine.

A Cochrane review on drug therapy for delirium in the terminally ill[80] concluded that haloperidol was the most suitable medication for the treatment of patients with delirium near the end of life, with chlorpromazine being an acceptable alternative.

The FDA has issued a warning against the risk of QTc prolongation and torsades de pointes with IV haloperidol, thus monitoring QTc intervals daily among medically ill patients receiving IV haloperidol has become the standard clinical practice.[82]

Atypical antipsychotic agents (i.e., risperidone, olanzapine, quetiapine, ziprasidone, and aripiprazole) are increasingly used in the treatment of delirium in cancer patients due to decreased risk of extrapyramidal adverse effects.[79]

Several researchers have published their open-label experience with treating delirium and agitation with atypical antipsychotics, including olanzapine, risperidone, quetiapine, ziprasidone, and aripiprazole.[17,79] A comprehensive review of these studies is available elsewhere.[79]

In a double-blind comparative delirium intervention study assessing the efficacy of haloperidol versus risperidone, Han and Kim demonstrated, in a small sample of 24 oncology patients, that there was no significant difference in clinical efficacy or response rate. The mean risperidone dose was 1.02 mg and the mean haloperidol dose was 1.71 mg. MDAS scores improved significantly in both groups. No significant difference was observed in adverse effects. However, despite the double-blind design in this study, authors acknowledged that they were not able to obtain identical looking tablets of haloperidol and risperidone.[75]

Breitbart and colleagues published an (n = 82) open trial of olanzapine for the treatment of delirium in hospitalized patients with advanced cancer.[44] Olanzapine was effective in the treatment of delirium, resolving delirium in 76% of patients with no incidence of extrapyramidal side effects. Several factors were found to be significantly associated with poorer response to olanzapine treatment for delirium, including age over 70, history of dementia, and hypoactive delirium. The average starting dose was in the 2.5–5 mg range and patients were given up to 20 mg per day of olanzapine. Sedation was the most common side effect.

A randomized controlled trial[76] comparing olanzapine (n = 75), haloperidol (n = 72), and placebo (n = 29) in the treatment of delirium among hospitalized patients (mean olanzapine dose of 4.5 mg/day, and a haloperidol dose of 7 mg/day) has demonstrated an improvement in DRS scores with olanzapine and haloperidol; significantly higher in the olanzapine (72%) and haloperidol (70%) groups compared with placebo (29.7%) (p <0.01). Increased rates of extrapyramidal symptoms (EPS) were observed in the haloperidol group. However, haloperidol was administered intramuscularly which makes it difficult to reliably interpret the study results.

A Cochrane review, comparing the efficacy and the incidence of adverse effects between haloperidol and atypical antipsychotics, concluded that, like haloperidol, selected newer atypical antipsychotics (risperidone, olanzapine) were effective in managing delirium.[78]

Haloperidol doses greater than 4.5 mg/day were more likely to result in increased rates of EPS compared with the atypical antipsychotics, but low-dose haloperidol (i.e., less than 3.5 mg/day) did not result in a greater frequency of extrapyramidal adverse effects.[75,76,78]

The APA guidelines[21] for treatment of delirium recommend use of low-dose haloperidol (i.e., 1–2 mg PO every 4 hours as needed or 0.25– 0.5 mg PO every 4 hours for the elderly) as the treatment of choice in cases where medications are necessary.

In the light of existing literature, risperidone may be used in the treatment of delirium, starting at doses ranging from 0.25 to 1 mg and titrated up as necessary with particular attention to the risk EPS, orthostatic hypotension and sedation at higher doses. Olanzapine can be started between 2.5 and 5 mg nightly and titrated up with the sedation being the major limiting factor, which may be favorable in the treatment of hyperactive delirium. The current literature on the use of quetiapine suggests a starting dose of 25–50 mg and a titration up to 100–200 mg a day (usually at twice daily divided doses). Sedation and orthostatic hypotension are the main dose-limiting factors.[79] Case reports suggest a starting dose of 10–15 mg daily for aripiprazole, with a maximum dose of 30 mg daily.[79]

Important considerations in starting treatment with any antipsychotic for delirium may include EPS risk, sedation, anticholinergic side effects, cardiac arrhythmias, and possible drug-drug interactions. The FDA has issued a "black box" warning of increased risk of death associated with the use of typical and atypical antipsychotics in elderly patients with dementia-related psychoses.[83]

Psychostimulants. Some clinicians have suggested that the hypoactive subtype of delirium may respond to psychostimulants such as methylphenidate, or combinations of antipsychotics and psychostimulants or antipsychotics and wakefulness agents such as modafinil.[17,84–87] However, studies with psychostimulants in treating delirium are limited to case reports and one open-label study.[85–87] The risks of precipitating agitation and exacerbating psychotic symptoms should be carefully evaluated when psychostimulants are considered in the treatment of delirium in cancer patients.[85–87]

Cholinesterase inhibitors. As detailed above, impaired cholinergic function has been implicated as one of the final common pathways in the neuropathogenesis of delirium.[30] Despite case reports of beneficial effects of donepezil and rivastigmine, a Cochrane review concluded that there is currently no evidence from controlled trials supporting use of cholinesterase inhibitors in the treatment of delirium.[88–90]

PREVENTION OF DELIRIUM

Several researchers studied both pharmacologic and nonpharmacologic interventions in the prevention of delirium among older patient populations, particularly in surgical settings.[73,74,91–94] The applicability of these interventions to the prevention of delirium in cancer patients has not been studied.

A Cochrane review of delirium prevention studies concluded that the evidence on effectiveness of interventions to prevent delirium is sparse.[92] A randomized, placebo-controlled, double-blind clinical trial in elderly hip-surgery patients, low-dose haloperidol (1.5 mg a day) prophylaxis was not found effective for the prevention of postoperative delirium; however, it markedly reduced the severity and duration of delirium, and no drug-related side effects were noted.[77] Two randomized placebo-controlled prevention trials with donepezil among surgical patients undergoing total joint replacement surgery failed to show a difference in the incidence of delirium and the duration of hospitalization.[73,74] A randomized controlled trial of proactive geriatric consultations in a population of patients undergoing surgery for hip fracture was found to be the only effective intervention in reducing incidence and severity of delirium.[93]

Inouye and colleagues[91] reported on a successful multicomponent intervention program to prevent delirium in hospitalized older patients, reducing the number and duration of episodes of delirium in this population.

CONTROVERSIES IN THE MANAGEMENT OF TERMINAL DELIRIUM

The use of antipsychotics and other pharmacologic agents in the management of delirium in the dying patient remain controversial.[3] Some researchers have argued that pharmacologic interventions are inappropriate in the dying patient. Delirium is viewed by some as a natural part of the dying process that should not be altered. Clearly, there are many patients who experience hallucinations and delusions during delirium that are pleasant and in fact comforting, and many clinicians question the appropriateness of intervening pharmacologically in such instances. Another concern is that these patients are so close to death that aggressive treatment is unnecessary, and antipsychotics or sedatives may be mistakenly avoided because of exaggerated fears that they might hasten death through hypotension or respiratory depression.

Clinical experience in managing delirium in dying patients suggests that the use of antipsychotics in the management of agitation, paranoia, hallucinations, and altered sensorium is safe, effective, and often quite appropriate. Management of delirium on a case-by-case basis seems wisest. The agitated, delirious dying patient should probably be given antipsychotics to help restore calm. A "wait-and-see" approach may be appropriate with some patients who have a lethargic or somnolent presentation of delirium or who are having frankly pleasant or comforting hallucinations. Such a wait-and-see approach must, however, be tempered by the knowledge that a lethargic or hypoactive delirium may very quickly and unexpectedly become an agitated or hyperactive delirium that can threaten the serenity and safety of the patient, family, and staff. It is important to remember that, by their nature the symptoms of delirium are unstable and fluctuate over time.[3]

Perhaps the most challenging clinical problem is the management of the dying patient with a terminal delirium that is unresponsive to standard pharmacologic interventions. Approximately 30% of dying patients with delirium do not have their symptoms adequately controlled by antipsychotic medications.[3,4,94–97] In studies of the use of palliative sedation for symptom control, delirium was identified as the target symptom in up to 36% of cases.[96,97] Clinicians are sometimes concerned that the use of sedating medications may hasten death via respiratory depression, hypotension, or even starvation. However, studies have found that the use of opioids and psychotropic agents in hospice and palliative care settings is associated with longer rather than shorter survival.[3,96–102]

The clinician must always keep in mind the goals of care and communicate these goals to the staff, patients, and family members when treating delirium in the terminally ill The clinician must weigh each of the issues in making decisions on how to best manage the dying patient with delirium that preserves and respects the dignity and values of that individual and family.[3]

THE CONTRIBUTION OF DELIRIUM TO PROGNOSIS

Delirium in the terminally ill cancer patients is a relatively reliable predictor of approaching death in the coming days to weeks.[66] The death rates among hospitalized elderly patients with delirium over the 3 month post-discharge period range from 22% to 76%.[21] In the palliative care setting several studies provide support that delirium reliably predict impending death in patients with advanced cancer. Bruera and colleagues[69] demonstrated a significant association between delirium and death within 4 weeks. In Japan, Morita and colleagues[103] found that delirium predicted poor short-term prognosis in patients admitted to hospice. Caraceni and colleagues[104] evaluated the impact of delirium on patients for whom chemotherapy was no longer considered effective and had been referred to palliative care programs. Length of survival of patients with delirium differed significantly from those without delirium. Compared with an overall median survival of 39 days in their study, delirious patients died, on average, within 21 days. Recognizing an episode of delirium, in the late phases of palliative care, is critically important in treatment planning and in advising family members on what to expect.

CONCLUSION

Psycho-oncologists commonly encounter delirium as a major complication of cancer and its treatments, particularly among hospitalized cancer patients. Proper assessment, diagnosis, and management of delirium are essential in improving quality of life and minimizing morbidity in cancer patients.

REFERENCES

1. Breitbart W, Gibson C, Tremblay A. The delirium experience: delirium recall and delirium-related distress in hospitalized patients with cancer, their spouses/caregivers, and their nurses. *Psychosomatics.* 2002;43(3):183–194.

2. Morita T, et al. Family-perceived distress from delirium-related symptoms of terminally ill cancer patients. *Psychosomatics.* 2004;45(2):107–113.

3. Breitbart W, Friedlander M. Confusion/Delirium. In: Bruera E, Higginson I, Ripamonti C, von Gunten C (eds). *Palliative medicine.* London, U.K. London Hodder Press; 2006:688–700.

4. Inouye SK. Delirium in older persons. *N Engl J Med.* 2006;354(11):1157–1165.

5. Gaudreau JD, Gagnon, et al. Psychoactive medications and risk of delirium in hospitalized cancer patients. *J Clin Oncol.* 2005;23(27):6712–6718.

6. Lawlor PG, Gagnon B, Mancini IL, et al. Occurrence, causes, and outcome of delirium in patients with advanced cancer: a prospective study. *Arch Intern Med.* 2000;160(6):786–794.

7. Ljubisavljevic V, Kelly B. Risk factors for development of delirium among oncology patients. *Gen Hosp Psychiatry.* 2003;25(5):345–352.

8. Morita T, Tei Y, Tsunoda J, Inoue S, Chihara S. Underlying pathologies and their associations with clinical features in terminal delirium of cancer patients. *J Pain Symptom Manage.* 2001;22(6):997–1006.

9. Spiller JA, Keen JC. Hypoactive delirium: assessing the extent of the problem for inpatient specialist palliative care. *Palliat Med.* 2006;20(1):17–23.

10. Bruera E, Fainsinger RL, Miller MJ, Kuehn N. The assessment of pain intensity in patients with cognitive failure: a preliminary report. *J Pain Symptom Manage.* 1992;7(5):267–270.

11. Coyle N, Breitbart W, Weaver S, Portenoy R. Delirium as a contributing factor to "crescendo" pain: three case reports. *J Pain Symptom Manage.* 1994;9(1):44–47.

12. Gagnon B, Lawlor PG, Mancini IL, Pereira JL, Hanson J, Bruera ED. The impact of delirium on the circadian distribution of breakthrough analgesia in advanced cancer patients. *J Pain Symptom Manage.* 2001;22(4):826–833.

13. Folstein MF, Bassett SS, Romanoski AJ, Nestadt G. The epidemiology of delirium in the community: the Eastern Baltimore Mental Health Survey. *Int Psychogeriatr.* 1991;3(2):169–176.

14. Massie MJ, Holland J, Glass E. Delirium in terminally ill cancer patients. *Am J Psychiatry.* 1983;140(8):1048–1050.

15. Pereira J, Hanson J, Bruera E. The frequency and clinical course of cognitive impairment in patients with terminal cancer. *Cancer.* 1997;79(4):835–842.

16. Ross CA, Peyser CE, Shapiro I, Folstein MF. Delirium: phenomenologic and etiologic subtypes. *Int Psychogeriatr.* 1991;3(2):135–147.

17. Breitbart W, Alici Y. Agitation and delirium at the end of life: "We Couldn't Manage Him." *JAMA.* 2008;300:2898–2910.

18. Gagnon P, Allard P, Mâsse B, DeSerres M. Delirium in terminal cancer: a prospective study using daily screening, early diagnosis, and continuous monitoring. *J Pain Symptom Manage.* 2000;19(6):412–426.

19. Minagawa H, Uchitomi Y, Yamawaki S, Ishitani K. Psychiatric morbidity in terminally ill cancer patients. A prospective study. *Cancer.* 1996;78(5):1131–1137.

20. American Psychiatric Association. *Diagnostic and statistical manual of mental disorders.* 4th ed, text revision. Washington, DC: American Psychiatric Association Press; 2000.

21. American Psychiatric Association. Practice guidelines for the treatment of patients with delirium. *Am J Psychiatry.* 1999;156:S1–S20.

22. Cole MG, Ciampi A, Belzile E, Zhong L. Persistent delirium in older hospital patients: systematic review of frequency and prognosis. *Age Ageing.* 2009 Jan;38(1):19–26.

23. Leonard M, Raju B, Conroy M, et al. Reversibility of delirium in terminally ill patients and predictors of mortality. *Palliat Med.* 2008;22(7):848–854

24. Engel GL, Romano J. Delirium, a syndrome of cerebral insufficiency. 1959. *J Neuropsychiatry Clin Neurosci.* 2004;16(4):526–538.

25. Jacobson S, Jerrier H. EEG in delirium. *Semin Clin Neuropsychiatry.* 2000;5(2):86–92.

26. Boettger S, Friedlander M, Breitbart W. Delirium. In: Blumenfeld M, Strain J (eds). *Textbook of psychosomatic medicine.* Lippincott Williams and Wilkins; 2006:493–512.

27. Yokota H, Ogawa S, Kurokawa A, Yamamoto Y. Regional cerebral blood flow in delirium patients. *Psychiatry Clin Neurosci.* 2003;57(3):337–339.

28. Lerner DM, Rosenstein DL. Neuroimaging in delirium and related conditions. *Semin Clin Neuropsychiatry.* 2000;5(2):98–112.

29. Trzepacz PT, Sclabassi RJ, Van Thiel DH. Delirium: a subcortical phenomenon? *J Neuropsychiatry Clin Neurosci.* 1989;1(3):283–290.

30. Trzepacz PT. Is there a final common neural pathway in delirium? Focus on acetylcholine and dopamine. *Semin Clin Neuropsychiatry.* 2000;5(2):132–148.

31. Dunne JW, Leedman PJ, Edis RH. Inobvious stroke: a cause of delirium and dementia. *Aust N Z J Med.* 1986;16(6):771–778.

32. Mullally WJ, Ronthal M, Huff K, Geschwind N. Chronic confusional state. *N J Med.* 1989;86(7):541–544.

33. Figiel GS, Krishnan KR, Doraiswamy PM. Subcortical structural changes in ECT-induced delirium. *J Geriatr Psychiatry Neurol.* 1990;3(3):172–176.

34. Trzepacz PT. Update on the neuropathogenesis of delirium. *Dement Geriatr Cogn Disord* 1999;10(5):330–334.

35. Gaudreau JD, Gagnon P. Psychotogenic drugs and delirium pathogenesis: the central role of the thalamus. *Med Hypotheses.* 2005;64(3):471–475.

36. Inouye SK, Ferrucci L. Elucidating the pathophysiology of delirium and the interrelationship of delirium and dementia. *J Gerontol A Biol Sci Med Sci.* 2006 Dec;61(12):1277–1280.

37. Hshieh TT, Fong TG, Marcantonio ER, Inouye SK. Cholinergic deficiency hypothesis in delirium: a synthesis of current evidence. *J Gerontol A Biol Sci Med Sci.* 2008 Jul;63(7):764–772.

38. Reischies FM, Neuhaus AH, Hansen ML, Mientus S, Mulert C, Gallinat J. Electrophysiological and neuropsychological analysis of a delirious state: the role of the anterior cingulate gyrus. *Psychiatry Res.* 2005;138(2):171–181.

39. Trzepacz P, van der Mast R. The neuropathophysiology of delirium. In: Lindesay J, Rockwood K, Macdonald A (eds). *Delirium in old age.* Oxford, England: Oxford University Press; 2002:51–90.

40. Adamis D, Treloar A, Martin FC, Gregson N, Hamilton G, Macdonald AJ. APOE and cytokines as biological markers for recovery of prevalent delirium in elderly medical inpatients. *Int J Geriatr Psychiatry.* 2007 Jul;22(7):688–694.

41. Meagher DJ, Trzepacz PT. Delirium phenomenology illuminates pathophysiology, management, and course. *J Geriatr Psychiatry Neurol.* 1998;11(3):150–156.

42. Meagher DJ, Moran M, Raju B, et al. Phenomenology of delirium: assessment of 100 adult cases using standardised measures. *Br J Psychiatry.* 2007;190:135–141.

43. Lipowski ZJ, *Delirium: Acute confusional states.* New York: Oxford University Press; 1990.

44. Breitbart W, Tremblay A, Gibson C. An open trial of olanzapine for the treatment of delirium in hospitalized cancer patients. *Psychosomatics.* 2002;43(3):175–182.

45. Meagher DJ, O'Hanlon D, O'Mahony E, Casey PR, Trzepacz PT. Relationship between symptoms and motoric subtype of delirium. *J Neuropsychiatry Clin Neurosci.* 2000;12(1):51–56.

46. Stagno D, Gibson C, Breitbart W. The delirium subtypes: a review of prevalence, phenomenology, pathophysiology, and treatment response. *Palliat Support Care.* 2004;2(2):171–179.

47. Mittal D, Majithia D, Kennedy R, Rhudy J. Differences in characteristics and outcome of delirium as based on referral patterns. *Psychosomatics.* 2006;47(5):367–375.

48. de Rooij SE, Schuurmans MJ, van der Mast RC, Levi M. Clinical subtypes of delirium and their relevance for daily clinical practice: a systematic review. *Int J Geriatr Psychiatry.* 2005 Jul;20(7):609–615.

49. Peterson JF, Pun BT, Dittus RS, et al. Delirium and its motoric subtypes: a study of 614 critically ill patients. *J Am Geriatr Soc.* 2006;54(3):479–484.

50. DiMartini A, Dew MA, Kormos R, McCurry K, Fontes P. Posttraumatic stress disorder caused by hallucinations and delusions experienced in delirium. *Psychosomatics.* 2007;48(5):436–439.

51. Buss MK, Vanderwerker LC, Inouye SK, Zhang B, Block SD, Prigerson HG. Associations between caregiver-perceived delirium in patients with cancer and generalized anxiety in their caregivers. *J Palliat Med.* 2007;10(5):1083–1092.

52. Kiely DK, Jones RN, Bergmann MA, Marcantonio ER. Association between psychomotor activity delirium subtypes and mortality among newly admitted postacute facility patients. *J Gerontol A Biol Sci Med Sci.* 2007;62(2):174–179.

53. Breitbart W, Marotta R, Platt MM, et al. A double-blind trial of haloperidol, chlorpromazine, and lorazepam in the treatment of delirium in hospitalized AIDS patients. *Am J Psychiatry.* 1996;153(2):231–237.

54. Foley KM. Pain syndromes in patients with cancer. *Med Clin North Am.* 1987;71(2):169–84.

55. Morita T, Tei Y, Inoue S. Impaired communication capacity and agitated delirium in the final week of terminally ill cancer patients: prevalence and identification of research focus. *J Pain Symptom Manage.* 2003;26(3):827–834.

56. Morrison RS, Meier DE, Fischberg D, et al. Improving the management of pain in hospitalized adults. *Arch Intern Med.* 2006;166(9):1033–1039.

57. Nicholas LM, Lindsey BA. Delirium presenting with symptoms of depression. *Psychosomatics.* 1995;36(5):471–479.

58. Smith M, Breitbart W, Platt M. A Critique of instruments and methods to detect, diagnose, and rate delirium. *J Pain Symptom Manage.* 1994;10:35–77.

59. Breitbart W, Rosenfeld B, Roth A. The Memorial Delirium Assessment Scale. *J Pain Symptom Manage.* 1997;13:128–137.

60. Lawlor P, Nekolaichuck C, Gagnon B, Mancini I, Pereira J, Bruera E. Clinical utility, factor analysis and further validation of the Memorial Delirium Assessment Scale (MDAS). *Cancer*. 2000;88:2859–2867.

61. Trzepacz PT, Mittal D, Torres R, Kanary K, Norton J, Jimerson N. Validation of the Delirium Rating Scale-revised-98: comparison with the delirium rating scale and the cognitive test for delirium. *J Neuropsychiatry Clin Neurosci*. 2001 Spring;13(2):229–242.

62. Inouye B, Vandyck C, Alessi C. Clarifying confusion: the confusion assessment method, a new method for the detection of delirium. *Ann Intern Med*. 1990;113:941–948.

63. Trzepacz P, Baker R, Greenhouse J. A symptom rating scale of delirium. *Psychiatry Res*. 1988;23:89–97.

64. Ryan K, Leonard M, Guerin S, Donnelly S, Conroy M, Meagher D. Validation of the confusion assessment method in the palliative care setting. *Palliat Med*. 2009;23(1):40–45.

65. Bruera E, Macmillan K, Hanson J, MacDonald RN. The cognitive effects of the administration of narcotic analgesics in patients with cancer pain. *Pain*. 1989;39(1):13–16.

66. Casarett DJ, Inouye SK, American College of Physicians-American Society of Internal Medicine End-of-Life Care Consensus Panel. Diagnosis and management of delirium near the end of life. *Ann Intern Med*. 2001;135(1):32–40.

67. Lawlor PG, Bruera ED. Delirium in patients with advanced cancer. *Hematol Oncol Clin North Am*. 2002;16(3):701–714.

68. Fainsinger R, Bruera E. Treatment of delirium in a terminally ill patient. *J Pain Symptom Manage*. 1992;7(1):54–56.

69. Bruera E, Miller L, McCallion J, Macmillan K, Krefting L, Hanson J. Cognitive failure in patients with terminal cancer: a prospective study. *J Pain Symptom Manage*. 1992;7(4):192–195.

70. Inouye SK, Zhang Y, Jones RN, Kiely DK, Yang F, Marcantonio ER. Risk factors for delirium at discharge: development and validation of a predictive model. *Arch Intern Med*. 2007;167(13):1406–1413.

71. Pitkala KH, Laurila JV, Strandberg TE, Kautiainen H, Sintonen H, Tilvis RS. Multicomponent geriatric intervention for elderly inpatients with delirium: effects on costs and health-related quality of life. *J Gerontol A Biol Sci Med Sci*. 2008;63(1):56–61.

72. Milisen K, Lemiengre J, Braes T, Foreman MD. Multicomponent intervention strategies for managing delirium in hospitalized older people: systematic review. *J Adv Nurs*. 2005;52(1):79–90.

73. Liptzin B, Laki A, Garb JL, Fingeroth R, Krushell R. Donepezil in the prevention and treatment of post-surgical delirium. *Am J Geriatr Psychiatry*. 2005 Dec;13(12):1100–1106.

74. Sampson EL, Raven PR, Ndhlovu PN, et al. A randomized, double-blind, placebo-controlled trial of donepezil hydrochloride (Aricept) for reducing the incidence of postoperative delirium after elective total hip replacement. *Int J Geriatr Psychiatry*. 2007 Apr;22(4):343–349.

75. Han CS, Kim Y. A double-blind trial of risperidone and haloperidol for the treatment of delirium. *Psychosomatics*. 2004;45(4):297–301.

76. Hu H, Deng W, Yang H. A prospective random control study comparison of olanzapine and haloperidol in senile delirium. *Chongging Med J*. 2004;8:1234–1237.

77. Kalisvaart KJ, de Jonghe JF, Bogaards MJ, et al. Haloperidol prophylaxis for elderly hip-surgery patients at risk for delirium: a randomized placebo-controlled study. *J Am Geriatr Soc*. 2005;53(10):1658–1666.

78. Lonergan E, Britton AM, Luxenberg J, Wyller T. Antipsychotics for delirium. *Cochrane Database Syst Rev*. 2007;(2):CD005594.

79. Boettger S, Breitbart W. Atypical antipsychotics in the management of delirium: a review of the empirical literature. *Palliat Support Care*. 2005;3(3):227–237.

80. Jackson KC, Lipman AG. Drug therapy for delirium in terminally ill patients. *Cochrane Database Syst Rev*. 2004;(2):CD004770.

81. Derogatis LR, Feldstein M, Morrow G, et al. A survey of psychotropic drug prescriptions in an oncology population. *Cancer*. 1979;44(5):1919–1929.

82. Information for healthcare professionals: haloperidol (marketed as Haldol, Haldol Decanoate and Haldol Lactate). US Food & Drug Administration Web page. 2007. Accessed on September 2, 2009. http://www.fda.gov/CDER/DRUG/InfoSheets/HCP/haloperidol.htm.

83. Information for healthcare professionals: antipsychotics. US Food & Drug Administration Web page. Accessed on September 2, 2009. http://www.fda.gov/cder/drug/InfoSheets/HCP/antipsychotics_conventional.htm

84. Lawlor PG, Fainsinger RL, Bruera ED. Delirium at the end of life: critical issues in clinical practice and research. *JAMA*. 2000;284(19):2427–2429.

85. Gagnon B, Low G, Schreier G. Methylphenidate hydrochloride improves cognitive function in patients with advanced cancer and hypoactive delirium: a prospective clinical study. *J Psychiatry Neurosci*. 2005;30(2):100–107.

86. Keen JC, Brown D. Psychostimulants and delirium in patients receiving palliative care. *Palliat Support Care*. 2004;2(2):199–202.

87. Morita T, Otani H, Tsunoda J, Inoue S, Chihara S. Successful palliation of hypoactive delirium due to multi-organ failure by oral methylphenidate. *Support Care Cancer*. 2000;8(2):134–137.

88. Mukadam N, Ritchie CW, Sampson EL. Cholinesterase inhibitors for delirium: what is the evidence? *Int Psychogeriatr*. 2008;20(2):209–218.

89. Overshott R, Karim S, Burns A. Cholinesterase inhibitors for delirium. *Cochrane Database Syst Rev*. 2008;(1):CD005317.

90. Kalisvaart CJ, Boelaarts L, de Jonghe JF, Hovinga IM, Kat MG. Successful treatment of three elderly patients suffering from prolonged delirium using the cholinesterase inhibitor rivastigmine. *Ned Tijdschr Geneeskd*. 2004;148(30):1501–1504.

91. Inouye SK, Bogardus ST Jr, Charpentier PA, et al. A multicomponent intervention to prevent delirium in hospitalized older patients. *N Engl J Med*. 1999;340(9):669–766.

92. Siddiqi N, Stockdale R, Britton AM, Holmes J. Interventions for preventing delirium in hospitalised patients. *Cochrane Database Syst Rev*. 2007;(2):CD005563.

93. Marcantonio ER, Flacker JM, Wright RJ, Resnick NM. Reducing delirium after hip fracture: a randomized trial. *J Am Geriatr Soc*. 2001 May;49(5):516–522.

94. Ventafridda V, Ripamonti C, DeConno F. Symptom prevalence and control during cancer patients' last days of life. *J Palliat Care*. 1990;6:7–11.

95. Fainsinger RL, Waller A, Bercovici M, et al. A multicentre international study of sedation for uncontrolled symptoms in terminally ill patients. *Palliat Med*. 2000 Jul;14(4):257–265.

96. Rietjens JA, van Zuylen L, van Veluw H, et al. Palliative sedation in a specialized unit for acute palliative care in a cancer hospital: comparing patients dying with and without palliative sedation. *J Pain Symptom Manage*. Apr 12, 2008. E-pub ahead of print.

97. Connor SR, Pyenson B, Fitch K, Spence C, Iwasaki K. Comparing hospice and nonhospice patient survival among patients who die within a three-year window. *J Pain Symptom Manage*. 2007 Mar;33(3):238–246.

98. Sykes N, Thorns A. Sedative use in the last week of life and the implications for end-of-life decision making. *Arch Intern Med*. 2003;163(3):341–344.

99. Morita T, Chinone Y, Ikenaga M, et al. Efficacy and safety of palliative sedation therapy: a multicenter, prospective, observational study conducted on specialized palliative care units in Japan. *J Pain Symptom Manage*. 2005;30(4):320–328.

100. Bercovitch M, Adunsky A. Patterns of high-dose morphine use in a home-care hospice service: should we be afraid of it? *Cancer*. 2004 Sep 15;101(6):1473–1477.

101. Vitetta L, Kenner D, Sali A. Sedation and analgesia-prescribing patterns in terminally ill patients at the end of life. *Am J Hosp Palliat Care*. 2005 Nov-Dec;22(6):465–473.

102. Lo B, Rubenfeld G. Palliative sedation in dying patients: "We turn to it when everything else hasn't worked." *JAMA*. 2005;294(14):1810–1816.

103. Morita T, Tsunoda J, Inoue S, Chihara S. Validity of the palliative performance scale from a survival perspective. *J Pain Symptom Manage*. 1999 Jul;18(1):2–3.

104. Caraceni A, Nanni O, Maltoni M, et al. Impact of delirium on the short term prognosis of advanced cancer patients. Italian Multicenter Study Group on Palliative Care. *Cancer*. 2000 Sep 1;89(5):1145–1149.

CHAPTER 46

Substance Abuse and Alcohol

Lauren J. Rogak, Tatiana D. Starr, and Steven D. Passik

INTRODUCTION

Substance abuse and addiction are among the most serious and complicated challenges faced by clinicians in an oncologic setting where opioid analgesics and other controlled substances are the cornerstones of care. For a small subset of cancer patients, exposure to opioids in the setting of their cancer care can potentially lead to the exacerbation or development of a set of problems that are becoming more and more common. This may be especially true for younger patients whose genetic and other vulnerabilities to addiction are not fully expressed by the time of their first opioid exposure during cancer treatments. The integration of pain management and addiction medicine has been slow in coming, and many psycho-oncologists lack specific training in these areas. There is a need to develop programs for managing the small, but labor intensive and difficult subset of higher addiction risk patients in cancer centers. Individualizing care for these patients is essential. Similarly, alcohol abuse complicates cancer care. For example, postsurgical withdrawal and delirium tremens (DTs) can be life threatening. Unfortunately many patients are recognized before surgery. Screening for alcoholism and doing offering detoxification ahead of surgery is an ongoing problem. This chapter will summarize and characterize the prescription opioid problem, clarify the relationship between opioid prescribing and prescription drug abuse, address the clinical aspects of alcoholism and cancer, examine issues of adherence in cancer pain patients and discuss some strategies for the higher risk subgroups. Furthermore, the need to address the high-risk problem by institutionalizing screening and employing recent improvements in urine screening and prescription monitoring programs, now commonplace in noncancer pain management, is discussed.

PREVALENCE

The backdrop for cancer pain management is a growing problem of prescription drug abuse. The incidence of prescription pain medication abuse has quadrupled over the past decade from 573,000 in 1990 to 2.5 million in 2002.[1] Furthermore, in 2004 the estimated number of new initiates to prescription drug abuse was 2.4 million, exceeding illicit drugs including marijuana (2.1 million) and cocaine (1 million).[2] The high prevalence of prescription drug abuse is a source of much concern in the medical setting, especially in the context of treating cancer pain, where it might not be the patient but, for example, the child who may be at risk. When working with patients with progressive life-threatening diseases who have a remote or current history of drug abuse, physical and psychosocial concerns that could potentially affect pain management and treatment must be addressed. The therapeutic use of such potentially abusable drugs and the abuse of these drugs is complex and must be understood to provide optimal patient care.[3]

The prevalence of substance abuse in the cancer population is relatively low. In 1990, only 3% of inpatient and outpatient consultations performed by the Psychiatry Service at Memorial Sloan-Kettering Cancer Center (MSKCC) included a request for management of issues related to substance abuse. This number is significantly lower than the overall prevalence of substance use disorders found in society, general medical populations, and emergency medical departments.[4–8] The Psychiatric Collaborative Oncology Group study assessed psychiatric diagnoses in ambulatory cancer patients from several tertiary care hospitals and also reported a similarly low-prevalence rate.[6] In a past study which followed structured clinical interviews, less than 5% of 215 cancer patients met the *Diagnostic and statistical manual for mental disorders* (DSM) 3rd edition criteria for a substance use disorder.[9] This study has yet to be replicated, and therefore the prevalence data have unclear relevance to today's cancer population, particularly those that are community based. The relatively low prevalence of substance abuse among cancer patients treated in tertiary care hospitals is not easily understood, considering the availability and accessibility to prescription pain medications. The fact that abuse rates are significantly lower in populations where individuals are actually exposed to potentially abusable medications more easily and frequently than the general population is in many ways counterintuitive, but is likely a result of many factors described below.

There have been relatively few studies that have examined the prevalence of alcoholism in an oncology population. The prevalence likely varies widely from one cancer to another with the highest rate found in the head and neck cancer population. One study found that greater than 25% of patients admitted to a palliative care unit were found to have problems with alcohol abuse.[10] The prevalence of alcoholism in major cancer centers is most likely underestimated. Socioeconomic barriers such as low income or unemployment, lack of health insurance, and possibly even attempts to self-medicate early signs of malignancies may preclude patients from seeking care at tertiary care centers. A study by Bruera and colleagues[10] of 100 terminally ill alcoholic cancer patients found that despite multiple hospital admissions and screenings, only one-third had documentation of alcoholism in their medical records.

The low-prevalence rates of alcohol and substance abuse may be a result from a variety of factors. First, there may be institutional biases or a tendency for patient underreporting in these settings. It has been shown that a high percentage of drug abusers fall into the lower socioeconomic bracket, feel alienated from the healthcare system, and may not seek care in tertiary centers, and therefore may show hesitation to acknowledge a history of drug abuse because of the potential for stigmatization. The fact that cancer patients are generally older, 50 and older, probably also explains the low-addiction rate. Most addictions are manifested by age 35.[11] If patients have never had problems with drugs or alcohol use before cancer in mid or late life, it is highly unlikely that a problem will develop de novo. In a survey of patients admitted to a palliative care unit, 25% had a current or remote history of alcohol abuse.[12] Additional studies are needed to clarify the epidemiology of substance abuse and addiction in cancer patients and other populations with progressive medical diseases. To adequately and successful treat a patient, the presence of a substance use disorder must be accurately assessed and diagnosed.

DEFINITIONS OF ABUSE AND ADDICTION

Among the most significant challenges of managing substance abuse within the cancer pain population is the lack of uniform terminology.[13] While epidemiologic studies and clinical management depend on an accepted, valid nomenclature for substance abuse and addiction, the current terminology is highly problematic. This is partially due to the fact that the pharmacologic phenomena of tolerance and physical dependence are commonly confused with abuse and addiction.[13] Defining abuse and addiction in medically ill populations, specifically oncology, has additional challenges because these terms were originally developed to assess the general population of addicts without the addition of a painful co-existing medical illness. Since many clinicians are not trained in and do not specialize in treating co-occurring substance abuse they may confuse behaviors associated with tolerance and dependence with those of abuse and addiction.[13] The presence of this additional barrier only furthers the need to accurately define this terminology in the context of oncology. The clarification of this terminology is a critical step toward improving the diagnosis and management of substance abuse as well as promoting pain management and overall patient care.

Tolerance. Tolerance is a pharmacologic phenomenon characterized by the need to increase doses to maintain the effect of the medication.[14,15] Tolerance has been associated with increasing pain or disease progression, and is not automatically a sign of abuse or addiction.[16–24] This has been a particular concern with use of opioid therapy. It is common for both clinicians and patients to express concerns that developing a tolerance to analgesics may compromise the benefits of therapy and lead to the requirement for progressively higher, and ultimately unsustainable, doses. Furthermore, the development of tolerance to the reinforcing effects of opioids, and the resulting need to escalate doses to maintain these effects, may be an important element in the pathogenesis of addiction.[25]

In the face of these concerns, extensive clinical experience with opioid drugs in the medical context has shown that tolerance rarely leads to substantial problems, including addiction.[17,20] Tolerance to a variety of opioid effects can be reliably observed in animal models,[26] and tolerance to nonanalgesic effects, such as respiratory depression and cognitive impairment,[27] occurs regularly in the clinical setting. However, analgesic tolerance does not appear to routinely interfere with the clinical efficacy of opioid drugs. Research has shown that most patients can manage stable doses of opioids and can demonstrate a balance between analgesia and side effects for prolonged periods. Tolerance to medication has shown to be indicative of escalating pain or disease progression. Unlike tolerance to the side effects of the opioids, clinically meaningful analgesic tolerance seems to be a rare phenomenon, and is infrequently the cause for dose escalation.[16,18,19,21–24]

Clinical observation lacks support for the conclusion that analgesic tolerance is a significant contributor to the development of addiction. Generally, addicts presenting without a co-occurring medical condition may or may not have any of the manifestations of analgesic tolerance. Occasionally, there are opioid-treated patients who present manifestations consistent with analgesic tolerance; however they typically do so without evidence of abuse or addiction.[3,26]

Physical dependence. Physical dependence is characterized by the occurrence of a withdrawal syndrome that follows a rapid decrease in dosage or administering an antagonist.[14,15,28] There is significant confusion among clinicians where the properties of physical dependence and addiction diverge. Similar to tolerance, physical dependence has been suggested to be an element of addiction,[29,30] such that the avoidance of withdrawal has been theorized to create behavioral contingencies that reinforce drug-seeking behavior.[25] Notably, the experience of physical dependence does not necessarily lead to impediments throughout the discontinuation of opioids in patients with nonmalignant pain,[31] and cessation of opioid therapy commonly occurs without difficulty in cancer patients, whose pain is diminished after completion of antineoplastic therapy. Circuitous evidence for a primary distinction between physical dependence and addiction has been provided by animal models of opioid self-administration, which have demonstrated that chronic drug-taking behavior can be maintained in the absence of physical dependence.[32]

Concerns over current definitions. The inconsistent definitions of tolerance and physical dependence emphasize deficiencies in the current nomenclature within the context of substance abuse. Specifically, the terms "addiction" and "addict" are exceptionally problematic. These labels have a tendency to be inadequately applied to describe both aberrant drug use (reminiscent of the behaviors that characterize active abusers of illicit drugs) and phenomena related to tolerance or physical dependence. Clinicians and patients may use the word "addicted" to describe compulsive drug taking in one patient and nothing more than the potential for withdrawal in another. This lack of universal understanding of these terms fosters concerns from patients, families, and staff about the outcome of opioid treatment when this term is applied.[33]

Patients who are perceived to have the capacity for an abstinence syndrome should never be labeled as "addicts" or having an "addiction." Rather, these patients should be identified as "physically dependent." Additionally, applying the label "dependent" alone also should be discouraged as it creates confusion between physical dependence and psychological dependence, which is a component of addiction. Similarly, the term "habituation" should not be used as to reduce any further confusion.[3]

CLINICAL ISSUES

There are many inpatient issues that impact the management of cancer patients with a history of addiction.

Co-morbid psychiatric disorders. Individuals who are alcoholics have been found to be at higher risk for other psychiatric disorders.[34] Christie and colleagues estimate that 78% of people with drug and alcohol problems have had a psychiatric disorder in their lifetime. The most common co-morbid mental disorders associated with alcoholism are anxiety disorders (19.4%), antisocial personality disorder (14.3%), affective disorder (13.4%), and schizophrenia (3.8%).[35] The occurrence of co-morbid mental disorders in alcoholics may contribute to poor treatment compliance and success due to cognitive limitations and premorbid (in relation to the diagnosis of cancer) pain and neurological deficits. The same is true of opioid abuse where 85% of addicts have a co-morbid, nondrug abuse related psychological disorder.[36] Thus, the psycho-oncologist assessing the cancer patient with addiction or alcoholism must identify and treat any co-morbid disorders present.

Aberrant drug-related behaviors. Treatment with potentially abusable medications, specifically opioids, may be complicated by concerns regarding aberrant drug-related behavior, addiction, and abuse. Such concerns are often complicated by the lack of empirical information that helps distinguish behaviors that signify abuse or addiction. As such, the problematic behaviors that are indicative of abuse and addiction are unclear to many clinicians, making the need to incorporate continuous assessment throughout treatment a critical part of pain management. Aberrant behavior can be described as any questionable drug-related behaviors exhibited by the patient that are suggestive of abuse.[33] Such behaviors vary significantly in severity or frequency, and should be viewed along a continuum that ranges from mild, or limited (e.g., use of a prescribed dose to self-medicate a problem not intended by the clinician, such as insomnia) to more severe or overwhelming behaviors (e.g., injection of an oral formulation) and have to potential to predict addiction[37] (see Table 46–1). Noncompliance must be discussed clearly and at length between patients and clinicians.

The identification of such aberrant behaviors should lead the clinician to formulate a differential diagnosis to guide a clinical response that will address the patient's behavior.[37] The main goal of such assessments is to determine the underlying nature of the problem which will foster development of an appropriate therapeutic intervention.[38,39]

The differential diagnosis may distinguish between a "true" addiction (a substance use disorder) and a "pseudo-addiction" (desperate behaviors motivated by unrelieved pain). Escalating drug-seeking behaviors may be exhibited in patients with addiction disorders as a result of untreated pain, reflecting both addiction and pseudo-addiction; this distinction is among the most confounding differential diagnoses.[40] Impulsive drug use may also be rooted in an underlying psychiatric disorder. For example, a patient with borderline personality disorder may engage in aberrant drug use to relieve boredom or to convey fear or anger. Likewise, patients suffering from depression, anxiety, or insomnia may self-medicate with their prescription drugs to obtain relief from the discomfort of their symptoms.[37] Additional explanations for aberrant drug use include criminal intent (drug diversion), or familial dysfunction (family members taking the patient's medication for their own use).[38,41]

Table 46–1. The spectrum of aberrant drug-related behaviors

Aberrant drug-related behaviors more suggestive of addiction	Aberrant drug-related behaviors less suggestive of addiction
Selling prescription drugs	Aggressive complaining about need for higher doses
Prescription forgery	Drug hoarding during periods of reduced symptoms
Stealing or borrowing another patient's drugs	Requesting specific drugs
Injecting oral formulation	Acquisition of similar drugs from other medical sources
Obtaining prescription drugs from nonmedical sources	Unsanctioned dose escalation, 1–2 times
Concurrent abuse of related illicit drugs	Unapproved use of the drug to treat another symptom
Multiple unsanctioned dose escalations	Reporting psychic effects not intended by the clinician
Recurrent prescription losses	

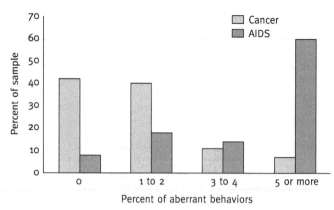

Fig. 46–1. Aberrant behaviors in cancer and AIDS. (Passik, Kirsh et al 2006).

ABBREVIATION: AIDS, acquired immunodeficiency syndrome.

Aberrant drug-related behaviors in medically ill populations. Investigating the prevalence and correlates of aberrant drug-related behavior in various populations (i.e., cancer and acquired immunodeficiency syndrome [AIDS]) will facilitate an understanding of these populations and behaviors. The following two studies illustrate the conceptual and assessment issues in substance abuse in medically ill populations with the presence of pain.

Passik and colleagues[33] examined self-reported attitudes toward aberrant drug taking and behaviors in a sample of cancer (n = 52) and AIDS (n = 111) patients using a questionnaire designed specifically for the purposes of their study. The authors found that patients in both groups reported past drug use and abuse more frequently than present drug use and abuse in, and current problematic drug-related behaviors were seldom reported. However, attitude items showed that in the context of unrelieved pain, patients would consider engaging in aberrant drug use, or conceivably excuse others engaging in these behaviors for the same reason. The authors also found that aberrant behaviors and attitudes were endorsed more frequently by women in the AIDS group than by the patients in the cancer group. Moreover, patients significantly overestimated addiction risk in pain treatment. Use of this questionnaire demonstrated a forthcoming and open response from, both, cancer and AIDS patients in regard to drug-related behaviors and attitudes. Experience with this questionnaire suggests these attitudes and behaviors may be relevant to the diagnosis and treatment of substance use disorders.

Another study by Passik and colleagues[42] looked at the prevalence and correlates of aberrant drug-taking behaviors in two populations: patients with HIV-related pain and a history of substance abuse (n = 73) and patients with cancer pain and no history of substance abuse (n = 100). This study employed a battery of questionnaires assessing substance abuse history, levels of pain depression, distress, and other related variables. The results showed, over both groups, that expressing anxiety or depression over recurrent symptoms and hoarding medications were the two most frequent aberrant behaviors seen. More specifically, the AIDS subgroup showed significant more use of potentially aberrant behaviors then the cancer group (see Fig. 46–1). Within the AIDS group, a low percentage of pain relief from to current analgesic therapy was found to be related to increased opioid doses without doctors orders, using more opioids then recommended, using opioids to treat other nonrelated symptoms, and admitting to family members they use other, street drugs to relieve pain. While in the cancer group, drinking alcohol to relieve pain was the only aberrant behavior significantly related to a low percentage of pain relief from current analgesic therapy. Additionally, the AIDS patients showed higher levels of psychological distress, depression, interference related to residual pain then cancer patients and less reported relief from current medications. Overall, the results of this study leads to the conclusion that aberrant behaviors seem connected to substance abuse and psychosocial distress than pain and analgesic variables.

These studies can be helpful in understanding the specific diagnostic meaning of different behaviors in different populations so that clinicians may identify which are the real "red flags" in a given population. Much too frequently, clinicians' perspective of these behaviors are shaped by anecdotal accounts. Some behaviors have been almost universally regarded as problematic despite limited systematic data to support this idea. An example of this is the patient who asks for a particular pain medication, or requests a specific route of administration or dose. These behaviors may appear to be aberrant based upon their face value; however, they may have limited predictive validity for true addiction. These behaviors may be more indicative of a patient who is knowledgeable about what works for them.

Primary or secondary abuse. The relationship between drug or alcohol abuse and co-existing psychiatric conditions is complex. While some patients' abuse is primary, creating mood and anxiety syndromes, for other patients it is secondary, reflecting out-of-control self-medication of mood and anxiety disorders.[43–45] Whether alcohol or substance use is primary or secondary, and whether it can be targeted for appropriate treatment is difficult to determine unless the patient's drug or alcohol use can be controlled. For example, a patient experiencing insomnia may experience it as a primary symptom or as a result of withdrawal or intoxication (secondary). The distinction between primary and secondary symptoms can only be made once control over patient's abusive behaviors can be obtained.[46]

NONMEDICAL USERS VERSUS CANCER PAIN PATIENTS

The rising tide of prescription drug abuse has created new dilemmas for cancer pain management. There is now a heterogeneous population of people who use prescription drugs, which can be broken down into two broad sections: nonmedical users and pain patients. Nonmedical users are comprised of people who aren't being prescribed the medications; often they are using someone else's, or acquiring them in other illegal ways (stealing, buying, etc.). The pain patients are patients living with chronic noncancer or cancer pain who require these medications to aid their quality of life. These broad groups can be broken down even further. Among the nonmedical users, those who are addicted, those who abuse, or those who use prescription drugs recreationally and those who are self-treaters. Among pain patients are the adherent pain patients, "chemical coping pain patients" (using medications to self-medicate bonafide problems) and those with substance abuse and addiction (see Fig. 46–2). In the following section, we will describe these subgroups and discuss the implications for clinicians when faced with these patients.

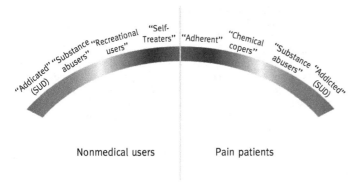

Nonmedical users   Pain patients

Fig. 46–2. Population of Rx opioid users is heterogeneous.

Cancer pain patients. When working with cancer pain patients, clinicians must learn how to recognize and manage patients who don't use medications as prescribed. Most cancer patients are adherent. These are patients who follow dosing schedules, do not increase or decrease doses without a doctors permissions. In other words, they adhere to the schedule their doctor implements, often one that can be quite flexible as a result.

Eduardo Bruera and colleagues coined the term "Chemical Copers." Chemical coping is a construct that was derived from the fine line between adherence and aberrancy[47] as a way to illustrate an archetype of maladaptive coping via substances.[48] This construct was first applied to a sample of cancer patients with high rates of historical substance abuse, which was furthered by the distress associated with cancer.[48] There are distinguishing traits associated with these patients who fall into the chemical copers category. These patients are guided by stress whereas when it becomes unmanageable, they are inclined to increase drug dose and deviate from the treatment path. Another trait of chemical copers is the lack of interest in nonpharmacological treatments.[47]

Within the construct of chemical coping, four associated features are seen: (1) self-medication,[49] (2) sensation seeking, (3) alexithymia, and (4) somatization. The first concept, the self-medication hypothesis, maintains that patients misuse substances to relieve feelings of physical or emotional distress as well as are drawn toward specific pharmacological substances.[49] Sensation seeking is defined as a proclivity to complicated and powerful experiences and will go outside the box to attain these feelings. The goal of sensation seeking is to find an alternative to everyday states of mind whereas chemical coping is a strategy used to avoid feelings of distress.[50] Alexithymia is characterized as the inability to manage and grasp emotions and feelings. These patients present with somatic complaints and have little to no emotional connection thereby solely relying on physical feelings.[51] The last associated feature, somatization, is a process where mental and emotional stresses are expressed by physical symptoms. These people are not always aware that they are misconstruing emotional distress as physical symptoms. The major problem is, the patients who actual believe these feelings are experiencing these physical pains and discomforts.[52]

Overall, these are patients under the onslaught of all the negative effects and fears and existential issues around cancer who don't cope well and seek out more centrally acting drugs and become overmedicated and can therefore not function. They are the prime candidates for psychiatric intervention coupled with the simplified drug regimens to learn to cope more efficiently and deal with their cancer in more adaptive ways.

Nonmedical users. Nonmedical users run the gamut from experimenters to self-medicators to true addicts. Starting in the 80s and 90s until the present pain relievers have become the single most sought after class of nonmedically used substances in our society and lead the way as first drugs for initiation by young users. According to the 2005 National Survey on Drug Use and Health, 2,193,000 people have reported the nonmedical use of prescription pain relievers, 526,000 of these people are new users of OxyContin.[53]

This subset of nonmedical users are not seen as pain patients, they are self-treating their diagnosed symptoms, conditions, and ailments with medications from nonmedical professionals that is, parents, sibling, grandparent, friends, and so on. According to the 2005 National Survey on Drug Use and Health 59.8% of nonmedical users obtain pain relievers from a friend or relative, 16.8% from one doctor, 4.3% from a dealer or stranger and 0.8% from the internet.[53]

The fast growing population of nonmedical users of prescription drugs are college-aged women.[54] They are often playing "arm chair pharmacist" with one another; that is, taking someone else's prescription sleeping pill because they are so stressed out and haven't slept, taking someone's methylphenidate because they have to stay up to study.[54] The existence of this phenomenon places new responsibilities on cancer pain clinicians and pain patients. Education about storage and not sharing medications is essential even in adherence patients.

CASE STUDY

This patient highlights issues surrounding drug selection. The patient is a male in his mid 50s who presented to the pain service with advanced bladder cancer via the urgent care center with his first pain crisis. Specifically was seen for "failure to thrive in need of pain control." Patient was assessed for depression and reported to have found religion 5 years prior. Patient is in recovery for a lifelong heroin addiction, currently in recovery. Notably, the patient is living in an unstable social situation: lives in a rented room in a flop house in a "tough part" of town, where there is a constant flow of younger men and women coming and going at all hours throughout the night. It is important to emphasize, that this is the patients first ever pain crisis. The first line of treatment presented is OxyContin, the most abused medicine on the street along with hydromorphone rescues. This represents the lack of concern in the forefront of most medical oncologists. They are focusing on alleviating the patient pain, not that the street value of the drug they are prescribing or the patients' social situation. This case study represents the need to education prescribing physicians about the increase in prescription drug abuse, and how to go about safely prescribing these medications.

ASSESSMENT

The first member of the medical team (often a nurse) to suspect drug or alcohol abuse should alert the team to begin the multidisciplinary assessment and management process. Too often, the fear of offending or stigmatizing the patient leaves signs of alcohol or drug abuse neglected. A physician should assess the potential of withdrawal or other pressing concerns and begin involving other staff (i.e., social work and/or psychiatry) to begin planning management strategies.

Successful treatment for ongoing pain management relies on the recognition of potentially dangerous drug-related behaviors. Extensive clinical experience has led to the development of guidelines specifically tailored to monitor chronic pain patients receiving opioid therapy, known as the "4 A's."[55] The "4 A's" incorporates the critical domains of pain management including: (1) Analgesia; (2) Activities of daily living; (3) Adverse side effects; and (4) Aberrant drug-taking behaviors. Continuous monitoring of these domains throughout treatment can provide clinicians with a useful framework that informs decision making and fosters compliance to the therapeutic use of controlled substances.[56]

Taking an accurate, detailed history from the patient is essential for the proper assessment and treatment of alcohol and drug abuse as well as any co-morbid psychiatric disorders. It is also important to ask information regarding duration, frequency, and desired effect of the drug or alcohol consumption. In the wake of current pressures to treat the majority of patients in the ambulatory setting, and to admit patients on the morning of major surgery, the quick identification of alcoholism and initiation of plans for social, medical, and physiological needs of the patient must begin upon initial contact. Alcohol and drug use is typically underreported, specifically in terms of frequency, quantity, and duration because of embarrassment, fear of stigmatization from the medical staff, and/or strong defense mechanisms, primarily denial.

When prescribing ongoing opioid therapy, particularly outside the context of ongoing cancer treatment (i.e., in long-term survivors), it is important to demonstrate that the 4 A's (Analgesia, Activities, Adverse Effects, and Aberrant Behavior)[57] are being assessed. Sufficient documentation is also especially helpful if the propriety of ongoing opioid therapy is ever questioned, however it is necessary for providing optimal treatment during the pain management process. Predesigned structured chart notes do exist[55] in the literature and can be utilized to guide clinicians toward better note writing and documentation.

Frequently, clinicians avoid asking patients about drug or alcohol abuse out of fear of an erroneous suspicion or that they will anger the patient. However, this approach will likely contribute to continued problems with treatment compliance and frustration among staff. Therefore, empathic and truthful communication is generally the best approach. The use of a careful, graduated interview approach can be instrumental in slowly introducing the patient's drug or alcohol use. The assessment interview should begin with broad questions about the patient's drug or alcohol use (e.g., nicotine or caffeine) in the patient's life and gradually becoming more specific in focus to include more aberrant drug and alcohol use. This type of approach is helpful in reducing denial and resistance that the patient may express.

Consultations with family members or close friends of the patient may be helpful in verifying the accuracy of the patient's reports and level of denial. However, the presence of co-dependent behavior (i.e., denial or enabling) should also be considered when interviewing family or friends of a drug- or alcohol-abusing cancer patient. In active abusers, time of last drug intake or alcohol consumption should be noted and the prevention of withdrawal should become first priority. This type of interview will also assist in identifying the presence of co-existing psychiatric disorders that may be present. Assessment and treatment of co-morbid psychiatric disorders can enhance management strategies and reduce the risk of relapse. Understanding the patient's desired effects from alcohol or drug use can often point to co-occurring psychiatric disorders (e.g., drinking to relieve panic symptoms).

Owing to the high prevalence of abuse of opioids, clinicians must be aware of the risk factors and vulnerabilities associated. As an aid in understanding which patients are at more risk, the opioid risk tool (ORT) is a screening tool comprised of five self-report items that evaluate risk potential for opioid abuse[58] (see Table 46–2). The ORT is designed to be administered to patients whose chronic pain is planned

to be treated with opioids at the clinical visit before initiation of treatment. This measure allows for evaluation of patients before the initiation of opioid therapy thereby allowing clinicians to classify patients into one of three categories; low risk, moderate risk, or high risk. The low risk (scoring 0–3) refers to those who are unlikely to abuse opioids; moderate risk (scoring 4–7) are seen as just as likely to abuse opioids as they are not to abuse; and high risk (greater than 8) refers to the group with highest likelihood to abuse.[58] The simplicity of the ORT allows the clinician to begin treatment while monitoring the underlying risk factors presented. Furthermore, the clinician is able to tailor treatment to meet the individual needs of each patient.[58,59]

Another assessment took to asses risk factors when initiating treatment with patients is the CAGE assessment tool. The CAGE is a four-question instrument that is been used primarily in clinical settings to identify people who have a history of alcohol dependency. The acronym CAGE aligns with the four questions: cut back, annoyance by critics, guilt about drinking, and eye-opening morning drinking. A positive response to two or more of the four a potential alcohol problem.[60] Using this cut off value, the CAGE's sensitivity in various populations ranges from 61% to 100%, and its specificity ranges from 77% to 96%.[61,62]

Alcohol withdrawal syndrome. All too frequently, alcoholism is not identified until the manifestations of alcohol withdrawal syndrome are present. According to the *Diagnostic statistical manual*, 4th edition, the alcoholic in withdrawal has decreased or stopped his or her prolonged ingestion of alcohol.[29]

Alcohol withdrawal is dangerous and can seriously complicate cancer treatment. In some instances, it is fatal. The first symptoms of withdrawal typically appear in the first few hours following the cessation of alcohol consumption and may consist of tremors, agitation, and insomnia. In cases of mild to moderate withdrawal, these symptoms tend to dissipate within 1–2 days without recurrence. However, in cases of severe withdrawal, autonomic hyperactivity, hallucinations, and disorientation may follow. The onset of DTs marks the individual's progression from the withdrawal state to a state of delirium that represents a serious medical emergency. DTs occur in approximately 5%–15% of patients in alcohol withdrawal typically within the first 72–96 hours of withdrawal and is characterized by agitation, hallucination, delusions, incoherence, and disorientation.[63] DTs is self-limiting and usually ends in 72 to 96 hours with the patient entering a deep sleep with amnesia for most of what had occurred. However, in the medically ill patients, the risk of further complications is high and the disorder must be treated.

Wernicke–Korsakoff's syndrome is indicative of a thiamine deficiency and represents a frequently underdiagnosed, debilitating disorder that causes permanent cognitive impairment. Although not a result of the development of DTs, the level of alcohol consumption required for the development of DTs is sufficient to cause thiamine depletion. Symptoms of Wernicke–Korsakoff syndrome may include a fixed upward gaze, alcoholic neuropathy, "stocking-glove" paresthesia, autonomic instability, and delirium encephalopathy.

Medical treatment of withdrawal. While a full discussion of the pharmacological approach to alcohol withdrawal is beyond the scope of this paper, a basic approach to the treatment of this syndrome is given. The use of hydration, benzodiazepines, and, in some cases, neuroleptics are appropriate for the management of alcohol withdrawal syndrome (see Table 46–3). The administration of a vitamin-mineral solution is indicated to counteract the effects of malnutrition that results from the alcohol itself and poor eating habits. Thiamine 100 mg administered intramuscularly or intravenously (IV) for 3 days before switching to oral administration for the duration of treatment to prevent the development of Karsakoff's syndrome and alcoholic dementia. A daily oral dose of folate 1 mg should also be given throughout the course of treatment. In cases of mild withdrawal, hydration alone may be sufficient. Benzodiazepines (lorazepam, midazolam, diazepam, and chlordiazepoxide) are the drugs of choice for the management of alcohol withdrawal because of their sedative effects (see Table 46–4).[64,65] Careful consideration must be given to route, absorption, potency, and dose of benzodiazepine prescribed. Dose should be based upon estimated

Table 46–2. Opioid risk tool

		Female	Male
Is there a history of substance abuse in your family?	Alcohol	[ ] 1	[ ] 3
	Illegal drugs	[ ] 2	[ ] 3
	Other	[ ] 4	[ ] 4
Have you had a history of substance abuse?	Alcohol	[ ] 3	[ ] 3
	Illegal drugs	[ ] 4	[ ] 4
	prescription drugs	[ ] 5	[ ] 5
Is your age between 16 and 45?		[ ] 1	[ ] 1
Is there a history of preadolescent (childhood) sexual abuse?		[ ] 3	[ ] 0
Do you have a history of any of the following conditions?	ADD, OCD, bipolar, scihzophrenia?	[ ] 2	[ ] 2
		[ ] 1	[ ] 1
	Depression?		
Low (0–3) Moderate (4–7) High (8+)	Total	[ ]	[ ]

ABBREVIATIONS: ADD, attention-deficit disorder; OCD, obsessive-compulsive disorder; ORT, opioid risk tool

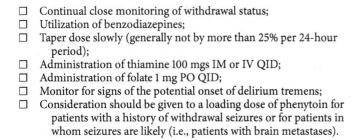

Table 46-3. Guidelines for the treatment of alcohol withdrawal

- ☐ Continual close monitoring of withdrawal status;
- ☐ Utilization of benzodiazepines;
- ☐ Taper dose slowly (generally not by more than 25% per 24-hour period);
- ☐ Administration of thiamine 100 mgs IM or IV QID;
- ☐ Administration of folate 1 mg PO QID;
- ☐ Monitor for signs of the potential onset of delirium tremens;
- ☐ Consideration should be given to a loading dose of phenytoin for patients with a history of withdrawal seizures or for patients in whom seizures are likely (i.e., patients with brain metastases).

ABBREVIATIONS: IM, intramuscular; IVM intravenous; PO, per oral; QID, quarter in die (Latin).

Table 46-4. Types and characteristics of benzodiazepines for treatment of alcohol withdrawal

Drug	Dose	Duration of action	Half-life (Hours)
Chlordiazepoxide	25–100 mg every 3 hours IV	Short	5–30
Diazepam	10–20 mg every 1–4 hours IV	Short	20–100
Lorazepam	1–2 mg every 1–4 hours IV	Intermediate	10–20
Midazolam	1–5 mg every 1–2 hours IV	Very short	1–4

alcohol consumption and the type of setting of detoxification (see below). Insufficient administration of benzodiazepines (too low dose; or too rapid taper) may allow the progression of withdrawal to a state of DTs. The development of seizures is life threatening and they may repeatedly recur in the patient while unconscious. The nonbenzodiazepine anticonvulsants are not prescribed prophylactically. In cases of severe withdrawal and confusion, neuroleptics (i.e., haloperidol 0.5–5.0 mg IV every 8 hours) are added to the treatment regimen. Commonly, alcoholic patients report to the hospital either intoxicated or in the early stages of withdrawal. From a surgical perspective, serious complications can arise from the presence of alcohol withdrawal and its acute management is the primary treatment goal. Unfortunately, clinicians are frequently provided insufficient lead time to properly detoxify the patient before surgery (typically less than 24 hours), the patient stands at an increased risk for the postoperative development of organic mental disorders, seizure, and DTs. Since alcoholic cancer patients are already at high risk for delirium postoperatively due to poor nutrition, prior head trauma, brain injury from excessive alcohol consumption, the development of seizures and DTs adds to the risk of fatality. It is important to note that since it desirable for the patient to be alert postoperatively for ambulation and use of pulmonary toilet, the amount of sedation required for detoxification is much lower than the desired level of sedation in a nonsurgical alcoholic patient.

TREATMENT MODALITIES

Alcohol and substance abuse is often a chronic, progressive disorder which can interfere with the treatment of a medical condition. As a result, the development of clear-cut treatment goals is crucial in treating alcoholism and substance abuse. Although, abstinence may be optimal, it is not necessarily a treatment goal for these patients in the oncology setting. Rather, the priority is a management plan that facilitates the effective implementation and continuation of cancer treatment. The most

common approaches to both alcoholism and substance abuse can be separated into psychotherapeutic and pharmacological interventions.

Psychotherapeutic approach. The most effective psychotherapeutic treatment approach with medically ill people appears to be one that focuses on the development of effective coping skills, relapse prevention, and most importantly, treatment compliance. Alcohol or the specific substance being abused, is representing one of the dependent patient's primary, albeit, maladaptive coping tools. As a result, the improvement of coping skills in these individuals is critical. When compounded with the stress associated with having cancer, the cessation can be overwhelming and contribute to noncompliance and discontinuation of treatment. Teaching specific, illness-related coping methods with an emphasis upon containing episodes of consumption is essential. Further, the recognition and treatment of anxiety and depression may decrease the patients need and desire for alcohol or substances. As an alternative to the abstinence approach, a harm reduction with crisis intervention as a central component should be utilized. The fundamental aims being enhancement of social support, maximization of treatment compliance, and to contain harm associated with episodic relapses. Further, minimizing the frequency and intensity of the patients use and consumption are the broad goals of treatment. Thereby, further damage to the patient will be reduced as well as the facilitation of treatment compliance.

Another psychotherapeutic approach that is beneficial for this population of patients is support groups and 12-step programs. The problem lies in that traditional 12 steps groups are based on an abstinence only policy. This poses a problem for the patients who are being treated with opioids for pain-related syndromes. More recently, support groups have been tailored for this specific population.

Pharmacological approach. Disulfiram (Antabuse) is a pharmacological agent that has been approved by the Food and Drug Administration (FDA) since 1951 for the treatment of alcoholism.[66] Antabuse serves as a deterrent by inducing an unpleasant physical state characterized by nausea or vomiting when alcohol is consumed, thus ideally leading to alcohol cessation.[66] The practicality and effectiveness of Antabuse is questionable; however, since its use has been limited by difficulties with patient adherence for continued use of the drug.[67]

There have been a number of studies that have shed light on subgroups of patients who have been shown to benefit the most from treatment with Antabuse. The findings have shown that patients with the following characteristics generally experience the most long-term benefits from Antabuse: (1) older than 40 years of age; (2) longer drinking histories; (3) socially stable; (4) highly motivated; (5) prior attendance of Alcoholics Anonymous; (6) cognitively intact; and (6) able to maintain and tolerate dependent or treatment relationships.[68–70] Further research is needed to ascertain what factors and patient characteristics will increase the likelihood of successful treatment. A greater understanding has the potential to significantly enhance clinicians' ability to select those patients who will experience optimal effectiveness.

Techniques such as supervised Antabuse treatment, or incentive-driven treatment has been shown to enhance adherence and have been associated with more positive outcomes including decreases in alcohol consumption and increased rate of abstinence.[71,72] Additionally, incorporating an adherence contract can be an effective tool to enhance treatment compliance. For example, patients can include in their contract to follow their prescribed Antabuse regimen under the supervision of a family member (e.g., spouse).[73]

Extensive clinical experience supports the current literature in that patients who will most likely benefit from Antabuse are those that are highly motivated. Patients wanting to preserve their ability to receive cancer treatment fit this bill. The use of long acting once a day alprazolam or clonazepam with Antabuse can help some make it through it.

CONCLUSION

Managing patients with drug and alcohol abuse and addiction is labor intensive and difficult. However, with a nonjudgmental structured approach can lead to satisfying outcomes in the most difficult of patients.

REFERENCES

1. Substance Abuse and Mental Health Services Administration (SAMHSA). Results from the 2003 national survey on drug use and health: national findings (NSDUH Series H-25, DHHS Publication No. SMA 04-3964). SAMHSA: Rockville, MD: Office of Applied Studies, Editor; 2004a.

2. Substance Abuse and Mental Health Services Administration (SAMHSA). Results from the 2004 national survey on drug use and health: national findings (NSDUH Series H-28, DHHS Publication No. SMA 05-4062). SAMHSA: Rockville, MD: Office of Applied Studies, Editor; 2005a.

3. Passik SD, Olden M, Kirsh KL, Portenoy RK.. Substance abuse issues in palliative care. In: Berger A, Portenoy RK, Weissman DE, (eds). *Principles and practice of palliative care and supportive oncology*. Lippincott Williams & Wilkins: PA; 2007:593–603.

4. Burton RW, Lyons JS, Devens M, Larson DB.. Psychiatric consultations for psychoactive substance disorders in the general hospital. *Gen Hosp Psychiatry*. 1991;13(2):83–87.

5. Colliver JD, Kopstein AN. Trends in cocaine abuse reflected in emergency room episodes reported to DAWN. Drug abuse warning network. *Public Health Rep*. 1991;106(1):59–68.

6. Derogatis LR, Morrow GR, Fetting J, et al. The prevalence of psychiatric disorders among cancer patients. *JAMA*, 1983;249(6):751–757.

7. Groerer J, Brodsky M, The incidence of illicit drug use in the United States, 1962–1989. *Br J Addict*. 1992;87(9):1345–1351.

8. Regier DA, Myers JK, Kramer M, et al. The NIMH Epidemiologic Catchment Area program. Historical context, major objectives, and study population characteristics. *Arch Gen Psychiatry*. 1984;41(10):934–941.

9. American Psychiatric Association. *Diagnostic and statistical manual for mental disorders III*. Washington DC: American Psychiatric Association; 1983.

10. Bruera E, Moyano J, Seifert L, et al. The frequency of alcoholism among patients with pain due to terminal cancer. *J Pain Symptom Manage*. 1995;10(8): 599–603.

11. Cloninger CR, Sigvardsson S, Bohman M. Childhood personality predicts alcohol abuse in young adults. *Alcohol Clin Exp Res*. 1988;12(4):494–505.

12. Bruera E, Moyano J, Seifert L, et al. The frequency of alcoholism among patients with pain due to terminal cancer. *J Pain Symptom Manage*. 1995;10(8):599–603.

13. Kirsh KL, Whitcomb LA, Donaghy L, Passik SD. Abuse and addiction issues in medically ill patients with pain: attempts at clarification of terms and empirical study. *Clin J Pain*. 2002;18:S52–S60.

14. Dole VP. Narcotic addiction, physical dependence and relapse. *N Engl J Med*. 1972;286(18):988–992.

15. Martin WR, Jasinski DR. Physiological parameters of morphine dependence in man—tolerance, early abstinence, protracted abstinence. *J Psychiatr Res*. 1969;7(1):9–17.

16. Chapman CR, Hill HF. Prolonged morphine self administration and addiction liability: evaluation of two theories in a bone marrow transplant unit. *Cancer*. 1989;63:1636–1644.

17. Foley KM. Clinical tolerance to opioids. In: Basbaum AU, Besson JM, (eds). *Towards a new pharmacotherapy of pain*. Chichester, UK: John Wiley and Sons; 1991:181.

18. France RD, Urban BJ, Keefe FJ. Long-term use of narcotic analgesics in chronic pain. *Soc Sci Med*. 1984;19:1379–1382.

19. Kanner RM, Foley KM. Patterns of narcotic drug use in a pacer pain clinic. *Ann N Y Acad Sci*. 1981;362:161–172.

20. Portenoy RK. Management of common opioid side effects during long-term therapy of cancer pain. *Ann Acad Med Singapore*. 1994;23(2):160–170.

21. Portenoy RK, Foley KM. Chronic use of opioid analgesics in non-malignant pain: report of 38 cases. *Pain*. 1986;25:171–186.

22. Twycross RG. Clinical experience with dia-morphine in advanced malignant disease. *Int J Clin Pharmacol Ther Toxicol*. 1974;7:187–198.

23. Urban BJ, France RD, Steinberger DL, Scott DL, Maltbie AA. Long term use of narcotic/antidepressant medication in the management of phantom limb pain. *Pain*. 1986;24:191–196.

24. Zenz M, Strumpf M, Tryba M. Long-term oral opioid therapy in patients with chronic nonmalignant pain. *J Pain Symptom Manage*. 1992;7(2):69–77.

25. Wikler A. *Opioid dependence: Mechanisms and treatment*. New York: Plenum Press; 1980.

26. Ling GS, Paul D, Simantov R, Pasternak GW.. Differential development of acute tolerance to analgesia, respiratory depression, gastrointestinal transit and hormone release in a morphine infusion model. *Life Sci*. 1989;45(18): 1627–1636.

27. Bruera E, Macmillan K, Hanson J, MacDonald RN. The cognitive effects of the administration of narcotic analgesics in patients with cancer pain. *Pain*. 1989;39(1):13–16.

28. Redmond DE Jr, Krystal JH. Multiple mechanisms of withdrawal from opioid drugs. *Annu Rev Neurosci*. 1984;7:443–478.

29. American Psychiatric Association. *Diagnostic and statistical manual for mental disorders IV*.Washington, D.C: American Psychiatric Association; 1994.

30. World Health Organization. Youth and Drugs. Report of a WHO Study Group. *Ann Intern Med*. 1974 Jan 1;80(1):133-c-.

31. Halpern LM, Robinson J. Prescribing practices for pain in drug dependence: a lesson in ignorance. *Adv Alcohol Subst Abuse*. 1985;5(1–2):135–162.

32. Dai SCorrigall WA, Coen KM, Kalant H. Heroin self-administration by rats: influence of dose and physical dependence. *Pharmacol Biochem Behav*. 1989;32(4):1009–1015.

33. Passik SD, Kirsh KL, McDonald MV, et al. A pilot survey of aberrant drug-taking attitudes and behaviors in samples of cancer and AIDS patients. *J Pain Symptom Manage*. 2000;19(4):274–286.

34. Helzer JE, Pryzbeck TM. The co-occurence of alcoholism with other psychiatric disorders in the general population and its impact on treatment. *J Stud Alcohol*. 1998;49:219–224.

35. Regier DA, Farmer ME, Rae DS, et al. Comorbidity of mental disorders with alcohol and other drug abuse. Results from the Epidemiologic Catchment Area (ECA) Study. *JAMA*. 1990;264(19):2511–2518.

36. Khantzian EJ, Treece C. DSM-III psychiatric diagnosis of narcotic addicts. Recent findings. *Arch Gen Psychiatry*. 1985;42(11):1067–1071.

37. Portenoy RK, Lussier D, Kirsh KL, Passik SD . Pain and addiction. In: Frances RJ, Miller SI, Mack AH, (eds). *Clinical textbook of addictive disorders*. New York: Guilford Press; 2005:367–395.

38. Passik SD, Portenoy RK. Substance abuse disorders. In: Holland JC (ed). *Psychooncology*. New York, Oxford University Press; 1998:576–586.

39. Passik SD, Kirsh KL, Whitcomb L, Dickerson PK, Theobald DE. Pain clinicians' rankings of aberrant drug-taking behaviors. *J Pain Palliat Care Pharmacother*. 2002;16(4):39–49.

40. Weissman DE, Haddox JD. Opioid pseudoaddiction—an iatrogenic syndrome. *Pain*. 1989;36(3):363–366.

41. Passik SD, Portenoy RK, Ricketts PL. Substance abuse issues in cancer patients. Part 1: prevalence and diagnosis. *Oncology (Williston Park)*. 1998;12(4): 517–521, 524.

42. Passik SD, , Kirsh KL, Donaghy KB, Portenoy RK. Pain and aberrant drug-related behaviors in medically ill patients with and without histories of substance abuse. *Clin J Pain*. 2006;22(2):173–181.

43. Brown SA, Inaba RK, Gillin JC, Schuckit MA, Stewart MA, Irwin MR. Alcoholism and affective disorder: clinical course of depressive symptoms. *Am J Psychiatry*. 1995;152(1):45–52.

44. Kushner MG, Sher KJ, Beitman BD. The relation between alcohol problems and the anxiety disorders. *Am J Psychiatry*. 1990;147(6):685–695.

45. Winokur G, Coryell W, Akiskal HS, et al. Alcoholism in manic-depressive (bipolar) illness: familial illness, course of illness, and the primary-secondary distinction. *Am J Psychiatry*. 1995;152(3):365–372.

46. Passik SD, Theobald DE. Managing addiction in advanced cancer patients: why bother? *J Pain Symptom Manage*. 2000;19(3):229–234.

47. Kirsh KL, Bennett JC DS, Hagen JE, Passik SD. Initial development of a survey tool to detect issues of chemical coping in chronic pain patients. *Palliat Support Care*. 2007 Sep;5(3):219–226.

48. Bruera E, Seifert L MJ, Fainsinger RL, Hanson J, Suarez-Almazor M. The frequency of alcoholism among patients with pain due to terminal cancer. *J Pain Symptom Manage*. 1995 Nov;10(8):599–603.

49. Khantzian EJ. The self-medication hypothesis revisited: the dually diagnosed patient. *Prim Care*. 2003;10:47–48, 53–54.

50. Kirsh KL, Jass C, Bennett DS, Hagen JE, Passik SD. Initial development of a survey tool to detect issues of chemical coping in chronic pain patients. *Palliat Support Care*. 2007;5(3):219–226.

51. Sifneos PE. Alexithymia: past and present. *Am J Psychiatry*. 1996;153 (Suppl 7):137–142.

52. Avila LA. Somatization or psychosomatic symptoms? *Psychosomatics*. 2006;47(2):163–166.

53. Substance Abuse and Mental Health Services Administration (SAMHSA). National survey on drug use and health: summary of methodological studies, 1971–2005. In Office of Applied Studies, (ed). *Methodology series M-6*. Dept. of Health and Human Services, Substance Abuse and Mental Health Services Administration, Office of Applied Studies: Rockville, MD; 2006:140.

54. Boyd CJ, McCabe SE. Coming to terms with the nonmedical use of prescription medications. *Subst Abuse Treat Prev Policy*. 2008;3:22.

55. Passik SD, , Kirsh KL, Whitcomb L, et al. A new tool to assess and document pain outcomes in chronic pain patients receiving opioid therapy. *Clin Ther*. 2004;26(4):552–561.

56. Kirsh KL, Passik SD. Managing drug abuse, addiction, and diversion in chronic pain. *Pharmacol Manage Pain Exp Col*. 2005.

57. Passik SD, Weinreb HJ. Managing chronic nonmalignant pain: overcoming obstacles to the use of opioids. *Adv Ther*. 2000;17(2):70–83.

58. Webster LR, Webster RM. Predicting aberrant behaviors in opioid-treated patients: preliminary validation of the opioid risk tool. *Pain Med*. 2005;6(6):432–442.

59. Webster LR. Assessing abuse potential in pain patients. *Medscape Neurol Neurosurg.* 2004;6(1).

60. Ewing JA. Detecting alcoholism. The CAGE questionnaire. *JAMA.* 1984;252(14):1905–1907.

61. Cherpitel CJ. Brief screening instruments for alcoholism. *Alcohol Health Res World.* 1997;21(4):348–351.

62. Cherpitel CJ. Gender and acculturation differences in performance of screening instruments for alcohol problems among U.S. hispanic emergency room patients. In: Paper presented at the Alcohol Epidemiology Symposium of the Kettil Bruun Society for Social and Epidemiological Research. Reykjavik, Iceland; 1997b.

63. Maxmen JS, Ward NG. Substance-related disorders. In: Jerrold S. Maxmen, Nicholas G. Ward (eds). *Essential psychopathology and its treatment.* W.W. Norton & Company: New York. 1995;132–172.

64. Erstad BL, Cotugno CL. Management of alcohol withdrawal. *Am J Health Syst Pharm.* 1995;52(7):697–709.

65. Newman JP, Terris DJ, Moore M. Trends in the management of alcohol withdrawal syndrome. *Laryngoscope.* 1995;105(1):1–7.

66. Suh JJ, Pettinati HM, Kampman KM, O'Brien CP. The status of disulfiram: a half of a century later. *J Clin Psychopharmacol.* 2006;26(3):290–302.

67. Weinrieb RM, O'Brien CP. (eds). Diagnosis and treatment of alcoholism. 2nd ed. *Current Psychiatric Therapy,* Dunner DL (ed). Philidelphia, PA: Saunders; 1997.

68. Fuller RK, Gordis E. Does disulfiram have a role in alcoholism treatment today? *Addiction.* 2004;99(1):21–24.

69. Banys P. The clinical use of disulfiram (Antabuse): a review. *J Psychoactive Drugs.* 1988;20(3):243–261.

70. Hughes JC, Cook CC. The efficacy of disulfiram: a review of outcome studies. *Addiction.* 1997;92:381–395.

71. Wright C, Moore RD. Disulfiram treatment of alcoholism. *Am J Med.* 1990;88(6):647–655.

72. Brewer C, Meyers RJ, Johnson J. Does disulfiram help to prevent relapse in alcohol abuse? *CNS Drugs.* 2000;14:329–341.

73. O'Farrell TJ, Allen JP, Litten RZ. Disulfiram (antabuse) contracts in treatment of alcoholism. *NIDA Res Monogr.* 1995;150:65–91.

CHAPTER 47

Posttraumatic Stress Disorder Associated with Cancer Diagnosis and Treatment

Michael A. Andrykowski and Maria Kangas

INTRODUCTION

Posttraumatic stress disorder (PTSD) is an anxiety disorder that occurs in response to a traumatic event. PTSD was first recognized as a formal psychiatric disorder in 1980 in the American Psychiatric Association's *Diagnostic and statistical manual of mental disorders*, third edition (DSM-III).[1] However, the notion that exposure to a significant stressor could trigger a severe and dysfunctional psychological response has a much longer history. Historically linked to warfare, PTSD has also been associated with significant civilian stressors such as assault, motor vehicle accidents (MVAs), and natural disasters. Beginning in 1994, the *Diagnostic and statistical manual of mental disorders*, fourth edition (DSM-IV),[2] specified a life-threatening illness, such as malignant disease, could also serve as a traumatic event capable of precipitating PTSD.

As a result of this change in the formal diagnostic criteria for PTSD, a large scientific literature has emerged examining PTSD associated with cancer diagnosis and treatment.[3–6] Initially, researchers focused on documenting the prevalence of PTSD symptoms and diagnoses in cancer patients and survivors, both children and adults.[7–9] Later, the focus of investigation broadened to include other individuals who, while not diagnosed with cancer themselves, might nevertheless be profoundly affected by cancer in a loved one. Thus, research examining the prevalence of PTSD in parental caregivers or family members (e.g., children, siblings) of individuals diagnosed and treated for cancer has also appeared in the literature.[10–14] Recently, the focus of investigation has broadened even further to include the possibility that PTSD might ensue following notification of carrier status in the context of genetic testing for a hereditary cancer syndrome.[15,16]

It is important to note that while the empirical literature examining PTSD in the context of malignant disease is quite large, only a small portion of this literature has actually employed formal diagnostic criteria to identify individuals with PTSD. The majority of extant studies have identified *putative* cases of PTSD based on responses to one or more questionnaires assessing symptoms associated with PTSD or have identified putative cases of PTSD based on the presence of some subset of formal PTSD diagnostic criteria. Obviously, the heterogeneity in how PTSD has been assessed and defined in the cancer literature represents a significant impediment to the understanding of this phenomenon, particularly as it is not always readily apparent whether formal DSM diagnostic criteria have been employed in a particular study to identify individuals with PTSD.

The remainder of this chapter will be devoted to a review and discussion of the literature regarding PTSD associated with cancer diagnosis and treatment. We will begin with a detailed review of the current diagnostic criteria for PTSD and a discussion of the conceptual and methodological difficulties encountered in applying these criteria to PTSD in the cancer setting. This will be followed by a review of the literature regarding cancer-related PTSD. We will focus our review on empirical investigations which have employed formal DSM diagnostic criteria for identifying cases of PTSD. Furthermore, we will restrict our review to studies which have examined PTSD in cancer patients and survivors, both pediatric and adult. Consequently, we will not review the literature which has examined PTSD in other individuals such as caregivers and family members, or in other cancer-related contexts, such as genetic testing or cancer screening. We will conclude the chapter with an identification of gaps in our current knowledge base and recommendations for future research.

DEFINITION AND DIAGNOSIS OF PTSD IN CANCER PATIENTS AND SURVIVORS

A summary of the DSM-IV and DSM-IV-TR[2,17] diagnostic criteria for PTSD and its specific application to cancer is presented in Table 47–1. In particular, an individual must satisfy all six criteria (A–F) to qualify for a diagnosis of PTSD. For the most part, these criteria are comparable for adults and children; although as outlined in Table 47–1, Criterion A2, B1–B3, C4, and D may be elicited in a variant format in young children due to developmental, maturation factors.

Criterion A is pertinent to the conceptualization of PTSD as a stress-response syndrome[18] and essentially requires an individual to have experienced (directly or indirectly) an event that threatened one's life and/or physical integrity. The number and types of potentially qualifying traumatic events that could precipitate PTSD has been expanded in DSM-IV.[19] As noted earlier, for the first time "life threatening illness" is explicitly included as a potentially traumatic event. This means individuals who are diagnosed with cancer can now be assessed for a diagnosis of PTSD resulting from their cancer experience. The mode of traumatization has also been broadened in DSM-IV to include individuals who "witnessed or confronted" the traumatic event. In particular, the DSM-IV PTSD guidelines explicitly include "learning that one's child has a life-threatening disease" as a traumatic event that could warrant a PTSD diagnosis.[2] More broadly, indirect/vicarious traumatization resulting in PTSD may also occur for persons who are family members or close friends of trauma survivors including partners, siblings, and offspring of cancer patients. However, direct or indirect exposure to cancer is not sufficient to meet Criterion A. This is because Criterion A consists of a conjunctive rule that requires an individual to satisfy *both* the objective and subjective subcomponents of this criterion. Hence, individuals must report experiencing "intense fear, helplessness or horror" in response to their personal or vicarious cancer experience to meet PTSD Criterion A.[2,17]

Cancer conceptualized as a traumatic event represents a unique stressor relative to other traumatic events that have traditionally been construed within the PTSD framework, such as combat, serious MVAs, assaults, and natural disasters.[4] Whereas nonmedical traumas (e.g., hurricane, MVA), tend to be discrete, externally induced events which have transpired, the stressor causing cancer-related PTSD is initially triggered by an internally induced event[9] that comprises a protracted and potentially complex experience. Specifically, cancer-related PTSD is multifaceted and may be due to traumatic experiences associated with the diagnosis itself, medical treatments, or disease and/or treatment side effects including complications, disfigurements, and dysfunctions.[4] To this end, the expression "*cancer experience*" will be used to convey the potential array of stressors associated with being diagnosed and treated for cancer (or witnessing this protracted experience), and the term "*cancer-related PTSD*" will be utilized to denote PTSD due to one's experience with cancer, either personal or vicarious. Moreover, there are a number of conceptual issues that need to be carefully considered when applying the PTSD framework to individuals with a cancer experience. Specific conceptual considerations pertaining to each specific PTSD Criterion are summarized in Table 47–1.

Table 47–1. Diagnostic criteria for posttraumatic stress disorder following cancer in accordance with DSM-IV guidelines and conceptual considerations

DSM-IV[a] criteria	Characteristic symptom profile	Conceptual issues to be considered
A	Objective (direct or indirect) exposure and subjective response to a traumatic event 1. *Objective Criterion*: Exposure to a traumatic event includes diagnosis of a life-threatening illness such as cancer that threatened one's life and/or their physical integrity and which involved *either* direct personal experience with the illness; or witnessing, confronting, or learning about this life-threatening illness experience by a family member (e.g., parent, spouse/partner, offspring) or close friend, and which may also pose a threat to the integrity of a significant other 2. *Subjective Criterion*: *Adults*: The individual's reaction to one's cancer experience involved feeling very frightened, and/or helpless, and/or horrified *Children*: A child's reaction to one's cancer experience may instead be elicited by disorganized or agitated behavior.	Criterion A consists of a conjunctive rule The individual must satisfy *both* Criterion A1 and A2 to be considered for a diagnosis of PTSD • Cancer as a traumatic stressor is a potentially protracted and multifaceted stressful experience. The stressor may be triggered by being informed of the diagnosis, or may occur in response to the disease and/or treatment side effects, complications, disfigurements, or dysfunctions, or other aversive medical experiences related to being treated for one's cancer • *Direct traumatization*: For individuals (child or adult) who are actually diagnosed with a malignancy. Although being diagnosed with a cancer is potentially life threatening, the life threat is future oriented. However, the threat to one's physical integrity may be more immediate due to disease and/or treatment side effects • *Indirect/vicarious traumatization*: For individuals who are informed that their child, or partner/spouse, or other family member is diagnosed with cancer • A person's subjective reaction to the cancer diagnosis and/or other cancer-related events involved feeling very frightened, and/or helpless or horrified. However, this criterion tends to be neglected by most self-report scales that assess PTSD symptoms • If the individual does not satisfy this criterion, need to consider alternative diagnosis, including Adjustment Disorder or another anxiety or mood disorder (see Table 47–2)
B	Persistent reexperiencing of one's cancer experience in at least one (or more) of the following five ways: 1. *Adults*: Intrusive and reoccurring distressing recollections of one's cancer experience that included intrusive thoughts or images *Children*: This symptom may be elicited as themes or aspects of one's cancer experience expressed in the form of repetitive play 2. *Adults*: Distressing recurrent bad dreams about one's cancer experience *Children*: May experience frightening dreams in which the content is not articulated or recognized as pertaining to one's cancer experience 3. *Adults*: An individual may experience a dissociative flashback episode (ranging from a few seconds up to several days) during which time they feel or act as if components of one's cancer experience were happening again *Children*: This symptom may be elicited by reenacting aspects of one's cancer experience (e.g., during play) 4. Exposure to internal cues (e.g., bodily symptoms) or external cues (e.g., oncology ward, cancer advertisements) that are associated or remind the individual of an aspect of one's cancer experience causes elevated emotional distress 5. Physiological symptoms (e.g., increased heart rate/palpitations, rapid breathing, sweating) occurred in response to exposure to internal cues (e.g., bodily symptoms) or external cues (e.g., oncology ward, cancer advertisements) that are associated or remind the person of an aspect of one's cancer experience	This Criterion implies that the distressing cancer event (or more specifically, aspects of the protracted cancer experience) has transpired as it pertains to *recollecting* distressing aspects of one's cancer experience. Hence, at the time of assessment the individual has at minimum been notified of the cancer diagnosis (for a minimum of 1 month prior—see also Criterion E) For an individual to meet Criterion B1, they must report feeling distressed in recalling components of one's cancer experience that have already occurred (e.g., recalling when they received news of diagnosis [for themselves or loved one] or recollecting treatment planning session) For an individual to meet Criterion B3, they must report experiencing flashback cancer-related experiences; that is, they report acting or feeling as though an aspect of their cancer experience which has already occurred; were about to happen again, even though it wasn't (e.g., reliving when they were notified of their own [or family member's] cancer diagnosis, or when they [or their family member] was undergoing treatment) For the individual diagnosed with cancer, depending on when the person is being assessed (e.g., at the time they are also undergoing medical treatment for their cancer) this criterion may be more salient for both internal and external cues, as it is more difficult to avoid exposure to cancer-related cues during acute stages of medical treatment(s) Same consideration as Criterion B4

(Continued)

Table 47–1. Continued

DSM-IV[a] criteria	Characteristic symptom profile	Conceptual issues to be considered
C	Persistent avoidance of external or internal cues related to one's cancer experience and/or numbing of one's responsiveness to this experience which is expressed by a minimum of three (or more) of the following seven symptoms:	For the person diagnosed with the cancer, contingent on when the person is being assessed [e.g., at the time they are also undergoing medical treatment for their cancer] it may be very difficult to avoid internal symptoms (i.e., somatic side effects due to the cancer itself and/or medical treatments) and external cancer-related cues (e.g., medical stimuli including daily or regular hospital visits)
	1. Regular, intentional attempts are made to avoid thoughts, feelings, or conversations associated with one's cancer experience	Although the individual diagnosed with the cancer may not be able to avoid somatic symptoms and external cancer-related cues (e.g., medical appointments), they may intentionally make an effort to avoid initiating or taking part in conversations pertaining to their cancer experience, and/or may deliberately avoid thinking or reflecting on their experience (i.e., they go through the motions of receiving medical treatment but avoid their thoughts and feelings related to this experience)
	2. Regular, conscious efforts are made to avoid situations, events, places, or people who remind the individual of one's cancer experience	Similar to considerations for Criterion C2, the individual may deliberately avoid situations or persons that remind them of their cancer experience. Although they may not be able to avoid the hospital setting (during active course of treatment), they may, however, avoid other cancer-related cues which they have more direct control over (e.g., avoiding viewing medical programs on TV or avoiding reading newspaper or magazine articles pertaining to cancer; and/or avoiding interacting with persons who continue to ask them about their cancer)
	3. Inability to remember an important aspect of one's cancer experience	This symptom is not directly due to somatic side effects (e.g., concentration difficulties) Rather, the individual diagnosed with the cancer reports amnesic symptoms related to an aspect of their cancer experience (e.g., cannot recall the day of their diagnosis), due to feeling heightened emotional distress by this experience
	4. *Adults*: Emotional numbing and/or a decline in responsiveness to one's external world that may be elicited by a substantial diminished interest or participation in activities previously enjoyed. *Children*: May not necessarily report withdrawal from activities; hence, this symptom could be verified by parental or teacher reports	Cancer patients undergoing medical treatment and/or recovering from acute treatment side effects may experience a diminished interest in engaging in regular social and recreational activities they previously enjoyed doing due to somatic symptoms (e.g., loss of energy/fatigue). In such instances, careful consideration needs to be taken in determining whether a person satisfies this criterion due to emotional reactivity to one's experience or primarily due to somatic disease and/or treatment side effects (the latter alone would not meet this criterion)
	5. Feeling alienated or detached from other people	
	6. Substantial decline in emotional affectivity, particularly related to "intimacy, tenderness, and sexuality"	For the individual diagnosed with cancer, disease and treatment side effects may cause a decline in libido and sexual functioning. Careful consideration therefore needs to be taken in differentiating between a decline in emotional affectivity that is primarily due to cancer-related side effects compared to psychological distress
	7. (*Unrealistic*) perception of a foreshortened future	For the individual diagnosed with cancer, contingent on one's medical prognosis, this criterion may not be applicable especially if a person's prognosis is determined to be poor
D	Persistent symptoms of physiological arousal and/or anxiety that was not present before one's cancer experience	For individuals diagnosed with cancer, Criterion D needs to be differentiated from pure somatic cancer-related side-effects. Differentiating disease and treatment side effects from more psychological induced physiological arousal may be more difficult when assessing patients during the acute stages of treatment as well as the initial treatment recovery period
	1. Sleeping disturbances that may include difficulty falling or staying asleep (and may be due to nightmares related to one's cancer experience)	For the individual with cancer, the sleeping disturbance is not explicitly and solely due to disease and medical side effects (e.g., pain).
	2. Feeling irritable or experiencing anger outbursts/loss of temper	Same consideration as Criterion D1
	3. Concentration difficulties	Same consideration as Criterion D1

DSM-IV[a] criteria	Characteristic symptom profile	Conceptual issues to be considered
	4. Hypervigilant; markedly increased awareness of external or internal stimuli due to increased concerns about danger	For individuals diagnosed with cancer, they may elicit more internal hypervigilant symptoms (e.g., being hyper-sensitive to changes in bodily symptoms such as skin texture, lumps which may be evidenced by ritualized scanning of body) than external symptoms. However individuals may also report heightened awareness of externally perceived threats. In the context of cancer, individuals may be externally hypervigilant toward stimuli that are perceived to pose medical/health-related threats (e.g., sitting near someone who is physically unwell)
	5. Exaggerated physiological, startle response (e.g., jumpy or easily startled by noises or movements) *Children*: In addition or in place of other Criterion D symptoms a child may report stomach pains and/or headaches which were not present before one's cancer experience	For children diagnosed with cancer, this alternate Criterion D is not explicitly due to disease and/or treatment side effects
E	An individual must exhibit the full PTSD symptom profile (Criteria B, C and D) for more than 1 month following the onset of the cancer stressor.	The cancer-related experience is typically perceived to be initiated when an individual is informed of their diagnosis (or the diagnosis of a family member). Hence an individual must exhibit the full PTSD symptom profile for a minimum of 4 weeks following cancer diagnosis
F	The PTSD symptoms lead to "clinically significant distress or impairment"[1,2] in important areas of one's life including interpersonal/social, occupational, and family functioning	This Criterion needs to be differentiated from impairment solely due to physical (disease and/or treatment) side effects This Criterion tends to be neglected by self-report scales for PTSD. However, for an individual to meet full diagnostic criteria for PTSD they must satisfy Criterion F
Specifications	(i) *Acute PTSD*: The individual meets full PTSD criteria for more than 1 month and less than 3 months (following the onset of the cancer stressor) (ii) *Chronic PTSD*: The individual meets full PTSD criteria for 3 months or more (following the onset of the cancer stressor) (iii) *Delayed onset*: Onset of full PTSD symptoms is at minimum 6 months after initial onset of cancer stressor	Same consideration as Criterion E

ABBREVIATION: PTSD, posttraumatic stress disorder.
[a]PTSD DSM-IV and DSM-IV-TR guidelines are comparable.

As Criterion A1 denotes the stressor precipitating the development of PTSD has already transpired, this means a person must have already experienced the relevant cancer-related event (or series of events) which initiated the PTSD response. Cancer as a traumatic stressor is further distinctive insofar as the threat to life is not necessarily immediate. Rather, contingent on the medical prognosis, the threat to one's life tends to be future oriented. Thus the subjective fear reaction is in the form of anticipatory anxiety (e.g., "*I am going to die*" or "*my child is going to die*") compared to a nonmedical discrete, traumatic event that has already elapsed, such as an MVA. For these events, the fear response is past oriented (e.g., "*I could have died*"). However, what is immediate in the context of cancer as a traumatic event is an ongoing "threat to physical integrity of self or others."[2]

PTSD Criteria B, C, and D represent the three main symptom clusters for PTSD that comprise reexperiencing symptoms (Criterion B), avoidance and numbing symptoms (Criterion C), and physiological arousal symptoms (Criterion D). Criterion B is likely the easiest symptom cluster to meet as an individual need only experience one out of a possible five types of reexperiencing symptoms (B1–B5). It should be noted both Criterion B1 and B3 further accentuate that the stressor is past oriented at the time of PTSD assessment as these symptoms involve "recollection" and a "sense of reliving/flashback" of the traumatic experience. Consequently, depending on when the assessment of PTSD occurs, it may be difficult for cancer patients or their family members to technically meet either of these two traditional PTSD reexperiencing symptoms. Furthermore, if an individual is assessed at the time they (or their family member) are still receiving active medical treatment or are undergoing frequent follow-up medical appointments in the initial stages of recovery, Criterion B4 and B5

are likely to be quite salient. This is because these individuals are exposed regularly to external reminders of their cancer experience. Moreover, given the internally induced nature of the cancer stressor, Criterion B4 and B5 are likely to be more pronounced in individuals who are most distressed by their own cancer diagnosis and/or treatment experience. For these individuals, the side effects and physical changes resulting from their disease and/or medical treatment may be a constant reminder of the ordeal they have been subjected to over a prolonged period.

The avoidance and emotional numbing symptoms (Criterion C) are the most stringent PTSD criteria to meet given an individual must elicit a minimum of three of seven specific symptoms (C1–C7). For individuals traumatized by cancer, four of the seven symptoms (i.e., C1–C3, C7) are problematic. Notably, avoidance of internal and external cancer-related cues (C1 and C2) may be difficult for cancer patients, particularly during the acute stages of their treatment and recovery. Additionally, the occurrence of dissociative amnesic symptoms (C3) may be difficult to ascertain in cancer patients due to disease (e.g., brain tumors) and treatment side effects (e.g., fatigue, concentration deficits) which may temporarily or permanently impair one's memory functioning. Furthermore, contingent on the cancer patient's medical prognosis, a "sense of foreshortened future" (Criterion C7) may be a realistic and quite common perspective.[4] Hence, the use of this latter criterion needs to be applied with caution, to prevent pathologizing realistic negative appraisals.

To meet PTSD Criterion D, an individual must exhibit two out of a potential five symptoms reflecting elevated physiological arousal. Three of these symptoms (D1–D3) need to be applied carefully, especially when assessing cancer patients during or soon after completing medical treatment. Sleep difficulties, irritability, and concentration deficits are common side effects resulting from malignant disease and/or its medical treatment. Hence the presence of these symptoms must be assessed in the context of whether an individual's emotional distress pertaining to their cancer experience directly contributes to disruptions in their sleep functioning, concentration, and ability to remain calm (e.g., worrying about one's cancer causes difficulties in falling asleep, and/or concentrating on tasks). Furthermore, whereas in nonmedical trauma survivors hypervigilance (D4) is expressed in terms of having heightened awareness of external, potentially dangerous trauma-related cues, cancer patients and survivors may be more hypervigilant to somatic features (such as changes in skin texture or appearance) in response to fears of a cancer recurrence or tumor progression.[4,9]

To meet full diagnostic criteria for PTSD, an individual must report having persistent symptoms for at least 1 month following one's experience with cancer (Criterion E). As a result, cancer-related PTSD could be diagnosed no earlier than 1 month after being informed of a cancer diagnosis and, given the protracted nature of cancer, could be diagnosed at any time thereafter. The sixth and final Criterion, Criterion F, is important as it assesses the effect that PTSD symptoms have on an individual's overall functioning. To merit a diagnosis of PTSD, symptoms not only must be present but also must be associated with clinically significant distress or impairment. Whether Criterion F is met is typically unknown when putative diagnoses of PTSD are made on the basis of questionnaires that simply ascertain whether a particular symptom pattern is present (e.g., PTSD Checklist[20]). Finally, DSM-IV PTSD guidelines stipulate diagnostic duration specifiers to indicate whether the individual is exhibiting "Acute PTSD" or "Chronic PTSD" at the time of assessment, and whether the diagnosis occurred "With Delayed Onset" (i.e., >6 months following the onset of the cancer experience). Use of these specifiers in the cancer setting is complicated by the difficulty noted previously in ascertaining precisely what constitutes the traumatic stressor when considering an individual's cancer experience.

Although the conceptual issues just noted relate to the application of DSM-IV PTSD criteria to cancer patients, survivors, and their family members, the past decade has seen an increasing discussion of the validity and utility of the application of DSM-IV PTSD criteria to a wide variety of trauma populations. This growing debate about the construct validity of PTSD diagnostic criteria, in general, has been examined recently in a special edition of the *Journal of Anxiety Disorders*.[21] So concerns about the application of DSM-IV PTSD criteria are not limited to the cancer setting, although the cancer setting does perhaps represent a more challenging context for their application.

In light of the difficulties just noted in applying DSM-IV PTSD diagnostic criteria in the cancer setting, it is imperative that DSM-IV diagnostic criteria are appropriately applied in full when attempting to identify "cases" of cancer-related PTSD for either clinical or research purposes. The reasons for this are threefold. First, the majority of studies that have examined PTSD symptoms in the cancer setting have *not* employed formal diagnostic criteria.[4] Rather, a variety of self-report questionnaires have been commonly employed to "diagnose" PTSD in cancer samples. However, these measures typically do not assess Criteria A2 and F. Diagnostic clinical interviews are the gold standard for identifying cases of PTSD in the cancer setting as they enable application of the full set of DSM-IV diagnostic criteria. Second, many studies in the cancer setting which purport to identify cases of PTSD have utilized questionnaires that are simply inappropriate diagnostic measures of PTSD; the most common measure being the impact of event scale (IES) or the revised version of this scale (IES-R). For the most part, researchers who have exclusively relied on the IES or IES-R acknowledge their data reflect the presence of "PTSD-like-symptoms" rather than frank PTSD diagnoses. However, this practice can misleadingly imply an individual is suffering from a formal clinical disorder[22] and can contribute to the problem of "conceptual bracket creep"[23] reflected in the application of the PTSD construct to potentially inappropriate populations and/or contexts. Third, in determining a diagnosis of PTSD following cancer, clinicians and researchers must take into account differential diagnostic considerations in determining whether an individual's symptom presentation meets full diagnostic criteria for PTSD or whether the symptom profile is better accounted for by another DSM-IV disorder. However, reliance on self-report assessments of PTSD hampers the ability to apply appropriate differential diagnostic considerations. Table 47–2 provides a summary outline of alternative diagnoses that need to be considered when assessing cancer-related PTSD. Notably, if an individual does not meet Criterion A2 and/or any other PTSD symptom cluster (i.e., Criteria B, C or D), then in accordance with DSM guidelines an assessment for adjustment disorder

Table 47-2. Differential diagnostic considerations in the assessment of cancer-related PTSD

DSM-IV-TR axis I disorders	Differential diagnostic issues
1. Acute stress disorder (ASD)	If an individual is assessed less than 4 weeks following cancer diagnosis (i.e., does not satisfy PTSD Criterion E), need to assess whether the individual meets diagnostic criteria for ASD. For the most part, the ASD criteria are similar to the PTSD criteria, with the exception that the ASD criteria have a heavy emphasis on dissociative symptoms
2. Adjustment disorder	Adjustment disorder needs to be considered in the following instances: (a) The individual does not meet full diagnostic criteria for PTSD, particularly not meeting Criterion A2; or if PTSD Criterion A2 is satisfied, the individual does not meet criteria for one of the three PTSD symptom clusters (i.e., B, C, or D) (b) The individuals' reported stress symptom profile does not meet diagnostic criteria for any other anxiety, depressive, or Axis I disorder, and the stress symptoms must occur within 3 months following onset of the cancer stressor (i.e., within 3 months following cancer diagnosis)
3. Major depressive disorder (MDD)	MDD needs to be considered if the individual reports a substantial decline in mood or disengaging from previously enjoyed activities due to low affect following one's cancer diagnosis (or diagnosis of family member) MDD may also occur concurrent with or secondary to a diagnosis of cancer-related PTSD
4. Anxiety disorders: (a) Panic disorder (b) Agoraphobia (c) Social phobia (d) Specific phobia	Other anxiety disorders also need to be considered, particularly in terms of whether the individual's stress symptoms are better accounted for by a nontrauma anxiety disorder Other Axis I anxiety disorders may also occur concurrent with or secondary to a diagnosis of cancer-related PTSD
6. Substance-related disorders	Substance-related disorders are commonly associated with PTSD in civilian and veteran populations. Therefore it is important to assess for primary or co-morbid substance disorders when screening for cancer-related PTSD, particularly in cancer populations that may be more prone to substance-related disturbances before their cancer diagnosis (e.g., head and neck, and lung cancer)

ABBREVIATION: PTSD, posttraumatic stress disorder.

as well as other affective disorders needs to be considered. Furthermore, although an individual may meet full diagnostic criteria for PTSD, they may also be suffering from a co-morbid, primary, or secondary psychological disturbance (particularly major depressive disorder, social and specific phobias)[24] as a result of their cancer experience.

In summary, in line with current DSM-IV PTSD criteria an individual may potentially qualify for a diagnosis of PTSD as a result of experiencing heightened trauma symptoms due to one's direct or indirect (e.g., familial) experience with cancer. To circumvent the "conceptual bracket creep" problem and identify appropriately the prevalence and predictors of PTSD in the cancer setting, it is imperative that appropriate DSM diagnostic methods are employed. Accordingly, our review of the cancer-related PTSD literature in the following section focuses explicitly on research that has utilized formal DSM diagnostic criteria to identify cases of PTSD in cancer patients or survivors.

PTSD IN CANCER PATIENTS AND SURVIVORS: A REVIEW OF THE LITERATURE

In general, the research literature regarding PTSD in cancer patients and survivors has focused on two questions: (1) What is the prevalence of PTSD in cancer patients and survivors? and (2) What clinical, demographic, and psychosocial factors are associated with risk for PTSD in cancer patients and survivors? Table 47–3 lists and summarizes studies which have employed formal DSM diagnostic criteria to identify cases of PTSD in samples of adult (≥18 years of age) cancer patients or survivors. Similarly, Table 47–4 summarizes studies which have employed formal DSM diagnostic criteria to identify cases of PTSD in samples of child and adolescent (<18 years of age) cancer patients or survivors.

PTSD in adult cancer patients and survivors. Table 47–3 summarizes findings from eighteen different reports of PTSD in adult cancer patients and survivors. Three of these reports[24-26] are based on the same longitudinal data set, leaving a total of 16 different studies which have furnished data relevant to issues regarding the prevalence of PTSD and its associated factors. As would be expected given life-threatening illness was only officially recognized as a potential traumatic stressor capable of triggering PTSD in the early 1990s, the literature is relatively young. The earliest report dates from 1996[7] with all but three reports[7-9] published since 2000. While all 18 studies report data from individuals who were adults (≥18 years of age) at the time of PTSD assessment, two studies are based on data from individuals who were initially diagnosed with cancer as a child or adolescent.[27,28] The remaining 16 studies examined samples of cancer patients and survivors diagnosed during adulthood. Of these 16 studies, exactly half focused exclusively on women with breast cancer.[7,9,15,29-33] The remaining eight studies included participants evidencing a mixture of cancer diagnoses.[7,24,27,28,34-37]

Sample sizes in the eight studies focusing exclusively on breast cancer patients and survivors range from 37 to 160 participants with a mean of 86 participants (median of 76). Prevalence rates for current cancer-related PTSD in these eight studies range from 0% to 6.5% with a mean of 3.3% (median of 2.8%). Five of these studies also reported prevalence rates for lifetime cancer-related PTSD ranging from 4% to 35% with a mean of 12.6% (median of 9%). Considered together, these estimates of current and lifetime PTSD prevalence rates suggest 10%–12% of women diagnosed with breast cancer might meet criteria for cancer-related PTSD at some point following their cancer diagnosis (i.e., lifetime cancer-related PTSD). At any single point in time, however, approximately 3% of women diagnosed with breast cancer might meet criteria for cancer-related PTSD (i.e., current cancer-related PTSD).

Sample sizes in the eight study samples that did not include breast cancer patients and survivors range from 27 to 251 participants with a mean sample size of 105 participants (median of 80). Prevalence rates for current cancer-related PTSD are reported for seven of these samples and range from 0% to 22% with a mean of 10.6% (median of 6.2%). Prevalence rates for lifetime cancer-related PTSD are reported for four of these samples and range from 4% to 22.5% with a mean of 18.3% (median of 13%). Considered together, these estimates of current and lifetime PTSD prevalence rates suggest 20% of cancer patients with diagnoses other than breast cancer might meet criteria for cancer-related PTSD at some point following their cancer diagnosis (i.e., lifetime cancer-related PTSD). At any single point in time, however, approximately 6% of these individuals might meet criteria for cancer-related PTSD (i.e., current cancer-related PTSD).

Twelve of the eighteen studies summarized in Table 47–3 examined factors associated with a diagnosis of cancer-related PTSD. Not surprisingly, individuals with PTSD are more likely to report distress in various forms[7,25,27,28,33,35] and/or evidence a co-morbid[24,30] or premorbid (before cancer diagnosis) psychiatric disorder[25,30,31] compared to individuals without PTSD. Females[25,28] and younger individuals[26] were also more likely to evidence cancer-related PTSD. Biochemical correlates of a PTSD diagnosis were examined in only a single study with lower morning cortisol levels associated with a diagnosis of PTSD.[29] Notably, objective characteristics associated with disease or treatment, such as stage of disease or type of treatment, were *not* linked to risk for PTSD in any study even though this relationship was examined in most of the 12 studies that examined correlates of PTSD. Rather, variables related to the *subjective* experience of disease and treatment, such as greater perceived life threat[35] and greater perceived treatment intensity,[28] were linked to greater likelihood of PTSD diagnosis. This, of course, is consistent with the subjective portion of PTSD Criterion A—the acknowledgement that an individual's subjective response to a stressor (i.e., fright, horror, helplessness) is more critical than simple exposure to that stressor.

PTSD in pediatric cancer patients and survivors. Table 47–4 summarizes findings from three reports of cancer-related PTSD in pediatric cancer patients and survivors. All respondents in these studies were <18 years of age at study assessment. Sample sizes range from 7 to 150 participants with a mean sample size of 60 participants (median of 23). Prevalence rates for current cancer-related PTSD range from 4.7% to 71% with a mean of 31% (median of 17%). However, the 71% figure comes from a study including only 7 "newly diagnosed" pediatric cancer patients[13] so there is some question regarding the appropriateness of applying PTSD diagnostic criteria to individuals who might have been <1 month postdiagnosis. Prevalence rates for lifetime cancer-related PTSD are reported in two of these studies. Kazak et al.[12] reported a lifetime prevalence rate of 8% while Pelcovitz et al.[38] reported a prevalence rate of 34.8%. Given the small number of studies to consider, we refrain from drawing any specific conclusion regarding prevalence rates for current and lifetime cancer-related PTSD in children and adolescents. However, apart from the Landolt et al. study,[13] the estimates furnished by the Kazak et al.[12] and Pelcovitz et al.[38] studies appear to be comparable to those from studies of adult cancer patients and survivors.

Only one of three studies of pediatric cancer patients and survivors examined factors associated with a PTSD diagnosis.[38] They found a diagnosis of cancer-related PTSD in the mother and the cancer survivor's perception their family was more "chaotic" were associated with a PTSD diagnosis. Obviously, there is a great deal that remains to be learned when considering factors associated with cancer-related PTSD in pediatric cancer patients and survivors.

SUMMARY

After reviewing the current literature regarding cancer-related PTSD in cancer patients and survivors, several points should be noted. First, of the 16 different study samples that have examined PTSD in adult patients and survivors, half included only women with breast cancer. So, as is quite typical for the psychosocial oncology literature, most of what we know about cancer-related PTSD is derived from study of breast cancer patients and survivors. So appropriate caution must be observed in generalizing findings from these studies to individuals with other cancer diagnoses. Second, given the often small sample sizes represented in Tables 47–3 and 47–4 and the relatively low prevalence of cancer-related PTSD, confidence intervals around PTSD prevalence rates reported in the majority of these studies are likely fairly large. Third, the vast majority of studies shown in Tables 47–3 and 47–4 employed cross-sectional designs with respondents evidencing a wide range of time since cancer diagnosis at time of study participation. The lone exception is

Table 47-3. Summary of studies of PTSD in adult cancer patients and survivors

Study	Design	Sample	Time of Assessment (mean, range, SD)	PTSD Prevalence	Factors Associated with CR PTSD (direction)
Akechi et al.[34]	Cross-sectional; in-person interview at registration with palliative care unit	n = 209; males and females; mixed cancer diagnoses	25 months post-dx (0–282 months; SD = 38 months)	0% current CR PTSD (only first 100 study participants assessed for PTSD)	Not examined
Alter et al.[7]	Cross-sectional; in-person interview	n = 27; females; mixed cancer diagnoses	5.4 years post-dx	4% current CR PTSD; 22% lifetime CR PTSD	SCL-90-R GSI scores (+)
Andrykowski et al.[8]	Cross-sectional; telephone interview	n = 82; females; stage 0-IIIA breast cancer	37 months post-tx (6–72 months; SD = 16.4 months)	6% current CR PTSD; 4% lifetime CR PTSD	Not examined
Green et al.[9]	Cross-sectional; in-person interview	n = 160; females; stage I-II breast cancer	6.5 months post-tx (4–12 months)	2.5% current CR PTSD; 5% lifetime CR PTSD	None
Hamann et al.[15]	Cross-sectional; in-person interview	n = 46; females with personal hx of breast cancer considering genetic testing	Not reported	6.5% current CR PTSD 10.9% lifetime CR PTSD	Not examined
Hobbie et al.[35]	Cross-sectional; in-person interview	n = 78; males and females; mixed childhood cancers	11 years post-tx (SD = 5.5 years)	20.5% lifetime CR PTSD	BSI scores (+), current life threat (+)
Kadan-Lottick et al.[36]	Cross-sectional; in-person interview	n = 251; males and females; mixed diagnoses of advanced cancer	not reported	2.4% current PTSD	Not examined
Kangas et al.[24]	Longitudinal; in-person interview	n = 82; males and females; stage I–IV head, neck, lung cancer	1, 6, and 12 months post-dx	22% current CR PTSD (6 months post-dx); 14% current CR PTSD (12 months post-dx)	Acute stress disorder (+), co-morbid anxiety, depression (+)
Kangas et al.[25]	Longitudinal; in-person interview	n = 82; males and females; stage I–IV head, neck, lung cancer	1 and 6 months post-dx	22% current CR PTSD (6 months post-dx)	Age (-), female (+), lung cancer (-), pre-dx psychiatric hx (+), peritraumatic dissociative response (+), MAC Hopeless, Anxious Preoccupation, BDI, STAI-Trait and State Anxiety scores (+), social support, EORTC emotional, cognitive function scores (−)
Kangas et al.[26]	Longitudinal; in-person interview	n = 82; males and females; stage I–IV head, neck, or lung cancer	1 and 6 months post-dx	22% current CR PTSD (6 months post-dx)	Age (−), female (+), emotional numbing, reliving, motor restlessness symptoms during acute trauma phase (+)
Kazak et al.[11]	Cross-sectional; in-person interview	n = 66; males and females; mixed cancer diagnoses	13 years post-tx (3–29 years; SD = 5.4 years)	6.2% current CR PTSD	Not examined
Luecken et al.[29]	Cross-sectional; in-person interview	n = 71; females; stage 0–III breast cancer	1–6 months post-dx	3% current CR PTSD	Morning plasma cortisol (−)
Meeske et al.[27]	Cross-sectional; in-person interview	n = 51; males and females; mixed childhood cancers	11 years post-tx (2.8–26.7 years; SD = 6 years)	22% current CR PTSD	Income (−), SF-36 QOL scores (−), BSI scores (+)
Mehnert and Koch[30]	Cross-sectional; in-person interview	n = 127; females; stage 0–IV breast cancer	15 days post-dx of initial (77%) or recurrent (23%) cancer (0–67days; SD = 13 days)	2.4% current CR PTSD; 9% lifetime PTSD	Co-morbid anxiety or depressive disorder (+), lifetime PTSD (+)
Mundy et al.[31]	Cross-sectional; in-person interview	n = 37; females; stage 0–IV breast cancer	>100 days post-tx (mean, range not reported)	0% current CR PTSD; 35% lifetime CR PTSD	Lifetime PTSD (+)

Study	Design	Sample	Time of Assessment (mean, range, SD)	PTSD Prevalence	Factors Associated with CR PTSD (direction)
Okamura et al.[32]	Cross-sectional; in-person interview	n = 50; females with recurrence of breast cancer	1–6 months post-dx of recurrent breast cancer	2% current PTSD (whether CR PTSD not reported)	None
Palmer et al.[33]	Cross-sectional; telephone interview	n = 115; females; stage I–IV breast cancer	32% >5 years post-dx 36%, 2–5 years post-dx, 13% 1–2 years post-dx, 19% <1 year post-dx	4% current CR PTSD	IES scores (+)
Rourke et al.[28]	Cross-sectional; in-person interview	n = 182; males and females; mixed childhood cancers	13.6 years post-tx (3–29 years; SD = 5.8 years)	14.3% current CR PTSD 15.9% lifetime CR PTSD	Female (+), late effect severity (+), perceived tx intensity (+), progress toward life goals (-), perceived negative effect of life events (+), QOL (–), distress (+)
Widows et al. [37]	Cross-sectional; telephone interview	n = 102; recipients of BMT for malignant disease	20.4 months post-BMT (3–62 months; SD = 14.3 months)	5% current CR PTSD; 4% lifetime CR PTSD	Not examined

ABBREVIATIONS: BDI, Beck Depression Inventory; BMT, bone marrow transplantation; BSI, Brief Symptom Inventory; CR PTSD, cancer-related posttraumatic stress disorder; EORTC, *European Organisation for Research and Treatment of Cancer*; GSI, Global Severity Index; IES, Impact of Events; MAC, Mental Adjustment to Cancer; STAI, State-Trait Anxiety Inventory; CR PTSD, "cancer-related" PTSD. Table includes only studies employing formal DSM diagnostic criteria and procedures to identify cases of PTSD.

Includes only studies where all respondents were ≥18 years of age at time of PTSD assessment.

Table 47–4. Summary of studies of PTSD in pediatric cancer survivors

Study	Design	Sample	Timeframe (average and range)	PTSD prevalence	Associated factors
Kazak et al.[12]	Cross-sectional; in-person interview	n = 150; males and females; mixed cancer diagnoses	5.3 years post-tx (SD = 2.9 years)	4.7% current CR PTSD 8.0% lifetime CR PTSD	Not examined
Landolt et al.[13]	Cross-sectional; in-person interview	n = 7; males and females; mixed cancer diagnoses	"newly diagnosed"	71% current PTSD	Not examined
Pelcovitz et al.[38]	Cross-sectional; in-person interview	n = 23; males and females; mixed cancer diagnoses	3.3 years post-tx (0–11 years)	17.4% current CR PTSD 34.8% lifetime CR PTSD	chaotic family (+), maternal dx of PTSD (+)

ABBREVIATION: PTSD, posttraumatic stress disorder.

CR PTSD refers to "cancer-related" PTSD. Table includes only studies employing formal DSM diagnostic criteria and procedures to identify cases of PTSD.

Includes only studies where all respondents were <18 years of age at time of PTSD assessment.

Kangas et al.[24] which employed a prospective, longitudinal research design with assessments 1, 6, and 12 months postcancer diagnosis. Use of a cross-sectional design precludes identification of *predictors* of PTSD, save for those demographic or clinical variables which are readily available from a medical chart review. So the reliance on cross-sectional research designs limits our understanding of the processes involved in the development of cancer-related PTSD. Furthermore, the lack of prospective research limits the ability to identify individuals at greatest risk for cancer-related PTSD early in their cancer experience—a hallmark of effective clinical management. Finally, the reliance upon cross-sectional research designs has precluded identification of the temporal trajectory of risk for cancer-related PTSD. Notably, Kangas et al.[24] found 22% of their sample of lung and head and neck cancer patients met criteria for current cancer-related PTSD 6 months postcancer diagnosis while 14% of her sample met PTSD criteria 12 months postcancer diagnosis. So the lone

longitudinal study in the literature suggests risk for a diagnosis of current PTSD varies as a function of time since diagnosis. This, of course, is not surprising. However, this makes comparison of current PTSD prevalence rates across studies difficult as the time since diagnosis when PTSD assessment occurs has varied widely in the research shown in Tables 47–3 and 47–4. Furthermore, cross-sectional research designs preclude identification of risk for delayed onset PTSD. So while it may be tempting to conclude from Kangas et al.'s[24] lone longitudinal study that risk for PTSD decreases with increasing time since cancer diagnosis, we know nothing at this time about risk for delayed onset PTSD in the cancer setting.

DIRECTIONS FOR FUTURE RESEARCH AND CONCLUSIONS

This chapter has outlined current DSM diagnostic criteria for identifying cases of cancer-related PTSD, identified a number of issues concerning the assessment of cancer-related PTSD, and reviewed the extant literature examining the prevalence and factors associated with cancer-related PTSD in patients and survivors. Several general points should be emphasized. First, construed within the PTSD framework, cancer represents a unique stressor. Individuals diagnosed with a potentially life-threatening malignant disease (as well as their close family members) are subjected to an array of medically related stressful experiences over a prolonged period of time. As a result, careful consideration needs to be taken in the assessment of cancer-related PTSD. The reason for this is twofold: (1) to prevent pathologizing "normal" transient stress-responses (especially if the individual is assessed during the acute stages of treatment or early recovery phase); and (2) to circumvent inappropriate utilization of a PTSD diagnosis for individuals who exhibit behavioral and emotional disturbances that are better accounted for by another DSM-IV-TR[2,17] Axis I disorder.

Second, since the inception of DSM-IV, many studies that have purported to investigate the prevalence, correlates, and/or predictors of cancer-related PTSD have failed to use appropriate measures to diagnosis cases of PTSD. Instead of using a clinical interview and applying DSM criteria, most studies in the literature have used self-report measures to assess PTSD symptoms or PTSD-like symptoms, inferring PTSD diagnoses based on this incomplete and/or inappropriate diagnostic information. While the use of such limited self-report measures is understandable given their greater economy relative to clinical interviews, their use can slow the growth of knowledge in this research area by broadening the meaning of what is considered cancer-related PTSD. We cannot overemphasize the importance of researchers and clinicians using appropriate measures in diagnosing cancer-related PTSD. We do recognize that practical considerations may warrant use of more limited self-report questionnaires to screen for PTSD in both research and clinical contexts. However, it is imperative that screening by self-report measures be followed by the use of a clinical interview and application of full DSM diagnostic criteria for PTSD.

Third, as shown in Tables 47–3 and 47–4, a total of 21 published studies based on 19 unique study samples have employed appropriate diagnostic methods to assess PTSD in cancer patients and survivors. Despite their limitations, these studies suggest up to 10% of women diagnosed with breast cancer and perhaps up to 20% of individuals diagnosed with a cancer other than breast cancer might meet criteria for a diagnosis of cancer-related PTSD at some point after their cancer diagnosis. The data for pediatric patients and survivors is much more limited but also suggests a lifetime prevalence rate of at least 10%. On the basis of this data, we conclude PTSD associated with cancer is a genuine phenomenon that can affect 10%–20% of cancer patients and survivors at some time after their cancer diagnosis. This conclusion has important therapeutic implications. Screening for PTSD should be incorporated into routine distress screening across the cancer trajectory. When diagnosed, appropriate treatment measures should be implemented. Unfortunately, there is a paucity of published treatment outcome studies which have been designed explicitly to treat cancer-related PTSD. While several studies of psychosocial intervention in the cancer setting have used traumatic stress symptoms as a clinical outcome[39-41] we could not find a single intervention study, controlled or otherwise, that specifically targeted individuals with cancer-related PTSD. Research examining clinical approaches to the management of cancer-related PTSD is needed as it should not be assumed that interventions shown efficacious in treating "distress" in cancer patients and survivors will be similarly efficacious in treating cancer-related PTSD. While research in this area can be guided by the evidence base accumulating for the efficacy of cognitive-behavioral therapy(CBT) for the treatment of PTSD in civilian, nonmedical traumatized populations,[42] there are a number of treatment issues that need to be considered in designing interventions specifically for the treatment of cancer-related PTSD. These include the timing of the implementation of the therapeutic program (i.e., acute phase following cancer diagnosis or following completion of medical treatment?) as well as the sequencing of specific therapeutic strategies during the acute phase of one's cancer experience (e.g., stress management, exposure, and cognitive strategies).[42]

In conclusion, while PTSD is a clinical disorder that can contribute to serious, chronic psychiatric disturbance if left untreated, the experience of subclinical levels of stress symptoms tends to be more transient in nature. This accentuates the necessity to curtail the intermingling of assessing clinical syndromes with nonclinical symptomatology in the assessment of cancer-related PTSD. This further reinforces the importance for clinicians and researchers working with cancer populations to adhere to appropriate assessment methods when considering a diagnosis of cancer-related PTSD. By doing so, this will improve the accuracy of determining the prevalence, profile, and determinants of PTSD in individuals directly or indirectly confronted by this potentially life-threatening disease.

REFERENCES

1. American Psychiatric Association. *Diagnostic and statistical manual of mental disorders*, 3rd ed. Washington, DC: American Psychiatric Association; 1980.
2. American Psychiatric Association. *Diagnostic and statistical manual of mental disorders*, 4th ed. Washington, DC: American Psychiatric Association; 1994.
3. Bruce M. A systematic and conceptual review of posttraumatic stress in childhood cancer survivors and their parents. *Clin Psychol Rev.* 2006;26:233–256.
4. Kangas M, Henry JL, Bryant RA. Posttraumatic stress disorder following cancer: a conceptual and empirical review. *Clin Psychol Rev.* 2002;22:499–524.
5. Smith MY, Redd WH, Peyser C, Vogl D. Post-traumatic stress disorder in cancer: a review. *Psychooncology.* 1999;8:521–537.
6. Taieb O, Moro MR, Baubet T, Revha-Levy A, Flament MF. Posttraumatic stress symptoms after childhood cancer. *Eur Child Adoles Psychiatry.* 2003;12:255–264.
7. Alter CL, Pelcovitz D, Axelrod A, et al. Identification of PTSD in cancer survivors. *Psychosomatics.* 1996;37:137–143.
8. Andrykowski MA, Cordova MJ, Studts JL, Miller TW. Posttraumatic stress disorder after treatment for breast cancer: prevalence of diagnosis and use of the PTSD Checklist—Civilian Version (PCL-C) as a screening instrument. *J Consult Clin Psychol.* 1998;66:586–590.
9. Green BL, Rowland JH, Krupnick JL, et al. Prevalence of posttraumatic stress disorder in women with breast cancer. *Psychosomatics.* 1998;39:102–111.
10. Boyer BA, Bubel D, Jacobs SR, et al. Posttraumatic stress in women with breast cancer and their daughters. *Am J Fam Ther.* 2002;30:323–328.
11. Kazak AE, Barakat LP, Alderfer M, et al. Posttraumatic stress in survivors of childhood cancer and mothers: development and validation of the impact of traumatic stressors interview schedule (ITSIS). *J Clin Psychol in Medical Settings.* 2001;8:307–323.
12. Kazak AE, Alderfer M, Rourke MT, Simms S, Streisand R, Grossman JR. Posttraumatic stress disorder (PTSD) and posttraumatic stress symptoms (PTSS) in families of adolescent cancer survivors. *J Pediatr Psychol.* 2004;29:211–219.
13. Landolt MA, Boehler U, Shallberger U, Nuessli R. Post-traumatic stress disorder in paediatric patients and their parents: an exploratory study. *J Paediatric Child Health.* 1998;34:539–543.
14. Manne SL, DuHamel K, Gallelli K, Sorgen K, Redd WH. Posttraumatic stress disorder among mothers of pediatric cancer survivors: diagnosis, comorbidity, and utility of the PTSD Checklist as a screening instrument. *J Pediatr Psychol.* 1998;23:357–366.
15. Hamann HA, Somers TJ, Smith AW, Inslicht SS, Baum A. Posttraumatic stress associated with cancer history and BRCA1/2 genetic testing. *Psychosom Med.* 2005;67:766–772.
16. Murakami Y, Okamura H, Sugano K, et al. Psychologic distress after disclosure of genetic test results regarding hereditary nonpolyposis colorectal carcinoma. *Cancer.* 2004;101:395–403.
17. American Psychiatric Association. *Diagnostic and statistical manual of mental disorders*, 4th ed. Text Revision. Washington, DC: American Psychiatric Association; 2000.
18. Weathers FW, Keane TM. The Criterion A problem revisited: controversies and challenges in defining and measuring psychological trauma. *J Trauma Stress.* 2007;20:107–121.
19. Spitzer RL, First MB, Wakefield JC. Saving PTSD from itself in DSM-V. *J Anx Disorders.* 2007;21:233–241.
20. Weathers FW, Litz B, Huska J, Keane T. *PTSD-checklist-civilian version.* Boston: National Center for PTSD, Behavioral Science Division; 1994.
21. Rosen GM, Frueh BC. Editorial: challenges to the PTSD construct and its database: the importance of scientific debate. *J Anx Disorders.* 2007;2:161–163.
22. Coyne JC, Thompson R. Posttraumatic stress syndromes: useful or negative heuristics? *J Anx Disorders.* 2007;21:223–229.
23. McNally RJ. Progress and controversy in the study of posttraumatic stress disorder. *Annu Rev Psychol.* 2003;54:229–252.
24. Kangas M, Henry JL, Bryant RA. The course of psychological disorders in the 1st year after cancer diagnosis. *J Consult Clin Psychol.* 2005;73:763–768.
25. Kangas M, Henry JL, Bryant RA. Predictors of posttraumatic stress disorder following cancer. *Health Psychol.* 2005;24:579–585.

26. Kangas M, Henry JL, Bryant RA. The relationship between acute stress disorder and posttraumatic stress disorder following cancer. *J Consult Clin Psychol.* 2005;73:360–364.

27. Meeske KA, Ruccione K, Globe DR, Stuber ML. Posttraumatic stress, quality of life, and psychological distress in young adult survivors of childhood cancer. *Oncol Nurs Forum.* 2001;28:481–489.

28. Rourke MT, Hobbie WL, Schwartz L, Kazak AE. Posttraumatic stress disorder (PTSD) in young adult survivors of childhood cancer. *Pediatr Blood Cancer.* 2006;49:177–182.

29. Luecken LJ, Dausch B, Gulla V, Hong R, Compas BE. Alterations in morning cortisol associated with PTSD in women with breast cancer. *J Psychosom Res.* 2004;56:13–15.

30. Mehnert A, Koch U. Prevalence of acute and post-traumatic stress disorder and comorbid mental disorders in breast cancer patients during primary cancer care: a prospective study. *Psychooncology.* 2007;16:181–188.

31. Mundy EA, Blanchard EB, Cirenza E, Gargiulo J, Maloy B, Blanchard CG. Postraumatic stress disorder in breast cancer patients following autologous bone marrow transplantation or conventional cancer treatments. *Behav Res Ther.* 200;38:1015–1027.

32. Okamura M, Yamawaki S, Akechi T, Taniguchi K, Uchitomi Y. Psychiatric disorders following first breast cancer recurrence: prevalence, associated factors and relationship to quality of life. *Jpn J Clin Oncol.* 2005;35:302–309.

33. Palmer SC, Kagee A, Coyne JC, DeMichele A. Experience of trauma, distress, and posttraumatic stress disorder among breast cancer patients. *Psychosom Med.* 2004;66:258–264.

34. Akechi T, Okuyama T, Sugawara Y, Nakano T, Shima YM, Uchitomi Y. Major depression, adjustment disorders, and post-traumatic stress disorder in terminally ill cancer patients: associated and predictive factors. *J Clin Oncol.* 2004;22:1957–1965.

35. Hobbie WL, Stuber M, Meeske K, et al. Symptoms of posttraumatic stress in young adult survivors of childhood cancer. *J Clin Oncol.* 2000;24:4060–4066.

36. Kadan-Lottick NS, Vanderwerker LC, Block SD, Zhang B, Prigerson HG. Psychiatric disorders and mental health service use in patients with advanced cancer: a report from the coping with cancer study. *Cancer.* 2005;104:2872–2881.

37. Widows MR, Jacobsen PB, Fields KK. Relation of psychological vulnerability factors to posttraumatic stress disorder symptomatology in bone marrow transplant recipients. *Psychosom Med.* 2000;62:873–882.

38. Pelcovitz D, Goldenburg Libov B, Mandel F, Kaplan S, Weinblatt M, Septimus A. Posttraumatic stress disorder and family functioning in adolescent cancer. *J Trauma Stress.* 1998;11:205–221.

39. Kazak A, Alderfer MA, Streisand R, et al. Treatment of posttraumatic stress symptoms in adolescent survivors of childhood cancer and their families: a randomized clinical trial. *J Fam Psychol.* 2004;18:493–504.

40. Levine EG, Eckhardt J, Targ E. Change in post-traumatic stress symptoms following psychosocial treatment for breast cancer. *Psychooncology.* 2005;14:618–635.

41. Winzelberg AJ, Classen C, Alpers GW, et al. Evaluation of an internet support group for women with primary breast cancer. *Cancer.* 2003;97:1164–1173.

42. Resick PA, Monson CM, Gutner C. Psychosocial treatments for PTSD. In: Friedman MJ, Keane M, Resick PA (eds). *Handbook of PTSD: Science and practice.* New York: Guilford Press; 2007:330–338.

Somatoform Disorders and Factitious Illness/ Malingering in the Oncology Setting

Lucy A. Epstein, Felicia A. Smith, and Theodore A. Stern

INTRODUCTION

The somatoform disorders have in common the unconscious production of physical symptoms for which no organic basis is found. These medically unexplained symptoms can be challenging for both oncologists and consulting psychiatrists. Although a medical condition, such as an underlying malignancy, may be the source of these varied complaints, a somatoform disorder must also be considered (especially in atypical presentations). In an oncology setting, physicians must differentiate between somatic *symptoms* (e.g., pain, fatigue, anorexia, or dyspnea) that may occur in a patient with cancer (but are out of proportion with what's expected) and those that occur in the context of a somatoform *disorder*. Somatizing patients account for up to 30% of all cases seen in outpatient clinics,[1,2] and they have twice the medical care utilization (and cost) of their nonsomatizing counterparts.[3] Moreover, somatizers have lower overall function than patients with chronic medical illness.[4,5] The etiology of somatoform disorders is multifactorial, involving a combination of biological, psychological, and social factors.[6-14]

Psychiatrists are likely to encounter patients with somatoform disorders in oncology clinics for a variety of reasons: they are common, they involve physical symptoms that mandate a full medical evaluation, they often come to light during times of stress (e.g., at the time of cancer diagnosis), and they are often associated with psychiatric illness (most often depression and anxiety).[15-20] Misdiagnosis is quite common; for example, up to 15% of patients diagnosed with conversion disorder are later found to have a neurological illness.[21,22] Treatment is focused on ruling out medical causes of symptoms, on fostering a treatment alliance with a primary provider, and on enhancing function.

PRESENTING CLINICAL FEATURES

Several subtypes of somatoform disorders are included in the *Diagnostic and Statistical Manual of Mental Disorders-IV* (DSM-IV).[23] *Somatization disorder* involves recurrent symptoms in at least four organ systems: gastrointestinal (e.g., with abdominal cramping); genitourinary (e.g., with dysuria); neurological (e.g., with unexplained headache); and pain (e.g., with pain in the absence of corroborating neurological signs).

CASE STUDY

A 55-year-old woman with a remote history of nonmetastatic breast cancer presents to her oncologist reporting a "diffusely positive" review of systems. The oncologist suspects her symptoms are somatoform in origin but is concerned about missing an obscure medical etiology. A review of the medical record reveals multiple visits for headache, abdominal pain, and vague somatic complaints over the preceding years, and that no obvious physical cause had ever been identified. The oncologist proceeds with a full medical evaluation in his office and encourages her to establish consistent follow-up with her primary care provider.

This disorder occurs more commonly in women than in men,[24-26] and it can co-exist with numerous psychiatric conditions (such as major depression, substance dependence, and Axis II disorders).

Another subset of somatoform disorders is *somatoform pain disorder*. In this condition, the patient has persistent pain that is the focus of clinical attention.[23] The pain has no clear medical basis, or, if it does, the experience of pain is out of proportion to what would be expected.[23] Patients describe the pain as severe and disabling, and they develop a significant loss of function. In the oncology setting, this pain may be related to the cancer itself (though significantly more than expected) or a result of a treatment (e.g., surgery or radiation therapy). Women are affected more commonly than are men, and patients may have co-morbid major depression. As with other somatoform disorders, somatoform pain disorder remains a diagnosis of exclusion and it may be difficult to distinguish it from cancer-related pain. In this situation, the psychiatrist should be particularly adept at delineating indicated uses for narcotics from use of narcotics for secondary gain. This may be complicated in the oncology setting, where indications for narcotic use are often clinically justified.

A patient with *conversion disorder* presents with acute physical symptoms (most often neurological) in the setting of psychological stress.[23]

CASE STUDY

A 32-year-old patient presents to her primary care physician with the sensation of a lump in her throat. She has been under tremendous stress at work. Her husband is concerned that she might have cancer. The patient (rather blandly) describes that she hasn't been eating much because of the feeling that she might choke. Her doctor initiates a work-up to rule out organic causes, but she suspects *globus hystericus*.

Symptoms often do not correspond to known neuroanatomical structures and may appear, and resolve, abruptly. Patients may demonstrate a striking lack of alarm at their symptoms (*la belle indifférence*). As with other somatoform disorders, conversion symptoms may be superimposed onto known medical illnesses (such as the appearance of pseudo-seizures in the setting of a known seizure disorder).[27] Functional brain imaging studies have implicated the anterior cingulate gyrus, orbitofrontal cortex, striatum, thalamus, and the primary sensorimotor cortex.[28,29] Several medical conditions, such as multiple sclerosis, can present with a similar array of disparate and perplexing symptoms. It may take several years and recurrent presentations before the correct diagnosis is made.

Hypochondriasis involves a worried preoccupation with the persistent belief that one has a serious medical illness, despite repeated evaluations and reassurances to the contrary.[28] Patients do not create symptoms, but rather they misattribute trivial symptoms to serious causes. They intensely fear disease and are preoccupied by bodily symptoms; the belief that one has cancer is quite common in this population. The prevalence of hypochondriasis is equal in women and men,[30-35] and patients may have had an early history of medical illness and/or abuse. As with other somatoform disorders, hypochondriasis does not protect against true medical illness. In fact, these individuals are at some risk of underdiagnosis, as physicians (after performing repeated negative evaluations) may not take the patient's symptoms seriously. Moreover, the presence of a true medical illness, such as cancer, and the concomitant increase in anxiety that accompanies it often causes an exacerbation in abnormal illness behavior in this population.

Body dysmorphic disorder is also relevant to the cancer population. In this condition, there is a preoccupation with an imagined defect with one's body. Commonly afflicted areas include the face, breasts, and genitals.[36] Such patients may repeatedly request consultations by plastic surgeons and dermatologists for correction of perceived defects. There may be substantial clinical overlap with obsessive-compulsive disorder and social phobia.[7]

Evaluation

History. The psychiatrist should attempt to gather a complete history from the patient, focusing on the presenting complaint. Typically, the primary physician or oncologist will have already asked about medical symptoms (including their pattern, quality, frequency, duration, and severity). The psychiatrist can add to the history by attempting to redress physical complaints with an ear tuned to the underlying affect. The psychiatrist should then conduct a full psychiatric interview, including the history of psychiatric symptoms and any temporal relationship to current physical symptoms. The consultant should also perform a psychiatric review of systems, covering symptoms from the affective, anxiety, and psychotic realms (and ruling out thoughts of suicide or homicide). Obtaining a history of substance abuse is important, as is any past trauma. Last, a psychiatric history (e.g., of suicide attempts, hospitalizations, medication trials, and current treaters) should be gathered.

Examination. The mental status examination is a detailed observation of a patient's behavior, speech, language, mood, affect, and cognition. With patients who somatize, there is often a noticeable disconnection between the stated severity of the symptoms and the affect displayed. The physical examination can also add important information. Among the most important physical findings are those that indicate frontal lobe dysfunction, as the frontal lobes govern executive function (e.g., decision making, planning, and inhibition of behavior). Tests that assess the status of the frontal lobes (by assessing the presence of frontal release signs and performing go-no-go tests) are brief and easily performed. Last, the patient's level of cognition can be screened with tests like the mini-mental state examination.[37]

Laboratory tests. A standard battery of tests includes a complete blood count, a metabolic panel, and levels of thyroid-stimulating hormone, B_{12}, folate, and rapid-plasma reagent. Specialized tests (e.g., an human immunodeficiency syndrome [HIV] test, an electrocardiogram, an electroencephalogram, a computed tomography or magnetic resonance scan, cancer-specific studies, or lumbar puncture) may also be appropriate, depending on the clinical situation.

Consultations. The psychiatrist may benefit from the results of neuropsychological testing. Neuropsychological tests are divided into two categories: objective (e.g., of cognitive function) and projective. Examples of cognitive screening include the 100-point mini-mental status examination (which follows a format similar to that used by Folstein et al.[37] but with more extensive questioning) and the trails making test B (which assesses frontal lobe function). Projective testing may provide a window into the patient's coping style, insight, and underlying psychiatric illnesses, which may contribute to physical complaints. Last, it may be useful for the psychiatric consultant to suggest that other services (such as Neurology) evaluate the patient, especially if symptoms span several domains.

Differential diagnosis. As somatoform disorders are diagnoses of exclusion, a broad differential diagnosis must be considered. The first priority is to rule out an acute medical illness. Psychological factors affecting medical illness, such as stress that worsens postchemotherapy nausea, must also be considered. Functional somatic symptoms (such as anorexia, fatigue, lethargy, or pain) can overlap with somatoform disorders, except that a sole organ system is most often the focus of the symptom. Factitious illness and malingering also may present with physical symptoms without an organic basis, for either primary or secondary gain. However, in these conditions, symptoms are consciously created

(as opposed to being derived from the subconscious, as in somatoform disorders). Other Axis I or Axis II disorders also need to be ruled out. In particular, affective disorders, anxiety disorders, and primary psychotic disorders can all include somatic complaints. Depression and anxiety are particularly common in the cancer population. Another important consideration is a substance dependence disorder, which commonly produces bodily complaints. Dissociative disorders, characterized by disruptions in consciousness, identity, perception, or memory, can result in an inconsistent or vague history that may not correlate with objective findings.[23] Last, it is important to remember that cultural components of psychiatric presentations often are somatic in nature,[38,39] and the somatoform diagnoses in general fit less well into cultures that have a more unified view of mind and body.[7] The cultural background of the physician may also influence how she or he interprets the symptom presented.[40]

Management. A three-step approach to somatoform disorders comprises the thorough evaluation of medical causes, a psychological approach that focuses on building and maintaining a treatment alliance, and the use of medications or psychotherapy.

Evaluation of medical causes. All potential medical causes should be evaluated fully. This is particularly true for patients who repeatedly seek care from their doctors. Although it may be tempting to dismiss these cases, one must remember that occult disease can be detected among those who persistently seek examinations and treatment. Medical illness can serve as a nidus around which somatization is built.[41] However, low probability conditions temper the desire to order extensive testing. Each procedure carries its own risks, and one needs to balance the investigation of a complaint with the potential risk of the test itself. This is especially true for patients with hypochondriasis; here, the physician's reassurance about a negative result is unlikely to produce a sense of relief.

Alliance-building. Throughout the medical evaluation, the physician should aim for an effective alliance with the patient.[42,43] Even when no organic basis is found, the patient's suffering may fail to improve. In some cases it is useful to tell the patient that negative tests are reassuring and that the physician realizes that symptoms may persist. An approach that combines validation of the patient's point of view (including emotional aspects of their situation in the discussion), and that emphasizes the connection among biological, psychological, and social factors can be useful.[6]

There is little to be gained from direct confrontation of the patient by denying the reality of their symptoms; moreover, it can be stigmatizing and frustrating.[6] However, much can be gained by displays of confidence (saying that symptoms can improve, even if we don't know their origin). Improvement in function should be the goal of all treatment. This is best done by referring the patient to a physician who can see the patient for time-limited, regular appointments.[38] Last, the persistence of the patient's complaint can lead to negative countertransference reactions (e.g., as manifest by hostility or contempt) on the part of the physician, who may feel that such patients waste their time and/or deplete resources. Physicians should remain cognizant of the patient's suffering and remember to use their countertransference reactions in the service of the patient.

Psychopharmacological/psychotherapeutic options. Medical management can be helpful in certain situations. For example, a patient with major depression and concurrent pain may benefit from a dual-acting agent, such as a tricyclic antidepressant (e.g., amitriptyline). Selective serotonin-reuptake inhibitors (SSRIs) and clomipramine have been shown to convey substantial benefits in those with body dysmorphic disorder.[38] Additionally, antidepressants are useful, both, in the treatment of medically unexplained symptoms and functional somatic syndromes.[44,45] However, it is wise to avoid polypharmacy in somatizing patients, who may become preoccupied with adverse effects. In addition, narcotics should be avoided so that additional problems (e.g., dependence, diversion, and the need for further presentations for secondary gain) do not develop. Lastly, behavior-based therapies, such as cognitive-behavioral therapy (CBT), can help the patient to address core beliefs around illness, to recognize cognitive distortions, to change maladaptive coping strategies, and to limit excessive use of medical care.[46,47]

FACTITIOUS ILLNESS AND MALINGERING

Patients who deliberately manufacture symptoms, as in factitious illness or malingering, create a perplexing and frustrating situation for the physicians who care for them. Patients with factitious illness create medical and/or psychiatric symptoms for primary gain, which is to occupy the sick role.[23] Malingering is driven by secondary gain, which is typically a material reward, such as disability payments.[23] These disorders violate an implicit contract of trust between doctor and patient, making them particularly frustrating for the provider. As with somatoform disorders, they are diagnoses of exclusion, and each presentation requires a full medical and psychiatric evaluation. They may occur in a patient who has a true underlying medical illness (e.g., a patient with chronic pain may also malinger to obtain opiates), and actual self-injury can result from them (e.g., by deliberate self-harm).[36] Treatment includes ruling out medical emergencies, offering psychiatric assistance, setting clear boundaries, thoroughly documenting the assessment and treatment, and managing intense countertransference reactions that these patients tend to elicit.

Presenting clinical features

Factitious illness

CASE STUDY

A 32-year-old woman presents to an outpatient oncology practice stating that due to her family history of cancer she needs a prophylactic double mastectomy and oophrectomy. She cites a long list of cancers in female relatives, including breast cancer in her mother and both sisters, and ovarian cancer in her maternal grandmother and another sister. She is unable to provide any documentation to support this request and refuses to submit to genetic testing. When her mother is contacted, she said that there was no such history of cancer in the family and that the patient had a long history of generating false medical reports.

Presentations may include an inconsistent history, false laboratory results, or self-injury.[48] At times, the results can be life-threatening (e.g., a patient who surreptitiously injects insulin and develops profound hypoglycemia).[49] See Table 48–1 for selected examples from the literature. The oncology literature describes several scenarios by which factitious illness presents in this setting. There are several examples of patients who fabricate personal or family histories of cancer to receive mastectomy or chemotherapy.[60–62] Patients have also used electronic resources to create false documents regarding a history of cancer.[63,64] In addition, the deliberate creation of symptoms consistent with pheochromocytoma

Table 48–1. Selected presentations of factitious illness

Cardiac: Acute chest pain[50]
Pulmonary: Cyanosis[51]
Vascular: Simulated aortic dissection[52]
Hematologic:
    Bleeding due to the injection of warfarin[53]
    Simulation of sickle cell crisis[54]
Infectious: False reports of HIV (+) status[55]
Toxic: Vomiting due to overingestion of ipecac[56]
Metabolic: Hypoglycemia due to self-injection with Insulin
Allergic: Factitious anaphylaxis to beestings[57]
Musculoskeletal: False reports of trauma[58]
Pain: Chronic cervical spine pain[59]

---

have been described (including using vanilla extract to create a false positive test result for vanillyl-mandelic acid).[65–68] A patient may also present with psychiatric complaints.[69,70] Munchausen's syndrome, defined by peregrination, *pseudologia phantastica* (embellishment of tales regarding symptoms), and feigning of illness, is a severe form of factitious illness.[71] It was named after Baron von Munchausen, an eighteenth century Prussian officer who traveled from inn to inn, telling tall tales of his journeys.[72] Psychiatrists should also be aware of Munchausen syndrome by proxy, a condition in which a caregiver generates a factitious illness in his or her child.

Unfortunately, it can be difficult to quantify the incidence of factitious illness, as the diagnosis is difficult to make, and physicians may be hesitant to document it in the medical record.[73] The prototypical patient is young and female (and may have had some training in healthcare), but highly variable demographics exist.[74,75] They tend to lead itinerant lives with few close contacts.[76] Patients may generate a narrative that contains detailed medical terminology, which unravels under close examination.[74,75] Such individuals may be vague and evasive when asked direct questions. They may have had an extensive history of medical examinations, and may appear oddly eager to undergo painful or invasive procedures.[76]

Malingering

CASE STUDY

A 47-year-old man with a history of heroin dependence and multiple jail sentences for illicit drug dealing presents to his oncologist with reports of chest wall pain. He has a history of metastatic lung cancer that has been unresponsive to surgery and chemotherapy. His oncologist becomes concerned when he reports he had lost his prescriptions for opiates several times in a row, and requests a rapidly escalating dose. The oncologist feels caught between her desire to treat his pain and her concern about the potential for drug diversion or abuse.

Malingering is not a formal psychiatric diagnosis on Axis I or II, but it can be a common reason for psychiatric consultation, especially when the patient's complaint is inconsistent with known medical or psychiatric illness.[74] Malingerers often provide a vague and unverifiable history, may have an extensive legal history, and describe symptoms that fail to correlate with objective findings.[76] Unlike the patient with factitious illness, a patient who is malingering may be uncooperative with objective tests or invasive procedures and may leave before such tests are conducted. There is a substantial overlap with antisocial personality disorder (defined by a lack of empathy, by lying, and by a flagrant disregard for social norms), and with substance dependence.[76]

Evaluation

History. The psychiatrist should aim to gather as complete a medical and psychiatric history from the patient as possible. Obtaining a history of substance dependence is critical (although it may be minimized). History gathering may be difficult, as the patient may present a "diffusely positive" review of systems; the interview may be rich with language, but short on detail.

Examination. The patient's mental status examination can provide crucial data. Patients may appear overly friendly in an effort to engage the interviewer. Alternatively, they may seem guarded, especially when certain topics (such as substance dependence or legal involvement) are broached. The psychiatrist may become internally aware of a growing mistrust and/or dislike of the patient. Observing the patient when the patient does not know he or she is not aware of being observed can also provide valuable information, as the patient may unwittingly exhibit the factitious behavior (such as heating up a thermometer to feign fever). In emergency circumstances, a search of a patient's belongings may be necessary.[76]

Laboratory tests and studies. In the case of factitious illness, spurious laboratory results may provide a clue to the diagnosis. For example, a finding of high serum insulin and a concurrent low C-peptide is diagnostic of the exogenous use of insulin.[77] Depending on the nature of the complaint other tests (such as HIV testing, computed tomography, magnetic resonance imaging, or electroencephalography) can be reasonable options. It can also be useful for the psychiatrist to refer patients for neuropsychological testing, although such individuals will be unlikely to agree to it. Psychological testing (such as with the Personality Assessment Inventory) can be particularly helpful.[78,79] Last, it may be appropriate to ask for consultations from other disciplines (such as neurology), especially when symptoms have a clinical overlap with psychiatric manifestations.

Differential diagnosis. Factitious illness and malingering are diagnoses of exclusion; extensive searches for other causes are warranted. However, there is often a complicated mix of motivations in these disorders, and at times more than one may be apparent. Differentiating among them (especially factitious illness from malingering) can be difficult.[80] As with somatoform disorders, underlying medical illness, functional somatic syndromes, and psychological factors affecting medical illness should all be ruled out. The psychiatrist should then consider another Axis I or Axis II disorder that could explain the presentation. Factitious illness may correlate most often with borderline personality disorder, while malingering is more often seen in the context of antisocial personality disorder.[46] The clinician should also rule out a substance dependence disorder, in particular with a patient for whom malingering is suspected. As with somatoform disorders, the clinician should consider how cultural aspects of psychiatric illness may influence the presentation.[81-83]

Management

Rule out and treat medical illness. Although it may be tempting to dismiss cases where factitious illness or malingering is clearly present, it is crucial to identify and treat self-injury, underlying prior disease, and/or occult illness in patients who repeatedly report medical or psychiatric symptoms.

Psychiatric treatment. For a patient with factitious illness, psychiatric assistance should be offered. Ideally, the treatment would address dependency needs and any underlying masochism (with pain and self-injury as a reflection of their need for care).[66] However, there has been little clinical success with interventions such as group psychotherapy, CBT, or psychodynamic psychotherapy.[66] In addition, the psychiatrist should be prepared for treatment refusal, as the patient may feel intensely angry and humiliated. Leaving the hospital against medical advice occur frequently.[66]

The role of confrontation is debated in the literature. In a retrospective case series of patients with factitious illness, 75% of cases resulted in confrontation; however, only 17% of patients acknowledged their problem.[65] Some clinicians advocate a therapeutic confrontation with related offers of assistance.[84] Others state that emphasis on a doctor-patient alliance should be promoted even if direct confrontation does not occur.[67,85] The psychiatrist can also play a valuable role by helping to contain staff's intense countertransference reactions (which may include feelings of hatred and contempt).[66]

Malingering is also difficult to treat, because the physician and patient have different goals. Physicians don't like to think of their patients as trying to create symptoms for personal gain, and they may fear legal ramifications if the patient in fact has a true medical illness.[64] However, physicians enter into an unwitting collusion with the patient's agenda if they fail to consider the diagnosis. Optimal management includes setting firm limits and clearly documenting care. There is no indication for the use of psychotropics or psychotherapy, and prescriptions for medications of any type should be avoided. Correlated conditions, such as substance dependence, can be treated. However, the psychiatrist should be prepared for rejection of offers of assistance.[66]

Limit setting. In the case of suspected factitious illness or malingering, setting limits and providing clear expectations is the key. Second,

a behavioral management plan can be beneficial for those who present frequently. Psychiatrists should do their best to consolidate care into one setting. Direct contact with a provider can be essential, so that they can be aware of a patient who is trying to obtain medications from multiple providers.

Careful documentation. It is also important to clearly and thoroughly document care, including the reason for the exclusion of medical or psychiatric illness. Additionally, if the psychiatrist has been able to contact collateral sources, this should be included in the notes as well. Electronic medical records that link affiliated hospitals can furnish a very useful database of a patient's presentation that can guide future management.[86]

REFERENCES

1. Bass C, Sharpe M. Medically unexplained symptoms in patients attending medical outpatient clinics. In: Weatherall DA, Ledingham JG, Warrell DA (eds). *Oxford textbook of medicine.* 4th ed. Oxford: Oxford University Press; 2003:1296–1303.

2. Escobar JI, Hoyos-Nervi C, Gara M. Medically unexplained physical symptoms in medical practice: a psychiatric perspective. *Environ Health Perspect.* 2002;110(S4):631–636.

3. Barsky AJ, Orav J, Bates DW. Somatization increases medical utilization and costs independent of psychiatric and medical comorbidity. *Arch Gen Psychiatry.* 2005;62:903–910.

4. Smith GR, Monson RA, Ray DC. Patients with multiple unexplained symptoms: their characteristics, functional health, and health care utilization. *Arch Intern Med.* 1986;146:69–72.

5. Kroenke K, Spitzer RL, Williams JBW, et al. Physical symptoms in primary care: predictors of psychiatric disorders and functional impairment. *Arch Fam Med.* 1994;3:774–779.

6. Stephenson DT, Price JR. Medically unexplained physical symptoms in emergency medicine. *Emerg Med J.* 2006;23:595–600.

7. Mayou R, Kirmayer LJ, Simon G, Kroenke K, Sharpe M. Somatoform disorders: time for a new approach in DSM-V. *Am J Psychiatry.* 2005;162(5):847–855.

8. Newman MG, Clayton L, Zuellig A, et al. The relationship of childhood sexual abuse and depression with somatic symptoms and medical utilization. *Psychol Med.* 2000;30(5):1063–1077.

9. Arnow BA, Hart S, Scott C, Dea R, O'connell, Taylor CB. Childhood sexual abuse, psychological distress, and medical use among women. *Psychosom Med.* 1999;61(6);762–770.

10. Drossman DA, Leserman J, Nachman G, et al. Sexual and physical abuse in women with functional or organic gastrointestinal disorders. *Ann Intern Med.* 1990;113(11):828–833.

11. Farley M, Patsalides BM. Physical symptoms, posttraumatic stress disorder, and healthcare utilization of women with and without childhood physical and sexual abuse. *Psychol Rep.* 2001;89(3):595–606.

12. Marsden CD. Hysteria—a neurologist's view. *Psychol Med.* 1986;16:277–288.

13. Williams DT, Ford B, Fahn S. Phenomenology and psychopathology related to psychogenic movement disorders. *Adv Neurol.* 1995;65:233–257.

14. Feinstein A, Stergiopoulos V, Fine J, Lang AE. Psychiatric outcome in patients with a psychogenic movement disorder: a prospective study. *Neuropsychiatry Neuropsychol Behav Neurol.* 2001;14:169–176.

15. Hamilton J, Campos R, Creed F. Anxiety, depression, and management of medically unexplained symptoms in medical clinics. *J R Coll Physicians Lond.* 1996;30:18–20.

16. Brown FW, Golding JM, Smith R. Psychiatric comorbidity in primary care somatization disorder. *Psychosom Med.* 1990;52:445–451.

17. Russo J, Katon W, Sullivan M, Clark M, Buchwald D. Severity of somatization and its relationship to psychiatric disorders and personality. *Psychosomatics.* 1994;35:546–556.

18. Kroenke K, Jackson JL, Chamberlin J. Depressive and anxiety disorders in patients presenting with physical complaints: clinical predictors and outcome. *Am J Med.* 1997;103:339–347.

19. Simon GE, VonKorff M, Piccinelli M, Fullerton C, Ormel J. An international study of the relation between somatic symptoms and depression. *N Engl J Med.* 1999;341:1329–1335.

20. Simon GE, VonKorff M. Somatization and psychiatric disorder in the NIMH epidemiologic catchment area study. *Am J Psychiatry.* 1991;148:1494–1500.

21. Hurwitz T, Prichard JW. Conversion disorder and fMRI. *Neurology.* 2006;67:1914–1915.

22. Hurwitz T. Somatization and conversion disorder. *Can J Psychiatry.* 2004;49:172–178.

23. American Psychiatric Association. *Diagnostic and statistical manual for mental disorders.* 4th ed. Washington, DC: APA; 1994.

24. Barsky AJ, Peekna HM, Borus JF. Somatic symptom reporting in women and men. *J Gen Intern Med.* 2001;16:266–275.

25. Swartz M, Blazer D, George L, Landerman R. Somatization disorder in a community population. *Am J Psychiatry.* 1986;143:1403–1408.

26. Smith GR, Monson RA, Livingston RL. Somatization disorder in men. *Gen Hosp Psychiatry.* 1985;7:4–8.

27. Alsaadi TM, Vinter Marquez A. Psychogenic nonepileptic seizures. *Am Fam Physician.* 2005;72(5):849–856.

28. Ballmaier M, Schmidt R. Conversion disorder revisited. *Funct Neurol.* 2005;20(3):105–113.

29. Ghaffar O, Staines WR, Feinstein A. Unexplained neurologic symptoms: an fMRI study of sensory conversion disorder. *Neurology.* 2006;67:2036–2038.

30. Kroenke K, Spitzer RL. Gender difference in the reporting of physical and somatoform symptoms. *Psychosom Med.* 1998;60:150–155.

31. Hibbard JH, Pope CR. Gender roles, illness orientation and the use of medical services. *Soc Sci Med.* 1983;17:129–137.

32. Hernandez J, Kellner R. Hypochondriacal concerns and attitudes toward illness in males and females. *Int J Psychiatry Med.* 1992;22:251–263.

33. Kirmayer LJ, Robbins JM. Three forms of somatization in primary care: prevalence, co-occurrence and sociodemographic characteristics. *J Nerv Ment Dis.* 1991;179:647–655.

34. Barsky AJ, Wyshak G, Klerman GL. Hypochondriasis: an evaluation of the DSM-III criteria in medical outpatients. *Arch Gen Psychiatry.* 1986;43:493–500.

35. Barsky AJ, Wyshak G, Klerman GL, Latham KS. The prevalence of hypochondriasis in medical outpatients. *Soc Psychiatry Psychiatr Epidemiol.* 1990;25:89–94.

36. Barsky AJ, Stern TA, Greenberg DB, Cassem NH. Functional somatic symptoms and somatoform disorders. In: Stern TA, Fricchione GL, Cassem NH, Jellinek MS, Rosenbaum JF (eds). *Massachusetts general hospital handbook of general hospital psychiatry.* 5th ed. Philadelphia: Mosby; 2004:269–312.

37. Folstein MF, Folstein SE, McHugh PR. "Mini mental state." A practical guide for grading the cognitive state of patients for the clinician. *J Pyschiatr Res.* 1975;12:189–198.

38. Goldberg DP, Bridges K. Somatic presentations of psychiatric illness in primary care settings. *J Psychosom Research.* 1988;32(2):137–144.

39. Lin KM, Cheung F. Mental health issues for Asian Americans. *Psychiatr Serv.* 1999;50(6):774–780.

40. Rabinowitz T, Lasek J. An approach to the patient with physical complaints or irrational anxiety about an illness or their appearance. In: Stern TA, (ed). *The ten-minute guide to psychiatric diagnosis and treatment.* New York: Professional Publishing Group; 2005:225–238.

41. Glick TH, Workman TP, Gaufberg SV. Suspected conversion disorder: foreseeable risks and avoidable errors. *Acad Emerg Med.* 2000;7:1272–1277.

42. McCahill ME. Somatoform and related disorders: delivery of diagnosis as the first step. *Am Fam Physician.* 1995;52(1):193–204.

43. Purcell TB. The somatic patient. *Emerg Med Clin North Am.* 1991;9(1):137–159.

44. O'Malley PG, Jackson JL, Santoro J, Tomkins G, Balden E, Kroenke K. Antidepressant therapy for unexplained symptoms and symptom syndromes. *J Fam Pract.* 1999;48:980–990.

45. Gruber AJ, Hudson JI, Pope HG. The management of treatment-resistant depression in disorders on the interface of psychiatry and medicine. Fibromyalgia, chronic fatigue syndrome, migraine, irritable bowel syndrome, atypical facial pain, and premenstrual dysphoric disorder. *Psychiatr Clin North Am.* 1996;19:351–369.

46. Kroenke K, Swindell R. Cognitive-behavioral therapy for somatization and symptoms syndromes: a critical review of controlled clinical trials. *Psychother Psychosom.* 2000;69:205–215.

47. Sharpe M, Peveler R, Mayou R. The psychological treatment of patients with functional somatic symptoms: a practical guide. *J Psychosom Res.* 1992;36:515–529.

48. Krahn LE, Hongzhe L, O'Connor MC. Patients who strive to be ill: factitious disorder with physical symptoms. *Am J Psychiatry.* 2003;160(6):1163–1168.

49. Bretz SW, Richards JR. Munchausen syndrome presenting acutely in the emergency department. *J Emerg Med.* 2000;18(4):417–420.

50. Mehta NJ, Khan IA. Cardiac Munchausen syndrome. *Chest.* 2002;122(5):1649–1653.

51. Kellner CH, Eth S. Code blue—factitious cyanosis. *J Nerv Ment Dis.* 1982;170(6):371–372.

52. Hopkins RA, Harrington CJ, Poppas A. Munchausen syndrome simulating acute aortic dissection. *Ann Thorac Surg.* 2006;81:1497–1499.

53. Lazarus A, Kozinn WP. Munchausen's syndrome with hematuria and sepsis: an unusual case. *Int J Psychiatry Med.* 1991;21(1):113–116.

54. Ballas SK. Factitious sickle cell acute painful episodes: a secondary type of Munchausen syndrome. *Am J Hematol.* 1996;53(4):254–258.

55. Ryan J, Taylor CB, Bryant GD, Nayagam AT, Sanders J. HIV malingering in the accident and emergency department. *J Accid Emer Med.* 1995;12(1):59–61.

56. Rashid N. Medically unexplained myopathy due to ipecac abuse. *Psychosomatics.* 2006;47(2):167–169.

57. Hendrix S, Sale S, Zeiss CR, Utley J, Patterson R. Factitious hymenoptera allergic emergency: a report of a new variant of Munchausen's syndrome. *J Allergy Clin Immunol.* 1981;67(1):8–13.

58. Meek SJ, Kendall J, Cornelius P, Younge PA. Munchausen syndrome presenting as major trauma. *J Accid Emerg Med.* 1996;13(2):137–138.

59. Elmore JL. Munchausen syndrome: an endless search for self, managed by house arrest and mandated treatment. *Ann Emer Med.* 2005;45(5):561–563.

60. Feldman MD, Hamilton JC. Mastectomy resulting from factitious disorder. *Psychosomatics.* 2007;48(4):361.

61. Feldman MD. Prophylactic bilateral radical mastectomy resulting from factitious disorder. *Psychosomatics.* 2001;42(6):519–521.

62. Grenga TE, Dowden RV. Munchausen's syndrome and prophylactic mastectomy. *Plast Reconstr Surg.* 1987;80(1):119–120.

63. Levenson JL, Chafe W, Flanagan P. Factitious ovarian cancer: feigning via resources on the internet. *Psychosomatics.* 2007;48(1):71–73.

64. Hadeed V, Trump DL, Mies C. Electronic cancer Munchausen syndrome. *Ann Intern Med.* 1998;129(1):73.

65. Spitzer D, Bongartz D, Ittel TH, Sieberth HG. Simulation of a pheochromocytoma—Munchausen syndrome. *Eur J Med Res.* 1998;3(12):549–553.

66. Stern TA, Cremens CM. Factitious pheochromocytoma. One patient history and literature review. *Psychosomatics.* 1998;39(3):283–287.

67. Kailasam MT, Parmer RJ, Stone RA, et al. Factitious pheochromocytoma: novel mimicry by Valsalva maneuver and clues to diagnosis. *Am J Hypertens.* 1995;8(6):651–655.

68. Keiser HR. Surreptitious self-administration of epinephrine resulting in 'pheochromocytoma'. *JAMA.* 1991;266(11):1553–1555.

69. Thompson CR, Beckson M. A case of factitious homicidal ideation. *J Am Acad Psychiatry Law.* 2004;32(3):277–281.

70. Waite S, Geddes A. Malingered psychosis leading to involuntary psychiatric hospitalization. *Australas Psychiatry.* 2006;14(4):419–421.

71. Asher R. Munchausen's syndrome. *Lancet.* 1951;1:339–341.

72. Rabinowitz T, Lasek J. An approach to the patient with physical complaints or irrational anxiety about an illness or their appearance. In: Stern TA (ed). *The ten-minute guide to psychiatric diagnosis and treatment.* New York: Professional Publishing Group; 2005:225–238.

73. Krahn LE, Hongzhe L, O'Connor MC. Patients who strive to be ill: factitious disorder with physical symptoms. *Am J Psychiatry.* 2003;160(6):1163–1168.

74. Stephenson DT, Price JR. Medically unexplained physical symptoms in emergency medicine. *Emerg Med J.* 2006;23:595–600.

75. Reich P, Gottfried LA. Factitious disorder in a teaching hospital. *Ann Intern Med.* 1983;99:240–247.

76. Ford CV, Abernethy V. Factitious illness: a multidisciplinary consideration of ethical issues. *Gen Hosp Psychiatry.* 1981;3:329–336.

77. Service FJ, Rubenstein A, Horwitz DL. C-peptide analysis in diagnosis of factitial hypoglycemia in an insulin-dependent diabetic. *Mayo Clin Proc.* 1975;50(12):697–701.

78. Hopwood CJ, Morey LC, Rogers R, Sewell K. Malingering on the Personality Assessment Inventory: identification of specific feigned disorders. *J Pers Assess.* 2007;88(1):43–48.

79. Edens JF, Poythress NG, Watkins-Clay MM. Detection of malingering in psychiatric unit and general population prison inmates: a comparison of the PAI, SIMS, and SIRS. *J Pers Assess.* 2007;88(1):33–42.

80. Turner MA. Factitious Disorders: reformulating the DSM-IV criteria. *Psychosomatics.* 2006;47(1):23–32.

81. Goldberg DP, Bridges K. Somatic presentations of psychiatric illness in primary care settings. *J Psychosom Research.* 1988;32(2):137–144.

82. Lin KM, Cheung F. Mental health issues for Asian Americans. *Psychiatr Serv.* 1999;50(6):774–780.

83. Mayou R, Kirmayer LJ, Simon G, et al. Somatoform disorders: time for a new approach in DSM-V. *Am J Psychiatry.* 2005;162(5):847–855.

84. Bass C, Murphy M. Somatisation, somatoform disorders and factitious illness. In: Guthrie E, Creed F (eds). *Seminars in liaison psychiatry.* London: Gaskell; 1996:150.

85. Eisendrath SJ, Rand DC, Feldman MD. Factitious disorders and litigation. In: Feldman MD, Eisendrath SJ (eds). *The spectrum of factitious disorders.* Washington, DC: APA; 1996:65–81.

86. Wright B, Bhugra D, Booth SJ. Computers, communication, and confidentiality: tales of Baron Munchausen. *J Accid Emerg Med.* 1996;13(1):18–20.

CHAPTER 49

Cancer Care for Patients with Schizophrenia

Linda Ganzini and Robert Socherman

INTRODUCTION

Patients with chronic psychotic disorders such as schizophrenia suffer disparities in healthcare throughout life and have special care needs and vulnerabilities at the end of life. Mental healthcare professionals, despite having cared for individuals with schizophrenia for many years, may be uncertain of their role in promoting wellness behaviors in their patients, or working collaboratively with other clinicians when their patients develop cancer. Oncologists and palliative care clinicians may lack comfort in communicating with mentally ill patients, negotiating a maze of mental health services, and prescribing for people already taking psychotropic medications. For patients with schizophrenia we will discuss preventing cancer, assessing pain, and decision-making capacity, prescribing antipsychotic medications, distinguishing delirium from psychosis, and caring for patients who are homeless. Because there are many gaps in our empirical understanding of the challenges that face patients with both schizophrenia and cancer, we will draw on our clinical experience in caring for these patients.

EPIDEMIOLOGY OF SCHIZOPHRENIA

Schizophrenia: In the United States, the prevalence of schizophrenia is approximately 1%. In the year 2000 there were an estimated 350,000 patients with schizophrenia over age 65.[1] There is great heterogeneity in the manifestations and functional impairment associated with schizophrenia. Some patients with decades of severe disease have spent many years in institutional care and never lived independently. Others, especially those whose symptoms first started in middle age, maintain normal affect, have preserved communication skills and cognitive ability, and display only mild residual symptoms between psychotic episodes.[2]

CLINICAL PRESENTATION AND BARRIERS TO CARE

The symptoms of schizophrenia influence health and healthcare practices at many levels. Both the positive symptoms of schizophrenia, including delusions, hallucinations, and paranoia; and the negative symptoms such as social withdrawal, poor eye contact, apathy, odd behaviors, and peculiar or impoverished speech, undermine patients' understanding of their medical illnesses and ability to collaborate with medical providers. Patients with disorganized speech may report physical symptoms in an idiosyncratic or muddled manner. Physical symptom assessment may either be confounded by bizarre somatic delusions or an apparent lack of awareness of gross physical pathology such as perforated bowel or fractures.[3–6] Patients with schizophrenia often admit to a sense of emptiness and appear to respond to distress in an emotionally inappropriate manner. Even a keenly empathic clinician may struggle to develop rapport and gauge her patient's emotional response to psychological stressors, such as knowledge of terminal illness, or to physical symptoms, such as pain.[7]

Patients with schizophrenia frequently demonstrate cognitive impairments, particularly in the attentional and executive systems, which prevent new learning, abstraction, and mental flexibility. Physicians may, at times, encounter maladaptive denial of disease. For example, approximately one-third of patients with schizophrenia do not believe that they have a psychiatric illness,[8] and some patients with schizophrenia continue to deny their cancer diagnosis even in the presence of obvious, and even grotesque physical signs.[4–6,9] These impairments hinder the ability to understand one's illness, make competent decisions regarding therapies, or adhere to rigorous or complicated treatment and medication regimens. Overall, faulty problem-solving abilities on the part of the patient lead to an unsophisticated use of the healthcare system.[10]

Despite these patient-related barriers, many mentally ill patients wish to be involved in and informed about their medical illnesses, and involved in making decisions, even though they perceive that their participation is limited. Their satisfaction with the amount of information they receive is low.[11,12] In one study, patients with psychotic disorders were about half as likely to identify a primary care physician; five times more likely to indicate they needed medical care, but were unable to obtain it; and seven times more likely to indicate they needed a prescription but were unable to secure one.[13]

MORBIDITY AND MORTALITY IN SCHIZOPHRENIA

Schizophrenia reduces life expectancy by at least 15 years.[14] Among patients with schizophrenia, the first decade of the illness is marked by high mortality from suicide and violence.[14,15] Subsequent premature medical morbidity is promoted by unhealthy lifestyles including: tobacco, drug, and alcohol abuse; sedentary activity and unhealthful diet that promotes obesity; and poor adherence to chronic disease regimens.[14,16] For example, over one-third, and in some studies as many as 92% of patients with schizophrenia use tobacco, and quit rates are substantially lower than nonmentally ill comparison groups.[17] As a result of these behaviors, patients with schizophrenia are at higher risk of developing diabetes mellitus and infectious, cardiovascular, and respiratory diseases when compared to age- and sex- matched controls.[18] Among patients with both cancer and schizophrenia, these co-morbidities may worsen overall outcomes. Age-adjusted mortality for patients with schizophrenia remains elevated throughout life, with excess deaths in middle and old age attributable to smoking-related illnesses such as chronic obstructive pulmonary disease, heart disease, and pneumonia.[10] Of great concern, the mortality gap—the gap between the age of death for people in the community without mental illness and those with schizophrenia—has increased over recent decades.[10]

SCHIZOPHRENIA AND CANCER RISK

Despite the aforementioned life style factors that predispose patients to cancer, several decades of research suggests that the risk of malignancy in patients with schizophrenia may be less than expected.[19] Two research groups reported that family members of people with schizophrenia are at reduced risk of developing cancer, suggesting a genetic protective component,[20,21] but this was not confirmed in a third study.[22] In contrast, some studies indicate an elevated risk of lung, breast, and digestive system cancers in patients with schizophrenia, and many develop cancer at a young age.[23–25] Irrespective of the true magnitude of risk, cancer remains one of the most common causes of death in patients with schizophrenia, ranging from 9% to 37%.[26–32]

The views expressed in this chapter are those of the authors and may not represent the views of the Department of Veterans Affairs or the U.S. Government.

PREVENTIVE CARE

Patients with schizophrenia are less likely to undergo routine screening for cancer than people without mental illness. For example, Lindamer and colleagues reported that older women in San Diego with schizophrenia were 25% less likely to undergo pelvic examinations and were 30% less likely to undergo mammograms.[33] Salsberry and coauthors found that among Medicaid-enrolled patients in the Midwest, those with schizophrenia were less likely to have cervical cancer screening when compared to patients with an affective disorder.[34] Carney and coauthors reported that women with psychotic disorders were half as likely to complete a mammography.[35] In addition, screening for colorectal cancer is particularly low among this population, ranging from 4% to 12%.[36,37] These disparities persist despite insurance status. For example, Druss and coauthors reported that Veterans with psychiatric disorders, but not substance abuse, had lower rates of cervical, breast, prostate, and colorectal cancer screening compared to Veterans without mental illness.[38] Lindamer and colleagues interviewed middle-aged and elderly women with schizophrenia. Only 41% had a mammogram in the previous year, though 89% had insurance and 91% had a primary care provider. In comparing patients with and without mammograms, there was no difference in knowledge about breast cancer or the benefits of a mammogram. Those without a mammogram, however, perceived more barriers to obtaining one, and had more negative attitudes about mammography, particularly if their doctor had performed a breast examination or expressed doubt about the need for a mammogram.[39]

CANCER DIAGNOSIS AND TREATMENT

Some patients with schizophrenia who develop cancer are diagnosed later in the course of disease and have fewer curative treatments available. Patients who present with very advanced disease or who have delayed evaluation despite signs of disease (i.e., fungating cancerous skin lesions) are often either severely mentally ill or cognitively impaired.[9] Laurence and colleagues reported higher case fatality rates for cancer among Australian patients with schizophrenia, particularly for skin, cervical, and breast cancer, suggesting a relative failure of secondary prevention. Little data is available on the degree to which mentally ill patients undergo biopsies or other diagnostic evaluations once cancer is suspected, or, avail themselves of chemotherapeutic, radiation or surgical treatments, or palliative interventions when diagnosed.[40] Iezzoni et al. reported that breast cancer patients with mental disability, as determined by social security status, were less likely to undergo surgery and radiotherapy compared to nondisabled people.[41] For these patients, all-cause mortality was higher, but cancer-specific mortality was not. Little is known about factors that facilitate or hinder delivery of cancer care in mentally ill patients. Vahia et al. found that among older patients with schizophrenia, medical treatment was facilitated by less severe positive symptom scores and more severe negative symptom scores.[42] In contrast, Inagaki reported that patients severely impaired by negative symptoms had poorer understanding of cancer treatments and were more likely to be uncooperative with care.[4]

SYMPTOM ASSESSMENT

There are many case reports of unusual pain insensitivity among patients with schizophrenia when severely injured, for example, by fractures, perforated bowel, or burns. This pain insensitivity may lead to delayed or missed diagnoses.[43,44] Sciolla, however, used the SF-36 to compare older patients with schizophrenia with normal controls[45] and found that the level of bodily pain was not different between the two groups, even though ratings of overall physical health by patients with schizophrenia were worse. Schizophrenia patients may also be at risk for undertreatment of pain if clinicians are concerned about prescribing medications, particularly opiates, to a group of patients already taking psychoactive medications. Though patients with schizophrenia have high rates of drug abuse, opiate abuse is relatively rare.[46,47] Descriptions of assessment of other common cancer symptoms, such as dyspnea or fatigue, in patients with schizophrenia are absent from the literature.

DECISION-MAKING CAPACITY AND ADVANCE CARE PLANNING

When a patient with schizophrenia refuses cancer treatments or is psychologically unable to tolerate it, the clinician may question the patient's decision-making capacity. Grisso and Appelbaum identify four legal standards relevant to decision-making capacity, including the abilities to (1) express a choice; (2) understand information relevant to treatment including risks, benefits and alternatives; (3) appreciate this information by applying it to ones own personal situation; and (4) use rational thinking processes, grounded in personal values and interests.[48] For example, patients with schizophrenia may have such disorganized speech or severe ambivalence that they are unable to communicate a stable choice. Cognitive impairments may undermine patients' abilities to weigh risks and benefits. Patients who deny that they have cancer are unable to apply information about options for cancer care to themselves. Psychotic symptoms may render a patient nondecisional if, for example, voices instruct the patient, severe paranoia impairs the patient's ability to work with care providers, or delusions develop around treatment needs. Studies indicate that approximately half of patients with schizophrenia, if applying one or more of these standards, have some difficulties with decision-making abilities. Only a small fraction, however, will have been adjudicated incompetent by a court of law.[49] These decision-making abilities may fluctuate with exacerbation and remission of psychiatric symptoms. Although actual legal standards vary by jurisdiction, clinicians caring for the patient have the de facto and often de jure authority to determine a patient's decision-making abilities without judicial intervention.[50]

Clinicians are granted some flexibility in applying these standards and thresholds in individual cases, and often use a sliding scale whereby as the risks of treatment refusal increase, so does the threshold for determining if the patient is decisional. For example, among patients with advanced cancer, the clinician may respect the patient's refusal of cardiopulmonary resuscitation, even when the patient's understanding of the risks and benefits is poor; however, clinicians may challenge the patient's refusal of this intervention among patients who are younger, are healthy, and are undergoing surgery. Although some ethicists have expressed concern that this sliding scale too easily allows the physician's values to trump the patient's choices, questioning capacity and decision making when a patient refuses beneficial treatments often leads to the involvement of mental health professionals and ethics committees with a more careful and rigorous review of the patient's abilities.[51]

Patients face decisions of varying levels of complexity, ranging from identifying a surrogate decision maker or determining overall goals of care, to deciding among specific treatments such as chemotherapy, surgery or radiation therapy. Patients with schizophrenia may be especially taxed by decisions that are complex in their trade offs between the goals of comfort and quality of life and the prolongation of life; with additional complexity from trade offs between short- and long-term benefits and burdens. Assessment of decision-making capacity should only occur after there have been attempts to educate the patient about the nature of the malignancy and the course of care recommended. Studies of research consent capacity have shown that enhanced consent procedures which include several reviews of the treatment options and tailored educational interventions can transform the level of understanding in nondecisional patients into that of people without mental illness.[52] Even patients with severe denial of cancer may gradually accept their diagnosis and be able to collaborate with the healthcare team. Educational efforts should continue as long as they do not result in worsening psychosis or agitation.

Some concern has been expressed regarding the ability of patients with serious mental illness to participate in advance care planning, including providing written advance directives and designating a healthcare proxy before decision-making capacity is completely lost.[53] Foti et al. interviewed 150 middle-aged patients with serious mental illness, two-thirds of whom had schizophrenic-spectrum disorders.[54] Although study participants had worse physical health than the general population, they reported little experience with advance care planning—only 5% had talked to their doctor about their care preferences for serious medical illness and only 2% had documented healthcare preferences. Over two-thirds expressed an interest in obtaining more information on how to formally designate a healthcare surrogate and most were able to specify at least one person who could act as a healthcare proxy. Only 4% of the study participants found completing information about advance care preferences very stressful, though the interviewer rated 70% of participants as uncomfortable with the conversation, suggesting that clinicians may overestimate the psychological difficulties and distress of patients making these decisions. Foti and coauthors suggest that mental health practitioners are one of the logical community resources for conducting advance care planning with patients with serious mental illness.[54]

For a patient who is nondecisional, the clinician will need to locate a surrogate. The clinician should first turn to the person named in an advance directive, followed by a guardian, if one is available. In the absence of an advance directive, many jurisdictions allow family, even friends, to make decisions regarding care; other jurisdictions will not allow any decision that withholds life-sustaining treatment for the patient without a legal process.[55] At times, the family may request that the clinician apply a therapeutic exception, whereby the physician declines to inform the patient of the cancer diagnosis for fear of a catastrophic psychological reaction. This is both ethically suspect and rarely warranted. Alternatively, patients may abdicate all decisions to family members, a preference clinicians can accept.

The presence of a mental disorder should not result in mandatory application of life-sustaining treatment, which may be at odds with comfort and palliation. Foti and colleagues reported that 59% of mentally ill individuals, when presented with the scenario of pain medication in the case of incurable cancer, indicated they would want increased dosage even if confusion or inability to communicate resulted.[54] Coercive treatments should be considered only in cases where there is high likelihood of improved survival or quality of life (or both).[56] Even then, treatments may be difficult to apply. Refusals by a nondecisional but continually resistive patient may be respected if the patient will never be able to appreciate the benefits of treatment, and the force required to treat the patient seems egregious.[6]

USE OF ANTIPSYCHOTICS IN ADVANCED CANCER

The last decade has been marked by an increased use of atypical or second-generation antipsychotic medications for the treatment of schizophrenia. A great deal of research has focused on the potential for improved efficacy of treatment and diminished adverse effects with these medications. The first atypical antipsychotic was clozapine, with convincing evidence for effectiveness of both positive and negative symptoms in treatment-resistant schizophrenia (see below for more on use of clozapine in terminally ill patients). Subsequent Food and Drug Administration (FDA) approvals were received for risperidone, olanzapine, quetiapine, ziprasidone, and aripiprazole. These medications are consistently associated with decreased rates of tardive dyskinesia (TD) compared to first-generation antipsychotics.[57] Subsequent studies suggested decreased rates of akathisia, improvements in negative symptoms, and improved quality of life. More recently two large government-funded studies did not show clear differences in effectiveness or quality of life ratings of the second-generation drugs compared to first-generation drugs, and highlighted substantial intolerance of second-generation drugs resulting from hyperglycemia.[58,59] Substantial research continues to support that there is a decreased risk of TD with the newer drugs.[57]

The most important potential adverse effects of antipsychotics for schizophrenia patients whose cancer is advanced, but who remain ambulatory, are anticholinergic adverse effects, drug-induced parkinsonism (DIP), and orthostatic hypotension. Orthostatic hypotension is prominent with any drug with α adrenergic receptor blockade including olanzapine, quetiapine, chlorpromazine, clozapine and risperidone.[60] Among patients who already may be somewhat dehydrated, orthostasis increases the risk of falls with injury and may facilitate confinement to bed, thus worsening patients' overall functional status.

Anticholinergic effects. Anticholinergic effects can be beneficial in terminal care and clinicians sometimes prescribe strong anticholinergics such as scopolamine, to dry secretions. These medications, however, can promote delirium, dry mouth, constipation, blurry vision, and urinary retention. Anticholinergic adverse effects are additive across medications with these properties.

Extrapyramidal adverse effects of antipsychotics. Antipsychotics are effective for the treatment of psychosis through their dopaminergic neuronal blocking effects. Dopaminergic blockade can also produce acute dystonia (which is rare in medically ill and older people), DIP, akathisia, and TD. Among patients on antipsychotics, initiating other medications with dopaminergic blocking effects, such as prokinetics like metoclopramide and antiemetics like prochlorperazine, may have additive effects.

Tardive dyskinesia. Tardive dyskinesia is a syndrome of irreversible, involuntary, choreoathetoid movements in the face, trunk, or limbs that develops after 3–6 months of antipsychotic treatment. TD is stigmatizing; can annoy caregivers who may not understand its involuntary nature; and when severe, can cause dental, gait and speech problems, and weight loss. In most cases, however, TD causes neither discomfort nor substantial functional impairment.[61,62] In fact, many patients with TD are unaware of their movements.[63] Although TD is a major concern in the treatment of schizophrenia, it is rarely relevant in decision making at the end of life: the risk for TD need not be considered in choosing an antipsychotic and surveillance for TD is not necessary among patients with a limited life expectancy. As such, a major benefit of second-generation antipsychotics is lost at the end of life.

Akathisia. Akathisia is a syndrome of motor restlessness in which patients complain of a very unpleasant need to move, aptly described as having "ants in the pants." Akathisia can be experienced as anxiety and dysphoria and patients can appear restless, agitated, and irritable. Akathisia will worsen the agitation associated with hyperactive delirium or psychosis, and can result in physical aggression.[60] The incidence of akathisia is between 20% and 30%.[64] Akathisia may be less common with some second-generation antipsychotics, particularly clozapine and olanzapine.[58] Lipophilic beta blockers, such as propranolol, are generally an effective and well-tolerated treatment at relatively low doses. Benzodiazepines are also modestly helpful in diminishing the subjective perception of akathisia.[60] Awareness and clinical suspicion for akathisia can result in improved quality of life and therefore should be systematically reviewed during treatment with antipsychotics, even among patients with advanced cancer.

Drug-induced parkinsonism. Drug-induced parkinsonism is common, age related and potentially reversible. Among ambulatory patients, DIP increases the risk of falls with injury and functional decline. Among bed-bound patients, it will lead to poor bed mobility, increased patient discomfort, and caregiver risk of injury. Compared to other second-generation antipsychotics, quetiapine and clozapine are the least likely to cause DIP.[60]

Metabolic syndrome Antipsychotics, particularly second-generation ones, are associated with increased risk of hyperglycemia, diabetes mellitus, and hyperlipidemia. These are rarely important in patients with advanced cancer though, at times, worsening hyperglycemia can cause symptoms that degrade quality of life.[60]

Clozapine. The adverse effects of clozapine, one of the earliest second-generation antipsychotics, represents an unusual treatment conundrum. Clozapine is used in people whose schizophrenia has not responded to other antipsychotics; approximately one-third of these treatment-resistant patients will have substantial improvement in both positive and negative symptoms of schizophrenia.[65] The life-threatening risk of neutropenia mandates hematological analysis regularly—clozapine's licensing company will not allow refills of the medication before a normal white blood cell count is demonstrated. Because of the risk of neutropenia, clozapine-treated patients with cancer may need to make decisions regarding cancer chemotherapy that could result in the need for either clozapine or cancer treatment discontinuation.[66,67] Clozapine-treated hospice patients who are not receiving any other life-sustaining treatments are still required to undergo periodic blood counts.

Choice of antipsychotics. Hospice medical directors may request that patients be switched to first-generation antipsychotics because of substantial cost savings; hospice providers are reimbursed on a per diem from which patients' medications are paid. Switching is acceptable as long as the patient is not put at increased risk of psychosis or adverse effects.

DISTINGUISHING DELIRIUM FROM WORSENING PSYCHOSIS

When a patient with schizophrenia and cancer develops worsening behavior, such as hallucinations or delusions, many clinicians may incorrectly assume that this represents a relapse of schizophrenia. In fact, delirium is the most common mental manifestation of serious illness including advanced cancer,[68] yet it is regularly mistaken for another mental disorder—patients with hypoactive delirium are often perceived as depressed, and patients with hyperactive delirium are often mistakenly diagnosed as psychotic or manic.[69] Schizophrenia, associated with neurodevelopmental abnormalities and polypharmacy, likely increases the risk of delirium at the end of life.[70] Alternatively, delirium may unmask preexisting psychosis in paranoid patients who can no longer maintain their guard.

Several aspects of the mental status examination may help the clinician distinguish between worsening psychosis of schizophrenia and delirium superimposed on schizophrenia. Attention and concentration are impaired in patients with delirium, but are usually normal in patients with schizophrenia.[71] The nondelirious patient with schizophrenia should be able to complete simple measures of attention without error, such as saying the days of the week backward, repeating at least five random numbers, and performing simple serial subtractions such as counting backward by 3 from 20. A decline of two or more points on the 30-item Folstein Mini-Mental State Examination was found to discriminate delirious from cognitively intact elderly patients.[72]

Hallucinations in schizophrenia are primarily auditory. In contrast, hallucinations in delirium are more frequently visual and tactile.[71] Patients with schizophrenia who are picking at things in the air or complaining of visions should be evaluated for delirium.

Delirious patients may have altered awareness and psychomotor abnormalities. For example, the hypomotoric apathy of delirium can be difficult to distinguish from DIP or emotional withdrawal. Typically, true sleepiness and difficulty with arousal are not symptoms of schizophrenia. Additionally, delirium severity fluctuates throughout the day, often worsening through the evening, whereas diurnal variations are seldom encountered in patients with schizophrenia. Overall, sleep disturbances with frequent nocturnal awakenings and worsening behavior at night are common in delirium, but unusual in schizophrenia. Agitation and physical aggression may be manifestations of either disorder.

The evaluation of delirium is no different in the patient with schizophrenia than the nonmentally ill patient. There is no reason to believe that the likely causes of delirium are any different in terminally ill patients with schizophrenia than other patients; infections, metabolic abnormalities, drugs, and dehydration are most commonly implicated with more than one of these factors usually present.[73] Clinician aggressiveness in pursuing a cause for delirium will depend more on the goals of care, the patient's setting (e.g., hospice vs. the acute care hospital), and estimated survival. For example, among patients with schizophrenia who are actively receiving chemotherapy, the clinician might fully evaluate the causes of a new delirium, whereas a patient in hospice with new hypoactive delirium might receive only limited and noninvasive evaluation.

Antipsychotics are the preferred medication for treating behavioral problems in patients with delirium.[73] In a paranoid, agitated, or aggressive patient with schizophrenia and delirium, the clinician has the option of increasing the patient's usual antipsychotic or temporarily adding a second agent. There are some advantages of temporarily adding haloperidol, as long as the patient does not have substantial problems with DIP or akathisia. Unlike second-generation medications, haloperidol

can be given by a variety of routes in patients with advanced disease who are unable to swallow, or in home hospice patients who do not have intravenous access. Haloperidol has a wide margin of safety lacking anticholinergic properties that may worsen confusion and antiadrenergic properties that may cause orthostatic hypotension in patients who are ambulatory. Finally, oncologists, palliative care physicians and other care providers are likely comfortable and familiar with prescribing haloperidol, as it is used in many settings for managing delirium.

CARING FOR HOMELESS PATIENTS WITH BOTH CANCER AND MENTAL ILLNESS

An estimated 2.3–3.5 million individuals in the United States are homeless; between one-fourth and one-third have a serious mental illness such as schizophrenia. Among people with a psychotic disorder, between 8% and 18% will have an episode of homelessness.[74,75] At the time of cancer diagnosis, homeless individuals are already struggling to secure food, housing, transportation, and basic medical care. Half have no health insurance. Homeless patients with mental illness are more likely to lack friends or family members to serve as surrogates. Short of legal guardianship, most states do not have legal processes for making decisions for such patients; though a few states allow the attending physician to make healthcare decisions in the absence of decisional capacity or surrogates.[75]

Homelessness compounds the difficulty of adhering to medication schedules. Such patients do best with once per day medication regimens. Clinicians may need to avoid prescribing unstable compounds requiring refrigeration. Prescribing small amounts of medications with abuse potential will reduce the risk medications will be sold, or that the client might be robbed. Clinicians should attempt to work with patients to reduce substance abuse, but should anticipate harm reduction associated with relapses, rather than complete remission.[75]

Many homeless individuals will either die in shelters or on the streets. Others die in hospital with long lengths of stay complicated by lack of surrogate decision makers. Innovative palliative care shelter programs for the homeless are described in the literature. For example, the Ottawa Inner City Health Project offers shelter-based palliative care for people who are homeless, have no caregivers, lack financial resources, and are diagnosed with a life-threatening illness. Forty percent of these clients have schizophrenia. Clients receive shelter, meals, daily nursing, 24-hour physician coverage, and transportation to hospital for appointments. Harm reduction is promoted in place of abstinence through clean needles, a smoking area outside the shelter, and dispensing 14 g of alcohol daily. Mean length of stay before death is 4 months. The authors point out that the clients of the program could not be placed in alternative palliative care settings because of disruptive behaviors or refusal of other placements based on suspiciousness of institutions and restrictions imposed on lifestyle.[76]

SUMMARY

The gap in life expectancy between people with schizophrenia and those without mental disorder has increased over recent decades; patients with schizophrenia appear to not have benefited from advances in disease prevention and disease management that have spurred steady increases in life expectancy among the population without mental illness. Key issues for improving cancer prevention and care may include greater integration of cancer screening into mental healthcare, individualizing and modifying cancer treatments for patients with schizophrenia by taking into account difficulty tolerating some types of care, developing systems for surrogate decision making for the "unbefriended," and examining the special palliative needs of patients with both schizophrenia and cancer at the end of life.

REFERENCES

1. McAlpine DD. Patterns of care for persons 65 years and older with schizophrenia. In: Cohen CI (ed). *Schizophrenia into later life: Treatment, research, and policy.* Washington DC: American Psychiatric Publishing; 2003:3–18.

2. Palmer B, Kayak G, Jeste D. A comparison of early- and late-onset schizophrenia. In: Cohen CI (ed). *Schizophrenia into later life: Treatment, research, and policy*. Washington DC: American Psychiatric Publishing; 2003:3–18.

3. Watson GD, Chandarana PC, Merskey H. Relationships between pain and schizophrenia. *Br J Psychiatry*. 1981;138:33–36.

4. Inagaki T, Yasukawa R, Okazaki S, et al. Factors disturbing treatment for cancer in patients with schizophrenia. *Psychiatry Clin Neurosci*. 2006;60: 327–331.

5. Schwartz CE, Steinmuller RI, Dubler N. The medical psychiatrist as physician for the chronically mentally ill. *Gen Hosp Psychiatry*. 1998;20(1):52–61.

6. Irvin TL. Legal, ethical and clinical implications of prescribing involuntary life-threatening treatment: the case of the Sunshine Kid. *J Forensic Sci*. 2003;48:856–860.

7. Craun MJ, Watkins M, Hefty A. Hospice care of the psychotic patient. *Am J Hosp Palliat Care*. 1997;14(4):205–208.

8. Pyne JM, Bean D, Sullivan G. Characteristics of patients with schizophrenia who do not believe they are mentally ill. *J Nerv Ment Dis*. 2001;189:146–153.

9. Kunkel EJS, Woods CM, Rodgers C, Myers RE. Consultations for 'maladaptive denial of illness' in patients with cancer: psychiatric disorders that result in noncompliance. *Psychooncology*. 1997;6:139–149.

10. Saha S, Chant D, McGrath J. A systematic review of mortality in schizophrenia: is the differential mortality gap worsening over time? *Arch Gen Psychiatry*. 2007;64:1123–1131.

11. Ruggeri M, Lasalvia A, Bisoffi G, et al. Satisfaction with mental health services among people with schizophrenia in five European sites: results from the EPSILON study. *Schizophr Bull*. 2003;29:229–245.

12. Hamann J, Cohen R, Leucht S, Busch R, Kissling W. Do patients with schizophrenia wish to be involved in decisions about their medical treatment? *Am J Psychiatry*. 2005;162:2382–2384.

13. Bradford DW, Kim MM, Braxton LE, et al. Access to medical care among persons with psychotic and major affective disorders. *Psychiatr Serv*. 2008;59(8):847–852.

14. Hennekens CH. Increasing global burden of cardiovascular disease in general populations and patients with schizophrenia. *J Clin Psychiatry*. 2007;68(Suppl 4):4–7.

15. Palmer BA, Pankratz VS, Bostwick JM. The lifetime risk of suicide in schizophrenia: a reexamination. *Arch Gen Psychiatry*. 2005;62:247–253.

16. Dickerson FB, Brown CH, Daumit GL, et al. Health status of individuals with serious mental illness. *Schizophr Bull*. 2006;32:584–589.

17. George T, Vessicchio J, Termine A. Nicotine and tobacco use in schizophrenia. In: Meyer JM, Nasrallah HA (eds). *Medical illness in schizophrenia*. Washington, DC: American Psychiatric Publishing; 2003:81–98.

18. Dixon L, Postrado L, Delahanty J, Fischer PJ, Lehman A. The association of medical comorbidity in schizophrenia with poor physical and mental health. *J Nerv Ment Dis*. 1999;187(8):496–502.

19. Leucht S, Burkard T, Henderson J, Maj M, Sartorius N. Physical illness and schizophrenia: a review of the literature. *Acta Psychiatr Scand*. 2007;116:317–333.

20. Lichtermann D, Ekelund J, Pukkala E, Tanskanen A, Lönnqvist J. Incidence of cancer among persons with schizophrenia and their relatives. *Arch Gen Psychiatry*. 2001;58(6):573–578.

21. Levav I, Lipshitz I, Novikov I, et al. Cancer risk among parents and siblings of patients with schizophrenia. *Br J Psychiatry*. 2007;190:156–161.

22. Dalton SO, Mellemkjaer L, Thomassen L, Mortensen PB, Johansen C. Risk for cancer in a cohort of patients hospitalized for schizophrenia in Denmark, 1969–1993. *Schizophr Res*. 2005;75(2–3):315–324.

23. Carney CP, Woolson RF, Jones L, Noyes R Jr, Doebbeling BN. Occurrence of cancer among people with mental health claims in an insured population. *Psychosom Med*. 2004;66(5):735–743.

24. Schoos R, Cohen C. Medical comorbidity in older persons with schizophrenia. In: Cohen CI (ed). *Schizophrenia into later life: Treatment, research, and policy*. Washington DC: American Psychiatric Publishing; 2003:113–138.

25. Hippisley-Cox J, Vinogradova Y, Coupland C, Parker C. Risk of malignancy in patients with schizophrenia or bipolar disorder: nested case-control study. *Arch Gen Psychiatry*. 2007;64(12):1368–1376.

26. Capasso RM, Lineberry TW, Bostwick JM, Decker PA, St Sauver J. Mortality in schizophrenia and schizoaffective disorder: an Olmsted County, Minnesota cohort: 1950–2005. *Schizophr Res*. 2008;98:287–294.

27. Tokuda Y, Obara H, Nakazato N, Stein GH. Acute care hospital mortality of schizophrenic patients. *J Hosp Med (Online)*. 2008;3:110–116.

28. Wood JB, Evenson RC, Cho DW, Hagan BJ. Mortality variations among public mental health patients. *Acta Psychiatr Scand*. 1985;72:218–229.

29. Copeland LA, Zeber JE, Rosenheck RA, Miller AL. Unforeseen inpatient mortality among veterans with schizophrenia. *Med Care*. 2006;44:110–116.

30. Buda M, Tsuang MT, Fleming JA. Causes of death in DSM-III schizophrenics and other psychotics (atypical group). A comparison with the general population. *Arch Gen Psychiatry*. 1988;45:283–285.

31. Brown S, Inskip H, Barraclough B. Causes of the excess mortality of schizophrenia. *Br J Psychiatry*. 2000;177:212–217.

32. Osby U, Correia N, Brandt L, Ekbom A, Sparen P. Mortality and causes of death in schizophrenia in Stockholm County, Sweden. *Schizophr Res*. 2000;45:21–28.

33. Lindamer LA, Buse DC, Auslander L, et al. A comparison of gynecological variables and service use among older women with and without schizophrenia. *Psychiatr Serv*. 2003;54:902–904.

34. Salsberry PJ, Chipps E, Kennedy C. Use of general medical services among Medicaid patients with severe and persistent mental illness. *Psychiatr Serv*. 2005;56:458–462.

35. Carney CP, Jones LE. The influence of type and severity of mental illness on receipt of screening mammography. *J Gen Intern Med*. 2006;21:1097–1104.

36. Xiong GL, Bermudes RA, Torres SN, Hales RE. Use of cancer-screening services among persons with serious mental illness in Sacramento County. *Psychiatr Serv*. 2008;59:929–932.

37. Folsom DP, McCahill M, Bartels SJ, et al. Medical comorbidity and receipt of medical care by older homeless people with schizophrenia or depression. *Psychiatr Serv*. 2002;53(11):1456–1460.

38. Druss BG, Rosenheck RA, Desai MM, Perlin JB. Quality of preventive medical care for patients with mental disorders. *Med Care*. 2002;40:129–136.

39. Lindamer LA, Wear E, Sadler GR. Mammography stages of change in middle-aged women with schizophrenia: an exploratory analysis. *BMC Psychiatry*. 2006;6:49.

40. Lawrence D, Holman CD, Jablensky AV, Threlfall TJ, Fuller SA. Excess cancer mortality in Western Australian psychiatric patients due to higher case fatality rates. *Acta Psychiatr Scand*. 2000;101(5):382–388.

41. Iezzoni LI, Ngo LH, Li D, et al. Treatment disparities for disabled Medicare beneficiaries with stage I non-small cell lung cancer. *Arch Phys Med Rehabil*. 2008;89:595–601.

42. Vahia IV, Diwan S, Bankole AO, et al. Adequacy of medical treatment among older persons with schizophrenia. *Psychiatr Serv*. 2008;59:853–859.

43. Singh MK, Giles LL, Nasrallah HA. Pain insensitivity in schizophrenia: trait or state marker? *J Psychiatr Pract*. 2006;12(2):90–102.

44. Rosenthal SH, Porter KA, Coffey B. Pain insensitivity in schizophrenia. Case report and review of the literature. *Gen Hosp Psychiatry*. 1990;12:319–322.

45. Sciolla A, Patterson TL, Wetherell JL, McAdams LA, Jeste DV. Functioning and well-being of middle-aged and older patients with schizophrenia: measurement with the 36-item short-form (SF-36) health survey. *Am J Geriatr Psychiatry*. 2003;11:629–637.

46. Margolese HC, Malchy L, Negrete JC, Tempier R, Gill K. Drug and alcohol use among patients with schizophrenia and related psychoses: levels and consequences. *Schizophr Res*. 2004;67(2–3):157–166.

47. Schneier FR, Siris SG. A review of psychoactive substance use and abuse in schizophrenia. Patterns of drug choice. *J Nerv Ment Dis*. 1987;175(11):641–652.

48. Grisso T, Appelbaum PS. *Assessing competence to consent to treatment: A guide for physicians and other health professionals*. New York: Oxford University Press; 1998.

49. Grisso T, Appelbaum PS. The MacArthur Treatment Competence Study. III: abilities of patients to consent to psychiatric and medical treatments. *Law Hum Behav*. 1995;19(2):149–174.

50. Ganzini L, Volicer L, Nelson WA, Fox E, Derse AR. Ten myths about decision-making capacity. *J Am Med Dir Assoc*. 2004;5(4):263–267.

51. Ganzini L, Volicer L, Nelson W, Derse A. Pitfalls in assessment of decision-making capacity. *Psychosomatics*. 2003;44:237–243.

52. Carpenter WT Jr, Gold JM, Lahti AC, et al. Decisional capacity for informed consent in schizophrenia research. *Arch Gen Psychiatry*. 2000;57(6):533–538.

53. Foti ME, Bartels SJ, Merriman MP, Fletcher KE, Van Citters AD. Medical advance care planning for persons with serious mental illness. *Psychiatr Serv*. 2005;56:576–584.

54. Foti ME, Bartels SJ, Van Citters AD, Merriman MP, Fletcher KE. End-of-life treatment preferences of persons with serious mental illness. *Psychiatr Serv*. 2005;56(5):585–591.

55. Karp N, Wood E. *Decision-makers of last resort: Trends in health care surrogacy for isolated elders; public guardianship*. Paper presented at: ABA Commission on Law and Aging; October 21, 2004; Washington DC.

56. Ganzini L, Goy E. Influence of mental illness on decision making at the end of life. In: Jansen L (ed). *Death in the clinic*. Lanham, MD: Rowman and Littlefield; 2006:81–96.

57. Correll CU, Leucht S, Kane JM. Lower risk for tardive dyskinesia associated with second-generation antipsychotics: a systematic review of 1-year studies. *Am J Psychiatry*. 2004;161(3):414–425.

58. Lieberman JA, Stroup TS, McEvoy JP, et al. Clinical Antipsychotic Trials of Intervention Effectiveness (CATIE) Investigators. Effectiveness of antipsychotic drugs in patients with chronic schizophrenia. *N Engl J Med*. 2005;353(12):1209–1223.

59. Jones PB, Barnes TR, Davies L, et al. Randomized controlled trial of the effect on quality of life of second- vs first-generation antipsychotic drugs in schizophrenia: cost utility of the latest antipsychotic drugs in schizophrenia study (CUtLASS 1). *Arch Gen Psychiatry.* 2006;63(10):1079–1087.

60. Janicak PG, Davis JM, Preskorn SH, et al. *Principles and practice of psychopharmacotherapy.* 3rd ed. Philadelphia, PA: Lippincott Williams & Wilkins; 2006.

61. Yassa R. Functional impairment in tardive dyskinesia: medical and psychosocial dimensions. *Acta Psychiatr Scand.* 1989;80(1):64–67.

62. Morley JE, Kraenzle D. Causes of weight loss in a community nursing home. *J Am Geriatr Soc.* 1994;42(6):583–585.

63. Macpherson R, Collis R. Tardive dyskinesia. Patients' lack of awareness of movement disorder. *Br J Psychiatry.* 1992;160:110–112.

64. Sachdev P. The epidemiology of drug-induced akathisia: Part I. Acute akathisia. *Schizophr Bull.* 1995;21(3):431–449.

65. Kane J, Honigfeld G, Singer J, Meltzer H. Clozapine for the treatment-resistant schizophrenic. A double-blind comparison with chlorpromazine. *Arch Gen Psychiatry.* 1988;45(9):789–796.

66. McKenna RC, Bailey L, Haake J, Desai PN, Prasad BR. Clozapine and chemotherapy. *Hosp Community Psychiatry.* 1994;45(8):831.

67. Miller PR. Clozapine therapy for a patient with a history of Hodgkin's disease. *Psychiatr Serv.* 2001;52(1):110–111.

68. Lawlor PG, Gagnon B, Mancini IL, et al. Occurrence, causes, and outcome of delirium in patients with advanced cancer: a prospective study. *Arch Intern Med.* 2000;160(6):786–794.

69. Farrell KR, Ganzini L. Misdiagnosing delirium as depression in medically ill elderly patients. *Arch Intern Med.* 1995;155(22):2459–2464.

70. Freudenreich O, Stern TA. Clinical experience with the management of schizophrenia in the general hospital. *Psychosomatics.* 2003;44(1):12–23.

71. First M, Pincus H, Frances A, Widiger T (eds). *Diagnostic and statistical manual of mental disorders,* 4th ed. (DSM-IV). Washington DC: American Psychiatric Association; 2000.

72. O'Keeffe ST, Mulkerrin EC, Nayeem K, Varughese M, Pillay I. Use of serial Mini-Mental State Examinations to diagnose and monitor delirium in elderly hospital patients. *J Am Geriatr Soc.* 2005;53(5):867–870.

73. Young J, Inouye SK. Delirium in older people. *BMJ.* 2007;334(7598):842–846.

74. Folsom DP, Hawthorne W, Lindamer L, et al. Prevalence and risk factors for homelessness and utilization of mental health services among 10,340 patients with serious mental illness in a large public mental health system. *Am J Psychiatry.* 2005;162:370–376.

75. Kushel MB, Miaskowski C. End-of-life care for homeless patients: "she says she is there to help me in any situation." *JAMA.* 2006;296:2959–2966.

76. Podymow T, Turnbull J, Coyle D. Shelter-based palliative care for the homeless terminally ill. *Palliat Med.* 2006;20(2):81–86.

CHAPTER 50

Difficult Personality Traits and Disorders in Oncology

John David Wynn

INTRODUCTION

A cancer diagnosis is a crisis. Many cancer patients experience extremes of emotional, cognitive, social, and spiritual strain. Many, perhaps most, patients cope effectively within their premorbid repertoire of responses, experiencing only transient dysfunction. They compensate effectively with the disruptions of their bodily functions, self-image, work, and relationships. They can accommodate the life changes without much strain. They have a flexible self-concept and supportive, understanding people to help them.

Some patients, however, are not so resilient. Their established ways of coping do not meet the challenge, and they respond to crisis with self-defeating, isolating, alienating strategies that stymie the most well-intentioned and sophisticated clinicians. They may be experienced by staff as aggravating, aggrandizing, chaotic, dramatic or odd, and their dysfunctional responses may appear as attempts to foil treatment or to monopolize resources.

Staff may experience feelings of anger, disinterest, neglect, and guilt, or even extreme feelings such as hatred. Despite their attempts to cope with such strong and "unprofessional" feelings, the staff may view the patient as unreachable, uncooperative, bizarre, dramatic, or demanding.

The question that arises is *why, in a setting of care and attention, when most patients are so compliant, would this person behave so badly? Furthermore, how could caring, thoughtful, hardworking clinicians be so angry, impatient, frustrated, or dismissive of a patient's suffering?*

As psycho-oncology consultants, our role is to identify dysfunctional working relationships between patients, family, and staff, and to facilitate quality care for all patients. This is an especially challenging task when working with the patients discussed in this chapter.

DEFINING DIFFICULT PERSONALITY TRAITS AND DISORDERS IN ONCOLOGY SETTINGS

Character rigidity. All patients long to trust someone who will understand their predicament and respond compassionately to their needs. Clinicians easily overlook how terribly stressful routine medical care can be for personality disorder patients. Close contact activates feelings of fear and at times desperate maneuvers to avoid emotional vulnerability and pain. Feelings of shame and guilt may interfere with expressing these needs, leading to fears of being forgotten, abandoned, or rejected. Interpersonal difficulties are caused by idiosyncratic perceptions, distorted cognitions, unstable or confusing affects, and troublesome behaviors. Labeling the patients and their distortions is of little value. Addressing their fears with care and reassurance, however, will go a long way to resolving conflict and supporting patients, families, and staff.

The essential presenting feature of a personality disorder is *character rigidity:* a limited ability to think about oneself and others in varied or new ways, combined with a limited repertoire of behaviors that may be counterproductive in challenging circumstances. Distorted cognitions—"ways of perceiving and interpreting self, others, and events"—surface as differences with staff, conflicts with family, or preoccupation with specialness, suspicions, guilty rumination, or self-criticism.[1]

By definition, the personality disorders of the Diagnostic Statistical Manual (DSM-IV-TR) are comprised of stable and enduring patterns of thinking, feeling, and behaving. In fact, however, personality features and Axis II disorders are not stable over time.[2–7] In longitudinal studies, many patients are found to meet other Axis II diagnostic criteria, or to have no diagnosis at all. In one study of college students, "change was typically and uniformly in the direction of decreasing personality disorder features over time."[5]

Clinicians must use caution assessing troubling behaviors occurring in difficult circumstances. Patterns of behavior that manifest in crisis may be mistaken for longstanding patterns of behavior.[3,5] Maladaptive responses may only represent an initial stumble in a steady march from diagnosis through treatment: Ms. Smith, admitted in October, may be very different from the Ms. Smith we met last May.

Properly managed, troubling behaviors often lead to maturation and emotional growth.[8] Clinicians often underestimate the potential for improvement over time.[9] A personality disorder diagnosis may be wrong, and yet indelibly, authoritatively inscribed in the patient's chart, only to mislead subsequent clinicians.

DSM-IV Axis II. DSM classifies personality disorders into three categories, or clusters, of disorders: A. *odd or eccentric;* B. *dramatic, emotional, or erratic;* and C. *anxious or fearful.*[1] These are listed in Table 50–1.

Axis II directs attention to "disorders that are frequently overlooked when attention is directed to the usually more florid Axis I disorder."[10] Personality disorders may establish the context in which Axis I disorders take place: schizoid and schizotypal patients are more vulnerable to psychosis; borderline and narcissistic patients are prone to depression, irritability, and egotism; and cluster C patients often develop anxiety disorders.[11–14] Personality disorders increase vulnerability, perhaps through a distortion of social perception and alienating interpersonal styles.[15–17] Distorted perceptions isolate patients, leaving them without social buffers against adverse life events. Solitary coping is less effective and reinforces aberrant patterns of thinking, feeling, and relating.

Alternatively, Axis I disorders may be precursors to personality disorder.[18,19] Chronic mood and anxiety disorders may restrict social interactions and obscure opportunities to learn social coping strategies. This restricted repertoire of interpersonal interactions constitutes the character rigidity that defines personality disorders.

In one large study, patients with schizotypal and borderline personality disorders were found to have significantly more impairment at work, in social relationships, and at leisure than patients with major depressive disorder.[20] Patients with co-occurring personality and mood disorders fare worse than those with mood disorder alone: spontaneous remission rates and treatment responses are worse when disorders co-occur.[15,17,18,21–28] In this light, personality disorder might be seen as a severity marker for Axis I disorders. Perhaps personality disorders are neither cause nor consequence of other mental illness, but merely occur beside the Axis I disorders, with overlapping symptoms or diatheses.[16] This co-morbidity alone may suffice to worsen patient outcomes.

The DSM-IV-TR personality disorders. Clinical characteristics of patients with personality disorders are listed in Table 50–1.

The Axis II diagnostic categories represent extremes that are rarely encountered—overlap syndromes are far more common than pure types.[29] *Note especially that the vast majority of uncooperative patients do*

Table 50–1. Personality disorders diagnostic features and typical interactions with clinical staff[1-3]

Diagnosis	Dominant features	Typical caregiver interactions	Helpful interventions	Diagnostic confounds, Rx options
Cluster A:				
Paranoid	Difficulties understanding others' actions, especially distrust and suspiciousness; others' motives are interpreted as malevolent. Deteriorate under stress.	Patient may make angry accusations, withdraw from staff. Staff has difficulty engaging and may feel misunderstood and wrongly accused.	Take extra time to explain and clarify problems and procedures, expect need for repetition and reassurance. Seek out patient's understanding of problems and procedures.	Consider schizophrenia, psychotic depression and mixed mania Autism spectrum disorders, limbic encephalitis, frontal abulia, steroid psychosis, or aphasia may be mistaken for the detachment and eccentricities seen in cluster A patients.
Schizoid and Schizotypal	Social detachment, restricted range of emotional expression masks shame and feelings of inadequacy. Acute discomfort in close relationships, cognitive or perceptual distortions, and eccentricities of behavior.	Patient perceived as odd, even frightening by staff who thus misinterpret patient's intent and needs and do not perceive intense anxiety and suffering.	Recognize diminished needs for interpersonal connection and lesser skills in relating to others. Explain restricted range to staff and reassure regarding unusual behaviors, especially "unfriendliness." Encourage simple, straightforward social interactions without humor, irony, or sarcasm. Beware of interpersonal over-stimulation.	Psychotic symptoms respond only weakly to neuroleptic treatment, but trial of an antidepressant or atypical neuroleptic may reduce comorbid depression and anxiety. Nonpsychotic patients are often more sensitive to neuroleptic side effects; *start low and go slow.*
Cluster B:				
Antisocial	Disregard for and violations of the rights of others.	Staff split between feeling special and rejected; patient has angry outbursts that exacerbate staff splits; staff feel seduced, deceived, loved, manipulated. Patient responds to confrontation with glib explanations of outrageous behavior or sham contrition.	Anticipate, educate, and address splitting. Encourage staff to discuss various impressions and to share information with one another. Reinforce clear task and role definitions, especially need for consistent, coherent responses to complaints, demands and threats.	Mood disorders, especially bipolar II (hypomania). Depressive disorders are common complications of all cluster B disorders, especially with threats of surgical disfigurement, diminished autonomy, and increased need to trust others.
Borderline	Unstable relationships, self-image, and affects, with marked impulsivity. Intense sensitivity to threats of rejection or abandonment.	Patient is panicky and needy, stimulating staff fantasies of specialness and rescuing the patient (e.g., from other staff). Staff reactions range from deep attachment to hatred and aggressive fantasies.	Clarify dysfunctional help-seeking style and disentangle (un)realistic expectations without blame. Be alert to bargaining, seduction, and manipulation. Reassure patient and facilitate staff alignment with role and task clarity.	Frontal disinhibition syndromes due to brain tumor, corticosteroids, drug abuse (intoxication), or delirium may cause marked impulsivity and socially inappropriate behavior.
Histrionic	Excessive emotionality and attention seeking.	Staff repelled by dramatic attention seeking, but may experience sexual attraction and arousal; splitting.	Help staff appreciate and discuss their own emotional responses, especially anger, neediness, and low self-worth.	Reduce polypharmacy when possible; consider episodic use of antidepressant, antipsychotic, and anxiolytic medication.

Diagnosis	Dominant features	Typical caregiver interactions	Helpful interventions	Diagnostic confounds, Rx options
Narcissistic	Grandiosity, need for admiration, and lack of empathy.	Angry outbursts, pitiful apologies, dramatic withdrawal. Staff feel special or worthless; patient "demanding & unreasonable" or "misunderstood & special."		
Cluster C: Avoidant	Social inhibition, feelings of inadequacy, and hypersensitivity to negative evaluation.	Patient seems fearful or uninterested, staff feel clumsy, intrusive, or unjustly accused of same.	Explain patient vulnerability and aversions to staff. Attend to dependency needs to the extent that they do not compromise staff or disrupt patient care.	Social anxiety disorder and obsessive-compulsive disorder are obvious overlap syndromes.
Dependent	Submissive, clinging behavior from excessive need to be taken care of, and terrible fear of being alone. Helpless, guilty, and indecisive.	Patient needy, demanding, childlike, and vulnerable. Staff feel protective or repelled by excessive demands for care and attention.	Describe and explain problems and procedures; give patient options and clear role in decision making as tolerated. Return locus of control to patient whenever possible.	Depression is common, as are generalized, phobic and obsessive-compulsive anxiety disorders. Mood, neurovegetative and disruptive anxiety symptoms strongly urge an antidepressant trial that may efface dependent or avoidant behavior.[2]
Obsessive-Compulsive	Preoccupation with orderliness, perfectionism, and control.	Patient may seem the ideal patient or staff may feel their performance is being monitored and harshly judged.	Encourage staff discussion of their own sensitivities, dependency needs, and meticulousness.	
Research criteria/appendix diagnoses				
Depressive	Pervasive depressive cognitions and behaviors, overly serious, self-critical, and pessimistic.	Staff feel criticized and helpless to engage with optimistic responses. Dissatisfaction is puzzling and may evoke staff anger, helplessness, or rejection.	Psychotherapy and medication directed at remoralization and depressive symptoms. Confront staff anger and clarify sources. Promote patient and family engagement. Encourage physical activation (PT, OT, exercise).	Dysthymic, depressive, and bipolar mood disorders; frontal or parietal lobe tumor: drug effects.
Passive-Aggressive (negativistic)	Passivity, complaints, unreasonable criticism, resentment, hostile defiance and apologies.	Patient is avoided by staff who feel unfairly judged and attacked.		

ABBREVIATIONS: OT, occupational therapy; PT, physical therapy.

[1] Shedler J, Westen D. Refining personality disorder diagnosis: integrating science and practice. *Am J Psychiatry.* Aug 2004;161(8):1350–1365.

[2] American Psychiatric Association, American Psychiatric Association. Task Force on DSM-IV. *Diagnostic and statistical manual of mental disorders : DSM-IV-TR.* 4th ed. Washington, DC: American Psychiatric Association; 2000.

[3] Fava M, Farabaugh AH, Sickinger AH, et al. Personality disorders and depression. *Psychol Med.* Aug 2002;32(6):1049–1057.

not have a personality disorder. Nevertheless, the DSM categories provide us with clear examples of personality dysfunction that strongly correlate with functional impairment and human suffering.[17,20,30–33] Understanding these types sensitizes us to their manifold presentations and strengthens our treatment strategies.

Cluster A. The odd or eccentric patients of cluster A all struggle with some degree of social discomfort. Interpersonal closeness may be unpleasant or simply of no interest, leading to avoidant and frankly odd behaviors.[34] Getting to know cluster A patients may be not only difficult, but actually alienating or frightening for the patient.

> *Like many patients, this 37 year old woman brought her favorite pillow and stuffed animal into the hospital with her. After several days staff became aware that she "consulted" her teddy bear regarding difficult treatment decisions and urged her husband to bring several other trusted plush toy "counselors" from home. She arranged the dolls at her bedside and grew angry if they were disturbed around bedtime.*

Social alienation can be increased by cluster A patients' unusual beliefs. Magical thinking and frankly paranoid ideas may be alarming to staff. Patients may experience others' judgments with blithe indifference, total ignorance, or dramatic secrecy breached only with selected staff. At times patients' unusual beliefs get in the way of proper care. Standard procedures are experienced as menacing, routine questions feel like threatening interrogation, and innocent jokes are deeply offensive. Uncovering these treatment-foiling beliefs or attitudes can be quite difficult, often requiring collateral interviews with family, friends, or trusted staff.

Cluster B. Cluster B patients may also be particularly vulnerable in medical settings, especially when circumstances demand high levels of stress tolerance, decision making, and shifting relationships. Uncomfortable with the passive role that many patients readily adopt, they need frequent reassurances that they are valued and safe. The subgroups—antisocial, borderline, narcissistic, and histrionic—are distinguished by their reactions to interpersonal ambiguity or strain.

Antisocial patients are often extraverted and manipulative: their focus is on establishing and maintaining interpersonal advantage. When secure they may be pleasantly thoughtful and ingratiating, even charming. They secure attachments not so much for security or affection, however, but for leverage and dominance; all relations are ultimately seen as instrumental, that is, as means to particular ends. Rageful, even violent reactions may occur when they feel disadvantaged or threatened. The change of attitude may be shocking (and frightening) to staff unaccustomed to the sudden appearance of rude, demanding, demeaning, or threatening behavior. Threats may escalate to physical violence that dissipate as soon as the desired result is obtained; the patient may then express surprise at others' angry, distancing reactions, as if their behavior were well within acceptable norms. Nonchalance in violating accepted norms is the hallmark of the disorder.

Borderline patients may exhibit many of the same behaviors, but tend to be less organized and less in control. They are more likely to be self-destructive than threatening to others, and tend to pursue relationship attachments for their own sake rather than interpersonal advantage per se. Under duress their perception of others is distorted by black-and-white thinking that sees only enemies and allies without nuance. They respond to distress with impulsive desperation that may include sexual adventurism, substance abuse, and self-mutilation. Offers of nurturance may be surprisingly sexualized, for example, a nurse's eagerness to provide physical comfort may be experienced as seductive, or a physician's concern may be seen as an offer of lifelong affection.

> *Margaret is an attractive 42 year old twice-divorced attorney with recurrent bronchitis. A recent chest x-ray revealed a small lung mass. Hours after a difficult meeting with her oncologist, she has paged the physician on call to ask more questions about the diagnosis and treatment. After a few minutes of conversation with the empathic doctor Margaret begins to cry and asks, "Can you meet me somewhere? I really need to talk this over."*

> *"I know you are worried about all of this, but I think you should talk things over with your oncologist," responds the doctor, a bit taken aback.*
> *"You seem so much more compassionate," she explains. "I feel like you really understand what I'm going through. Your office is right next door to my doctor's, isn't it? I saw you earlier today. You have such a warm smile, such a kind way with everyone around you. Are you married?"*

Borderline and antisocial patients' dramatic behavior may be seen as instrumental, but for the borderline patient it is more often simply an immature, ineffective way of expressing extreme distress. It is striking to see the disparate responses of involved clinicians to these behaviors: some will be angry and alienated, while others are moved to tears and desperate rescue. Conflict between staff may ensue. This staff splitting is a commonplace in work with borderline patients: *multiple clinicians working on the same team experience the patient very differently.* Productively responding to the patient can tax even the most experienced clinicians.

Histrionic and narcissistic patients are far more predictable and less threatening than either antisocial or borderline patients. Like the borderline, they are motivated by a need for love and security rather than simple interpersonal advantage. Unlike the borderline, who will be whatever the person before her demands, histrionic and narcissistic patients have a much more solidly established personality and sense of self. Histrionic patients are pervasively attention seeking: it is their dominant mode of relating to others whether or not they are in distress. Rather than feeling manipulated, staff tend to feel entertained, exhausted or, eventually, bored and annoyed. The histrionic will elaborate dramatic stories, offer fantastic rewards, and look for special treatment. Both borderline and histrionic patients may be highly intolerant of being alone; the former needs to be reassured that she is loved, the latter to be reminded that she is still alive.

The narcissistic patient is least likely of the cluster B patients to elicit psychiatric consultation. The setting of medical care, with numerous resources directed towards the patient's comfort and well-being, may be experienced as supremely reassuring. The feelings that narcissistic patients arouse in staff—including guilt, shame, and inadequacy—are often very hard for staff to identify as emanating from the patient rather than originating in themselves. The narcissist responds to interpersonal threat by highlighting the deficits of others.

Although instrumentally oriented like the antisocial patient, seeing others as means to their own esteem and gratification, the narcissist feels and often gets others to feel that he deserves whatever he wants. When ill, he is whiney and demanding, even infantile and petulant. Mature nursing staff will quickly identify the narcissist and simply become more efficient in meeting his needs while dismissing his unreasonable behaviors and demands. Less sophisticated clinicians, however, may find themselves feeling the low self-esteem, guilt, and self-doubt that reside at the core of the narcissistic personality.[35]

Cluster C. **Avoidant** patients experience extremes of social inhibition that may extend to all interpersonal relations. Some patients with avoidant personality disorder will avoid all human touch whenever possible. Inpatient care is thus extremely difficult. The patient may freeze, panic, or dissociate. Puzzled staff responses may reveal extreme hypersensitivity to negative evaluation, manifest as withdrawal, depression, or overt anger.

Dependent patients tend to be extremely compliant and submissive and are thus less likely to elicit staff complaint. Their high degree of deference, clinging behavior, and intense need for direct care may overtax clinicians, especially nurses running interference for physicians. In extremis these patients demonstrate regressive, childlike neediness that may elicit or repel staff attention.

Obsessive-compulsive personality disorder (OCPD) must be distinguished from obsessive-compulsive disorder (OCD). OCD manifests with ritualized thoughts and behaviors that interfere with daily activities. OCPD presents as a preoccupation with orderliness, perfectionism, and control that clinicians may find endearing, inspiring, or maddening. For the most part these patients are not clinically problematic; they are more likely to be seen as ideally organized, adherent, and predictable.

Etiology. The personality disorders encompass very heterogeneous groups of people with wide varieties of family makeup, developmental history, traits, and disease course. No single cause will suffice to create adult traits or disorder. Genetic endowment, parental influences, social learning, and trauma are well-established contributors.[36,37] The cluster B disorders, for example, may be seen as resulting from an amalgam of genetic predisposition, childhood neglect, and lack of developmental resources.[38]

Genetic influences may impact regulation of affects, impulse/action patterns, cognitive organization, and anxiety/inhibition.[14,39,40] Heritable traits may include deficits "in recruitment of brain mechanisms of emotion regulation, and this process may be potentiated by...particularly stressful or negative contexts."[41] Compelling epigenetic studies link genetic endowment and early life experience to phenotypic expression in adrenal reactivity, stress tolerance, and other personality traits.[35,38,42] This may explain the stymied maturation of brain mechanisms regulating impulse control and identity formation.

These mechanisms may be impacted more acutely as well. Orbitofrontal insult from trauma or surgery may be associated with new onset of personality disorder features,[43] reflecting, for example, regional dysfunction in antisocial and borderline disorders.[14,41,44,45]

Epidemiology. Personality disorders are infrequent in the general population, but far more common in general medical outpatient and inpatient populations.[46–49] The low frequency may reflect stringent criteria that demand extreme forms of disorder to reach diagnostic threshold—or the reluctance of such troubled people to participate in surveys. Medical care invites some behaviors, including dependency, passivity, and attention seeking, perhaps reinforcing them in cancer patients with preexisting personality pathology.

The association of substance abuse disorders with head and neck and esophageal cancers suggests that they may be more frequently associated with personality disorder.[50] Adequate studies have not been done to substantiate these suspicions, however.

Diagnostic challenges. The distinction between normality, major mental disorder, and personality disorder has vexed clinicians for over a century.[37] Kraepelin observed that *"wherever we try to mark out the frontier between mental health and disease, we find a neutral territory, in which the imperceptible change from the realm of normal life to that of obvious derangement takes place"* (p. 295).[51] This statement is especially true of personality disorders, which present on a continuum with normal adaptive behavior, and yet often overlap genetically and phenomenologically with Axis I disorders.[36,37,52–55]

Establishing a personality disorder diagnosis presents multiple challenges. Rapport with such patients is by definition difficult, and is often the reason for consultation. Much time may be required to avoid premature diagnostic closure, to sort through the range of traits, assess their stability over time, and link them to significant dysfunction. The presence of longstanding dysfunction is clearly not enough: concomitant mood, anxiety or psychotic disorder, substance abuse, and circumstantial chaos may be more causative than the patient's personality traits per se. The traits must be the cause of "significant functional impairment or subjective distress."[1]

Akiskal argues forcefully that careful assessment of many borderline personality disorder patients will reveal a bipolar mood disorder.[11] Gunderson provides strong biologic and phenomenologic data in rebuttal, however.[56] This controversy, along with much data regarding the evanescence of personality disorder diagnoses, cautions us regarding the hazards of superficial assessment and premature diagnostic closure.[57] There is no substitute for a detailed history, sensitively elicited, and supplemented by collateral sources.

Cultural determinants of coping behavior must also be addressed, including beliefs that might be mistaken for magical thinking, fastidiousness misconstrued as compulsive neatness, or dramatic self-expression confused with histrionics.[58]

Hazards and value of diagnostic labeling in oncology settings. It

is not surprising that some patients are hard to engage in complex cancer treatment. But clinicians' fear, ignorance, and frustration may lead to pejorative labeling and a downward spiral of clinician frustration, mutual avoidance, and patient deterioration. A personality diagnosis may be less a guide to diagnosis and treatment than a dismissive shorthand applied to a difficult patient.

Skillfully used, however, the diagnosis will help staff recognize the morbidity and suffering of patients with personality disorders. A named illness with established treatments can demystify and destigmatize the patient, and reduce staff helplessness, frustration, and anger.[59] Diagnostic clarity often gives staff permission to express frustration, anger, or guilt over their own feelings and behaviors. Awareness of avoidant, paranoid, shame-prone, or rejection-sensitive vulnerabilities allows staff to address their own feelings of rejection, guilt, or sadism that personality disorder patients may engender. Above all, the diagnosis should help to shape patient-clinician interactions around a set of problems and solutions.[60,61]

MANAGEMENT OF PATIENTS WITH DIFFICULT PERSONALITY TRAITS AND DISORDERS

Diagnostic assessment of disruptive behavior should be approached with an emphasis on interactions between patients and staff. Most difficult patient encounters may be organized into a small number of such interactions.

General principles in working with personality disorder patients

Cluster A: patients who are odd or eccentric

- Seek out the patient's understanding of what is happening.
- Take extra time to clarify problems and procedures, expect need for repetition and reassurance.
- Recognize diminished needs for interpersonal connection and lesser skills in relating to others. Beware of interpersonal overstimulation.
- Explain restricted range to staff and reassure regarding unusual behaviors, especially "unfriendliness."
- Encourage simple, straightforward social interactions without humor, irony, or sarcasm.

Cluster B: patients who are dramatic, emotional, or erratic

- Anticipate, address, and educate staff about splitting.
- Encourage staff to share information and discuss differing impressions with one another.
- Reinforce clear task and role definitions, especially need for consistent, coherent responses to complaints, demands and threats.
- Clarify dysfunctional help-seeking style and disentangle (un)realistic expectations without blame.
- Be alert to bargaining, seduction, and manipulation.
- Reassure patient and facilitate staff alignment with role and task clarity.
- Help staff appreciate and discuss their own emotional responses, especially anger, neediness, and low self-worth.

Cluster C: patients who are anxious or fearful

- Describe and explain problems and procedures; give patient options and clear role in decision making as tolerated.
- Return locus of control to patient whenever possible.
- Explain patient vulnerability and aversions to staff.
- Attend to dependency needs to the extent that they do not compromise staff or disrupt patient care.
- Encourage staff discussion of their own sensitivities, dependency needs, and meticulousness.

Problematic patient encounters. Regardless of the DSM diagnosis, clinical personnel find patients to be...

- overwhelmed and chaotic;
- thoughtful, misguided, and uncooperative;

- superficially agreeable but foiling care;
- needy or overentitled;
- odd, confusing, or daunting;
- perplexing, frightening, or repellent.

Overwhelmed and chaotic. Some patients may disagree with the care plan because they do not understand explanations of the disease or the treatments, or because the information is so overwhelming they cannot collaborate effectively with the care team. We may see them as overwhelmed and chaotic:

Roberta was 29 years old when her suspicious mammogram led to an abnormal biopsy and, the day after her son's first birthday, a diagnosis of cancer. The oncologist explained to this intelligent, thoughtful, bewildered woman that she had a ductal carcinoma in situ that would require lumpectomy and a brief course of radiation therapy. An excellent outcome was all but assured.

Roberta's response was to sit down and make a list of women for her husband to date after her death. She became irritable, tearful, and angry. She consulted megavitamin gurus and researched alternative treatments on the web. She refused to return to the oncologist's office. Anguished and desperately suicidal, she drafted a farewell letter to each of her family members, including one to be read to her son on his thirteenth birthday. Despite her minimal disease and excellent prognosis, no matter who tried to reassure her, all she could hear was the first thing her oncologist had told her: you have cancer.

Roberta demonstrates extreme narcissistic vulnerability and fears of abandonment, along with unstable identity, mood, and impulse control. These borderline traits are dramatically expressed, leaving those around her as bewildered as she is. But Roberta's frantic behavior diminished as she gradually yielded to the pleas of her family and friends to again review her diagnosis and treatment plan. The oncologist patiently reexplained what to expect, and an oncology social worker helped Roberta meet other breast cancer survivors who demonstrated better coping strategies.

Overwhelmed and confused patients like Roberta foil care because they cannot take in the information and work with the team. They experience the diagnosis and plan as "too much, too fast," and they panic. We err by using jargon or otherwise missing the level at which a particular patient should be approached. Or we may simply misread a superficially agreeable, compliant patient.

The clinician may take time to carefully and thoroughly present information, leaving ample room for questions, only to find that the patient adamantly refuses to cooperate. These patients are hard to read, because they appear calmer than they feel, they have difficulty relating to authority figures, or they simply fear or detest the patient role. They demand our best clinical communication skills. We have to repeatedly back-up and make sure we understand what we heard us say, not just the factual details, but especially the meanings and consequences. Eye contact, body language, and patience are essential.[62] And check at each step for signs of miscommunication and mistrust.

Thoughtful, misguided, and uncooperative. Oncology patients are increasingly educated by a growing array of information sources. Disagreements with the care plan may stem from differences in "expert opinion" or from the intrusion of unproved (or disproved) therapies. The patients feel they have valuable information that contradicts what the care team is offering. They rationally disagree with the care plan, demand care the team feels is not indicated, or refuse treatments considered essential to survival. Oncology staff may see them as thoughtful and misguided, or odd and irksome. Such patients may prefer complementary or alternative cancer treatments with clinicians they find less threatening or more reassuring.

Sometimes we are arguing with folk beliefs that have great currency in certain ethnic groups. For example, "you should never have surgery for cancer, because when the air hits the tumor it spreads everywhere."[63,64]

Such "uncooperative patients" are often thoughtful, rational, and misinformed. Their ignorance is sometimes misread as a refusal to cooperate with care when in fact it is precisely the opposite: they are trying to join the treatment team and collaborate. When treated with consideration and respect they routinely come around—or get the medical team to reconsider their recommendations.

Superficially agreeable, but foil care. Patients may agree with the care plan but not behave the way staff expect: they may miss scheduled appointments, lab draws, examinations, and consultations. They don't stick to the treatment plan, even after they appear to understand and agree. The cues we expect when people disagree never surface. Everything looks fine until they have to follow through.

Overwhelmed by the facts, these mistrustful, fearful, or anxious patients may anticipate disapproval or punishing responses to their questions or problems. Lengthy, detailed conversations may be entirely forgotten, because anxiety prevents them from taking in the information. And the odd patient, preoccupied with unusual beliefs and fears, just has a different, often unpredictable way of hearing and responding that the clinician may not fully appreciate.

The "perfect patient" is an interesting variant. Passively cooperative, they never complain or object. Uncertain of how staff will react to their disagreement, they smile and go their own way or obey with mounting anxiety. These ideal patients may do worst at the end of treatment, when they find the reward for their obedience is not cure, but long-term surveillance.

Again, we may be misreading their understanding of the facts and consequences of care, or we may be under-appreciating how much their emotional responses are interfering with their ability to act on the information. These patients should be carefully questioned about the treatment plan, with special attention paid to their reluctance to disclose unspoken fears: the emphasis must be on shared understanding, rather than the shared commitment that will hopefully follow.

Needy, demanding, clinging, or overentitled. Some patients understand, agree, participate with care-as-planned, and drive the staff batty: they talk at great length, call frequently, and ask infinite questions—or the same questions over and over. Others do everything as clinically expected, but the rest of their life takes over and complicates the clinician-patient relationship beyond recognition. Clinicians find these patients needy and demanding, clinging, or overentitled.

Such patients run the gamut from the anxious-but-endearing elderly woman to the obsessive-compulsive young man who always has just one more question. They may be anxious worriers or odd ducks with magical thinking, but often, with time and familiarity, what emerges is that they are terribly lonely and scared.

The treatment team is their newfound and only social outlet, and they have a difficult time managing the attachments. Every test, every drug, every side effect, risk-benefit ratio, or research controversy is another opportunity to engage and not let go. The technical aspects of the medical setting are tickets to the world of clinical care.

These patients cry out for reassurance and constancy: they need to know that the team will stand by them. Every superfluous question is another plea for a reliable caretaker; any rebuff is an affirmation of their worst fears, namely, that you will not be there when they really need you. Such patients generally respond well to clear, compassionate boundaries, as long as they are accompanied by calm, reassuring office visits. They are brilliant readers of body language, so the clinician's words and actions must be consistent. Remember to use lots of eye contact (they're used to being avoided), and keep your hand off the doorknob until the visit is officially (and explicitly) over.

Alternatively it may be the patients' advocates—family members, well-intentioned friends, or clergy—who frustrate clinical staff. The patient may express helpless frustration or passive acquiescence, but however they handle things the family is now your problem.

Presence, clarity and consistency, reassurance, and clear boundaries—when you are available, what you can offer, and what you cannot—will go a long way to engaging without overengaging or alienating these patients and caregivers.

Patients who perplex, frighten or repel. Some patients do everything we require of them, but they do other things that perplex, frighten or repel. They may threaten, alienate, or seduce us, leaving us feeling like the vulnerable person in need of specialized care. These patients, because of their dramatic presentations and emotionally challenging engagements, can bring out the worst in us. We feel a need to fight or flee, to put them in their place or take them home with us, to kick them out or kick ourselves. We may label them out of frustration or anger: crock, kook, borderline, crazy.

The seductive patient presents a more sophisticated version of the previous clinging, demanding group. Rather than clinging with infinite questions or requests, such patients invite us into their life's drama. They convince you that you are very special, that you are the only one who understands their dilemmas and that only your powers will suffice. Of course once you sit down with your team you realize that everyone gets that message from the patient: *only you can help me!* We feel drawn in and may not realize how involved we are until we wake up in the middle of the night, wondering how to extricate ourselves without giving up our values of gracious, compassionate care. Recalling the story of Margaret, above:

> *Margaret is obviously frightened and in need; she is asking for comfort and reassurance; you dole out comfort and reassurance all day. You're still at the office, you haven't had dinner yet, she is only a short drive away....what could it hurt?*

The answer is to be mindful of your position and your limitations. Consider the role(s) you have taken on, the tasks you perform, and the constraints of time and place that define your roles and tasks. Are you responding to requests beyond these roles, tasks, and situations? Are you the only one who can fulfill these requests? *Generally speaking, the more unique you feel the more the patient needs a team approach.* If you find yourself increasingly drawn to special care arrangements with the patient, consider transferring care to a colleague. Your worst fantasies about the patient's reaction to your rejection are still better than the path to increasing entanglement, confusion, and catastrophe. At the very least, if you are uncomfortable or preoccupied with a clinical relationship, discuss it with a colleague who can help you think it through.

Threats and instances of self-harm should be seen as "a means of managing emotional pain and not as a deliberate attempt to control others"[59] Oncology staff focused on survival may feel betrayed by such behavior, and it is important to distinguish amongst dramatic help-seeking, despondent suicidality, and rational euthanasia.[65,66] Confusion in such situations should prompt rapid peer or clinical ethics consultation.

The unresponsive, distant, or passive patient. While not exactly uncooperative, some patients still do not meet staff demands or expectations. They may appear "distant" or "needy" in ways that are oddly unresponsive, incurious, or passive. This inert, unreactive style sometimes alternates with prolonged, disproportionate distress that demands additional time from nursing and physicians. The staff winds up feeling confused, disoriented, and guilty, incapable of connecting through collaboration or consolation.

Clinicians often overread such odd patients. Their distance may be interpreted as a retreat or withdrawal while in fact it is just their comfort level to stay apart. Their emotional storms are confusing, overvalued, or underappreciated. They don't know how to use the interpersonal supports offered by staff; their habit and skills are in righting their own ships without ballast or direction from others. Only trial and error can reveal and repair the mismatches of expectations and understanding.

The consultant's role: enhancing resilience of patients with personality disorders

As with all patients, the consulting psycho-oncologist must use and provide a biopsychosocial perspective (see Table 50–2):

- ***identify destabilizing biological influences***: medication, tumor effect, infection, sleep deprivation, malnutrition, and physical deconditioning;
- ***clarify psychological dysfunction***: depression, hopelessness, psychosis, emotional lability, cognitive distortions, irritability, impulsivity, and passive resistance;

Table 50–2. Biopsychosocial dimensions of clinical care

Destabilizing biological influences	Infection (*CNS or systemic*)
	Malnutrition (*global or nutrient deficiency*)
	Medication
	Physical deconditioning
	Sleep disruption
	Tumor effect (*direct or paraneoplastic*)
Psychological vulnerabilities	Anxiety
	Cognitive distortions
	Depression
	Emotional lability
	Hopelessness
	Impulsivity, irritability, aggression
Social complexity	Distortions of social perception
	Isolation (*chronic or recent onset*)
	Family challenge, criticism, chaos
	Staff conflicts
Spiritual crisis	Existential guilt or despair
	Loss of faith
	Persecutory or grandiose preoccupations

- ***address social complications***: legal or financial problems, family chaos, staff conflicts, and distortions of social perception; and
- ***give voice to spiritual needs***: loss of faith, despair, preoccupations with persecution abandonment.

Personality disorders are treatable conditions. Multiple treatment modalities can reduce symptoms of depression and anxiety, enhance global functioning, and improve social adjustment.[9,26,67-69] Even with adequate skills, however, treatment can be challenging, frustrating, and prolonged.[20,70]

Proper care of patients with personality disorders demands patience and creativity. Regardless of the patient's diagnosis, interpersonal problems are generally most prominent at the time of consultation. An empathic, supportive approach demands attention to the stage of treatment and essential areas in which the patient needs immediate assistance. This will often require attention to biological, psychological and social dimensions, any of which may be threatened throughout the course of cancer care.[71]

Psychotherapy and medication strategies developed to prevent or diminish trauma-related symptoms may be helpful in cancer-related distress, particularly hyper-arousal and dysphoric mood.[72-74] Medication benefits in cluster B personality disorder may be limited, although antidepressants do have some supporting evidence.[75] Meditation, including imagery, relaxation, and mindfulness strategies are helpful for many patients alone or in conjunction with structured psychotherapy.[68,76]

Psychotherapy should be problem-focused and activate psychosocial strengths. Social complications, including family conflict, financial and legal concerns must be addressed as precipitants of distress and disruptive behavior. Individual, family, and group therapies may powerfully assist with relating to caregivers, strengthening outside sources of nurturance, and self-esteem.[8,26,77-79] (See Interventions section.)

Beyond the problem focus that consultation initially demands, we must anticipate pitfalls, bolster mature defenses, and encourage productive coping. Diagnostic assessment that clarifies the patient's personality features, even without a formal DSM label, will facilitate predicting the patient's reactions to each stage of treatment. An appreciation of the patient's strengths and limitations will help build rapport and support remoralization.[80]

The same may be said of clinicians working with these patients, who need clarity and encouragement for such challenging work. We can greatly enhance patients' resilience by supporting the staff and families that care for them.

REFERENCES

1. American Psychiatric Association. Task Force on DSM-IV. *Diagnostic and statistical manual of mental disorders : DSM-IV-TR*. 4th ed. Washington, DC: American Psychiatric Association; 2000.

2. Drake RE, Vaillant GE. A validity study of axis II of DSM-III. *Am J Psychiatry*. 1985 May;142(5):553–558.

3. Ferro T, Klein DN, Schwartz JE, Kasch KL, Leader JB. 30-month stability of personality disorder diagnoses in depressed outpatients. *Am J Psychiatry*. 1998 May;155(5):653–659.

4. Johnson JG, Williams JB, Goetz RR, Rabkin JG, Lipsitz JD, Remien RH. Stability and change in personality disorder symptomatology: findings from a longitudinal study of HIV+ and HIV- men. *J Abnorm Psychol*. 1997 Feb;106(1):154–158.

5. Lenzenweger MF, Johnson MD, Willett JB. Individual growth curve analysis illuminates stability and change in personality disorder features: the longitudinal study of personality disorders. *Arch Gen Psychiatry*. 2004 Oct;61(10):1015–1024.

6. Loranger AW, Lenzenweger MF, Gartner AF, et al. Trait-state artifacts and the diagnosis of personality disorders. *Arch Gen Psychiatry*. 1991 Aug;48(8):720–728.

7. Jorm AF, Duncan-Jones P, Scott R. An analysis of the re-test artefact in longitudinal studies of psychiatric symptoms and personality. *Psychol Med*. 1989 May;19(2):487–493.

8. Perry J, Banon E, Ianni F. Effectiveness of psychotherapy for personality disorders. *Am J Psychiatry*. 1999;156:1312–1321.

9. Zanarini MC, Frankenburg FR, Hennen J, Silk KR. The longitudinal course of borderline psychopathology: 6-year prospective follow-up of the phenomenology of borderline personality disorder. *Am J Psychiatry*. 2003 Feb;160(2):274–283.

10. American Psychiatric Association. *Diagnostic and statistical manual of mental disorders: DSM-III*. 3rd ed. Washington, DC: American Psychiatric Association; 1980:23.

11. Akiskal HS. Demystifying borderline personality: critique of the concept and unorthodox reflections on its natural kinship with the bipolar spectrum. *Acta Psychiatr Scand*. 2004 Dec;110(6):401–407.

12. Orstavik RE, Kendler KS, Czajkowski N, Tambs K, Reichborn-Kjennerud T. The relationship between depressive personality disorder and major depressive disorder: a population-based twin study. *Am J Psychiatry*. 2007 Dec 1;164(12):1866–1872.

13. Ramklint M, Ekselius L. Personality traits and personality disorders in early onset versus late onset major depression. *J Affect Disord*. 2003 Jun;75(1):35–42.

14. Skodol AE, Siever LJ, Livesley WJ, Gunderson JG, Pfohl B, Widiger TA. The borderline diagnosis II: biology, genetics, and clinical course. *Biol Psychiatry*. 2002 Jun 15;51(12):951–963.

15. Viinamaki H, Tanskanen A, Koivumaa-Honkanen H, et al. Cluster C personality disorder and recovery from major depression: 24-month prospective follow-up. *J Personal Disord*. 2003 Aug;17(4):341–350.

16. Gamez W, Watson D, Doebbeling BN. Abnormal personality and the mood and anxiety disorders: implications for structural models of anxiety and depression. *J Anxiety Disord*. 2007;21(4):526–539.

17. Morse JQ, Pilkonis PA, Houck PR, Frank E, Reynolds CF, IIIrd. Impact of cluster C personality disorders on outcomes of acute and maintenance treatment in late-life depression. *Am J Geriatr Psychiatry*. 2005 Sep;13(9):808–814.

18. Fava M, Farabaugh AH, Sickinger AH, et al. Personality disorders and depression. *Psychol Med*. 2002 Aug;32(6):1049–1057.

19. Kasen S, Cohen P, Skodol AE, Johnson JG, Smailes E, Brook JS. Childhood depression and adult personality disorder: alternative pathways of continuity. *Arch Gen Psychiatry*. 2001 Mar;58(3):231–236.

20. Skodol AE, Gunderson JG, McGlashan TH, et al. Functional impairment in patients with schizotypal, borderline, avoidant, or obsessive-compulsive personality disorder. *Am J Psychiatry*. 2002 Feb;159(2):276–283.

21. Brieger P, Ehrt U, Bloeink R, Marneros A. Consequences of comorbid personality disorders in major depression. *J Nerv Ment Dis*. 2002 May;190(5):304–309.

22. Fournier JC, Derubeis RJ, Shelton RC, Gallop R, Amsterdam JD, Hollon SD. Antidepressant medications v. cognitive therapy in people with depression with or without personality disorder. *Br J Psychiatry*. 2008 Feb;192:124–129.

23. Grilo CM, Sanislow CA, Shea MT, et al. Two-year prospective naturalistic study of remission from major depressive disorder as a function of personality disorder comorbidity. *J Consult Clin Psychol*. 2005 Feb;73(1):78–85.

24. Hirschfeld RM. Personality disorders and depression: comorbidity. *Depress Anxiety*. 1999;10(4):142–146.

25. Iacovides A, Fountoulakis KN, Fotiou F, Fokas K, Nimatoudis I, Kaprinis G. Relation of personality disorders to subtypes of major depression according both to DSM-IV and ICD-10. *Can J Psychiatry*. 2002 Mar;47(2):196–197.

26. Joyce PR, McKenzie JM, Carter JD, et al. Temperament, character and personality disorders as predictors of response to interpersonal psychotherapy and cognitive-behavioural therapy for depression. *Br J Psychiatry*. 2007 Jun;190:503–508.

27. Kool S, Dekker J, Duijsens IJ, de Jonghe F. Major depression, double depression and personality disorders. *J Personal Disord*. 2000 Fall;14(3):274–281.

28. Shea MT, Pilkonis PA, Beckham E, et al. Personality disorders and treatment outcome in the NIMH Treatment of Depression Collaborative Research Program. *Am J Psychiatry*. 1990 Jun;147(6):711–718.

29. Coid J, Yang M, Tyrer P, Roberts A, Ullrich S. Prevalence and correlates of personality disorder in Great Britain. *Br J Psychiatry*. 2006 May;188:423–431.

30. Ansell EB, Sanislow CA, McGlashan TH, Grilo CM. Psychosocial impairment and treatment utilization by patients with borderline personality disorder, other personality disorders, mood and anxiety disorders, and a healthy comparison group. *Compr Psychiatry*. 2007 Jul-Aug;48(4):329–336.

31. Kunkel EJ, Woods CM, Rodgers C, Myers RE. Consultations for 'maladaptive denial of illness' in patients with cancer: psychiatric disorders that result in noncompliance. *Psychooncology*. 1997;6(2):139–149.

32. Skodol AE, Gunderson JG, Pfohl B, Widiger TA, Livesley WJ, Siever LJ. The borderline diagnosis I: psychopathology, comorbidity, and personality structure. *Biol Psychiatry*. 2002 Jun 15;51(12):936–950.

33. Skodol AE, Oldham JM, Bender DS, et al. Dimensional representations of DSM-IV personality disorders: relationships to functional impairment. *Am J Psychiatry*. 2005 Oct;162(10):1919–1925.

34. Spitzer RL, Endicott J, Robins E. Research diagnostic criteria: rationale and reliability. *Arch Gen Psychiatry*. 1978 Jun;35(6):773–782.

35. Kraus G, Reynolds DJ. The "A-B-C's" of the cluster B's: identifying, understanding, and treating cluster B personality disorders. *Clin Psychol Rev*. 2001 Apr;21(3):345–373.

36. Reichborn-Kjennerud T, Czajkowski N, Torgersen S, et al. The relationship between avoidant personality disorder and social phobia: a population-based twin study. *Am J Psychiatry*. 2007 Nov 1;164(11):1722–1728.

37. Sass H, Junemann K. Affective disorders, personality and personality disorders. *Acta Psychiatr Scand Suppl*. 2003(418):34–40.

38. Caspi A, McClay J, Moffitt TE, et al. Role of genotype in the cycle of violence in maltreated children. *Science*. 2002 Aug 2;297(5582):851–854.

39. Coccaro EF, Bergeman CS, McClearn GE. Heritability of irritable impulsiveness: a study of twins reared together and apart. *Psychiatry Res*. 1993 Sep;48(3):229–242.

40. Goldsmith H, Buss K, KS L. Toddler and childhood temperament: Expanded content, stronger genetic evidence, new evidence of the importance of environment. *Dev Psychobiol*. 1997;33:891–905.

41. Siegle GJ. Brain mechanisms of borderline personality disorder at the intersection of cognition, emotion, and the clinic. *Am J Psychiatry*. 2007;164(12):1776–1779.

42. Fish EW, Shahrokh D, Bagot R, et al. Epigenetic programming of stress responses through variations in maternal care. *Ann N Y Acad Sci*. 2004 Dec;1036:167–180.

43. Meyers CA, Berman SA, Scheibel RS, Hayman A. Case report: acquired antisocial personality disorder associated with unilateral left orbital frontal lobe damage. *J Psychiatry Neurosci*. 1992 Sep;17(3):121–125.

44. Damasio H, Grabowski T, Frank R, Galaburda AM, Damasio AR. The return of Phineas Gage: clues about the brain from the skull of a famous patient. *Science*. 1994 May 20;264(5162):1102–1105.

45. Silbersweig D, Clarkin JF, Goldstein M, et al. Failure of frontolimbic inhibitory function in the context of negative emotion in borderline personality disorder. *Am J Psychiatry*. 2007 Dec;164(12):1832–1841.

46. Casey PR, Dillon S, Tyrer PJ. The diagnostic status of patients with conspicuous psychiatric morbidity in primary care. *Psychol Med*. 1984 Aug;14(3):673–681.

47. Casey PR, Tyrer PJ, Platt S. The relationship between social functioning and psychiatric symptomatology in primary care. *Soc Psychiatry*. 1985;20(1):5–9.

48. Reich J, Boerstler H, Yates W, Nduaguba M. Utilization of medical resources in persons with DSM-III personality disorders in a community sample. *Int J Psychiatry Med*. 1989;19(1):1–9.

49. Lyons MJ, Jerskey BA. Personality disorders: epidemiological findings, methods and concepts. In: Tsuang MT, Tohen M (eds). *Textbook in psychiatric epidemiology*. 2nd ed. New York: Wiley-Liss; 2002:563–599.

50. Grant BF, Hasin DS, Chou SP, Stinson FS, Dawson DA. Nicotine dependence and psychiatric disorders in the United States: results from the national epidemiologic survey on alcohol and related conditions. *Arch Gen Psychiatry*. 2004 Nov;61(11):1107–1115.

51. Kraepelin E. *Lectures on clinical psychiatry*. 3rd ed. New York: William Wood; 1917.

52. Maser JD, Patterson T. Spectrum and nosology: implications for DSM-V. *Psychiatr Clin North Am*. 2002 Dec;25(4):855–885.

53. Tyrer P. Personality diatheses: a superior explanation than disorder. *Psychol Med*. 2007 Nov;37(11):1521–1525.

54. Lenzenweger MF. Schizotaxia, schizotypy, and schizophrenia: Paul E. Meehl's blueprint for the experimental psychopathology and genetics of schizophrenia. *J Abnorm Psychol.* 2006 May;115(2):195–200.

55. Tsuang MT, Stone WS, Gamma F, Faraone SV. Schizotaxia: current status and future directions. *Curr Psychiatry Rep.* 2003 Jun;5(2):128–134.

56. Gunderson JG, Weinberg I, Daversa MT, et al. Descriptive and longitudinal observations on the relationship of borderline personality disorder and bipolar disorder. *Am J Psychiatry.* 2006 Jul;163(7):1173–1178.

57. Zimmerman M, Ruggero CJ, Chelminski I, Young D. Is bipolar disorder overdiagnosed? *J Clin Psychiatry.* 2008;6:e1–e6.

58. Bhugra D, Bhui K. *Textbook of cultural psychiatry.* Cambridge ; New York: Cambridge University Press; 2007.

59. Nadine N. Borderline personality disorder: the voice of patients. *Res Nurs Health.* 1999;22(4):285–293.

60. Schwartz H. A person is a person and a shpos is not. *Man Med.* 1980;5(3):226–228.

61. Strauss A. "Shpos". *South Med J.* 1983 Aug;76(8):981–984.

62. Lee SJ, Back AL, Block SD, Stewart SK. Enhancing physician-patient communication. *Hematology Am Soc Hematol Educ Program.* 2002:464–483.

63. Kaptchuk TJ, Eisenberg DM. Varieties of healing. 2: a taxonomy of unconventional healing practices. *Ann Intern Med.* 2001 Aug 7;135(3):196–204.

64. Kaptchuk TJ, Eisenberg DM. Varieties of healing. 1: medical pluralism in the United States. *Ann Intern Med.* 2001 Aug 7;135(3):189–195.

65. Chochinov HM, Wilson KG, Enns M, Lander S. Depression, hopelessness, and suicidal ideation in the terminally ill. *Psychosomatics.* 1998;39(4):366–370.

66. Breitbart W, Rosenfeld B, Pessin H, et al. Depression, hopelessness, and desire for hastened death in terminally ill patients with cancer. *JAMA.* 2000 Dec 13;284(22):2907–2911.

67. Clarkin JF, Levy KN, Lenzenweger MF, Kernberg OF. Evaluating three treatments for borderline personality disorder: a multiwave study. *Am J Psychiatry.* 2007 Jun;164(6):922–928.

68. Linehan MM, Comtois KA, Murray AM, et al. Two-year randomized controlled trial and follow-up of dialectical behavior therapy vs therapy by experts for suicidal behaviors and borderline personality disorder. *Arch Gen Psychiatry.* 2006 Jul;63(7):757–766.

69. Binks CA, Fenton M, McCarthy L, Lee T, Adams CE, Duggan C. Psychological therapies for people with borderline personality disorder. *Cochrane Database Syst Rev.* 2006(1):CD005652.

70. Bender DS, Dolan RT, Skodol AE, et al. Treatment utilization by patients with personality disorders. *Am J Psychiatry.* 2001 Feb;158(2):295–302.

71. Holland JC. Improving the human side of cancer care: psycho-oncology's contribution. *Cancer J.* 2001 Nov-Dec;7(6):458–471.

72. Bennett WRM, Zatzick D, Roy-Byrne P. Can medications prevent PTSD in trauma victims? *Curr Psychiatry Online.* 2007;6(9):47–55.

73. Davidson JR, Payne VM, Connor KM, et al. Trauma, resilience and saliostasis: effects of treatment in post-traumatic stress disorder. *Int Clin Psychopharmacol.* 2005 Jan;20(1):43–48.

74. Yen S, Shea MT, Battle CL, et al. Traumatic exposure and posttraumatic stress disorder in borderline, schizotypal, avoidant, and obsessive-compulsive personality disorders: findings from the collaborative longitudinal personality disorders study. *J Nerv Ment Dis.* 2002 Aug;190(8):510–518.

75. Binks CA, Fenton M, McCarthy L, Lee T, Adams CE, Duggan C. Pharmacological interventions for people with borderline personality disorder. *Cochrane Database Syst Rev.* 2006(1):CD005653.

76. McMain S. Dialectic behaviour therapy reduces suicide attempts compared with non-behavioural psychotherapy in women with borderline personality disorder. *Evid Based Ment Health.* Feb 2007;10(1):18.

77. de Figueiredo JM. Demoralization and psychotherapy: a tribute to Jerome D. Frank, MD, PhD (1909–2005). *Psychother Psychosom.* 2007;76(3): 129–133.

78. Dimeff L, Koerner K. Overview of dialectical behavior therapy. In: Dimeff L, Koerner K, (eds). *Dialectical behavior therapy in clinical practice: Applications across disorders and settings.* New York: The Guilford Press; 2007:1–18.

79. Lacy TJ, Higgins MJ. Integrated medical-psychiatric care of a dying borderline patient: a case of dynamically informed "practical psychotherapy". *J Am Acad Psychoanal Dyn Psychiatry.* 2005 Winter;33(4):619–636.

80. Slavney PR. Diagnosing demoralization in consultation psychiatry. *Psychosomatics.* 1999 Jul-Aug;40(4):325–329.

CHAPTER 51

Psychotropic Medications in Cancer Care

Ilana M. Braun and William F. Pirl

INTRODUCTION

Psychiatric medications have wide-ranging utility in oncology. Although these medications primarily address psychiatric conditions, from mood disorders to delirium, they may also be helpful in managing nonpsychiatric symptoms and side effects including cancer-related fatigue, sleep disturbances, nausea, anorexia, weight loss, pain, and hot flashes. Over half of all cancer patients receive at least one psychiatric medication during their cancer treatment.[1] A competent psycho-oncologist must have some knowledge of these medications, in terms of possible benefits and side effects.

This chapter provides a general overview of psychiatric medications, reviewing major classes of psychiatric drugs in terms of on- and off-label uses, mechanisms, time-courses of action, side effects, risks, and important pharmacokinetic and pharmacodynamic drug-drug interactions. It is meant to supplement the chapters on particular disorders and symptoms, which include more specific information on psychiatric medication uses. For purposes of this chapter, pharmacokinetic interactions are defined as those that alter the amount and duration of a drug's availability; pharmacodynamic interactions as the antagonistic, additive, or synergistic clinical effects of concomitantly administered agents.

ANTIDEPRESSANTS

Several classes of antidepressant medications exist. Although some, like monoamine oxidase inhibitors, may be prescribed in general psychiatry, the possibility of drug interactions with common oncologic agents often precludes use of monoamine oxidase inhibitors in cancer patients. This section will focus on antidepressant medications commonly used in the cancer setting such as selective serotonin-reuptake inhibitors (SSRIs), selective serotonin and norepinephrine reuptake inhibitors (SNRIs), tricyclic antidepressants, and agents that are considered "atypical" antidepressants. The specific medications reviewed in this section are outlined in Table 51–1.

Indications for use. Although the Food and Drug Administration (FDA) has approved antidepressant use in depressive syndromes such as adjustment disorder and major depression, and anxiety disorders such as general anxiety disorder, panic disorder, obsessive compulsive disorder, and posttraumatic stress disorder, few randomized, double-blind, placebo-controlled trials have been carried out specifically in people with cancer.[2] In the absence of such studies, general psychiatry guides psycho-oncology standard of care.

In addition to use for psychiatric indications, antidepressants are sometimes employed for their side effects, which can be advantageous in the cancer setting. Sedating antidepressants, such as mirtazepine, nortriptyline, and trazodone, can serve as soporifics. The appetite stimulating effects of mirtazepine might be used to address poor food intake and cachexia. Antidepressant medications may also have some efficacy for other cancer-related symptoms. Neuropathic pain might respond to duloxetine, mirtazepine, tricyclics, or venlafaxine. Hot flashes induced by some cancer treatments might respond to SSRIs and venlafaxine.[3–5]

Mechanism and time-course of action. For the most part, antidepressants exert their effects by modulating the serotonin and/or norepinephrine systems. Serotonergic drugs are primarily the SSRIs which include citalopram, escitalopram, fluoxetine, paroxetine, and sertraline. Buproprion and mirtazapine are mainly norepinephrinergic agents and venlafaxine and duloxetine dual action on both systems. Although antidepressants have traditionally been thought to take between 4 and 6 weeks to show some effect, recent evidence suggests that the time course of action may be more rapid.[6] However, their full effect can still take between 6 and 8 weeks to manifest.

Side effects and risks. Specific antidepressant side effects vary by class of medication. Common side effects can include headache, gastrointestinal disturbances, nausea (particularly with duloxetine), sedation, weight gain (particularly with fluoxetine, mirtazapine, and paroxetine), sexual dysfunction, restlessness, blood pressure increases (particularly with venlafaxine), dry mouth, and lowering of the seizure threshold (particularly with buproprion). As previously mentioned, some of these side effects can be harnessed to help with co-morbid symptoms, such as using a sedating medication in patients with insomnia and a weight-inducing one in patients with poor appetite. In individuals with underlying bipolar disorder, antidepressants can trigger mania. For this reason, they should be avoided if possible in this population in favor of mood stabilizers with antidepressant effects such as lamotrigine (see under Anticonvulsants/Mood Stabilizers in this chapter).

Long-term antidepressant use carries few known risks. There is some evidence to suggest that antidepressants increase the incidence of fracture among the elderly.[7,8] Certain antidepressant medications, such as SSRIs, may also slightly increase bleeding risk.[9] These vulnerabilities purportedly arise through antidepressants' serotoninergic effects on bone and platelets, respectively. Although some (mainly older generation) antidepressants have been shown to promote tumor growth in animal studies, epidemiological research has not concluded that newer agents such as SSRIs have similar effects in humans.[10]

Antidepressant withdrawal may be associated with a discontinuation syndrome that can include malaise, light-headedness, dizziness, and lightning-like pains in extremities. This syndrome is most pronounced in antidepressants with short half-lives or with abrupt drug cessation. Agents with notable withdrawal reactions include paroxetine, venlafaxine, and duloxetine. If possible, discontinuation of any antidepressant should be gradual over the course of several weeks to months.

Very rarely, antidepressants trigger excess serotoninergic activity in the central nervous system, a condition known as serotonin syndrome. The hallmarks of this illness include acute onset autonomic instability, mental status changes, and neuromuscular signs including clonus, myclonus, and hyperreflexia. Although serotonin syndrome may occur in individuals on a single serotoninergic agent at a therapeutic level, it typically occurs in the setting of multiple serotinergic agents at high doses. Examples of serotinergic agents outside of the psychiatric medicine chest include analgesics such as fentanyl, meperidine, and tramadol, and the antibiotic linezolid. At least theoretically, the presence of serotonin-secreting carcinoid tumors can also predispose individuals to the condition. Management of serotonin syndrome involves the removal of all offending agents and the institution of supportive care.

A similar process can also be seen with the use of antidepressant medications in patients with pheochromocytomas. Antidepressants that are noradrenergic may precipitate even higher levels of epinephrine which could lead to a hypertensive crisis. Although there have some case reports of SSRIs also causing the same results, they have been thought to

Table 51–1. Antidepressants commonly used in the cancer setting

Drug	Dose (mg/day po)	Possible unique benefits	Possible side effects
Buproprion/ Buproprion ER	75–450	May be helpful for concentration and low energy; fewer sexual side effects	Seizures, headache, nausea, likely impedes tamoxifen's efficacy
Citalopram	10–40	Few P450 interactions	Headache, diarrhea, constipation, restlessness, sexual dysfunction
Duloxetine	20–60	Neuropathic pain and possibly hot flashes	Worsening of narrow-angle glaucoma and hepatic insufficiency, nausea, dizziness, fatigue, sexual dysfunction
Escitalopram	10–20	Few P450 interactions	Headache, diarrhea, constipation, restlessness, sexual dysfunction
Fluoxetine	10–80	Long-acting so (1) may be dosed once weekly at 90 mg and (2) least likely to trigger discontinuation syndrome	Nausea, nervousness, weight gain, headache, insomnia, strong inhibition of tamoxifen and other CYP 2D6 substrates
Mirtazapine	15–45	Sleep aid at low doses; appetite stimulant; antiemetic; less gastrointestinal side effects; minimal sexual dysfunction	Dry mouth, sedating at low doses, weight gain, cholesterol and triglyceride increases
Paroxetine/ Paroxetine CR	5–60 (62.5, if CR)		Headache, somnolence, dizziness, sexual dysfunction, gastrointestinal upset, dry mouth, prominent discontinuation syndrome, strong inhibition of tamoxifen and other 2D6 substrates
Sertraline	25–200		Headache, diarrhea, constipation, restlessness, sexual dysfunction
Trazodone	25–250	Sleep aid	Sedation, orthostasis, priapism, sexual dysfunction
Venlafaxine/ Venlafaxine SR	37.5–300	Possibly helpful for hot flashes and neuropathic pain; least interaction with tamoxifen; few P450 interactions	Blood pressure increases, sexual dysfunction, prominent discontinuation syndrome

be safer and might be prescribed with caution and close monitoring in patients with pheochromocytomas.[11]

Drug-drug interactions. Because polypharmacy is the norm for cancer patients, attention to possible pharmacokinetic and pharmacodynamic drug-drug interactions is essential when considering the addition of a psychotropic medication. A single agent can disrupt the balance of an established pharmaceutical regimen. In general, one should select an agent with few drug-drug interactions and rely on its lowest effective dose. Antidepressants that carry risk of significant pharmacokinetic drug interactions and that should probably be avoided in the cancer setting include fluoxetine and paroxetine. These agents are inhibitors of the cytochrome 2D6 (CYP 2D6), a pathway responsible for metabolism of many antidepressants, antipsychotics, β-blockers, and narcotics including codeine, oxycodone, and methadone. Concomitant administration of these antidepressants and CYP 2D6 substrates can theoretically lead to dangerous accumulation of the latter in the body. Buproprion might also inhibit CYP 2D6, but less seems to be known about its metabolism.

Caution should also be taken when prescribing duloxetine in the medically ill. In addition to undergoing CYP 2D6 metabolism, this agent is metabolized along a cytochrome 1A2 (CYP 1A2) pathway. Drugs that inhibit this pathway, including cimetidine and fluoroquinolones, can significantly increase duloxetine blood levels, placing patients at risk for hepatotoxicity. Similarly, CYP1A2 inducers such as cigarette smoking and omeprazole can significantly reduce duloxetine blood levels and, by extension, its effect.

A pharmacokinetic drug-drug interaction worthy of special mention is the potential interaction between many antidepressants and tamoxifen. Antidepressants are frequently prescribed in the setting of tamoxifen for their effectiveness both in treating psychiatric side effects and in ameliorating hot flashes exacerbated by the hormone antagonist. Unfortunately, fluoxetine, paroxetine, and, to a lesser extent, other antidepressants are metabolized along a shared cytochrome P450 pathway with tamoxifen. This pathway is of the 2D6 isoenzyme. By impeding conversion of tamoxifen to its active metabolite, antidepressants may decrease tamoxifen's efficacy. In the setting of depression and tamoxifen use, the antidepressant of choice is venlafaxine, followed closely by escitalopram and citalopram. Fluoxetine, paroxetine, and sertraline should best be avoided and there is little to no data for buproprion, duloxetine, mirtazapine, and trazodone.

ANXIOLYTICS

Anxiolytics fall under two broad classes: barbiturates and benzodiazepines. Because of their potential for drug-drug interactions and side effects, barbituates are rarely used in the cancer setting. Benzodiazepines, however, are very commonly used for both psychiatric and nonpsychiatric reasons. Some of the more widely prescribed benzodiazepines are described in Table 51–2.

Indications for use. In contrast to antidepressants that take weeks to exert their full effects, benzodiazepines rapidly curb psychic distress and promote sleep. In the cancer setting, they are frequently used to manage acute anticipatory anxiety, for instance before chemotherapy or magnetic resonance imaging, and in the case of specific phobias, for instance to needle sticks or the radiation mask in head and neck

Table 51–2. Benzodiazepines commonly used in the cancer setting

Drug	Dose (mg/day)	Half-life (hours)	Possible unique benefits	Possible side effects and risks
Alprazolam	0.125–2 PO	6–20	Helpful in the management of anxiety; no cross-tolerance with other benzodiazepines Higher potential for dependence and abuse; no cross-tolerance with other benzodiazepines	Sedation, dizziness, ataxia (or other psychomotor impairment), memory impairment, irritability, rebound anxiety, sexual dysfunction, disorientation, abuse, tolerance, dependence, withdrawal on abrupt discontinuation, multiple CYP3A4-based drug interactions
Clonazepam	0.25–4 PO	20–50	Helpful in the management of anxiety, seizure disorders, nocturnal sleep disorders, neuralgia, mania; may have less abuse liability than shorter-onset agents	Sedation, dizziness, ataxia (or other psychomotor impairment), memory impairment, irritability, sexual dysfunction, disorientation, abuse, tolerance, dependence, withdrawal on abrupt discontinuation
Diazepam	1–20 PO, IV, IM	30–60	Helpful in the management of anxiety, alcohol withdrawal, muscle spasm, seizure disorders	Sedation, dizziness, ataxia (or other psychomotor impairment), memory impairment, irritability, sexual dysfunction, disorientation, abuse, tolerance, dependence, withdrawal on abrupt discontinuation, bradycardia and respiratory depression
Lorazepam	0.5–5 PO, IV, IM	10–18	Helpful in the management of anxiety, depression, seizure disorders, alcohol withdrawal, and as an antiemetic; preferable in those with liver disease as not subject to Phase I metabolism	Sedation, dizziness, ataxia (or other psychomotor impairment), memory impairment, irritability, sexual dysfunction, disorientation, abuse, tolerance, dependence, withdrawal on abrupt discontinuation, bradycardia and respiratory depression
Oxazepam	5–30 PO	6–12	Helpful in the management of anxiety and alcohol withdrawal; preferable in those with liver disease as not subject to Phase I metabolism; may have less abuse liability than shorter-onset agents	Sedation, dizziness, ataxia (or other psychomotor impairment), memory impairment, irritability, sexual dysfunction, disorientation, abuse, tolerance, dependence, withdrawal on abrupt discontinuation, blood dyscrasias
Temazepam	7.5–15 PO	10–12	Helpful in the management of anxiety, depression, insomnia; preferable in those with liver disease as not subject to Phase I metabolism; may have less abuse liability than shorter-onset agents	Sedation, dizziness, ataxia (or other psychomotor impairment), memory impairment, irritability, sexual dysfunction, disorientation, abuse, tolerance, dependence, withdrawal on abrupt discontinuation
Triazolam	0.125–.25 PO	2–6	Helpful in the short-term management of insomnia	Sedation, dizziness, ataxia (or other psychomotor impairment), memory impairment, irritability, sexual dysfunction, disorientation, abuse, tolerance, dependence, withdrawal on abrupt discontinuation, tachycardia, GI upset, multiple CYP3A4-based drug–drug interactions
Midazolam	1–10 IV/IM	1–6	Conscious sedation in the terminally ill; short acting so easily reversible	Respiratory depression, hypotension, multiple CYP3A4-based drug-drug interactions

ABBREVIATIONS: GI, gastrointestinal; IM, intramuscular; IV, intravenous; PO, per oral.

cancers. They serve as useful adjuncts to antidepressants in quelling acute anxiety and as sleep aids. Because they do little to prevent future episodes of anxiety, however, they should not be used in lieu of antidepressants in the setting of major depression or an enduring anxiety disorder.

Benzodiazepines have far-reaching medical utility. They are often used as skeletal muscle relaxants, antiemetics, and anticonvulsants.[12] Midazolam, a benzodiazepine derivative, boasts sedative and amnestic properties that render it ideal for palliative sedation.[13] Finally benzodiazepines are commonly used in the management and prevention of alcohol withdrawal. Alcohol-dependent patients might abruptly decrease or cease alcohol consumption in the setting of a hospital admission and a life-threatening syndrome can ensue, marked by profound autonomic instability, sensorium alterations, and agitation. Benzodiazepines mimic binding of alcohol to its receptor. When administered in doses large enough to block autonomic instability these medications dampen signs of withdrawal and can be slowly tapered, often to lifesaving benefit.

Mechanism and time-course of action Like alcohol, benzodiazepines bind to the benzodiazepine binding site of gamma-amino butyric acid (GABA)$_A$ receptors, enhancing the binding of the inhibitory neurotransmitter, GABA, to the receptor. The set of interactions leads to inhibitory effects on the central nervous system.

Onset and duration of action vary widely among agents. Such differences are of clinical significance as benzodiazepines with rapid onset of action, for instance alprazolam and diazepam, are more likely to trigger euphoria and substance abuse than agents with slower onset of action, for instance clonazepam and oxazepam. Longer acting agents such as clonazepam and diazepam, are more likely than shorter acting agents such as alprazolam or lorazepam to accumulate in the system, risking amplification of side effects described below.

Table 51–3. Stimulants commonly used in the cancer setting

Drug (generic name in bold followed by trade name)	Duration of action (hours)	Dose (mg/day)	Possible unique benefits	Possible side effects
Amphetamine/ Dextroamphetamine			Appetite suppression, insomnia, anxiety, irritability as medication wears off, abuse potential, increase in blood pressure, elevated heart rate, sudden death	Appetite suppression, insomnia, anxiety, irritability as medication wears off, abuse potential, increase in blood pressure, elevated heart rate, sudden death
Adderall	4–6	2.5–40		
Adderall XR	8+	5–20		
***d*-Amphetamine**			May improve symptoms of common cold	Appetite suppression, insomnia, anxiety, irritability as medication wears off, abuse potential, increase in blood pressure, elevated heart rate, sudden death
Dexedrine, Dextrostat	4–5	2.5–40		
Dexedrine spansules	8	5–40		
***dl*-Methylphenidate**			Daytrana is a trans-dermal system; both Metadate CD and Ritalin LA capsules have beads that can be sprinkled; Methylin ER is available in solution	Appetite suppression, insomnia, anxiety, irritability as medication wears off, abuse potential, increase in blood pressure, elevated heart rate, sudden death
Concerta	12	18–72		
Daytrana	12	10–30		
Metadate CD, Ritalin LA	8	10–60		
Metadate ER	3–8	10–60		
Methylin, Ritalin	3–4	2.5–60		
Methylin ER	8	2.5–60		
Ritalin SR	3–8	20–60		
***d*-Methylphenidate**			*d*-methylphenidate is touted as having less of a "crash" than dl-methylphenidate	Appetite suppression, insomnia, anxiety, irritability as medication wears off, abuse potential, increase in blood pressure, elevated heart rate, sudden death
Focalin	3–5	1.25–20		
Modafinil	8–18	25–200	Low abuse potential; DEA schedule IV drug; marketed as gentler and less likely than other stimulants to trigger insomnia	Headache; mild GI distress; anxiety; insomnia

ABBREVIATIONS: DEA, Drug Enforcement Administration; GI, gastrointestinal; IV, intravenous.

Side effects and risks. Benzodiazepines can trigger central nervous system side effects, including sedation, dizziness, ataxia and frequent falling, anterograde amnesia, irritability, and disorientation. As sleep aids, they can have adverse effects on respiration and on sleep architecture, with decreases in both slow wave sleep and rapid eye movements.[14] The above-mentioned side effects may be particularly pronounced in the elderly and in those with central nervous system fragility, for instance, as a result of cerebral vascular accident, traumatic brain injury, or mass. They should be used with caution, if at all, in these populations. Because benzodiazepines carry abuse liability, they should also be used with caution in individuals with histories of substance abuse, particularly of alcohol. Agents with the greatest risk for abuse include alprazolam, diazepam, and lorazepam.[15]

After prolonged use, benzodiazepines should be discontinued very gradually over the course of weeks to months. Abrupt cessation may lead to a powerful and potentially life-threatening withdrawal reaction akin to alcohol withdrawal and characterized by hyperthermia, autonomic arousal, sweating, neuromuscular irritability, paranoia, and hallucinations.

Drug-drug interactions. In general, anxiolytics boast few pharmokinetic drug-drug interactions. Three exceptions are alprazolam, midazolam, and triazolam. The cytochrome P450 3A (CYP 3A) pathway metabolizes these drugs, rendering them sensitive to a wide array of CYP 3A inhibitors and inducers that raise and lower their concentrations, respectively. CYP 3A inhibitors include macrolide antibiotics, several antifungals, cimetidine, fluoxetine, and grapefruit juice. CYP 3A inducers include several antiepileptic medications and, important to the practice of oncology, dexamethasone. Because of the pharmacologic complexity of many cancer treatment regimens, anxiolytics with fewer P450 interactions are preferable in this setting.

The sedating effects of benzodiazepines are additive with those of other sedating medications including antidepressants such mirtazapine and trazodone, certain antipsychotics, and narcotics.

STIMULANTS

Although traditionally associated with use in children, stimulants are also often employed in medically ill patients. The stimulant medications detailed in this section are outlined in Table 51–3.

Indications for use. Food and Drug Administration-approved for the management for attention deficit disorder and narcolepsy, stimulants such as amphetamine and methylphenidate have several important off-label uses in the cancer setting. First, like benzodiazepines, methylphenidate and amphetamine can bolster a depressed patient in the period before an antidepressant takes full clinical effect. The medications may increase energy, stimulate appetite and concentration, and provide a sense of well-being. Although stimulants are frequently used as monotherapy for depression in cancer, there is no data to support this practice and stimulant monotherapy has been shown to not be effective in noncancer populations. Second, stimulants might help with cancer-related fatigue, one of the most debilitating symptoms of cancer and its treatment.[16] In the instances in which fatigue persists after reversible causes have been addressed, stimulants, along with behavioral modifications, could potentially improve functionality (although randomized clinical trials have not yet been convincing).[17] Third, stimulants can combat the sedating effects of narcotics, which may be necessary for adequate pain control. Finally, these medications may have some utility in the management of cancer-related cognitive difficulties, colloquially referred to as "chemo-brain" or "chemo-fog."[18,19]

Modafinil, a newer FDA-approved agent for excessive sleepiness caused by narcolepsy, obstructive sleep apnea, and shift work sleep disorder, improves wakefulness and may help with fatigue, sedation from narcotics, and cancer-related cognitive difficulties in the cancer setting.[20]

Table 51–4. Antipsychotics commonly used in the cancer setting

Drug	Dose (mg/day)	Half-life (hours)	Possible unique benefits	Possible side effects
Aripiprazole	2–30 PO	75 (active metabolite: 94)	Little sedation	Metabolic syndrome, orthostasis, cognitive and motor impairment, increased mortality risk in elderly
Haloperidol	0.25–15 PO/IM 0.25–100 IV (upper limits only in cases of severe agitation)	12–36	No metabolic syndrome risk; IV preparation with fewer extrapyramidal side effects as compared to PO or IM; useful as sleep aid	Cardiac arrhythmia; extrapyramidal side effects, hypotension, worsening of narrow-angle glaucoma
Olanzapine	2.5–20 PO/SL/IM	21–54	Useful as sleep aid and antiemetic	Metabolic syndrome, orthostasis, sedation, headache, dry mouth, constipation, increased mortality risk in elderly
Quetiapine Quetiapine XR	12.5–750 PO	6	Useful as sleep aid; only atypical antipsychotic approved for management of depressive episodes in bipolar patients	Metabolic syndrome, sedation, headache, orthostasis, cataracts, QT prologation, increased mortality risk in elderly
Risperidal	0.25–12 PO	3–20	Useful as sleep aid	Metabolic syndrome, orthostasis, extrapyramidal side effects at high doses, arrhythmias, sedation, blood dyscrasias, dry mouth, constipation, increased mortality risk in elderly
Ziprasidone	20–160 PO 40 IM	2–5		Metabolic syndrome, QT prolongation, bradycardia, orthostasis, somnolence, increased mortality risk in elderly

ABBREVIATIONS: IM, intramuscular; IV, intravenous; PO, per oral.

Mechanisms and time course of action. The primary actions of amphetamine and methylphenidate are two-fold: to promote neuronal release of dopamine, as well as to prevent the neurotransmitter's reuptake. While amphetamine and methylphenidate exert their effects in several brain areas, modafinil acts specifically on excitatory histamine projections to the hypothalamus. The discrete nature of its effect has led some experts to view it as a gentler medication as compared to other stimulants in terms of both effect and side effects.[21]

Stimulants vary widely in their duration of action. The effects of immediate release methylphenidate and amphetamine wear off in several hours necessitating twice daily dosing. Extended-release versions of these medications, as well as of modafinil, persist for much of the day.

Side effects and risks. Although generally well tolerated, amphetamine and methylphenidate use can result in untoward side effects including appetite suppression, insomnia, anxiety, and a "crash" characterized by irritability as their effect wane late in the day. They are considered abuse-able and for this reason classified by the Drug Enforcement Agency as Schedule II substances. Finally, they possess cardiovascular effects including elevations in blood pressure and heart rate that, in patients with underlying heart abnormalities, can lead to arrhythmia and in rare cases sudden death. In April, 2008, the American Heart Association recommended that children on such medications undergo a thorough cardiac work-up, including an electrocardiogram (EKG), before beginning stimulants. By contrast, both the American Academy of Pediatrics and the American Psychiatric Association assert that EKGs are costly and unnecessary. As the standard of care debate continues in the attention deficit arena, we recommend that healthcare providers wishing to start a cancer patient on stimulant medication follow a complete physical examination, as well as careful personal and family history, with a screening EKG in worrisome cases. We also recommend relying on the lowest effective dose of medication.

Modafinil can commonly trigger headache, mild gastrointestinal (GI) distress, and anxiety. Less common side effects include insomnia, heart rate increases, and blood pressure elevations. It has not been extensively studied in populations with cardiac disease. Rarely (in <1% of users), it can cause rash that can progress to Stevens–Johnson syndrome.

Drug-drug interactions. Modafinil is an inducer of the CYP 3A enzyme and can lead to overmetabolism of CYP 3A substrates, including oral contraceptives, steroids, cyclosporine, and some anxiolytics, tricyclic antidepressants, and anticonvulsants. Other stimulants do not have significant pharmacokinetic drug-drug interactions.

ANTIPSYCHOTICS

Since the first generation of antipsychotics were known to carry risks of neurologic and cardiac side effects, these agents waned in popularity with the arrival of the newer antipsychotic medications that were considered safer in these respects. Second generation antipsychotics, known as atypicals, are now understood to have the potential for their own concerning side effects such as glucose intolerance and metabolic syndrome. Although both types of antipsychotic medications can have serious side effects, they remain important and essential medications in the treatment of psychiatric disorders and symptoms. The following section reviews the pharmacology of both newer agents such as aripiprizole, olanzapine, quetiapine, risperidal, and ziprasidone, and of haloperidol, a first generation antipsychotic that remains the gold standard for delirium management. These medications are described in Table 51–4.

Indications for use. In general psychiatry, antipsychotics are used in the management of bipolar disorder and psychotic disorders such as schizophrenia, schizoaffective disorder, and depression with psychotic features. In medical settings, they are also used in the management of delirium. Although the primary treatment for delirium is the identification and correction of the underlying medical cause, antipsychotics are used for the distress and agitation that often accompany confusion. At low doses, antipsychotics improve sensorium, alertness, and perhaps even cognition. At higher doses, they are sedating. Antipsychotics also have utility in nondelirious patients. The more sedating of these medications—haloperidol, olanzapine, and quetiapine—are used as sleep aids, particularly in substance abusers for whom traditional hypnotics may be contraindicated. They can be used for anxiety that is refractory to benzodiazepines or in patients in whom benzodiazepines are contraindicated. They may be particularly useful in managing the side effects of glucocorticoid steroids, including irritability, sleep disturbance, and some mood symptoms. Finally, some antipsychotics may have antiemetic properties including haloperidol, perphenazine, and olanzapine. These effects may be similar to prochlorperazine and metocloperamide, which can make them useful agents with chemotherapy regimens.[12] In addition, olanzapine increases appetite, which can be useful in patients with cachexia.

Mechanism and time course of action. A crucial action of both first and second generation antipsychotics is to tamp the dopamine neurotransmitter system which becomes overactive in both psychotic illness and delirium. Many atypical antipsychotics including aripiprizole, olanzapine, quetiapine, and risperidone also act on the serotonin system, but affect different receptors than SSRIs. Most antipsychotics have half-lives of a day to several days. Exceptions include quetiapine with a half-life of approximately 6 hours and ziprasidone with a half-life of 2–5 hours. The makers of quetiapine have recently released a long-acting version, with a half-life of 9–12 hours.

Side effects and risks. First generation antipsychotics such as haloperidol are associated with cardiac and neurologic side effects. Hypotension and QT prolongation occur frequently, the latter placing individuals at risk for a very rare but potentially fatal torsade de pointes arrhythmia. Neuroleptic-induced movement disorders, referred to as extrapyramidal symptoms, include Parkinson-like movements, dystonia, and a subjective sense of restless referred to as akithesia. The side effects usually remit with medication withdrawal. Occasionally, first generation antipsychotics trigger tardive dyskinesia: uncontrollable, repetitive, and purposeless movements such as lip smacking, blinking, or arm flailing. These movement disorder can persist for months to years after the agent has been withdrawn and, in some instances, may become permanent. First generation antipsychotics should be used at their lowest effective doses and avoided, if possible, in patients with Parkinson's disease or who are on other medications that prolongate QT.

Newer antipsychotics have a different side-effect profile. With exception of ziprasidone and quetiapine, they do not cause significant QT prolongation. In addition, atypical antipsychotics more infrequently cause extrapyramidal symptoms or tardive dyskinesia. They are, however, not completely without risk. Atypicals have the potential to cause signs of metabolic syndrome including weight gain, elevations in blood glucose and cholesterol levels. They are also associated with increased risk for stroke and even premature death in the elderly.

Very rarely, antipsychotics trigger dose-dependent excess dopamine blockade in the central nervous system, known as neuroleptic malignant syndrome (NMS). The hallmarks of this dangerous condition include muscle rigidity, fever, autonomic instability, and cognitive changes. Laboratory assessment in the setting of the illness is notable for elevated creatinine phosphokinase. Particularly since exhaustion, dehydration, malnutrition, and polypharmacy are risk factors for this condition, cancer patient, at least theoretically, represent a high-risk group.[22] Medications outside of the psychiatric medicine chest with anti-dopaminergic action include antiemetics such as metocloperamide and prochlorperazine. One should be cautious with patients receiving antiemetic and antipsychotic polypharmacy. NMS management includes withdrawal of the offending agent and supportive measures.

Drug-drug interactions. Antipsychotics are vulnerable to a variety of pharmacokinetic drug-drug interactions. The CYP 3A4 enzyme metabolizes aripiprizole, quetiapine, and ziprasidone. CYP 3A inhibitors include macrolide antibiotics, several antifungals, cimetidine, fluoxetine, and grapefruit juice. CYP 3A inducers include several antiepileptic medications and, important to the practice of oncology, dexamethasone. Aripiprizole, haloperidol, olanzapine, and risperidone are

CYP 2D6 enzyme substrates. Inhibitor of the CYP 2D6 enzyme that may significantly increase levels of these drugs include fluoxetine, paroxetine, haloperidol, and quinidine. Finally, olanzapine is metabolized in part along the cytochrome CYP 1A2 pathway. Inhibitors of this pathway that increase olanzapine's blood concentration include fluoroquinolones and cimetidine; CYP 1A2 inducers that lower blood concentration of the drug include cigarette smoking and omeprazole.

Antipsychotics are also subject to several pharmacodynamic drug-drug interactions. Several of their potential side effects are additive with those of other agents. The QT-prolonging effects of first generation antipsychotics, as well as ziprasidone and quetiapine, are additive with those of other QT-prolonging medications including erythromycin, methadone, pentamidine, and amiodarone.[23] The sedating effects of antipsychotics such as olanzapine and quetiapine are compounded by those of central nervous system depressants including benzodiazepines and narcotics. Finally, the hypotensive effects of atypical antipsychotics and haloperidol can significantly magnify the actions of traditional antihypertensives.

ANTICONVULSANTS/MOOD STABILIZERS

Although lithium is widely used for mood stabilization in general psychiatry, its narrow therapeutic window, sensitivity to subtle fluctuations in fluid balance, and many adverse effects make it less frequently used in the setting of cancer treatment. The following section focuses on other mood stabilizers that are commonly used in cancer patients, such as lamotrigine, gabapentin, pregabalin, and valproic acid (Table 51–5).

Indications for use. Many anticonvulsants are used as mood stabilizers in bipolar disorder and as medications for neuropathic pain syndromes.[24] Carbamazepine, lamotrigine, and valproic acid (as well as divalproex sodium and sodium valproate) can quell manic episodes; lamotrigine protects individuals against depressive ones. Some psychiatrists include gabapentin in their management of bipolar disorder, particularly in mild cases.[25] However, there is little data to support this and the FDA has not approved it for this indication. These medications are also sometimes used for manic-like presentations in the context of cancer or cancer treatment such as steroid use and brain metastases.

Mechanisms and onset of action. Lamotrigine stabilizes neuronal membranes by blocking the glutamate neurotransmitter system. Gabapentin, pregabalin, valproic acid, and sodium valproate all exert their effects by amplifying the inhibitory GABA neurotransmitter system. The exact mechanisms by which they achieve this end are poorly elucidated. Carbamazepine also exerts inhibition effects through its effects on sodium channels. Anticonvulsants have relatively short half-lives and ideally should be dosed 2–3 times daily.

Side effects. Common side effects of anticonvulsants include sedation, dizziness, nausea, ataxia, headache, tremor, visual changes, and rash. Over the long term, these medications, and particularly valproic acid and pregabalin, can lead to significant weight gain. Pregabalin should be avoided in patients with severe renal impairment, in the elderly, and in the setting of severe congestive heart failure It should be tapered slowly. Valproic acid and sodium valproate are associated with rare idiosyncratic toxicities including hemorragic pancreatitis and agranulocytosis. Although generally very well tolerated, lamotrigine is associated with a rash in 10% of its users. Very rarely, such a rash progresses to the life-threatening Stevens–Johnson syndrome. To reduce risk for a serious rash, the medication should be started at low dose and titrated upward quite gradually, for instance, by 25 mg every 2 weeks. Individuals on the medication should be encouraged to maintain stable drug levels by not missing doses and should stop the drug at the first appearance of any rash.

Drug-drug interactions. Lamotrigine is metabolized solely by glucuronidation and does not affect the P450 hepatic enzymes itself. When taken in conjunction with lamotrigine, valproic acid (as well as

Table 51–5. Mood stabilizers commonly used in the cancer setting

Drug	Dose (mg/day)	Possible unique benefits	Possible side effects
Gabapentin	100–2400 PO	May serve as sleep aid, analgesic in neuropathic pain syndromes, anticonvulsant, antianxiety medication, and antiemetic in intractable cases	Somnolence, dizziness, ataxia, peripheral edema
Lamotrigine	25–200 PO	Anticonvulsant and mood stabilizer that prophylaxes against depression in bipolar disorder	Rash that rarely progresses to Stevens–Johnson syndrome, photosensitivity, headache, gastrointestinal upset, dizziness, ataxia
Pregabalin	50–300 PO	May serve as analgesic in neuropathic pain syndromes; anticonvulsant; antianxiety medication	Dizziness, drowsiness, dry mouth, peripheral edema, blurred vision, weight gain, difficulty concentrating
Divalproex sodium, Sodium valproate, Valproic Acid	250–60 mg/kg/day PO	May have utility as sleep aid; allows for therapeutic blood level monitoring	Somnolence, dizziness, GI upset, double vision, ataxia, thrombocytopenia, hepatitis, alopecia, weight gain, thrombocytopenia, agranulocytosis

ABBREVIATIONS: GI, gastrointestinal; PO, per oral.

Table 51–6. Hypnotics commonly used in the cancer setting

Drug	Dose (mg/day)	Possible unique benefits	Possible side effects
Eszopiclone	1–3	Low potential for tolerance and withdrawal; short half-life (~1 hour) renders it ideal for patients with sleep initiation difficulties	Headache, dry mouth, somnolence, dizziness, hallucinations, rash, unpleasant metallic taste after ingestion
Zaleplon	5–20	Low potential for tolerance and withdrawal; short half-life (~1 hour) renders it ideal for patients with sleep initiation difficulties	Headache, somnolence, amnesia, photosensitivity, edema; should be used with caution in patients with hepatic or renal insufficiency
Zolpidem Zolpidem CR	Zolpidem: 2.5–10 Zolpidem CR: 6.25–12.5	Helpful in the short-term management of insomnia; low potential for tolerance and withdrawal; tends not to impair nocturnal respiratory and sleep architecture	Headache, dizziness, drowsiness, nausea, myalgia, sleep eating syndrome, hallucination addiction

sodium valproate) significantly increases lamotrigine blood concentrations, ostensibly by competing for a particular step in the glucuronidation pathway. In the setting of combined therapy with lamotrigine and valproic acid, the former should be titrated to its target dose extremely slowly, for instance by 12.5 mg every 2 weeks, to minimize the risk for serious rash. Gabapentin and pregabalin boast minimal pharmacokinetic drug-drug interactions. The sedating effects of anticonvulsants may be pharmacodynamically additive with other sedating medications.

HYPNOTICS

Hypnotics are medications that induce sleep. The hypnotics detailed in this section are outlined in Table 51–6.

Indications for use. Hypnotic drugs aid in both sleep induction and maintenance, and can be extremely helpful to individuals with insomnia in both the active and surveillance stages of their treatments. The causes of insomnia vary widely between people, however, and an understanding the etiologies of a particular sleep disturbance may lead to a more targeted treatment approach. Over the long term, one might best manage insomnia due to: (1) depression or anxiety with an antidepressant medication (not even necessarily a sedating one) (2) steroids with their reduction or cessation (3) menopausal symptoms with the antidepressant venlafaxine or the anticonvulsant gabapentin (4) obstructive sleep apnea with a positive airway pressure machine (5) restless legs syndrome with gabapentin or mirapex and (6) a pain disorder with appropriate analgesia. In the short term, however, hypnotics can be useful sleep promoting agents and, at least in the case of zolpidem, do so without affecting normal sleep architecture or breathing patterns.[14,26]

Mechanisms and time-course of action. Like sedatives, hypnotics act on the GABAergic system. They tend to have short half-lives. Eszopiclone and zalepon with half-lives of 1 hour are ideal for patients with sleep initiation difficulties. The intermediate acting zolpidem with a half-life of 2–3 hours and long-acting zolpidem CR with half-life of 7 hours are preferable in individuals with mid-cycle awakenings and shortened total sleep duration.

Side effects and risks. For the most part, hypnotics tend to have benign side-effect profiles. Most commonly, individuals may experience a mild hangover following their use, particularly with longer acting agents. Eszopiclone has gained some notoriety for a metallic taste following its ingestion. Zolpidem has received attention for its uncommon association with sleep-related disorders such as sleep walking, eating, and even driving. It has also been associated with and hallucinations.

Although hypnotics have low potential for tolerance and withdrawal, abrupt hypnotic cessation following prolonged use may lead to a brief period of rebound insomnia. Unlike anxiolytics, they are not dependency-forming; however, they do carry some abuse liability. For this reason, hypnotics are best avoided in individuals with strong histories of substance abuse or dependence. Finally, in delirious patients, a sedating antipsychotic such as olanzapine or quetiapine is preferable to a hypnotic; in a manner similar to an anxiolytic, the latter can worsen an underlying encephalopathy.

Drug-drug interactions. Hypnotics have minimal pharmacokinetic drug-drug interactions. Other sedating medications can compound their sedating effects.

CONCLUSION

In oncology, psychotropic medications are used to treat both psychiatric and cancer-related symptoms as well as cancer-related symptoms. Although many of these medications are FDA-approved for specific psychiatric disorders, there are very few clinical trials in cancer patients for these same indications. Individuals with cancer are usually much more complicated than the typical participant in a general psychiatry clinical trial in terms of both medical co-morbidity and psychosocial challenges. While general psychiatry can guide the use of these medications, there may be special issues in cancer patients, particularly with tolerability, drug interactions, and timeframe for onset of action.

Cancer-related symptoms such as fatigue, nausea, pain, cachexia, and hot flashes might also be relieved by some psychotropic medications. However, almost all of these uses are off-label and not approved by the FDA. The increasing interest in cancer-related symptom management may lead to the accumulation of clinical trial data that supports the use of some of these agents. Until then, clinicians must weigh the impact of the potential benefits against the potential side effects. Some of these symptoms may not have standards treatments and a medication trial may represent some possible relief.

REFERENCES

1. Coyne JC, Palmer SC, Shapiro PJ, Thompson R, DeMichele A. Distress, psychiatric morbidity, and prescriptions for psychiatric medication in a breast cancer waiting room sample. *Gen Hosp Psychiatry.* 2004;26(2):121–128.

2. Pirl WF. Evidence report on the occurrence, assessment, and treatment of depression in cancer patients. *J Natl Cancer Inst Monogr.* 2004;32:32–39.

3. Cankurtaran ES, Ozalp E, Soygur H, Akbiyik DI, Turhan L, Alkis N. Mirtazapine improves sleep and lowers anxiety and depression in cancer patients: superiority over imipramine. *Support Care Cancer.* 2008 Feb 26. Epub ahead of print.

4. Durand JP, Alexandre J, Guillevin L. Clinical activity of venlafaxine and topiramate against oxaliplatin-induced disabling permanent neuropathy. *Anticancer Drugs.* 2005;16:587–591.

5. Kim HF, Fisch MJ. Antidepressant use in ambulatory cancer patients. *Curr Oncol Rep.* 2006;8(4):275–281.

6. Mitchell A. Two-week delay in onset of action of antidepressants: new evidence. *Br J Psychiatry.* 2006;188:105–106.

7. Richards JB, Papaioannou A, Adachi JD, et al. Effect of selective serotonin reuptake inhibitors on risk of fracture. *Arch Intern Med.* 2007;167(2):188–194.

8. Spangler L, Scholes D, Brunner RL, et al. Depressive symptoms, bone loss, and fractures in postmenopausal women. *J Gen Intern Med.* 2008;23(5):567–574.

9. Opatrny L, Delaney JA, Suissa S. Gastro-intestinal haemorrhage risks of selective serotonin receptor antagonist therapy: a new look. *Br J Clin Pharmacol.* 2008;66(1):76–81.

10. Oksbjerg Dalton S, Johansen C, Mellemkjaer, et al. Antidepressant medication and risk for cancer. *Epidem.* 2000;11:171–176.

11. Kashyap AS. Pheochromacytima unearthed by fluoxetine. *Postgrad Med.* 2000;76:303.

12. Lohr L. Chemotherapy-induced nausea and vomiting. *Cancer J.* 2008;14(2):85–93.

13. Elsayem A, Curry IE, Boohene J. Use of palliative sedation for intractable symptoms in the palliative care unit of a comprehensive cancer center. *Support Care Cancer.* 2008. Epub ahead of print.

14. Barbera J, Shapiro C. Benefit-risk assessment of zaleplon in the treatment of insomnia. *Drug Saf.* 2005;28(4):301–318.

15. Griffith RR, Wolf B. Relative abuse liability of different benzodiazepines in drug abusers. *J Clin Psychopharmacol.* 1990;10:237–243.

16. Lower E, Fleishman S, Cooper A, et al. A phase III, randomized placebo-controlled trial of the safety and efficacy of d-MPH as new treatment of fatigue and "chemobrain" in adult cancer patients. *Asco Annual Meeting.* 2005. (Abstract 8000).

17. Minton O, Stone P, Richardson A, et al. Drug therapy for the management of cancer related fatigue. *Cochrane Database Syst Rev.* 2008;23(1):CD006704.

18. Daly BP, Brown RT. Scholarly literature review: management of neurocognitive late effects with stimulant medication. *J Pediatr Psychol.* 2007;32(9):1111–1126.

19. Sood A, Barton DL, Loprinzi, CL. Use of methylphenidate in patients with cancer. *Am J Hosp Palliat Care.* 2006;23(1):35–40.

20. Prommer E. Modafinil: is it ready for prime time? *J Opioid Manag.* 2006;2(3):130–136.

21. Jasinski DR. An evaluation of the abuse potential of modafinil using methylphenidate as a reference. *J Psychopharmacol.* 2000;14(1):53–60.

22. Kawanishi C, Onishi H, Kato D, et al. Neuroleptic malignant syndrome in cancer treatment. *Palliat Support Care.* 2005;3(1):51–53.

23. Roden D. Drug therapy: drug induced prolongation of the QT interval. *NEJM.* 2004;350(10):1013–1022.

24. Stacey BR, Swift JN. Pregabalin for neuropathic pain based on recent clinical trials. *Curr Pain Headache Rep.* 2006;10(3):179–184.

25. Mack A. Examination of evidence for off-label use of gabapentin. *J Managed Care Pharm.* 2003;9(6):559–568.

26. Girault C, Muir JF, Mihaltan F, et al. Effects of repeated administration of zolpidem on sleep, diurnal and nocturnal respiratory function, vigilance and physical performance in patients with COPD. *Chest.* 1996;110:1203–1211.

PART IX

Interventions

Matthew J. Loscalzo, ED

CHAPTER 52

Screening Procedures for Psychosocial Distress

Alex J. Mitchell

OVERVIEW OF PSYCHOSOCIAL DISTRESS, DEPRESSION AND ANXIETY

Prevalence of depression, anxiety, and distress. In the 12 years since the last edition of "Psycho-oncology" there has been a burgeoning of evidence pertaining to screening and related diagnostic procedures. Before 1990 the focus was mainly on attempts to summarize the prevalence of depression following cancer with few systematic attempts to develop validated methods to assess anxiety or broadly defined distress and no implementation studies (Textbox 52–1).[1]

It has taken a long time to come to the conclusion that there is no single rate of depression in cancer but rather different rates depending on background risk factors such as early and late stage disease.[2-6] A number of rating scales have been used to supplement unassisted clinical skills although only a handful have been specifically designed for this population.[3] The Hospital Anxiety and Depression Scale (HADS) has been employed in three large scale (n = ≥500) studies.[4,5] For example, Sharpe's group in Edinburgh (2007) surveyed 3071 patients using a touch-screen adaptation of the HADS.[5] Twenty-two percent had distress (defined by a total HADS score ≥15), 23% had anxiety, and 16% had depression.[5] Two equally large studies used the Brief Symptom Inventory (BSI). The BSI was originally a 53-item measure of psychological distress that contains three global scales and nine subscales (Derogatis and Melisaraatos, 1983).[6] Zabora and colleagues (2001) used the original BSI, and found prevalence rates of 35% for distress, 24% for anxiety, and 19% for depression.[7] Carlson and colleagues (2004) used the shorter BSI-18 in 2776 patients. Pooling data from these two studies shows that individuals with lung, brain, and pancreatic cancer tend to be most distressed but differences between cancers are modest (Fig. 52–1).[8] The mean level of distress from the BSI studies was 37.8% almost identical to that found by Fallowfield et al., 2001, in 2297 patients using the General Health Questionnaire (GHQ-12) (36.4%).[9]

Looking beyond major depression. We now recognize that many patients who struggle emotionally don't meet criteria for *Diagnostic statistical manual* (DSM)-IV major depression. This has led, both, to the development of the concept of distress as the 6th vital sign[10] (and hence ultra-short screens) and also to a more precise delineation of mood disorders including minor and subsyndromal variants.[11] Each method serves a different purpose. Those who want to identify and classify emotional disorders as accurately as possible might use a structured psychiatric interview.[5] Health professionals wanting to detect emotional difficulties as simply as possible might use one or two simple questions (ultra-short screens).

The long-standing debate about the prevalence of depression (or anxiety) in cancer has also been refined. Although summary rates of distress, anxiety, and depression have been produced (see Fig. 52–2) it is important to remember that cancer is not a homogenous condition, with significant differences between the early and late stages. Sufferers with early cancer, typically those undergoing first episode chemotherapy have a low to moderate risk of emotional complications[12] whereas those in the late stages, such as those with metastases have a higher risk of emotional complications.[13] Research is beginning to examine whether screening methods should differ for low and high-prevalence settings. In addition new research has attempted to examine what methods might best distinguish major depression from those without major depression, major + minor depression from those with subsyndromal symptoms alone and

healthy controls and those with any form of depressive symptoms from those without. Results are awaited with interest.

SUMMARY OF CLINICAL ACCURACY AND SCREENING HABITS OF HEALTH PROFESSIONALS

Detection studies (clinical accuracy). There have been several studies examining the unassisted ability of cancer clinicians to identify depression.[14-18] These provide an important baseline to any future attempts to improve detection through screening. One study used the BSI-18 on 2776 patients.[8] Of those who met criteria for clinically significant distress almost half had not sought professional psychosocial support and surprisingly neither did they intend to seek help in the future (see section: Toward a help paradigm). Robust detection studies have now examined detection sensitivity as well as detection specificity, which is the ability to rule-in a case and rule-out a noncase. Sollner et al. (2001) examined the accuracy of eight oncologists who had evaluated 298 cancer patients.[15] Against moderate or severe distress on the HADS$_T$ (a 12v13 cut off), oncologists' sensitivity was 80.2% and their specificity was 32.8%. Using a HADS$_T$ cut off 18 to represent severe distress, sensitivity was only 36.7%, but specificity increased to 87.6%. This study suggests that oncologists are likely to identify only a minority of those with severe distress. Fallowfield's group (2001) compared cancer clinicians' ratings using visual-analogue scales with an independent GHQ-12 score (cut off 3v4).[16] In this high-prevalence sample, detection sensitivity was only 28.9%. Notably patients who were identified had longer consultations than did those who were missed (Textbox 52–2).

There are many possible reasons for underrecognition. For example, just as not all health professionals ask about emotional difficulties, not

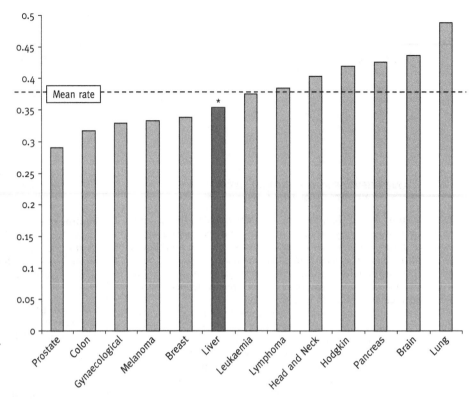

Fig. 52–1. Pooled rates of Distress by Cancer Site from 7272 individuals with cancer.

SOURCE: Data from Carlson LE, Angen M, Cullum J et al. High levels of untreated distress and fatigue in cancer patients. British Journal of Cancer. 90:2297–2304; Zabora J, et al The prevalence of distress by cancer site. Psychooncology. 2001;10:19–28. * = data from Zabora, et al only.

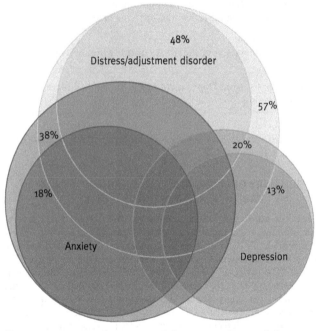

Fig. 52–2. Meta-analytic rates of distress, anxiety, and depression by interview (inner circle) and self report (outer circle).

SOURCE: Adapted from Mitchell AJ. Pooled results from 38 analyses of the accuracy of distress thermometer and other ultra-short methods of detecting cancer-related mood disorder. J Clin Oncol. 2007;25:4670–4681.

all patients want to talk about their problems.[17] Clinician-related factors linked with low detection include the willingness to look for emotional problems, clinical confidence/skills, and consultation time. Patient factors include confidence in the clinician, willingness to discuss personal difficulties, and belief that help is available. Several groups have examined whether clinician training might improve recognition of emotional problems.[18]

Screening habits of health professionals. Given these concerns it is surprising that only two studies have examined how cancer professionals look for depression or anxiety. The first examined 134 doctors working palliative medicine.[19] Seventy-three percent said they routinely assessed patients for depression but 50% said they never used a formal method, 10% used a simple one-question test ("are you depressed?") and 27% used HADS. In the second study, 63.3% of multidisciplinary cancer clinicians "always or regularly" screened for distress/depression whereas 36.7% only occasionally asked about emotional problems or relied on patients mentioning a problem first. Only 5.9% of all staff reported using a formal questionnaire with the majority (62.2%) relying on their own clinical judgment. About one-third attempted to remember and use one, two, or three simple questions. The main barriers to screening in this sample were lack of time, lack of training on screening methods and low personal skills or confidence about diagnosis. Much more evidence from primary care reinforced that most health professionals do not use a scale to diagnose or quantify depression and many do not ask about emotional issues routinely.

CLINICAL VALUE OF EXISTING SCREENING METHODS FOR EMOTIONAL DISORDERS

Accuracy of existing approaches. Most depression screening studies in cancer are not "screening" in the strict epidemiological sense but rather case-finding attempts using one or many conventional depression scales. There are over 50 validated depression scales but only a handful are in everyday use (Textbox 52–3). Nearly all classic depression severity tools published before 1980 have had validation attempts in cancer. These include the HAM-D, the MADRS, the BDI, the SDS, and the CES-D. Of the new scales developed since 1980 two have been particularly successful. These are the HADS and the Patient Health Questionnaire (PHQ9). In addition, tools examining more general psychopathology including the GHQ, and the Hopkins Symptom Checklist (SCL) family (SCL90, SCL-25, and SCL-8) have been validated.[20,21]

Many authors have advised caution when using conventional scales in those with physical illness. The main concern is of contamination from somatic symptoms generated by the physical illness and leading to false positives. Whilst this is a potential hazard, there is also the issue of underrecognition if reported somatic symptoms are assumed to be due solely to physical illness. In fact a series of studies in cancer and general medicine examining this issue systematically have found that somatic symptoms retain diagnostic significance even in depression with underlying physical disease.[22] For example, Van Wilgen et al. (2006) analyzed the influence of somatic symptoms on the CES–D in 509 cancer patients compared with 223 depressed patients without cancer.[23] They found that somatic items do not interfere with the diagnosis of depression measured with the CES–D.

What then does the evidence suggest from diagnostic validity studies and do any particular scales emerge with superior accuracy? With numerous self-report questionnaires and visual-analogue scales and a mixture of outcomes (distress, anxiety, and depression) it is difficult to reach a consensus.[24] Leaving aside acceptability and licensing costs, the accuracy of such scales is best compared against the optimal references standard, usually a semi-structured psychiatric interview. Studies reporting multiple comparisons in head-to-head studies would be particularly informative. To date studies using the Zung (against the MINI)[25] and CES-D (against DSMIIIR)[26] have shown modest success. Of all methods, the most commonly studied tool has been the HADS which was introduced in 1983 (appendix 1). A meta-analysis of the HADS scale studies in cancer has been conducted and is useful to illustrate the potential advantages of using a scale over and above the performance of clinicians when unassisted. From nine diagnostic validity studies using the HADS, sensitivity was 0.52 and specificity 0.89 (prevalence 0.22). Comparing this level of performance against the unassisted clinician data from Fallowfield et al. (2001), corrected for prevalence, shows a significant difference (Fig. 52–3). Whereas clinicians were able to detect 6.3 out of 22 true cases, HADS-assisted clinicians diagnosed 11.4, a gain of 23%. Similarly, when unassisted clinicians correctly ruled out 32.3 out of 78 nondepressed cases compared with 69.2 using the HADS, a gain of 47.3%. Thus, assuming the HADS (or similar scales) came to be used routinely by cancer clinicians, there is the potential to improve detection. However, it is not necessarily the case that quality of care would improve. For this, implementation studies are needed (see Fig. 52–3).

Regarding head-to-head comparisons of screening methods, Le Fevre administered the HADS and GHQ-12–79 hospice inpatients against a Revised Clinical Interview Schedule. In this study the HADS performed better than the GHQ-12 for identifying depression.[27] In a small study Katz et al. (2007) diagnosed major and minor depression according to Research Diagnostic Criteria using the Schedule for Affective Disorders and Schizophrenia (SADS).[28] All methods were found to be equally accurate including the BDI, the HADS, and the CES-D scale. In a larger study from Singer et al. (2008) involving 250 individuals diagnosed according to DSM-IV. Again the HADS, the subscale "Emotional Functioning" of the European Organization for Research and Treatment of Cancer Quality of Life Core Questionnaire (EORTC QLQ-C30) and a single-item visual analogues scale (VAS) were all highly accurate. The best levels of sensitivity and specificity were associated with the total score of the HADS. Baker Glenn and colleagues (2008) recently examined several screening tools in a sample of 217 chemotherapy attendees who had early cancer.[29] The prevalence of major and minor depressions was 11.1% and 6.9%, respectively. Accuracy of the PHQ2 question 1 (interest), PHQ2 question 2 (depression), PHQ Q1 OR Q2, PHQ9, HADS-T, HADS-D are show in Table 52–1. The PHQ2 emerged as the optimal strategy for detection of DSM-IV defined major or minor depressions.

Acceptability of existing approaches. Given that existing scales can be used, is there any merit in formulating new methods? Recent screening research has moved away from accuracy alone towards accuracy and acceptability. Some groups have begun to develop economic models of screening success. An ideal scale is very brief, highly acceptable, highly accurate, easily accessible, and highly used. At the same time it must be long enough to measure severity (unless another scale is used for this purpose) and measure change. Currently, it is unclear exactly how brief a scale can become before significant value is lost. Short versions of every major scale have been released comprising 10 items or less. A good example is the 10-item Edinburgh Depression Scale recently

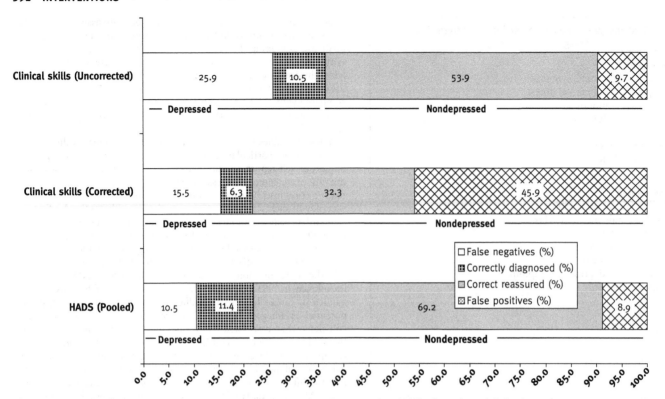

Fig. 52–3. Real number analysis from 100 consecutive Screens using the HADS (pooled data) or Clinical skills alone. ABBREVIATION: HADS, Hospital Anxiety and Depression Scale.

Table 52–1. Head-to-head comparison of multiple screening methods for major or minor depression

Test	Sensitivity	Specificity	PPV	NPV	Predictive summary index	Youden
PHQ2 Q2 Alone (Depressed)	0.51	1.00	1.00	0.90	0.90	0.51
PHQ2 Q1 or Q2	0.95	0.98	0.90	0.99	0.89	0.93
PHQ9	0.82	0.89	0.63	0.96	0.59	0.71
HADS-Depression (7v8)	0.62	0.89	0.55	0.91	0.46	0.50
HADS–Total (14v15)	0.72	0.69	0.33	0.92	0.25	0.40
Distress thermometer (3v4)	0.72	0.74	0.38	0.92	0.30	0.46

ABBREVIATIONS: HADS, Hospital Anxiety and Depression Scale; NPV, negative predictive value; PHQ, Patient health questionnaire; PPV, positive predictive value.

refined into an 8-item version.[30] Of course, eight items might not be short enough and in the extreme example there are single-item scales which can be applied by pen and paper, verbally "are you depressed?" or in visual-analogue form. This process has been assisted by work which began in the 1970s developing and testing visual-analogue methods of rating mood.[31] Since then many other groups have also noted the value of similar methods.[32–34] The accuracy of these "ultra-short" methods has been summarized. Generally single-item tests have high rule-out (reassurance) accuracy but limited rule-in (case-finding) ability.[34]

Implementation studies for detection of cancer-related distress.
Ultimately a scale may be capable of accurate detection of depression (or anxiety or distress) when compared with a gold standard but this does not imply that quality of care will be improved by its use. Improvements in care require that any increase in detection is accompanied by improvements in treatment and follow-up care. Thus, despite great enthusiasm developing questionnaires to detect emotional complications of cancer, few groups have produced evidence to show successful implementation of a screening program for mood disorders.

Taenzer and colleagues (2000) asked patients to complete a computerized version of the EORTC QLQ-C30 questionnaire.[35] Patients were assigned patients to either a usual care control group who completed the EORTC QLQ-C30 paper version after the clinic appointment and an experimental group, which completed the questionnaire before their first clinic appointment with feedback to staff. Patients reported being equally satisfied with the treatment in both groups but more quality of life issues were identified by the intervention patients (48.9% vs. 23.6%). McLachlan et al. (2001) collected data on self-reported needs, quality of life and psychosocial symptoms from 450 people with cancer. For a randomly chosen two-thirds, this information was made available to the healthcare team and for the remaining one-third not revealed. In addition, in the intervention arm a nurse was also present during this consultation and formulated an individualized management plan based on the issues raised in the summary report and prespecified expert psychosocial guidelines. Six months after randomization there were no significant differences between the two arms in any domain or regarding satisfaction with care. However, for the subgroup of patients who were moderately or severely depressed at baseline, there was a significant reduction in depression for the intervention arm.[36] Detmar and colleagues in the Netherlands (2002) Design Prospective, randomized clinicians to receive summaries of the EORTC QLQ-C30 score before appointments.[37] It was found that

HROOL issues were discussed significantly more frequently in the intervention than in the control group and in subgroup analysis there was better identification in some but not all HRQOL domains. Boyes and colleagues in Australia (2006) asked patients to complete a computerized screen assessing their psychosocial well-being while waiting to see the oncologist during each visit. This included the HADS scale. Responses were immediately scored and summary reports were placed in each patient's file for oncologist's attention.[38] There was no effect on levels of anxiety, depression, and perceived needs among those who received the intervention but only three intervention patients reported that their oncologist discussed the feedback report with them. Velikova and colleagues in Leeds (2006) recruited 28 oncologists treating 286 cancer patients and randomly assigned them to an intervention group with feedback of results to physicians, an attention-control group who completion of questionnaires without feedback and a control group with no questionnaires.[39] The questionnaires of choice were the EORTC QLQ and touch-screen version of the HADS. A positive effect on emotional well-being was associated with feedback of data but not with instrument completion. Although more frequent discussion of chronic nonspecific symptoms was found in the intervention group (without prolonging encounters), there was no detectable effect on patient management. Recently, Rosenbloom and colleagues (2007) randomly assigned 213 patients with metastatic breast, lung, or colorectal cancer were to usual care; quality of life assessment or HRQOL assessment followed by a structured interview (with presentation to the treating nurse). There were no significant differences in HRQOL and treatment satisfaction outcomes at 3 and 6 months.

These studies suggest that screening for psychosocial issues in cancer settings may not be sufficient even when accompanied by feedback of results to clinicians and that additional steps are probably required to demonstrate an effect on well-being. Further, any potential benefit is likely to be limited by the perceived value to cancer clinicians and their willingness to use the suggested method. In the context of a research trial the use of a questionnaire is closely monitored. In routine practice a vital consideration is whether the screening procedure is acceptable to patients and staff alike.[40]

RECOMMENDATIONS FOR SCREENING METHODS IN CLINICAL PRACTICE

Depression, anxiety, and broadly defined distress are common emotional complications of cancer that deserve clinicians attention. Despite much useful data on a variety of scales and tools few authors have applied a rigorous trial format to evaluate how screening can improve patient outcomes. Tools have improved over the last 20 years mostly in terms of acceptability rather than accuracy. Tools can be administered in the waiting room or via computer increasing the uptake where routine application is planned. In addition, algorithm approaches are possible

in which screening methods begin simply and become more complex (and accurate) only if needed. In fact the two can be combined using computer-adaptive testing, essentially an item bank of questions and an evidence-based decisional algorithm that adjusts the next question depending on the answer received.[41–43] Despite these innovations there remains a gap between those identified as distressed and currently untreated (that is those with unmet need) and those who want help for these concerns. In a study from New South Wales, Australia, amongst a total of 888 consecutive patients the mean number of unmet needs reported by cancer patients was 10.9. However, lung cancer patients reported a higher mean number of unmet psychological needs (7.6 vs. 5.0) and physical and daily living unmet needs (2.8 vs. 1.4), compared to the other cancer patients.[44] This and other research has led to a focus the concept of help as an important accompaniment of screening.

Toward a help paradigm. There have been several attempts to use problem checklists to support simple ratings of distress. One such study indicated the most common problems in cancer were fatigue (48.5%), followed by pain (26.4%), managing emotions/stress (24.8%), depression (24.0%), and anxiety (24.0%).[8] However, this has been refined further by asking which problems require professional help. The Moores UCSD

Textbox 52–4. Top ten concerns from the Moores UCSD cancer center		
Biopsychosocial problems	*% concerns*	*% wanting help*
Fatigue (feeling tired)	41.90	9.60
Sleeping	32.50	8.10
Finances	31.10	7.80
Pain	29.40	7.90
Controlling my fear and worry about the future	28.20	6.00
Me being dependent on others	27.50	3.50
Being an anxious or nervous person	27.40	5.40
Feeling down, depressed, or blue	27.40	5.40
Understanding my treatment options	23.10	15.00
Managing my emotions	22.90	4.40

SOURCE: Adapted from: Loscalzo M, Clark KL. Problem-related distress in cancer patients drives requests for help: a prospective study. *Oncology.* 2007;21(9): 1133–1138.

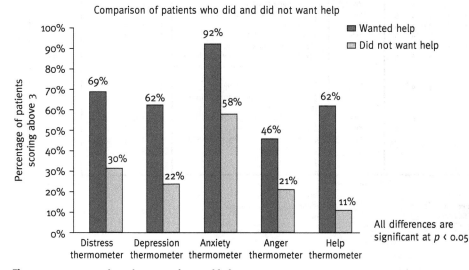

Fig. 52–4. Reasons for refusing professional help.
SOURCE: Data from Baker-Glenn, et al 2008.

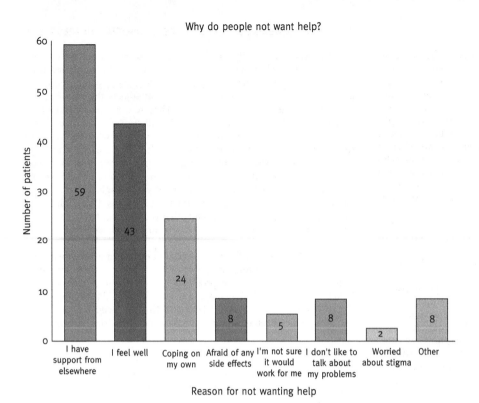

Fig. 52–5. Reasons for refusing professional help.
SOURCE: Data from Baker-Glenn, et al 2008.

How Can We Help You and Your Family?
By completing this form you will tell us how we can best work together with you as an effective team.
Pleasse take a few moments to:

1. Rate <u>each and every</u> problem by circling a number 1 thru 5. [1 means this is Not A Problem At All To Me 2 Mild Problem, 3 Moderate Problem, 4 Severe Problem, 5 means Very Severe].

2. Then, please circle (Yes) to indicate problems you would like to discuss with a member of our staff.

Ask at the Front Desk if you would like help completing this form.

Problems	Rating [1–5]					(Yes)		*Problems*	Rating [1–5]					(Yes)
1. Transportation	1	2	3	4	5	Yes		20. Ability to have children	1	2	3	4	5	Yes
2. Finances	1	2	3	4	5	Yes		21. Being an anxious or nervous person	1	2	3	4	5	Yes
3. Needing someone to help coordinate my medical care	1	2	3	4	5	Yes		22. Losing control of things that matter to me	1	2	3	4	5	Yes
4. Sleeping	1	2	3	4	5	Yes		23. Feeling down, depressed or blue	1	2	3	4	5	Yes
5. Talking with the doctor	1	2	3	4	5	Yes		24. Thinking clearly	1	2	3	4	5	Yes
6. Understanding my treatment options	1	2	3	4	5	Yes		25. Me being dpendent on others	1	2	3	4	5	Yes
7. Talking with the health care team	1	2	3	4	5	Yes		26. Someone else totally dependent on me for their care	1	2	3	4	5	Yes
8. Talking with family, children, friends	1	2	3	4	5	Yes		27. Fatigue (feeling tired)	1	2	3	4	5	Yes
9. Managing my emotions	1	2	3	4	5	Yes		28. Thoughts of ending my own life	1	2	3	4	5	Yes
10. Solving problems due to my illness	1	2	3	4	5	Yes		29. Pain	1	2	3	4	5	Yes
11. Managing work, school, home life	1	2	3	4	5	Yes		30. Sexual Function	1	2	3	4	5	Yes
12. Controlling my anger	1	2	3	4	5	Yes		31. Recent weight change	1	2	3	4	5	Yes
13. Writing down my choices about medical care for the medical team and my family if I ever become too ill to speak for myself	1	2	3	4	5	Yes		32. Having people nearby to help me or needing more practical help at home	1	2	3	4	5	Yes
14. Controlling my fear and worry about the future	1	2	3	4	5	Yes		33. Nausea and vomiting	1	2	3	4	5	Yes
15. Questions and concerns about end of life	1	2	3	4	5	Yes		34. Substance abuse (drugs, alcohol, nicotine, other)	1	2	3	4	5	Yes
16. Finding community resources near where I live	1	2	3	4	5	Yes		35. My ability to cope	1	2	3	4	5	Yes
17. Getting medicines	1	2	3	4	5	Yes		36. Abandonment by my family	1	2	3	4	5	Yes
18. Spiritual Concerns	1	2	3	4	5	Yes		37. Any other Problems you would like to tell us about	1	2	3	4	5	Yes
19. Fear of medical procedures (needles, enclosed places, surgery).								*(Please specify):*						

PLEASE CHECK ONE :

<u>Present Relationship -</u>
Married ☐   Single ☐
Living with Partner ☐   Widowed ☐
Divorced ☐

PLEASE CHECK ONE :

Race-
African American ☐
Asian/Pacific Islander ☐
Caucasian ☐
Hispanic ☐

Multi-racial ☐
Native American/Native Alaskan ☐
Unknown ☐
Other_____

[Stick-on Patient Info
Label here]
(For Office Use Only)

Fig. 52–6/Appendix 1. How can we help you and your family instrument.

<u>Instructions</u> In the first four columns, plese mark the number (0 –10) that best describes how much emotional upset you have been experiencing in the past two weeks, including today. In the next three columns please indicate how much impact this has had on you.

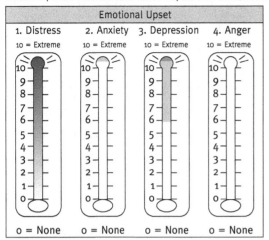
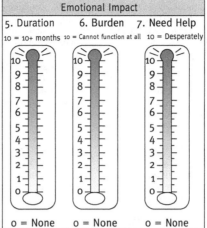

Fig. 52–7/Appendix 2. Emotion thermometer revised.
SOURCE: Adapted from the NCCN Distress Thermometer. Alex Mitchell ©

Cancer Center has implemented this approach using a 36-item problem list in 2071 patients. The five most common causes of problem-related distress were fatigue, sleeping, finances, pain, and controlling my fear and worry about the future. The five most common problems for which patients wanted assistance were understanding my treatment options, fatigue, sleeping, pain, and finances.

Two recent studies have shown that only about a third of those scoring as significantly distressed on the distress thermometer actually want professional help for emotional problems (Textbox 52–4).[45,46] For example, Baker-Glenn and colleagues (2008) used an innovative verbal and visual-analogue help tool to assess desire for professional help in 130 chemotherapy attendees.[46] Only 3/26 of those wanting help had no identifiable condition compared with 40/104 of those who declined help. Of those who indicated that they wanted help, 35% scored above 3 on all four domains of the Emotion Thermometers tool (Fig. 52–4). Similarly, 54% scored above 14 on HADS, and 27% met the DSM-IV criteria for a major depressive episode. Of those individuals saying that they didn't want help, 22% scored above 14 on HADS and 8% met the DSM-IV criteria for a major depressive episode. The most popular requests for sources of help were face-to-face psychological support (62%) and complementary therapies (58%). This study also examined why people refused help when offered. The most common reasons were "getting help elsewhere" (57%), "feel well" (41%), and "coping on my own" (31%) (Fig. 52–5).

CONCLUSION

There is evidence that clinical care for emotional complications of cancer has improved with annual depression screening among veterans with cancer increasing from 42% in 2000 to 81% in 2003.[47] National guidance on screening is available in several countries although a unified approach to emotional problems have not been seen.[48] The critical question has moved from one of clarifying prevalence to one of improving quality of care, namely "How can individuals with cancer-related emotional complications be helped?" The next step in screening is to follow a robust methodological approach to examine whether screening improves the outcomes for patients with cancer. Essentially this involves incorporating screening into randomized control trials where the comparator arm is "diagnosis as usual." It is useful to remember that improvements in distress identification will not be effective in isolation and must be linked with physician communication skills and subsequent interventions.[49] Pairing evidence-based detection with evidence-based treatment is an essential step to improve clinical care.

APPENDICES

See Appendix Figs. 52–6 and 52–7.

REFERENCES

1. Carroll BT, Kathol RG, Noyes R Jr, Wald TG, Clamon GH. Screening for depression and anxiety in cancer-patients using the hospital anxiety and depressions scale. *Gen Hosp Psychiatry*. 1993;15(2):69–74 Published: MAR 1993.

2. Van't Spijker A, Trijsburg RW, Duivenvoorden HJ. Psychological sequelae of cancer diagnosis: a meta-analytical review of 58 studies after 1980. *Psychosom Med*. 1997;59:280–293.

3. Herschbach P, Book K, Brandl T, et al. Psychological distress in cancer patients assessed with an expert rating scale. *Br J Cancer*. 2008;99(1):37–43.

4. Ibbotson T, Maguire P, Selby T, Priestman T, Wallace L. Screening for anxiety and depression in cancer patients: the effects of disease and treatment. *Eur J Cancer*. 1994;30A: 37–40.

5. Strong V, Waters R, Hibberd C, et al. Emotional distress in cancer patients: the Edinburgh Cancer Centre symptom study. *Br J Cancer*. 2007;96:868–874.

6. Derogatis LR, Melisaraatos N. The Brief Symptom inventory (BSI): an introductory report. *Psychol Med*. 1983;13:595–606.

7. Zabora J, Brintzenhofeszoc K, Curbow B, Hooker C, Piantadosi S. The prevalence of distress by cancer site. *Psychooncology*. 2001;10:19–28.

8. Carlson LE, Angen M, Cullum J, et al. High levels of untreated distress and fatigue in cancer patients. *Br J Cancer*. 2004;90:2297–2304.

9. Fallowfield L, Ratcliffe D, Jenkins V, Saul J. Psychiatric morbidity and its recognition by doctors in patients with cancer. *Br J Cancer*. 2001;84:1011–1015.

10. Holland, Jimmie C, Bultz, Barry D. The NCCN guideline for distress management: a case for making distress the sixth vital sign. *J Natl Compr Canc Netw*. 2007;5(1):3–7.

11. Mitchell AJ, Elena Baker-Glen E. Clinical significance of DSMIV major, minor & sub-syndromal depression in cancer: preliminary report of chemotherapy attendees. *Psychooncology*. 2008; 17 (suppl 19): S1–S348.

12. Love AW, Kissane DW, Bloch S, Clarke D. Diagnostic efficiency of the Hospital Anxiety and Depression Scale in women with early stage breast cancer. *Aust N Z J Psychiatry*. 2002;36(2):246–250.

13. Love AW, Grabsch B, Clarke DM, Bloch S, Kissane DW. Screening for depression in women with metastatic breast cancer: a comparison of the Beck Depression Inventory Short Form and the Hospital Anxiety and Depression Scale. *Aust N Z J Psychiatry*. 2004;38(7):526–531.

14. Hardman A, Maguire P, Crowther D The recognition of psychiatric morbidity on an oncology ward. *J Psychosom Res*. 1989;33:235–239.

15. Söllner W, DeVries A, Steixner E, et al. How successful are oncologists in identifying patient distress, perceived social support, and need for psychosocial counselling? *Br J Cancer*. 2001;84(2):179–185.

16. Fallowfield L, Ratcliffe D, Jenkins V, Saul J. Psychiatric morbidity and its recognition by doctors in patients with cancer. *Br J Cancer*. 2001;84(8):1011–1015.

17. Kvale K. Do cancer patients always want to talk about difficult emotions? A qualitative study of cancer inpatients communication needs. *Eur J Oncol Nurs.* 2007;11(4):320–327.

18. Merckaert I, Libert Y, Delvaux N, et al. Factors that influence physicians' detection of distress in patients with cancer - Can a communication skills training program improve physicians' detection? *Cancer.* 2005;104(2):411–421.

19. Lawrie I, Lloyd-Williams M, Fiona T. How do palliative medicine physicians assess and manage depression. *Palliat Med.* 2004;18(3):234–238.

20. Derogatis LR, Lipman RS, Covi L. SCL-90: an outpatient psychiatric rating scale, preliminary report. *Psychopharmacol Bull.* 1973;9:13–28.

21. Fink P, Ørbøl E, Hansen MS, Søndergaard L, De Jonge P. Detecting mental disorders in general hospitals by the SCL-8 scale. *J Psychiatr Res.* 2004;56(3):371–375.

22. Babaei F, Mitchell AJ. Screening for depression in physical disease: the case for somatic symptoms when detecting comorbid mood disorders. In Mitchell AJ, Coyne JC. (eds). *Screening for depression in clinical practice.* Oxford: Oxford University Press; 2009.

23. van Wilgen CP, Dijkstra PU, Stewart RE, Ranchor AV, Roodenburg JLN. Measuring somatic symptoms with the CES–D to assess depression in cancer patients after treatment: comparison among patients with oral/oropharyngeal, gynecological, colorectal, and breast cancer. *Psychosomatics.* 2006;47:465–470.

24. Carlson LE, Bultz BD. Cancer distress screening—Needs, models, and methods. *J Psychosom Res.* 2003;55(5):403–409.

25. Passik SD, Kirsh KL, Donaghy KB, et al. An attempt to employ the Zung self-rating depression scale as a "Lab Test" to trigger follow-up in ambulatory oncology clinics: criterion validity and detection. *J Pain Symptom Manage.* 2001;24:273–281.

26. Schein RL, Koenig HG. The center for epidemiological studies-depression (CES-D) scale: assessment of depression in the medically ill elderly. *Int J Geriat Psychiatry.* 1997;12:436–446.

27. Le Fevre P, Devereux J, Smith S, Lawrie SM, Cornbleet M. Screening for psychiatric illness in the palliative care inpatient setting: a comparison between the Hospital Anxiety and Depression Scale and the General Health. Questionnaire-12. *Palliat Med.* 1999;12:399/407.

28. Katz MR, Kopek N, Waldron J, Devins GM, Tomlinson G. Screening for depression in head and neck cancer *Psychooncology.* 2004;13(4):269–280.

29. Baker-Glenn E, Mitchell AJ, Symonds P. Screening using the emotion thermometers: a useful extension to the distress thermometer when identifying major and minor depression? *Psychooncology.* 2008 (Supplement IPOS 2008).

30. Lloyd-Williams M, Shiels C, Dowrick C. The development of the Brief Edinburgh Depression Scale (BEDS) to screen for depression in patients with advanced cancer. *J Affect Disord.* 2007;99(1–3):259–264.

31. Folstein MF. Reliability, validity, and clinical application of visual analog mood scale. *Psychiatr Med.* 1973;3:479.

32. Kertzman S, Aladjem Z, Milo R, et al. The utility of the Visual Analogue Scale for the assessment of depressive mood in cognitively impaired patients. *Int J Geriatr Psychiatry.* 2004;19(8):789–796.

33. Mccormack HM, Horne DJD, Sheather S. Clinical applications of visual analog scales—a critical-review. *Psychiatr Med.* 1988;18(4):1007–1019 Published: NOV 1988.

34. Mitchell AJ. Pooled results from 38 analyses of the accuracy of distress thermometer and other ultra-short methods of detecting cancer-related mood disorder. *J Clin Oncol.* 2007;25:4670–4681.

35. Taenzer P, Bultz BD, Carlson LE, et al. Impact of computerized quality of life screening on physician behaviour and patient satisfaction in lung cancer outpatients. *Psychooncology.* 2000 May-Jun;9(3):203–213.

36. McLachlan SA, Allenby A, Matthews J, et al. Randomized trial of coordinated psychosocial interventions based on patient self-assessments versus standard care to improve the psychosocial functioning of patients with cancer. *J Clin Oncol.* 2001;19(21):4117–4125.

37. Detmar SB, Muller MJ, Schornagel JH, Wever LDV, Aaronson NK. Health-related quality-of-life assessments and patient-physician communication—a randomized controlled trial. Author(s). *JAMA.* 2002 Dec 18;288(23):3027–3034.

38. Boyes A, Newell S, Girgis A, Mcelduff P, Sanson-Fisher R. Does routine assessment and real-time feedback improve cancer patients' psychosocial well-being? *Eur J Cancer Care (Engl).* 2006;15(2):163–171.

39. Velikova G, Booth L, Smith AB, et al. Measuring quality of life in routine oncology practice improves communication and patient well-being: a randomized controlled trial. *J Clin Oncol.* 2004;22(4):714–724.

40. National Screening Committee. *The UK National Screening Committee's criteria for appraising the viability, effectiveness and appropriateness of a screening programme.* London: HMSO; 2003. www.nsc.nhs.uk/pdfs/criteria.pdf. Accessed August 12, 2009.

41. Fliege H, Becker J, Walter OB, Bjorner JB, Klapp BF, Rose M. Development of a computer-adaptive test for depression (D-CAT). *Qual Life Res.* 2005;14:2277–2291.

42. Lai J, Dineen K, Reeve B, et al. An item response theory-based pain item bank can enhance measurement precision. *J Pain Symptom Manage.* 2005;30:278–288.

43. Smith AB, Rush R, Velikova G, et al. The initial development of an item bank to assess and screen for psychological distress in cancer patients. *Psychooncology.* 2007;16:724–732.

44. Li J, Girgis A. Supportive care needs: are patients with lung cancer a neglected population? *Psychooncology.* 2006;15(6):509–516.

45. Graves KD, Arnold SM, Love CL, Kirsh KL, Moore PG, Passik SD. Distress screening in a multidisciplinary lung cancer clinic: prevalence and predictors of clinically significant distress. *Lung Cancer.* 2007;55(2):215–224.

46. Baker-Glenn EA, Mitchell AJ. Screening for perceived need for help using the latest screening tools—what do we know about who wants help? *Psychooncology.* 2008;17:S1-S348:14S-3.

47. Jones LE, Doebbeling CC. Suboptimal depression screening following cancer diagnosis. *Gen Hosp Psychiatry.* 2007;29:547–554.

48. Jacobsen PB. Screening for psychological distress in cancer patients: challenges and opportunities. *J Clin Oncol.* 2007 Oct 10;25:29.

49. Merckaert I, Libert Y, Delvaux N, et al. Factors that influence physicians' detection of distress in patients with cancer—Can a communication skills training program improve physicians' detection? *Cancer.* 2005;104(2):411–421.

Principles of Psychotherapy

E. Alessandra Strada and Barbara M. Sourkes

INTRODUCTION

As the understanding of psychological morbidity associated with a diagnosis of cancer has increased, so has the need for access to psychological care for patients, families, and caregivers. Mental health professionals, including psychologists, psychiatrists, and social workers, as well as other allied health professionals with formal training in psychotherapy have become an increasingly important part of the oncology treatment team. Psychotherapeutic and psychosocial interventions have been developed and implemented for diverse patient populations with cancer. They are representative of a variety of theoretical frameworks and approaches. The most commonly utilized interventions are psychodynamically oriented individual psychotherapy, supportive expressive therapy, group interventions, and cognitive-behavioral interventions.

While different therapeutic interventions are inspired by different theoretical frameworks, there are basic clinical issues related to the delivery, management, and outcome of psychotherapy shared by every professional working in psycho-oncology.

This chapter will review and discuss essential clinical principles of individual psychotherapy that should be considered in every approach. The discussion addresses patient selection, conceptual framework, setting, goals and objectives, the therapeutic relationship, and cultural issues.

THE CONTINUUM OF CARE: PSYCHOEDUCATION, COUNSELING, AND PSYCHOTHERAPY

A diagnosis of cancer inevitably causes significant distress for the individual patient as well as for the entire family system. It disrupts the personal and shared narrative of health and well-being and may transform it into one of fear, loss of control, and chaos.[1] Professional psychosocial interventions are optimally provided by clinicians with formal training in this area. At a minimum, a competent therapist will be familiar with types of neoplasms, stages of disease, and medical interventions available to patients at different stages of illness. An accurate understanding of the psychological implications of the stages of the illness will allow the therapist to accompany the patient through diagnosis, treatment, the cycles of remissions and recurrences, and, in some instances, palliative care.

Assessment of the patient's ability to assimilate and integrate the diagnosis of cancer requires significant clinical skills. It is a necessary first step to offer patients an adequate level of psychological support. Accurate assessment reveals the patient's coping skills, risk level, and willingness to explore emotions elicited by the diagnosis.

Psychosocial interventions in cancer care can be conceptualized as a continuum, along which treatments can be differentiated on the basis of structure, frequency, and depth. Psychoeducation, at one end of the continuum, was originally developed with the goal of providing education and support to patients with mental illness and their families, minimizing the impact of the illness on relationships and quality of life.[2] Psychoeducation maintains a focus on the present and on the development of skills that can be used by patients to decrease stress, improve interpersonal communication, and improve overall quality of life.[3] In the context of psycho-oncology, psychoeducation often takes the form of a structured or semistructured approach that can include health education, stress management classes, and teaching coping skills to newly

diagnosed patients.[4] It maintains a strong focus on the "here and now" of the patient's reality and usually does not address past experience or old conflicts. The time-limited nature of this approach and its focus on problem solving makes psychoeducation appropriate for patients at all stages of the illness.

Counseling is a short-term approach appropriate for individuals who wish to focus on improving their problem-solving ability and coping skills. As in psychoeducation, counseling is primarily focused on the present, with the individual and counselor working toward achieving concrete goals. Counseling may occasionally identify and address deeper and older issues in the patient's life. However, it remains focused on concrete and achievable goals. Counseling does not commonly address defense mechanisms, old intrapsychic conflicts, or significant psychological distress.[5] The frequency of both psychoeducation and counseling sessions may vary, depending on patients' needs.

Traditionally, psychotherapy involves a specific theoretical framework and targets patient with or without prior or current psychiatric history and symptoms. Even though there are several therapeutic schools, they all share the following basic principles: emphasis on the importance of the therapeutic alliance; a setting where the therapy takes place; an explanatory model for the patient's symptoms and distress; a structured set of interventions aimed at resolving psychopathology and improving psychological well-being.[6] It must be pointed out that not all therapists believe there is a difference between counseling and psychotherapy. As a result, the two terms are sometimes used interchangeably.[7] Still, most therapists would agree that different psychotherapeutic interventions target symptoms to a various degree of depth. It is important that the intervention offered to the patient matches the degree of distress and individual styles.

INDICATIONS FOR PSYCHOTHERAPEUTIC TREATMENT

The distressing impact of a diagnosis of life-threatening illness has been recognized and has provided impetus for the development and growth of the field of psycho-oncology.[8-10] The growth of psycho-oncology research over the last decade has promoted attention to the psychological and emotional needs of patients with cancer. As psychotherapy research has improved and become more sophisticated, valuable studies have explored issues of patient selection and outcome in an effort to identify which patients may benefit from specific interventions.[11-13]

Early investigative efforts demonstrated that not every patient diagnosed with cancer will accept the offer of psychotherapeutic or psychosocial support. The assumption that psychotherapy is inherently helpful and should be provided to all patients with cancer has been replaced by a modern research-based approach aimed at identifying patients at-risk and attempting to apply evidence-based interventions selectively.[14,15] One might speculate that early adaptation to a diagnosis of cancer does not necessarily mean that patients will not have difficulty later on in the process. Therefore, it is important to convey the message that psychological support is available at all stages of illness.

In an important early study, Worden and Weissman[16,17] found that in a sample of 372 patients newly diagnosed with cancer, only approximately one-third of those identified at high-risk accepted the offer for psychological support. Patients who did not accept psychological support tended to minimize the implications of the illness and were concerned that psychotherapy could release emotions successfully coped with or suppressed. Patients who accepted psychotherapy were less able to minimize the implications of the illness and were less hopeful. They were also more likely to frame the diagnosis in existential terms. When accepted, benefit from the intervention was demonstrated.

Other recent studies have attempted to link patients' characteristics to their acceptance or rejection of participation in psychosocial interventions. Boesen et al.[18] found that higher socioeconomic status predicted melanoma patients' acceptance of participation in a psychosocial randomized control trial that was based on interventions developed by Fawzy et al.[19] Conversely, lower socioeconomic status, high levels of social support and low levels of distress predicted a decline from participation. Research on patients' preferences regarding group interventions has shown that intervention modalities focused on health promotion and medical education were preferred over interventions focused on emotional support.[20]

The stage of the disease at the moment of diagnosis may also impact on patients' ability to cope and receptivity to psychological support. Often a diagnosis of stage I cancer, with good prospect for cure, creates different implications and distress than an initial diagnosis of metastatic disease with a more limited prognosis. Additionally, the ability to minimize the implications of the illness will likely be affected by the presence of pain and other distressing symptoms.

THE IMPORTANCE OF A FLEXIBLE FRAMEWORK

The term "patient" is usually applied to identify the recipient of medical or psychosocial interventions. In this context, a "patient" can be an adult individual, a child, a family, a couple, or a group of individuals. The identity of the patient is generally determined at the onset of the therapeutic relationship and it becomes part of the "therapeutic contract." In traditional psychotherapy, there is usually no room for modifications to the contract; individual therapy does not become couples therapy, or family therapy. However, providing psychotherapy to patients with cancer often requires the therapist to adopt a more flexible framework.[21] The basic structure of the therapy may be impacted by the patient's health status, the patient's relationship with family and caregivers, as well as system issues related to the delivery of care. A diagnosis of cancer affects not only the patient, but the entire system around the patient, including family and support network. As a life-threatening illness becomes a family issue[22] it has the potential to destabilize family dynamics and the equilibrium of relationships. Usually, working with an individual who is physically sick often requires the therapist to obtain some access to the entire family system. Adopting a flexible modality does not necessarily mean that all individual therapy will become family therapy. However, as the illness progresses, the need to include other family members or caregivers in the session often becomes more prominent. Patients who are parents may ask the therapist for assistance communicating with children and spouses. The therapist may be asked by the patient to join the family and the medical team in discussions regarding goals of care.

A flexible contract does not relieve the therapist from the responsibility to adhere to the highest ethical standards possible, including confidentiality.[23,24] However, the therapist should share pertinent information regarding the patient's adjustment level and emotional functioning with other team members. This is especially important as symptoms of depression or anxiety may affect medical treatment and need to be addressed pharmacologically, in conjunction with psychotherapy.

While the goals and objectives of therapy are negotiated between the therapist and patient at the beginning of the relationship, these goals may change significantly during the process of therapy and become the object of frequent negotiation between patient and therapist. Soon after being diagnosed with cancer, many patients may benefit from help adjusting to the diagnosis and coping with treatment. Patients may need assistance processing grief, reframing the meaning of the illness, relieving symptoms of depression and anxiety, and communicating effectively with family members and significant others. Some patients may develop a significant fear of death, regardless of disease severity, as soon as they hear the word "cancer" and want to address their fears in therapy. Other

patients prefer to adopt a very pragmatic problem solving approach and tend to avoid expressing deeper emotions and fears. It is important that the therapist allow the patient to take the lead in the therapeutic process, constantly assessing for the need for more direct interventions. This becomes urgently important for patients who develop increasing anxiety, suicidal ideation, and major depression.[25,26]

PSYCHOTHERAPY CASE FORMULATION AS EXPLANATORY MODEL

The delivery of both short and long-term psychotherapy often requires a comprehensive case formulation of the underlying causes of the patient's difficulty.[27] This conceptualization provides both theoretical and clinical understanding of the psychological diagnosis and a guide to treatment. Many individuals with cancer who receive psychotherapy do not meet criteria for a formal psychiatric diagnosis. However, careful conceptualization that can be shared with the treatment team facilitates the implementation of an overall treatment plan that addresses the patient's goals.

Sim et al.[28] identified five aspects of case formulations: integrative, explanatory, prescriptive, predictive, and therapist. According to this model, a case formulation highlights and summarizes the most important clinical issues (integrative), helps to understand the development of symptoms in patients and caregivers (explanatory), guides treatment and addresses goal setting and treatment plan (prescriptive), and allows for evaluation and redirection of treatment (predictive). The "therapist" component addresses the nature of the therapeutic relationship. The goal is to identify and address ruptures that may negatively affect the therapeutic alliance.

THE PSYCHOTHERAPEUTIC SETTING

Time. In a traditional outpatient psychotherapy framework, sessions occur usually at the same time on the same day of the week. This structure is based on the belief that having sessions at the appointed time allows for better containment of the psychotherapy process. Additionally, while patients' lives may often be characterized by significant unpredictability, maintaining a clear structure in psychotherapy allows patient and therapist to create a therapeutic space that is relatively unaffected by outside changes.[29] This element, in of itself, may have a calming influence on the patient and allow for an improved sense of control. While adherence to time is often possible in an outpatient setting, if patients become more debilitated, the appointment time may need to be frequently changed to accommodate their needs. Controlling time may become increasingly challenging if the patient's illness progresses and hospitalizations occur. The need to adapt to the schedule of an inpatient unit may alter the appointment time even if the therapist works in the same hospital where the patient is being treated. Patients' reactions to changes in scheduled appointment time have not been systematically studied. However, clinical experience suggests that most patients can successfully adapt to schedule changes, as long as they are kept informed as promptly as possible. As their illness progresses, especially if the emotional environment becomes more ambiguous and fearful, it becomes even more important that patients not be kept guessing about the availability of their therapists.

As patients' illness progresses, they may become unable to sustain a customary 50-minute session. Fatigue, pain, and other distressing symptoms often interfere with their ability to concentrate and interact with the therapist. Additionally, as patients enter a terminal state, they may experience physical and psychological withdrawal. Therefore, they may progressively or sometimes suddenly lose interest in the content of the psychotherapy session. Experienced clinical assessment is required to differentiate this natural withdrawal from clinical depression. Even asking the patient about the presence of depression can be appropriate in this context. It is not uncommon for patients to say they do not feel depressed, but rather less interested in engaging in the outside world. Asking patients how they feel about their level of disengagement and whether they would like to feel more energetic is also a helpful assessment tool. If patients report that they would like to have more physical and emotional energy to continue interact with family and other caregivers, consideration should be given to cognitive-behavioral interventions, antidepressants, or psychostimulants. If, however, patients report that they feel comfortable with their decreased level of engagement and report being peaceful, the therapist may support this process.

Physical space. In a traditional psychotherapy framework, great importance is placed on preserving the therapeutic space, usually the therapist's office, as free from change and distracting elements as possible. The rationale for this approach can be traced in the history and development of psychoanalysis. The physical space was conceptualized as a symbolic container of the patient's unconscious and as such was supposed to be immutable.

As long as patients are ambulatory and can physically go to the therapist's office a certain level of immutability in the physical space can be achieved. As illness progresses and patients spend more time in the hospital, the physical space of the therapy session may change repeatedly. Continuity of treatment takes precedence over immutability of the physical space. The session can take place in various locations including the chemotherapy infusion suite, the examination room of a palliative care clinic, the hospital room, the patient's home, or the inpatient hospice setting. Psychotherapy interventions at the bed side can effectively provide patients with needed support.[30] Dealing with the instability of the therapeutic setting can be burdensome for the patient and therapist. The therapist can facilitate this process by noting that unpredictability of the setting is expected. Additionally, the therapist should emphasize the primary importance of the stability of their relationship.

THERAPEUTIC CONTENT AND PROCESS

In psychodynamic-oriented psychotherapy, therapeutic content and process are expected to flow in a relatively unstructured manner, without setting specific time limitation to the organic unfolding of the process. However, a diagnosis of life-threatening illness will often create a heightened sense of awareness of the importance of time both in the therapist and the patient. The theme of time itself with associated questions related to the course of the disease may dominate the focus of the sessions. Psychotherapy provides patients with a space where present, past, and future can be perceived separately or in a framework based not only on the "here and now" but on a parallel dimension of intrapsychic reality. In such space, patients can hold both the awareness of probable or imminent death and hope for cure. Sometimes patients need permission to hold both a life narrative and a death narrative and will test the therapist's experience and personal level of comfort and skill accepting both temporal dimensions.

A man with advanced cancer in an inpatient hospice facility had previously spent every Thursday night of the past thirty years playing poker with a group of friends. During those years, while a few of the group had become ill and died the surviving members continued to meet. During a psychotherapy session the patient said his friends had invited him to join the group for the Thursday game, one more time. He told the therapist that he did not feel like going. Sensing ambivalence from the patient the therapist gently explored the reasons for his decision, asking first if it was primarily physical. The patient replied with surprise asking, "Isn't this what I am supposed to do? Aren't I supposed to let go and accept my dying? How can I go play poker and let go at the same time?"

During this important session the patient's perceptions were explored and he became comfortable embracing both the reality of imminent death, as well as the ability to engage in pleasurable activities. The patient decided to play poker that night and treat it as a normal event. He did not say final goodbyes to his friend, nor did he focus his emotional energy on whether that poker game was going to be his last. During the following psychotherapy session he told the therapist "I was just living; just doing what I would normally do, and it was a relief."

The themes of separation, loss, and grief are also often closely related to the theme of time. As the therapist allows these themes to unfold during the session, following the patient's lead, there is an opportunity to explore patients' personal grieving styles and personal history of loss. The balanced combination of supportive psychotherapy, timely interpretation, and careful assessment will allow the therapist to identify patients at risk for the development of complicated grief, major depression, or anxiety. A patient's personal grieving style is the result of longstanding cultural, familiar, and more general interpersonal patterns that can originate with the first exposure to death. Subsequent exposure to other grieving styles exhibited by important figures in the patient's life will also affect how patients process loss and separation.

In recent years, significant attention has been given to the importance of existential and spiritual themes for the process of making meaning of the experience of illness.[31] As they are now widely recognized as having a fundamental impact on patients' adaptation to illness, therapists need to recognize the potential importance of exploring existential and spiritual aspects of the patient's intrapsychic reality. This can be especially challenging as there is a wide variation in the depth of personal exploration of these matters in patients and therapists.

Psychotherapy for patients with a life-threatening illness necessitates providing a literal and symbolic container where expectations, perceptions, fears, and anxieties can be safely expressed by the patient. However, during the psychotherapeutic relationship patients may never utter the word "cancer" or "death." This should not be necessarily interpreted by the therapist as a sign of unhealthy denial or lack of coping. Clearly, a skilled therapist would want to gently explore the patient's level of awareness, and how decisions about communication regarding the disease are supportive or unsupportive of the patient's therapeutic process. An important aspect of psychotherapy with patients who have cancer is that it is aimed at "preserving" life, even as the illness progresses. From the original Latin meaning, preserving life in the context of patients with cancer means safeguarding them from psychological harm, helping them adjust to the diagnosis, coping with the illness, and fostering healing and growth.[32] It should be recognized that certain patients may exhibit what could be described as self-directed disclosure, or acceptance. In this self-directed process, patients may have an internal and clear awareness of the severity of their prognosis and, at the same time, might decide not to disclose this awareness or share it with family members or staff, including the therapist. Whether this approach is deleterious to the patient's psychological well being should be assessed in the context of the therapeutic relationship.

THE IMPORTANCE OF CULTURALLY SENSITIVE PSYCHOTHERAPY

The importance of providing culturally sensitive psychotherapy cannot be overemphasized. Simply applying Western psychotherapeutic approaches to culturally diverse patients without an understanding of their background and world view will negatively impact the therapeutic alliance and outcome. The therapist must negotiate these differences without minimizing or trivializing them. This is important to achieve in the initial phase of psychotherapy, sometimes referred to as engagement, as it is often crucial in determining whether the patient will continue treatment.[33] In a larger sense, every psychotherapeutic encounter is cross-cultural.[34] Even when patient and therapist belong to the same racial or ethnic group, their personal world view is shaped by unique elements, such as family, community, as well as spiritual and religious beliefs. Therefore, psychotherapy should always include a through exploration of the patient's world view, the patient's explanatory model for the illness, and specific cultural elements that may impact on decisions about medical treatment.[35] A good therapeutic alliance is the main predictor of patient's compliance with treatment, regardless of the therapist's theoretical framework or ethnicity.[36,37] In traditional outpatient psychotherapy patients have the option to meet several therapists to find a "good match." Patients with cancer who are in need of psychotherapy often do not have the luxury to explore several therapeutic relationships before they commit to one therapist. Not only are patients especially vulnerable due to the diagnosis of life-threatening illness; they may not have the option to search for a culturally competent therapist. Research has demonstrated the need for therapists to develop generic and specific cultural competence.[38] Generic competence refers to qualities and skills that are necessary any time a therapist works with a patient, whether from a different cultural background or one similar to the therapist's. A therapist who has developed generic cultural sensitivity will not assume that apparent similarities in cultural backgrounds necessarily translate into similarity of values and practices. Specific cultural competence refers to the therapist knowledge and understanding of the particular culture the patient belongs to. The ways patients integrate a cancer diagnosis, make meaning of their diagnosis, and conceptualize how and why the illness was developed is culturally determined. A sense of curiosity, freshness, and deep respect for the patient's cultural values and practices will allow the therapist to promote therapeutic alliance and increase the likelihood of obtaining positive outcomes.

THE THERAPEUTIC RELATIONSHIP

In the midst of the illness narrative, the relationship with the therapist should bring a sense of stability and safety in the patient's life. With illness threatening many aspects of life, including the very sense of body integrity and survival, the stability and predictability of the relationship with the therapist can promote a sense of hope.

A hospitalized patient heard from his therapist that she would be away for a week to present at a conference. In an attempt to express his deep disappointment he stated "I feel as if I was on a sinking ship, and the life vest has just been taken away from me."

Transference. In traditional psychodynamically oriented psychotherapy, transference is the primary vehicle of communication and exploration between the therapist and the patient and is regarded as not limited by the constraints of real time and space.[39] Once conceptualized exclusively as a projection of the patient's development and ego function, it is now understood as a result not only of the patient's feelings, but also of the therapist' countertransference. When working with patients with cancer, the luxury to operate exclusively within the transference metaphor does not exist.[40]

Countertransference. The term countertransference refers to the collection of feelings and emotional reactions evoked in the therapist during the course of the therapeutic relationship. It is the result of the patient's behavior, the therapist's past or current situation or, most often, by a combination of the three.[41] Fear of death and feelings related to loss and bereavement are commonly experienced by patients at various stages of the illness and can often represent most of the content of the session. As a result, the therapist may be vicariously "forced" to become more in touch with his or her own feelings about mortality and past or current losses. Working with certain individuals, or those with certain diagnoses, may be more emotionally challenging than others. The quality and intensity of the emotions developed in the therapist are often modulated by the losses and deaths experienced and the degree to which grief has been processed. If the patient's illness progresses during the course of therapy, the therapist must be able to discuss the possibility of death. The importance of self-assessment for therapists cannot be emphasized enough. For example, if the patient feels helpless and afraid of dying, the therapist may regress to a helpless position with the patient. Or, the therapist may also engage in anxious avoidance of the patient. At times, the personal reality of the therapist may even mirror the patients' experience; the therapist may lose a loved one to cancer, or the therapist may be diagnosed with a life-threatening illness.[42] Successful management of this type of countertransference involves deciding whether to disclose, and the extent of the disclosure, as well as managing potential ruptures in the relationship.[43] If the therapist has strong feelings of distress working with a particular patient, consultation with colleagues is crucial. And, if the therapist feels that it may be important to refer the patient to a colleague, there needs to be an awareness of abandonment feelings that will likely be evoked in the patient. Referring a patient to a colleague because the therapist's countertransference is negatively impacting on the therapeutic relationship is a difficult scenario, both for the patient and for the therapist. However, it is the best option when it becomes clear that the countertransference has become unmanageable.[44]

Termination. Termination is a crucial and delicate part of every therapeutic relationship and process. It is a carefully planned process by which therapist and patients review the work done together and acknowledge the completion of that particular therapeutic relationship. While termination marks the end of a therapeutic segment it does not necessarily mean therapy is complete. The importance of addressing termination in a proactive manner, following clinical and ethical principles, may create significant challenges for the therapist and the patient.[45]

Termination of therapy with a physically healthy patient may allow the therapist to project a scenario in which the patient continues to live her life with a higher level of satisfaction. When working with patients with cancer, especially patients with advanced disease, the therapist must be aware that an unplanned interruption may occur at any point and termination may be relatively abrupt. This is problematic for the patient and therapist as each session may need to be considered as a potential form of termination. Depending on the health status of the patient and the staging of the disease, saying good-bye can take on different meanings. The ability to effectively direct termination of therapy with a cancer patient challenges the therapist's clinical experience, judgment, and intuition.

Psychotherapy interventions based on a time-limited approach may be more likely to offer patient and therapist the opportunity to review the work done and say good-bye, thus openly acknowledging the end of the therapeutic relationship. When psychotherapy is provided within a long-term model, it may start at any point during the course of the patient's illness, and it may continue until the patient's death.

Issues of countertransference may have an unexpected and important impact on the therapist's behavior and emotional responses during the termination phase. The therapist may experience significant grief, sadness, or relief that the therapy is over. At the same time the patient, however, may focus on expressing gratitude for the help received and may not want to recognize or acknowledge any further feelings related to loss or sadness. For successful termination it is important that the therapist hold any agenda or expectation lightly and not impose them on the patient. Therapist and patient may be aware and openly acknowledge that the sadness they are experiencing is not only the result of the end of the therapeutic relationship, but also due to the shared awareness that the patient may not likely survive the disease. While the awareness of the progressive decline of the patient's health may prompt the therapist's desire to begin saying good-bye to the patient, clinical experience suggests that this process should not be started or imposed on the patient who is not ready. If the patient appears unwilling or unable to share any negative emotions related to the end of the relationship, the therapist should respect this choice. However, the therapist may express his or her feelings, modeling the expression of emotions for the patients. The patient may or may not choose to follow the therapist's implicit invitation to share feelings of sadness. Thus, for example, a therapist may gently raise the issue by saying "I have been thinking about what it would be like for us to say good-bye." The patient may decide to accept or ignore the invitation and it is essential that the therapist respects the patient's boundaries. In this context termination, whether due to the end of therapy, or to the end of the patient's life, must follow the same principle of preserving the integrity of patients' emotional life, safeguarding them from suffering.

SUMMARY

Patients with cancer often present a unique situation for therapists, because of the uncertainties of their lifespan and the profound emotional and physical impact of their diagnosis and medical treatment. Therapists with extended knowledge of both theory and practice of individual psychotherapy can help patients and their caregivers cope with the diagnosis and progression of the illness, promoting healing and growth. The presence of professionally trained therapists, expert in assessment and provision of individualized interventions represents an invaluable asset for institutions that treat patients with cancer. A flexible theoretical framework will allow the therapist to adapt the therapeutic model to the changes in setting often imposed by the clinic or hospital environment. Working with patients who have cancer can be emotionally very demanding, especially as the illness progresses and they may approach death. Such emotional intensity can elicit strong feelings in the therapist who may develop death anxiety, fear, desire to protect and "save" the patient, or avoidance of the patient. Awareness and adequate management of countertransference through peer consultation and supervision can allow the therapist to minimize the negative impact of such feelings on the therapeutic relationship and allow it to continue to be a predictable and supportive element in the patient's life.

As they accompany patients during their difficult journey, therapists will need to mobilize skills and sensitivity in complex settings that will test their tolerance for ambiguity and their ability to offer predictable, skillful, and compassionate presence.

REFERENCES

1. Frank AW. *The wounded storyteller: Body, illness, and ethics*. Chicago, CA: The University of Chicago Press; 1995.

2. Goldman CR. Toward a definition of psycho-education. *Hosp Community Psychiatry*. 1988;39(6):666–668.

3. Karasu TB. The specificity versus non-specificity dilemma: toward identifying therapeutic change agents. *Am J Psychiatry*. 1986;143:687–695.

4. Fawzy FI. A short-term psycho-educational intervention for patients newly diagnosed with cancer. *Supp Care Cancer*. 1995;3:325–328.

5. Tyler LE. Counseling. *Annu Rev Psychol*. 1958;9:375–390.

6. Messer SB, Watchel PL. The contemporary psychotherapeutic landscape: issues and prospects. In: Watchel PL, Messer SB (eds). *Theories of psychotherapy: Origins and evolution*. Washington, DC: American Psychological Association; 1997.

7. Arbuckle DS. *Counseling and psychotherapy: An overview*. New York: McGraw Hill; 1967.

8. Creech RH. The psychological support of the cancer patient: a medical oncologist viewpoint. *Sem Oncol*. 1975;2:285–292.

9. Postone N. Psychotherapy with cancer patients. *Am J Psychother*. 1998;52(4):412–424.

10. Holland JC. American Cancer Society award lecture. Psychological care of patients: psycho-oncology's contributions. *J Clin Oncol*. 2003;21:253–265.

11. Holland JC. IPOS Sutherland Memorial Lecture: an international perspective on the development of psychosocial oncology: overcoming cultural and attitudinal barriers to improve psychosocial care. *Psycho-oncology*. 2004;13(7):445–459.

12. Massie M, Holland JC, Straker N. Psychotherapeutic interventions. In: Holland JC, Rowland JR (eds). *Handbook of psychooncology: Psychological care of the patient with cancer*. New York: Oxford University Press; 1990:455–469.

13. Owen JE, Klapow JC, Hicken B, Tucker DC. Psychosocial Interventions for cancer: review and analysis using a three-tiered outcomes model. *Psychooncology*. 2001;10(3):218–230.

14. Rehse B, Pukrop R. Effects of psychosocial interventions quality of life in adult cancer patients: meta analysis of 37 published controlled outcome studies. *Patient Educ Couns*. 2003;50(2):179–186.

15. LeMay K, Wilson KG. Treatment of existential distress in life-threatening illness: a review of manualized interventions. *Clin Psychol Rev*. 2008;28(3):472–493.

16. Worden JW, Weisman AD. Do cancer patients really want counseling? *Gen Hosp Psychiatry*. 1980;2:100–103.

17. Worden JW, Weisman AD. Preventive psychosocial interventions with newly diagnosed cancer patients. *Gen Hosp Psychiatry*. 1984;6:243–249.

18. Boesen E, Boesen D, Christensen S, Johansen C. Comparison of participants and non-participants in a randomized psychosocial intervention study among patients with malignant melanoma. *Psychosomatics*. 2007;48:510–516.

19. Fawzy FI. A short-term psychoeducational intervention for patients newly diagnosed with cancer. *Supp Care Cancer*. 1995;3:325–328.

20. Sherman AC, Pennington J, Latif U, Farley H, Arent, L, Simonton S. Patient preferences regarding cancer group psychotherapy interventions: a view from the inside. *Psychosomatics*. 2007;48:426–432.

21. Sourkes BM. *The deepening shade: Psychological aspects of life-threatening illness*. Pittsburgh: University of Pittsburgh Press; 1982.

22. McGoldrick M, Walsh F. Death and the family cycle. In: Carte B, McGoldrick M (eds). *The expanded family life cycle: Individual, family, and social perspectives*. Needham Heights, MA: Allyn and Bacon; 1999

23. Younggren JN, Harris EA. Can you keep a secret? Confidentiality in psychotherapy. *J Clin Psychol*. 2008;64(5):589–600.

24. Sourkes BM. *The deepening shade: Psychological aspects of life-threatening illness*. Pittsburgh: University of Pittsburgh Press; 1982.

25. Akechi T, Okuyama T, Onishi J, Morita T, Furukawa TA Psychotherapy for depression among incurable cancer patients (Review). *Cochrane Collab*. 2008.

26. Pitman RK, Lanes DM, Williston SK, et al. Psychophysiologic assessment of posttraumatic stress disorder in breast cancer patients. *Psychosomatics*. 2001;42:133–140.

27. Eels TD, ed. *Handbook of psychotherapy case formulation*. New York: The Guilford Press; 1997.

28. Sim K, Peng Gwee K, Bateman A. Case formulation in psychotherapy: revitalizing its usefulness as a clinical tool. *Acad Psychiatry*. 2005;289–292.

29. Sourkes BM. *The deepening shade: Psychological aspects of life-threatening illness*. Pittsburgh: University of Pittsburgh Press; 1982.

30. Griffith JL, Gaby L. Brief psychotherapy at the bedside: countering demoralization from medical illness. *Psychosomatics*. 2005;46(2):109–116.

31. Lee V, Robin Cohen S, Edgar L, Laizner AM, Gagnon AJ. Meaning-making intervention during breast or colorectal cancer treatment improves self-esteem, optimism, and self-efficacy. *Soc Sci Med*. 2006;62(12):3133–3145.

32. Strada EA. Preserving life at the end of life: shifting the temporal dimension of hope. *J Palliat Support Care*. 2008;6(2):187,188.

33. Lo HT, Fung KP. Culturally competent psychotherapy. *Can J Psychiatry*. 2003;48(3):161–170.

34. Sue DW. *Counseling the culturally different: Theory and practice*. 3rd ed. New York: John Wiley and Sons; 1999.

35. Kleinman A. Culture, illness and cure: clinical lesions from anthropologic and cross-cultural research. *Ann Intern Med*. 1978;88:251–258.

36. Sue S. In search of cultural competence in psychotherapy and counseling. *Am Psychol*. 1998;53:440–448.

37. Reis BF, Brown LG. Reducing psychotherapy dropouts: maximizing perspective convergence in the psychotherapy dyad. *Psychother Theor*. 1999;36:123–136.

38. Cross T, Bazron B, Dennis K, and Isaacs M. *Towards a culturally competent system of care*. Washington (DC): CASSP Technical Assistance Center; 1989.

39. Jung CG. *The practice of psychotherapy: Essays of the psychology of transference and other subjects*. (Collected Works, Vol.16). Princeton, NJ: Princeton University Press; 1995.

40. Sourkes BM. *The deepening shade: Psychological aspects of life-threatening illness*. Pittsburgh: University of Pittsburgh Press; 1982.

41. McWilliams N. *Psychoanalytic diagnosis: Understanding personality structure in the clinical process*. New York: The Guilford Press; 1994.

42. Counselman EF, Alonso A. The ill therapist: therapists' reactions to personal illness and the impact of psychotherapy. *Am J Psychother*. 1999;47(4):591–602.

43. Omer H. Troubles in the therapeutic relationship: a pluralistic perspective. *J Clin Psychol*. 2000;56(2):201–210.

44. Sourkes BM. *The deepening shade: Psychological aspects of life-threatening illness*. Pittsburgh: University of Pittsburgh Press; 1982.

45. Vasquez MJ, Bingham RP, Barnett JE. Psychotherapy termination: clinical and ethical responsibilities. *J Clin Psychol*. 2008;64(5):653–665.

Cognitive Therapy

Stirling Moorey

WHAT IS COGNITIVE THERAPY?

The term cognitive-behavior therapy (CBT) refers to a broad range of psychological approaches that have in common an interest in the role of thoughts and behaviors in creating and maintaining psychological distress. Problem solving therapies, stress management and coping skills training are all examples of cognitive behavior therapies which have been applied in cancer.[1-3] This chapter will describe a therapy for helping cancer patients cope which is based on Beck's cognitive therapy.[4,5] Cognitive therapy was originally developed as a treatment for depression, but has since been extended to the anxiety disorders, eating disorders, chronic fatigue, and psychosis.[6-8] One of cognitive therapy's strengths is its insistence on rigorous scientific investigation of its theory and treatment; this has contributed to a large body of outcome research supporting its efficacy.

Cognitive therapy is a structured, problem-focused treatment that places cognition, or consciously accessible thoughts and beliefs, at its centre. A cognitive formulation of a problem will stress how thoughts, behaviors, emotions, and physical sensations interact together to maintain the problem. For instance, in panic disorder the cognitive model asserts that normal autonomic arousal (often as a result of stress or anxiety) is catastrophically misinterpreted as a sign of impending disaster.[9] There is a clear link between the sensation that is perceived as threatening and the catastrophic cognition—so a feeling of breathlessness may lead to a belief that one is about to suffocate, or tightness in the chest to a belief that a heart attack is imminent. These thoughts can then create a vicious cycle of increasing fear, physical reactions, and negative cognitions. The panic patient's behavior is again in keeping with the meaning ascribed to the situation; so a person who fears they cannot breathe may open windows to get more air, or if they think they are having a heart attack may sit down to rest. Another common behavioral reaction is to avoid situations where the panic has occurred. These reactions are called "safety seeking behaviours" and confirm the negative belief, because they prevent the person from being exposed to the feared consequence and so learning that their fear is misplaced. Similar maintenance models have been applied to other anxiety disorders. They share a number of features: a personal meaning of perceived threat, selective attention to the threatening stimulus, and safety behaviors that paradoxically reinforce the anxiety. Although cognitive therapy is sometimes seen as a cookbook therapy, the specific formulation of a presenting problem and how it is maintained is essential in constructing a treatment program, which will help the person correct their distorted thinking and test the impact of their behavioral reactions. In depression Beck's model describes how negative thoughts about the self, the world, and the future trap the depressed person in a helpless and hopeless view of the world, and result in reduced activity and social withdrawal that further deepen the depression. One of the important assumptions here is that although the thoughts may be distorted, the emotional and behavioral responses are perfectly natural given the interpretation of the situation: we are all doing our best within our view of reality. Therapy is about helping people to question whether their current view is accurate or helpful and to explore alternatives.

In distinction from some of the other cognitive behavior therapies mentioned already, Beck's cognitive therapy pays attention to cognitive factors that might predispose to mental distress. The underlying beliefs or rules we have about our self, other people, and the world in general make us vulnerable or protect us from emotional disorder. So, if we have strong beliefs that to be happy we have to be successful at everything we do, we may feel fine until we fail at something, but once this happens we may conclude that we are inadequate and become depressed. The cognitive model therefore allows therapists to understand both the maintenance and predisposition to a particular disorder, and it allows flexibility in deciding how "deep" you dig. For many problems the maintenance conceptualization and treatment is sufficient to effect significant and lasting change, but at other times a developmental model focusing on core beliefs is required.

There are two ways in which cognitive therapy can make a contribution to coping with cancer. Firstly, many of the psychological problems experienced by people with cancer share similarities with problems for which we have effective cognitive-behavioral treatments. In cancer the prevalence of depression varies from 15% to 25% across studies.[10] Nearly half of all cancer patients report some anxiety and this may be clinically significant in 23%.[11,12] In addition to treatments for these syndromes of depression, generalized anxiety, panic, and health anxiety, cognitive therapy also has change methods for common cancer symptoms like fatigue and insomnia.[13,14] Second, the general theory and therapeutic approach of cognitive therapy with its emphasis on normalizing stress reactions, collaboration, and problem solving may be particularly helpful in understanding and treating adjustment reactions.

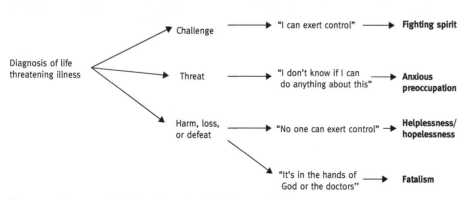

Fig. 54-1. The appraisal of the diagnosis of life-threatening illness.

THE COGNITIVE MODEL OF ADJUSTMENT TO LIFE-THREATENING ILLNESS

The personal meaning of illness and death. As we have seen, the fundamental principle of any cognitive model is that our interpretation of events determines how we feel and how we act. Lazarus and Folkman's model of coping is particularly relevant to the case of life-threatening illness.[15–17] Many people, after an initial period of distress and confusion, perceive cancer as a challenge, and are able to call upon a range of coping strategies. Others focus on the uncertainty inherent in the diagnosis of a life-threatening illness and understandably feel anxious, while other people may see the diagnosis in terms of loss of a hoped-for future. This broad appraisal of the diagnosis as a challenge, threat, or loss then leads to a secondary appraisal of the resources available to the individual for coping with the illness that is, what can be done about it?

If the diagnosis is seen as a challenge that can be met by the individual with the help of health professionals and the prognosis is seen as hopeful, a positive adjustment style that has been termed by some as a "fighting spirit" develops. On the other hand, if the diagnosis is seen as a loss or defeat which no one has the power to affect and death is seen as inevitable, a "helpless/hopeless" adjustment results. A person who focuses on the uncertainty inherent in their situation and the unpredictability of their future will become anxiously preoccupied with their disease and how to deal with it. Two further patterns of interpretation and coping may be found: fatalism and denial. People who respond to the question "what can be done about this?" by externalizing responsibility—giving it up to the doctors, fate, or God—will tend to have a stoic acceptance of their illness. For some people the threat may be so great that they minimize or even deny its severity and so the response to the questions about how to cope and what the future holds become less salient. Outright denial of the diagnosis of a life-threatening illness is relatively rare these days, but the tendency to minimize the seriousness or the impact of disease is quite common and many patients practice varying levels of avoidance. "Denial" is a complex psychosocial reaction which is not always simply a defense mechanism; the effects of education and knowledge about the disease, information received from health professionals, family influences, and adaptive decisions to be positive about adversity all interact with minimization of threat to produce the overall coping response. Fig. 54-1 shows these adjustment styles diagrammatically. Studies have consistently found that patients with helpless/hopeless and anxious adjustment styles have greater emotional distress than those who see their illness as a challenge.[18,19]

A diagnosis of cancer not only challenges our hopes about our life and survival and our confidence in our ability to cope; but also may challenge our view of ourselves and our world. For instance, someone may be hopeful that they can be cured of their illness, but the side effects of treatment such as radical surgery may be so difficult for them to bear that they become depressed. Here again the cognitive model would state that it is the personal meaning of symptoms, treatment, or side effects that determines the emotional reaction. And the reverberations of a serious illness do not stop with its physical effects. The reactions of others and the general social perception of the disease will also influence the person's coping behavior. A heavy smoker who develops lung cancer may be highly critical of himself for contributing to the development of his illness, but this may be compounded by a partner who feels let down and blames him for getting ill, not to mention the social stigma that may also be involved.

One important difference between cognitive therapy with people who have serious physical illness and those with psychiatric disorders is the reality of the dangers and disturbances they face. As we will see when we discuss therapeutic interventions, it is important to distinguish between appraisals that are unrealistic (e.g., a woman with early stage primary breast cancer who becomes depressed because she believes she will inevitably die within a short time) and realistic ones (such as a woman with metastatic breast cancer who is sad about not living to see her children grow up). Where thinking is clearly unrealistic standard methods of challenging negative thoughts can be used, but where thoughts are more realistic the focus moves more to problem solving and coping strategies (Fig 54-2).

When coping fails the person with cancer can become trapped in vicious circles of thoughts, feelings, and behaviors (Fig. 54-3). Unhelpful

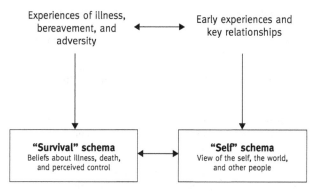

Fig. 54-2. Past experience and core beliefs.

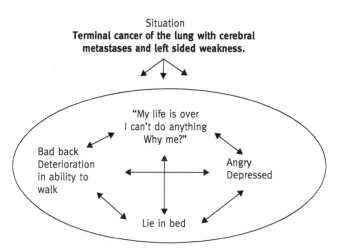

Fig. 54-3. The cognitive model.

Table 54-1. The interaction of negative thoughts and behaviors

Automatic thought	Unhelpful behavior	Consequence
"If I can't do what I used to do, my life's over."	Give up, ruminate about loss	Loss of pleasurable activities, depression
"I'm different."	Avoid people	Reinforces feeling of being an outsider
"I'm no longer attractive."	Neglect appearance	Confirms negative self-image

thoughts may lead to unhelpful behavior that often has the consequence of confirming the initial negative appraisal (Table 54-1). Effective therapy breaks these vicious circles.

The influence of underlying beliefs on adjustment. We often live our lives with an implicit assumption that we are going to live forever and that bad things will somehow not happen to us. Cancer challenges these implicit beliefs about invulnerability and immortality.[20] It may also challenge our beliefs that we are competent and able to cope, and that the world is a predictable, fair, and controllable place. How someone appraises the impact of cancer will depend on their underlying system of beliefs about themselves, other people, and the world around them, as well as more specific beliefs about illness and its treatment. The cognitive model proposes that early experiences shape our core beliefs.[5] If those core beliefs are overly positive and rigid they may be shattered by the trauma of a diagnosis of a terminal illness. Beliefs that the world is just and predictable make it hard for some people to accommodate their beliefs in the face of trauma.[20] For some people a life-threatening illness may confirm their secret fears and so activate core beliefs like "I am vulnerable," "The world is dangerous, unpredictable, hostile," "Others are abusive, unavailable." The individual may have more conditional beliefs and coping strategies to mitigate these unconditional negative beliefs. With a diagnosis of a life-threatening illness the person will often try unsuccessfully to use the same strategies they have used in the past. For instance, someone who has had significant separations or abuse during their childhood may have core beliefs that the world is a dangerous and unpredictable place where they are helpless and vulnerable, and where people let you down. To cope with this they may have developed a belief like "*If I can control my life I will be safe,*" and used compensatory strategies of perfectionism and self-reliance (Fig. 54–4). With a diagnosis of cancer their fears that the world is dangerous and unpredictable may be confirmed as will their sense of vulnerability, but there may be more limited scope to exert their usually controlling strategies; moreover, they will be forced to become dependent on others for their treatment and care. So their negative beliefs may be activated along with feelings of anxiety and depression.

Adjustment and coping across the course of chronic illness. Most people will have their positive beliefs challenged by the diagnosis of a life-threatening illness and will feel vulnerable, unable to cope, and hopeless about the future temporarily, but then find strength and resources to deal with the stress. It may be that most people adapt by integrating the news of their diagnosis into their preexisting belief system and there is some evidence that cancer patients may actually be more optimistic than healthy controls.[21] This adaptation is not static but will vary across the course of the disease. There is much more uncertainty over the course of the disease and prognosis and there may be periods of remission before a relapse. After the initial diagnosis and treatment of cancer there may be a period of hope that the disease has been cured which is then dashed if there is a recurrence.

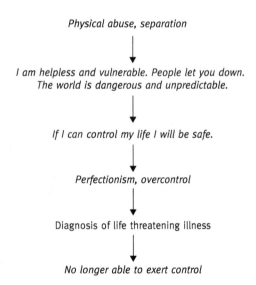

Fig. 54–4. Longitudinal or developmental model.

Basic principles of cognitive therapy in serious illness. Cognitive therapy encourages the patient to become their own therapist by learning to identify and modify their unhelpful thoughts, beliefs, and behavior.[5] Therapist and patient work collaboratively to agree a set of target problems and develop a shared conceptualization of how the problems are being perpetuated. Patients are helped to see their negative beliefs as hypotheses about themselves, their illness, and the world, which are then tested through the use of cognitive and behavioral techniques. This reality testing approach has been termed "collaborative empiricism."[4] Sessions usually follow an agenda set by patient and therapist and will include the setting and review of homework assignments to test beliefs and practice new ways of coping (Textbox 54–1).

Modifications of cognitive therapy in cancer. Because cognitive therapy for life-threatening illness often addresses emotional problems such as anxiety and depression it is very similar to standard cognitive therapy for these conditions.[4,6,22] However, a number of modifications to therapy may be required to accommodate the effects of physical illness and the process of adjustment that many patients will be going through (Textbox 54–2).

As with CBT for older people therapy may need to be delivered in healthcare settings or patients' homes rather than in the traditional outpatient clinic.[23] It is often difficult to pursue a typical course of therapy with patients with active physical illness. Fluctuations in the disease, demands of physical treatment may disrupt the flow of weekly therapy. This means that therapy in this setting is often shorter and has more circumscribed goals. The aim with ill patients is to achieve the maximum change with minimum intervention and wherever possible the therapist works to regain and enhance previous coping strategies.

While cognitive therapy always pays attention to emotional and interpersonal issues, these considerations are particularly important with this patient group. Many may be going through an adjustment process and the therapist needs to achieve a balance between encouraging and supporting adjustment and promoting effective problem solving. Identifying and managing maladaptive interactions with carers and fostering adaptive social support is a significant factor in working with these patients.

Textbox 54–1. Characteristics of cognitive therapy in cancer

- Based on a cognitive model of adjustment
- Structured
- Short-term (6–12 sessions)
- Focused and problem-oriented
- Educational
- Collaborative
- Makes use of homework assignments
- Uses a variety of treatment techniques including nondirective methods, behavioral techniques, cognitive techniques, and interpersonal techniques.

Textbox 54–2. Modifications of cognitive therapy in cancer

- Sessions less formal, more flexible, and more supportive
- Sessions may be briefer and adjusted to patient's physical status
- Therapy may need to be delivered in healthcare settings or patients' homes
- Techniques are adjusted to patients' physical status
- Therapy includes family and health professionals
- Goals of therapy are more circumscribed
- Primary goal of therapy is to promote maximum change with minimum intervention

Phase 1: Engagement and conceptualization. In the first session the therapist will need to make a judgment about the length and intensity of therapy and then establish a contract with the patient. In some cases time may be limited (terminal illness, severe fatigue, time restraints of a liaison consultation) and the aims of therapy will be consequently less ambitious. In other cases (early stage disease, less debility) there may be more time available which will allow a full course of therapy and perhaps even time to work on underlying beliefs that have made the person vulnerable. In the early sessions the therapist will also need to establish rapport, engage and "socialise" the patient into the therapy, and develop a shared conceptualization. These tasks are common to CBT in any setting. With patients facing death there may also be a need to facilitate the adjustment process. This can often be done simply by letting the patient tell their story, including what symptoms first led them to seek help, how the diagnosis was made, how treatment has progressed and so on. The therapist may be the first person to listen in this way. Developing a "compassionate case conceptualisation" helps this process and also helps to make sense of the confusing set of feelings experienced by the patient. At this stage a simple conceptualization using the "five areas model" is very useful (Fig. 54–3). Goals are established that are appropriate for the stage and severity of disease. Some basic self monitoring of thoughts and/or behavior can be set at this stage to clarify the conceptualization and start to demonstrate the model to the patient.

Phase 2: Cognitive and behavioral interventions. These should arise naturally from the conceptualization. In Fig. 54–3 we can see how a woman with terminal cancer has become locked into a vicious circle of negative thinking and withdrawal. Her ruminations about her disease and death have led her to feel depressed, hopeless, and angry. She has physical symptoms of weakness and pain and these together with the hopelessness have led her to take to her bed. Unfortunately the consequence of this is that she feels more isolated, and becomes more physically debilitated. The five areas model or "hot cross bun" is an effective nonstigmatizing way of showing the patient how these different systems interact. In the alternative ABC model, which has a linear form situation → thoughts → feelings → there is a risk that people with physical illness will feel that the seriousness of the situation is not being adequately recognized. The five areas model does not assume that any of the systems is primary. So in cancer it is possible to start with the physical state (e.g., fatigue or pain) as a given and then examine the patient's thoughts and behaviors in response to the physical reality of the illness. Once this maintenance conceptualization is agreed, the therapist now has a number of options:

1. She could use emotional techniques to facilitate anticipatory grieving.
2. She could use cognitive techniques to test the patient's belief that her life is over and she can't do anything.
3. She could set up a behavioral experiment to test this negative belief. This might involve the patient spending some time out of bed and engaging in some small tasks which used to give her a sense of achievement. She can then monitor her mood, fatigue, and pain. This will usually demonstrate that these are not made worse by activity but may actually improve and this may start to introduce a more positive cycle.

COGNITIVE TECHNIQUES

The threat of cancer to survival generates many realistic and sometimes catastrophic negative thoughts (Textbox 54–3). The cognitive techniques used will differ depending on the stage of the disease and prognosis. Patients with early stage disease and a good chance of cure or remission can be helped to see that their hopeless thoughts are unrealistic through *looking at the evidence* for and against their beliefs that the future is hopeless. Patients with a poor prognosis may be helped more by techniques that address the usefulness rather than the rationality of their thinking. A *cost benefit analysis* of realistic negative thoughts often reveals them to be ruminative in nature rather than helpful in solving problems or moving anticipatory grieving forward. If the patient accepts that recurrent thoughts about death are not productive it may be possible to schedule

> **Textbox 54-3. Questioning automatic thoughts**
> - What is the evidence?
> - Is there an alternative way of looking at the situation?
> - What is the worst that could happen?
> - What is the effect of thinking this way?
> - What would I say to a friend if I were in this situation?

some *worry time* during the day when they can allow themselves to ruminate, but at other times to schedule more constructive activities that give them a sense of control over their life. Sometimes these apparently realistic thoughts may overlie other fears for example, fears about what will happen to your family when you die. Uncovering these fears may allow the process of anticipatory grieving to take place or allow more effective problem solving (see under behavioral techniques).

Many negative thoughts are centered not on death but on the implications of the disease, regarding a person's self-esteem or competence. People may feel stigmatized by their illness and so "buy into" perceived social rejection. They may sometimes feel guilty and blame themselves for developing their condition. Often their sense of powerlessness comes from all or nothing thinking such as "If I can't be the person I used to be, I'm nothing." This leads them to selectively attend to the areas of their life they have lost rather than the areas where they still have some control. These themes of guilt and shame, anger toward self or others, and perceived helplessness are often distorted cognitions. Cognitive techniques can be used to test the validity and functionality of these thoughts.

BEHAVIORAL TECHNIQUES

In cognitive therapy, behavioral techniques usually arise out of a cognitive conceptualization and intervention. Negative beliefs are turned into hypotheses. For instance the belief that "If I can't do what I used to do my life's over" (Table 54–1) can be rephrased as a prediction "If I engage in activities I won't get any pleasure." The therapist asks the patient to rate the likelihood that she will get pleasure from doing some small things over the next week. In the following session the results of the *behavioral experiment* are reviewed. In most cases, the patient finds that she got more pleasure than she predicted, and the vicious cycle of inactivity begins to be broken. For helpless/hopeless patients simply *scheduling activities* can be very helpful in overcoming inactivity and demoralization. For more depressed or more physically ill patients, large tasks will need to be broken down into small steps (*graded task assignment*). Some ingenuity may be needed to find activities that are meaningful to patients who are very disabled or bedridden. Family members can sometimes be recruited to make suggestions based on their knowledge of the patient. For anxious patients behavioral experiments can be set up to test feared situations. Much of this behavioral work centers on establishing a sense of control. It is helpful to work within an individual's value and belief system to find empowering behavioral tasks. The message to the patient is to focus on what you can control, not what you can't ("you can't control your death, but you can control your life.").

Problem solving is another very powerful behavioral technique and has been applied as a therapy in its own right.[1,24] When the appraisal of the stress is accurate, rather than trying to change the thoughts about it, finding effective ways of coping or removing obstacles may be the best policy. For instance, in the case of a mother worrying about what will happen to her family when she dies, the problem solving may take the form of discussions with her partner about how to plan the future. The patient can make her own wishes for the children's future clear through writing advice to the partner on how to handle situations he may not have had so much experience in managing. Other examples of problem solving would be preparing and rehearsing how to talk to oncologists and be more involved in your treatment; preparing puzzles, music and so on to take with you during chemotherapy; making a will; working out and rehearsing a way to tell people you have cancer. More detailed description of cognitive and behavioral techniques for cancer can be found in Moorey and Greer and Sage.[17,25]

Phase 3: Consolidating coping and ending therapy. The length and form of this phase will depend on the nature of the therapeutic contract. In liaison settings time is often scarce. If the therapist can see the patient for 12 or more sessions it may be possible to do some work on underlying beliefs. This can be an opportunity for psychological growth: the impact of the illness on the person's life can be more fully assessed, the limitations of their more rigid beliefs and coping strategies evaluated, and alternative beliefs generated and tested. Briefer therapies will be more concerned with enhancing coping in the here and now. At the end of any course of cognitive therapy the therapist develops a "blueprint" collaboratively with the patient. This contains a summary of what the patient has learned in therapy, what strategies he or she needs to continue using, what might be factors that could cause a set back and how they can be managed.

EFFECT OF CBT ON QUALITY OF LIFE

In cancer cognitive-behavioral approaches have usually been delivered in a group coping skills format, though some researchers have applied a more formulation-based individual treatment as described in this article.[3,17] The usual outcome measures have been distress, anxiety, and depression. When CBT has been compared with no treatment or treatment as usual all trials have demonstrated the superiority of CBT.[3,26–28] These differences have been shown to persist for at least a year.[29] The majority of trials have demonstrated a superiority of CBT over treatment as usual when all patients are entered into the trial, but the effect size of this intervention is small compared to that with psychologically distressed patients. A smaller number of trials have compared CBT with other treatments, usually nondirective therapy. Some of these found CBT to be more effective at the end of therapy while others found the two therapies to be equally effective.[3,26,28,30–33]

A meta-analysis by Osborn et al. concluded that CBT was effective for depression (ES = 1.2; 95% CI = 0.22–2.19), anxiety (ES = 1.99; 95% CI = 0.69–3.31), and quality of life (ES = 0.91; 95% CI = 0.38–1.44).[34] Quality of life was improved at short-term follow-up and (ES = 1.45, 95% CI = .43–2.47) but the effect size reduced to 0.26 (95% CI = .06–.46) at long-term follow-up. Reviews have tended to support the idea that individual interventions were more effective than group, and that therapy is more effective when directed at patients with high levels of distress rather than all patients. Recently Lepore and Coyne have questioned the methodological rigor of both the original studies and reviews.[35,36] There is a challenge to carry out larger, more methodologically sound multicentre trials that have sufficient power to establish the efficacy of psychological interventions.

Trials have mainly used patients with early stage disease but three trials using a cognitive therapy approach have now been carried out with patients with advanced disease. Edelman et al. used a group approach and Savard et al. used individual cognitive therapy, both for women with metastatic breast cancer.[31,37] Cognitive therapy proved more effective than a control group. Moorey et al. taught cognitive and behavioral techniques to palliative care nurses and demonstrated an effect on levels of anxiety in people with terminal illness treated in their own homes.[38]

CONCLUSIONS

Cognitive therapy is a treatment that has substantial evidence for its effectiveness with a range of psychological problems. Because it is brief, problem-focused, and collaborative it has the potential to be a useful tool for liaison psychiatrists and psychologists, and in a "first aid" form may even be useful to nonmental healthcare workers.[38,39] There are encouraging signs from randomized controlled trials that it can be effective in the cancer setting both for early and advanced disease. Most work so far has been done on quality of life and emotional distress but targeting specific cancer-related symptoms such as fatigue, pain, or insomnia may help to refine the treatment in the future.[14,40] As with all psychological therapies, the challenge is to identify what works for whom, and to find ways to disseminate skills so that as many people as possible have access to evidence-based therapy.

REFERENCES

1. Nezu AM, Nezu CM, Friedman SH, Faddis S, Houts PS. *Helping cancer patients cope.* Washington DC: American Psychological Association; 1998.

2. Antoni MH, Bagget L, Ironson G, et al. Cognitive-behavioral stress management intervention buffers distress responses and immunological changes following notification of HIV-1 seropositivity. *J Consult Clin Psychol.* 1991;59:906–915.

3. Telch CF, Telch MJ. Group coping skills instruction and supportive group therapy for cancer patients: a comparison of strategies. *J Consult Clin Psychol.* 1986;34:802–808.

4. Beck AT, Rush AJ, Shaw BF, Emery G. *Cognitive therapy for depression.* New York, Guilford; 1979.

5. Beck JS *Cognitive therapy: Basics and beyond.* New York: Guilford Press; 1995.

6. Wells A. *Cognitive therapy of anxiety disorders: A practical guide.* London: Wiley; 1997.

7. Fairburn CG. *Cognitive behaviour therapy and eating disorders.* London: Guilford; 2008.

8. Fowler DG, Garety P, Kuipers E. *Cognitive behaviour therapy for psychosis: Theory and practice.* Chichester: John Wiley & Sons; 1995.

9. Clark DM. A cognitive approach to panic. *Behav Res Ther.* 1986;24:461–470.

10. Bodurka-Bevers D, Basen-Engquist K, Carmack CL, et al. Depression, anxiety, and quality of life in patients with epithelial ovarian cancer. *Gynecol Oncol.* 2000;78:302–308.

11. Schag CA, Heinrich RL. Anxiety in medical situations: adult cancer patients. *J Clin Psychol.* 1989;45:20–27.

12. Stark D, Kiely M, Smith A, et al. Anxiety disorders in cancer patients: their nature, associations, and relation to quality of life. *J Clin Oncol.* 2002;20:3137–3148.

13. Gielissen MF, Verhagen S, Witjes F, Bleijenberg G. Effects of cognitive behavior therapy in severely fatigued disease-free cancer patients compared with patients waiting for cognitive behavior therapy: a randomized controlled trial. *J Clin Oncol.* 2006;24:4882–4887.

14. Savard J, Simard S, Ivers H, Morin CM. Randomized study on the efficacy of cognitive-behavioral therapy for insomnia secondary to breast cancer, part II: Immunologic effects. *J Clin Oncol.* 2005;23:6097–6106.

15. Lazarus RS, Folkman S. *Stress, appraisal, and coping.* New York: Springer; 1984.

16. Folkman S, Greer, S. Promoting psychological well-being in the face of serious illness: when theory, research, and practice inform each other. *Psychooncology.* 2000;9:11–19.

17. Moorey S, Greer S. *Cognitive behaviour therapy for people with cancer.* Oxford: Oxford University Press; 2002.

18. Watson M, Greer S, Young J, Inayat Q, Burgess C, Robertson B. Development of a questionnaire measure of adjustment to cancer: the MAC scale. *Psychol Med.* 1988;18:203–209.

19. Schnoll RA, Harlow LL, Brandt U, Stolbach LL Using two factor structures of the Mental Adjustment to Cancer (MAC) scale for assessing adaptation to breast cancer. *Psychooncology.* 1998;7:424–435.

20. Janoff-Bulman R. *Shattered assumptions: Towards a new psychology of trauma.* New York: Free Press; 1992.

21. Stiegelis HE, Hagedorn M, Sanderman R, van der Zee KI, Buunk BP, van den Bergh AC. Cognitive adaptation: a comparison of cancer patients and healthy references. *Br J Health Psychol.* 2003;8:303–318.

22. Westbrook D, Kennerley H, Kirk J. *An introduction to cognitive behaviour therapy: Skills and applications.* London: Sage; 2007.

23. Evans C. Cognitive–behavioural therapy with older people. *Adv Psychia Treat.* 2007;13:111–118.

24. Nezu AM, Nezu CM, Weiner IB, Geller PA. Problem solving. In: Nezu AM, Nezu CM, Weiner IB, Geller PA (eds). *Handbook of psychology: Health psychology.* Chichester: John Wiley & Sons; 2003.

25. Sage N, Sowden M, Chorlton E. *CBT for chronic illness and palliative care: a workbook and toolkit.* London: Wiley; 2008.

26. Evans RL, Connis RT. Comparison of brief group therapies for depressed cancer patients receiving radiotherapy. *Public Health Rep.* 1995;110:306–311.

27. Greer S, Moorey S, Baruch JDR, et al. Adjuvant psychological therapy for cancer patients: a prospective randomised trial. *Br Med J.* 1992;304:675–680.

28. Moorey S, Greer S, Bliss J, Law M. A comparison of adjuvant psychological therapy and supportive counselling in patients with cancer. *Psychooncology.* 1998;7:218–228.

29. Moorey S, Greer S, Watson M, et al. Adjuvant psychological therapy for patients with cancer: outcome at one year. *Psychooncology.* 1994;3:39–46.

30. Cunningham AJ, Toccom EK. A randomized trial of group psychoeducational therapy for cancer patients. *Pat Ed Couns.* 1989;14:101–114.

31. Edelman S, Bell DR, Kidman A. A group cognitive-behaviour therapy programme with metastatic breast cancer. *Psychooncology.* 1999;8:295–305.

32. Bottomley A, Hunton S, Roberts G, et al. A pilot study of cognitive-behavioural therapy and social support group interventions with newly diagnosed cancer patients. *J Psychosoc Oncol.* 1996;14:65–83.

33. Edmonds CVI, Lockwood GA, Cunningham AJ. Psychological response to long term group therapy: a randomized trial with metastatic breast cancer patients. *Psychooncology.* 1999;8:74–91.

34. Osborn RL, Demoncada AC, Feuerstein M. Psychosocial interventions for depression, anxiety, and quality of life in cancer survivors: meta-analyses. *In J Psychiat Med.* 2006;36:13–34.

35. Lepore SJ, Coyne JC. Psychological interventions for distress in cancer patients: a review of reviews. *Ann Behav Med.* 2006;32:85–92.

36. Coyne JC, Lepore SJ, Palmer SC. Efficacy of psychosocial interventions in cancer care: evidence is weaker than it first looks. *Ann Behav Med.* 2006;32:104–110.

37. Savard J, Simard S, Giguère I, et al. Randomized clinical trial on cognitive therapy for depression in women with metastatic breast cancer: psychological and immunological effects. *Palliat Support Care.* 2006;4:219–237.

38. Moorey S, Cort E, Kapari M, et al. A cluster randomised controlled trial of cognitive behaviour therapy for common mental disorders in patients with advanced cancer. *Psychol Med.* 2009;39:713–723.

39. Mannix A, Blackburn IM, Garland A, et al. Effectiveness of brief training in cognitive behaviour therapy techniques for palliative care practitioners. *Palliat Med.* 2006;20:579–584.

40. Armes J, Chalder T, Addington-Hall J, Richardson A, Hotopf M. A randomized controlled trial to evaluate the effectiveness of a brief, behaviorally oriented intervention for cancer-related fatigue. *Cancer.* 2007;110:1385–1395.

CHAPTER 55

Group Psychotherapy for Persons with Cancer

James L. Spira and Danielle R. Casden

Group psychotherapy specifically designed for persons with cancer may very well be the most powerful psychosocial intervention available for the vast majority of patients. Beyond the scope of individual therapy, group therapy can address the major issues of cancer patients by garnering the emotional support of persons with similar experiences and using the experiences of others to buffer the fear of future unknowns. Yet beyond its effectiveness, group therapy is also extremely time and cost-efficient.[1] In terms of direct costs, group therapy for cancer patients has not been found to significantly reduce healthcare utilization costs,[2] Although the indirect savings to patients and society are difficult to calculate, this approach is associated with improved patient quality of life[3] which affects mood, job performance, marital functioning and child-rearing—all contributors to a healthy society.

For decades, group psychotherapy has been utilized effectively with patients facing a variety of psychosocial issues.[4] Several professional societies and journals have been founded specifically to advance the discipline of group psychotherapy (e.g., International Group Therapy Association [Gilford Press] American Psychological Association, Division of Group Psychology and Group Psychotherapy). During the past 10 years, groups specifically designed for cancer patients have also been utilized, described, and researched in increasing numbers[5–7] and the reader is directed to these sources for an explanation of clinical method. This chapter is intended to summarize the burgeoning effort that has been accomplished in this field, and describes the type of patients most likely to benefit from group intervention, the formats that best serve them, therapeutic guidelines for a successful intervention, and suggestions for how to recruit and retain group member. Before addressing clinical implementation, however, psychosocial factors addressed by group psychotherapy for cancer patients and the therapeutic groups which have demonstrated improvement in cancer patients' health will be discussed.

THE BENEFITS OF GROUP THERAPY FOR PERSONS WITH CANCER

Certainly, group formats are extremely cost effective for the patient, and time efficient for the therapist. Efficacy of time is especially noticed when teaching specific information or skills in psychoeducational classes, in person or via the web. Most importantly, group therapy is highly effective in improving quality of life.

Not surprisingly, persons diagnosed with cancer undergo substantial changes in mood, psychophysical functioning, and existential aspects of their lives. Fortunately, all these psychosocial factors can be improved through the group psychotherapy format. Many descriptions of group therapy for medically ill patients[8] and specifically cancer patients exist in the literature.[5–7] Therefore, we limit ourselves here to a review of expected outcomes for group therapy with cancer patients, as well as which patients might benefit from which approaches.

Beginning in the late 1970s, research has consistently demonstrated the benefits of group therapy for improving cancer patient's quality of life (such as mood, coping, psychophysical distress, and physical functioning). Most reported studies of group therapy have been short term (less than twelve meetings), typically following a cognitive-behavioral format combining educational information, coping skills, and emotional/social support.[5,6,8] A notable exception was a research group based on the traditional group therapy style of Irvin Yalom,[9] which met weekly for the entire year, and emphasized more on traditionally interactive, emotionally supportive therapeutic style.[10] Since briefer meetings require greater structure, longer groups can afford to allow patients to generate topics and exert relatively less therapeutic direction. Although not strictly group psychotherapy in the "traditional" sense, psychoeducational groups for recently diagnosed patients and those at risk for developing disease focus on information, improving compliance with treatment, and prevention, and although do not attempt to directly impact on mood or family functioning, this approach can hold great promise for improving the effectiveness of medical treatment or preventing future disease.[11–14]

Several studies have attempted to separate interventional styles to determine which methods might be most effective. Cain and associates[14] found that both individual and group therapies were equally beneficial compared to a control group in gynecological cancer patients' psychological adjustment 6 months after treatment. Telch and Telch[15] reported improved coping and self-efficacy for cancer patients attending a cognitive-behavior style group compared to an unstructured and nontherapeutically led support group. Cunningham and Tocco[16] also found that short-term cognitive-behavioral group was superior to unstructured support groups where patients were encouraged to express emotions, although both groups benefited from their respective interventions. In contrast, Evan and Connis[17] found that while cognitive-behavioral and supportive group therapy were both beneficial for depressed cancer patients, supportive therapy was superior in the long-run.

Several studies have attempted to determine if group therapy may also be effective for improving physical health. The year-long group therapy based on Yalom's approach to group psychotherapy found in a retrospective follow-up that patients who had been randomly assigned to receive group therapy lived an average of 18 months longer from study entry than did control patients.[18] However, Fox has pointed out that the treatment group lived only as long as the national and local average whereas the control group died at a faster than expected rate, suggesting that statistical sampling error accounted for the survival effect.[19] Further, several large and well conducted studies based on this method, including one conducted by the original team, failed to find a survival effect.[20,21] This approach encouraged confronting distress in an open and honest manner rather than avoidance of feelings and thoughts, and quality of life was consequently improved compared to subjects not receiving group therapy.

Family groups. Family groups have also been found to be effective for spouses, young siblings, and other family members of cancer patients.[22,23] Just as distress among the patient influences the family members' stress, similarly distress among the family members will in turn influence the patient. Thus, groups specifically designed for family members will help the family members, the cancer patient, and the family unit as a whole.

Technology-based groups. Over the past 10 years there has been a surge in the use of technology-based therapy groups, including on-line support groups with real-time discussion in chat-rooms, video conferencing groups, and web-blogging groups, where members can log-on at their convenience and post a message or solicit support at a time of need. These groups are unique as they provide access to therapy and support that otherwise may not be feasible due to problems with transportation, being home bound or other functional restrictions. Additional attractions for participation in distance-based support may include reduced stigma, or connecting individuals with rare diagnoses.[24] In fact, these types of groups often cater to cancer patients who simply have access to and familiarity with computers. Reviews of Internet Cancer Support Groups (ICSG) on the web have found that the majority of participants using on-line support groups are older women of an upper socio-economic status.[25]

Peer groups. The attraction of peer support offered to people with cancer by cancer patients and survivors is undeniable.[26] When two individuals share the unique experience of cancer, they perceive each other as able to empathize and identify with each other in a way that a healthcare professional or family member may be unable to grasp. When cancer patients come together in a group, they often form quick bonds and a sense of belonging, share information, coping strategies, offer encouragement and support, resulting in reduced feelings of isolation, stress, anxiety, and depression. Some groups that have formed to offer this type of support have been without professional leadership, or even without any identified leader whatsoever. Unfortunately, even for those groups with an identifiable peer-support leader, such facilitators rarely are provided sufficient training or supervision to adequately facilitate the complexities a cancer support group. Taken together with other research, these studies point to the benefits of therapeutically led groups versus unstructured support groups that are not therapeutically guided by a skilled facilitator, and appear to be at least as beneficial as individual therapy for cancer patients.[27,28]

Which group therapy approach is best? Given the preponderance of evidence for group therapy improving quality of life for cancer patients and their families, researchers have turned to explore what type of therapy is most effective for which patients. For example, Helgeson and colleagues[29] found that those lacking social support benefited from an interpersonal group format, whereas, those seeking information benefited more from a psychoeducational approach, and patients lacking coping skills improved from a cognitive-behavioral therapy (CBT)-oriented group. Clearly, therapists should select the style of intervention which will best facilitate the desired outcome.[29] The next section explores in greater detail the types of groups that are likely to be most appropriate for various patient characteristics.

GROUP THERAPY FOR CANCER PATIENTS COMPARED TO OTHER FORMATS

Understanding how group therapy for cancer patients differs from both individual therapy as well as group psychotherapy for persons with psychosocial disturbance will lay a foundation for understanding the power as well as the limits of this treatment.

Group versus individual treatment. Certainly individual psychotherapy is indicated for certain cancer patients, especially those with personality characteristics that interfere with adjusting to living with cancer and coping with treatment. Yet group therapy is considered by many to be the "treatment of choice" for most cancer patients, since group formats provide equal psychosocial benefit to individual therapy,[30] but at a reduced cost to the patient and provider. In contrast to the usual emphasis on examining and modifying personality patterns prevalent in individual therapy, group therapy for the persons with cancer emphasizes living more fully in each moment, and garnering supportive experiences from others regarding ways to handle the stresses faced in coping with life as a cancer patient. Certainly individual therapy can assist patients with such adjustments, and group therapy can emphasize personality patterns. Still, each is better suited to different therapeutic processes due to their special contextual circumstances. An individual therapist can focus on the complex puzzle that comprises each person's life, whereas a group setting is better suited to utilize the invaluable experience of others in coping with and adjusting to issues common to most cancer patients. The power of the group is therefore especially beneficial when utilized with the medically ill.[31]

Group therapy for persons with psychosocial disturbance versus persons with cancer. Typically, group psychotherapy is conducted for persons with various levels of psychosocial dysfunction, yet members are selected to participate on the basis of similar levels of ego functioning.[31] Group therapy for the medically ill is very different, however. A serious illness can affect anyone at any time. Therefore, these groups are typically comprised of persons with a wide range of past experiences, personal and external resources, and personality styles. Nonetheless, they have much in common. Typical themes discussed in groups of cancer patients include communication with medical professionals; relationships with family, friends, and co-workers; coping with medical treatment and ill effects of the disease; adjusting to living with a cancer diagnosis; existential issues such as addressing the possibility of dying, examining one's priorities, and shifting self-image[10,31] Although there is much in common among issues addressed by cancer patients, the range of personality types in these groups are as varied as those who can develop cancer—that is, the general population.

Group therapy for persons with psychosocial dysfunction most typically follows an interpersonal format.[9] Group therapy for cancer patients includes a variety of formats, including drop-in meetings with a cancer patient serving as coordinator, educational/didactic class format with a oncology clinical nurse specialist or social worker, or a supportive-expressive therapy group led by a psychologist or other experienced mental health professional, that provides a combination of coping skills training, expression of emotion, peer support, and education.[8] Naturally, the style of facilitating groups depends upon group format, patient make-up, stated goals, and therapist training.

FACILITATING GROUP PSYCHOTHERAPY FOR CANCER PATIENTS

Clearly, psychosocial support is of great value for persons with cancer. Yet the type of support offered depends to a great extent upon the stage of illness and the goals of therapy. Styles of group therapy and structure of groups which optimally facilitate various populations in their psychosocial development are considered below. Nevertheless, there are commonalities which exist across most types of groups, such as basic group facilitation methods, choice of topics, and dealing with special problems which are bound to arise in group formats.

Topics discussed in groups. The focus of the group should address the most relevant issues affecting the patients' quality of life and physical health. Two perspectives can be followed with regard to what is addressed in the groups: scientifically determined risk factors for worsening quality of life and physical health, and personal concerns as stated by the patient (Table 55–1).

Table 55–1. Examples of deductive (therapist-driven) and inductive (patient-driven) topics of discussion

Scientifically determined topics	Patients' personal concerns
Social support/ isolation	Psychophysical (pain, nausea, sleeplessness)
Confronting fears/ avoidance	Psychological (negative mood; intrusive thoughts)
Emotional expression/ suppression	Functional changes (physical fatigue, disability)
Active coping/ helplessness	Appearance (cosmetics, prosthesis, reconstruction)
	Communication (doctor, family, friends, coworkers)

SOURCES: Reprinted from Spira JL, "Group Therapies," Chapter 61 from Holland JC, *Psycho-oncology*, 1st ed. New York: Oxford University Press, 1999. With permission from Oxford University Press.

Topics generated by the patients stem directly from patients' immediate needs and concerns, such as coping with pain, nausea, sleeplessness, negative mood, intrusive thoughts, fatigue, appearance and body image, and communication with doctors, family, and friends.[10,32] Addressing these issues early and often will go far in establishing rapport with the patients. And as Maslow so well describes, one must take care of basic functional concerns before one is able to adequately address existential issues.[33]

Topics chosen by the therapists are often emotionally difficult for the patients to pursue at the time, even though they may well feel better afterward. These include issues of establishing meaningful social support, confronting fears, expressing negative emotions, and seeking control over what can be improved, while letting go of what cannot be controlled. Although patients may not choose to discuss or express negative emotions or issues of death and dying, it ends up being very beneficial and appreciated by the patients. It appears that by discussing these difficult issues in the groups, patients are able to focus on living more fully in each moment without as much distraction the rest of the week. Moreover, directly addressing the difficult issues of illness and dying assists patients to reexamine the way they live, with the result of choosing to spend more time in activities that are more meaningful and valuable to them. In short-term CBT-oriented groups, topics typically drive the discussion. In interpersonally-oriented groups, rather than *what* is discussed, it is often the therapeutic *style* that leads patients to examine these aspects of their lives. When therapists lead patients into exploring difficult realms, they must do so gently, lest they meet resistance and lose the trust of the group. The best leader is usually one who can follow the patient, gently introducing new ideas within the context of the patient's relevant experience.

Exactly what, how, and when topics are discussed will vary greatly, depending on the special issues faced by each population. Yet the therapeutic goals, methods, and structure of the group will also structure the discussion of topics. Some forms of group treatment are more inductive in nature while others are almost entirely deductive. The style will lead to differing results, and so should be selected with specific goals in mind.

Styles of therapeutic facilitation. Three fundamental styles of therapeutic intervention can be described, each of which may be suited to a different therapeutic population or structure. The manner with which any topic is discussed can be *deductive,* didactically directed by the therapist, *inductively* facilitated, with patient-generated topics subtly facilitated by therapists, or a balanced *interaction* between therapist and patients' raising of issues (see Table 55–2).

No matter which approach to group therapy one pursues, it is advisable to facilitate discussion in a manner that leads to authentic expression of participants; that is, drawing them out in a way that leads to personal, specific, and affective content, helping them to develop active coping skills, interpersonal support, and focusing on topics that are of greatest meaning, purpose, and value to each participant (Table 55–3).

DETERMINING THE FORMAT FOR THERAPEUTIC GROUPS

There is little question that group therapy is useful for cancer patient's quality of life. Current efforts are focusing on which types of groups are beneficial for which types of patients.[29] The therapeutic style utilized for helping cancer patients will depend upon the specific population seen in any particular group and the structure employed to serve these patients special needs. These factors are reviewed subsequently (Table 55–4).

Structure of the group. Thoughtful choices must be made in organizing a group for cancer patients, including the therapeutic intention, method of facilitation, populations comprising the group, and size and time-course of the group. These are each considered subsequently.

Therapeutic intent. Three basic structures of group therapy can be considered: informational education, coping skills training, and those offering social and emotional support, as well as combinations of these. Each of these structured formats is best served by a different therapeutic style. In general, informational education is best delivered through a deductive presentation, coping skills training by an interactive therapeutic style, and social and emotional support in an inductive facilitative style.

Table 55–2. Styles of therapeutic facilitation

Deductive	Interactive	Inductive
Lecture about set topics for education	Lecture about set topics Provide exercise to personalize Facilitate discussion for integration into patients' lives.	Discussion of any topic of concern raised by patients is facilitated by the therapist to enable authentic expression, stimulate active coping, and provide group support

SOURCES: Reprinted from Spira JL, "Group Therapies," Chapter 61 from Holland JC, *Psycho-oncology*, 1st ed. New York: Oxford University Press, 1999. With permission from Oxford University Press.

Table 55–3. Facilitating group discussion

Lead	Quality of expression *from inauthentic*		Therapeutic leads *to authentic*
Subject	Impersonal/external	*"How does that affect you personally?"*	Personal/internal
Object	Abstract/general	*"Can you give a specific example of that problem?"*	Concrete/specific
Affect	Intellectual/repressed	*"How does that make YOU feel?"*	Emotional/expression
Relationship	Solipsistic/isolated	*"Has anyone else had that type of experience?"*	Supportive/interactive
Coping	Passive/helpless	*"What can you do to handle the situation in a way that works better for YOU?"*	Active/appropriate control
Existential	Routine/meaningless	*"What could you do that would bring more meaning and value to your life?"*	Meaningful/living more fully

When needed, therapists ask open-ended questions to elicit more authentic patient expression. For example, in response to "Doctors never care what's going on with *you*, only what's going on with the *tumor!*" therapist might ask one or several of the above questions, depending on patients' subsequent responses.
SOURCE: Reprinted from Spira JL, "Group Therapies," Chapter 61 from Holland JC, *Psycho-oncology*, 1st ed. New York: Oxford University Press, 1999. With permission from Oxford University Press.

Table 55-4. Comparing the therapeutic emphasis of major facilitory styles

Facilitory style	Therapeutic emphasis		
	Therapeutic intent	Advice	Direct experience
Deductive (Educational)	Informational knowledge	Mostly given	None
Interactive (Cognitive behavioral)	Functional coping skills	Sometimes given	Reflection about problems occurring throughout one's life; practice specific skills through special exercises
Inductive (process facilitation)	Social/emotional support of existential concerns	Rarely given	Directly experience alternative ways of active coping through naturally arising interactions

SOURCE: Reprinted from Spira JL, "Group Therapies," Chapter 61 from Holland JC, *Psycho-oncology*, 1st ed. New York: Oxford University Press, 1999. With permission from Oxford University Press.

Informational-education. Informational groups are useful for those concerned with preventing cancer and early detection, and may focus on smoking cessation, breast self-examination, timely cancer screenings, the benefits of low-fat diets and exercise, and the like. An educational focus is also commonly offered for those recently diagnosed who wish to learn more information about their disease, treatment options, rehabilitative choices following surgery (physical therapy, cosmetic surgery, prosthetics etc.), and what, if any, preventive measures they can take in the future (sun exposure, skin creams, and self-examinations for melanoma patients). Typically brief (1–4 meetings), these groups are either lecture-oriented, with patients merely asking questions of the professional (arguably *not* group therapy), or with more of an active educational focus (e.g., teaching prevention skills as in smoking cessation or self-examination). Such groups are frequently coordinated by social workers with clinical nurse specialists as guest speakers, and are usually offered at no charge to participants.[34]

Coping skills. The most common type of group for cancer patients teaches active coping strategies focusing on specific and immediate concerns for the patient. These concerns include identifiable stressors and stress reactions, communication issues, practicing health behaviors such as diet and exercise, specific self-help techniques for reducing pain and nausea, and so on. Such groups are usually short-term (6–10 meetings), run 90–120 minutes per session, and most commonly utilize a cognitive-behavioral orientation. Typically, a therapist will present a topic for the first few minutes of a group, followed by a paper and pencil exercise or an interaction with a partner to practice a strategy. The rest of the group will be taken up with discussion on how one can implement and maintain these active coping strategies in one's life. Many times such groups will begin and end with a brief physical relaxation or cognitive-meditation training. Most often run by psychologists, social workers, or mental health nurse specialists trained in behavioral medicine techniques, these groups are effective for patients who have specific concerns about a recent cancer diagnosis.[35]

Social and emotional support. Persons with more advanced disease, or who are having difficulty adjusting to having cancer can benefit from longer-term therapy (3 months–1 year or longer). Since longer groups have the opportunity to form intimate bonds of support, patients are able to discuss virtually any issue of personal concern related to their living with cancer. Specific topics rarely need to be introduced by the therapists as all topics will eventually be raised by the patients. Such groups have the potential to address both immediate issues of coping with distress, as well as deeper existential considerations of changing priorities, self-image, and directly confronting issues of death and dying. In these groups, the patients are most active, with the therapists typically taking a back seat, only to emerge to keep the patients "on track" and to facilitate interactions. These types of groups are most similar to traditional group psychotherapy, with the modifications made for cancer patients rather than patients with strictly psychosocial dysfunction.

Combinations of educational coping skills and social-emotional support. Combinations of two or three of these major approaches are certainly not uncommon. Clearly, a health educator may provide mainly lecture, but then ask participants to practice a skill, and then facilitate discussion among the participants. A psychologist in a coping skills class may tend to focus on lecturing about and practice of specific skills, or else spend more time in facilitation of discussion, depending upon therapeutic orientation or persons in the group. Or, a typical 12-session group for new breast cancer patients may include (1) basic education of prosthesis or reconstructive surgery, (2) relaxation skills and pain management, and (3) discussion of how to communicate needs and desires to one's spouse, and so on. When resources permit, a different therapist may present different aspects of such mixed-orientation groups.

Open or closed groups. *Closed groups* are those which require all patients to join the group at the same time, and remain in the group for a committed duration (e.g., 16 weekly meetings), during which time no other patients can join. *Open groups,* in contrast are those which allow members to join at any time, for any length, as is common in *American Cancer Society* monthly drop-in support groups. Effective groups intending therapeutic improvement are either closed or semi-closed groups.

Semi-closed groups allow members to join when there is an opening in the group (member leaves, dies, or completes their commitment), but the patient must make a commitment for a specified duration.

Advantages of closed group are primarily in the consistency and ease of treatment. Disadvantages of closed groups are found in several areas. Often times recruiting new members for a group is challenging, so beginning a group with six patients while requiring newly interested patients to wait for months until the present group ends may be impractical. Short-term groups which have a specific agenda to cover may be able to demand a closed group. Yet in a long-term group with recurrent cancer patients, illness and death will reduce the size of the group to a point where it is difficult to continue effectively. Therefore, semi-closed groups are often utilized in longer-term formats.

Experiential methods. The incorporation of relaxation, meditation, and self-hypnosis into groups can be highly beneficial. Such methods introduced at the beginning and end of each group, can not only assist with tolerating side effects and reducing anxiety,[36] but can encourage fuller participation in the group, knowing that, however, much they bring up during the group, they can return to a state of mental and physical calmness before they leave.

APPLICATIONS TO SPECIFIC POPULATIONS

In deciding which therapeutic structures and styles to employ, it is necessary to consider factors associated with the patients being served. These factors include stage of disease, disease type, and the personal characteristics of those who make-up the groups.

Table 55–5. Therapeutic goals, methods, and structures useful for addressing the special issues of specific cancer populations

Stage of illness	Special issues	Goals	Methods	Structure
Prevention	At increased risk for disease incidence or recurrence	Education	Deductive: Didactic information	Brief Class (1–4 meetings)
Diagnosis	Distress over diagnosis Confusion about cancer	Education Coping in the moment Emotional Support	Interactive: Didactic information Experiential skills Inductive: Supportive discussion	Brief Group (1–6 weeks)
Treatment	Discomfort: nausea, pain, fatigue, etc. Reality of illness sets in	Coping with treatment Adjusting to life with cancer Emotional support	Interactive: Experiential skills Inductive: Supportive discussion	Brief to Short-term Group (4–12 weeks)
Recovery	Self-image (cancer patient) Questioning life activities Relationships Sense of control Possible recurrence or death Attitudes/behavior affecting Health	Active coping Emotional/social support Reexamining life values, beliefs, priorities Considering one's future Living a healthy lifestyle	Interactive: Cognitive therapy Experiential skills Inductive: Supportive discussion	Short-term Group (8–12 weeks to ongoing)
Recurrence and dying	Emotional distress Death and dying Coping with treatment Loss of control Family and friends Physical discomfort/ fatigue	Active coping Pain and stress management Emotional/social support Existential issues Living fully in the moment	Inductive: Supportive discussion Interactive: Experiential skills	Long-term Group (24 weeks to ongoing)
Family members and bereavement	Emotional distress Existential issues Guilt	Emotional support Work through distress Living more in the moment Planning for the future	Inductive: Supportive discussions Interactive: Experiential skills	As needed: Brief formats, weekly or monthly Support persons attend with patient Longer formats: Support and bereaved members meet separately for the most part

SOURCE: Reprinted from Spira JL, "Group Therapies," Chapter 61 from Holland JC, *Psycho-oncology*, 1st ed. New York: Oxford University Press, 1999. With permission from Oxford University Press.

Disease stage. Each stage of illness has its own special challenges which psychotherapists must be sensitive to determine appropriate therapeutic goals and select optimal methods and group structures to achieve these goals. The various group structures and therapeutic methods discussed above can be appropriately utilized to assist various types of persons with cancer (see Table 55–5).

Prevention. Individuals at increased risk for cancer incidence or recurrence are frequently interested in education about preventive and monitoring measures; however, learning skills to manage the stress of uncertainty is often just as important. The group method of education for these individuals is didactic which most often occurs in a brief format (between one and six weekly meetings).

Diagnosis. Patients who have recently received a first diagnosis of cancer are naturally distressed over the diagnosis, and may be confused about cancer, its etiology, treatment, and prognosis. Goals for this population should include basic education, stress management to attend more to the present and cope with immediate decisions regarding treatment, and emotional support. While some deductive intervention is useful for

offering basic information, therapeutic facilitation is primarily interactive for developing active coping skills, with some inductive facilitation for supportive discussion. It is difficult to mix didactic and interactive formats, since, once they have been lectured to, patients find it difficult to engage in discussion or open emotionally. Therefore, many therapists find it most beneficial to separate the didactic education from the interactive components. Different meetings, different parts of meetings separated by a break, or even different facilitators, can help patients to get the most out of each type of method.

Treatment. Special issues for persons undergoing treatment may include the need to deal with recovery from surgery and discomfort from chemotherapy and radiotherapy which often includes fatigue, nausea, dry or sore mucus membranes, weight changes, flu-like symptoms, and so on. Changes in appearance (e.g., hair loss) and daily functioning are also common. With these changes occurring, the urgency of dealing with the initial diagnosis and treatment decisions passing, and the initial shock subsiding, the reality of the illness begins to set-in. Patients at this stage are concerned with coping with treatment, adjusting to a lifestyle of being a cancer patient, and receiving emotional support. An interactive therapeutic style which offers emotional support and discussion along with experiential skills is therefore appropriate, and can be delivered effectively for most patients in a brief (4–12 week) group, at least initially.

Recovery. Once treatment is completed, a patient's concerns turn to changes in self-image (*"Am I a cancer patient?"*), changes in relationships, questioning and reprioritizing daily activities, wanting more control over one's health and course of disease, wondering whether personality or behavior affects their health, and considering the possibility of disease recurrence and death. Therapeutic goals for this stage include training in active coping strategies, offering emotional and social support, reexamining life values, beliefs, priorities, considering one's optimal future way of living, and learning to live a mentally and physically healthy lifestyle. Utilizing an interactive therapeutic style with a CBT orientation, teaching experiential coping skills, and then switching to an inductive therapeutic style allowing for supportive discussion will help achieve these skills, usually in a short-term (8–16 week) group format.

Recurrence and dying. Patients who have disease recurrence face substantial emotional distress (quite likely reexperiencing distress from the initial diagnosis, protracted and intensive treatment, greater loss of control, physical discomfort and fatigue, reduced daily functioning and decisions regarding retirement and disability, new ways of relating to family and friends, and also more directly confronting the likelihood of dying. Learning to cope more actively, managing pain and stress, receiving emotional support, addressing existential issues, and living more fully in each moment are goals that are extremely beneficial to patients at this stage of illness. An inductive approach allowing for supportive discussion and occasional interactive facilitation of experiential skills (relaxation, self-hypnosis) can facilitate these goals in a longer format (24 weeks to ongoing).

Family members and bereavement. Families of cancer patients should not be neglected. Assisting family members to cope better goes a long way in supporting the patient. Often times family members suffer many of the same issues as the patient. Therefore, a similar style of therapy may be appropriate for family members. In early stages of care (for patients who tested positive for genetic mutations, recently received a cancer diagnosis, or those coping with treatment), it is valuable to have family members present in the groups. However, for longer-term groups (greater than 4 weeks), patients and family members are better served in separate groups, so that they can each discuss their own concerns and not worry about distressing the other. Resources permitting, it can be convenient to have patients and family members meet at the same time, in adjacent rooms. Of course, not all patients have family members in the area, or who can attend such groups, and this lack of support should be addressed in the patient groups.

When a cancer patient dies, their surviving family members may face considerable emotional distress, existential considerations, and possibly guilt. Offering emotional support to work through grief requires an inductive, interactive format, along with teaching experiential skills (i.e., relaxation, self-hypnosis). Family members who have been involved in family groups while the patient was alive should be invited to stay on in the group for as long as they like. However, for many individuals a group specific to bereavement may provide a more appropriate means for processing the grief.

Disease type. In the same way that stages of disease can be broken down to address specific issues, type of cancer needs to be considered as well. Cancer patients, no matter what organ is affected, have many issues in common that should be addressed in groups. However, women with breast cancer have some very different concerns than do men with prostate cancer. Members of mixed-gender groups may find it difficult to discuss issues of prosthesis, reconstruction, or sexuality. Our clinical experience has shown that lung cancer patients often discuss issues related to the stigma and severity of the disease, while Hodgkin patients frequently try and put the disease behind them and learn to move on.

Demographic and cultural differences. Age, race, income, education, and so on all need to be considered when developing groups. For example, groups designed specifically to educate poor minority women about the need to receive regular Pap-smears and follow-up in case of cervical dysplasia[65] will be very different than a group of women in a wealthy community who meet to discuss the implications of cervical dysplasia. Another thing to consider is that ethnic minorities with cancer are less likely than Caucasian Americans to seek out and participate in group therapies. Lack of services, trust issues, and inadequate cultural competence of oncology professionals, is often pointed to as the culprit. However, investigations have revealed that minorities prefer to receive support from within their families, religious and communities groups, and are not likely to participate in groups unless they are encouraged by family or community members. This was found to be especially true for Latino Women[37] and Asian Americans.[38] Similarly, African-American men tend to underutilize online support groups preferring other avenues for receiving psychological and social support.[39] Therapists should consider these cultural factors when creating groups both in their composition and in their marketing.

Appropriate training for therapists. Although group psychotherapy for persons with cancer appears to be a subspecialty of group psychotherapy, this type of facilitation in fact requires more breadth of training than many other groups. Therapists should be familiar with psychotherapeutic methods including cognitive therapy (active coping skills), behavioral skills (relaxation, pain management), facilitation of social support and emotional expression (as outlined above), and existential considerations. While training and experience in these psychotherapeutic methods is essential, additional training in group therapy is also a prerequisite for effective group treatment. Finally, experience with medically ill patients is also useful. Until sufficient experience is obtained, co-leading groups with an experienced therapist can serve as excellent "on the job training." At the very least, these criteria should be achieved between two co-therapists.

Working with cancer patients can be extremely rewarding, as long as one is willing to confront issues of death and dying or strong negative emotions in an open and honest way. Fear of such issues and feelings will lead the therapist to avoid the patients' distress, which in turn may encourage patients to flee from their own emotions. It is normal to want to rush away from strong negative emotions and thoughts. However, if the therapist can lead the discussion therapeutically then the patients will be better able to tolerate their experiences, and cope more effectively with their emotions. A balance between accepting negative thoughts and feelings and considering ways to moderate them is far more effective than rushing into positive solutions, which can be a form of denial of the feelings and avoidance of issues the patient lives with constantly.

SUMMARY

Group therapy is a potent effective modality for giving psychosocial support to cancer patients and their families. Research over the past 30 years has shown repeated efficacy. Since there are now several excellent sources describing clinical methods of therapeutic intervention for a variety of types of cancer groups,[5,6,8] this chapter focused on the types of cancer groups that abound, especially those that have been shown to be effective for improving quality of life. Although many different approaches to group therapy for cancer patients are possible, it is clear that every effort to assist these patients and their families is warranted.

REFERENCES

1. Hellman CJ, Budd M, Borysenko J, McClelland DC, Benson H. A study of the effectiveness of two group behavioral medicine interventions for patients with psychosomatic complaints. *Behav Med.* 1990;16(4):165–73.

2. Lemieux J, Topp A, Chappell H, Ennis M, Goodwin PJ. Economic analysis of psychosocial group therapy in women with metastatic breast cancer. *Breast Cancer Res Treat.* 2006 Nov;100(2):183–190.

3. Hoey LM, Ieropoli SC, White VM, Jefford M. Systematic review of peer-support programs for people with cancer. *Patient Educ Couns.* 2008 Mar;70(3):315–337.

4. Corsini R, Rosenber B. Mechanisms of group psychotherapy: processes and dynamics. *J Abnorm Psychol.* 1955 Nov;51(3):406–11.

5. Spira JL, Reed GM. *Group psychotherapy for women with breast cancer.* 1st ed. Washington, DC: American Psychological Association; 2003.

6. Spiegel D, Classen C. *Group therapy for cancer patients a research-based handbook of psychosocial care.* New York: Basic Books; 2000.

7. Antoni MH, Smith R. *Stress management intervention for women with breast cancer.* Washington, DC: American Psychological Association; 2003.

8. Spira JL. *Group therapy for medically ill patients.* New York: Guilford Press; 1997.

9. Yalom ID. *The theory and practice of group psychotherapy.* New York: Basic Books; 1970.

10. Speigel D, Spira J. *Supportive expressive group therapy: A treatment manual of psychosocial intervention for women with recurrent breast cancer.* Stanford, CA: Stanford University School of Medicine Department of Psychiatry; 1991.

11. Fawzy FI, Fawzy NW, Wheeler JG. A post-hoc comparison of the efficiency of a psychoeducational intervention for melanoma patients delivered in group versus individual formats: an analysis of data from two studies. *Psychooncology.* 1996 Jun;5(2):81–89.

12. Jonhson J. The effects of a patient education course on persons with a chronic illness. *Cancer Nurs.* 1982;5(117):123.

13. Lerman C, Lustbader E, Rimer B, et al. Effects of individualized breast-cancer risk counseling—a randomized trial. *J Natl Cancer Inst.* 1995 Feb 15;87(4):286–292.

14. Cain EN, Kohorn EI, Quinlan DM, Latimer K, Schwartz PE. Psychosocial benefits of a cancer support group. *Cancer.* 1986 Jan 1;57(1):183–189.

15. Telch CF, Telch MJ. Group coping skills instruction and supportive group therapy for cancer patients: a comparison of strategies. *J Consult Clin Psychol.* 1986;54(6):802–808.

16. Cunningham AJ, Tocco EK. A randomized trial of group psychoeducational therapy for cancer-patients. *Patient Educ Couns.* 1989 Oct;14(2):101–14.

17. Evans RL, Connis RT. Comparison of brief group therapies for depressed cancer-patients receiving radiation treatment. *Public Health Rep.* 1995 May;110(3):306–311.

18. Spiegel D, Bloom JR, Kraemer HC, Gottheil E. Effect of psychosocial treatment on survival of patients with metastatic breast cancer. *Lancet.* 1987;2(8668):888–891.

19. Fox B. The role of psychological factors in cancer. *Incidence Prognosis Oncol.* 1995;9:245–52.

20. Goodwin PJ. Support groups in breast cancer: when a negative result is positive. *J Clin Oncol.* 2004 Nov 1;22(21):4244–4246.

21. Spiegel D, Butler LD, Giese-Davis J et al. Effects of supportive-expressive group therapy on survival of patients with metastatic breast cancer—a randomized prospective trial. *Cancer.* 2007 Sep 1;110(5):1130–1138.

22. Sidhu R, Passmore A, Baker D. The effectiveness of a peer support camp for siblings of children with cancer. *Pediatr Blood Cancer.* 2006 Oct 15;47(5):580–588.

23. Carter PA. A brief behavioral sleep intervention for family caregivers of persons with cancer. *Cancer Nurs.* 2006 Mar;29(2):95–103.

24. Collie K, Kreshka MA, Ferrier S, et al. Videoconferencing for delivery of breast cancer support groups to women living in rural communities: a pilot study. *Psychooncology.* 2007 Aug;16(8):778–782.

25. Im EO, Chee W, Liu Y, et al. Characteristics of cancer patients in internet cancer support groups. *Comput Inform Nurs.* 2007 Nov;25(6):334–343.

26. Hoey LM, Ieropoli SC, White VM, Jefford M. Systematic review of peer-support programs for people with cancer. *Patient Educ Couns.* 2008 Mar;70(3):315–337.

27. Sheard T, Maguire P. The effect of psychological interventions on anxiety and depression in cancer patients: results of two meta-analyses. *Br J Cancer.* 1999 Jul 9;80(11):1770–1780.

28. Kissane DW, Bloch S, Smith GC, et al. Cognitive-existential group psychotherapy for women with primary breast cancer: a randomised controlled trial. *Psychooncology.* 2003 Sep;12(6):532–546.

29. Helgeson VS, Cohen S, Schulz R, Yasko J. Group support interventions for women with breast cancer: who benefits from what? *Health Psychol.* 2000 Mar;19(2):107–114.

30. Sheard T, Maguire P. The effect of psychological interventions on anxiety and depression in cancer patients: results of two meta analyses. *Br J Cancer.* 1999 Aug;80(11):1770–1780.

31. Spira J, Spiegel D. Group psychotherapy of the medically ill. In: Stoudemire A, Fogel BS (eds). *Psychiatric care of the medical patient.* 2nd ed. New York: Oxford University Press; 1993:31–50.

32. Roberts CS, Cox CE, Reintgen DS, Baile WF, Gibertini M. Influence of physician communication on newly-diagnosed breast patients psychologic adjustment and decision-making. *Cancer.* 1994 Jul 1;74(1):336–341.

33. Maslow AH. *Toward a psychology of being.* 2d ed. Princeton, NJ: Van Nostrand; 1968.

34. Mooney S, Greer S, Watson M, et al. Adjuvant psychological therapy for patients with cancer: outcome at one year. *Psychooncology.* 1994;3:39–47.

35. Mitchell JT, Everly GS. *Critical incident stress debriefing—(CISD) an operations manual for the prevention of traumatic stress among emergency services and disaster workers.* Ellicott City, MD: Chevron Pub; 1993.

36. Kabat-Zinn J, Massion AO, Herbert JR, Rosenbaum E. Meditation. In: Holland JC, Breitbart W (eds). *Psychooncology.* New York: Oxford University Press; 1998.

37. Napoles-Springer AM, Ortiz C, O'Brien H, az-Mendez M, Perez-Stable EJ. Use of cancer support groups among Latina breast cancer survivors. *J Cancer Surviv.* 2007 Sep;1(3):193–204.

38. Ashing KT, Padilla G, Tejero J, Kagawa-Singer M. Understanding the breast cancer experience of Asian American women. *Psychooncology.* 2003 Jan;12(1):38–58.

39. Fogel J, Ribisl KM, Morgan PD, Humphreys K, Lyons EJ. Underrepresentation of African Americans in online cancer support groups. *J Natl Med Assoc.* 2008 Jun;100(6):705–712.

CHAPTER 56

Cognitive and Behavioral Interventions

Brittany M. Brothers, Lisa M. Thornton, and Barbara L. Andersen

A diagnosis of cancer can be devastating. Patients may be overwhelmed with the necessities of the diagnosis, such as choosing physicians, making treatment decisions, coping with side effects of treatment, navigating financial strain, and managing the disruption to the family. Added to this burden may be depressive and anxiety disorders—a prevalence exceeding 20% among the newly diagnosed. In this chapter we focus on these patients, who have been underserved by psychological/psychiatric and the oncology communities. It is also important that the second generation of psychological intervention trials for cancer patients focus on those patients in greatest need, whether the needs be psychological or other needs which result in poorer biobehavioral morbidity or disease mortality.

Depressive and anxiety disorders among adults are common. More than 19 million Americans experience these disorders annually, with 50% of patients with major depressive disorder (MDD) also having a co-morbid anxiety disorder.[1,2] With aging, adults become vulnerable to physical illnesses such as cancer, and medical illness, disability, and functional decline are risk factors for mental disorders.[3] Despite the added risk that chronic illness poses, there has been a dearth of research on co-morbidity of psychiatric disorders among cancer patients and no determination of which therapies might be suitable and efficacious.

FACING CANCER WITH THE BURDEN OF PSYCHOPATHOLOGY

Mood and anxiety disorders are common, disabling, and unremitting. Over 16% of people will experience a MDD in their lifetime, with 6.6% meeting criteria for depression within a 12-month period.[4] For anxiety disorders, lifetime estimates are currently 16.6%, with 12-month prevalence of 10.6%.[5] Generalized anxiety disorder (GAD) is one of the most common of the anxiety disorders. Lifetime prevalence estimates of GAD range from 4% to 7%, with 12-month estimates ranging from 3% to 5%. Both MDD and GAD are associated with substantial functional impairment.[6–9] Unfortunately, circumstances are made even more difficult by the fact that, for the individual, co-morbidity of psychopathology tends to be the rule, not the exception. Of those with MDD, it is likely that within 12 months, 58% of them will also meet criteria for an anxiety disorder.[4] Of the comorbidities, MDD/GAD is the most common. In fact, there is evidence that genetic risk for MDD and GAD is largely shared.[10] Finally, both GAD and MDD are more common for women than men; depression, in fact, is the leading cause of disease-related disability among women.[11]

Rates for mood and anxiety disorders are high, but they increase further for the medically ill. For example, rates of depression range from 9% in outpatient clinics to 30% or more among the hospitalized.[12] Not surprisingly, the diagnosis of a life threatening illness can be a risk factor for a depressive episode or an anxiety attack.[13] Indeed, the lifetime prevalence of any psychiatric disorder for those with chronic illness is higher—42%—than is found for the general population (i.e., 33%[14]). With the two most common killers—heart disease and cancer—mental disorders among patients are well above the base rate[15] and are linked to disease course, morbidity, and death. The greatest study has focused on depression, anxiety, and coronary heart disease.[16–19] By contrast, much less is known about depression and anxiety in the context of cancer, even though both disorders are more prevalent among cancer patients than among coronary heart disease patients (or *any other* chronic illnesses patient, (e.g., respiratory or cerebrovascular disease, diabetes[20]).

The absence of study of psychopathology among cancer patients is alarming. In both early and recent surveys, 30%–50% of patients studied meet criteria for mood or anxiety disorders,[21–23] with depression being the most common.[24,25] Estimates for MDD are 22%–29% for patients with early-stage (stage I) disease,[26] 8%–40% for patients with advanced disease,[27] and the rates increase further with recurrence.[21] The numbers of patients with anxiety disorders are somewhat lower, approximately 18%, with GAD among the most common.[28] As is the case for those without concurrent physical illness, depression and anxiety co-occur among cancer patients. Thirty-eight percent (38%) of cancer patients found to have anxiety disorders by Stark et al.[28] also had MDD.

With such a high base, one might expect that patients with co-morbidity would be readily identified, but they are not. For example, among 112 women with major depression undergoing cancer treatment, Ell[29] found that few were being treated: only 12% were receiving anti depressants and only 5% receiving psychological therapy. Excepting the most obvious symptoms (e.g., suicidal ideation[30]), diagnostic criteria for psychopathology may not be known or recognized by a busy oncology team, symptoms may be trivialized as a "normal" reaction, or interpreted as due only to impaired physical status.[20] Indeed, studies show that oncologists and nurses detect depressive symptoms in only a third of the patients who have them and then under estimate their severity.[31–33] Even when recognized and antidepressant medication is prescribed, patients may not receive an adequate dose.[34,35] But it should be noted that many with anxiety or depression without co-morbid physical illness also go untreated.[3,36–38] In addition to lack of symptom relief, however, the absence of treatment brings added sequelae—more symptom distress,[39–41] less meaning in life,[42,43] less social support,[44,45] maladaptive coping,[46] and employment absenteeism,[47] among others.

EFFICACIOUS PSYCHOLOGICAL TREATMENTS FOR MOOD AND ANXIETY DISORDERS

Fortunately, efficacious treatments exist, with the primary options being medication[48] or psychotherapy,[49] and testing their relative efficacy has been a priority.[50] Among psychotherapies, the most extensively studied, with over 325 outcome studies, is cognitive-behavioral therapy (CBT[51,52]), and it is an effective treatment for both mood and anxiety disorders. In randomized controlled trials (RCTs), CBT has generally been found to be as effective as antidepressant medication.[53] Even among the severely depressed, Hollon and colleagues[54] found that both produced comparable results (approximately 58% treatment responders in both arms) during the acute phase, but when discontinued, patients treated with CBT were at lower risk for relapse than those treated with medication, even for as long as 2 years. Overall, when effect sizes for CBT are examined across trials, they are large. For short-term posttreatment outcomes, median effect sizes have been 0.61 for depressive disorders and 0.69 for anxiety disorders.[55–60] Few studies have followed patients beyond 12–18 months, however. The available effect size estimates for long term outcomes are roughly half the magnitude of the short-term effects.[59–61]

Cognitive-behavioral therapy for depression has three components.[62] *Behavioral activation* involves efforts to increase patients' engagement in activities and contexts that may allow them to experience pleasure or a sense of accomplishment; behavioral activation is also done to promote cognitive change.[63] Second, *correcting negative automatic thoughts* is a collaborative process when therapist and client work together to identify and evaluate depressive thinking accompanying patients' negative mood states. Once patients have mastered these and other basic skills (e.g., problem solving, assertive communication), therapists assist clients to *identify and change core beliefs and schema, which*, more generally, underlie a depressed patient's pervasive, negative beliefs. Research suggests that all three components are important, although some studies show the contrary.[64]

The efficacy of CBT for GAD is also strong. Unlike the depression trials, many fewer RCTs have compared medications to CBT, but in them, CBT outperforms medications.[65] This conclusion is tempered, however, by the limiting factor of benzodiazepines being the primary drug with which CBT has been compared. Relative to other treatments/conditions, however, meta-analytic reviews show CBT for GAD to be superior to wait-list conditions, no treatment control conditions, non-directive therapy, and pill placebo conditions.[57,65] CBT for GAD clearly produces significant improvements in the acute phase of treatment as it does for MDD, but the strongest findings are from studies showing its long-term effects. Durham and colleagues[66] found that GAD patients who received CBT (compared to those receiving medication, placebo, or analytic psychotherapy) had lower symptom severity and were less likely to have sought additional treatment during the next 8–14 years, suggesting enduring effects. CBT for GAD involves several components. As worry is pathognomonic, patients are first taught to attend the internal and external cues that precede their worry. Second, patients are taught progressive muscle relaxation training and encouraged to use it for preventing and/or reducing daily symptoms. Thirdly, patients are taught cognitive coping skills, as is done in CBT for depression. Patients learn to identify and correct their automatic worries and perception of future threats (rather than correcting negative self-relevant views as is done for depression). To practice their new coping strategies, in-session imagery rehearsal is used[67] and then out-of-session homework follows. Earlier research suggested that the cognitive elements of treatment were essential for efficacy.[68] More recent RCTs suggest that cognitive therapy, applied relaxation with self-control desensitization condition, and the combination are similarly efficacious.[69]

While having strong empirical support for the treatment of MDD and GAD, it is unclear if CBT would be efficacious with cancer patients with MDD or GAD. The available data with unscreened patients is encouraging. Some psychological intervention studies with cancer patients[70-75] have included components of CBT (e.g., relaxation training, assertiveness training, thought monitoring). Other RCTs have tested the efficacy of a single component, such as cognitive reappraisal[76,77] or problem solving.[78-80] Across studies with unscreened patients, there is a predominance of positive, significant findings at posttreatment[72-74,77-79] rather than null.[71,75,76] Three trials, however, tested a comprehensive CBT intervention and/or tested CBT with screened patients and confirmed its efficacy in comparison to no treatment, and further, found CBT to be equivalent to[74,81] if not superior to[78,82] a traditional cancer support group at posttreatment. Few studies have included follow-up data (which is critically important for psychopathology outcomes), and it is unclear if patients maintain their gains. Two studies reported patients doing so[77,78] and three did not[72,73,83] for intervals ranging from 4 to 12 months posttreatment.

In summary, the findings are suggestive that CBT may be efficacious for cancer patients with psychopathology. There are components of CBT that seem well suited for cancer patients coping with depression. The cognitive diathesis implicated in cognitive models of depression[84,85] may be readily activated with the cancer stressor. Most patients are thrust into an unfamiliar, complex medical environment and life trajectories are suddenly uncertain. Depressed patients without cancer tend to view their environment as overwhelming, obstacle laden, and for some, there is hopelessness. Cancer patients, in general, respond to the diagnostic period with similar judgments.[86] Thus, CBT's direct treatment of distorted cognitions, feelings of helplessness, and/or pessimism about the future would be timely and appropriate. Similarly, the magnitude of stress accompanying cancer may be so significant that it may trigger depressed patients core beliefs ("I am worthless, inadequate, unlovable, deficient."), and CBT directly identifies, challenges, and attempts to change these recurrent, negative, self views. Similar advantages for

CBT would be expected for cancer patients diagnosed with GAD. For those who have gone untreated, GAD is oftentimes a lifelong disorder,[87] and the chronic, anxious apprehension characterizing these individuals would be easily activated with a cancer diagnosis. For them, CBT would identify specific worries and address their typical overestimation of the likelihood of negative events and/or catastrophizing. The relaxation therapy component of CBT for GAD would be particularly helpful for cancer patients, as it has been shown to be so in other contexts.[88]

Yet, CBT may have limitations because it is the context of cancer. Behavioral activation is a component important to treatment efficacy. However, activities typically prescribed as homework would need to be significantly modified for patients undergoing or recovering from cancer treatment. Helping patients' cope with side effects or physical morbidities is not a part of cognitive therapy, nor is assistance in coping with practical, cancer-specific issues such as understanding how the cancer treatments work or choosing treatments,[89] for example. In a related manner, it may be difficult for patients to identify unrealistic or exaggerated negative views of the self when there are emergent, immediate, and multiple cancer-relevant stressors and negative sequelae. Thus, as one of the most extensively researched forms of psychotherapy, it would be important to know the efficacy CBT with depressed and/or anxious cancer patients.

PSYCHOSOCIAL TREATMENTS FOR DISTRESS IN CANCER PATIENTS

Psychological interventions tailored to the context of cancer are efficacious for reducing cancer stress and distress.[90-92] Unlike the psychopathology research literature which has advanced to compare components to the CBT "package,"[69] interventions with cancer patients have varied from study to study and there have been few replications.[93,94] RCTs in cancer have primarily contrasted intervention and control arms (e.g., no intervention, waitlist, usual care), with many fewer multiarm studies. In the latter, significant differences often do not emerge,[95-99] likely due to reduced power from small and/or heterogeneous samples. Meta-analyses suggest that interventions may be more effective in treating symptoms of anxiety rather than depression,[100] but again, the majority of studies have included unscreened samples.

Many treatments are cognitive behavioral in orientation with added stress management. In contrast to CBT for psychopathology, however, cognitive change and behavioral activation are rarely central. Common treatment components are some form of active di/stress reduction (e.g., progressive muscle relaxation, guided imagery), information about the disease and treatment, an emotionally supportive context for treatment (with the "component" often being treatment in a support group format), behavioral coping strategies (e.g., seeking information), cognitive-coping strategies (e.g., cognitive reframing), and tailored, site specific interventions (e.g., sun protection for melanoma patients). While such components are based in CBT, they are included at the discretion of the trial investigator or individual therapist, rather than routinely administered. It is infrequent for interventions to include components for improving health behaviors[98,101] or adherence.[96]

The efficacy of these same interventions for cancer patients with comorbid depressive or anxiety disorders is unclear. To our knowledge, only 9 of 200+ RCTs either screened patients for clinical levels of distress or, did not screen, but did assess for psychiatric diagnoses. Across studies, the interventions were varied. Five interventions included one or more of the "core" CBT components. A methodologically strong, early study was that by Telch and Telch[82] who screened patients for high distress and compared CBT to support group and control arms. The 6-week intervention included behavioral activation and "constructive thinking" in addition to relaxation, stress management, assertive communication, problem solving, and feelings management. The CBT group was most effective, and this is one of the few studies in the literature showing the control group to actually worsen. Moorey et al.[79] accrued patients diagnosed with an adjustment reaction and found problem-focused CBT to significantly reduce depressive and anxiety symptoms compared to supportive counseling. The intervention had 6–8 sessions with the patient and, optionally, the spouse. Cognitive change

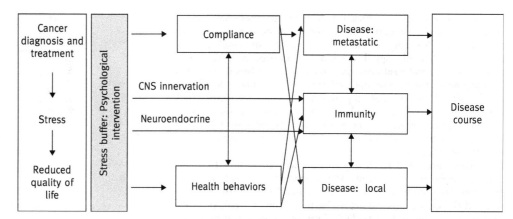

Fig. 56–1. The biobehavioral model of cancer stress and disease course.
ABBREVIATION: CNS, central nervous system.
SOURCE: Reference 109.

was achieved through identification of automatic thoughts, as is done in classic CBT for depression. Behavioral activation was also included, along with progressive muscle relaxation, spousal communication strategies, and fostering a "fighting spirit." To treat insomnia among breast cancer patients (56% of whom had psychiatric disorders), Savard et al.[77] offered stimulus control/sleep hygiene and cognitive restructuring in an 8-session group intervention and significantly improved patients sleep patterns and also reduced depressed moods. Education and behavioral strategies for sleep hygiene were also included. While not determining *Diagnostic and Statistical Manual* of Mental Disorders (DSM) diagnoses, Nezu and colleagues[78] accrued only patients scoring within the clinical range on the Hamilton Rating Scale of Depression.[102,103] They found individual problem solving therapy to have robust, positive effects across depression, distress, and quality of life outcomes. Like Savard et al., Nezu included cognitive restructuring only in service to a specific aim: to modify dysfunctional cognitions, which interfered with effective problem solving. Finally, a recent pilot by Hopko[104] found pre- to post-CBT treatment gains for 18 patients, all with MDD. Hopko's intervention was unique in using behavioral activation as the central treatment component. Nine individual sessions were focused on increasing activities that foster a sense of pleasure or mastery.

An additional four interventions targeting distressed individuals did not include core CBT components. Simpson et al.[105] provided group treatment combining stress management and goal setting to breast cancer patients (26% of whom had depressive or anxiety disorders) and found no significant improvement. This 6-week group intervention did not include cognitive change or behavioral activation components, but did include progressive muscle relaxation, self-hypnosis, mental imagery, stress management, goal setting, and planning/achieving change. Petersen and Quinlivan[106] effectively reduced anxious and depressive symptoms in gynecologic patients through relaxation training. Finally, Kissane and colleagues tested supportive expressive group therapy (based on an existential, rather than cognitive-behavioral perspective) in two studies. In the first,[107] stage I/II breast cancer patients (36% of whom had depressive or anxiety disorders) showed no improvement in depressive symptoms but a trend toward reductions in anxiety symptomatology. Kissane reported positive findings, however, with supportive-expressive group therapy offered to breast cancer patients with metastasis (32% of whom had a mood disorder)[108]; the intervention significantly reduced hopelessness and traumatic stress, improved social functioning, and prevented new depressive disorders.

In summary, there is suggestive support for general psychosocial interventions as effective for cancer patients with psychopathology. Psychosocial interventions are tailored to help the patient with the immediate, overwhelming stressor—cancer. Such interventions normalize patients' worries, fears, and concerns. They offer active, behavior change strategies to cope, such as seeking information to answer disease relevant questions. Coping strategies to reduce both the psychological and physiologic manifestations of anxiety and treat symptoms (e.g., chemotherapy nausea/vomiting) are often included. To the extent that these elements have efficacy equaling (if not exceeding) disorder-specific elements of CBT, psychological interventions for cancer patients might be at least (if not more) efficacious.

BIOBEHAVIORAL INTERVENTION (BBI) FOR CANCER STRESS: APPLICABILITY TO PATIENTS WITH PSYCHIATRIC CO-MORBIDITY

The Biobehavioral Model of Cancer Stress and Disease Course, detailed in Andersen, Kiecolt-Glaser and Glaser[109] (see Fig. 56–1), has guided our previous research, and we offer that it has applicability to cancer patients with co-morbid psychiatric disorders. According to the model, severe, acute stress occurs at the time of cancer diagnosis.[110–112] Diagnostic stress can contribute to a stable, lower quality of life,[113] depressive symptoms,[114] and less meaning in patients' lives.[115] We suggest there would be an even more difficult trajectory for cancer patients with co-morbid psychiatric disorders.

Cancer stress also triggers biological effects. We have confirmed that stress at diagnosis covaries with immune downregulation.[116] Stress-related alterations could, in turn, affect mood or elicit symptoms consistent with depressive or anxiety disorders. Immune activation has been hypothesized as a causal factor in depression, as proinflammatory cytokines have been shown to produce "sickness behaviors," that is, fatigue, lethargy, anorexia, and low mood.[117] Anxiety, too, is correlated with immune and endocrine function.[118] Finally, both depression and anxiety are believed to contribute to further dysregulation of the hypothalamic-pituitary-adrenal (HPA) axis, an overactive inflammatory response, and decreased cellular immunity.[118–121] Thus, we would expect a robust down regulation of immunity for cancer patients facing diagnosis with a co-morbid psychiatric disorder.

The biobehavioral model suggested that stress at diagnosis also produces important behavioral sequelae. Regarding health behaviors, negative ones (e.g., dietary changes, caffeine use) can intensify the physiologic effects of stress, such as increasing catecholamine release.[122] Conversely, positive health behaviors, such as regular physical exercise, may decrease in frequency or be abandoned.[123,124] Negative health behaviors covary with a downward trend in immunity (e.g., smoking[125,126]), but if they are reduced, immunity may rebound or even be enhanced.[127] Positive health behaviors, such as exercise, may enhance immunity and additionally have a positive impact on mood,[6] even for those with major depression.[128,129] Another important behavioral factor is compliance or cancer treatment adherence. Depression, in fact, is a correlate of noncompliance.[130,131] Thus, patients with co-morbid disorders would be at greater risk for high rates of negative and low rates of positive health behaviors and lowered treatment adherence. Moreover, patients with co-morbidity would be at greater risk for poorer health, including slower recovery, higher levels of morbidity, and perhaps, poorer survival.

A randomized trial, the Stress and Immunity Breast Cancer Project (SIBCP), was designed to test the model and the hypothesis that provision of a psychological intervention would not only reverse the negative pathways in the model but also improve survival. The biobehavioral intervention (BBI) that was developed produced some of the most robust effects yet documented in the psychosocial cancer literature. Intervention patients were found to have significant gains at the end of both the intensive (4 month[132]) and maintenance phases (12 month[133]). Compared to the Assessment only arm, patients in the Biobehavioral

Intervention arm had significant reductions in emotional distress, increases in social support from family members, improved dietary behaviors (i.e., lowering fat intake, reductions in smoking), reduced variability in chemotherapy dose intensity, improved immunity, fewer signs/symptoms and treatment toxicities, and higher functional status. Mechanisms of the intervention's effectiveness have been identified.[134] Finally, the BBI intervention improved survival. After a median of 11 years, analyses showed, as predicted, that the Intervention arm had a reduced risk of breast cancer recurrence (Hazard ratio [HR] 0.55, $p = 0.034$) and breast cancer death (HR 0.44, $p = 0.016$) compared to the Assessment only arm.

We have conducted secondary analyses with the SIBCP to test its potential applicability to patients with co-morbid psychopathology. We determined that approximately 25% (n = 56 of 227) of the SIBCP sample reported clinically significant depressive (i.e., Center for Epidemiologic Studies Depression Scale [CES-D][135] short form scores ≥10) or anxiety symptoms (scores ≥20 on both the intrusion and avoidance subscales of the Impact of Event Scale (IES)[136]). Thirty patients (54%) were randomized to the assessment arm and the remaining 26 (44%) to the intervention arm. Using linear mixed effects models and controlling for baseline levels, the BBI significantly reduced anxious ($p = 0.001$; Cohen's D=. 63; Fig. 56–2, top) and depressed moods ($p = 0.012$; Cohen's D = .48; Fig. 56–2, middle and bottom) as assessed with the Profile of Mood States and the CES-D.[137] Also, response rates, defined as a change of 1.96 or greater on the reliable change index,[138] were higher in the BBI arm than in the Assessment only arm (71% vs. 45%). These data suggest that significant symptom relief would occur for patients with depressive or anxiety disorders who receive the BBI treatment.

An important test of the model is to examine whether intervention-related improvements in psychological outcomes would trigger improvements in associated biological outcomes. Mediation analyses suggest that reduction of emotional distress during the intervention lead to better health outcomes (functional status, physical symptoms) 12 months after diagnosis.[133] For patients with significant depressive symptomatology, reducing depressive and associated symptoms (pain, fatigue) lead to reductions in indicators of inflammation (e.g., white blood cell counts).[139] These data support the causal paths in the model by showing that an intervention which can effectively improve psychological functioning can have salutary downstream effects on health and disease.

SUMMARY

Depressive and anxiety disorders of cancer patients are prevalent, unrecognized, and untreated. In general, little is known, even though both depression and anxiety are more prevalent among cancer patients than among those with *any other* chronic illness,[13] and there is now evidence of higher suicide rates in cancer patients as well.[140] Breast cancer patients have received significant psychosocial study, but it is painfully ironic that it has not prevented the worst of depression's outcomes: suicide. Breast cancer patients have an increased risk of suicide for as long 25 years following diagnosis.[141]

Plausible, efficacious treatments exist. To the extent that both CBT for MDD and GAD and the psychosocial treatments have independent active ingredients, a combination treatment may be most effective overall. It is the "cognitive" component (i.e., addressing the disorder-specific cognitive diathesis, identifying and evaluating depressive/anxious cognitions, etc.) of CBT that has been most often missing from psychosocial interventions. To the extent that psychosocial treatments additionally address the cognitive diatheses underlying psychopathologies and to the extent that CBT might additionally include disease-specific elements, a combination treatment might be more efficacious than either treatment alone. The BBI provided significant psychological, behavioral, immune, health, and survival benefits, with suggestive effectiveness for symptoms of psychopathology. Regardless of the therapeutic model(s) chosen for study, what is important is that the professional community begins to address needs of patients with co-morbid psychopathology.

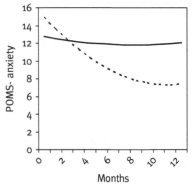

Group X time effect $p = 0.001$

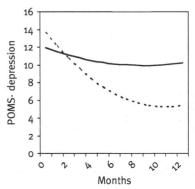

Group X time effect $p = 0.012$

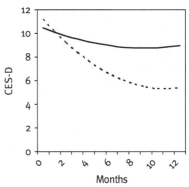

Group X time effect $p = 0.069$

Fig. 56–2. Biobehavioral Intervention reduced emotional distress for patients with clinically significant depressive or anxiety symptoms (n=56).
ABBREVIATIONS: POMS, Profile of Mood States; CES-D, Center for Epidemiological Studies-Depression Scale.
NOTE: *P* values refer to the fixed interaction effect in a mixed effects model; Solid line = Assessment only group Dotted line = Intervention group

ACKNOWLEDGMENT

Sources of support: National Cancer Institute (R01CA92704, K05 CA098133), National Institute of Mental Health (R01MH51487), with additional support from the American Cancer Society (PBR-89, PF-07-169-01-CPPB), the Longaberger Company-American Cancer Society (PBR-89A), and the U.S. Army Medical Research Acquisition Activity (DAMD17-94-J-4165, DAMD17-96-1-6294, and DAMD17-97-1-7062). We thank the patients for their participation and guidance.

REFERENCES

1. Massie MJ. Prevalence of depression in patients with cancer. *J Natl Cancer Inst Monogr.* 2004;32:57–71.

2. Grady-Weliky TA. *Comorbidity and its implication on treatment: Change over the life span.* Syllabus and Proceedings Summary, American Psychiatric Association, 2002, Annual Meeting. Philadelphia, PA; 2002:295.

3. Kessler RC, Berglund P, Demler O, Jin R, Walters EE. Lifetime prevalence and age-of-onset distributions of DSM-IV disorders in the National Comorbidity Survey Replication. *Arch Gen Psychiatry.* 2005;62:593–602.

4. Kessler R. Depression is a timely topic. *Comp Health Prac Rev.* 2003;8:6–8.

5. Somers JM, Goldner EM, Waraich P, Hsu L. Prevalence and incidence studies of anxiety disorders: a systematic review of the literature. *Can J Psychiatry.* 2006;100–113.

6. Trivedi MH, Greer TL, Grannemann BD, Endicott J. Exercise as an augmentation strategy for treatment of major depression. *J Psychiatr Pract.* 2006;12:205–211.

7. Lyness JM, Kim J, Tang W, et al. The clinical significance of subsyndromal depression in older primary care patients. *Am J Geriatr Psychiatry.* 2007;15:214–223.

8. Rapaport MH, Clary C, Fayyad R, Endicott J. Quality-of-life impairment in depressive and anxiety disorders. *Am J Psychiatry.* 2005;162:1171–1178.

9. Kessler RC, DuPont RL, Berglund P, Wittchen H-U. Impairment in pure and comorbid generalized anxiety disorder and major depression at 12 months in two national surveys. *Am J Psychiatry.* 1999;156:1915–1923.

10. Kendler KS, Gardner CO, Gatz M, Pedersen NL. The sources of co-morbidity between major depression and generalized anxiety disorder in a Swedish national twin sample. *Psychol Med.* 2007;37:453–462.

11. Murray CJL, Lopez AD. *The global burden of disease: a comprehensive assessment of mortality and disability from diseases, injuries, and risk factors in 1990 and projected to 2020, Global burden of disease and injury series.* Cambridge, MA, Harvard School of Public Health on behalf of the World Health Organization and the World Bank; 1996.

12. Katon W, Sullivan MD. Depression and chronic medical illness. *J Clin Psychiatry.* 1990;51:3–11.

13. Evans DL, Charney DS, Lewis L, et al. Mood disorders in the medically ill: Scientific review and recommendations. *Biol Psychiatr.* 2005;58:175–189.

14. Wells KB, Golding JM, Burnam MA. Psychiatric disorder in a sample of the general population with and without chronic medical conditions. *Am J Psychiatry.* 1988;145:976–981.

15. Rudisch B. Epidemiology of comorbid coronary artery disease and depression. *Biol Psychiatr.* 2003;54:227–240.

16. Wulsin LR, Singal BM. Do depressive symptoms increase the risk for the onset of coronary disease? A systematic quantitative review. *Psychosom Med.* 2003;65:201–210.

17. Barefoot JC, Schroll M. Symptoms of depression, acute myocardial infarction, and total mortality in a community sample. *Circulation.* 1996;93:1976–1980.

18. Frasure-Smith N, Lesperance F. Depression—a cardiac risk factor in search of a treatment. *JAMA.* 2003;289:3171–3173.

19. Bush DE, Ziegelstein RC, Tayback M, et al. Even minimal symptoms of depression increase mortality risk after acute myocardial infarction. *Am J Cardiol.* 2001;88:337–341.

20. Evans DL, Charney DS, Lewis L, et al. Mood disorders in the medically ill: scientific review and recommendations. *Biol Psychiatr.* 2005;58:175–189.

21. Burgess C, Cornelius V, Love S, Graham J, Richards M, Ramirez A. Depression and anxiety in women with early breast cancer: five year observational cohort study. *BMJ.* 2005;330:1–4.

22. Derogatis LR, Melisaratos N. The Brief Symptom Inventory: an introductory report. *Psychol Med.* 1983;13:595–605.

23. Zabora JR, Brintzenhofeszoc K, Curbow B, Hooker C, Piantadosi S. The prevalence of psychological distress by cancer site. *Psychooncology.* 2001;10:19–28.

24. van't Spijker A, Trijsburg RW, Duivenvoorden HJ. Psychological sequelae of cancer diagnosis: a meta-analytical review of 58 studies after 1980. *Psychosom Med.* 1997;59:280–93.

25. Massie MJ, Greenberg DB. Oncology. In: Levenson JL (ed). *The American psychiatric publishing textbook of psychosomatic medicine.* Chicago: American Medical Association; 2005:517–534.

26. Raison CL, Miller AH. Depression in cancer: new developments regarding diagnosis and treatment. *Biol Psychiatr.* 2003;54:283–294.

27. Hotopf M, Chidgey J, Addington-Hall J, Ly KL. Depression in advanced disease: a systematic review Part 1. Prevalence and case finding. *Palliative Medicine.* 2002;16:81–97.

28. Stark D, Kiely M, Smith A, Velikova G, House A, Selby P. Anxiety disorders in cancer patients: their nature, associations, and relation to quality of life. *J Clin Oncol.* 2002;20:3137–3148.

29. Ell K, Sanchez K, Vourlekis B, et al. Depression, correlates of depression, and receipt of depression care among low-income women with breast or gynecologic cancer. *J Clin Oncol.* 2005;23:3052–3060.

30. Oquendo MA, Galfalvy H, Russo S, et al. Prospective study of clinical predictors of suicidal acts after a major depressive episode in patients with major depressive disorder or bipolar disorder. *Am J Psychiatry.* 2004;161:1433–1441.

31. Keller MB, McCullough JP, Klein DN, et al. A comparison of nefazodone, the cognitive behavioral-analysis system of psychotherapy, and their combination for the treatment of chronic depression. *N Engl J Med.* 2000;342:1462–1470.

32. McDonald MV, Passik SD, Dugan W, Rosenfeld B, Theobald DE, Edgerton S. Nurses' recognition of depression in their patients with cancer. *Oncol Nurs Forum.* 1999;26:593–599.

33. Newell S, Sanson-Fisher RW, Girgis A, Bonaventura A. How well do medical oncologists' perceptions reflect their patients' reported physical and psychosocial problems? Data from a survey of five oncologists. *Cancer.* 1998;83:1640–1651.

34. Ashbury FD, Madlensky L, Raich P, et al. Antidepressant prescribing in community cancer care. *Support Care Cancer.* 2003;11:278–285.

35. Sharpe M, Strong V, Allen K, et al. Major depression in outpatients attending a regional cancer centre: screening and unmet treatment needs. *Br J Cancer.* 2004;90:314–320.

36. Olfson M, Marcus SC, Druss B, Elinson L, Tanielian T, Pincus HA. National trends in the outpatient treatment of depression. *J Am Med Assoc.* 2002;287:203–209.

37. Dietrich AJ, Oxman TE, Williams JW, et al. Going to scale: re-engineering systems for primary care treatment of depression. *Ann Fam Med.* 2004;2:301–304.

38. Oxman TE, Dietrich AJ, Williams JW, Kroenke K. A three-component model for reengineering systems for the treatment of depression in primary care. *Psychosomatics.* 2002;43:441–450.

39. Mystakidou K, Tsilika E, Parpa E, Katsouda E, Galanos A, Vlahos L. Assessment of anxiety and depression in advanced cancer patients and their relationship with quality of life. *Qual Life Res.* 2005;14:1825–1833.

40. Sadler IJ, Jacobsen PB, Booth-Jones M, Belanger H, Weitzner MA, Fields KK. Preliminary evaluation of a clinical syndrome approach to assessing cancer-related fatigue. *J Pain Symptom Manage.* 2002;23:406–416.

41. Smith EM, Gomm SA, Dickens CM. Assessing the independent contribution to quality of life from anxiety and depression in patients with advanced cancer. *Palliat Med.* 2003;17:509–513.

42. Simonelli LE, Fowler JM, Maxwell GL, Andersen BL. Physical sequelae and depressive symptoms in gynecologic cancer survivors: meaning in life as a mediator. *Ann Behav Med.* 2008;35:275–284.

43. Carver CS, Antoni MH. Finding benefit in breast cancer during the year after diagnosis predicts better adjustment 5 to 8 years after diagnosis. *Health Psychol.* 2004;23:595–598.

44. Parker PA, Baile WF, De Moor C, Cohen L. Psychosocial and demographic predictors of quality of life in a large sample of cancer patients. *Psychooncology.* 2003;12:183–193.

45. Schroevers MJ, Ranchor AV, Sanderman R. The role of social support and self-esteem in the presence and course of depressive symptoms: a comparison of cancer patients and individuals from the general population. *Soc Sci Med.* 2003;57:375–385.

46. Carver CS, Pozo C, Harris SD, et al. How coping mediates the effect of optimism on distress: a study of women with early stage breast cancer. *J Pers Soc Psychol.* 1993;65:375–390.

47. Shelby RA, Golden-Kreutz DM, Andersen BL. PTSD diagnoses, subsyndromal symptoms, and comorbidities contribute to impairments for breast cancer survivors. *J Trauma Stress.* 2008;21:165–172.

48. Rapaport MH, Gharabawi GM, Canuso CM, et al. Effects of risperidone augmentation in patients with treatment-resistant depression: results of open-label treatment followed by double-blind continuation. *Neuropsychopharmacology.* 2006;31:2505–2513.

49. Pedro L. Delgado PZ. Treatment of mood disorders. In: J. Panksepp (ed). *Textbook of biological psychiatry.* Hoboken, NJ: Wiley-Liss; 2004;231–266.

50. Marangell LB. Augmentation of standard depression therapy. *Clin Ther.* 2000;22(Suppl A):A25.

51. Butler AC, Chapman JE, Forman EM, Beck AT. The empirical status of cognitive-behavioral therapy: a review of meta-analyses. *Clin Psychol Rev.* 2006;26:17–31.

52. Hollon SD, Stewart MO, Strunk D. Enduring effects for cognitive behavior therapy in the treatment of depression and anxiety. *Annu Rev Psychol.* 2006;57:285–315.

53. Strunk DR, DeRubeis RJ. Cognitive therapy for depression: a review of its efficacy. *J Cognit Psychother.* 2001;15:289–297.

54. Hollon SD, DeRubeis RJ, Shelton RC, et al. Prevention of relapse following cognitive therapy vs medications in moderate to severe depression. *Arch Gen Psychiatry.* 2005;62:417–422.

55. Dobson KS. A meta-analysis of the efficacy of cognitive therapy for depression. *J Consult Clin Psychol.* 1989;57:414–419.

56. Scogin F, McElreath L. Efficacy of psychosocial treatments for geriatric depression: a quantitative review. *J Consult Clin Psychol.* 1994;62:69–73.

57. Gould RA, Otto MW, Pollack MH, Yap L. Cognitive behavioral and pharmacological treatment of generalized anxiety disorder: a preliminary meta-analysis. *Behav Ther.* 1997;28:285–305.

58. Engels GI, Vermey M. Efficacy of nonmedical treatments of depression in elders: a quantitative analysis. *J Clin Geropsychol.* 1997;3:17–35.

59. Westen D, Morrison K. A multidimensional meta-analysis of treatments for depression, panic, and generalized anxiety disorder: an empirical examination of the status of empirically supported therapies. *J Consult Clin Psychol.* 2001;69:875–899.

60. Haby MM, Donnelly M, Corry J, Yap L. Cognitive behavioural therapy for depression, panic disorder and generalized anxiety disorder: a meta-regression of factors that may predict outcome. *Aust N Z J Psychiatry.* 2006;40:9–19.

61. Seidler GH, Wagner FE. Comparing the efficacy of EMDR and trauma-focused cognitive-behavioral therapy in the treatment of PTSD: a meta-analytic study. *Psychol Med.* 2006;36:1515–1522.

62. Beck AT, Rush AJ, Shaw BF, Emery G. *Cognitive therapy of depression.* New York, Guilford Press; 1979.

63. Jacobson NS, Martell CR, Dimidjian S. Behavioral activation treatment for depression: returning to contextual roots. *Clin Psychol: Sci Prac.* 2001;8:255–270.

64. Dimidjian S, Hollon SD, Dobson KS, et al. Randomized trial of behavioral activation, cognitive therapy, and antidepressant medication in the acute treatment of adults with major depression. *J Consult Clin Psychol.* 2006;74:658–670.

65. Mitte K. Meta-analysis of cognitive-behavioral treatments for generalized anxiety disorder: a comparison with pharmacotherapy. *Psychol Bull.* 2005;131:785–795.

66. Durham RC, Chambers JA, MacDonald RR, Power KG, Major K. Does cognitive-behavioural therapy influence the long-term outcome of generalized anxiety disorder? An 8–14 year follow-up of two clinical trials. *Psychol Med.* 2003;33:499–509.

67. Steketee G, Lam JN, Chambless DL, Rodebaugh T, McCullough C. Effects of perceived criticism and sensitivity to criticism on processes during behavioral treatment for anxiety disorders. *Behav Res Ther.* 2007;45:11–19.

68. Borkovec TD, Costello E. Efficacy of applied relaxation and cognitive-behavioral therapy in the treatment of generalized anxiety disorder. *J Consult Clin Psychol.* 1993;61:611–619.

69. Borkovec TD, Newman MG, Pincus AL, Lytle R. A component analysis of cognitive-behavioral therapy for generalized anxiety disorder and the role of interpersonal problems. *J Consult Clin Psychol.* 2002;70:288–298.

70. Given C, Given B, Rahbar M, et al. Does a symptom management intervention affect depression among cancer patients: results from a clinical trial. *Psychooncology.* 2004;13:818–830.

71. Antoni MH, Lehman JM, Klibourn KM, et al. Cognitive-behavioral stress management intervention decreases the prevalence of depression and enhances benefit finding among women under treatment for early-stage breast cancer. *Health Psychol.* 2001;20:20–32.

72. Marchioro G, Azzarello G, Checchin F. The impact of a psychological intervention on quality of life in non-metastatic breast cancer. *Eur J Cancer (Oxford, England: 1990).* 1996;32A:1612–1615.

73. Greer S, Moorey S, Baruch JD, et al. Adjuvant psychological therapy for patients with cancer: a prospective randomised trial. *BMJ (Clinical Research ed.).* 1992;304:675–80.

74. Edelman S, Bell DR, Kidman AD. A group cognitive behaviour therapy programme with metastatic breast cancer patients. *Psychooncology.* 1999;8:295–305.

75. Edmonds CV, Lock wood GA, Cunningham AJ. Psychological response to long-term group therapy: a randomized trial with metastatic breast cancer patients. *Psychooncology.* 1999;8:74.

76. Edgar L, Rosberger Z, Nowlis D. Coping with cancer during the first year after diagnosis. Assessment and intervention. *Cancer.* 1992;69:817–828.

77. Savard J, Simard S, Ivers H, Morin CM. Randomized study on the efficacy of cognitive-behavioral therapy for insomnia secondary to breast cancer, part I: sleep and psychological effects. *J Clin Oncol.* 2005;23:6083–6096.

78. Nezu AM, Nezu CM, Felgoise SH, McClure KS, Houts PS. Project genesis: assessing the efficacy of problem-solving therapy for distressed adult cancer patients. *J Consult Clin Psychol.* 2003;71:1036–1048.

79. Moorey S, Greer S, Bliss J, Law M. A comparison of adjuvant psychological therapy and supportive counselling in patients with cancer. *Psychooncology.* 1998;7:218–228.

80. Rosberger Z, Edgar L, Collet J-P, Fournier MA. Patterns of coping in women completing treatment for breast cancer: a randomized controlled trial of Nucare, a brief psychoeducation workshop. *J Psychosoc Oncol.* 2002;20:19–37.

81. Evans RL, Connis RT. Comparison of brief group therapies for depressed cancer patients receiving radiation treatment. *Public Health Rep (Washington, DC, 1974).* 1995;110:306–311.

82. Telch CF, Telch MJ. Group coping skills instruction and supportive group therapy for cancer patients: a comparison of strategies. *J Consult Clin Psychol.* 1986;54:802–808.

83. Edelman S, Lemon J, Bell DR, Kidman AD. Effects of group CBT on the survival time of patients with metastatic breast cancer. *Psychooncology.* 1999;8:474–481.

84. Alloy LB, Abramson LY, Francis EL. Do negative cognitive styles confer vulnerability to depression? *Curr Dir Psychol Sci.* 1999;8:128–132.

85. O'Hara MW. The cognitive diathesis for depression. In: Miller GA, (ed). *The behavioral high-risk paradigm in psychopathology.* New York, Springer-Verlag; 1995:250–270.

86. Andersen BL, Shapiro CL, Farrar WB, Crespin T, Wells-Digregorio S. Psychological responses to cancer recurrence. *Cancer.* 2005;104:1540–1547.

87. Brown TA, O'Leary TA, Barlow DH. *Generalized anxiety disorder, clinical handbook of psychological disorders: a step-by-step treatment manual.* New York, Guilford Press; 2001:154–178.

88. Luebbert K, Dahme B, Hasenbring M. The effectiveness of relaxation training in reducing treatment-related symptoms and improving emotional adjustment in acute non-surgical cancer treatment: a meta-analytical review. *Psychooncology.* 2001;10:490–502.

89. Whelan T, Sawka C, Levine M, et al. Helping patients make informed choices: a randomized trial of a decision aid for adjuvant chemotherapy in lymph node-negative breast cancer. *J Natl Cancer Inst.* 2003;95:581–587.

90. Andersen BL. Psychological interventions for cancer patients to enhance the quality of life. *J Consult Clin Psychol.* 1992;60:552–568.

91. Andersen BL. Biobehavioral outcomes following psychological interventions for cancer patients. *J Consult Clin Psychol.* 2002;70:590–610.

92. Meyer TJ, Mark MM. Effects of psychosocial interventions with adult cancer patients: a meta-analysis of randomized experiments. *Health Psychol.* 1995;14:101–108.

93. Spiegel D, Bloom J, Kraemer H, Gottheil E. Effect of psychosocial treatment on survival of patients with metastatic breast cancer. *Lancet.* 1989;2:888–891.

94. Goodwin PJ, Leszcz M, Ennis M, et al. The effect of group psychosocial support on survival in metastatic breast cancer. *N Engl J Med.* 2001;345:1719–1726.

95. Syrjala KL, Donaldson GW, Davis MW, Kippes ME, Carr JE. Relaxation and imagery and cognitive-behavioral training to reduce pain during cancer treatment: a controlled clinical trial. *Pain.* 1995;63:189–198.

96. Richardson JL, Marks G, Johnson CA, et al. Path model of multidimensional compliance with cancer therapy. *Health Psychol.* 1987;6:183–207.

97. Helgeson VS, Cohen S, Schulz R, Yasko J. Education and peer discussion group interventions and adjustment to breast cancer. *Arch Gen Psychiatry.* 1999;56:340–347.

98. Lepore SJ, Helgeson VS, Eton DT, Schulz R. Improving quality of life in men with prostate cancer: a randomized controlled trial of group education interventions. *Health Psychol.* 2003;22:443–452.

99. Richardson MA, Post-White J, Grimm EA, Moye LA, Singletary SE, Justice B. Coping, life attitudes, and immune responses to imagery and group support after breast cancer treatment. *Altern Ther Health Med.* 1997;3:62–70.

100. Sheard T, Maguire P. The effect of psychological interventions on anxiety and depression in cancer patients: results of two meta-analyses. *Br J Cancer.* 1999;80:1770–1780.

101. Fawzy FI, Kemeny ME, Fawzy NW, et al. A structured psychiatric intervention for cancer patients. II. Changes over time in immunological measures. *Arch Gen Psychiatry.* 1990;47:729.

102. American Psychiatric Association. *Diagnostic and statistical manual disorders: DSM-IVTR.* 4th ed., text revision ed. Washington, DC: American Psychiatric Association; 2000.

103. Hamilton M. A rating scale for depression. *J Neurol Neurosurg Psychiatry.* 1960;23:56–62.

104. Hopko DR, Bell JL, Armento M, et al. Cognitive-behavior therapy for depressed cancer patients in a medical care setting. *Behav Ther.* 2008;2:126–136.

105. Simpson JSA, Carlson LE, Beck CA, Patten S. Effects of a brief intervention on social support and psychiatric morbidity in breast cancer patients. *Psychooncology.* 2002;11:282–294.

106. Petersen RW, Quinlivan JA. Preventing anxiety and depression in gynaecological cancer: a randomised controlled trial. *BJOG.* 2002;109:386–394.

107. Kissane DW, Bloch S, Smith GC, et al. Cognitive-existential group psychotherapy for women with primary breast cancer: a randomized controlled trial. *Psychooncology.* 2003;12:532–546.

108. Kissane DW, Grabsch B, Clarke D, et al. Supportive-expressive group therapy for women with metastatic breast cancer: survival and psychosocial outcome from a randomized controlled trial. *Psychooncology.* 2007;16:277–286.

109. Andersen BL, Kiecolt-Glaser JK, Glaser R. A biobehavioral model of cancer stress and disease course. *Am Psychol.* 1994;49:389–404.

110. Andersen BL, Anderson B, deProsse C. Controlled prospective longitudinal study of women with cancer: II. psychological outcomes. *J Consult Clin Psychol.* 1989;57:692–697.

111. Andersen BL, Anderson B, deProsse C. Controlled prospective longitudinal study of women with cancer: I. sexual functioning outcomes. *J Consult Clin Psychol.* 1989;57:683–691.

112. Epping-Jordan JE, Compas BE, Osowiecki DM, et al. Psychological adjustment in breast cancer: processes of emotional distress. *Health Psychol.* 1999;18:315–326.

113. Golden-Kreutz DM, Thornton LM, Wells-Di Gregorio SM, et al. Traumatic stress, perceived global stress, and life events: prospectively predicting quality of life in breast cancer patients. *Health Psychol.* 2005;24:288–296.

114. Golden-Kreutz DM, Andersen BL. Depressive symptoms after breast cancer surgery: relationships with global, cancer-related, and life event stress. *Psychooncology.* 2004;13:211–220.

115. Jim HS, Richardson SA, Golden-Kreutz DM, Andersen BL. Strategies used in coping with a cancer diagnosis predict meaning in life for survivors. *Health Psychol.* 2006;25:753–761.

116. Andersen BL, Farrar WB, Golden-Kreutz D, et al. Stress and immune responses after surgical treatment for regional breast cancer. *J Natl Cancer Inst.* 1998;90:30–36.

117. Anisman H, Merali Z. Cytokines, stress and depressive illness: brain-immune interactions. *Ann Med Psychol.* 2003;35:2–11.

118. Stein M, Keller SE, Schleifer S. Immune system: relationship to anxiety disorders. *J Psych Clin Nr Am.* 1988;11:349–360.

119. Zorrilla EP, Luborsky L, McKay JR, et al. The relationship of depression and stressors to immunological assays: a meta-analytic review. *Brain Behav Immun.* 2001;15:199–226.

120. Pace TWW, Hu F, Miller AH. Cytokine-effects on glucocorticoid receptor function: relevance to glucocorticoid resistance and the pathophysiology and treatment of major depression. *Brain Behav Immun.* 2007;21:9–19.

121. Elenkov IJ, Iezzoni DG, Daly A, Harris AG, Chrousos GP. Cytokine dysregulation, inflammation and well-being. *Neuroimmunomodulation.* 2005;12:255–269.

122. Grunberg NE, Popp KA, Bowen DJ, Nespor SM, Winders SE, Eury SE. Effects of chronic nicotine administration on insulin, glucose, epinephrine, and norepinephrine. *Life sciences.* 1988;42:161–170.

123. Stetson BA, Rahn JM, Dubbert PM, Wilner BI, Mercury MG. Prospective evaluation of the effects of stress on exercise adherence in community-residing women. *Health Psychol.* 1997;16:515–520.

124. Rosch PJ. Stress and sleep: some startling and sobering statistics. *Stress Med.* 1996;12:207–210.

125. McAllister-Sistilli CG, Caggiula AR, Knopf S, Rose CA, Miller AL, Conny EC. The effects of nicotine on the immune system. *Psychoneuroendocrinology.* 1998;23:175–187.

126. Jung W, Irwin M.: Reduction of natural killer cytotoxic activity in major depression: interaction between depression and cigarette smoking. *Psychosom Med.* 1999;61:263–270.

127. Fairey AS, Courneya KS, Field CJ, Mackey JR. Physical exercise and immune system function in cancer survivors: a comprehensive review and future directions. *Cancer.* 2002;94:539–551.

128. Stathopoulou G, Powers MB, Berry AC, Smits JAJ, Otto MW. Exercise interventions for mental health: a quantitative and qualitative review. *Clin Psychol: Science and Practice.* 2006;13:179–193.

129. Blumenthal JA, Babyak MA, Moore KA, et al. Effects of exercise training on older patients with major depression. *Arch Intern Med.* 1999;159:2349–2356.

130. Lebovits A, Strain J, Schleifer S, Tanaka J, Bhardwaj S, Messe M. Patient noncompliance with self-administered chemotherapy. *Cancer.* 1990;65:17–22.

131. McDonough EM, Boyd JH, Varvares MA, Maves MD. Relationship between psychological status and compliance in a sample of patients treated for cancer of the head and neck. *Head and Neck.* 1996;18:269–276.

132. Andersen BL, Farrar WB, Golden-Kreutz DM, et al. Psychological, behavioral, and immune changes following a psychosocial intervention: a clinical trial. *J Clin Oncol.* 2004;17:3570–3580.

133. Andersen BL, Farrar WB, Golden-Kreutz DM, et al. Distress reduction from a psychological intervention contributes to improved health for cancer patients. *Brain Behav Immun.* 2007;21:953–961.

134. Andersen BL, Shelby RA, Golden-Kreutz DM. Results from an RCT of a psychological intervention for patients with cancer: I. mechanisms of change. *J Consult Clin Psychol.* 2007;75:927–938.

135. Radloff LS. The CES-D Scale: a self-report depression scale for research in the general population. *Appl Psychol Meas* 1977;1:385–401.

136. Horowitz MJ, Wilner N, Alvarez W. Impact of event scale: a measure of subjective stress. *Psychosom Med.* 1979;41:209–218.

137. Curran S, Andrykowski M, Studts J. Short form of the Profile Mood States (POMS-SF): psychometric information. *Psychol Assess.* 1995;7:80–83.

138. Jacobson NS, Truax P. Clinical significance: a statistical approach to defining meaningful change in psychotherapy research. *J Consult Clin Psychol.* 1991;59:12–19.

139. Thornton LM, Andersen BL, Schuler TA, Carson WE. A psychological intervention reduces inflammatory markers by alleviating depressive symptoms: secondary analysis of a randomized controlled trial. *Psychosom Med,* 2009;71:715–724.

140. Miller M, Mogun H, Azrael D, Hempstead K, Solomon DH. Cancer and the risk of suicide in older Americans. *J Clin Oncol.* 2008;26:4720–4724.

141. Schairer C, Brown LM, Chen BE, et al. Suicide after breast cancer: an international population-based study of 723810 women. *J Natl Cancer Inst.* 2006;98:1416–1419.

CHAPTER 57

Art Therapy and Music Therapy

Paola M. Luzzatto and Lucanne Magill

Art Therapy

Paola M. Luzzatto

Art therapy has its roots in art and psychoanalysis, and it is based on the notions that imagination is an essential part of mental functioning, and that individuals may project their internal world, both consciously and unconsciously, into visual images.[1] The first pioneers of art therapy, in the 1940s and 1950s, were artists who introduced image making to traumatized soldiers, to psychiatric patients, to children with emotional problems. The influence of psychoanalysis helped art therapy to develop in the direction of art-psychotherapy: promoting insight, and facilitating change in the patients' inner world.

INTRODUCTION

In *art therapy* the mental content is objectified in *external images*, transforming the setting into a triangular field (patient; therapist; image), where communication may be activated on three levels: (1) A silent creative communication between patient and image *(Expressive Dimension)*. (2) The symbolic work, to understand and elaborate the image, using free association, fantasy, and narrative *(Symbolic Dimension)*. (3) Direct communication between therapist and patient *(Interactive Dimension)*.[2]

In connection with these three types of communication, there are three main types of art therapy interventions:

Studio-based art therapy. This is the ideal structure to activate the Expressive Dimension. It is based on the provision of a safe and nonjudgmental environment, with a variety of art materials, to facilitate concentration, creativity, and the development of personal imagery.

Group art therapy. There are many forms of group art therapy and in all of them the art therapist helps patients to reach a certain degree of symbolic self-expression and to develop a certain degree of interaction within the group.

Individual art therapy. Individual art therapy is a most flexible type of intervention. According to each patient's needs, the art therapist may privilege the expressive, the symbolic, or the interactive approach.

MEDICAL ART THERAPY

The term *medical art therapy* refers to the use of art therapy with physically ill patients, experiencing trauma to the body, undergoing aggressive or long-term medical treatments.[3] The general aim of medical art therapy is to improve the quality of life of medically ill patients. Attention must be given to the whole range of human needs, from physical to spiritual, and the greatest challenge is the attempt to integrate somatic, psychological, and existential themes such as pain, loss, and death. Adrian Hill[4] is the first pioneer who started to work with medically ill patients. He worked with patients treated for tuberculosis in a sanatorium, to help them reach a sense of life and hope. The number of art therapists who work with medically ill people is growing, and many of them now work in the field of psycho-oncology.

Evidence-based research is still scarce in the field of medical art therapy, but randomized and controlled studies on the effectiveness of art therapy with cancer patients that began being carried out showed an improvement in coping resources, in comparison to controlled groups.[5,6] A number of books on medical art therapy, and art therapy in cancer care have been published in the last 10 years.[7-11] Many clinical reports of art therapists working with cancer patients have been published in professional journals *(Oncology, Nursing, Art Therapy)*.[12]

WORKING WITH CHILDREN: PLAY AND REALITY

Many art therapists[13,14] describe the concept of *therapeutic play* to reach young patients. This is a playful approach to hospital environment and medical procedures, which includes making up stories about people and animals who are in similar situations. Rode has made videos where children film each other and interview medical staff, the filming itself is an innovative form of art therapy. To facilitate emotional expression, Sourkes[15] has created a structured intervention, based on three steps: (1) The Color-Feeling Wheel; (2)The Change-In-Family Drawing; (3) The Scariest Drawing, where the child can work symbolically. Favara-Scacco[16] has described a number of effective art therapy interventions used for children with leukemia during painful procedures. Art therapy interventions may also be useful during terminal stages of disease.[17,18] It seems that children feel less depressed when they can communicate their concerns about death and the artwork may function as a bridge between the children and their family. The inclusion of the art therapist as part of the pediatric team is a unique humanizing influence during the child's illness.

DEALING WITH PAIN, FATIGUE, AND STRESS

Interventions focused on pain may range from giving colors and shape to the pain and distancing from it, to an existential integration of the pain into the meaning of life.[19,20] Art therapy has been used effectively with patients *during chemotherapy* to decrease levels of fatigue,[21] and with patients *during radiotherapy*, to improve coping resources.[5] Pain is both a physical and an emotional experience. At Memorial Sloan-Kettering Cancer Center in New York City, the art therapist offered a small outline of the body on a white page to 70 hospitalized patients, and the majority used the outline to express a combination of physical pain, emotions, and spiritual beliefs.[22] Lusebrink and Scifres[23] conduct brief art therapy for stress reduction with mastectomy patients: (1) the patients build their "world" in a sand tray, reflecting the stressful situations and their coping style; (2) the tactile aspects of the sand facilitates relaxation; (3) the use of the sand tray provides the opportunity to explore alternative ways of coping. In this way, art therapy integrates the two basic aspects of stress reduction: *tension-release* and *problem-solving*, within a creative approach.

ART THERAPY WITH PATIENTS IN ISOLATION

Cancer patients may feel isolated in hospital for different reasons. Connell[24] describes one technique to overcome feelings of isolation of hospitalized cancer patients: she collects their drawings, poems, and stories into a "Big Book of Memories and Reflections," which she takes from room to room. This silent nonintrusive interaction may be comforting and stimulating. Art therapy with bone marrow transplant patients in isolation is described by Gabriel et al.[25] Although physically very weak and often unable to get up and talk, these patients were able to move from the pleasure of using art material, to sharing thoughts about their family, to symbolic imagery about life and death. Greece[26] provides a case study of an art therapy process with a war veteran in isolation for bone marrow transplantation. Some cancer patients withdraw from communicating due to impaired self-worth, after traumatizing surgery, and this is particularly so for laryngectomy patients, whose capacity to speak may be lost, transiently or permanently. Art therapy has been used as an effective therapeutic adjunct for laryngectomy patients at the University of Mississippi Medical Center.[27]

PSYCHOLOGICAL, EXISTENTIAL, AND SPIRITUAL ISSUES

Frequently cancer patients decide to deal with personal and emotional issues, which may also be old unresolved conflicts, and this may happen in two very different moments: (1) when they feel better at the end of treatment; (2) when they are aware that the end of life is approaching. Posttreatment patients usually respond well to short-term group art therapy, where they can express themselves symbolically; the search for new internal strength is often the main theme for these groups.[28,29] For some of these patients individual art-psychotherapy may be more appropriate.[30] Art therapy may be combined effectively with music therapy and movement therapy, with creative writing and with meditation practices, for personal growth.[6,11,31] Art therapy offers a unique way of dealing with death. Images about death may emerge freely during an art therapy group. They may be images from dreams or about the death of loved relatives or symbolic images of one's mortality. It is always striking for the art therapist to see how patients may choose to make images about death and feel relieved about it.[32] As hospices rapidly become part of our culture, the development of art therapy in hospice care is becoming more and more relevant, because of its unique combination of being very private and facilitating in-depth experiences. Art therapists often feel much moved by working with terminal patients who can use imagery to communicate and explore the experience of approaching death.[33-35]

WORKING WITH CAREGIVERS AND HEALTH PROFESSIONALS

The use of art therapy to support family caregivers, and to prevent burnout among health professionals, has been developed in recent years.[36] Belfiore was among the first art therapists who provided a group for nurses and doctors caring for terminally ill patients in Italy.[37] An art therapy program was led by an art therapist in Alabama, for highly stressed workers in a clinic for terminally ill patients: the participants planned to nurture themselves, to free up their energy and rechannel it to help their patients.[38] Bertman[39] describes an educational process for healthcare professionals using visual images of illness and death from the art world, to elicit personal feelings and reactions to dying and grief.

ART THERAPY SERVICE IN CANCER CENTERS: WHY, WHERE, AND HOW

In conclusion, the literature supports the idea that an effective psycho-oncology service should include art therapy.

Why. Evidence-based research and clinical reports from art therapists working with cancer patients strongly suggests these five positive outcomes: (1) reduction in reports of physical pain; (2) cathartic release of emotional issues; (3) improved positive coping strategies; (4) new insight into their own behavior; (5) increased ability to confront existential issues. More research should be carried out on each of these points.

Where. Art therapy seems to be especially effective in these following areas: (1) pediatric oncology; (2) patients in isolation; (3) patients during chemotherapy and radiotherapy treatment; (4) posttreatment cancer patients; (5) hospices; (6) staff support.

How. All three basic art therapy interventions may be helpful to cancer patients, at different times during their illness: (1) In the Open Studio, patients seem to benefit from the silent creative endeavor, to repair an internal feeling of damage and loss; (2) In Art Therapy Groups, patients use their symbolic image making to share and elaborate their emotions, to strengthen their identity and positive core; (3) Some patients may need individual sessions, where the art therapist may employ very flexible combinations of intrapsychic symbolic work and verbal interaction.

References

1. Waller D. *Becoming a profession*. London: Tavistock; 1991.
2. Luzzatto P. On the relationship between art and therapy. *Inscape*. 1989;12(2):53.
3. Malchiodi CA. Art and medicine. *Art Ther*. 1993;10(2):66–69.
4. Hill A. *Art versus illness*. London: Allen & Unwin; 1945.
5. Oster I, Svensk AC, Magnusson E, et al. Art therapy improves coping resources: a randomized, controlled study among women with breast cancer. *Palliat Support Care*. 2006;4(1):57–64.
6. Monti DA, Paterson C, Kunkel EJ, et al. A randomized, controlled trial of mindfulness-based art therapy for women with cancer. *Psychooncology*. 2006;15(5):363–373.
7. Pratt M, Wood M (eds). *Art therapy in palliative care*. London: Routledge; 1998.
8. Malchiodi CA (ed). *Medical art therapy with children*. London: Jessica Kingsley; 1999a.
9. Malchiodi CA (ed). *Medical art therapy with adults*. London: Jessica Kingsley; 1999b.
10. Waller D, Sibbett C (eds). *Art therapy and cancer care*. New York: McGrow Hill; 2005:82–101.
11. Hartley N, Payne M (eds). *The creative arts in palliative care*. London: Jessica Kingsley; 2008.
12. Wood M. Shoreline: the realities of working in cancer and palliative care. In: Waller D, Sibbett C (eds). *Art therapy and cancer care*. New York: McGrow Hill; 2005:87–89.
13. Rode D. Building bridges within the culture of pediatric medicine. *Art Ther*. 1995;2:104–110.
14. Walker C. Use of art and play therapy in pediatric oncology. *J Pediatr Oncol Nurs*. 1989;6:121–126.
15. Sourkes BM. Truth to life: art therapy with pediatric oncology patients and their siblings. *J Psychosoc Oncol*. 1991;9(2):81–96.
16. Favara-Scacco C, Smirne G, Schiliro' G, DiCataldo A. Art therapy as support for children with leukemia during painful procedures. *Med Pediatr Oncol*. 2001;36(4):474–480.
17. Councill T. Art therapy with pediatric cancer patients. *Art Ther*. 1993;10(2):78–87.
18. Rollins J. Helping children cope with hospitalization. *Imprint*. 1990;37(4):79–83.
19. Halliday D. My art healed me. *Inscape*. 1988;11(1):18–22.
20. Ronen R, Packman W, Field NP, Davies B, Kramer R, Long JK. The relationship between grief adjustment and continuing bonds for parents who have lost a child. *OMEGA, Journal of Death and Dying*. 2009;60(1):1–31.
21. Bar-Sela G, Atid L, Danos S, Gabay N, Epelbaum R. Art therapy improved depression and influenced fatigue levels in cancer patients on chemotherapy. *Psychooncology*. 2007;16(11):980–984.
22. Luzzatto P, Sereno V, Capps R. A communication tool for patients with pain: the art therapy technique of the body outline. *Palliat Support Care*. 2003;1(2):135–142.
23. LusebrinkVB. Dreamwork and sandtray therapy with mastectomy patients. In: Malchiodi CA (ed). *Medical art therapy with adults*. London: Jessica Kingsley; 1999b: 87–111.
24. Connell C. Art therapy as part of a palliative care programme. *Palliat Med*. 1992;6:18–25.

25. Gabriel B, Bromberg E, Vandenbovenkamp J, Walka P, Kornblith AB, Luzzatto P. Art therapy with adult bone marrow transplant patients in isolation: a pilot study. *Psychooncology.* 2001;10:114–123.

26. Greece M. Art therapy on a bone marrow transplant unit: the case study of a Vietnam veteran fighting myelofibrosis. *Arts Psychother.* 2003;30:229–238.

27. Anand S, Anand V. Art therapy with laryngectomy patients. *Art Ther.* 1997;14(2):109–117.

28. Luzzatto P, Gabriel B. The creative journey: a model for short-term group art therapy with post treatment cancer patients. *Art Ther.* 2000;17:265–269.

29. Goll Lerner E. The healing journey: a ten-week group focusing on long-term healing processes. In: Waller D, Sibbett C (eds). *Art therapy and cancer care.* New York: McGrow Hill; 2005:149–162.

30. Stone Matho E. A woman with breast cancer in art therapy. In: Waller D, Sibbett C (eds). *Art therapy and cancer care.* New York: McGrow Hill; 2005:102–118.

31. Collie K, Bottorff JL, Long BC. A narrative view of art therapy and art making by women with breast cancer. *J Health Psychol.* 2006;11(5):761–775.

32. Luzzatto P. Musing with death in group art therapy with cancer patients. In: Waller D, Sibbett C (eds). *Art therapy and cancer care.* New York: McGraw Hill; 2005:163–171.

33. Duesbury T. Art therapy in the hospice: rewards and frustrations. In: Waller D, Sibbett C (eds). *Art therapy and cancer care.* New York: McGraw Hill; 2005:199–209.

34. Bocking M. A 'don't know' story: art therapy in an NHS medical oncology department. In: Waller D, Sibbett C (eds). *Art therapy and cancer care.* New York: McGrow Hill; 2005:210–222.

35. Thomas G. What lies within us: individuals in a Marie Curie Hospice. In: Pratt M, Wood MJM (eds). *Art therapy in palliative care: The creative response.* London: Routledge; 1998:64–74.

36. Italia S, Favara-Scacco C, Di Cataldo A, Russo G. Evaluation and art therapy treatment of the burnout syndrome in oncology units. *Psychooncology.* 2008;17(7):676–680.

37. Belfiore M. The group takes care of itself: art therapy to prevent burn out. *Arts Psychother.* 1994;21(3):119–126.

38. Elkinson-Griff A. Let me wipe my tears so I can help with yours. *Art Ther.* 1995;12(1):67–69.

39. Bertman S. *Facing death: Images, insights and interventions.* Bristol, PA: Taylor & Francis; 1991.

Music Therapy

Lucanne Magill

Music therapy is a well-established profession that offers treatment approaches found efficacious in addressing a range of needs and issues presented by cancer patients and families.[1] In oncology settings, music therapy is identified as a nonpharmacologic modality offering soothing and expressive benefits to those receiving this care. Specific music therapy strategies are provided by board certified music therapists to facilitate meaningful changes in physiological, psychosocial, and spiritual processes. In the following, the use of music therapy in this context will be summarized, including a review of methods, common approaches and specialized areas of practice.

INTRODUCTION

Music therapy has become widely incorporated into healthcare and medical services around the world, and is an established profession that can enhance the quality of life of patients, families, and staff.[2] Music therapy is the purposeful use of music to address physical, emotional, cognitive, social, and spiritual needs of individuals of all ages.[3] It became formalized in both the United States and Europe in the mid-twentieth century and was originally used for treating ailing veterans returning from war. The profession expanded to services in psychiatric and medical institutions, especially as education and training became standardized and degree programs were established world wide. Currently, those music therapists who have fulfilled national education and certification requirements are employed internationally in a wide variety of medical, rehabilitative, psychiatric, long-term care, and wellness settings.[3]

Music therapy in cancer care has been found to provide multiple benefits.[1] Music is intricately woven into the fabrics of life and takes on deeper significance during times of transition, loss, and grief. Music therapists strive to assist patients, families, and staff in finding ways to integrate the medium of music to ameliorate grief and suffering, as well as to relieve stress, anxiety, depression, and isolation.[1,4,5]

Over the past three decades in particular, music therapists have been conducting empirical studies to further explore and document the use of music therapy in oncology. Literature describes the effectiveness of music to promote relaxation,[5–8] alter mood,[9–12] improve communication,[13,14] and to break the cyclical nature of pain.[6,15,16] Music therapists have skilled approaches for treating anxiety in children[17–20] and adults.[4,8,12,21–25] Music therapists and healthcare professionals are continuing to research the impact of music on the various components of the human experience during life threatening and terminal illnesses, that is, physiological (improved cardiac, respiratory, and adrenal functioning as well as decreased symptoms of nausea, insomnia, or fatigue), psycho-emotional (alteration in mood and enhanced coping styles) social (enhanced communication), and spiritual (improved sense of meaning, connectedness, and faith).[1,26–30]

METHODOLOGY

As the needs and issues of cancer patients and their families are multifaceted and often complex, music therapists practice thorough assessment skills and offer strategies to help improve comfort, overall coping skills, and enhance personal well being.

Assessment. Assessment is ongoing and is done on a moment-by-moment and session-by-session basis.[4] The initial and ongoing assessment of patients and families includes a review of the comprehensive needs presented, such as disease status; overall mood; cognitive functioning abilities; prior musical experiences; cultural and spiritual values; and preferences, familial/social issues, coping skills, and the degree of emotional vulnerability.[4,31] Ongoing assessment is done through close observation, gentle questioning, and collaboration with the medical team. The music therapist is trained to be highly sensitive to the needs of patients and families so as to provide appropriate music and individualized creative techniques aimed to enhance comfort and sense of control. When patients are particularly vulnerable and not capable of contending with emotional expression, music therapists may offer gently uplifting music with peaceful, hopeful lyrics. Likewise, there may be times during sensory overload when music needs be especially modified or perhaps temporarily omitted. Generally, appropriate music aimed to improve ability to cope can bring relief to a wide range of symptoms, as music has the unique potential to function multidimensionally.

Role of therapist. As the aims of music therapy are to facilitate well-being and improve quality of life through music-therapeutic relationships, music therapy relies on the therapeutic benefits of human contact and the supportive, caring presence of the music therapist.[32] Thus, a significant aspect of music therapy is the role assumed by the therapist in establishing a compassionate, attentive, and creative milieu within which patients and caregivers can regain a sense of dignity and existential meaning.[22,31–33] Music therapists strive to offer an empathetic, accepting, and caring presence as they listen, observe, and provide individualized approaches in sessions. Within this context, patients and families may regain sense of personal identity and life meaning, as well as have opportunities for creative expression and the processing of thoughts, feelings, or issues.

Common procedures and techniques. Music therapists are generally referred to patients by medical professionals. Individual and group sessions range in length of time and are organized depending on patient needs and location. Hospitalized patients are generally seen at the bedside, however, are also seen in intensive care units, in perioperative settings or treatment/procedure areas, such as radiation therapy waiting rooms or chemotherapy units. Sessions are often characterized by gentle, yet prompt approaches. Thus the music therapist must maintain the ability to assess and address predominant issues upon contact with patient and caregivers. Live music is generally used in sessions, such as guitar, voice, harp, acoustic string instruments, or hand instruments when appropriate. Commonly, pre-composed songs are offered in the beginning, and patients are invited to select music of their preference. The music therapist aims to find simple ways to help patient and family become engaged, such as through selecting preferred imagery, singing lyrics, playing instruments, or personalizing songs with their words. Whenever possible, music therapists work with patients and family members on an ongoing basis to offer continual supportive care.

Techniques are offered based on patients' needs, their expressed preferences, and the music therapist's assessment. Each of these patient-centered techniques has been found to help restore sense of control, as patients are offered opportunities to participate in ways suitable to their capabilities and personal desires.

Examples of common techniques used in music therapy sessions:

- Songs: Song content may be used to express that which is difficult to express.[26,33,34] Previously composed songs in sessions may be selected by the patient, family members, or at times by the music therapist to reflect themes of importance. As lyrics can help guide thoughts and images, songs can provide form, structure, and a pertinent frame of reference during times of doubt, fear, apprehension, or episodic pain. Singing in sessions involves the intimate presence of the human voice, an element that can help reduce anxiety and sense of isolation.[26] Likewise, singing can provide various physiological benefits.[1]
- Song writing: The personalized use of lyrics in sessions fosters self-expression and communication. The music therapist commonly assists patients and families in creating songs with their own words. Such songs are often provided for or dedicated to their loved ones as "gifts"; or they may be written with special messages for others; or may be testimonials regarding their life stories.
- Chants: The use of common chants to verbalize prayers or meditations often provides further opportunities for patients and families to substitute lyrics with their own words. Likewise, chants may support cultural or spiritual themes of significance. Repetition of vocal intonations, with or without words, is a way to focus attention and can reduce fatigue, increase relaxation, improve breath flow, and enhance expression.[22,35]
- Toning: The use of nonlyrical vocalizations to enhance expression through the making of sounds with patient and family members.
- Music listening: Often patients elect to listen to soft music for relaxation during sessions. The therapist provides them with live harmonic and melodic instrumental music, or with lyrical music reflecting desired images. This music is often improvised at the patient's side, as the mood, rhythm, and timbre of music may be adapted spontaneously to meet patient needs. Therapists often guide patients into relaxation and listening techniques and offer recorded music for use after sessions. This technique can serve to help refocus attention during times of pain, fatigue, agitation, or insomnia.[36,37]
- Music meditation: Music can be used to create a mood of peace.[36] Patients may select mantras or words that refer to affirmations or to peace as a way to focus thoughts and/or regain sense of personal value. This technique can redirect thoughts, improve sense of control, and enhance comfort and relaxation.[22]
- Improvisation by therapist to meet patient and support needs: The music therapist improvises music, finding tempos and melodies that create the mood desired.
- Improvisation with patient: The music therapist provides the patient with instruments to facilitate creative expression through instruments.
- Audio recording: Special songs or complete sessions may be recorded and given by patients to families as "gifts." Such audio recordings are generally designed by the patients and are presented to loved ones as memoirs and tokens of affection. Patients sometimes also use these recordings to return to feelings and states of comfort, pleasure, and peace.

AREAS OF SPECIALIZATION

Music therapists have been furthering the development of specialized skills to address multifaceted issues; and theoretical models and methods of treatment are being used with children, adults, and caregivers. These current trends in areas of specialization exist: pain management, neurological sciences, music psychotherapy, integrative medicine, and various population specializations.

Pain management. Music therapists provide strategies to help ameliorate symptoms of pain. The music therapist aims to assuage pain by using music relaxation techniques while attending to the psychospiritual components of the pain experience.[4] The therapist's skill for assessing the overall aspects of the patient's pain plays a vital role in the treatment approaches used. While the music can enhance relaxation, alter mood, and provide cognitive stimulation, the expressive nature of music can also facilitate relief from suffering.[6] Some music therapists use techniques, such as entrainment, the use of sound stimuli to match and then alter responses.[37] Other therapists use physioacoustic therapy, the use of pure sinusoidal sound waves[38]; and the use of nonrhythmic, slow tempos, and low frequencies.[39]

Neurological sciences. In patients with neurological impairments, music therapy can be helpful in diminishing symptoms of fear, anxiety, depression, frustration and loneliness.[40] Research in neurological medicine further demonstrates the implications for the use of music with patients with related diseases, such as brain tumors, central nervous system (CNS) lymphoma, and metastatic illness.[13,41] As hearing is the first sense to be developed and the last sense to deteriorate,[42] music is a particularly effective stimulus to reach and make contact with patients who are otherwise not responding to words or touch. Also, music therapists use music for those with communication challenges, such as disease-related expressive aphasia.[43] Music stimulates the language centers of the brain and can facilitate expression and articulation within the context of music.[13] Likewise, music stimulates memory functioning and is used as a "retrieval mechanism" to help patients with memory impairment recall significant events.[39]

Integrative medicine. As an evidence-based complementary therapy, music therapy follows the principles of integrative medicine in considering the mind-body connections and whole-person care.[7] Music therapists work as collaborative members of multidisciplinary teams and aim to achieve the broader goals of music therapy in oncology, such as improved personal well-being and quality of life. Clinical work often includes individual and group sessions aimed at promoting wellness, stress reduction, recovery, and cancer survivorship,[7] as well as sessions supporting patients, families, and staff through grief, loss, and times of transition.[22]

Music psychotherapy. Music therapists are applying psychotherapeutic skills in the care and treatment of cancer patients. Analytic music therapy has been found to benefit some children and adult cancer patients through the uncovering of issues surrounding symptoms, some of which are psychosomatically based.[44] Music therapists in oncology settings, as well as in other areas of healthcare, often base clinical work in various models of psychotherapy as they attend to the psycho-emotional and existential issues presented by patients and caregivers.

Spirituality and existentiality. Often patients contending with life threatening or advanced illness seek support with existential issues, such as faith or the larger meaning of life. Music therapy naturally provides the means to sustain these quests, as music has innate associations with nature, infinity and humanity across borders and throughout history.[2] Various music therapy strategies acknowledge spiritual customs and values and also facilitate sense of hope, connection, transcendence, meaning, and faith.[28]

Population specializations

1. Pediatric oncology: Music therapists working with children in the oncology setting use music as a means to address medical and psychosocial needs.[18] They commonly use songs and improvisational techniques to enhance creative self-expression while aiming to relieve the distress and anxiety frequently experienced during hospitalizations and out patient procedures. Pediatric patients and their families are given opportunities to play small instruments, participate in improvisational song-story writing, sing familiar songs, or listen to calming music as needed.[20] Such techniques provide a less threatening means of expression for withdrawn or agitated children, while also helping familiarize and normalize medical setting environments. In hospitals and clinics, children may receive individual sessions or may participate in small groups, depending on assessed needs and pertinent issues. Music therapists are often present during difficult procedures to offer the distracting and engaging medium of music within the context of therapeutic support.[19,45]

2. Adult oncology: In working with adult patients and caregivers, music therapists aim to treat symptoms and provide for moments of comfort, respite, meaning and reflection. A range of creative strategies to address emergent psychosocial and existential issues are provided; and therapists encourage family involvement, offering individual and family sessions as desired. Likewise theme-based patient and caregiver groups are held in hospitals and oncology clinics.

3. Gerontology/oncology: Patients in the 65+ age group may have co-morbid medical conditions that can compound and exacerbate symptoms related to cancer. Thus, this age group can have added difficulties in coping with stress related to the impact of disease. Patients may experience increased emotional vulnerability, isolation, fatigue, and memory loss.[46] Music therapists working with this age group provide strategies to address these multifaceted symptoms, as this therapy has been found to improve memory,[47] communication,[13] sense of meaning,[28] and social integration[16] in this age category.

4. Family caregivers: It is well know that caregivers of cancer patients often carry burden and need psycho emotional and social support. Music therapy can provide benefits to caregivers, as evidenced by its potential to address multiple issues Music therapists often spend time in sessions offering family caregivers,[48] including children,[49] psycho-emotional support, as well as teach them simple stress reduction techniques and methods for administering comfort care to themselves and to their loved ones.

5. Staff caregivers: As oncology staff often experience stress and burnout, therapies such as music therapy can be helpful. Literature has documented the benefits of music therapy for oncology staff.[50] Music therapists often offer classes in stress reduction, such as healing through the voice, movement, and relaxation through guided imagery.

CONCLUSION

Music therapy in the oncology setting can provide patients, family members, and staff with multiple psycho emotional, physiological, and spiritual benefits that can enhance coping and disease management. Through interactive and personalized approaches, music therapy has been found efficacious in (1) helping reduce adverse symptoms and restore relaxation and personal well-being; (2) offering a means for self-expression; (3) facilitating the processing of existential and spiritual issues; and in (4) providing channels for communication and social engagement. Music therapy embraces the therapeutic benefits of human contact and the compassionate presence of the music therapist. Thus, it can offer a supportive milieu within which patients and caregivers may potentially find healing.

REFERENCES

1. Dileo C, Bradt J. *Medical music therapy: A meta-analysis.* Cherry Hill, NJ: Jeffrey Books; 2005.

2. Aldridge D. *Music therapy in palliative care: New voices.* London: Jessica Kingsley Publishers; 1999.

3. American Music Therapy Association. 2008. www.musictherapy.org. Accessed July 21, 2009.

4. Magill L. The use of music therapy to address the suffering in advanced cancer pain. *J Palliat Care.* 2001;17:166–72.

5. Gallagher LM, Lagman R, Walsh D, Davis MP, Legrand SB. The clinical effects of music therapy in palliative medicine. *J Support Care Cancer.* 2006;14(8):859–866.

6. Magill Levreault L. Music therapy in pain and symptom management. *J Palliat Care.* 1993;9(4):42–48.

7. Deng G, Vickers A, Cassileth B. *PDQ integrative oncology: Complementary therapies in cancer care.* Hamilton, ON Canada: B.C. Decker; 2005.

8. Burns SJ, Harbuz MS, Hucklebridge F, Bunt L. A pilot study into the therapeutic effects of music therapy at a cancer help center. *Altern Ther Health Med.* 2001;7(1):48–56.

9. Ferrer AJ. The effect of live music on decreasing anxiety in patients undergoing chemotherapy treatment. *J Music Ther.* 2007;44(3):242–255.

10. Bailey L. The effects of live music versus tape-recorded music on hospitalized cancer patients. *Music Ther.* 1983;3(1):17–28.

11. Burns DS. The effect of the bonny method of guided imagery and music on the mood and life quality of cancer patients. *J Music Ther.* 2001;38(1):51–65.

12. Cassileth BR, Vickers AJ, Magill L. Music therapy for mood disturbance during hospitalization for autologous stem cell transplantation: a randomized controlled trial. *Cancer.* 2003;98:2723–2729.

13. O'Callaghan C. Communicating with brain-impaired palliative care patients through music therapy. *J Palliat Care.* 1993;9(4):53–55.

14. Cortes A. The use of music in facilitating emotional expression in the terminally ill. *Am J Hosp Palliat Med.* 2004;21:255–260.

15. Porchet-Munro S. Music therapy. In: Doyle D, Hanks G, MacDonald N (eds). *Oxford textbook of palliative medicine*, 2nd ed. Oxford: Oxford University Press; 1998:855–860.

16. Krout RE. The effects of single-session music therapy interventions on the observed and self-reported levels of pain control, physical comfort, and relaxation of hospice patients. *Am J Hosp and Palliat Care.* 2000;18(6):383–390.

17. Kemper KJ, Hamilton CA, McLean TW, Lovato J. Impact of music on pediatric oncology outpatients. *Pediatr Res.* 2008;64(1):105–109.

18. Robb SL, Clair AA, Watanabe M, et al. Randomized controlled trial of the active music engagement (AME) intervention on children with cancer. *Psychooncology.* 2008;17(7):699–708.

19. O'Callaghan C, Sexton M, Wheeler G. Music therapy as a non-pharmacological anxiolytic for paediatric radiotherapy patients. *Australas Radiol.* 2007;51(2):159–162.

20. Daveson BA, Kennelly J. Music therapy in palliative care for hospitalized children and adolescents. *J Palliat Care.* 2000;16(1):35–38.

21. O' Callaghan C. Bringing music to life: a study of music therapy and palliative care experiences within a cancer hospital. *J Palliat Care.* 2001;17(3).

22. Magill L. Role of music therapy in integrative oncology. *J Soc Integrat Oncol.* 2006;4(2):79–81.

23. Clark M, Isaacks-Downton G, Wells N, et al. Use of preferred music to reduce emotional distress and symptom activity during radiation therapy. *J Music Ther.* 2006;43(3):247–265.

24. Hanser S. Research issues: music therapy in adult oncology. *J Soc Integrat Oncol.* 2006;4(2):62–66.

25. O'Callaghan CC. Clinical issues: music therapy in an adult cancer inpatient treatment setting. *J Soc Integrat Oncol.* 2006;4(2):57–61.

26. Bailey L. The use of songs in music therapy with cancer patients and their families. *Music Ther.* 1984;4:5–17.

27. Hilliard RE. Music therapy in hospice and palliative care: a review of the empirical data. *Evid Based Complement Altern Med.* 2005;2(2):173–178.

28. Magill L. The spiritual meaning of pre-loss music therapy to bereaved caregivers of advanced cancer patients. *J Palliat Support Care.* 2009 Mar;7(1):97–108.

29. Daykin N, McClean S, Bunt L. Creativity, identity and healing: participants' accounts of music therapy in cancer care. *Heath (London).* 2007;11(3):349–370.

30. Hanser SB. Music therapy to enhance coping in terminally ill cancer patients. In: Dileo C, Loewy J (eds). *Music therapy and end-of-life.* Cherry Hill, NJ: Jeffrey Books; 2005:33–42.

31. Burns DS, Sledge RB, Fuller LA, Daggy JK, Monahan PO. Cancer patients' interest and preferences for music therapy. *J Music Ther.* 2005;42(3):185–199.

32. Magill L. Music therapy: enhancing spirituality at the end-of-life. In: Dileo C, Loewy J (eds). *Music therapy and end-of-life.* Cherry Hill, NJ: Jeffrey Books; 2005:3–18.

33. Dileo C. Final moments: the use of songs in relationship completion. In: Dileo C, Loewy J (eds). *Music therapy and end-of-life.* Cherry Hill, NJ: Jeffrey Books; 2005:43–56.

34. O'Callaghan CC. Lyrical themes in songs written by palliative care patients. *J Music Ther.* 1996;33:74–92.

35. Tamplin J. A pilot study into the effect of vocal exercises and singing on dysarthric speech. *Neuro Rehabilitation.* 2008;23(3):207–216.

36. Aldridge D, Fachner J (eds). *Music and altered states: Consciousness, transcendence, and addiction.* London: Jessica Kingsley Publishers; 2006.

37. Dileo C, Bradt J. Entrainment, resonance and pain-related suffering. In: Dileo C (ed). *Music therapy in medicine: Theoretical and clinical applications.* Silver Spring, MD: American Music Therapy Association; 1999:181–188.

38. Butler CF, Butler PJ, Physioacoustic therapy with cardiac surgery patients. In: Wigram T, Dileo C (eds). *Music vibration and health.* Cherry Hill, NJ: Jeffrey Books; 1997:197–207.

39. Tomaino C. Active music therapy approaches for neurologically impaired patients. In: Dileo C (ed). *Music therapy in medicine: Theoretical and clinical applications.* Silver Spring, MD: American Music Therapy Association; 1999:115–122.

40. Magill L, Berenson S. The conjoint use of music therapy and reflexology with hospitalized advanced stage cancer patients and their families. *J Palliat Support Care.* 2008;6(3):289–296.

41. Sacks O. The power of music. *Brain.* 2006;129(pt 10):2528–2532.

42. Schwartz F, Ritchie R. Music listening in neonatal intensive care units. In: Dileo C (ed). *Music therapy in medicine: Theoretical and clinical applications.* Silver Spring, MD: American Music Therapy Association; 1999:13–22.

43. Ozdemir E, Norton A, Schlaug G. Making non-fluent aphasics speak: sing along! *Brain.* 2006;129(pt 10):2571–2584.

44. Scheiby B. "Better trying than crying": analytical music therapy in a medical setting. In: Dileo C (ed). *Music therapy in medicine: Theoretical and clinical applications.* Silver Spring, MD: American Music Therapy Association; 1999:95–106.

45. Caprilli S, Anastasi F, Grotto RP, Abeti MS, Messeri A. Interactive music as a treatment for pain and stress in children during venipuncture: a randomized prospective study. *J Dev Behav Ped.* 2007;28(5):399–403.

46. Derby S, O'Mahoney S. Elderly patients. In: Ferrell BR, Coyle N (eds). *Textbook of palliative nursing,* 2nd ed. New York: Oxford University Press, Inc; 2006:635–659.

47. Aldridge D (ed). *Music therapy in dementia care.* London: Jessica Kingsley Publishers; 2000.

48. Kemper KJ, Danhauer SC. Music as therapy. *South Med J.* 2005; 98(3):282–288.

49. Slivka HH, Magill L. Working with children of cancer patients. *Caring.* 1993;12(2):90–95.

50. O'Callaghan CC, Magill L. The effect of music therapy on oncologic staff bystanders: a substantive theory. *J Palliat Support Care.* 2009 Jun;7(2):219–228.

CHAPTER 58

Meditation and Yoga

Linda E. Carlson

INTRODUCTION

Most people have some familiarity with the concepts of meditation and yoga. In the context of healthcare meditation is considered a form of mind training, a skill that anyone can develop gradually over time that may have the potential to facilitate coping with a host of stressors endemic in the fast-pace of modern society. Yoga, too, includes a philosophy, ethics, and meditation practice which complement the familiar postures or *asanas* practiced in most mainstream studios. Both the physical postures and meditation practices of yoga have been utilized in healthcare settings. This chapter will review the growing body of literature that has utilized practices derived from meditation and yoga traditions for the purpose of helping people with cancer cope with a wide range of symptoms and issues concomitant with the disease, its treatment, and recovery. Although there is significant overlap between meditation and yoga, each practice will be described separately and its basic assumptions outlined, followed by a critical review of the empirical literature in each area, focusing on applications in psycho-oncology settings. Finally, results will be summarized and directions for future research suggested.

MEDITATION

While meditation may evoke images of swamis sitting in the lotus position in high Himalayan caves or 1960s hippies repeating secret mantras to reach altered mind-states, meditation in healthcare settings is comparatively mundane. Meditation refers to both a state of being, and a variety of techniques or practices for secular mind training. It has been defined broadly in contemporary research, for example:

A family of self-regulation practices that focus on training attention and awareness in order to bring mental processes under greater voluntary control and thereby foster general mental well-being and development and/or specific capacities such as calm, clarity, and concentration.[1]

Any procedure that comprises: (a) a specific, clearly defined technique, i.e., a "recipe" for meditation; (b) muscle relaxation in some moment of the process; (c) "logic relaxation" (not to intend to analyze, judge or create any expectation of practice); (d) a self-induced state; and (e) a "self-focus" skill or anchor.[2]

As can be seen from these two examples, there are many ways to define the key characteristics of meditation; applying one definition over another may result in some techniques being ruled out as bona fide meditation practices. Most meditation practices do have one thing in common—the purposive direction of attention towards a specific target. Attention can be directed towards one particular chosen object (for example, repeating a sound or mantra, following the breath) which is often known as *concentration meditation*, or on all mental events that enter the field of awareness, which is called *mindfulness meditation*. This distinction is useful, although it is not the only one that can be made, and in practice these forms of meditation are not always mutually exclusive.

In the past three decades, there has been growing clinical and research interest in the practice of mindfulness meditation, due in large part to the pioneering work of Jon Kabat-Zinn, at the University of Massachusetts Medical Centre. The program he devised in the late 1970s, based on intensive secular training in mindfulness meditation techniques, is now known as Mindfulness-based stress reduction (MBSR),[3] described in the next section. With this growing interest in the application of mindfulness meditation in medical settings, significant effort has been applied to operationally defining the concept of mindfulness. Kabat-Zinn defined mindfulness as "The awareness that emerges through paying attention on purpose, in the present moment, and nonjudgmentally to the unfolding of experience moment to moment"[4]: Bishop and colleagues described a two-factor model of mindfulness[5]: the first component involves the self-regulation of attention to maintain focus on immediate experience, which allows for increased recognition of mental events in the present moment. The second involves adopting an orientation toward one's experience that is characterized by curiosity, openness, and acceptance. This is similar to a model proposed by Shapiro et al.,[6] which stresses the importance of Intention, Attention, and Attitude (IAA) in mindfulness practices. Meditation is a complex concept referring to a wide variety of self-regulation practices and states of mind. The ultimate goal of meditation practice varies, depending on the type of practice, its history, and application. In a Westernized medical context, the goal of meditation is often reducing stress and helping individuals to cope with difficulties inherent in living with sometimes life-threatening illnesses and uncomfortable symptoms.

A comprehensive review of mediation in healthcare applications was recently published by the National Centre for Complementary and Alternative Medicine (NCCAM)[7]—this 472-page report includes a broad range of meditation-based interventions and should be consulted for an overview of the wider field of research. For the remainder of this section, focus will be on research applying the MBSR program to cancer patients, which is the primary modality that has been investigated in the scientific oncology literature.

Mindfulness-based stress reduction. Mindfulness-based stress reduction is an 8-week structured group program that incorporates intensive training in mindfulness meditation with group reflection and mindful Hatha yoga practice. The foundations of MBSR stem from Buddhist philosophy and practice, but it is free from any religious context. Participants learn fundamentals of the mind-body connection and how their interpretations of the world can cause both physical and mental suffering. The concept of mindfulness is introduced as learning to be present in life as it is occurring, applying attitudes of kindness, patience, curiosity, acceptance, letting go, and nonjudging. MBSR participants begin to recognize that the amount of mental energy spent regretting the past or worrying about the future, has resulted in missing the present moment and can cause depression and anxiety. Through the application of careful attention in this way, a process of "re-perceiving" can occur whereby the world view that had perpetuated suffering is abolished.

The primary meditation techniques used to cultivate mindfulness in the MBSR program are the body scan, sitting meditation, walking meditation, and loving-kindness meditation, in conjunction with mindful yoga postures. The body scan is a sensate focus meditation practice in which participants are guided to direct attention to successive body parts, moving systematically through the body. At each point of focus they are directed to take in whatever sensory experience is accessible, along with any emotions or associations with that body part, without expectation or judgment—then simply let go and move on to the next region. Sitting meditation begins with awareness of the breath passing in and out of the body, paying attention to sensations of rising and falling in the belly or the rushing of air in and out through the nostrils. Eventually, the focus widens to encompass any aspect of present-moment experience that may arise, from sensation to emotion, sounds, thoughts, and so on... all are seen with awareness as passing events simply rising and falling in consciousness. Walking meditation is similar to sitting, but in this case the awareness is typically directed towards some aspect of the body walking—the rising and falling of the feet, shifting of the weight from foot to foot, or a sense of the whole body moving through space. As with all forms of mindfulness meditation, when the attention wanders to thinking of the past, planning the future, desiring or pushing away elements of experience, or discursive analysis, it is gently redirected to the raw experience of each passing moment. Finally, loving-kindness meditation is a purposive practice that focuses on generating feelings of compassion and care for oneself, loved ones, and eventually all living beings. These practices form the core of the formal meditation practice in MBSR, which is learned in conjunction with mindful yoga postures.

For people dealing with cancer, many of the issues that arise are amenable to an MBSR approach. Fears of an uncertain future, pain, and death are common reactions to a cancer diagnosis. Mindfulness training can offer one venue for coping with these often uncomfortable and difficult emotions in a safe and controlled container of one's own making. By adopting a stance of observer to the overwhelming thoughts and emotions, patients can take a step back and allow themselves to process these experiences at their own pace, seeing their experience as constantly changing, and their distressing thoughts as simply mind-events that are often untrue. Ultimately, they begin to see that they are more than a cancer patient; they are connected to, and supported by, everyone else who shares this human condition.

Hence, there are theoretical reasons to believe that meditation training in general, or MBSR in particular, has potential to be beneficial to people going through a cancer experience.[8,9] There is also a growing empirical literature that is beginning to lend support to these ideas (Table 58–1).

Psycho-oncology Research in MBSR. There is a significant body of work investigating the efficacy of MBSR for patients with various types of cancer. This literature itself has been reviewed on several occasions since 2005.[8-13] All of the studies published to date, including abstracts and dissertations available through Medline, SCOPUS and PsychINFO, and through secondary searching of reference lists and contacting authors, are summarized chronologically in Table 58–1. Twenty-two studies are included; all of which have been published since the year 2000; 11 stem from our research program at the Tom Baker Cancer Centre in Calgary, Canada, with the rest primarily in the United States. Given this relatively small number, studies were not excluded based on quality or design. Fifteen of the 22 studies were uncontrolled trials, usually simple pre-post assessments of one group of MBSR participants on a range of outcome measures, or qualitative interview studies. The other 7 studies were randomized controlled trials (RCTs) that compared MBSR (or a variation of it) to either a waiting list (5/7) or some other active form of therapy (2/7). Sample sizes ranged from 9 to 157, but most were in the 20–60 range. Research in this area is just beginning to move beyond showing simple benefit to investigating specificity compared to other active treatments and the passage of time.

Psychological Outcomes. A range of psychological outcomes have been assessed in uncontrolled trials, often focusing on anxiety and mood symptoms. Tacon and colleagues conducted a small pre-post study of 27 women diagnosed with breast cancer who showed improvements over the MBSR course on measures of stress, anxiety, hopelessness, internal locus of control, and anxious preoccupation about cancer.[14] Similar improvements were found in a larger study of 40 women which also included less pain and distress related to symptoms.[15] In other uncontrolled trials, Spahn found improvements in role function and fatigue in 18 MBSR program participants,[16] and Brown and Ryan[17] found decreases in mood disturbance and stress levels that were associated with higher levels of mindfulness in 41 breast and prostate cancer patients. Garland et al.[18] assessed posttraumatic growth, spirituality, stress symptoms, and

mood disturbance in 104 patients participating in either MBSR or a Healing Arts program. All of the outcomes improved pre-post MBSR in 60 patients with a variety of cancer diagnoses, and when compared to the Healing Arts program, the MBSR participants improved more on spirituality, anxiety, anger, stress reduction, and mood symptoms.

Some qualitative interview work has also been conducted in this area. Mackenzie et al. conducted qualitative interviews with a specific subgroup of MBSR participants who attended weekly drop-in meditation practice groups following the 8-week program.[19] Five major themes were identified in the interviews, labeled as follows: (1) Opening to Change; (2) Self-Control; (3) Shared Experience; (4) Personal Growth; and (5) Spirituality. Analyses suggested that the participants developed qualities of positive health beyond initial symptom reduction, which focused more on finding meaning and purpose in life and feeling increasingly interconnected with others. Themes similar to those discovered by Mackenzie et al. were found in a mixed method study conducted with 13 women who had completed breast cancer treatment.[20] The women experienced decreases in perceived stress and medical symptoms as well as improvements on a measure of mindfulness. Themes identified by the women were as follows: (1) acceptance; (2) regaining and maintaining mindful control; (3) taking responsibility for what could change; and (4) cultivating a spirit of openness and connectedness.

In the first published RCT in cancer patients, 89 participants with a variety of cancer diagnoses were randomized to MBSR or a waitlist control condition.[21] Patients in the MBSR program improved significantly more on mood states and symptoms of stress than those in the control condition. They reported less tension, depression, anger, concentration problems, and more vigor, as well as fewer peripheral manifestations of stress (e.g., tingling in hands and feet), cardiopulmonary symptoms of arousal (e.g., racing heart, hyperventilation) central neurological symptoms (e.g., dizziness, faintness), gastrointestinal symptoms (e.g., upset stomach, diarrhea), habitual stress behavioral patterns (e.g., smoking, grinding teeth, overeating, insomnia), anxiety/fear, and emotional instability compared to those still waiting for the program. Both the immediate treatment group and the waitlist control group maintained these benefits 6-months following program completion.[22] Overall, more home practice was associated with greater decreases in mood disturbance; the largest improvements were seen on anxiety, depression, and irritability.

Biological and Sleep Outcomes. A number of uncontrolled studies have also been conducted investigating biological outcomes and health behaviors following MBSR. Carlson et al.[22-26] looked at measures of immune, endocrine, and autonomic function in addition to similar psychological variables as in the aforementioned RCT in 59 breast and prostate cancer survivors. Improvements were seen in overall quality of life, symptoms of stress, and sleep quality. Immune function was investigated by looking at the counts and function of a number of lymphocyte subsets, including T cells and natural killer (NK) cells, through secretion of cytokines in response to cell stimulation. Although there were no significant changes in the overall number of lymphocytes or cell subsets, T cell production of interferon-gamma (IFN-λ), a proinflammatory cytokine, decreased. Patterns of change were also assessed over a full year following program participation, and levels of pro-inflammatory cytokines continued to decrease.[26] Although the exact meaning of theses changes in relation to cancer progression is not known, in some studies elevated proinflammatory cytokines have been associated with poorer cancer outcomes.[27]

Carlson et al. also looked at salivary cortisol levels in response to MBSR. Daily salivary cortisol levels have been related to stress and health, and dysregulated levels have been associated with shorter survival time in cancer patients.[28] Cortisol profiles also shifted following the intervention. Fewer evening cortisol elevations were found post-MBSR and some normalization of initially abnormal diurnal salivary cortisol profiles occurred.[25] Over the year of follow-up, continuing decreases in overall cortisol levels were seen, mostly due to decreases in evening cortisol levels.[26] This is significant as higher cortisol levels, particularly in the evening, are considered to be an indicator of dysregulated cortisol secretion patters and poorer clinical outcomes. In this same study, overall resting systolic blood pressure (SBP) decreased significantly from

Table 58–1. Studies of MSBR in oncology samples

Study	Design	Sample	Measures	Results
Speca et al. (2000)[21]	Pre-post RCT to MBSR or waitlist	89 mixed dx both in and out of treatment 51 Stage I and II and 38 Stage III or IV Average age 51 years; 82% of sample female	Mood (POMS), Stress symptoms (SOSI), Homework logs	Greater decreases in 5 of 6 POMS subscales and TMD and 6 of 10 SOSI subscales and SOSI total score in treatment compared to control Home practice minutes correlated with decreases in POMS TMD and sessions attended correlated with decreases in SOSI total
Carlson et al. (2001)[22]	Pre-post 6-month follow-up on Speca et al. (2000)	Used original Speca et al. (2000) sample after wait-list group completed intervention. 89 at baseline, 80 after intervention and 54 follow-up	Mood (POMS), Stress symptoms (SOSI), Homework logs	Decreases pre-to-post on all 6 POMS subscales and TMD and on 9 of 10 SOSI subscales and total score Largest standardized changes on POMS anxiety, depression and anger, and SOSI depression, irritability, and muscle tension No further significant changes occurred over the follow-up
Hebert et al. (2001)[23]	Pre-post RCT comparing MBSR, nutrition education and usual care with 1 year follow-up	157 women with Stage I or II breast cancer	Dietary fat intake Complex carbohydrate intake, fibre intake, BMI, Anxiety (BAI), depression (BDI), self-esteem (RSES), psychiatric symptoms (SCL-90-R)	Nutrition group had greater reduction in BMI and fat consumption than MBSR and usual care at 4 months and 1 year Scores on psychological measures were not reported
Saxe et al. (2001)[36]	Pre-post UCT, combined MBSR with nutrition education	10 men with locally advanced prostate cancer and their partners	PSA levels, 7-day dietary recall	Decrease in PSA in 8 of 10 men Reduction in fate intake, BMI, and weight; increase in fiber and physical activity
Brown and Ryan (2003)[17]	Pre-post UCT of MBSR	32 breast and 9 prostate patients; subsample of Carlson et al. (2003; 2004)	Quality of life (EORTC-QLQ C-30), mood (POMS), stress (SOSI), mindfulness (MAAS)	Higher levels of mindfulness on MAAS was related to lower levels of mood disturbance and stress both before and after MBSR intervention
Carlson et al. (2003)[24]	Pre-post UCT of MBSR	59 early-stage patients completed treatment at least 3 months previously; 49 breast and 10 prostate cancer	Quality of life (EORTC-QLQ C-30), mood (POMS), stress (SOSI), Lymphocyte counts, cytokine production Weekly meditation logs Health behavior form	Improvements in EORTC and SOSI scores pre-post; improved sleep quality; no change in lymphocyte counts but cytokine production (IFN-γ) shifted towards anti-inflammatory pattern
Shapiro et al. (2003)[32]	Pre-post RCT to MBSR or "free choice" stress management group	Stage II breast cancer 62 at baseline; 54 post; 41 3-month f/u; 49 9-month f/u	Mood (POMS), depression (BDI), worry (PENN), anxiety (STAI), quality of life (FACT-B), sense of coherence (SOC), control (SCI), sleep diary	Only reported sleep results in this paper Higher baseline distress was related to lower sleep quality in both groups No group difference in sleep changes over time; within the MBSR group informal mindfulness practice was related to feeling more refreshed upon awakening
Spahn et al. (2003)— abstract[16]	Pre-post UCT, MBSR plus diet, self-care, complementary therapies, exercise	24; 23 female Variety of cancer diagnoses Full data on 18	Quality of life (EORTC-QLQ C-30), fatigue	Improvement in role function and fatigue

(Continued)

Table 58-1. Continued

Study	Design	Sample	Measures	Results
Carlson et al. (2004)[25]	Pre-post UCT of MBSR	Same sample as Carlson (2003)	Quality of life (EORTC-QLQ C-30), mood (POMS), stress (SOSI), Salivary cortisol DHEAS Melatonin	Improvements in quality of life correlated with decreases in afternoon cortisol pre- to post-MBSR Patients with elevated cortisol levels before intervention showed decreases after intervention and overall normal-ization of cortisol slopes
Tacon et al. (2004)[14]	Pre-post UCT of MBSR	27 breast cancer patients	Stress on 0–10 scale, anxiety (STAI), coping (MAC), locus of control (MHLC)	Reduction in stress, state anxiety, help-less/hopeless and anxious preoc-cupation coping styles, internal and chance health locus of control pre-post intervention
Bauer-Wu et al. (2004)[33]	Pre-post UCT, individualized mindfulness meditation sessions 1–2/week during hospitalization	20 patients undergoing stem-cell or bone marrow transplantation	Psychological and physical symptom VAS completed pre-post each ses-sion; HR and RR	Improvements in relaxation, pain, happiness, comfort, HR and RR on average pre-post each session
Carlson et al. (2005)[31]	Pre-post UCT of MBSR	63 patients with mixed can-cer diagnoses, both in and out of treatment	Sleep (PSQI), stress symptoms (SOSI), mood (POMS)	Improvements in sleep quality and effi-ciency, less sleep disturbance, longer duration of sleep, decreased stress, mood disturbance, and fatigue Decreases in stress symptoms were related to improvements in sleep quality and decreases in fatigue
Horton-Duetsch (2005)[34]	Pre-post UCT of individualized mindfulness meditation— 6–8 total sessions offered 2x/ week during hospitalization	24 patients undergoing BMT, 15 available for follow-up after discharge	Anxiety and depres-sion (HADS), affect (PANAS), Mastery/perceived control scale, symptom experi-ence scale	Negative affect decreased over the interven-tion but all other changes were ns Participants found the live intervention more helpful than the CDs provided for between-session practice Symptoms such as nausea and lack of appetite increased over the course of hospitalization
Monti et al. (2005)[35]	Pre-post waitlist RCT of MBAT	93 mixed cancer: 51 breast; 13 hematologic; 19 gyne; 9 neuro; 23 other	Psychiatric symp-toms (SCL-90-R); quality of life (SF-36)	All subscales and the GSI of the SCL improved more in MBAT participants compared to controls Greater improvements were also seen on the mental health, general health, social, and vitality subscales of the SF-36
Van Wielingen et al. (2006)–abstract[29]	Pre-post non-randomized trial of MBSR versus waitlist	10 MBSR participants and 7 waitlist controls	Stress test (TSST)— laboratory mea-sures of BP, HR, salivary cortisol, and weekly home BP monitoring	Preliminary findings: greater systolic BP recovery following a public speaking laboratory stress task in the MBSR group compared to waitlist controls
Van Wielingen et al. (2007) abstract[30]	Pre-post non-randomized trial of MBSR versus waitlist	29 female cancer patients completed treatment 18 in immediate MBSR and 11 waitlist	Weekly home rest-ing BP, stress (SOSI), depression (CES-D), rumina-tion and mindful-ness (MAAS)	Participants with relatively high levels of baseline systolic BP in the MBSR program had decreases in resting systolic BP over the 8 weeks, decreased symptoms of stress, depression, rumination, and increased mindfulness compared to wait-ing controls
Mackenzie et al. (2007)[19]	Qualitative Interviews with grounded theory analysis of MBSR graduates attending continuing drop-in groups	9 patients with mixed diag-noses; 7 women and 2 men	Qualitative inter-views with open-ended questions asking about their experience learn-ing MBSR during and after cancer	Five themes were identified: (1) opening to change; (2) self-control; (3) shared experi-ence; (4) personal growth; and (5) spirituality A theory was developed regarding the process of how for cancer patients the application of MBSR may evolve over time from focusing on symptom control to personal growth

Study	Design	Sample	Measures	Results
Carlson et al. (2007)[26]	Pre-post 6-month and 1-year follow-up UCT of MBSR	Same sample as Carlson (2003); N = 59, 51, 47, 41 for pre, post, 6-month and 1-year assessments	Quality of life (EORTC-QLQ C-30), mood (POMS), stress (SOSI), salivary cortisol, lymphocyte counts, cytokine function, BP and HR	Pre-post improvements in symptoms of stress were maintained over the follow-up Cortisol levels decreased systematically over 1 year A reduction in pro-inflammatory cytokines continued over the year Systolic BP decreased from pre- to post-intervention HR was correlated with stress symptoms
Garland et al. (2007)[18]	Between group pre-post non-randomized comparison of MBSR versus Healing Arts (HA)	104 patients; 60 in MBSR and 44 in HA Mixed cancer diagnoses both in and out of treatment	mood (POMS), stress (SOSI), post-traumatic growth (PTGI-R), spirituality (FACIT-Sp)	Both groups improved on the PTGI subscales of ability to relate to others, discover new possibilities, and recognize personal strengths, as well as depression and confusion on the POMS and on 7 of 10 SOSI subscales MBSR participants improved more than the HA group on spirituality, anxiety, anger, overall TMD, and total SOSI.
Tacon (2007)[15]	Pre-post UCT of MBSR	40 breast cancer patients	Depression (CES-D), pain (SF-MPQ), symptom distress (SDS), anxiety (STAI)	Pre-post improvements seen on measures of depression, state anxiety, pain, and symptom distress
Dobkin (2008)[20]	Pre-post UCT of MBSR with a focus group	13 breast cancer patients completed treatment	Depression (CES-D), medical symptoms (MSCL), stress (PSS), coping (CHIP), coherence (SOC), mindfulness (MAAS), qualitative focus group	Improvements pre-post on perceived stress (PSS), medical symptoms (MSCL) and mindfulness (MAAS) Themes from the focus group were: acceptance; regaining and sustaining mindful control; taking responsibility for what can change and developing a spirit of openness and connectedness
Carmody (2008)[37]	Pre-post RCT with 3-month follow-up comparing 11-week dietary change and mindfulness program to waitlist (based on Saxe et al., 2001 pilot study)	36 men with prostate cancer completed treatment and their partners	PSA levels, PSA doubling time, QL (FACT-P), dietary intakes, BMI, amount of meditation home practice	Greater reductions in saturated fat, animal protein, and increases in vegetable protein, fiber, lycopene, carotenoid consumption and QL in intervention group compared to control. PSA doubling time after intervention slowed to 59 versus 19 months in control Over half of men practiced meditation 3x/week or more Meditation practice correlated with more vegetable protein and less animal protein consumption

ABBREVIATIONS: BAI, Beck Anxiety Inventory; BDI, Beck Depression Inventory; BMI, body mass index; BMT, Bone Marrow Transplantation; BP, blood pressure; CES-D, Centre for Epidemiologic Studies Depression questionnaire; CHIP, coping with health injuries and problems; DHEAS, dehydroepiandrosterone-sulfate; EORTC-QLQ C-30, European Organization for Research and Treatment of Cancer Quality of Life Questionnaire—30 Item Version; FACIT-Sp, Functional Assessment of Chronic Illness Therapy Spirituality Scale; FACT-B, functional assessment of cancer treatment—breast module; FACT-P, functional assessment of cancer treatment—prostate module; GSI, General Severity Index of the SCL-90-R; HADS, Hospital Anxiety and Depression Scale; HR, heart rate; IFN-γ, interferon-gamma; MAAS, Mindful Attention Awareness Scale; MAC, mental adjustment to cancer; MBSR, mindfulness-based stress reduction; MHLC, multidimensional health locus of control; MSCL, medical symptoms checklist; PANAS, Positive and Negative Affect Scale; PENN, Penn State Worry Questionnaire; POMS, profile of mood states; PSA, prostate-serum antigen; PSQI, Pittsburg Sleep Quality Index; PSS, Perceived Stress Scale; PTGI-R, Post-traumatic Growth Inventory-Revised; QL, quality of life ; RCT, randomized controlled trial; RR, respiratory rate; RSES, Rosenberg Self-Esteem Scale; SCI, Shapiro Control Index; SCL-90-R, Symptom Checklist 90 Item-Revised; SDS, Symptom Distress Scale for Cancer; SF-36, Medical Outcomes Survey Short Form Quality of Life Questionnaire—36 item version; SF-MPQ, Short Form McGill Pain Questionnaire; SOC, Sense of Coherence Scale; SOSI, Symptoms of Stress Inventory; STAI, State-Trait Anxiety Inventory; TMD, total mood disturbance; TSST, Trier Social Stress Test; UCT, uncontrolled trial.

pre- to post-MBSR.[26] This is desirable as high blood pressure (hypertension) is the most significant risk factor for developing cardiovascular disease, and cancer patients who have received some common forms of chemotherapy (CT) are already at higher risk for developing cardiac problems due to treatment-related cardiotoxicity.

Using a laboratory social stress paradigm and a waiting list trial design, Van Wielingen et al. subjected women registered in the MBSR program to the Trier Social Stress Test (public speaking task and mental arithmetic).[29] Women in the immediate group were retested post-MBSR while those still waiting were tested a second time prior to MBSR participation. Measures of cardiovascular reactivity and recovery were compared. Women who had taken MBSR showed greater SBP recovery following the public speaking task, but both groups had similar reactivity to the stressors. This suggests that while they still reacted physiologically to stress-provoking stimuli, mindfulness training may have helped these women recover more quickly to baseline, an ability that has been related to decreased risk for cardiovascular disease. In a larger sample of women from the same study, Van Wielingen et al. found that home blood pressure measured weekly decreased significantly only for those women who were currently taking the program.[30] For those with initially elevated SBP, an average decrease of 15 mm Hg was reported, which is similar in magnitude to decreases resulting from blood pressure medication, suggesting that these improvements were likely to have clinically meaningful repercussions.

Finally, in an uncontrolled pre-post trial, Carlson et al. found a very high proportion of cancer patients with disordered sleep (approximately 85%) in a general sample of 63 patients before attending the MBSR program.[31] In these patients, sleep disturbance was closely associated with levels of self-reported stress and mood disturbance, and when stress symptoms declined over the course of the MBSR program, sleep also improved. On average, sleep hours increased by ½ to 1 hour per night. Shapiro et al. also examined the relationship between participation in an MBSR program and sleep quality/efficiency in a sample of 54 breast cancer patients.[32] Women were randomly assigned to either MBSR or a free choice stress reduction intervention where they could choose what techniques they wished to use (e.g., books, social support). The women were followed for 9 months after the intervention. There were no statistically significant relationships between participation in an MBSR group and sleep quality; however, within the MBSR group those who practiced more informal mindfulness reported feeling more rested.

Adaptations of MBSR. There have also been adaptations of the traditional 8-week group MBSR program for special populations of cancer patients, particularly two studies that looked at mindfulness meditation for hospitalized patients undergoing bone marrow or stem-cell transplantation (BMT/SCT). Bauer-Wu and Rosenbaum found immediate decreases in levels of pain and anxiety following meditation sessions.[33] Horton-Duetsch et al. provided 6–8 bi-weekly 20- to 40-minute individual sessions consisting of one-on-one training in mindfulness with an experienced instructor, based on an adaptation of the group MBSR curriculum.[34] Less negative affect was reported after the intervention despite increasing symptoms of nausea and appetite loss, and patients found the program feasible, although they felt training in mindfulness before hospitalization would have been preferable.

A unique modification on MBSR that has been applied to cancer patients is called Mindfulness-based art therapy (MBAT), which combines the principles of MBSR with other creative modalities. Patients practice meditation and then express their experience through a number of visual arts outlets such as painting and drawing. In an RCT (N = 111), researchers compared the 8-week MBAT intervention to a wait list control in a heterogeneous cohort of women with mixed cancer types receiving usual oncology care. MBAT participants had less depression, anxiety, somatic symptoms of stress, and less hostility than control participants after the intervention.[35]

In another study of biological outcomes using a modified program, an innovative project by Carmody et al. looked at the effects of combining a dietary intervention with MBSR on prostate-specific antigen (PSA) levels, an indicator of the level of activity of prostate cancer cells in men with biochemically recurrent prostate cancer.[36] They found the combined program resulted in a slowing of the rate of PSA increase in a pilot sample of 10 men. In 2008 they published a larger RCT of this intervention (36 men), measuring dietary intake of various nutrients, and quality of life as well as PSA outcomes and time spent meditating.[37] Although there were no overall group differences in PSA levels, those in the intervention group had increased their PSA doubling time from 18 to 59 months, while the waitlist participants remained steady around 19 months. It is impossible to determine the specific roles that meditation practice and dietary change may have played in this outcome, but it may be that the meditation practice allowed the men to be more vigilant

and mindful of their dietary choices, as time spent in mediation practice correlated with intake of vegetable protein.

In summary, the work to date on MBSR in cancer patients supports its usefulness for decreasing a wide range of psychological outcomes such as symptoms of stress, anxiety, anger, depression and mood disturbance, and improving quality of life and sleep outcomes. It may be effective both for patients undergoing treatment (including BMT/SCT) or completed treatment protocols. Effects on biological outcomes such as cortisol and immune function are suggested, but more research with controlled comparison groups is required. Few studies have compared MBSR directly to other supportive care interventions, so it is impossible to know which of these effects are specific to MBSR or if many different types of interventions would produce similar positive results.

YOGA

The term "Yoga" is derived from the Sanskrit word *yug*, meaning "union."[38] This, according to traditional yoga philosophy, is the ultimate intent of a yoga practice—to unite the individual with the totality of the universe—giving yoga students a deeper awareness of life, one where they no longer experience living as separate, but instead as part of the larger whole.[38] The techniques of yoga include ethical practice for daily living, physical exercise, breathing techniques, and meditation training. Over the centuries, the practice of yoga postures has evolved to exercise every muscle, nerve, and gland in the body.[38] They provide a combination of static and active stretching; isometric and dynamic strengthening which enables practitioners to gain flexibility and develop stability, strength, and balance.[39]

The type of yoga widely practiced at mainstream studios typically consists of Hatha postures, but many subtypes are practiced. One such modality that is commonly used with cancer patients is known as *Yoga therapy*, or restorative yoga. Yoga therapy has been defined as:

the adaptation and application of Yoga techniques and practices to help individuals facing health challenges at any level manage their condition, reduce symptoms, restore balance, increase vitality, and improve attitude…it comprises a wide range of mind/body practices, from postural and breathing exercises to deep relaxation and meditation. Yoga therapy tailors these to the health needs of the individual (International Association of Yoga Therapists: http://www.iayt.org/).

Other yoga techniques used in studies with cancer patients focus on meditation-like exercises and breathing, such as Sudarshan Kriya yoga (SKY), which combines breathing exercises with meditation and chanting. The breathing exercises range from slow breathing against airway resistance at 3 cycles/min to a quick and forceful exhalation at 20–30 cycles/min, and rhythmic, cyclical breathing in increasing frequencies from slow to medium to fast cycles.

As can be seen from these brief descriptions, the term "yoga" by no means refers to a uniform package of practices, so it is important in this type of research to specify exactly which aspects of the broad yoga portfolio were focused on in any given intervention.

Psycho-oncology research in yoga. Recent interest in specific yoga-based interventions for cancer patients has resulted in the publication of a number of studies solely focused on various yoga practices. Bower[40] reviewed the literature in 2005, identifying six studies on yoga in cancer patients.[41-46] Since that time five other RCTs[47-51] and several uncontrolled trials have been published[52-54] (Table 58–2). Of the 14 studies reviewed, 10 were RCTs, but only 2 compared yoga to one or more other active interventions; the other 8 used waitlist groups as the comparison.

These studies utilized a variety of yoga interventions, some of which focused more on yogic meditation and relaxation than physical postures. An early nonrandomized study in India compared yoga to transcendental meditation (TM) and group supportive therapy with prayer.[41] The TM group was found to be the most beneficial, although formal statistical group comparisons were not made. Other uncontrolled trials evaluated various yoga programs. Rosenbaum[52] conducted a one-time evaluation of patient satisfaction with a variety of complementary medicine programs, including a restorative yoga program. Of those who

Table 58–2. Studies of yoga interventions in oncology samples

Study	Design	Sample	Measures	Results
Joseph (1983)[55]	Pre-post UCT 90-min class 2x/week Yoga versus TM versus group therapy (patient choice) Yogic relaxation exercises 2x/week but no strenuous postures	125 cancer patients, type not specified, undergoing RT Yoga: n = 50; TM n = 25; group therapy n = 50	Postprogram questionnaire administered via interview	No statistical analyses conducted Yoga: improved appetite (n = 11/50), sleep (11/50) peace and tranquility (10/50), bowel habits (13/50); TM: improved peace and tranquility (23/25), vigor and energy (15/25); group therapy: 45/50 felt better after group, 30/50 reported less fear of cancer
Cohen (2004)[42]	Pre-post RCT to Tiebetan yoga or waitlist 7 weekly yoga classes	38 lymphoma patients stage I–IV 24 women 19 patients in waitlist group	Distress (IES), Anxiety (STATE), depression (CES-D), sleep (PSQI), fatigue (BFI)	No group differences on any psychological measures Subjective sleep quality, latency, duration, use of medications, and overall sleep score improved more in the yoga group
Rosenbaum (2004)[52]	Program evaluation of the Stanford Cancer Supportive Care Program—one-time assessment Program includes restorative yoga 2x/week	380 yoga program participants completed forms (of a total of 1183 evaluations—785 provided incomplete data)	Self-report on 5- or 10-point linear analogue scales for pain relief, stress and anxiety, and coping	96% reported reduced stress, 94% felt an increased sense of well-being, 74% felt an increase in energy, 65% reported more restful sleep, and 51% noted some improvement in pain
Moadel (2004) - abstract[44]	Pre-post RCT to Hatha yoga or waitlist 12 weekly 90-min classes	76 Breast cancer patients stages I–II on treatment—primarily African-American and Hispanic Compared 25 controls, 24 low adherence to yoga and 27 high adherence to yoga	quality of life (FACT-B)	Control group had increased physical symptoms and decreased social well-being, yoga patients with higher compliance had increased emotional well-being and no significant deterioration in physical function
Cohen et al. (2005) abstract[45]	Pre-post RCT to Tiebetan Yoga or waitlist with 3-month follow-up 7 weekly classes	58 stage I–III breast cancer patients Approximately half in active treatment	Distress (IES), cancer-related symptoms (M. D. Anderson Symptom Inventory), mood, sleep, QL	Compared to controls, the yoga group reported fewer cancer-related symptoms at the 1-week follow-up and lower cancer-related distress at the 3-month follow-up No effects on sleep, mood, or quality of life
Blank (2005)[50]	Pre-post RCT to yoga or waitlist Iyengar yoga 2x/week for 8 weeks	18 breast cancer patients stage I–III on hormonal therapy (9 in yoga, 9 on waitlist)	3I-question self-report survey about stress, level of physical and mental effort during class sessions, and perceptions about how yoga had influenced their awareness	25% said yoga practice relieved joint aches and shoulder stiffness All felt less stressed immediately after class, compared with when they arrived 88% felt more relaxed in their daily lives, were more aware of their body posture, and had improved body image 63% reported improved mood and less anxiety Ability to relax the body was rated as 8.5 ±1.8 on a 1–10 scale, ability to relax the mind was rated as 8.4 ±1.4, and ability to achieve inner quiet was rated as 8.9 ±1.3 No statistical comparisons with the waitlist group were reported
Carlson et al. (2005) abstract[46]	Pre-post RCT to yoga therapy or waitlist 7 weekly 75-min classes	20 participants with mixed cancer dx. (subsample of Culos-Reed et al. 2006)	Salivary cortisol (CRT) at 8 AM, 2 PM and 8 PM. Mood (POMS), stress symptoms (SOSI), quality of life (EORTC-QLQ C-30),	Higher CRT associated with higher fatigue, stress symptoms, mood disturbance, and lower QL Yoga group had better QL and less mood disturbance following the intervention No group differences in mean CRT or slopes after intervention Less variance in morning CRT scores in the yoga group after intervention, indicating extreme low or high levels had normalized, but not for the control group

(Continued)

435

Table 58–2. Continued

Study	Design	Sample	Measures	Results
Culos-Reed (2006)[43]	Pre-post RCT to yoga therapy or waitlist 7 weekly 75-min classes	38 patients, 95% women, 85% breast cancer, all completed treatment	Mood (POMS), stress symptoms (SOSI), quality of life (EORTC-QLQ C-30), BMI, grip strength, flexibility, functional capacity (6-min walking test)	Improved quality of life, emotional function, irritability, GI symptoms, confusion, tension, depression and overall mood disturbance in yoga compared to the waitlist participants No differential improvements on the physical outcomes
Warner (2006) - dissertation[54]	Pre-post UCT Art of Living Program Daily Sudarshan Kriya yoga (SKY) classes for 8 days with 5-weeks maintenance Assessed four times: 2 weeks before the program, 1st day, last day, 5 weeks	26 breast cancer patients stages 0–III	Quality of life (FACT-B), spirituality (FACIT-Sp), stress (PSS), mood (PSOM) Qualitative interviews with thematic analysis	Improvement in quality of life, spiritual well-being, positive states of mind, and perceived stress scores by the end of the 8-day course, maintained following the 5-week maintenance period Participants described decreased fears of recurrence, self-care, and healing of body image issues; feelings of peace, love, joy, gratitude, and mental clarity; feelings of interconnectedness, release and cleansing, and being in the present moment, and enhanced spirituality
Carson (2007)[56]	Pre-post UCT of Yoga of Awareness program 8 weekly 120 min class	13 metastatic breast cancer patients	Daily diaries with 10 cm VAS for pain, fatigue, distress, invigoration, acceptance, and relaxation during two preintervention weeks and the final two weeks of the intervention, plus a focus group after program	Significant improvements pre-to-post in daily invigoration and acceptance, along with trends for improvement in pain and relaxation On the day after a day with more yoga practice, significantly lower levels of pain and fatigue, and higher levels of invigoration, acceptance, and relaxation were reported Program perceived as very helpful in addressing the specific needs of metastatic breast cancer patients
Banerjee (2007)[47]	Pre-post RCT to an integrative yoga program or supportive counseling with light exercise 6 weeks of 90-min classes Yoga consisted of meditation, gentle postures, imagery, and chanting	58 stage II–III breast cancer patients 23 randomized to control All received RT over the course of the program	Anxiety and depression (HADS), stress (PSS), measure of DNA damage	Larger decreases on anxiety, depression, and perceived stress in yoga group than control DNA damage due to RT was less in the yoga group
Raghavendra et al. (2007)[49]	Pre-post RCT to an integrative yoga program or supportive-expressive therapy with coping skills Yoga (breathing and relaxation) practiced for 30-min before each CT infusion and home practice (mostly meditation) for 3–6 hr/week between infusions	62 breast cancer patients receiving CT	Nausea and vomiting (MANE), anxiety (STAI), depression (BDI), quality of life (FLIC), checklist of 31 items assessing symptoms and treatment side-effects evaluated on two dimensions: severity and distress Treatment toxicity on the WHO Toxicity Criteria	Yoga group had less post-CT and anticipatory nausea severity and frequency, less anticipatory vomiting Less anxiety, depression, and better quality of life in yoga group Less CT-related toxicity in yoga group

Study	Design	Sample	Measures	Results
Moadel (2007)[48]	Pre-post RCT to Hatha yoga or waitlist 12 weekly 90-min classes	128 breast cancer patients on CT or RT 44 in waitlist Final results of Moadel 2004 abstract	Quality of life (FACT-G), fatigue (FACT-F), spirituality (FACIT-Sp), mood (Distressed mood index from 19 POMS items)	Primary analysis showed more decline in social functioning only in control group Secondary analysis of only patients NOT on CT (yoga = 45; control = 26) showed more improvement in global QL, emotional, social, and spiritual well-being, distressed mood, anxiety/sadness and irritability in yoga compared to control
Cohen et al. (2008)[51] abstract	Pre-post RCT of Hatha yoga or waitlist with 1 week, and 1 and 3-month f/u 6 weeks of bi-weekly classes of postures, breathing, relaxation and meditation	61 stage 0–III breast cancer patients undergoing RT	Distress (IES), depression (CES-D), sleep (PSQI), fatigue (BFI), quality of life (SF-36), and benefit finding (FM)	The yoga group had higher SF-36 physical scores 1 week after the end of RT, higher intrusive thoughts 1 month after RT and higher benefit finding scores 3 months after RT No other group differences Intrusive thoughts scores at 1 month were a significant predictor of FM scores at 3 months, suggesting that intrusive thoughts mediated the effects of group on FM scores

ABBREVIATIONS: BDI, Brief Depression Inventory; BFI, Brief Fatigue Inventory; BMI, body mass index; CES-D, Centre for Epidemiologic Studies Depression questionnaire; CRT, cortisol, ; CT, Chemotherapy; EORTC-QLQ C-30, European Organization for Research and Treatment of Cancer Quality of Life Questionnaire—30 Item Version; FACIT-Sp, Functional Assessment of Chronic Illness Therapy Spirituality Scale; FACT-B, Functional Assessment of Cancer Treatment—Breast Module; FACT-G, Functional Assessment of Cancer Treatment—General Quality of Life; FACT-F, Functional Assessment of Cancer Treatment—Fatigue; FLIC, Functional Living Index for Cancer; FM, finding meaning in cancer; GI, gastrointestinal; HADS, Hospital Anxiety and Depression Scale; IES, Impact of Events Scale; MANE, Morrow Assessment of Nausea and Emesis; POMS, Profile of Mood States; PSOM, Positive States of Mind; PSQI, Pittsburgh Sleep Quality Index; RT, radiation therapy; PSS, Perceived Stress Scale; QL, quality of life; SKY, Sudarshan Kriya yoga; SOSI, Symptoms of Stress Inventory; STAI, State-Trait Anxiety Inventory; STATE, Spielberger State Anxiety Inventory; TM, transcendental meditation; VAS, Visual Analogue Scales; WHO, World Health Organization.

returned the surveys regarding yoga, 96% reported reduced distress and 94% felt increased well-being. Warner evaluated an 8-day intensive SKY intervention which combined the SK breathing exercises with "yoga-based aspects of cognitive-behavioral therapy and psychoeducation in human values of acceptance, social responsibility, and community service" (p.49). Improvements were found in the 28 participants with breast cancer on quality of life (QL), spirituality, positive mind states, and stress. Many advantages of the practice were also identified through the qualitative interviews. One other uncontrolled trial offered a Yoga of Awareness program to women with metastatic breast cancer.[53] This 8-week program incorporated gentle Hatha postures, breathing exercises, meditation techniques (awareness of breath and mindfulness meditation), didactic study of topics such as how one can bring awareness into everyday life, and group discussions. The 13 women who participated reported feeling more invigorated and relaxed, and had less pain and fatigue after the program.

The RCTs also evaluated a variety of yoga interventions. Blank reported on a fairly rigorous program of Iyengar yoga postures in 18 breast cancer patients.[50] Although this was an RCT, they reported results only for women in the yoga treatment group (not the waitlist group), citing decreased feelings of stress, more relaxation, and improved mood. Culos-Reed and colleagues[43] used a waitlist RCT design to evaluate a 7-week yoga therapy program in groups of mixed-diagnosis patients. The yoga participants had scores indicating more improvement than the controls after intervention on global QL, stress symptoms, emotional function, emotional irritability, tension, depression, anger, and confusion. They also had greater cardiovascular endurance and lower resting heart rates. A subsample of this group were also assessed on salivary cortisol levels with results showing modulation or normalization of cortisol levels towards healthier patterns.[46] Moadel, in two studies, evaluated a Hatha yoga program of 12 weekly 90-minute classes in low income, ethnically diverse women with breast cancer.[44,48] The first study reported on 76 women, comparing QL in the control group to participants low and high in compliance with the yoga intervention.[44] The control group had increased physical symptoms and decreased social well-being over time, while yoga patients with higher compliance had increased emotional well-being and no significant deterioration in physical function. Only when a subgroup of patients not on CT during the intervention (n = 71) were examined did the yoga group show more improvement overall than controls on global QL, emotional, social and spirituality well-being, mood, anxiety, and irritability.[48]

In three other RCTs of slightly different yoga programs, Cohen studied patients with lymphoma[42] and breast cancer.[45,51] The first two studies of Tibetan yoga incorporated controlled breathing, visualization, mindfulness techniques, and low-impact postures. In the lymphoma trial, patients in the yoga group reported significantly lower sleep disturbance scores during follow-up compared with patients in the waitlist control group, including better subjective sleep quality, faster sleep latency, longer sleep duration, and less use of sleep medications. They did not show any other differential improvements on measures of distress, anxiety, depression, or fatigue.[42] In contrast, the same intervention in breast cancer patients resulted in fewer cancer-related symptoms after the intervention and lower cancer-related distress at a 3-month follow-up, but no beneficial effects on sleep.[45] The most recent study investigated a modified intervention based on Hatha yoga for women with breast cancer undergoing radiation therapy (RT).[51] Results showed no group differences in sleep, depression, or QL, but those in the yoga group reported more intrusive thoughts 1 month after the intervention and more finding of benefit or meaning in the cancer experience 3-months after the intervention. Intrusive thoughts at 1 month, in fact, mediated the relationship between group membership and benefit finding at 3-months, suggesting that active processing of the trauma associated with breast cancer diagnosis and treatment may lead to beneficial outcomes some time later for these patients in the yoga program.

Two RCTs compared yoga to other active interventions. Banerjee compared 6-weeks of yoga classes to individual supportive counseling in a sample of 58 women with breast cancer undergoing RT.[47] Clinically significant improvements were found in the yoga group compared to the supportive care group on measures of anxiety, depression, and stress. The women were also undergoing RT at the time, and damage to DNA related to the RT was compared between groups. The yoga participants had less evidence of cellular damage than those in the counseling group. Another similar RCT examined an integrative yoga program compared to individual supportive-expressive therapy for 62 women undergoing CT for breast cancer—the women practiced yogic breathing and meditation prior to each CT infusion and at home between treatments.[49] The yoga group had less post-CT and anticipatory nausea, lower CT-related toxicity and less anticipatory vomiting than the control condition.

In summary, although the literature is still nascent in this area and rapidly growing, a variety of yoga interventions do hold potential for overall symptom reduction and improvements in quality of life, mood, and sleep. In addition, yoga appears to have the potential to help to control treatment-related symptoms such as nausea and vomiting and to help with physical rehabilitation from cancer treatments. It is important to highlight the specific details of different yoga interventions, since some focus more heavily on meditation and breathing practices, whereas others focus on the more physical postures. Outcomes of these different focuses of practice may be quite specific, so making across-the-board comparisons is not always advisable.

SUMMARY AND FUTURE DIRECTIONS

In summary, the literature on the effects of both meditation and yoga in cancer patients provides promising preliminary data on the efficacy of these interventions. The majority of the studies in MBSR used uncontrolled designs with small sample sizes; therefore the specificity of benefits has not been well-established. In yoga research, more evidence supports its efficacy compared to waiting list control conditions, but this only controls for the passage of time and not for patient expectancy or any other nonspecific factors associated with the interventions. The bulk of the research has also been conducted on women with breast cancer; therefore generalizability to other groups of patients is poor. The research universally suffers from selection bias as most participants were self-referred volunteers, further impacting the ability to generalize any positive findings to the larger population of cancer patients. Conclusions are thus limited to stating that benefits are reported across a wide range of psychological, quality of life and some physical outcomes, including reduced pain, fatigue, and better sleep for people who are interested in and seek out mediation or yoga programs.

Future research in this area should focus on determining the specificity of the interventions being studied compared to other proven efficacious active interventions for cancer patients. Determining the specificity of outcomes and the optimal timing of programs to enhance desired outcomes should also be a focus of future research. A broader range of outcomes including not only psychological and quality of life indicators, but objective measures of physical functioning and rehabilitation should be included. There is also a great deal of interest in determining the mechanisms through which these multidimensional programs may engender change, such as through the development of mindfulness skills, enhanced emotion regulation, decreased rumination, social support and group processes, or time spent in home practice. Studies designed to dismantle various program aspects such as these would be welcome.

ACKNOWLEDGMENTS

Dr. Linda E. Carlson holds the Enbridge Research Chair in Psychosocial Oncology at the University of Calgary, co-funded by the Canadian Cancer Society Albert/NWT Division and the Alberta Cancer Foundation. Thanks to Joshua Lounsberry for assistance with editing and referencing.

REFERENCES

1. Walsh R, Shapiro SL. The meeting of meditative disciplines and western psychology: a mutually enriching dialogue. *Am Psychol.* 2006;61:227–239.
2. Cardoso R, De Souze E, Camano L, Roberto-Leite J. Meditation in health: an operational definition. *Brain Res Brain Res Protoc.* 2004;14:60.
3. Kabat-Zinn J. *Full catastrophe living: Using the wisdom of your body and mind to face stress, pain and illness.* New York: Delacourt; 1990.
4. Kabat-Zinn J. Mindfulness based interventions in context: past, present and future. *Clin Psychol.* 2003;10:144–156.
5. Bishop SR, Lau M, Shapiro S,. Mindfulness: a proposed operational definition. *Clin Psychol.* 2004;11:230–241.
6. Shapiro SL, Carlson LE, Astin JA, Freedman B. Mechanisms of mindfulness. *J Clin Psychol.* 2006;62:373–386.
7. Ospina MB, Bond TK, Karkhaneh M, et al. *Meditation practices for health: State of the research.* Rockville, MD: Agency for Healthcare Research and Quality; 2007; Evidence Report/Technology Assessment No. 155.
8. Mackenzie MJ, Carlson LE, Speca M. Mindfulness-based stress reduction (MBSR) in oncology: rationale and review. *Evid Base Integr Med.* 2005;2:139–145.
9. Carlson LE, Speca M. Managing daily and long-term stress. In: Feurrestein M (ed). *Handbook of cancer survivorship.* New York: Springer; 2007:339–360.
10. Ott MJ, Norris RL, Bauer-Wu SM. Mindfulness meditation for oncology patients. *Integr Cancer Ther.* 2006;5:98–108.
11. Smith JE, Richardson J, Hoffman C, Pilkington K. Mindfulness-based stress reduction as supportive therapy in cancer care: systematic review. *J Adv Nurs.* 2005;52:315–327.
12. Matchim Y, Armer JM. Measuring the psychological impact of mindfulness meditation on health among patients with cancer: a literature review. *Oncol Nurs Forum.* 2007;34:1059–1066.
13. Lamanque P, Daneault S. Does meditation improve the quality of life for patients living with cancer? *Can Fam Physician.* 2006;52:474–475.
14. Tacon AM, Caldera YM, Ronaghan C. Mindfulness-based stress reduction in women with breast cancer. *Fam Syst Health.* 2004;22:193–203.
15. Tacon AM. Mindfulness effects on symptoms of distress in women with cancer. *J Cancer Pain Symp Palliat.* 2007;2:17–22.
16. Spahn G, Lehmann N, Franken U, et al. Improvement of fatigue and role function of cancer patients after an outpatient integrative mind-body intervention. *Focus Alternative Compl Ther.* 2003;8:540.
17. Brown KW, Ryan RM. The benefits of being present: mindfulness and its role in psychological well-being. *J Pers Soc Psychol.* 2003;84:822–848.
18. Garland SN, Carlson LE, Cook S, Lansdell L, Speca M. A non-randomized comparison of mindfulness-based stress reduction and healing arts programs for facilitating post-traumatic growth and spirituality in cancer outpatients. *Support Care Cancer.* 2007;15(8):949–61.
19. Mackenzie MJ, Carlson LE, Munoz M, Speca M. A qualitative study of self-perceived effects of mindfulness-based stress reduction (MBSR) in a psychosocial oncology setting. *Stress Health: J Int Soc Invest Stress.* 2007;23:59–69.
20. Dobkin PL. Mindfulness-based stress reduction: what processes are at work? *Complement Ther Clin Pract.* 2008;14:8–16.
21. Speca M, Carlson LE, Goodey E, Angen M. A randomized, wait-list controlled clinical trial: the effect of a mindfulness meditation-based stress reduction program on mood and symptoms of stress in cancer outpatients. *Psychosom Med.* 2000;62:613–622.
22. Carlson LE, Ursuliak Z, Goodey E, Angen M, Speca M. The effects of a mindfulness meditation based stress reduction program on mood and symptoms of stress in cancer outpatients: six month follow-up. *Support Care Cancer.* 2001;9:112–123.
23. Hebert J, Ebbeling C, Olendzki D, et al. Change in women's diet and body mass following intensive intervention for early-stage breast cancer. *J Am Diet Assoc.* 2001;101:421–431.
24. Carlson LE, Speca M, Patel KD, Goodey E. Mindfulness-based stress reduction in relation to quality of life, mood, symptoms of stress, and immune parameters in breast and prostate cancer outpatients. *Psychosom Med.* 2003;65:571–581.
25. Carlson LE, Speca M, Patel KD, Goodey E. Mindfulness-based stress reduction in relation to quality of life, mood, symptoms of stress and levels of cortisol, dehydroepiandrosterone-sulfate (DHEAS) and melatonin in breast and prostate cancer outpatients. *Psychoneuroendocrinology.* 2004;29:448–474.
26. Carlson LE, Speca M, Faris P, Patel KD. One year pre-post intervention follow-up of psychological, immune, endocrine and blood pressure outcomes of mindfulness-based stress reduction (MBSR) in breast and prostate cancer outpatients. *Brain Behav Immun.* 2007;21(8):1038–1049.
27. Costanzo ES, Lutgendorf SK, Sood AK, Anderson B, Sorosky J, Lubaroff DM. Psychosocial factors and interleukin-6 among women with advanced ovarian cancer. *Cancer.* 2005;104:305–313.
28. Sephton SE, Sapolsky RM, Kraemer HC, Spiegel D. Diurnal cortisol rhythm as a predictor of breast cancer survival. *J Natl Cancer Inst.* 2000;92:994–1000.
29. Van Wielingen LE, Carlson LE, Campbell TS. Mindfulness-based stress reduction and acute stress responses in women with cancer. *Psychooncology.* 2006;15:S42.
30. Van Wielingen LE, Carlson LE, Campbell TS. Mindfulness-based stress reduction (MBSR), blood pressure, and psychological functioning in women with cancer. *Psychosomatic Medicine.* 2007;69:A43.

31. Carlson LE, Garland SN. Impact of mindfulness-based stress reduction (MBSR) on sleep, mood, stress and fatigue symptoms in cancer outpatients. *Int J Behav Med.* 2005;12:278–285.

32. Shapiro SL, Bootzin RR, Figueredo AJ, Lopez AM, Schwartz GE. The efficacy of mindfulness-based stress reduction in the treatment of sleep disturbance in women with breast cancer: an exploratory study. *J Psychosom Res.* 2003;54:85–91.

33. Bauer-Wu SM, Rosenbaum E. Facing the challenges of stem cell/bone marrow transplantation with mindfulness meditation: a pilot study. *Psychooncology.* 2004;13:S10-S11.

34. Horton-Deutsch S, O'Haver Day P, Haight R, Babin-Nelson M. Enhancing mental health services to bone marrow transplant recipients through a mindfulness-based therapeutic intervention. *Complement Ther Clin Pract.* 2007;13:110–115.

35. Monti DA, Peterson C, Kunkel EJ, et al. A randomized, controlled trial of mindfulness-based art therapy (MBAT) for women with cancer. *Psychooncology.* 2005; 15(5):363–73.

36. Saxe GA, Hebert JR, Carmody JF, et al. Can diet in conjunction with stress reduction affect the rate of increase in prostate specific antigen after biochemical recurrence of prostate cancer? *J Urol.* 2001;166:2202–2207.

37. Carmody J, Olendzki B, Reed G, Andersen V, Rosenzweig P. A dietary intervention for recurrent prostate cancer after definitive primary treatment: results of a randomized pilot trial. *Urology.* 2008;72(6):1324–1328.

38. Iyengar, B. K. S. *Light on yoga.* New York: Allen and Irwin; 1976.

39. Raub JA. Psycho-physiologic effects of hatha yoga on musculo-skeletal and cardiopulmonary function: a literature review. *J Complement Med.* 2002;8:7–12.

40. Bower JE, Woolery A, Sternlieb B, Garet D. Yoga for cancer patients and survivors. *Cancer Control.* 2005;12:165–171.

41. Joseph CD. Psychological supportive therapy for cancer patients. *Indian J Cancer.* 1983;20:268–270.

42. Cohen L, Warneke C, Fouladi RT, Rodriguez MA, Chaoul-Reich A. Psychological adjustment and sleep quality in a randomized trial of the effects of a Tibetan yoga intervention in patients with lymphoma. *Cancer.* 2004;100:2253–2260.

43. Culos-Reed SN, Carlson LE, Daroux LM, Hately-Aldous S. A pilot study of yoga for breast cancer survivors: physical and psychological benefits. *Psychooncology.* 2006;15:891–897.

44. Moadel A, Shah C, Shelov D, Wylie-Rosett J, Sparano J. Effects of yoga on quality of life among breast cancer patients in Bronx, New York. *Psychooncology.* 2004;13(Suppl 8): S107.

45. Cohen L, Thornton B, Perkins G. A randomized trial of a Tibetan yoga intervention for breast cancer patients. *Psychosom Med.* 2005;67:A-33.

46. Carlson LE, Culos-Reed SN, Daroux LM. The effects of therapeutic yoga on salivary cortisol, stress symptoms, quality of life and mood states in cancer outpatients: a randomized controlled study. *Psychosom Med.* 2005;67:A-41.

47. Banerjee B, Vadiraj HS, Ram A, et al. Effects of an integrated yoga program in modulating psychological stress and radiation-induced genotoxic stress in breast cancer patients undergoing radiotherapy. *Integ Cancer Ther.* 2007;6:242–250.

48. Moadel AB, Shah C, Wylie-Rosett J, et al. Randomized controlled trial of yoga among a multiethnic sample of breast cancer patients: effects on quality of life. *J Clin Oncol.* 2007;25:4387–4395.

49. Raghavendra RM, Nagarathna R, Nagendra HR, et al. Effects of an integrated yoga programme on chemotherapy-induced nausea and emesis in breast cancer patients. *Eur J Cancer Care (Engl).* 2007;16:462–474.

50. Blank SE, Kittel J, Haberman MR. Active practice of Iyengar yoga as an intervention for breast cancer survivors. *Int J Yoga Ther.* 2005;15:59.

51. Cohen L, Chandwani G, Perkins B, et al. Randomized trial of yoga in women with breast cancer undergoing radiation treatment: long-term effects. ASCO Annual Meeting Proceedings Part I. Abstract #9639: *J Clin Oncol.* 2008;26:S20.

52. Rosenbaum E, Gautier H, Fobair P, et al. Cancer supportive care, improving the quality of life for cancer patients. A program evaluation report. *Support Care Cancer.* 2004;12:293–301.

53. Carson JW, Carson KM, Porter LS, Keefe FJ, Shaw H, Miller JM. Yoga for women with metastatic breast cancer: results from a pilot study. *J Pain Symptom Manage.* 2007;33:331–341.

54. Warner AS. *Exploration of psychological and spiritual well-being of women with breast cancer participating in the Art of Living Program.* [Doctoral]. Institute of Transpersonal Psychology; 2006.

55. Joseph CD. Psychological supportive therapy for cancer patients. *Indian J Cancer.* 1983;20:268–270.

56. Carson JW, Carson KM, Porter LS, Keefe FJ, Shaw H, Miller JM. Yoga for women with metastatic breast cancer: results from a pilot study. *J Pain Symptom Manage.* 2007;33:331–341.

CHAPTER 59

The Role of Religion/Spirituality in Coping with Cancer: Evidence, Assessment, and Intervention

George Fitchett and Andrea L. Canada

INTRODUCTION

Religion plays an important role in the lives of many people. Surveys conducted in the United States in 2006 indicate that 84% of Americans reported that religion was very important or fairly important in their own life, a proportion that has been remarkably stable over the past 15 years.[1] A similar proportion of the U.S. population (87%) report that they believe God exists, and 60% believe that religion "can answer all or most of today's problems."[1] Religion is not only important to many people, but also appears to play a role in helping people stay healthy[2] and is often one of the most important resources people use in coping with illness or other stressful life events.[3]

In the past 30 years there has been a dramatic increase in research about the relationship between religion and health. Koenig, McCullough, and Larson's *Handbook of religion and health*[2] provides a useful overview of this research, summarizing the results of over 1200 studies of religion and health. Academic and professional journals have also published special issues about religion and health, including *Psycho-Oncology*, 1999 and *Annals of Behavioral Medicine*, 2002.

In this chapter we begin with a review of research about religion and spirituality (R/S) and a variety of cancer outcomes, including screening behavior, coping and adjustment to cancer, and quality of life (QOL). We then describe several approaches to assessment of R/S in the clinical context and to their measurement in the research context. Our final section summarizes research about R/S interventions designed to improve coping with cancer.

Before proceeding to the research, it is important to clarify two key terms, religion and spirituality. In current health research, the term religion is usually employed to refer to the beliefs and practices associated with affiliation with a formal religious organization such as a church, synagogue, or mosque. In contrast, "spirituality is concerned with the transcendent, addressing ultimate questions about life's meaning, with the assumption that there is more to life than what we see or fully understand" ([4], p. 2). While there are important distinctions to be made between R/S, until recently, most health-related research has focused on religion rather than spirituality. Miller and Thoresen[5] provide a helpful discussion of this issue.

It is important to emphasize that both R/S are best considered as multidimensional.[4] Important dimensions include private and group devotional activities, beliefs, behavioral norms and values that may stem from R/S beliefs, relationships with others, such as members of one's congregation, and R/S experiences, including direct experiences with the divine or transcendent.

We also wish to mention that in recent years there has been a debate about what the research about religion and health shows. On one side of the debate are investigators, such as Harold Koenig, who argue that the evidence indicates that religion is "consistently associated with better health and predicted better health over time" ([2], p. 591). On the other side of the debate is the health psychologist Richard Sloan, and his colleagues, who argue, "the evidence is generally weak and unconvincing, since it is based on studies with serious methodological flaws, conflicting findings, and data that lack clarity and specificity" ([6], p. 1913). A middle ground in this debate has been suggested by Powell and colleagues who write, "A relationship between religion or spirituality and physical health does exist but…it may be more limited and more complex than has been suggested by others" ([7], p. 50).

It should also be noted that in recent years a growing number of professional organizations have issued guidelines and statements that recognize the importance of attending to the R/S dimension of life. For example, in the U.S., the standards of the Joint Commission, a major healthcare accrediting agency, require hospitals and other healthcare institutions to include a spiritual assessment in their general patient evaluations.[8] Other important statements include the National Comprehensive Cancer Network's Clinical Practice Guidelines on "Distress Management"[9] and the National Consensus Project for Quality Palliative Care, Clinical Practice Guidelines.[10]

ESTABLISHING THE LINK: RELIGION/SPIRITUALITY AND CANCER OUTCOMES

There is a remarkably large and growing body of research about the relationship between R/S and many different cancer outcomes. In this review we give an overview of the research, describing studies of outcomes such as cancer incidence and mortality, cancer screening behavior, and QOL and adjustment to the disease. Other helpful reviews are available.[2,11,12] Also see the National Cancer Institute's Physician Data Query, "Spirituality in Cancer Care."[13]

The research suggests that the vast majority of individuals with cancer view R/S as personally important. For example, Balboni and colleagues[14] surveyed 230 patients with advanced cancer; 68% of patients indicated that religion was "very important" and an additional 20% endorsed religion as "somewhat important." Only 12% of respondents reported that religion was "not important." Similarly, in a study of 290 patients diagnosed with multiple myeloma, 90% indicated religion as "important."[15] The importance of R/S may be higher in minority populations. In one study, African-Americans and Hispanics rated religion as more important than whites, 89%, 79%, and 56%, respectively.[14]

Several studies have investigated change in the importance of religion/religious involvement following a diagnosis of cancer. Feher and Maly[16] found that, among breast cancer patients, roughly half reported their faith had strengthened during the health crisis. No women reported that their faith had weakened. In a community-dwelling sample of elderly people, a diagnosis of cancer was associated with becoming more religious over a 3-year period.[17] This pattern of religious mobilization was also reported in a study of 1600 mostly rural and poor Muslim cancer patients from Morocco.[18] The investigators reported that among the 51% of the sample who were nonpracticing Muslim's, almost all (95%) began to observe religious practices such as wearing a headscarf (Hijab) among the women. After receiving a diagnosis of cancer, more religiously observant patients maintained their religious practices and interpreted their illness as a test from God.

Investigators have used both qualitative and quantitative methods to explore the R/S needs of cancer patients and their family caregivers. On the basis of interviews with 21 patients in active treatment, Taylor[19] reported seven different categories of R/S needs, including those relating to God, maintaining hope and positive attitudes, giving and receiving love from others, and reconsidering religious beliefs and finding meaning in light of one's illness. The R/S needs of seven family caregivers were found to be similar to those of the cancer patients. A research team in Scotland reported similar findings.[20]

Data from several cross-sectional surveys provide additional information about the R/S needs experienced by cancer patients and their family caregivers. Among 248 ethnically diverse cancer patients, Moadel and colleagues[21] found 51% of participants felt a need for help to overcome fear, and 40% felt a need for hope and meaning. In a study of 369 cancer outpatients with early stage and advanced disease, 73% of participants reported at least one R/S need and 18% reported unmet R/S needs.[22] Further research is needed to understand the determinants of R/S needs as well as their trajectory over the course of the disease.

There is a small body of evidence that suggests a lower incidence of cancer among more religious people (e.g., see reference 23), but this association can be explained by the health behavior of the more religious individuals in the study. However, in a case-control study conducted in Melbourne Australia, involving 715 colorectal cancer patients and 727 healthy controls, patients were 30% less likely to be religious; a finding that remained after adjustment for established risks.[24]

There have been two large studies of worship attendance and mortality from cancer.[25,26] In their review of these studies, Powell and colleagues[7] concluded the evidence was "inadequate" to support an association between religion and cancer mortality.

Powell and colleagues[7] also reviewed seven studies that examined the association between R/S and survival among people with cancer. They report that for 6 of the studies there was no univariate association. In the seventh study,[27] the protective effect of religious affiliation (Seventh-day Adventist) became nonsignificant when stage at diagnosis was taken into account. In their review, Powell and colleagues conclude there was sufficient evidence from well-designed studies to conclude there was a "consistent failure" to find an association between R/S and cancer survival.

Although some studies suggest otherwise (e.g. see reference 28), studies with large, representative samples point to a positive association between R/S involvement and use of cancer screening in men as well as women.[29,30]

Studies have identified R/S as a key strategy in the adaptive coping repertoire of many patients with cancer. In several investigations with breast cancer patients, R/S faith were found to be important sources of emotional support in dealing with the disease[31] and provided patients with the ability to find meaning in everyday life.[16] R/S also helps to provide a sense of hope. Among women diagnosed with gynecological cancers, 93% reported that their faith had increased their ability to be hopeful.[32] The relationship between R/S and hope may be even stronger in the cancer palliative care setting, where R/S was shown to offer protection against end-of-life despair.[33] Qualitative interviews with 19 Muslim women in Iran, with newly diagnosed breast cancer, also found that R/S beliefs played a central role in their coping with their illness.[34]

Research indicates that prayer is the most prevalent R/S means with which cancer patients cope with their illness. In a large study of patients with different types of cancer, 77% reported using prayer to assist them in coping with diagnosis/treatment.[35] Additional studies report the prevalence of prayer in coping with cancer to range from 49% to 76% of participants.[36,37]

Studies suggest that R/S coping is significantly associated with measures of adjustment and the management of disease-related symptoms. As examples, R/S factors have been related to various aspects of adaptation to cancer including self-reported physical well-being,[38] general QOL[39,40] self-esteem and optimism,[41] positive appraisals and nonreligious coping,[42] and life satisfaction.[43] R/S coping in patients with cancer has also been associated with lower levels of patient discomfort, reduced

hostility, and less social isolation[44] as well as decreased anxiety.[45] These positive effects on QOL and adjustment have been observed not only in North America, but also in studies among breast cancer patients in Croatia,[46] and 309 patients with diverse cancers in Montevideo, Uruguay.[47]

It has been suggested that R/S resources may serve multiple functions in long-term adjustment to cancer including maintaining confidence, providing a sense of meaning or purpose, giving comfort, reducing emotional distress, increasing inner peace, and engendering a positive attitude toward life.[48,49] In one study, spiritual well-being, particularly a sense of meaning and peace, was significantly associated with an ability of cancer patients to continue to enjoy life despite high levels of pain or fatigue.[50] Some survivors who had drawn on spiritual resources to cope with cancer even reported substantial personal growth as a consequence of their illness experience.[51]

As suggested above, many individuals find the consolation they seek in R/S during times of emotional turmoil (i.e., following a health crisis). However, there are some patients for whom illness may precipitate a brief, or prolonged, period of R/S struggle including feeling punished or abandoned by God.[52] A growing body of evidence, including studies from outside the United States, indicates that R/S struggle is associated with poorer outcomes in the oncology population.[53-55] For example, among 213 multiple myeloma patients, those with greater religious struggle had greater levels of general distress and depression and, to a lesser extent, higher indices of pain and fatigue, and more difficulties with daily physical functioning.[56]

A few studies have examined R/S and coping with cancer in the experience of patients with advanced disease. In a study of 160 patients in a palliative care hospital, with an average life expectancy of less than 3 months, in adjusted models, higher levels of spiritual well-being were associated with less hopelessness, less suicidal ideation, and less desire for a hastened death.[33] In contrast, among 230 advanced-cancer patients, many reported low levels of support for their R/S needs from their religious community (47%) and from the "medical system," defined as "doctors, nurses, chaplains" (72%).[14] In this sample, in adjusted models, spiritual support was positively, and religious struggle, negatively, associated with QOL.

While a substantial literature has developed describing the role of R/S in coping with serious illness among adults, there are very few studies of the R/S coping of children or adolescents who are diagnosed with a serious illness.[57] One study of 114 adolescents who were admitted to an inpatient unit with diverse diagnoses, including cancer, found those who were more seriously ill reported more interest in religion and more frequent prayer and 15% of these teens requested help with R/S concerns.[58]

A small body of research has begun to describe the role of R/S in the coping and adjustment of spouses or informal caregivers of cancer patients. Among caregivers of 162 terminally ill cancer patients, in demographically controlled models, positive religious coping was associated with greater caregiver burden, but also more satisfaction.[59] Among these caregivers, higher levels of religious struggle were associated with worse QOL and greater likelihood of depression and anxiety.

Having a child diagnosed with a serious illness is a stressful time for their parents. Limited existing research indicates that religion is an important resource for parent's coping with this stress.[60] One study of fathers of children diagnosed with cancer reported that prayer was one of their two most common coping activities.[61] Another study of 27 mothers of children diagnosed with cancer found that 74% reported increased levels of religious activity after their child's diagnosis; 11% reported decreased activity.[62]

The evidence we just reviewed for the link between R/S and cancer outcomes is, largely, not theory driven. However, a number of models have been proposed to explain the relationship between R/S and cancer outcomes. These models often include behavioral (e.g., R/S influences on health-relevant conduct, such as diet and high-risk behaviors), social (e.g., R/S congregations provide tangible and/or emotional support), psychological (e.g., R/S beliefs and cognitions affect appraisal, coping, and QOL), and physiological (e.g., R/S practices, such as quieting behaviors, that affect the stress response) factors. Fig. 59–1 outlines one such model.

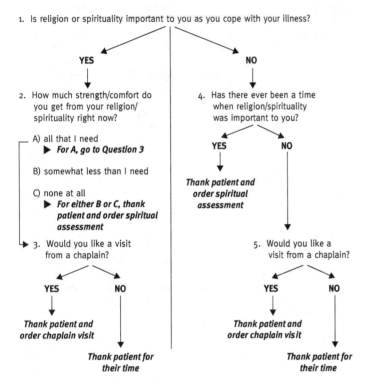

Dimensions of religion/spirituality · Pathways · Outcomes

- Values
- Beliefs
- Ritual/devotional practices
- Experiences
- Relationships

Health behaviors

Social/instrumental support

Coping appraisals/strategies

Physiological states

Adjustment and quality of life

Fig. 59–1. Model of religion/spirituality and cancer outcomes.

1. Is religion or spirituality important to you as you cope with your illness?

YES

NO

2. How much strength/comfort do you get from your religion/spirituality right now?

A) all that I need
▶ *For A, go to Question 3*

B) somewhat less than I need

C) none at all
▶ *For either B or C, thank patient and order spiritual assessment*

4. Has there ever been a time when religion/spirituality was important to you?

YES

NO

Thank patient and order spiritual assessment

3. Would you like a visit from a chaplain?

YES NO

Thank patient and order chaplain visit

Thank patient for their time

5. Would you like a visit from a chaplain?

YES NO

Thank patient and order chaplain visit

Thank patient for their time

Fig. 59–2. Religious struggle screening protocol.

CAPTURING THE LINK: ASSESSMENT AND MEASUREMENT OF RELIGION/SPIRITUALITY

We have seen that R/S is associated with a number of important cancer outcomes, including psychological adjustment and QOL. We now turn our attention to resources for clinicians and researchers who want to address R/S in their practice or in their investigations. We begin with resources for assessment of R/S in clinical practice. When clinicians think about assessment of R/S in their practice we think it is helpful to distinguish among three levels of inquiry: spiritual screening, spiritual history taking, and spiritual assessment.

Spiritual screening or triage is a quick determination of whether a person is experiencing a serious spiritual crisis. Spiritual screening can help identify which patients may benefit from a more in-depth spiritual assessment. Earlier in the chapter we described research that suggests R/S struggle is associated with poorer QOL and poorer psychological adjustment for cancer patients and others. R/S screening can be used to identify patients who may be experiencing R/S struggle and who may benefit from a referral for more in-depth R/S assessment. Fig. 59–2 describes one approach to R/S screening.[63]

Another approach to screening for acute R/S distress is the distress thermometer developed by the National Comprehensive Cancer Network.[9] In this instrument, "Spiritual/religious concerns" can be checked as specific

Table 59–1. Possible areas for religious spiritual concern

Grief
Concerns about death and afterlife
Conflicted or challenged belief system
Loss of faith
Concerns with meaning/purpose of life
Concerns about relationship with deity
Isolation from religious community
Guilt
Hopelessness
Conflict between religious beliefs and recommended treatments
Ritual needs

SOURCE: Adapted from Algorithm DIS-19 with permission from The NCCN 1. 2008 Distress Management Clinical Practices Guidelines in Oncology. © National Comprehensive Cancer Network, 2008. Available at: http://www.nccn.org. Accessed September 23, 2008. To view the most recent and complete version of the guideline, go online to www.nccn.org.

Table 59–2. FICA model for religious spiritual history taking

F—Faith, belief, meaning
What is your faith or belief?
Do you consider yourself spiritual or religious?
What things do you believe give meaning to your life?

I—Importance and influence
Is it important in your life?
What influences does it have on how you take care of yourself?
How have your beliefs influenced your behavior during this illness?
What role do your beliefs play in regaining your health?

C—Community
Are you part of a spiritual or religious community?
Is this of support to you and how?
Is there a person or group of people you really love or who are really important to you?

A—Address/action in care
How would you like me, your healthcare provider, to address these issues in your healthcare?

SOURCE: Puchalski C, Romer AL. Taking a spiritual history allows clinicians to understand patients more fully. *J Palliat Med.* 2000;3(1):129-137.
Copyright Christina M. Puchalski, MD, 1996. Reprinted with permission.

sources of distress. Table 59–1 lists 11 additional areas of R/S concerns that are included in this protocol. Another approach to screening for R/S distress is the nursing diagnosis, spiritual distress.[64] Fitchett[65] reviews other screening models developed by chaplains and others.

Spiritual history taking is the process of interviewing a patient to come to a better understanding of their R/S needs and resources. In recent years, a number of models for R/S history taking have been published, including Maugans'[66] SPIRIT model, and Anandarajah and Hight's[67] HOPE model. Table 59–2 shows the FICA model, a popular model developed by Christina Puchalski.[68] Compared to screening, R/S history taking employs a broader set of questions, usually asked in the context of a comprehensive examination, to capture salient information about R/S needs and resources. The information from the R/S history permits the clinician to understand how R/S concerns could either complement or complicate the patient's overall care.

Spiritual assessment refers to a more extensive process of listening to a patient's story as it unfolds in a professional relationship, and summarizing the R/S needs and resources that emerge in that process. It is a more in-depth, on-going process of evaluating the R/S needs and resources of people to whom we provide care. Unlike R/S history taking, the major models for R/S assessment are not built on a set of questions that can be employed in an interview. Rather, the models are interpretive

Table 59-3. Paul Pruyser's "Guidelines for Pastoral Diagnosis"

1. Awareness of the holy
   What if anything is sacred, revered
   Any experiences of awe or bliss, when, in what situations
   Any sense of mystery, of anything transcendent
   Any sense of creatureliness, humility, awareness of own limitations
   Any idolatry, reverence displaced to improper symbols

2. Providence
   What is God's intention toward me
   What has God promised me
   Belief in cosmic benevolence
   Related to capacity for trust
   Extent of hoping versus wishing

3. Faith
   Affirming versus negating stance in life
   Able to commit self, to engage
   Open to world or constricted

4. Grace or gratefulness
   Kindness, generosity, the beauty of giving and receiving
   No felt need for grace or gratefulness
   Forced gratitude under any circumstances
   Desire for versus resistance to blessing

5. Repentance
   The process of change from crookedness to rectitude
   A sense of agency in one's own problems or ones response to them
   versus being a victim versus being too sorry for debatable sins
   Feelings of contrition, remorse, regret
   Willingness to do penance

6. Communion
   Feelings of kinship with the whole chain of being
   Feeling embedded or estranged, united or separated in the world,
   in relations with one's faith group, one's church

7. Sense of Vocation
   Willingness to be a cheerful participant in creation
   Signs of zest, vigor, liveliness, dedication
   Aligned with divine benevolence or malevolence
   Humorous and inventive involvement in life versus grim and
   dogmatic

SOURCE: Reproduced from *The minister as diagnostician* by Paul Pruyser. ©1976 The Westminster Press. Used by permission of Westminster John Knox Press.

frameworks that are applied based on listening to the patient's story as it unfolds in the clinical relationship. An early and influential model for R/S assessment was developed by the psychologist Paul Pruyser.[69] In his model Pruyser suggested clergy attend to seven aspects of a person's religious life (see Table 59–3).

Another model for R/S assessment is the 7×7 model, developed by Fitchett[70] and colleagues. The 7×7 model employs a functional and multidimensional approach to R/S assessment. As can be seen in Table 59–4, the 7×7 model for R/S assessment has two broad divisions, a holistic assessment and a multidimensional R/S assessment.

Work on models for R/S assessment continues. The R/S assessment proposed by Lucas[71] focuses on the patient's concept of the holy, meaning, hope and community. Some models, such as Shulevitz and Springer's model[72] for assessment of Jewish patients, were designed for use with people from one specific faith or tradition. Recently a model for R/S screening in children and adolescents has been published.[73] Research that tests the effectiveness of all our models for R/S screening, history taking, and assessment is needed.

Measurement of R/S in clinical research is primarily accomplished through the administration of standardized measures to consenting patients. In this section, we briefly describe four of the more widely used and/or psychometrically sound instruments. Other excellent reviews of measures of R/S are available.[2,11,74,75]

Table 59-4. The 7×7 model for spiritual assessment

Holistic assessment	*Spiritual assessment*
Medical dimension	Belief and meaning
Psychological dimension	Vocation and obligations
Family systems dimension	Experience and emotions
Psychosocial dimension	Courage and growth
Ethnic, racial, or cultural dimension	Ritual and practice
Social issues dimension	Community
Spiritual dimension	Authority and guidance

SOURCE: Reprinted with permission from Fitchett G. *Assessing spiritual needs: A guide for caregivers.* Lima, OH: Academic Renewal Press; 2002.

The *Brief Multidimensional Measure of Religiousness/Spirituality (BMMR/S)* is a 33-item, multidimensional measure of R/S, developed by an expert panel, explicitly for research about R/S and health.[4] The measure was tested in the nationally representative 1998 General Social Survey which found acceptable internal consistency reliability estimates (minimum Cronbach's alpha of 0.64; most reliabilities >0.70). Strengths of the BMMR/S include that it is multidimensional, allowing for investigation of multiple possible mechanisms of R/S effects on health; it is brief enough to be included in clinical or epidemiological surveys; it is inclusive of both traditional religiousness and noninstitutionally based spirituality.[76]

The *Functional Assessment of Chronic Illness Therapy–Spiritual Wellbeing* (FACIT-Sp), developed by Peterman and colleagues,[77] is a 12-item scale designed to assess spiritual well-being in patients with chronic illness. This measure was validated with 1617 oncology and human immunodeficiency virus (HIV) patients, 75.5% of whom were Black or Hispanic. Factor analysis revealed two factors: meaning/peace and faith. Cronbach's alpha in the initial sample was 0.87 for the total score, and 0.81 and 0.88 for the respective subscales. In subsequent studies, the FACIT-Sp score was found to be a unique predictor of general QOL in oncology patients.[50] A recent study among 240 women, 81.7% of whom were White, found support for three factors with meaning and peace forming separate factors.[78] Investigators may wish to be aware of racial/ethnic differences in the R/S constructs underlying this, and perhaps other, measures of R/S. A 23-item version, the FACIT-Sp-Ex, which includes items concerning love, thankfulness, hope, and forgiveness, is also available.[79]

The *Brief RCOPE*[52] is an efficient, theoretically meaningful measure for health researchers seeking to integrate religious dimensions of coping into models of stress and health. The 14 items assess positive and negative religious coping. The participant's score on "negative religious coping" reflects the degree of religious struggle present. Cronbach's alpha was estimated at 0.87 for positive and 0.69 for negative religious coping. In initial studies, the Brief RCOPE also demonstrated discriminant validity.

The *Systems of Belief Inventory-15R (SBI-15R)*[80] measures a combination of R/S beliefs and practices and the social support derived from a community sharing those beliefs. The SBI-15R has high internal consistency (Cronbach's alpha = 0.93) as well as high test-retest reliability ($r = 0.95$). In addition, it demonstrated good convergent, divergent, and discriminant validity. The SBI-15R has also been validated in Hebrew[81] and German.[82]

FACILITATING THE LINK: RELIGIOUS/SPIRITUAL INTERVENTIONS

The literature suggests that many patients experience R/S needs during the course of the illness. However, the R/S concerns/needs of patients may often go unaddressed. As we noted earlier, Balboni and colleagues[14] reported that among patients with advanced cancer (N = 230), 72% reported that their spiritual needs were supported minimally or not at all by the medical system and nearly half reported the same lack of support by their religious community To date, only a few studies have examined the value of explicitly R/S intervention in patients with cancer. Among the scant evidence are two studies[83,84] that, although in need of replication, suggest R/S intervention in patients with cancer would likely be well-received and efficacious.

Cole and Pargament[83] designed an intervention for patients with cancer that integrates psychotherapy and spirituality. The goals of this intervention were to facilitate general adjustment to cancer, enhance spiritual coping, and resolve spiritual strain and struggle. The specific components of this intervention were formulated around four existential issues: control, identity, relationships, and meaning. The intervention incorporates some of the coping components of documented efficacious cognitive-behavioral group interventions for patients with cancer.

A nonrandomized pilot trial of this protocol was conducted with 16 cancer patients, 81% female, all Caucasian, with an average age of 53 years.[85] The sample was diverse with regards to diagnosis, time since diagnosis, and treatment status. Participants in the intervention group had relatively stable levels of pain and depression; while those in the no treatment control group experienced greater pain ($p = 0.02$) and increased depression ($p = 0.05$) from before to after treatment and 2-month follow-up.

In another study, the *OASIS Project*,[84] oncologists were trained to deliver a semistructured, manualized spirituality intervention to their patients during a regular office visit. In this intervention, the oncologist introduced the issue of spirituality to his/her patients in a neutral inquiring manner. After the initial exchange, the oncologist continued to explore the issue, inquiring about the patient's R/S concerns and resources. Finally the oncologist closed the intervention by stating, "I appreciate you discussing these issues with me. May I ask about it again?"

The intervention was tested with 118 cancer patients being seen by three community oncologists and one oncologist at a medical school cancer center. From baseline to 3-week follow-up, intervention patients reported greater reductions in depressive symptoms ($p < 0.01$), more improvement in health-related QOL ($p < 0.05$), and an improved sense of interpersonal caring from their physician ($p < 0.05$) in comparison to the control group. In addition, greater than 80% of the time, oncologists rated themselves as being "quite" or "very" confident and comfortable in delivering the intervention.

Breitbart[86] has developed a spiritual intervention, "Meaning Centered Group Psychotherapy (MCGP)," based on Viktor Frankl's logotherapy, for use with advanced cancer patients. The purpose of MCGP is to help patients sustain or enhance a sense of meaning, peace, and purpose in their lives even as they approach the end of life. The manualized intervention is delivered in a group format over an 8-week period (one 1–1/2 hr session per week). The group sessions include a mixture of didactics, discussion, and experiential exercises focused around particular themes related to meaning and advanced cancer. A pilot group was conducted in a cohort of advanced cancer patients to establish the feasibility, practicality, applicability, and acceptance of such an intervention.[87] No randomized clinical trial of MCGP has yet been published.

Which professionals should provide R/S interventions? Gordon and Mitchell[88] have helpfully described a multilevel framework of knowledge and skills for R/S care in the (Scottish) palliative care context that could be applied in other clinical contexts. At the first level, all staff and volunteers who have casual contact with patients and families are expected to understand that patients have R/S needs and be able to refer patients' R/S concerns to others on the care team. As a staff member's professional responsibilities increase, they are expected to have increased ability to assess and refer complex R/S and ethical issues. Chaplains and others with primary responsibility for R/S care are expected to have the most advanced level of knowledge and skill in this area.

IDEAS FOR FUTURE RESEARCH

Research on the associations between R/S and cancer has grown significantly over the last three decades, and associated methodology is becoming increasingly refined and rigorous. Although not without

debate, a good deal of evidence suggests that most dimensions of R/S have salutary effects on cancer outcomes (e.g., improved psychological well-being, better health-related QOL). Despite these advances, many important questions remain to be addressed.

As the literature review in this chapter has shown, much of the research about R/S and coping with cancer has been empirically driven. Relatively few studies have tested theoretically derived hypotheses. Important next steps in this research include examining how R/S is linked to coping with cancer as well as other outcomes. The relationships between R/S dimensions and cancer outcomes are likely to be strongly influenced by demographic (e.g., age, ethnicity, gender, religious affiliation) and disease-related (e.g., diagnosis, prognosis, length of survivorship) factors. Further research is needed to clarify associations between R/S and cancer outcomes within such demographic- and disease-specific contexts. This research also needs to be extended to include populations that have, thus far, received little attention. These include studies of the role of R/S among children with cancer, as well as studies of the role of R/S in the lives of family caregivers, including parents and partners, of people living with cancer. It will be important for all of these next steps in the research to be guided by strong conceptual frameworks.

Although a number of investigations demonstrate a link between R/S and improved health outcomes in cancer, very few studies have attempted to test explanatory biological mechanisms for such associations. Only one investigation in the cancer literature reports a relationship between R/S and immune indices.[89] The field is in great need of further exploration regarding the associations between R/S and physiologic, immune, and endocrine parameters as they relate to cancer outcomes.

Future research should also explore how the associations between R/S and cancer outcomes change over time. Most of the research in this area has been limited to cross-sectional data and analyses. Therefore, our understanding of how R/S change or evolve over the course of cancer treatment/ survivorship and how R/S affect long-term changes in cancer outcomes are in need of further research. Finally, in light of the evidence that some aspects of R/S are beneficial for people living with cancer, and some aspects of R/S (e.g., religious struggle) are detrimental, additional work is needed to develop and test R/S interventions, for both individuals and groups.

REFERENCES

1. The Gallup Poll. Religion 2007. http://www.galluppoll.com/. Accessed February 3, 2007.

2. Koenig HG, McCullough ME, Larson DB. *Handbook of religion and health.* New York: Oxford University Press; 2001.

3. Pargament KI. *The psychology of religion and coping.* New York: Guilford; 1997.

4. Fetzer Institute/National Institute on Aging Working Group. *Multidimensional measure of religiousness/spirituality for use in health research.* Kalamazoo, MI: Fetzer Institute; 1999.

5. Miller WR, Thoresen CE. Spirituality, religion, and health: an emerging research field. *Am Psychol.* 2003;58(1):24–35.

6. Sloan RP, Bagiella E, VandeCreek L, et al. Should physicians prescribe religious activities? *N Engl J Med.* 2000;342(25):1913–1916.

7. Powell LH, Shahabi L, Thoresen CE. Religion and spirituality: linkages to health. *Am Psychol.* 2003;58(1):36–52.

8. Joint Commission. Evaluating your spiritual assessment process. *Source.* 2005;3(2):6–7.

9. National Comprehensive Cancer Network 2007. Distress Management V.1.2008. http://www.nccn.org. Accessed April 1, 2008.

10. National Consensus Project for Quality Palliative Care. Clinical practice guidelines for quality palliative care; 2007. http://www.nationalconsensusproject. org. Accessed April 2, 2008.

11. Stefanek M, McDonald PG, Hess SA. Religion, spirituality, and cancer: current status and methodological challenges. *Psychooncology.* 2005;14(6):450–463.

12. Sherman AC, Simonton S. Spirituality and cancer. In: Plante TG, Thoresen CE (eds). *Spirit, science, and health: How the spiritual mind fuels physical wellness.* Westport, CT: Praeger; 2007:157–175.

13. National Cancer Institute. Spirituality in cancer care (PDQ); 2007. http://www.cancer.gov/cancertopics/pdq/supportivecare/spirituality/healthprofessional. Accessed April 1, 2008.

14. Balboni TA, Vanderwerker LC, Block SD, et al. Religiousness and spiritual support among advanced cancer patients and associations with end-of-life treatment preferences and quality of life. *J Clin Oncol.* 2007;25(5):555–560.

15. Silberfarb PM, Anderson KM, Rundle AC, Holland JCB, Cooper MR, McIntyre OR. Mood and clinical status in patients with multiple myeloma. *J Clin Oncol.* 1991;9(12):2219–2224.

16. Feher S, Maly RC. Coping with breast cancer in later life: the role of religious faith. *Psychooncology.* 1999;8(5):408–416.

17. Musick MA, Koenig HG, Hays JC, Cohen HJ. Religious activity and depression among community-dwelling elderly persons with cancer: the moderating effect of race. *J Gerontol B Psychol Sci Soc Sci.* 1998;53(4):S218-S271.

18. Errihani H, Mrabti H, Boutayeb S, et al. Impact of cancer on Moslem patients in Morocco. *Psychooncology.* 2008:17(1):98–100.

19. Taylor EJ. Spiritual needs of patients with cancer and family caregivers. *Cancer Nurs.* 2003;26(4):260–266.

20. Murray SA, Kendall M, Boyd K, Worth A, Benton TF. Exploring the spiritual needs of people dying of lung cancer or heart failure: a prospective qualitative interview study of patients and their carers. *Palliat Med.* 2004;18(1):39–45.

21. Moadel A, Morgan C, Fatone A, et al. Seeking meaning and hope: self-reported spiritual and existential needs among an ethnically-diverse cancer patient population. *Psychooncology.* 1999;8(5):378–385.

22. Astrow AB, Wexler A, Texeira K, He MK, Sulmasy DP. Is failure to meet spiritual needs associated with cancer patients' perceptions of quality of care and their satisfaction with care? *J Clin Oncol.* 2007;25(36):5753–5757.

23. Gardner JW, Sanborn JS, Slattery ML. Behavioral factors explaining the low risk for cervical carcinoma in Utah Mormon women. *Epidemiology.* 1995;6(2):187–189.

24. Kune GA, Kune S, Watson LF. Perceived religiousness is protective for colorectal cancer: data from the Melbourne Colorectal Cancer Study. *J R Soc Med.* 1993;86(11):645–647.

25. Hummer RA, Rogers RG, Nam CB, Ellison CG. Religious involvement and US adult mortality. *Demography.* 1999;36(2):273–285.

26. Oman D, Kurata JH, Strawbridge WJ, Cohen RD. Religious attendance and cause of death over 31 years. *Int J Psychiatry Med.* 2002;32(1):69–89.

27. Zollinger TW, Phillips RL, Kuzma JW. Breast cancer survival rates among Seventh-day Adventists and non-Seventh-day Adventists. *Am J Epidemiol.* 1984;119(4):503–509.

28. Schwartz MD, Hughes C, Roth J, et al. Spiritual faith and genetic testing decisions among high-risk breast cancer probands. *Cancer Epidemiol Biomarkers Prev.* 2000;9(4):381–385.

29. Benjamins MR, Brown C. Religion and preventative health care utilization among the elderly. *Soc Sci Med.* 2004;58(1):109–118.

30. Van Ness PH, Kasl SV, Jones BA. Are religious women more likely to have breast cancer screening? *J Relig Health.* 2002;41(4):333–346.

31. Heim E, Augustiny KF, Shaffner L, Valach L. Coping with breast cancer over time and situation. *J Psychosom Res.* 1993;37(5):523–542.

32. Roberts JA, Brown D, Elkins T, Larson DB. Factors influencing views of patients with gynecological cancer about end-of-life decisions. *Am J Obstet Gynecol.* 1997;176(1):166–172.

33. McClain CS, Rosenfeld B, Breitbart W. Effect of spiritual well-being on end-of-life despair in terminally-ill cancer patients. *Lancet.* 2003;361(9369): 1603–1607.

34. Taleghani F, Yekta ZP, Nasrabadi AN. Coping with breast cancer in newly diagnosed Iranian women. *J Adv Nurs.* 2006;54(3):265–272.

35. Yates JS, Mustian KM, Morrow GR, et al. Prevalence of complementary and alternative medicine use in cancer patients during treatment. *Support Care Cancer.* 2005;13(10):806–811.

36. Lengacher CA, Bennett MP, Kip KE, Berarducci A, Cox CE. Design and testing of the use of a complementary and alternative therapies survey in women with breast cancer. *Oncol Nurs Forum.* 2003;30(5):811–821.

37. VandeCreek L, Rogers E, Lester J. Use of alternative therapies among breast cancer outpatients compared with the general population. *Altern Ther Health Med.* 1999;5(1):71–76.

38. Highfield MF. Spiritual health of oncology patients: nurse and patient perspectives. *Cancer Nurs.* 1992;15(1):1–8.

39. Canada AL, Parker PA, de Moor JS, Basen-Engquist K, Ramondetta LM, Cohen L. Active coping mediates the association between religion/spirituality and quality of life in ovarian cancer. *Gynecol Oncol.* 2006;101(1):102–107.

40. Tarakeshwar N, Vanderwerker LC, Paulk E, Pearce MJ, Stanislav VK, Prigerson HG. Religious coping is associated with quality of life of patients with advanced cancer. *J Palliat Med.* 2006;9(3):646–657.

41. Gall TL, Miguez de Renart RM, Boonstra B. Religious resources in long-term adjustment to breast cancer. *J Psychosoc Oncol.* 2000;18(2):21–38.

42. Gall TL. Integrating religious resources within a general model of stress and coping: long-term adjustment to breast cancer. *J Religion Health.* 2000;39:167–182.

43. Yates JW, Chalmer BJ, James P St, Follansbee M, McKegney FP. Religion in patients with advanced cancer. *Med Pediatr Oncol.* 1981;9:121–28.

44. Acklin MW, Brown EC, Mauger PA. The role of religious values in coping with cancer. *J Relig Health.* 1983;22(4):322–333.

45. Kaczorowski JM. Spiritual well-being and anxiety in adults diagnosed with cancer. *Hosp J.* 1989;5(3–4):105–116.

46. Aukst-Margetić B, Jakovljević M, Margetić B, Bišćan M, Šamija M. Religiosity, depression and pain in patients with breast cancer. *Gen Hosp Psychiatry.* 2005;27(4):250–255.

47. Dapueto JJ, Servente L, Francolino C, Hahn EA. Determinants of quality of life in patients with cancer: a South American study. *Cancer.* 2005;103(5):1072–1081.

48. Jenkins RA, Pargament KI. Religion and spirituality as resources for coping with cancer. *J Psychosoc Oncol.* 1995;13(1/2):51–73.

49. Johnson SC, Spilka B. Coping with breast cancer: the role of clergy and faith. *J Relig Health.* 1991;30(1):21–33.

50. Brady MJ, Peterman AH, Fitchett G, Mo M, Cella D. A case for including spirituality in quality of life measurement in oncology. *Psychooncology.* 1999;8(5):417–428.

51. Carpenter JS, Brockopp DY, Andrykowski MA. Self-transformation as a factor in the self-esteem and well-being of breast cancer survivors. *J Adv Nurs.* 1999;29(6):1402–1411.

52. Pargament KI, Smith B, Koenig HG, Perez L. Patterns of positive and negative religious coping with major life stressors. *J Sci Study Relig.* 1998;37:710–724.

53. Boscaglia N, Clarke DM, Jobling TW, Quinn MA. The contribution of spirituality and spiritual coping to anxiety and depression in women with a recent diagnosis of gynecological cancer. *Int J Gynecol Cancer.* 2005;15(5):755–761.

54. Fitchett G, Murphy PE, Kim J, Gibbons JL, Cameron JR, Davis JA. Religious struggle: prevalence, correlates and mental health risks in diabetic, congestive heart failure, and oncology patients. *Int J Psychiatry Med.* 2004;34(2):179–196.

55. Zwingmann C, Wirtz M, Muller C, Korber J, Murken S. Positive and negative religious coping in German breast cancer patients. *J Behav Med.* 2006;29(6):533–547.

56. Sherman AC, Simonton S, Latif U, Spohn R, Tricot G. Religious struggle and religious comfort in response to illness: health outcomes among stem cell transplant patients. *J Behav Med.* 2005;28(4):359–367.

57. Cotton S, Zebracki K, Rosenthal SL, Tsevat J, Drotar D. Religion/spirituality and adolescent health outcomes: a review. *J Adolesc Health.* 2006;38(4):472–480.

58. Silber TJ, Reilly M. Spiritual and religious concerns of the hospitalized adolescent. *Adolescence.* 1985;20(77):217–224.

59. Pearce MJ, Singer JL, Prigerson HG. Religious coping among caregivers of terminally ill cancer patients: main effects and psychosocial mediators. *J Health Psychol.* 2006;11(5):743–759.

60. Spilka B, Zwartjes WJ, Zwartjes GM. The role of religion in coping with childhood cancer. *Pastoral Psychology.* 1991;39(5):295–304.

61. Cayse LN. Fathers of children with cancer: a descriptive study of their stressors and coping strategies. *J Pediatr Oncol Nurs.* 1994;11(3):102–108.

62. Elkin TD, Jensen SA, McNeil L, Gilbert ME, Pullen J, McComb L. Religiosity and coping in mothers of children diagnosed with cancer: an exploratory analysis. *J Ped Oncol Nurs.* 2007;24(5):274–278.

63. Fitchett G and Risk JL. Screening for spiritual struggle. *J Pastoral Care Counsel.* [Online] 63:1,2.

64. NANDA International. *NANDA-I nursing diagnoses: Definitions and classification, 2007–2008.* Philadelphia, PA: NANDA International; 2007.

65. Fitchett G. Selected resources for screening for spiritual risk. *Chap Today.* 1999;15(1):13–26.

66. Maugans TA. The SPIRITual history. *Arch Fam Med.* 1996;5(1):11–16.

67. Anandarajah G, Hight E. Spirituality and medical practice: using the HOPE questions as a practical tool for spiritual assessment. *Am Fam Physician.* 2001;63(1):81–89.

68. Puchalski C, Romer AL. Taking a spiritual history allows clinicians to understand patients more fully. *J Palliat Med.* 2000;3(1):129–137.

69. Pruyser PW. *The minister as diagnostician.* Philadelphia, PA: Westminster Press; 1976.

70. Fitchett G. *Assessing spiritual needs: A guide for caregivers.* Lima, OH: Academic Renewal Press; 2002.

71. Lucas AM. Introduction to the discipline for pastoral care giving. In: VandeCreek L, Lucas AM (eds). *The discipline for pastoral care giving.* Binghamton, NY: Haworth Press, Inc.; 2001:1–33.

72. Shulevitz S, Springer M. Assessment of religious experience—a Jewish approach. *J Pastoral Care.* 1994;48(4):399–406.

73. Grossoehme DH. Development of a spiritual screening tool for children and adolescents. *J Pastoral Care Counsel.* 2008;62(1–2):71–85.

74. Hill PC, Hood RW Jr, eds. *Measures of religiosity.* Birmingham, AL: Religious Education Press; 1999.

75. Hill PC, Pargament KI. Advances in the conceptualization and measurement of religion and spirituality: implications for physical and mental health research. *Am Psychol.* 2003;58(1):64–74.

76. Idler EL, Musick MA, Ellison CG, et al. Measuring multiple dimensions of religion and spirituality for health research: conceptual background and findings from the 1998 General Social Survey. *Res Aging.* 2003;25(4):327–365.

77. Peterman AH, Fitchett G, Brady MJ, Hernandez L, Cella D. Measuring spiritual well-being in people with cancer: the functional assessment of chronic illness therapy—Spiritual Well-being Scale (FACIT-Sp). *Ann Behav Med.* 2002;24(1):49–58.

78. Canada A, Murphy P, Fitchett G, Peterman A, Schover L. A 3-factor model for the FACIT-Sp. *Psychooncology.* 2008;17(9):908–916.

79. Brady MJ, Peterman AH, Fitchett G, Cella D. The expanded version of the Functional Assessment of Chronic Illness Therapy-Spiritual Well-Being Scale (FACIT-Sp-Ex): initial report of psychometric properties. *Ann Behav Med.* 1999;21:129.

80. Holland JC, Kash KM, Passik S, et al. A brief spiritual beliefs inventory for use in quality of life research in life-threatening illness, *Psychooncology.* 1998;7(6):460–469.

81. Baider L, Holland JC, Russak SM, De-Nour AK. The System of Belief Inventory (SBI-15): a validation study in Israel. *Psychooncology.* 2001;10(6):534–540.

82. Albani C, Bailer H, Grulke N, Geyer M, Brahler E. Religiosity and spirituality in the elderly [German]. *Z Gerontol Geriatr.* 2004;37(1):43–50.

83. Cole B, Pargament K. Re-creating your life: a spiritual/psychotherapeutic intervention for people diagnosed with cancer. *Psychooncology.* 1999;8(5):395–407.

84. Kristeller JL, Rhodes M, Cripe LD, Sheets V. Oncologist assisted spiritual intervention study (OASIS): patient acceptability and initial evidence of effects. *Int J Psychiatry Med.* 2005;35(4):329–347.

85. Cole BS. Spiritually-focused psychotherapy for people diagnosed with cancer: a pilot outcome study. *Ment Health Religion Cult.* 2005;8(3):217–226.

86. Breitbart W. Spirituality and meaning in supportive care: spirituality- and meaning-centered group psychotherapy interventions in advanced cancer. *Support Care Cancer.* 2002;10(4):272–280.

87. Greenstein M. The house that's on fire: meaning-centered psychotherapy pilot group for cancer patients. *Am J Psychotherapy.* 2000;54(4):501–511.

88. Gordon T, Mitchell D. A competency model for the assessment and delivery of spiritual care. *Palliat Med.* 2004;18:646–651.

89. Sephton SE, Koopman C, Schaal M, Thoresen C, Spiegel D. Spiritual expression and immune status in women with metastatic breast cancer: an exploratory study. *Breast J.* 2001;7(5):345–353.

CHAPTER 60

Integrative Oncology

Lorenzo Cohen, Nancy Russell, M. Kay Garcia, Kelly Biegler, and Moshe Frenkel

INTRODUCTION

Integrative medicine seeks to combine conventional medicine with the safest and most effective complementary therapies. The Consortium of Academic Health Centers for Integrative Medicine has defined "integrative medicine" term as

the practice of medicine that reaffirms the importance of the relationship between practitioner and patient, focuses on the whole person, is informed by evidence, and makes use of all appropriate therapeutic approaches, healthcare professionals and disciplines to achieve optimal health and healing.[1]

This definition makes clear that there is an important psychosocial component to integrative medicine, whereby the connection between practitioner and patient becomes an important part of the therapeutic process. Although applying the concept of integrative medicine to cancer care is relatively new, a number of comprehensive cancer centers in the United States have incorporated this discipline into their care plans. This chapter reviews the role of integrative medicine in cancer care, with an emphasis on effective communication, an overview of the evidence, a review of integrative-based information resources to guide healthcare providers and patients, and suggestions for how to effectively incorporate integrative medicine into cancer care.

DEFINITIONS

The National Center for Complementary and Alternative Medicine (NCCAM) has defined complementary and alternative medicine (CAM) as "…diverse medical and healthcare systems, practices, and products that are not presently considered to be part of conventional medicine."[2] Although some CAM modalities are supported by scientific evidence, it may not be sufficient to bring them into *conventional* medical practice, and other CAM modalities may be unsupported for use in conventional settings. *Alternative* medicine, by definition, is when a patient makes use of a nonconventional treatment modality in place of conventional medicine regardless of whether there is evidence for its efficacy. *Complementary* medicine is when a patient makes use of a CAM modality in combination with conventional medicine.

The term *integrative* medicine, the preferred term in the field, is a philosophy of medical practice that utilizes both conventional and complementary medicine. Integrative medicine makes use of both conventional and complementary treatment modalities, constituting a multidisciplinary approach to healthcare. In the practice of integrative medicine, practitioners of conventional and nonconventional therapies are knowledgeable and aware of all treatment options and are open to communication with each other. When this is done effectively, patients receive complementary treatment modalities through an integrative medicine approach. The practice of integrative medicine is the ideal that we strive to achieve daily, relieving patients of the additional stress of fractionated health care, whereby conventional and complementary treatment modalities are completely independent and uncoordinated. Throughout this chapter we use the term complementary and integrative medicine (CIM) in favor of CAM or other terms.

Complementary therapies include mind-body approaches such as meditation, guided imagery, music, art, and other expressive arts and behavioral techniques; body-manipulative approaches such as massage

and reflexology; whole medical systems such as traditional Chinese medicine, homeopathy, and Ayurveda; biologically based approaches such as those centered on nutrition, herbs, and/or other plant, animal, or mineral products; and energy-based therapies that seek to affect proposed bio-energy fields, whose existence is not yet experimentally proven, that surround and penetrate the human body. Energy therapies can be administered through self-practice (e.g., yoga, tai chi, or internal qigong), manipulation of electromagnetic waves through the use of magnets, or the use of the energy of individual practitioners (e.g., external qigong, reiki, healing touch). There is overlap between some of these different practices. For example, traditional Chinese medicine and other whole medical systems use biologically active botanicals. Yoga and tai chi/qigong have mind-body and manipulative components and theory from Ayurvedic medicine and traditional Chinese medicine, respectively. Several different types of specialty healthcare providers offer CIM therapies; these may include physicians, nurses, physical therapists, psychiatrists, psychologists, chiropractors, massage therapists, and naturopaths, all of whom are operating within the guidelines of their licenses or accrediting organizations.

As a result of the growing interest in integrative medicine in cancer care, the National Cancer Institute (NCI) formed the Office of Cancer Complementary and Alternative Medicine (OCCAM), the American Cancer Society (ACS) dedicated a portion of its web site to assessment of complementary therapies, the Consortium of Academic Health Centers for Integrative Medicine formed an oncology working group, and the Society for Integrative Oncology (SIO) was founded along with its publication *Journal of the Society for Integrative Oncology* (www.integrativeonc.org).

UTILIZATION

A 1997 survey of U.S. adults found CIM use (excluding self-prayer) varied from 32% to 54%.[3] A 2002 survey by the U.S. Centers for Disease Control and Prevention found that 36% of adults had used CIM therapies (62% when prayer was included) during the past 12 months.[4]

When we examine CIM use specifically in people battling cancer the numbers are even higher than in the general population. An estimated 48%–69% of U.S. patients with cancer use CIM therapies[5,6] and the percentage increases if spiritual practices are included.[6] Complementary therapies are used in 70% of all oncology departments engaged in palliative care in Britain.[7] A survey of five clinics within a U.S. comprehensive cancer care center found that CIM therapies (excluding psychotherapy and spiritual practices) were used by 68.7% of patients.[6] A later survey in the breast and gynecologic clinics within that same cancer center found that CIM therapies, defined as herbs, supplements, and mega doses of vitamins, were used by 48% of patients.[5] Most estimates are that at least 50% of cancer patients utilize CIM at some point in their treatment or into survivorship.

People who use CIM are typically not disappointed or dissatisfied with conventional medicine but want to do everything possible to regain health and improve their quality of life.[8,9] Patients turn to CIM to reduce side effects and organ toxicity, to improve quality of life, to protect and stimulate immunity, or to prevent further cancers or recurrences. Regardless of whether patients with cancer use CIM therapies to treat the disease or its effects, they may use such modalities to treat other chronic conditions such as arthritis, heart disease, diabetes, or chronic pain.

COMMUNICATION

The use of CIM by patients with cancer can be a challenge to healthcare professionals. Although some types of complementary practices have a place in the treatment of cancer and the side effects of therapy, many complementary therapies carry risks, and thus it is important that oncologists be aware of complementary therapies their patients are using. This is particularly true for ingestibles such as herbs, supplements, and megadoses of vitamins, highlighting the importance of knowing what substances patients are taking and understanding their potential physiologic effects. It is, therefore, necessary for patients and healthcare professionals to openly discuss all treatments being used, both conventional and nonconventional. A significant proportion of patients with cancer (38%–60%) are taking complementary medicines along with conventional treatment without informing any member of their healthcare team.[5,6]

There are a variety of reasons why open communication about complementary treatments is not taking place in oncology clinics. Cancer clinicians typically have limited knowledge of this "new" area and limited time to reeducate themselves, and as such they may be reluctant to raise the topic. At the same time, patients may become frustrated if they cannot discuss CIM with their healthcare team. This bilateral frustration can result in a communication gap, which damages the patient–clinician interaction. The most common reason patients give for not bringing up the topic of CIM, even if they have questions or are taking CIM, is that it just never came up in the discussion; that is, no one asked them, and they did not think it was important.[5,9] Patients may fear that the topic will be received with indifference or dismissed without discussion[10] and healthcare professionals may not want to initiate a time-consuming discussion or may fear that they won't know how to respond to questions. Another challenge to effective communication is that patients and healthcare professionals have disparate views on why patients use CIM.[9] This lack of discussion is of grave concern, especially for ingestible substances.

The failure of the healthcare team to communicate effectively with patients about CIM may result in a loss of trust within the therapeutic relationship. In the absence of professional guidance, patients may choose harmful, useless, or ineffective (and costly) complementary therapies when effective complementary or conventional therapies are available. The erosion in trust due to lack of communication can lead to decreased compliance with conventional medicine and certainly to not following advice about CIM use. Poor communication also may lead to a diminution of patient autonomy and sense of control over their treatment, thereby interfering with potential self-healing responses.[10] Moreover, arguing with the patient that they should not try an unproven therapy which they are convinced will be helpful is not very productive: it is likely to damage the therapeutic relationship and drive the communication process underground.

Research suggests that the majority of cancer patients desire communication with their doctors about CIM,[11] and there is general agreement within the oncology community that oncologists must be aware of CIM use and be able to guide patients' use of all therapeutic approaches to provide effective patient care.[12] A number of strategies can be used to increase the chance of a worthwhile dialogue. Underlying these specific strategies should be an open attitude combined with a willingness to review evidence-based references and consult with other healthcare professionals.[13]

An initial step in effective communication is understanding the patient's viewpoint. Psychological, social, and spiritual dimensions of care may be ignored if the clinician cannot adapt to the individual needs of the patient or provides care without sensitivity. Successful integration of complementary therapies with conventional treatments is dependent upon many different aspects of effective communication. Communication is defined as the giving or exchange of information, but patient–clinician communication is not unilateral and is not limited to the transfer of information. This type of communication is an interactive process and usually more than a concise, focused dialogue of questions and answers.

Communication relating to complementary therapy use can be introduced related to previous visits, family and caregiver involvement, other

Table 60–1. For health care professionals to help cancer patients be appropriately informed and autonomous, the following steps may be useful[16]

1. For each patient, learn about conventional treatments that have been tried, have failed, or have been rejected because of safety, quality of life, cost, or other issues
2. Discover the levels of support that the patient relies on from family, community, faith, and friends
3. Ask each patient about their use of CIM or interest in using CIM
4. Identify each patient's beliefs, fears, hopes, and expectations about CIM and experience with CIM
5. Acknowledge the patient's spiritual and religious values and beliefs, including views about quality of life and end-of-life issues, and seek to understand how these issues affect their healthcare choices

ABBREVIATION: CIM, complementary and integrative medicine.

healthcare providers, and personal and professional experiences of the clinician and the patient. Family and employment concerns, emotions, desires and wants, hidden wishes and concerns, health beliefs, and social, religious, and spiritual issues all may be necessary topics of this communication.

The issue of a patient's CIM use surfaces quite frequently, and clinicians need to develop an empathetic communication strategy that addresses the patient's needs while maintaining clinical objectivity to provide the best care for that patient without compromising the healthcare professionals' clinical practice. Because of the threat posed by cancer and the uncertain outcome of treatment, most patients require much information about their disease and its treatment.[14] As such, patients need reliable information on CIM, adequate time to discuss this information, and access to reliable resources that they can refer to easily.

Patient–clinician communication is complicated, and the use of CIM by the patient may cause additional confusion. That some CIM therapies are administered by a CIM practitioner can complicate communication even more because of the triangular relationship that develops between the patient, the clinician, and the CIM practitioner. A productive and fruitful communication process requires that all three relationships be addressed.[15]

Ultimately, clinicians should encourage patients to make their own choices after advising them to the best of their knowledge. It is appropriate for clinicians to ask patients about their use of CIMs and for a patient and members of the healthcare team to decide together on therapeutic management options at each stage of cancer care, from prevention to acute care (radiation, chemotherapy, or surgery) to follow-up care (survivorship issues, follow-up visits, and prevention of recurrence). The main purpose of this early patient–clinician discussion is not to prove or disprove the efficacy of CIM treatments but to sharpen and refine the answers to questions that may come up when the patient and healthcare professionals are faced with uncertainties about therapies. Asking the right questions at the right time, particularly when definitive answers are not available, leads to improved patient–clinician communication and to a rational strategy to address the patient's needs and expectations in the face of uncertainty. See Table 60–1 for suggestions on facilitating communication regarding CIM between healthcare professionals and patients.

THE EVIDENCE

Integrative oncology represents a number of different areas of research, and the evidence is constantly changing over time. The evidence quickly becomes dated as new modalities for specific conditions are found to be either effective or ineffective and either incorporated into conventional medicine or dismissed. There has been a dramatic increase in research in integrative oncology. There are now peer-reviewed journals with a focus on CIM, including two journals specifically dedicated to integrative oncology: the *Journal of the Society for Integrative Oncology* and *Integrative Cancer Therapies*. Both of these journals are indexed in Medline (PubMed) and are dedicated to publishing original research and to education within the field of integrative oncology.

Although scientific evidence for the efficacy of a treatment is necessary to gain its acceptance within the conventional medical arena, evidence alone is usually not sufficient; several political steps are often necessary. An example of this is the role of acupuncture in treating chemotherapy-induced nausea and vomiting (CINV). An NIH consensus statement in 1997 supported the use of acupuncture as a treatment for CINV, stating that the level of evidence was sufficient.[17] Further research has substantiated this claim, and the ACS now states that clinical studies have found that acupuncture may help treat nausea caused by chemotherapy drugs or surgical anesthesia.[18] In addition, neuroimaging research has delineated some of the neural mechanisms of action of this therapy.[19] Even so, acupuncture is still not accepted within conventional medicine as standard care for CINV.

Even though many CIM treatments are safe and effective, some are associated with risks. When people use herbal or other biological therapies with conventional treatments, adverse interactions may occur. For example, ginger[20] and garlic[21] may increase a tendency to bleed in people who are taking blood thinners or are thrombocytopenic. St. John's wort affects multiple cytochrome P450 liver enzymes that speed up metabolism of certain medications.[22] Adverse interactions with conventional medicines also can occur with grapefruit juice, caffeine, alcohol, nicotine, and vitamin and mineral supplements taken in large quantities.[23]

There are other risks associated with certain CAM therapies. Herbs that have prohormonal properties, such as red clover, could be problematic in patients with breast cancer.[24] Other herbs may contribute to immune stimulation or modulation, with positive, negative, or unknown effects.[25] Herbs and isolated antioxidants may be beneficial in preventing heart disease and even cancer, but the free radicals that they sometimes target are not necessarily all bad, and many cancer chemotherapies produce free radicals that attack cancer cells.[26] The issues are complex, however; the rationale for and evidence supporting a therapeutic role for antioxidants have been published, and the debate continues today.[27]

To complicate matters further, some herbs and other supplements may be contaminated with toxins from the environment or from the manufacturing process.[28] Safety and quality control challenges for natural products are similar to those for foods and food products. "Good manufacturing practices" have been adopted by regulatory agencies and major herb producers. Organizations such as ConsumerLab (www.consumerlab.com) can test products upon request. Of course, herbs, foods, and other natural products do not usually undergo the rigorous testing that conventional medicines do, so efficacy and safety remain in question.

Many natural products are understood to be safe for patient use, however, and some physicians may be comfortable with the preponderance of evidence for them in terms of quality of life or even disease-related outcomes. For example, St. John's wort has been found to be effective for moderate mood regulation,[29] ginger has been found to be effective for nausea in pregnancy, but not after surgery and ongoing research is examining the benefits for chemotherapy-induced nausea,[30] and valerian has been shown to be safe to use as a sleep aid, although the evidence demonstrating its efficacy is mixed.[31,32] On the basis of safety and anticancer effects observed in cellular and animal studies, additional herbs, mushrooms, and their extracts are now in the process of human trials. Agents now undergoing examination in clinical trials include, but are not limited to, β-glucan, *Boswellia serrata*, curcumin, flaxseed, ginseng, green tea, lycopene, mistletoe, modified citrus pectin, pomegranate, resveratrol, selenium, oleander, and silibinin.[33]

The current literature is often not sufficient to answer questions about CIM use with a high level of certainty from the perspective of evidence-based medicine. So the challenge for healthcare professionals is how to manage a therapeutic issue that has a high level of uncertainty. We suggest a rational strategy for approaching CIM use by patients who suffer from cancer. The first step is for the professional to increase his or her knowledge about the therapy in question, mainly by searching reliable web sites and Medline (details on authoritative web sites are provided later in this chapter). Information on CIM is now widely available in medical journals, texts, reliable web sites, and databases. Patients and healthcare professionals alike need to seek information from reputable and reliable resources and make shared decisions on what to incorporate into treatment plans (and what to avoid) based on each person's level of comfort.[34–37] Frank, nonjudgmental discussion with the patient is necessary to inform them effectively about the known risks and benefits of the therapies under consideration. When a CIM treatment is contraindicated, it is critical that the patient be advised to avoid the treatment. The patient's receptivity and compliance will ultimately depend on effective communication techniques and how the message is delivered. If a therapy is ineffective, but known to be safe, the patient must be appropriately informed.

If it seems that the therapy is safe and there are clinical clues that it may have some effectiveness, the next step is to discuss the level of uncertainty of the treatment's efficacy with the patient. A realistic view may be that more complete information will not be available in the near future and that a decision that balances risk and benefit is needed. The higher the patient's expectations, the higher the degree of disappointment when the course of care does not go as expected. An informed discussion should provide the available information on the therapy to minimize unrealistic expectations. This discussion can be used as a tool to improve communication and empower the patient in his own care at a critical juncture in the cancer care journey. If a decision is reached to add a complementary therapy to the treatment of cancer, the healthcare professional's role has not ended. Regular follow-up is needed to monitor adverse effects and effectiveness and make adjustments, as with any other conventional treatment.[38]

The remainder of this section describes some of the key findings on CIM therapies for which there is sufficient evidence to recommend them in integrative oncology: mind-body treatments, massage, and acupuncture. The important roles of physical activity, exercise, and energy-balance/nutrition are discussed thoroughly in Chapters 3 and 4. Although there is ongoing research in many other CIM areas, such as healing touch, homeopathy, natural products, and special diets, there is insufficient evidence to recommend these at this time. The SIO Integrative Oncology Practice Guidelines state that "…until there is evidence for the safety and efficacy of the substance, they should not be used as alternatives to mainstream care."[36]

Mind-body practices. The belief that what we think and feel can influence our health and healing dates back thousands of years.[39] The importance of the role of the mind, emotions, and behaviors in health and well-being is central to traditional Chinese, Tibetan, and Ayurvedic medicine and other medical traditions of the world. Many cancer patients believe that stress plays a role in the etiology and progression of their disease. Although the role of stress in the etiology of cancer remains controversial, there is substantial evidence showing the negative health consequences of sustained stress on health and well-being through profound psychological, behavioral, and physiological effects.[40,41] There is also evidence to suggest that chronic stress has a role in the progression of disease[42] and that it may contribute to overall mortality.[43] The clinical significance of stress-related physiological changes and changes in the tumor microenvironment has not been widely studied. These changes may be significant enough to affect not only the immediate health of the patient, but also the course of the disease and thus the future health of the patient.[41] Decreasing distress and maintaining the functional integrity of the immune system and other physiological systems are therefore important in helping patients adjust to cancer treatment, recovery, treatment complications, and possibly metastatic growth. Although this area of research is relatively new, it has been demonstrated that psychological factors can result in behavioral and regulatory system changes that, in turn, may affect future health.[40,41] This has helped to legitimize what is called the mind-body connection and mind-body medicine research, and has lead to an increased interest in mind-body therapies as a way to manage stress.

Extensive research has documented that mind-body interventions appear to address many of the issues mentioned in the Institute of Medicine report. Some techniques are discussed in this chapter; further details on the more conventional behavioral techniques can be found in Chapters 53 through 56.

Mind-body practices are defined as a variety of techniques designed to enhance the mind's capacity to affect bodily function and symptoms.[2] Mind-body techniques include relaxation, hypnosis, visual imagery, meditation, biofeedback, cognitive-behavioral therapies, group support, autogenic training, and therapies involving spirituality or expressive arts such as visual art, music, or dance. Therapies such as yoga, tai chi, and qigong often fall into the CIM category of energy medicine, as they are intended to work with bodily "energetic fields," such as meridians and *qi* (pronounced chee, China), *lung* (pronounced long, Tibet), *prana* (India), and *ki* (pronounced kee, Japan). Such therapies are also likely, however, to exert strong effects through a mind-body connection, and as such can also be included in the mind-body medicine category. Some of these therapies are no longer considered "alternative" and are well integrated into conventional medicine and most medical settings; examples include hypnosis, biofeedback, cognitive-behavioral therapy, and group support. As research continues, it is hoped that the treatments that are found to be beneficial will become integrated into conventional medical care.

Research has shown that after a diagnosis of cancer, patients try to bring about positive changes in their lifestyle, indicating a tendency to take control of their healthcare.[44] Techniques of stress management that have proven helpful include progressive muscle relaxation, diaphragmatic breathing, guided imagery, social support, supportive expressive group therapy, and meditation.[45,46] Participating in stress management programs before treatment has enabled patients to tolerate therapy with fewer reported side effects.[45] For more details on supportive care see Chapters 53 through 59.

A meta-analysis of 116 studies found that mind-body therapies could reduce anxiety, depression and mood disturbance in cancer patients, and assist their coping skills.[47] Newell and colleagues reviewed psychological therapies for cancer patients and concluded that interventions involving self-practice and hypnosis for managing nausea and vomiting could be recommended, whereas further research was suggested to examine the benefits of relaxation training and guided imagery.[48] Further research was also warranted to examine the benefits of relaxation and guided imagery for managing general nausea, anxiety, and overall physical symptoms and improving quality of life.[48] More recently, Ernst et al. examined changes in the state of the evidence for mind-body therapies for various medical conditions between 2000 and 2005 and found that, over that period, maximal evidence had appeared for the use of relaxation techniques for anxiety, hypertension, insomnia, and nausea due to chemotherapy.[49]

Research examining yoga, tai chi, and meditation incorporated into cancer care suggests that these mind-body practices help to improve aspects of quality of life, including improved mood, sleep quality, physical functioning, and overall feeling of well-being.[50,51] For more details see Chapter 58. Hypnosis, especially self-hypnosis, has been found beneficial in helping to reduce distress and discomfort during difficult medical procedures.[52] An NIH Technology Assessment Panel found strong evidence that hypnosis can alleviate cancer-related pain.[53] Hypnosis effectively treats anticipatory nausea in pediatric[54] and adult cancer patients[55] reduces postoperative nausea and vomiting,[56] improves hot flashes,[57] and improves adjustment to invasive medical procedures.[58]

Mounting evidence suggests that impaired cognitive function can result from having cancer and/or undergoing treatment,[59] joining the list of cancer-related sequelae such as distress, nausea, and sleep difficulties. Converging lines of evidence from a number of recent empirical studies investigating mind-body practices suggest that a mindfulness-based practice such as meditation may help to alleviate cancer-related cognitive impairment by engaging the individual in an attention-based mental activity. This "mental practice" has been shown to employ the frontal-subcortical circuits that have been reported to be impaired in cancer-related cognitive dysfunction (see reference 60 for a review). Only a small number of studies have specifically examined the efficacy of meditation in improving self-reported cognitive function in cancer patients,[61] and no study has investigated its efficacy in improving objective cognitive function as assessed by standardized neuropsychological tests. Given the extant data demonstrating an association between meditation practice and improved cognitive function in both clinical[62] and nonclinical[63,64] populations, further examination of meditation as an intervention for cancer-related cognitive impairment is warranted.

Massage. Physical touch and massage are therapies that have been used for thousands of years. Massage is used for relaxation, to help manage pain and discomfort, and as a physiotherapeutic intervention. There are various forms of massage; all typically apply some degree of pressure to muscle and connective tissue, and some work with specific pressure points. A clinical form of massage known as manual lymph drainage has been shown to decrease lymphedema when combined with elastic sleeves or bandaging for patients with arm edema after breast cancer surgery.[65] This is a detailed and lengthy process, however, and self-massage with this technique has not been found to be as effective as either that done by a trained therapist or simulation by a specially designed pump.[66]

Research findings suggest that massage is helpful in relieving pain, anxiety, fatigue, and distress and in increasing relaxation.[67,68] Conducting massage therapy research is especially challenging in terms of selecting an appropriate control group with comparable treatment and symptom status while controlling for attention and physical contact, and thus design of a conventional placebo-controlled trial is difficult. Regardless of some of the imperfections in research design, however, the findings are encouraging, and there is no question that patients derive benefits such as relaxation and an increased sense of general well-being from various types of massage. Even massage limited to the feet, hands, or head can be beneficial.[67,68] Moreover, massage is generally safe in the hands of a licensed practitioner who has had training in an oncology setting. In general, cancer patients should not receive deep tissue massage, and patients at increased risk of bleeding should receive only light touch. Obviously, areas of the body that have been subject to recent surgery or radiation exposure should be avoided.

Acupuncture. According to the World Health Organization acupuncture is used in at least 78 countries around the world.[69] The underlying theory of acupuncture is based on the premise that the placement of needles, heat, or pressure at specific body sites can help regulate the flow of qi (vital energy) within the body.

The most common form of acupuncture involves the placement of solid, sterile, stainless steel needles into points on the body thought to have reduced bioelectrical resistance and increased conductance.[70] Different techniques, such as manual or electrical manipulation, can be used to stimulate the needles,[70] causing vasodilation and release of various neurohormones/neurotransmitters. Stainless steel or gold (semipermanent) needles, or "studs," are also sometimes placed at specific points on the ears and left in place for several days.[71] Other techniques include application of heat, electrical stimulation through pads placed on the skin, or pressure to acupuncture points; however, the therapeutic benefit is thought to be greater when needles are inserted.

The strongest evidence for the efficacy of acupuncture in cancer care is for symptom management of nausea, vomiting, and some types of pain. Furthermore, good evidence supports its use in the management of nausea and vomiting from various causes (i.e., CINV, postoperative nausea and vomiting, and pregnancy).[16,72] It should be noted, in one systematic review comparing acupuncture with antiemetics, stimulation of acupoint P6 reduced the risk of nausea but not vomiting.[73] Although there is good evidence for the use of acupuncture to control some types of pain, research findings specific to the cancer setting are still limited. One well-designed randomized, blinded, placebo-controlled trial among cancer patients, however, did find that auricular acupuncture decreased pain scores by 36% in the active treatment group, while scores remained stable in two placebo groups (auricular acupuncture or ear seeds at non-acupuncture points).[71]

Another indication for which evidence is highly promising involves the use of acupuncture to treat radiation-induced xerostomia.[74] A number of controlled and uncontrolled studies have been conducted, but methodological rigor is still lacking. A large, definitive randomized clinical trial is needed. The initial research does suggest, however, that acupuncture is beneficial and in some cases can have a lasting effect. Studies to evaluate the efficacy of acupuncture in preventing radiation-induced xerostomia are currently underway.

Table 60–2. Recommended web sites for evidence-based information on complementary and alternative therapies

Organization/Web site (alphabetical order)	Address/URL	Description
Bandolier[80]	http://www.jr2.ox.ac.uk/bandolier/booth/booths/altmed.html	A monthly journal about evidence-based healthcare produced by scientists at Oxford University, provides a subset of in-depth analyses, commentaries, and meta-analyses on complementary therapies found in searches of the Cochrane Library and PubMed
Cochrane Review Organization[88,94]	www.cochrane.org	Founded in 1993 as an international nonprofit independent organization, Cochrane now provides over 2000 systematic reviews and has recently added the complementary therapies of massage, acupuncture, and chiropractic
		Its review process includes searches of multiple bibliographic databases by professional librarians
		At least two blinded independent reviewers evaluate studies according to standard sets of questions; discrepancies are resolved through conferences with attempts to contact authors for resolution of remaining questions
		A statistician and an editorial board join with reviewers for development and summation of final conclusions. Abstracts of Cochrane reviews are free, but completed reviews require either individual or institutional subscription
Memorial Sloan-Kettering Cancer Center[33]	http://www.mskcc.org/aboutherbs	Memorial Sloan-Kettering Cancer Center provides over 200 evidence-based reviews on its web site
		These are written by either an oncology-trained pharmacist with expertise in botanicals or a cancer nutrition specialist, and are accompanied by secondary reviews by at least two other editors or panel advisors
Natural Medicines Comprehensive Database[90]	http://www.naturaldatabase.com/	Natural Medicines Comprehensive Database provides the largest number of evidence-based reviews of complementary therapies with over 1000 reviews
		The majority of its authors and editors hold a doctorate in pharmacy, and their reviews include scientific names, uses, safety, effectiveness, mechanisms of action, adverse reactions, interactions, dosage, and administration
		Full access requires an individual or institutional subscription
		The one- to two-page reviews do not provide background or in-depth assessments of the evidence on which their conclusions are based
Natural Standard[89]	http://www.naturalstandard.com/	Modeling itself upon the Cochrane organization, Natural Standard formed a multidisciplinary, multiinstitutional initiative dedicated to the review of complementary and alternative therapies
		It follows a process similar to that of Cochrane to build in-depth evidence and consensus-based analysis of scientific data in addition to historic and folkloric perspectives
		It now provides over 700 authoritative reviews
		Access requires an institutional subscription, but some subscribing institutions have purchased summaries of reviews for public access (see www.mdanderson.org/cimer)
NCI Office of Cancer Complementary and Alternative Medicine[81]	http://www.cancer.gov/cam	The NCI OCCAM has reviewed about a dozen complementary therapies
		These PDQ Cancer Information Summaries provide extensive details and citations for healthcare professionals, including background, history of development, proposed mechanisms of action, and relevant laboratory, animal, and clinical studies
The University of Texas M. D. Anderson Cancer Center Complementary/Integrative Medicine Education Resources[34]	www.mdanderson.org/CIMER	M. D. Anderson Cancer Center's web site provides over 90 reviews that include in-depth assessments of the background and evidence by its own staff, purchased summaries of some of the previously described reviews by Natural Standard and the Cochrane Library, and access to all reviews by the NCI and Memorial Sloan-Kettering
		M. D. Anderson's methodology includes searches by library personnel; reviews by staff with expertise in laboratory, clinical, and population studies; and secondary reviews by appropriate faculty members or outside advisors

For other treatment- or cancer-related symptoms, the evidence is not as strong as that for pain and nausea. Nevertheless, there is evidence to suggest that acupuncture may be useful in helping to treat or manage symptoms such as constipation, loss of appetite, peripheral neuropathy, hot flashes, fatigue, insomnia/sleep disorders, dyspnea, anxiety/depression, and leucopenia.[75,76] The quality of the research for these symptoms remains weak, however, and further investigation is needed.

Many studies have found that acupuncture, when performed correctly, is a safe, minimally invasive procedure with very few side effects. The side effects most commonly reported are fainting, bruising, and mild pain. Although uncommon, infection is also a potential risk.[77]

Acupuncture should be performed only by a healthcare professional with an appropriate license, and when treating cancer patients, it is preferable for the practitioner to have experience treating patients with malignant diseases.

Although the underlying mechanisms of action for relieving symptoms such as chemotherapy-related and postoperative nausea, vomiting, and pain are not completely understood, there is evidence to support the use of acupuncture as an adjunct in their management. Data are currently lacking for the control of other disease and cancer treatment-related symptoms, but as a very low-risk and cost-effective option, acupuncture should be considered as a potential complementary therapy for patients in whom conventional approaches have failed or for those suffering from uncontrolled symptoms or treatment-related side effects.[78]

EDUCATIONAL RESOURCES

The rapidity with which a comprehensive review can become out of date and the ease of Internet publishing have fostered the growth of comprehensive scientific review organizations that provide electronic access to information on CIM. An assessment of web sites with reviews of CIM therapies for oncology was published in 2004 by Schmidt and Ernst.[79] They used eight popular search engines to search for the terms "complementary" or "alternative medicine" and "cancer" and identified the first 50 web sites that appeared on at least three engines. Their final list of 32 web sites was evaluated for (1) quality based upon a Sandvik score of 0–5 points as "poor," 6–10 points as "medium," and 11–14 points as "excellent"; (2) reliability, based on whether it displayed the Health on the Net (HON) code; and (3) risk to patients, based on an overall score and type of CIM discussed (curative, preventative, or palliative). Web sites were also downgraded for discouraging the use of conventional medicine or clinician's advice, or for providing commercial details. Ten web sites received a score of 12 or better. Seven of these top ten web sites were sponsored by either a government or academic institution and three were sponsored by individuals or private businesses.[79]

We evaluated 15 web sites for recommendations to healthcare professionals: the ten web sites recognized by Schmidt and Ernst with a score of 12 or better, which included Quackwatch[80]; Oxford University's *Bandolier*[81]; NCI Fact Sheets[82]; Rosenthal Center of Columbia University[83]; Holistic online[84]; International Health News—yourhealthbase[85]; Oncolink sponsored by the Abramson Cancer Center of the University of Pennsylvania[86]; University of Virginia Medical Center[87]; NCI OCCAM Physician Data Query (PDQ) summaries[82]; and The University of Texas M. D. Anderson Cancer Center Complementary/Integrative Medicine Education Resources (CIMER),[35] plus five others that were not identified by Schmidt and Ernst: the American Cancer Society,[88] Memorial Sloan-Kettering Cancer Center,[34] the Cochrane Review Organization,[89] Natural Standard,[90] and Natural Medicines Comprehensive Database.[91]

Eight of these fifteen web sites provide generally reliable information for patients and the general public, but are not adequate for health professionals due to bias (positive or negative) or a lack of comprehensive, organized, up-to-date information, detailed study results, or systematic reviews from peer-reviewed journals. The seven remaining web sites provide valuable resources for healthcare professionals (see Table 60-2).

These web sites may be searched efficiently by both physicians or to appropriate clinic personnel. Patients or caregivers can be given specific recommendations, printed summaries, or the names of these or other prescreened web sites. Questions generated from this information can then be brought back for discussion with the physician or other clinic professional.

Although the NCI, ACS, and M. D. Anderson Cancer Center web sites provide links to other reliable web sites, patients or caregivers may wish to investigate independently. If so, they should be encouraged to look for web sites that subscribe to the principles of the Health on the Net Foundation and carry its "HONcode" seal. This nongovernmental organization is supported by the State of Geneva in Switzerland, the Swiss Institute of Bioinformatics, and the University Hospitals of Geneva. It screens web sites for compliance with its eight principles of authority: medically trained and qualified professionals, support of the patient/site visitor and his/her physician, confidentiality, clear references to source data, claims supported by appropriate and balanced evidence, transparency of authorship, transparency of ownership, and honesty in advertising and editorial policy.[92] The HONcode is displayed by two of the seven web sites described here for healthcare professionals: those of the NCI and M. D. Anderson Cancer Center.

EFFECTIVE INTEGRATION

To provide patients with appropriate management of their cancer and cancer-related morbidity, it is likely that complementary medicine therapeutic modalities will need to be integrated into the treatment plan. This makes clinical sense when the evidence for safety and efficacy is strong. Conversely, it makes clinical sense to avoid therapies and discourage therapies when the evidence for safety and efficacy is weak.[93] This will result in the safer delivery of medicine as a whole. When patients receive their conventional medical treatments independently from their complementary medical treatments, the consequent lack of communication between patient and conventional practitioner and between the practitioners of conventional and nonconventional therapies increases the risk of adverse events.

Integrative oncology is a rapidly expanding discipline that holds tremendous promise for providing a greater range of treatment options and more effective symptom control. Many comprehensive cancer centers have integrative medicine established within their conventional care system, including Dana Farber Cancer Institute, Memorial Sloan-Kettering Cancer Center, M. D. Anderson Cancer Center, and others.[94] An integrative approach provides patients with a more personalized system of care for meeting their needs. The majority of patients are either using complementary therapies or want to know about them, so it is incumbent on the conventional medical system to provide appropriate education and clinical services. The clinical model for integrative care requires a patient-centered approach with attention to patient concerns and enhanced communication. It is essential that practitioners of conventional and nonconventional therapies work together in developing an integrative model. In this way, cancer patients will receive the best available medical care making use of all appropriate treatment modalities.

REFERENCES

1. Consortium of Academic Health Centers for Integrative Medicine. http://www.imconsortium.org/cahcim/about/home.html. Accessed June 24, 2008.
2. National Center for Complementary/Alternative Medicine. What is complementary and alternative medicine? http://nccam.nih.gov/health/whatiscam/. Accessed June 24, 2008.
3. Eisenberg DM, Davis RB, Ettner SL, et al. Trends in alternative medicine use in the United States, 1990-1997: results of a follow-up national survey. *JAMA*. 1998;280(18):1569–1575.
4. Barnes P, Powell-Griner E, McFann K, Nathin R. CDC Advance Data Report #343: complementary and alternative medicine use among adults: United States, 2002. 2004 May 27; Report No: 343.
5. Navo MA, Phan J, Vaughan C, et al. An assessment of the utilization of complementary and alternative medication in women with gynecologic or breast malignancies. *J Clin Oncol*. 2004;22(4):671–677.
6. Richardson MA, Sanders T, Palmer JL, Greisinger A, Singletary SE. Complementary/alternative medicine use in a comprehensive cancer center and the implications for oncology. *J Clin Oncol*. 2000;18(13):2505–2514.
7. Ernst E. *The desktop guide to complementary and alternative medicine: An evidence-based approach*. London: Harcourt Publishers Ltd; 2001.
8. Eisenberg DM, Kessler RC, Van Rompay MI, et al. Perceptions about complementary therapies relative to conventional therapies among adults who use both: results from a national survey. *Ann Intern Med*. 2001;135(5):344–351.
9. Richardson MA, Masse LC, Nanny K, Sanders C. Discrepant views of oncologists and cancer patients on complementary/alternative medicine. *Support Care Cancer*. 2004;12(11):797–804.
10. Tasaki K, Maskarinec G, Shumay DM, Tatsumura Y, Kakai H. Communication between physicians and cancer patients about complementary and alternative medicine: exploring patients' perspectives. *Psychooncology*. 2002;11(3):212–220.
11. Verhoef MJ, White MA, Doll R. Cancer patients' expectations of the role of family physicians in communication about complementary therapies. *Cancer Prev Control*. 1999;3(3):181–187.
12. Berk LB. Primer on integrative oncology. *Hematol Oncol Clin North Am*. 2006;20(1):213–231.
13. Cohen L, Cohen MH, Kirkwood C, Russell NC. Discussing complementary therapies in an oncology setting. *J Soc Integ Oncol*. 2007;5(1):18–24.
14. Jenkins V, Fallowfield L, Saul J. Information needs of patients with cancer: results from a large study in UK cancer centres. *Br J Cancer*. 2001;84(1):48–51.
15. Frenkel M, Ben-Arye E. Communicating with patients about the use of complementary and integrative medicine in cancer care. In: Cohen L, Markman M (eds). *Incorporating complementary medicine into conventional cancer care*. Totowa: Humana Press; 2008:33–46.
16. NIH Consensus Conference. Acupuncture. *JAMA*. 1998;280:1518–1524.
17. American Cancer Society: Acupuncture. http://www.cancer.org/docroot/ETO/content/ETO_5_3X_Acupuncture.asp?sitearea=ETO. Accessed June 15, 2008.

18. Wu MT, Hsieh JC, Xiong J, et al. Central nervous system pathway for acupuncture stimulation: localization of processing with functional MR imaging of the brain-preliminary experience. *Radiology*. 1999;212:133–141.

19. Backon J. Ginger as an antiemetic: possible side effects due to its thromboxane synthetase activity [comment]. *Anaesthesia*. 1991;46(8):705–706.

20. Jain RC. Effect of garlic on serum lipids, coagulability and fibrinolytic activity of blood. *Am J Clin Nutr*. 1977;30(9):1380–1381.

21. Jiang X, Williams KM, Liauw WS, et al. Effect of St John's wort and ginseng on the pharmacokinetics and pharmacodynamics of warfarin in healthy subjects. *Br J Clin Pharmacol*. 2004;57(5):592–599.

22. McCabe BJ. Prevention of food-drug interactions with special emphasis on older adults. *Curr Opin Clinl Nut Met Care*. 2004;7(1):21–26.

23. Umland EM, Cauffield JS, Kirk JK, Thomason TE. Phytoestrogens as therapeutic alternatives to traditional hormone replacement in postmenopausal women. *Pharmacotherapy*. 2000;20(8):981–990.

24. Spelman K, Burns J, Nichols D, Winters N, Ottersberg S, Tenborg M. Modulation of cytokine expression by traditional medicines: a review of herbal immunomodulators. *Altern Med Rev*. 2006;11(2):128–150.

25. Hileman EO, Liu J, Albitar M, Keating MJ, Huang P. Intrinsic oxidative stress in cancer cells: a biochemical basis for therapeutic selectivity. *Cancer Chemother Pharmacol*. 2004;53(3):209–219.

26. Lawenda BD, Kelly KM, Ladas EJ, et al. Should supplemental antioxidant administration be avoided during chemotherapy and radiation therapy? *JNCI*. 2008;100(11):773–783.

27. Saper RB, Kales SN, Paquin J, et al. Heavy metal content of Ayurvedic herbal medicine products. *JAMA*. 2004;292(23):2868–2873.

28. Gastpar M, Singer A, Zeller K. Comparative efficacy and safety of a once-daily dosage of hyericum extract STW3-VI and citalopram in patients with moderate depression: a double-blind, randomized, multicentre, placebo-controlled study. *Pharmacopsychiatry*. 2006;39:66–75.

29. Borrelli F, Capasso R, Aviello G, et al. Effectiveness and safety of ginger in the treatment of pregnancy-induced nausea and vomiting. *Obstet Gynecol*. 2005;105:849–856.

30. Bent S, Padula A, Moore D, Patterson M, Mehling W. Valerian for sleep: a systematic review and meta-analysis. *Am J Med*. 2006;119(12):1005–1012.

31. Taibi DM, Landis CA, Petry H, Vitiello MV. A systematic review of valerian as a sleep aid: safe but not effective. *Sleep Med Rev*. 2007;11(3):209–230.

32. National Cancer Institute. Clinical trials. www.cancer.gov. Accessed September 26, 2008.

33. Memorial Sloan-Kettering Cancer Center. About Herbs. http://www.mskcc.org/aboutherbs. Accessed June 15, 2008.

34. The University of Texas M. D. Anderson Cancer Center: Complementary/Integrative Medicine Education Resources (CIMER). http://www.mdanderson.org/cimer. Accessed June 15, 2008.

35. Deng GE, Cassileth BR, Cohen L, et al. Integrative oncology practice guidelines. *J Soc Integr Oncol*. 2007;5(2):65–84.

36. Weiger WA, Smith M, Boon H, et al. Advising patients who seek complementary and alternative medical therapies for cancer. *Ann Intern Med*. 2002;137(11):889–903.

37. Frenkel M, Ben-Arye E, Baldwin CD, Sierpina V. Approach to communicating with patients about the use of nutritional supplements in cancer care. *South Med J*. 2005;98(3):289–294.

38. Shankar K, Liao LP. Traditional systems of medicine. *Phy Med Rehab Clin Nr Am*.2004;15(4):725–747.

39. Antoni MH, Lutgendorf SK, Cole SW, et al. The influence of bio-behavioural factors on tumour biology: pathways and mechanisms. *Nat Rev Cancer*. 2006;6(3):240–248.

40. Glaser R, Kiecolt-Glaser JK. Stress-induced immune dysfunction: implications for health. *Nat Rev. Immunol*. 2005;5(3):243–251.

41. Thaker PH, Han LY, Kamat AA, et al. Chronic stress promotes tumor growth and angiogenesis in a mouse model of ovarian carcinoma. *Nat Med*. 2006;12(8):939–944.

42. Steel JL, Geller DA, Gamblin TC, Olek MC, Carr BI. Depression, immunity, and survival in patients with hepatobiliary carcinoma. *J Clin Oncol*. 2007;25(17):2397–2405.

43. Blanchard CM, Denniston MM, Baker F, et al. Do adults change their lifestyle behaviors after a cancer diagnosis? *Am J Health Behav*. 2003;27(3):246–256.

44. Jacobsen PB, Jim HS. Psychosocial interventions for anxiety and depression in adult cancer patients: achievements and challenges. *CA Cancer J Clin*. 2008;58(4):214–230.

45. Lepore SJ, Coyne JC. Psychological interventions for distress in cancer patients: a review of reviews. *Ann Behav Med*. 2006;32(2):85–92.

46. Devine EC, Westlake SK. The effects of psychoeducational care provided to adults with cancer: meta-analysis of 116 studies. *Oncol Nurs Forum*. 1995;22(9):1369–1381.

47. Newell SA, Sanson-Fisher RW, Savolainen NJ. Systematic review of psychological therapies for cancer patients: overview and recommendations for future research. *J Natl Cancer Inst*. 2002;94(8):558–584.

48. Ernst E, Pittler MH, Wider B, Boddy K. Mind-body therapies: are the trial data getting stronger? *Altern Ther Health Med*. 2007;13(5):62–64.

49. Bower JE, Woolery A, Sternlieb B, Garet D. Yoga for cancer patients and survivors. *Cancer Control*. 2005;12(3):165–171.

50. Gordon JS. Mind-body medicine and cancer. In: Cohen L, Frenkel M (eds). *Integrative medicine in oncology: Hematology/oncology clinics of North America (vol. 22)*. Philadelphia: W. B. Saunders Co-Elsevier, Inc. 2008:683–708.

51. Spiegel D, Moore R. Imagery and hypnosis in the treatment of cancer patients. *Oncology (Williston Park)*. 1997;11(8):1179–1189. Discussion 1189–1195.

52. National Institutes of Health Technology Assessment Panel on Integration of Behavioral and Relaxation Approaches into the Treatment of Chronic Pain and Insomnia. Integration of behavioral and relaxation approaches into the treatment of chronic pain and insomnia. *JAMA*. 1996;276:313–318.

53. Zeltzer LK, Dolgin MJ, LeBaron S, LeBaron C. A randomized, controlled study of behavioral intervention for chemotherapy distress in children with cancer. *Pediatrics*. 1991;88(1):34–42.

54. Morrow GR, Morrell C. Behavioral treatment for the anticipatory nausea and vomiting induced by cancer chemotherapy. *N Engl J Med*. 1982;307(24):1476–1480.

55. Faymonville ME, Mambourg PH, Joris J, et al. Psychological approaches during conscious sedation. Hypnosis versus stress reducing strategies: a prospective randomized study. *Pain*. 1997;73(3):361–367.

56. Elkins G, Marcus J, Stearns V, et al. Randomized trial of a hypnosis intervention for treatment of hot flashes among breast cancer survivors. *J Clin Oncol*. 2008;26(31):5022–6.

57. Montgomery GH, Bovbjerg DH, Schnur JB, et al. A randomized clinical trial of a brief hypnosis intervention to control side effects in breast surgery patients. *J Natl Cancer Inst*. 2007;99(17):1304–1312.

58. Vardy J, Wefel JS, Ahles T, Tannock IF, Schagen SB. Cancer and cancer-therapy related cognitive dysfunction: an international perspective from the Venice cognitive workshop. *Ann Oncol*. 2008;19(4):623–629.

59. Biegler K, Chaoul A, Cohen L. Cancer, cognitive impairment, and meditation *Acta Oncologica*. 2009;48:18–26.

60. Carlson LE, Speca M, Patel KD, Goodey E. Mindfulness-based stress reduction in relation to quality of life, mood, symptoms of stress, and immune parameters in breast and prostate cancer outpatients. *Psychosom Med*. 2003;65(4):571–581.

61. Zylowska L, Ackerman DL, Yang MH, et al. Mindfulness meditation training in adults and adolescents with ADHD: a feasibility study. *J Atten Disord*. 2008;11:737–46.

62. Jha AP, Krompinger J, Baime MJ. Mindfulness training modifies subsystems of attention. *Cogn Affect Behav Neurosci*. 2007;7(2):109–119.

63. Slagter HA, Lutz A, Greischar LL, et al. Mental training affects distribution of limited brain resources. *PLoS Biol*. 2007;5(6):e138.

64. Thomas RC, Hawkins K, Kirkpatrick SH, et al. Reduction of lymphedema using complete decongestive therapy: roles of prior radiation therapy and extent of axillary dissection. *J Soc Integr Oncol*. 2007;5(3):87–91.

65. Wilburn O, Wilburn P, Rockson SG. A pilot, prospective evaluation of a novel alternative for maintenance therapy of breast cancer-associated lymphedema. *BMC Cancer*. 2006;6:84–693.

66. Russell NC, Sumler SS, Beinhorn CM, Frenkel MA. Role of massage therapy in cancer care. *J Altern Complement Med*. 2008;14(2):209–214.

67. Myers CD. The value of massage therapy in cancer care. In: Cohen L, Frenkel M (eds). *Integrative medicine in oncology: Hematology/oncology clinics of North America*; New York: Elsevier BV 2008:649–660.

68. World Health Organization. *WHO traditional medicine strategy 2002-2005*. WHO: Geneva. 2002.

69. Helms JM. *Acupuncture energetics: A clinical approach for physicians*. Berkeley, CA: Medical Acupuncture Publishers; 1997.

70. Alimi D, Rubino C, Pichard-Leandri E, et al. Analgesic effect of auricular acupuncture for cancer pain: a randomized, blinded, controlled trial. *J Clin Oncol*. 2003;21(22):4120–4126.

71. Ezzo J, Vickers A, Richardson MA, et al. Acupuncture-point stimulation for chemotherapy-induced nausea and vomiting. *J Clin Oncol*. 2005;23(28):7188–7198.

72. Lee A, Done ML. Stimulation of the wrist acupuncture point P6 for preventing postoperative nausea and vomiting. *Cochrane Database Syst Rev*. 2004;3:CD003281.

73. Jedel E. Acupuncture in xerostomia—a systematic review. *J Oral Rehabil*. 2005;32(6):392–396.

74. Filshie J, Hester J. Guidelines for providing acupuncture treatment for cancer patients—a peer-reviewed sample policy document. *Acupunct Med*. 2006;24(4):172–182.

75. Lewith G, Berman B, Cummings M, et al. Systematic review of systematic reviews of acupuncture published 1996–2005. *Clin Med*. 2006;6(6):623–625; Author reply 625–626.

76. Ernst E, White AR. Prospective studies of the safety of acupuncture: a systematic review. *Am J Med*. 2001;110(6):481–485.

77. Lu W, Dean-Clower E, Doherty-Gilman A, Rosenthal DS. The value of acupuncture in cancer care. *Hematol Oncol Clin North Am*. 2008;22(4):631–648, viii.

78. Schmidt K, Ernst E. Assessing websites on complementary and alternative medicine for cancer. *Ann Oncol*. 2004;15(5):733–742.

79. Barrett S. Quackwatch. http://www.quackwatch.org. Accessed June 15, 2008.

80. Oxford University—Bandolier: evidence based thinking about health issues. http://www.jr2.ox.ac.uk/bandolier/booth/booths/altmed.html. Accessed June 15, 2008.

81. National Cancer Institute. Office of cancer complementary & alternative medicine: CAM information. http://www.cancer.gov/cam/. Accessed June 15, 2008.

82. Rosenthal Center for Complementary and Alternative Medicine: HerbMedPro. http://rosenthal.hs.columbia.edu. Accessed June 15, 2008.

83. Mathew J. HolisticHealth.Com. http://holisticonline.com/hol_about.htm. Accessed June 15, 2008.

84. Larsen H. International Health News. http://www.yourhealthbase.com. Accessed June 15, 2008.

85. Abramson Cancer Center of the University of Pennsylvania: Oncolink. http://www.oncolink.com/. Accessed June 15, 2008.

86. University of Virginia: Center for the study of complementary and alternative therapies (CSCAT). http://www.healthsystem.virginia.edu/internet/cscat/. Accessed June 15, 2008.

87. American Cancer Society. Complementary and alternative therapies. http://www.cancer.org/docroot/eto/eto_5.asp?sitearea=eto. Accessed June 15, 2008.

88. Cochrane Collaboration Steering Group: The Cochrane Collection. http://www.cochrane.org. Accessed June 15, 2008.

89. Basch E, Ulbricht C. Natural standard. http://www.naturalstandard.com. Accessed June 15, 2008.

90. Jellin JM. Natural medicines comprehensive database. http://www.naturaldatabase.com. Accessed June 15, 2008.

91. Health on the Net Foundation. About health on the net : about health on the net. http://www.hon.ch/. Accessed June 15, 2008.

92. Cohen MH, Eisenberg DM. Potential physician malpractice liability associated with complementary and integrative medical therapies. *Ann Intern Med*. 2002;136(8):596–603.

93. Frenkel M, Cohen L. Incorporating complementary and integrative medicine in a comprehensive cancer center. *Hematol Oncol Clin North Am*. 2008;22(4):727–736, ix.

94. Dickersin K, Manheimer E. The Cochrane Collaboration: evaluation of health care and services using systematic reviews of the results of randomized controlled trials. *Clin Obstet Gynecol*. 1998;41(2):315–331.

CHAPTER 61

Physical Activity and Exercise Interventions in Cancer Survivors

Kerry S. Courneya

Improved survival and more tolerable treatments have generated interest in behavioral strategies that might further improve quality of life (QOL) and reduce the risk of disease recurrence and early mortality in cancer survivors. One lifestyle factor that has received significant research attention in recent years is physical activity (PA). PA is defined as any bodily movement produced by the skeletal muscles that results in a substantial increase in energy expenditure.[1] Leisure-time PA refers to activity undertaken during discretionary time based on a personal choice and is usually contrasted with occupational and/or household activity. Exercise is a form of leisure-time PA that is performed on a repeated basis over an extended period of time with the intention of improving fitness, performance, or health.[1] The purpose of this chapter is to provide an overview of the latest research on PA and exercise in cancer survivors.

IMPORTANT DISTINCTIONS IN EXERCISE RESEARCH WITH CANCER SURVIVORS

Research studies on exercise in cancer survivors can be organized in many different ways but three of the most important distinctions are (1) the cancer survivor group being studied, (2) the timing of the intervention, and (3) the primary endpoint of interest. The cancer survivor group being studied is relevant because cancer includes many different diseases that can vary dramatically based on the pathophysiology of the disease, the prognosis, the types of treatments received, the side effects experienced, the demographic profile (e.g., age range, sex distribution), the medical profile (e.g., obesity rates, co-morbidities), and even the behavioral profile (e.g., smoking history, alcohol consumption, past exercise). Although early exercise research sometimes included participants with different cancer diagnoses, most recent studies have focused on a single cancer survivor group, mostly breast cancer survivors.

The timing of the exercise intervention postdiagnosis can be divided into pretreatment, treatment, survivorship, and end-of-life phases.[2] Pretreatment includes the period after a definitive cancer diagnosis until treatment is first initiated. Although this period is often short for many cancers (i.e., days to a few weeks), there are several situations in which it may last for months or even years (e.g., active surveillance or "watchful waiting" for non-Hodgkin lymphoma or prostate cancer survivors). The treatment time period is usually defined as receiving the "primary" cancer treatments such as surgery, radiation therapy, chemotherapy, and biologic therapies. The amount of time spent in the treatment phase may last for months or even years. Survivorship is the disease-free period after primary treatment until the development of a cancer recurrence or death. It is probably useful to make a further distinction between an early survivorship phase focused on recovery (e.g., within 6–12 months after treatment) and a longer term survivorship phase focused on health promotion and disease prevention.[2] The end of life phase refers to the situation when the disease is incurable and progressive, and the primary focus is on palliative care. Although some early exercise studies included participants at different phases of the cancer experience, most recent studies have focused on a single phase with the two most common being the treatment phase and the early survivorship phase.

The primary endpoint of interest in exercise studies can be categorized as (1) a supportive care endpoint, (2) a clinical or disease endpoint, (3) an exercise behavior endpoint, or (4) a proposed mechanism for one of these endpoints (Fig. 61–1). Supportive care endpoints are those that are primarily indicators of the *quality* of a cancer survivor's life and include measures such as generic and disease-specific QOL, happiness, self-esteem, patient-rated physical functioning, psychosocial functioning, existential well-being, fatigue, and other symptoms and side effects. Clinical or disease endpoints are those that are primarily indicators of the *quantity* of expected life for a cancer survivor such as treatment completion rates, disease-free survival, cancer-specific mortality, and overall survival. Exercise behavior endpoints are those that are focused on the behavior itself and may include indicators such as the type of exercise being performed, the volume of exercise, and the intensity of exercise. Finally, biopsychosocial mechanisms refer to indicators that are considered along the causal pathway to supportive care, disease, and/ or exercise behavior endpoints. In exercise research, these mechanisms may include biologic markers, physical fitness, objective physical functioning, body composition, and psychosocial markers (e.g., self-efficacy, social support). Most exercise studies to date have focused on supportive care endpoints and their associated mechanisms. More recently, there has been a growing interest in the disease endpoints and exercise behavior endpoints as well as their associated mechanisms. Many studies have included multiple endpoints from more than one of these categories.

These three factors—the cancer survivor group being studied, the timing of the exercise intervention, and the primary endpoints of interest—are useful in organizing research results from exercise studies in cancer survivors. The following sections provide an overview of exercise research in cancer survivors organized by the main endpoints—supportive care, disease/treatment, and exercise behavior. Relevant biopsychosocial mechanisms are also reviewed with each endpoint category. The timing of the exercise intervention and the particular cancer survivor group studied are noted within each endpoint category.

EXERCISE STUDIES WITH SUPPORTIVE CARE ENDPOINTS AND MECHANISMS

As noted earlier, most research studies on exercise in cancer survivors have focused on supportive care endpoints such as QOL, physical functioning, emotional well-being, and fatigue. Many of these studies have also included possible mechanisms for improvements in these endpoints such as aerobic fitness, muscular strength, body composition, and objective physical functioning. The majority of these studies have focused on breast cancer survivors. McNeely et al.[3] conducted a systematic review and meta-analysis of 14 randomized controlled trials (RCT) of exercise interventions involving 717 breast cancer survivors aged 35–72 years. The overall pooled data from these trials showed significant positive effects of exercise on QOL, cardiorespiratory fitness, and objective physical functioning. The pooled data also demonstrated a statistically significant effect of exercise on fatigue reduction but only during the survivorship phase as compared to the treatment phase.

Several recent large exercise trials have been reported since McNeely et al.'s[3] systematic review and meta-analysis. The largest study to date is the Supervised Trial of Aerobic versus Resistance Training (START) which compared aerobic exercise training (AET) and resistance exercise training (RET) to usual care (UC) in breast cancer patients receiving adjuvant chemotherapy.[4] The trial demonstrated that exercise training during chemotherapy improved self-esteem, aerobic fitness, muscular strength, lean body mass, body fat levels, and chemotherapy completion rate.[4] The benefits were particularly pronounced for breast cancer patients that preferred RET (Fig. 61–2), were unmarried (Fig. 61–3),

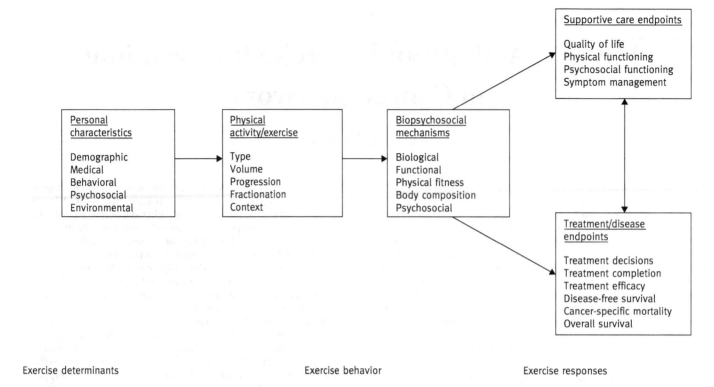

Fig. 61–1. Organizational model of exercise in cancer survivors.

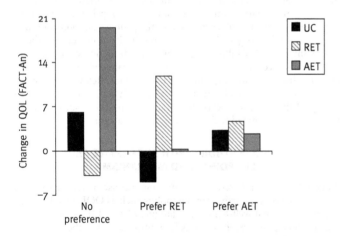

Fig. 61–2. Effects of exercise on quality of life by patient preference from the start trial.

ABBREVIATIONS: AET, aerobic exercise training; RET, resistance exercise training; UC, usual care.

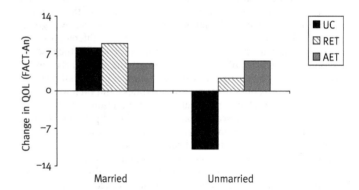

Fig. 61–3. Effects of exercise on quality of life by marital status from the START trial.

ABBREVIATIONS: AET, aerobic exercise training; RET, resistance exercise training; UC, usual care.

under age 50 (Fig. 61–4), received nontaxane chemotherapies (Fig. 61–5), and presented with more advanced disease stage (Fig. 61–6).[5] Moreover, intention-to-treat analysis revealed significant positive effects on self-esteem and anxiety at 6-month follow-up.[6] In correlational analyses, it was noted that improvements in aerobic fitness were associated with improvements in QOL, fatigue, anxiety, and depression. Increases in lean body mass were associated with improvements in QOL, self-esteem, and depression.[4]

In other recent large trials, Mutrie et al.[7] compared 12 weeks of combined aerobic and resistance exercise to UC in 201 breast cancer patients receiving mixed chemotherapy and/or radiation treatments. Results showed postintervention effects on aerobic fitness, shoulder mobility, breast cancer-specific symptoms, depression, and positive mood that

were largely maintained at 6-month follow-up. Daley et al.[8] examined the effects of 8 weeks of either aerobic exercise or flexibility exercise compared to UC in a trial of 108 breast cancer survivors 12–36 months posttreatment and reported postintervention effects on QOL, fatigue, self-worth, aerobic fitness, and depression with the effect on depression being maintained at 6-month follow-up.

In one of the few trials to date to directly test for statistical mediation, Courneya et al.[9] examined potential mechanisms of improvement in supportive care endpoints in breast cancer survivors. The Rehabilitation Exercise for Health After Breast cancer (REHAB) trial was a RCT designed to determine the effects of a 15-week exercise training program on cardiovascular fitness and QOL in 53 postmenopausal breast cancer survivors during the early survivorship phase. Significant improvements were noted for various indices including peak oxygen consumption, peak power output, QOL, fatigue, happiness, and self-esteem. Mediation analyses indicated that changes in peak oxygen consumption mediated the effects of

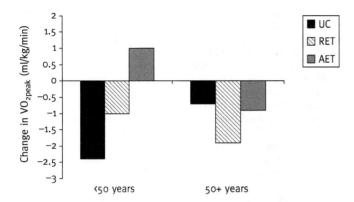

Fig. 61–4. Effects of exercise on aerobic fitness by age from the START trial.
ABBREVIATIONS: AET, aerobic exercise training; RET, resistance exercise training; UC, usual care.

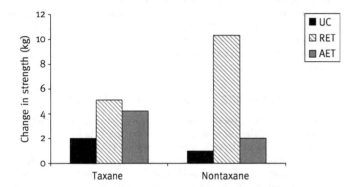

Fig. 61–5. Effects of exercise on muscular strength by chemotherapy regimen from the START trial.
ABBREVIATIONS: AET, aerobic exercise training; RET, resistance exercise training; UC, usual care.

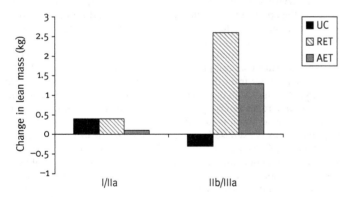

Fig. 61–6. Effects of exercise on lean body mass by disease stage from the START trial.
ABBREVIATIONS: AET, aerobic exercise training; RET, resistance exercise training; UC, usual care.

exercise on cancer-specific QOL and the trial outcome index (an indicator of physical and functional well-being). Moreover, changes in peak power output mediated the effects of exercise on fatigue and the trial outcome index. These data suggest that aerobic fitness may be one mechanism that mediates the effects of exercise on important supportive care endpoints in breast cancer survivors during the early survivorship phase.

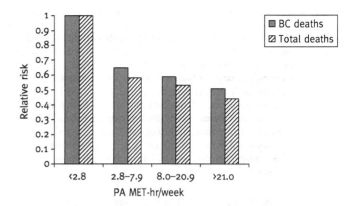

Fig. 61–7. Associations Between Physical Activity and Risk of Death from Breast Cancer and All Causes in the Collaborative Women's Longevity Study.
ABBREVIATIONS: BC, breast cancer; PA MET-hours/week, physical activity metabolic equivalent task-hours per week.

EXERCISE STUDIES WITH DISEASE/TREATMENT ENDPOINTS AND MECHANISMS

Several recent large epidemiologic studies have provided promising evidence of an association between postdiagnosis PA levels and disease endpoints in breast and colon cancer survivors. Holmes et al.[10] followed 2987 women from the Nurses Health Study for a median of 8 years who were diagnosed with stage I-III breast cancer between 1984 and 1998. PA was assessed by self-report every 2 years. After adjusting for known prognostic factors, including body mass index (BMI), analyses showed that women reporting 9–15 metabolic equivalent task (MET)-hours of PA per week (equivalent to 3–5 hours of average speed walking) had a 50% lower risk of breast cancer-specific mortality compared to women reporting less than 3 MET-hours per week (equivalent to 1 hour of walking). At 10 year follow-up, women with greater than 9 MET-hours/week had an absolute survival advantage of 6% (92% vs. 86%) compared to women reporting less than 9 MET-hours/week. Similar risk reductions were observed for breast cancer recurrence and all-cause mortality.

Holick et al.[11] examined the association between postdiagnosis recreational PA and risk of breast cancer death in 4482 breast cancer survivors enrolled in the Collaborative Women's Longevity Study. Participants were aged 20–79 years and were a median of 5.6 years postdiagnosis at the time of enrollment. PA was assessed by self-report of six recreational activities over the past year and women were followed for a maximum of 6 years. After adjusting for known prognostic factors including age, family history of breast cancer, disease stage, hormone therapy use, treatments, energy intake, and BMI, women engaging in more PA had a lower risk of breast cancer death and all-cause death by 40%–50% (Fig. 61–7). The association was similar regardless of age and disease stage.

Meyerhardt et al.[12] conducted a prospective observational study of 573 women from the Nurses' Health Study diagnosed with stage I to III colorectal cancer. Leisure-time PA was self-reported before diagnosis (median 6 months) and 1–4 years postdiagnosis (median 22 months). Analyses adjusted for known prognostic factors, including BMI, indicated a significant negative linear association between the volume of PA performed and the risk of both colorectal cancer-specific mortality and overall mortality. In a companion study, Meyerhardt et al.[13] presented a prospective observational study of 832 patients with stage III colon cancer enrolled in a randomized adjuvant chemotherapy trial and followed for a median of 3.8 years from trial entry. Leisure-time PA was self-reported approximately 6 months after completion of chemotherapy. Analyses adjusted for known prognostic factors, including BMI, indicated a significant negative linear association between the volume of PA and disease-free survival, recurrence-free survival, and overall mortality.

Several biological mechanisms have been hypothesized to explain the associations between PA and cancer prognosis including general and site-specific mechanisms. General effects include the modification of metabolic hormones and growth factors, improvements to the immune system, regulation of energy balance and fat distribution, and antioxidant defense and DNA repair. Site-specific mechanisms include alterations in sex steroid hormones, decreased gastrointestinal transit time, and improved pulmonary ventilation and perfusion. Interestingly, the observational data reviewed earlier indicate that the association between PA and cancer prognosis is independent of BMI or obesity, suggesting other mechanisms may be active. A small number of clinical exercise trials have examined intermediate biological markers in cancer survivors and have reported some positive effects on markers such as insulin, insulin-like growth factors, natural killer cell cytotoxic activity, and c-reactive protein.[14–18]

EXERCISE STUDIES WITH EXERCISE BEHAVIOR ENDPOINTS AND MECHANISMS

Exercise motivation and behavior change is a major challenge in any population but it is especially challenging for cancer survivors. Cancer survivors often endure long and difficult medical treatments that may make exercise participation more difficult and also make the potential benefits of exercise seem less relevant. Given the preliminary positive findings concerning the benefits of exercise in cancer survivors, research has begun to examine the determinants of exercise in cancer survivors and strategies to promote exercise in this population.[19]

Several recent RCTs have examined the effects of exercise behavior change interventions in cancer survivors.[20–23] Jones et al.[24] examined the effects of an oncologist's recommendation to exercise. During the initial treatment consultation, breast cancer patients were randomized to receive either: (1) an oncologist's recommendation to exercise, (2) an oncologist's recommendation to exercise plus a referral to an exercise specialist for an exercise test and prescription, or (3) UC (i.e., no recommendation). Results showed that participants receiving one of the two exercise recommendations reported more exercise during the 6-week follow-up. The authors concluded that an oncologist's recommendation to exercise may be an important component in promoting exercise to cancer patients. In a follow-up paper, Jones et al.[25] reported that perceived behavioral control from the theory of planned behavior mediated the effects of the oncologist's recommendation on self-reported exercise behavior.

The Activity Promotion (ACTION) trial was a RCT designed to determine the effects of distance-based breast cancer-specific print materials, a step pedometer, or their combination, on PA and QOL in 377 breast cancer survivors during the survivorship phase.[23] At the 3-month postintervention assessment, all three intervention groups reported approximately 40–60 min/wk more moderate-to-vigorous PA than a group that received a recommendation to exercise. There was also some evidence that the behavior change was maintained at 6-month follow-up.[26] Moreover, the researchers were able to demonstrate that at least some of the behavior change was mediated by social cognitive variables from the theory of planned behavior.[27]

FUTURE RESEARCH DIRECTIONS

Despite the recent progress in understanding the role of exercise in cancer survivors, a significant amount of research remains to be done. The most progress has been made in understanding the effects of exercise on supportive care endpoints. Future directions in this area include examining the effects of exercise on: (1) understudied endpoints (e.g., sleep quality, pain, symptom management, cognitive function), (2) understudied time points (e.g., pretreatment, end of life), (3) understudied cancer survivor groups, including those that exclusively or disproportionately affect men (e.g., prostate, testicular, bladder, head and neck), and (4) understudied treatments (e.g., radiation, biologic therapies, hormone therapies). There is also a need to determine the optimal type, amount, periodization, and progression of exercise in each of these contexts.

Research on PA and disease/treatment endpoints in cancer survivors is just beginning. We have good epidemiologic research with valid self-report measures of PA and good control of potential confounders. One

major challenge to this research, however, is the difficulty of accurately quantifying exposure to short-term and long-term PA in population-based samples. All epidemiologic studies to date have relied on self-report measures of PA with their well known measurement issues. One possible approach to this limitation is to assess cardiovascular fitness as an objective indicator of recent exercise, although this approach is also not without limitations.

There is also a strong need for RCTs to examine the effects of exercise on the purported biologic mechanisms of recurrence and mortality in cancer survivors (e.g., immune function, sex steroid hormones, peptide hormones, energy balance). These studies will help provide the rationale for large-scale RCTs that will examine the effects of exercise on the clinical cancer endpoints. Ultimately, large scale RCTs with disease endpoints are needed.

Research into exercise motivation and behavior change in cancer survivors is also needed to answer many basic questions. In terms of descriptive behavioral epidemiology, we need more studies documenting the exercise patterns and prevalence rates of cancer survivors including the type, frequency, duration, and intensity of the activities. In terms of exercise determinants research, we need a greater appreciation of the factors that influence the various components of exercise behavior (e.g., type, intensity). In terms of exercise behavior change research, we need to apply rigorous RCT methodology. Finally, it will ultimately be very important to conduct research on knowledge translation to determine how best to put these exercise behavior change interventions into practice to benefit cancer survivors.

CLINICAL AND PUBLIC HEALTH IMPLICATIONS

On the basis of the current evidence, the American Cancer Society has recommended regular exercise to cancer survivors.[28] As indicated in the present review, the evidence is most compelling for breast cancer survivors. In general, exercise during adjuvant therapy will be a struggle for cancer survivors but it is still feasible and likely that benefits can be realized. Depending on fitness level and treatment toxicities, low-to-moderate intensity exercise performed 3–5 days per week for 20–30 minutes each time should be useful. Most cancer survivors prefer walking and this activity will likely be sufficient to meet the recommended intensity for most cancer survivors on adjuvant therapy. Exercise periodization during adjuvant therapy is unpredictable and does not always follow a linear course given the accumulating side effects of most cancer therapies. Cancer survivors should be encouraged to exercise to tolerance during adjuvant therapy, including reducing intensity and performing exercise in shorter durations (e.g., 10 minutes) if needed. RET may be particularly helpful to cancer survivors during adjuvant therapy.

After treatments, when most of the acute toxicities have dissipated, most cancer survivors can probably be recommended the public health exercise guidelines from the American College of Sports Medicine and the United States Centers for Disease Control.[29] These guidelines propose two different exercise prescriptions for general health. The more traditional prescription is to perform at least 20 minutes of continuous vigorous intensity exercise (i.e., ≥75% of maximal heart rate) on at least 3 days per week. An alternative prescription is to accumulate at least 30 minutes of moderate intensity exercise (i.e., 50%–75% of maximal heart rate) in durations of at least 10 minutes on most (i.e., at least 5), preferably, all days of the week. Exercise trials in cancer survivors have generally tested the traditional prescription and there is some evidence that QOL benefits may be enhanced if cardiovascular and strength adaptations occur. Nevertheless, in the absence of clinical trials comparing the two prescriptions in cancer survivors, it seems reasonable to expect both exercise prescriptions to yield similar health benefits. The key issue is developing an exercise program that cancer survivors are able and willing to follow.

SUMMARY

Longer survival for some cancer survivor groups has created an opportunity to examine the potential role of lifestyle factors in further improving QOL and reducing the risk of recurrence and extending survival.

Research on PA and exercise has increased dramatically in the past decade and is producing compelling results. In addition to improvements in supportive care endpoints, there are several recent large prospective observational studies that have reported an inverse association between postdiagnosis PA and disease recurrence, cancer-specific mortality, and all-cause mortality in breast and colorectal cancer survivors. To date, however, there are no RCTs demonstrating that adopting a PA program after a cancer diagnosis can alter the course of the disease or extend overall survival. Nevertheless, fitness and cancer care professionals should feel comfortable recommending exercise to cancer survivors during and after treatments based on evidence for supportive care benefits.

ACKNOWLEDGMENTS

Kerry S. Courneya is supported by the Canada Research Chairs Program and a Research Team Grant from the National Cancer Institute of Canada with funds from the Canadian Cancer Society and the Sociobehavioral Cancer Research Network. I would like to thank the many colleagues, students, and study participants that have contributed to this research.

REFERENCES

1. Bouchard C, Shephard RJ. Physical activity, fitness and health: the model and key concepts. In: Bouchard C, Shephard RJ, Stephens T (eds). *Physical activity, fitness and health: international proceedings and consensus statement.* Champaign, IL: Human Kinetics; 1994:77–78.

2. Courneya KS, Friedenreich CM. Physical activity and cancer control. *Semin Oncol Nurs.* 2007;23:242–252.

3. McNeely ML, Campbell KL, Rowe BH, Klassen TP, Mackey JR, Courneya KS. Effects of exercise on breast cancer patients and survivors: a systematic review and meta-analysis. *Can Med Assoc J.* 2006;175:34–41.

4. Courneya KS, Segal RJ, Mackey JR, et al. Effects of aerobic and resistance exercise in breast cancer patients receiving adjuvant chemotherapy: a multicenter randomized controlled trial. *J Clin Oncol.* 2007;25:4396–4404.

5. Courneya KS, Segal RJ, Gelmon K, et al. Moderators of the effects of exercise training in breast cancer patient receiving chemotherapy. a randomized controlled trial. *Cancer.* 2008;112:1845–1853.

6. Courneya KS, Segal RJ, Gelmon K, et al. Six-month follow-up of patient-rated outcomes in a randomized controlled trial of exercise training during breast cancer chemotherapy. *Cancer Epidemiol Biomarkers Prev.* 2007;16:2572–2578.

7. Mutrie N, Campbell A, Whyte F, et al. Benefits of supervised group exercise program for women being treated for early stage breast cancer: pragmatic randomised controlled trial. *Br Med J.* 2007;334:517–523.

8. Daley AJ, Crank H, Saxton JM, Mutrie N, Coleman R, Roalfe A. Randomized trial of exercise therapy in women treated for breast cancer. *J Clin Oncol.* 2007;25:1713–1721.

9. Courneya KS, Mackey JR, Bell GJ, Jones LW, Field CJ, Fairey AS. Randomized controlled trial of exercise training in postmenopausal breast cancer survivors: cardiopulmonary and quality of life outcomes.[see comment]. *J Clin Oncol.* 2003;21:1660–1668.

10. Holmes MD, Chen WY, Feskanich D, Kroenke CH, Colditz GA. Physical activity and survival after breast cancer diagnosis. *J Am Med Assoc.* 2005;293:2479–2486.

11. Holick CN, Newcomb PA, Trentham-Dietz A, et al. Physical activity and survival after diagnosis of invasive breast cancer. *Cancer Epidemiol Biomarkers Prev.* 2008;17:379–386.

12. Meyerhardt JA, Giovannucci EL, Holmes MD, et al. Physical activity and survival after colorectal cancer diagnosis. *J Clin Oncol.* 2006;24:3527–3534.

13. Meyerhardt JA, Heseltine D, Niedzwiecki D, et al. Impact of physical activity on cancer recurrence and survival in patients with stage III colon cancer: findings from CALGB 89803. *J Clin Oncol.* 2006;24:3535–3541.

14. Fairey AS, Courneya KS, Field CJ, Bell GJ, Jones LW, Mackey JR. Effects of exercise training on fasting insulin, insulin resistance, insulin-like growth factors, and insulin-like growth factor binding proteins in postmenopausal breast cancer survivors: a randomized controlled trial. *Cancer Epidemiol Biomarkers Prev.* 2003;12:721–727.

15. Fairey AS, Courneya KS, Field CJ, et al. Effect of exercise training on C-reactive protein in postmenopausal breast cancer survivors: a randomized controlled trial. *Brain, Behav Immun.* 2005;19:381–388.

16. Fairey AS, Courneya KS, Field CJ, Bell GJ, Jones LW, Mackey JR. Randomized controlled trial of exercise and blood immune function in postmenopausal breast cancer survivors. *J Appl Physiol.* 2005;98:1534–1540.

17. Schmitz KH, Ahmed RL, Hannan PJ, Yee D. Safety and efficacy of weight training in recent breast cancer survivors to alter body composition, insulin, and insulin-like growth factor axis proteins. *Cancer Epidemiol Biomarkers Prev.* 2005;14:1672–1680.

18. Ligibel JA, Campbell N, Partridge A, et al. Impact of a mixed strength and endurance exercise intervention on insulin levels in breast cancer survivors.[see comment]. *J Clin Oncol.* 2008;26:907–912.

19. Courneya KS, Karvinen KH, Vallance JKH. Exercise motivation and behavior change. In: Feuerstein M (ed). *Handbook of cancer survivorship.* New York, NY: Springer; 2007:113–132.

20. Demark-Wahnefried W, Clipp EC, Morey MC, et al. Lifestyle intervention development study to improve physical function in older adults with cancer: outcomes from Project LEAD. *J Clin Oncol.* 2006;24:3465–3473.

21. Demark-Wahnefried W, Morey MC, Clipp EC, et al. Leading the way in exercise and diet (Project LEAD): intervening to improve function among older breast and prostate cancer survivors. *Control Clin Trials.* 2003;24:206–223.

22. Jones LW, Courneya KS. Exercise counseling and programming preferences of cancer survivors. *Cancer Pract.* 2002;10:208–215.

23. Vallance JK, Courneya KS, Plotnikoff R, Mackay JR. Randomized controlled trial of the effects of print materials and step pedometers on physical activity and quality of life in breast cancer survivors. *J Clin Oncol.* 2007;25:2352–2359.

24. Jones LW, Courneya KS, Fairey AS, Mackey JR. Effects of an oncologist's recommendation to exercise on self-reported exercise behavior in newly diagnosed breast cancer survivors: a single-blind, randomized controlled trial. *Ann Behav Med.* 2004;28:105–113.

25. Jones LW, Courneya KS, Fairey AS, Mackey JR. Does the theory of planned behavior mediate the effects of an oncologist's recommendation to exercise in newly diagnosed breast cancer survivors? Results from a randomized controlled trial. *Health Psychol.* 2005;24:189–197.

26. Vallance JK, Courneya KS, Plotnikoff RC, Dinu I, Mackey JR. Maintenance of physical activity in breast cancer survivors after a randomized trial. *Med Sci Sports Exerc.* 2008;40:173–180.

27. Vallance JK, Courneya KS, Plotnikoff RC, Mackey JR. Analyzing theoretical mechanisms of physical activity behavior change in breast cancer survivors: results from the activity promotion (ACTION) Trial. *Ann Behav Med.* 2008;35:150–158.

28. Doyle C, Kushi LH, Byers T, et al. Nutrition and physical activity during and after cancer treatment: an American Cancer Society guide for informed choices. *CA: Cancer J Clin.* 2006;56:323–353.

29. Haskell WL, Lee I, Pate RR, et al. Physical activity and public health: updated recommendation for adults from the American college of sports medicine and the American heart association. *Med Sci Sports Exerc.* 2007;39:1423–1434.

Rehabilitation Medicine in Oncology

Lisa M. Ruppert, Michael D. Stubblefield, Jessica Stiles, and Steven D. Passik

A central focus for patients after cancer diagnosis and treatment is the return of normalcy in day to day life; this constitutes the return of normal function in a wide range of life domains: physical, psychological, vocation, social, and sexual. Rehabilitation medicine aims to restore function with the ultimate goal of functional independence. This area of medicine has become increasingly important as patient-centered medicine has evolved interest in health-related quality of life (HRQOL). In addition, advances in medicine have markedly increased cancer survival rates, with more people who will require rehabilitation services to reach optimal function.

Rehabilitation is a growing and expanding subdiscipline of oncology today. However, it has been slow to develop, similar to the psychological aspects of oncology that were neglected until approximately 30 years ago.[1] This historical picture relates in part to the fact that a cancer diagnosis was considered to a death sentence for many years. The assumption was that since all patients with cancer would die quickly there was no need for rehabilitation efforts. In the mid-twentieth century, patients with an amputation would not be given a prosthesis until at least 1 year later. The emotional stress of cancer was equally stigmatized- patients were not to ask questions about diagnosis or prognosis- and asking for psychological help was considered a sign of moral weakness. Today, these issues are managed better and are more prominent, relatively, but still take a back seat to more traditional oncology treatment modalities.

The progression of the field rehabilitation medicine is reflected in a shift in the World Health Organization's classification of functioning and disability. In 1980, the framework for classification in the *International classification of impairments, disabilities and handicaps* was based on "consequences of disease,"[2] whereas the current version, *International Classification of Functioning, Disability, and Health (ICF)* focuses on "components of health." It distinguishes two parts of the disabling process: *body structures* and *functions* (anatomic and physiologic aspects) and *activities* and *participation* (completion of task and involvement in life situation). From this distinction, the ICF defines *impairments* as significant deviation or loss in body function or structure, shifts disability and handicap towards *activity and participation limitations*. In addition, there is recognition of the facilitative and destructive role the environment can play for people with disabilities. Figure 62–1 shows the ICF's model of the dynamic interactions of the components of health.[3]

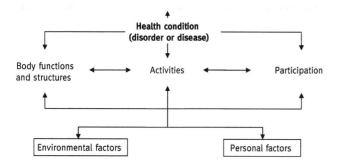

Fig. 62–1. International classification of functioning, disability and health interactions between components of health.[4]

SOURCE: World Health Organization: International Classification of Functioning, Disability, and Health: ICF. Geneva, Switzerland, World Health Organization, 2001.

The WHO definitions are applicable to a broad range of rehabilitation issues, but are particularly relevant to cancer. The nature of many neoplasms and their treatments, the number of patients and survivors, and the need for rehabilitation in all stages of disease and treatment require the presence of a rehabilitation team across the disease continuum: outpatient clinics, inpatient units, and palliative care. In this chapter, we focus on the issues of the cancer patient in the rehabilitation setting, common therapeutic techniques used, and the role of the psycho-oncologist as part of a multidisciplinary rehabilitation team.

THE REHABILITATION TEAM

Due to the multifaceted nature of cancer and its treatment, the rehabilitation team must be multidisciplinary.[5] A team requires the following:

- Physiatrist—a physician trained in rehabilitation medicine that does the comprehensive assessment and oversees the team. The physiatrist is trained to assess functional disability.
- Rehabilitation nurse (RN)—an RN who works closely with the physiatrist and represents the "front line." Often the first to mobilize the patient and assist in activities of daily living (ADL).
- Physical therapist—concentrates on the patient's gross motor function and mobility.
- Occupational therapist—focuses on fine motor function, skills of daily activity, and cognitive and perceptual abilities. Also provides exercises for limb and hand impairment, and may be requested to help with functional impairments of swallowing.
- Speech/language pathologists—specialized in the anatomic and physiologic impairments of speech and swallowing.
- Prosthetist/orthotist—fits and constructs braces and limb prostheses.
- Prosthodontist—responsible for oral prostheses
- Psycho-oncologist—important for assuring psychosocial liaison and a range of psychological and psychopharmacological interventions which may be provided by a psychologist, psychiatrist, or social worker; the latter also helping coordinate discharge. Psychologic intervention may consist of helping the discouraged or depressed patient to set goals that are challenging enough to boost self-esteem, but not so difficult as to result in a sense of failure.

A rehabilitation team should also have services available of a recreational therapist, a vocational counselor, and a chaplain.

REHABILITATION AND CANCER

It is particularly important in oncology for the physiatrist to evaluate the specific symptoms with which the patient presents. The effect of the cancer on function will vary greatly, based on size and location. For example, a mass in the upper lobe of a lung may be silent until it increases in size enough to manifest as dyspnea upon significant exertion. As the mass continues to grow, the amount of physical activity necessary for the patient to experience shortness of breath may decrease. Other symptoms will depend on the direction of tumor growth. If the tumor increases upward, it may lead to impaired function of the arm as a result of direct pressure on the neurovascular bundle entering the arm. Pain, motor and sensory deficits, and edema may begin to interfere with the patient's ADLs. Lack of use will lead to joint stiffness and contracture.

There are several sites of metastasis that require rehabilitation intervention: bone, central nervous system, and the cardiopulmonary system. Weight bearing is a problem when a metastasis to bone threatens the matrix resulting in threat of or actual fracture. Indication of an impending fracture requires a recommendation for change in weight-bearing. Tumors of the spine or cranium produce neurologic sequelae which can require urgent intervention.

Cancer treatments can cause functional impairment which requires rehabilitation management. Surgical resection of a tumor may be at the expense of neurologic, muscular, bony, or other tissues. Chemotherapeutic agents result in specific neurologic, cardiac and pulmonary toxicities. Radiation affects healthy tissue and produces late effects. (See chapters related to sites of cancer.)

Cancer and treatment may result in prolonged periods of bed rest with weakness and muscle wasting, after even a short period of immobility. Decreased aerobic capacity of muscle compromises endurance[6]; pressure ulcers result from confinement to bed; and venous stasis increases risk for deep vein thrombosis and pulmonary embolism.[7]

Dietz, the founder of the field, described four levels of cancer rehabilitation.[8] In each, active collaboration of the rehabilitation team and psycho-oncologist is needed.

1. *Preventative rehabilitation* is implemented in an attempt to limit anticipated functional impairment, such as deconditioning from prolonged bed rest. The psycho-oncologist helps the patient to anticipate and minimize the psychological and physical effects of immobility, plan coping strategies, and helping with setting realistic goals.
2. *Restorative rehabilitation* is used to restore premorbid function when permanent impairment is not anticipated. Patients may become frustrated, depressed, or discouraged by their state and encouragement in the continuation of rehabilitation is important by providing support and helping to set reachable intermediate goals.
3. *Supportive rehabilitation* seeks to maximize function when a permanent impairment exists, such as with amputation. Amputees must adapt to a prosthesis and learn to use the prosthesis in daily life. The patient with cancer requiring above-knee amputation for osteogenic sarcoma is usually much younger than the typical amputation patient. "Phantom limb" pain and grieving the loss are problems.
4. *Palliative rehabilitation* serves to reduce distressing symptoms by a range of physical therapeutic interventions, which are ideally accompanied by psychological support.

There are often special rehabilitation considerations with cancer patients that are not seen with other rehabilitation candidates.

Malignancies of the central nervous system require a dynamic rehabilitation approach, as the lesions are changing. This is seen in epidural metastatic disease causing spinal cord compression where initial aggressive management minimizes permanent neurological sequelae.[9] Epidural disease may be present in other areas of the spine, so the patient may later experience episodes of paraparesis or tetraparesis, requiring a rapid and radically changing rehabilitation plan.

The psychological needs of the patient with cancer should be considered within the context of the illness, and the level of optimal rehabilitation intervention. Psychological factors influence rehabilitation and the ultimate level of functioning the patient is able to attain. When patients are unable to follow rehabilitation recommendations due to psychological factors, it is crucial to determine the cause and to correct it. Medical issues such as brain metastases, high dose corticosteroids, and electrolyte imbalances impede attempts at rehabilitation. They are common problems and should be ruled out before considering a psychological basis for a mood disorder. The most common distress in the rehabilitation setting relate to anxiety and depression. In addition, inability to attain rehabilitation goals may contribute to a patient's depressed mood. Activities such as exercise tend to boost a patient's sense of self confidence and diminish anxiety and depression. Because of their effect on compliance, and therefore the ultimate success of rehabilitation efforts, the diagnosis and treatment of these common psychiatric disorders is crucial. In our clinical experience at Memorial Sloan Kettering Cancer Center, inpatient oncology requests for rehabilitation are often for patients with advanced disease, as disease progression increases physical impairments. This is a time in the course of the disease when psychiatric

co-morbidity is high and intensifies the need for collaboration between physiatrists and psycho-oncologists.

REHABILITATION INTERVENTIONS

Several categories of intervention are described below. They should not be viewed in isolation from one another. Not only is rehabilitation a multidisciplinary approach but it is also multifaceted. The effects of interventions are often complementary and interdependent.

Therapeutic exercise is most commonly used to strengthen weakened musculature. Aerobic exercise and other activities that increase endurance are of equal importance.[10] Devices used to assist in exercise are elastic bands with low to moderate resistance, bicycle pedals with variable resistance, weights for progressive resistive exercises, and isokinetic devices in the later stages of rehabilitation of specific joints. Active range of motion exercises prevent loss of muscle strength, endurance, and maintain range of motion in the involved joints. Neuromuscular reeducation techniques are helpful when increased muscle tone interferes with motor movement. Antispasticity agents, as well as physical modalities such as ice, electrical stimulation, and electromyographic biofeedback, may be beneficial.[11,12] Sustained stretching of muscles are useful in cases of spasticity when joint contracture has occurred.[13]

Muscle incoordination, particularly in disorders involving the cerebellum or its tracts, requires physical rehabilitation. Coordination exercise is a type of neuromuscular reeducation which is helpful. The use of a weighted walker or the use of weights on the lower limbs is helpful in gait training.[14]

In the debilitated, bedridden patient, mobility training is useful. Activities as simple as changing position in bed are initiated and prevent pressure sores. Training the patient to be able to transfer from one surface to another (eg. bed to chair) helps to achieve independence. An over-bed trapeze or other device such as a sliding board or walker may be necessary. For the patient who has difficulty tolerating an upright posture or is prohibited from sitting, a tilt table may be employed. This allows gradual movement from a supine posture to an inclined and eventually, standing posture.[15]

Initial ambulation training should utilize a support for the patient such as a walker, an IV pole, or walking behind a wheelchair. As the patient improves, assistive devices are helpful to widen the patient's base of support and involve the arms in weight-bearing.[16] In the case of sensory ataxia, an assistive device allows the upper limb to receive sensory information from the surface upon which the patient is walking.

Various orthoses may be used to maintain proper limb positioning and thus enhance function. Thoracic and lumbar spine orthoses are helpful in preventing pain provoked by movement.[17] Mechanical pain is often provoked by forward flexion because the weight bearing portion of the vertebrae is most commonly affected by bone metastases. Thus, discouraging forward flexion may discourage vertebral compression deformity and fracture. Lumbosacral corsets and lumbosacral and thoracolumbosacral orthoses are used. Lower limb prostheses following amputation are fabricated in hopes of returning the patient to independent ambulation. In general, the more proximal the level of amputation, the greater the energy expenditure required for a normal gait. Today's lighter weight components, "energy-storing feet," and improved socket designs have improved available prostheses.[18,19] Adequate training with the prosthesis is absolutely necessary to maximize the patient's new compensated gait. Upper limb amputations are much less common than lower limb. The terminal devices of an upper limb prosthesis may be cosmetic or volitionally controlled by the patient. Extensive therapy is necessary to integrate the prosthesis into the patient's ADLs.

Activities of daily living training by an occupational therapist relies on a combination of therapeutic exercise, compensatory technique, and adaptive equipment. Bimanual activities may be helpful, and fine motor retraining may be required. If there is severe weakness or amputation of the dominant arm, the patient will require dominance retraining.

Various physical modalities are used in management of pain. When pain is of muscular or myofascial origin, ice or heat, electrical stimulation, massage and treatment of trigger points may all be utilized. Heat increases local blood flow and metabolic rates.[20] Superficial heat and cold may serve as local counter-stimulants, inhibiting transmission of pain signals up the spinal cord. Various forms of manual stimulation may be used.[21]

Neurogenic bladder or bowel disorders are commonly addressed by the rehabilitation team. Initial indwelling catheters for urinary incontinence are often gradually replaced by either clean intermittent catheterization techniques or bladder retraining.[22] The latter is managed by developing a scheduled voiding regimen. Pharmacologic intervention may be helpful.[23] Constipation is by far the most common form of bowel dysmotility. Increased mobility often enhances bowel motility. Initial management of constipation begins with increased fluid or fiber intake, stool softeners, and oral laxatives.[24] Suppositories, digital stimulation, or enemas may be required, and digital extraction may be necessary for fecal impaction.[25,26]

Swallowing disorders result from anatomic disruption or neurologic dysfunction which are common following surgical treatment for head and neck cancers. Interventions for dysphagia vary from simply limiting the texture and bolus of food or liquids, or altering head or body position to improve swallowing. Therapeutic swallowing techniques are carried out by therapists trained in management of dysphagia.[27]

Disorders of language occur following lesions of the central language processing areas of the brain. Resulting aphasias, or less common verbal apraxia, are addressed by the speech therapist using techniques such as melodic intonation therapy and different communication devices.[28,29]

Chest physical therapy enhances gas exchange in the lungs by assisting in mobilization of secretions. Postural drainage, often in combination with chest vibration or percussion, assist in clearing specific areas of the lungs.[30] Secretions may be loosened before therapy with the use of a nebulizer. Reconditioning exercises for the muscles of ventilation may also be helpful.[31]

Lymphedema is limb swelling which most frequently follows mastectomy. Static compression garments help contain limb volume and enhance the "muscle pump" action of muscle contraction of the limb. Gradient pressure elastic sleeves or stockings are most commonly employed. Bandaging techniques and specific therapeutic exercises are helpful with the "muscle pump."[32,33] Pneumatic compression pumps deliver dynamic limb compression; more contemporary pumps inflate in a distal to proximal direction, thus "milking" the limb.[34-36] Manual lymph drainage facilitates the flow of lymph fluid through residual lymphatic channels. Bandaging the limb between sessions helps to maximize treatment results.[37,38]

THE INTERFACE OF REHABILITATION AND PSYCHO-ONCOLOGY

Assessment and treatment of psychiatric disorders. The psycho-oncologist plays an integral liaison role in the multidisciplinary approach to the rehabilitation of the cancer patient. At Memorial Sloan Kettering Cancer Center, a significant number of requests for physical rehabilitation are for complications related to advanced disease. Upon consultation, these patients are typically found to be badly deconditioned and experiencing significant symptoms. These conditions may be attributable to prolonged bed rest, aggressive treatment modalities, and/ or advanced stage of disease, which increases the risk of a psychiatric disorder. Our experience at Memorial Sloan Kettering is that depression and delirium are the most prevalent psychiatric disorders among hospitalized patients with advanced disease. These patients are likely to be fatigued, mildly confused with mild to severe memory deficiencies. Successful rehabilitation efforts will be limited without management of the delirium. Stimulants and neuroleptics, alone or in combination, are useful in decreasing levels of fatigue and improving mental status. (See chapters on delirium and depression.)

In addition to pharmacologic approaches, there are psychotherapeutic interventions which should be utilized by the psycho-oncologist and the team in facilitating compliance with rehabilitation. The patient's motivation for rehabilitation is a critical component of a successful rehabilitation plan. Psychotherapeutic and behavioral interventions help to maximize compliance and minimize frustration. In addition, involving the family in the program is very helpful.

Disease-related complications and treatment side effects frequently impact upon the patient's quality of life and require the implementation of restorative rehabilitation. Collaboration between the rehabilitation team and a mental health liaison person helps to assure success. Psychiatric consultation that provides assessment, support, and treatment contributes to compliance with rehabilitative treatment and therefore assures more likely success in reaching rehabilitation goals.

REFERENCES

1. Holland J. History of psycho-oncology: overcoming attitudinal and conceptual barriers. *Psychosom Med.* 2002;64:206–221.

2. World Health Organization. Internal classification of impairments, disabilities, and handicaps. Geneva: World Health Organization; 1980.

3. Fann JR, Kennedy R, Bombadier CH. Physical medicine and rehabilitation. In: Levenson JL (ed). *Textbook of psychosomatic medicine,* 1st ed. Washington, DC: American Psychiatric Publishing; 2005:787–825.

4. World Health Organization. *World Health Organization: International classification of functioning, disability and health: ICF.* Geneva, Switzerland; 2001.

5. DeLisa JA, Martin GM, Currie DM. Rehabilitation medicine past, present and future. In: DeLisa JA (ed). *Rehabilitation medicine—principles and practice,* 2nd ed. Philadelphia, pa: JB Lippincott; 1993:3–27.

6. Halar EM, Bell KR. Rehabilitation's relationship to inactivity. In: Krusen FH, Kottke FJ, Lehmann JF (eds). *Krusen's handbook of physical medicine and rehabilitation.* 4th ed. Philadelphia, PA: WB Saunders; 1990:1113–1133.

7. Taylor HL, Henschel A, Brozek J, Keys A. Effects of bed rest on cardiovascular function and work performance. *J Appl Physiol.* 1949;2:223–239.

8. Deitz JH Jr. *Rehabilitation oncology.* New York: Wiley; 1981.

9. Rodichok LD, Harper GR, Ruckdeschel JC, et al. Early diagnosis of spinal epidural metastases. *Am J Med.* 1981;70:1181–1188.

10. DeLorme TL. Restoration of muscle power by heavy resistance exercises. *J Bone Joint Surg.* 1945;27:645–667.

11. Bajd T, Gregoric M, Vodovnik L, Benko H. Electrical stimulation in treating spasticity resulting from spinal cord injury. *Arch Phys Med Rehabil.* 1985;66:515–517.

12. Basmajian JV. Biofeddback in rehabilitation medicine. In: DeLisa JA, (ed). *Rehabilitation medicine—principles and practice,* 2nd ed. Philadelphia, PA: JB Lippcott; 1993:425–439.

13. Steinberg FU. *The immobilized patient: Functional pathology and management.* New York: Plenum Medical Books; 1980.

14. Hewer RL, Cooper R, Morgan MH. An investigation into the value of treating intention tremor by weighting the affected limb. *Brain.* 1972;95:579–590.

15. Nagler W. *Manual for physical therapy technicians.* Chicago: Year Book Medical Publishers; 1974.

16. Joyce BM, Kirby RL. Canes, crutches and walkers. *Am Fam Physician.* 1991;43:535–542.

17. Fidler MW, Plasmans CM. The effect of four types of support on the segmental mobility of the lumbosacral spine. *J Bone Joint Surg Am.* 1983;65:943–947.

18. Micheal J. Energy storing feet: a clinical comparison. *Clin Prosthet Orthop.* 1987;11:154–68S.

19. Leonard JA Jr, Meier RH III. Upper and lower extremity prostetics. In: DeLisa JA (ed). *Rehabiliation medicine—principles and practice,* 2nd ed. Philadelphia, PA: JB Lippincott; 1993:507–525.

20. Lehmann JF, deLateur BJ. Diathermy and superficial heat, alser, and cold therapy. In: Krusen FH, Kottke FJ, Lehmann JF (eds). *Krusen's handbook of physical medicine and rehabilitation.* 4th ed. Philadelphia, PA: Saunders; 1990: 283–267.

21. Melzack R, Wall PD. Pain mechanisms: a new theory. *Science.* 1965;150:971–979.

22. Cardenas DD. Neurogenic bladder evaluation and management. *Phys Med Rehabil Clin North Am.* 1992;3:751–763.

23. Wein AJ. Practical uropharmacology. *Urol Clin North Am.* 1991;18: 269–281.

24. Portenoy RK. Constipation in the cancer patient: causes and management. *Med Clin North Am.* 1987;71:303–311.

25. Lennard-Jones JE. Clinical aspects of laxatives, enemas, and suppositories In: Kamm Ma, Lennard-Jones JE (eds). *Constipation.* Petersfield: Wrightson Biomedical; 1994:327–341.

26. Wrenn K. Fecal impaction. *N Engl J Med.* 1989;321:658–662.

27. Davis JW. Prosthodontic management of swallowing disorders. *Dysphagia.* 1989;3:199–205.

28. Sparks RW. Melodic intonation therapy. In: Chapey R (ed). *Language intervention strategies in adult aphasia.* 2nd ed. Baltimore: Williams & Wilkins; 1981:265–282.

29. Bennett J. Talking about low technology. In: Enderby PM, (ed). *Assistive communication aids, for the speech impaired.* Edinburgh; New York: Churchill Livingstone; 1987:112–132.

30. Helmholz HF Jr, Stonnington HH. Rehabilitation for respitory dysfunction. In: Krusen FH, Kottke FJ, Lehmann JF (eds). *Krusen's handbook of physical medicine and rehabilitation* 4th ed. Philadelphia: Saunders; 1990:858–873.

31. Coffin Zadai C. Terhapeutic exercises in pulmonary disease and disability. In: Basmajian JV, Wolf SL (eds). *Therapeutic exercise.* 5th ed. Baltimore: Williams & Wilkins; 1990:405–427.

32. Casley-Smith JR. Modern treatment of lymphedema. *Mod Med Aust.* 1992;32:70–83.

33. Vernick SH, Shapiro D, Shaw FD. Legging orthosis for venous and lymphatic insufficiency. *Arch Phys Med Rehabil.* 1987;68:459–461.

34. Zanolla R, Monzeglio C, Balzarini A, Martino G. Evaluation of the results of three different methods of postmastectomy lymphedema treatment. *J Surg Oncol.* 1984;26:210–213.

35. Zelikovski A, Haddad M, Reiss R. The "Lympha-Press" intermittent sequential pneumatic device for the treatment of lymphoedema: five years of clinical experience. *J Cardiovasc Surg (Torino).* 1986;27:288–290.

36. Klein MJ, Alexander MA, Wright JM, Redmond CK, LeGasse AA. Treatment of adult lower extremity lymphedema with the Wright linear pump: statistical analysis of a clinical trial. *Arch Phys Med Rehabil.* 1988;69:202–206.

37. Weiselfish S. Manual lymph drainage: a total body approach. *Phys Ther Forum.* 1987;6:2–4.

38. Foldi E, Foldi M, Weissleder H. Conservative treatment of lymphoedema of the limbs. *Angiology.* 1985;36:171–180.

CHAPTER 63

Self-Management Support

Edward H. Wagner and Ruth McCorkle

"I need information so I know how to take care of myself, including what to expect and what resources are available to help me and my family." 56 year old woman with stage III ovarian cancer

More than 50 years ago, the sociologist Talcott Parsons coined the term "sick role" to describe and explain the very different social expectations of an ill person. Ill individuals were exempted from social obligations, and expected to passively do what the professionals ordered so as to recover from the illness and resume their usual roles.[1] This paradigm reflected the epidemiologic and social realities of the time, and the dominance of acute illness and the hospital in medical care. It continues to have a major hold on the attitudes of health professionals and the design of healthcare systems. Patients cede control to the professionals, and the professionals feel responsible for solving patient problems.[2] Most chronic illnesses are a poor fit for this paradigm as was recognized by Freidson.[3] Most chronically ill patients want and are able to remain fully engaged in all aspects of their lives, and must balance professional recommendations with other competing demands. They can not surrender control because living effectively with chronic illness requires skillful self-monitoring, and management of medications, lifestyle, and symptoms. It challenges patients with a daily barrage of decisions about what to eat, how much to exercise, whether to take a medicine, what to do in response to stress or a symptom, or whether to keep a doctor's appointment. The competence with which these decisions are made influences one's health and other important outcomes.[4]

The terms "self-care" and "self-management" have been used interchangeably to describe the actions and decisions that individuals take in dealing with their health and illnesses. Self-management has been defined as "the individual's ability to manage the symptoms, treatment, physical and social consequences, and lifestyle changes inherent in living with a chronic condition. Efficacious self-management encompasses (the) ability to monitor one's condition and to effect the cognitive, behavioral and emotional responses necessary to maintain a satisfactory quality of life."[5] Corbin and Strauss list three goals or tasks of self-management: taking care of the body and illness; adapting to carry out normal activities and roles; and managing emotional changes including uncertainty about the future.[6] The breadth of these definitions reflects the broad array of physical, social, and emotional challenges that major chronic illnesses add to an individual's life. While the challenges pertain to all chronic conditions, their prevalence and severity will vary from condition to condition. On the one hand, lifestyle changes are a major focus of diabetes and coronary heart disease management, but may be less urgent for the patient with cancer. Managing emotional changes, on the other hand, is a critical aspect of living with cancer, but may be less salient in other conditions. Another perspective on what self-management encompasses is to look at the curriculum of the best tested self-management support program, which, unlike most programs, is not disease specific. Developed by Lorig and colleagues at Stanford University, the Chronic Disease Self-Management Program (CDSMP) is a lay person-led group program for individuals with any chronic illness, including cancer.[7] In randomized trials, program participants demonstrated significant improvements in exercise, cognitive symptom management, communication with physicians, self-reported general health, health distress, fatigue, disability, and social/role activities

limitations compared to controls.[8–11] The course consists of six weekly 2½-hour workshops given in community settings such as senior centers, churches, libraries, and hospitals. The material covered in each session includes (1) dealing with problems such as frustration, fatigue, and pain; (2) appropriate exercise; (3) appropriate use of medications; (4) communicating effectively with family, friends, and health professionals; (5) nutrition; and (6) how to evaluate new treatments. The appropriateness of these topics for the cancer patient is obvious.

Medical care's traditional approach to assisting patients addresses the challenges of living with chronic conditions has been varying combinations of information and exhortation. Didactic patient education, often modeled on professional education, was the norm. Its premise was that if patients understood the relationship between their decisions and behaviors and the pathophysiology of their illness, they would change their behaviors accordingly, especially if accompanied by dire warnings and strong recommendations from their physicians. Considerable research demonstrated conclusively that this premise was incorrect—didactic information alone had minimal effects on behavior change and disease outcomes.[8] We needed a new approach and new premises. Pioneers such as Glasgow,[12] Orem,[13] Clark,[14] Anderson,[15] and many others recognized that effective or competent patient self-management was a strong determinant of health outcomes in illnesses such as diabetes, asthma and chronic obstructive pulmonary disease (COPD), depression, arthritis, and other conditions. They also appreciated that patients are really in control, and that professional support must acknowledge and reinforce the patient's primary role through true collaboration. Despite the fact that different theories were invoked or created (e.g., social learning, self-regulation and self-care deficit theories) to guide the development of self-management support, the resulting programs share a common set of principles:

- collaborative definition of problems,
- collaborative goal setting, and problem solving,
- providing a continuum of self-management training and support services, and
- active, sustained follow-up.

The word that best differentiates modern self-management support from traditional provider–patient interactions is *collaboration* as manifest by active patient participation in defining problems, making decisions affecting their treatment, setting goals, and developing plans to achieve goals.[16] Social learning theory and more patient-centric counseling approaches such as motivational interviewing problem solving often provide the theoretical foundation and interaction model. Active patient involvement is not just politically or philosophically correct; it is associated with better decisions, greater adherence with treatment plans, higher patient satisfaction, and better health outcomes.[17] Patients who understand the nature and importance of their involvement in their care facilitate collaboration. Such patients are said to be empowered or activated. Funnell and Anderson describe empowered patients as having "the knowledge, skills, attitudes, and self-awareness necessary to influence their own behavior and that of others to improve the quality of their lives."[18] "Others" obviously include healthcare professionals. Table 63–1 summarizes the differences between collaborative self-management support and traditional medical care.[19]

Table 63–1. Comparison of traditional and collaborative care in chronic illness

Issue	Traditional care	Collaborative care
What is the relationship between patient and health professionals?	Professionals are the experts who tell patients what to do. Patients are passive	Shared expertise with active patients. Professionals are experts about the disease and patients are experts about their lives
Who is the principal caregiver and problem solver? Who is responsible for outcomes?	The professional	The patient and professional are the principal caregivers; they share responsibility for solving problems and for outcomes.
What is the goal?	Compliance with the instructions. Noncompliance is a personal deficit of the patient	The patient sets goals and the professional helps the patient make informed choices. Lack of goal achievement is a problem to be solved by modifying strategies
How is behavior changed?	External motivation	Internal motivation. Patients gain understanding and confidence to accomplish new behaviors
How are problems identified?	By the patient, e.g., pain or inability to function; and by the professional	By the professional, e.g., changing unhealthy behaviors
How are problems solved?	Professionals solve problems for patients	Professionals teach problem-solving skills and help patients in solving problems

SOURCE: Reprinted with permission from Bodenheimer T, Lorig K, Holman H, Grumback K. Patient self-management of chronic disease in primary care. *JAMA.* 2002 Nov 20;228(19):2469–2475.

SELF-MANAGEMENT AND CANCER

Much of the seminal work on self-management and self-management support involved patients with diabetes or asthma. The important role of patients and/or their families in the management of these two conditions is clear. They exercise considerable control over drug therapy. Lifestyle choices have significant impacts on metabolic control and health outcomes in diabetes, and environmental changes in the home may substantially impact asthma severity. The prevailing view of self-management tends to be related to these and related conditions in which patients and families, of necessity, have considerable influence over treatment and outcomes. At first glance, the role of patients in the management of most cancers appears to be less pivotal. Historically professionals have not thought of self-management as a critical component of cancer care because drugs have been largely provider administered, and lifestyle changes appear to be less critical to outcomes. But, as the use of oral chemotherapy has increased in prevalence and continued as outpatient care, and most drugs to prevent or ameliorate symptoms are self-administered, attitudes are changing. Behavior changes such as the promotion of increased physical activity demonstrated pioneering results and have important impacts on cancer patient functioning and quality of life.[20] In addition, the definitions of self-management mentioned above make it clear that more than drug manipulation and lifestyle behavior change are involved in managing "the symptoms, treatment, physical and social consequences, and lifestyle changes inherent in living with a chronic condition". As more patients with cancer are surviving the disease, these survivors have formed advocacy groups who have championed for information for treatment options and services for management. Consequently, as survivors become more knowledgeable, the demand for quality cancer care including strategies for self-management support has increased. The Institute of Medicine's Committee on Psychosocial Services to Cancer Patients' Families in a Community Setting recognized the importance of competent self-management for cancer patients.[21]

Given the diverse physical, psychological, and social challenges posed by cancer, its treatment, and its sequelae, providing patients and their caregivers with knowledge, skills, abilities, and support in managing the psychosocial and biomedical dimensions of their illness and health is critical to effective health care and health outcomes for these patients.[21]

The Committee intensively reviewed the literature on the psychosocial needs of cancer patients, and the availability and effectiveness of services to meet those needs. Psychosocial needs were defined broadly as outlined in Table 63–2. Most of the needs identified by the Committee

Table 63–2. IOM-defined psychosocial needs of cancer patients and self-management tasks[21]

IOM-defined psychosocial needs	Self-management tasks
Information about illness, treatment, health, and services	X
Help in coping with emotions	X
Help in managing the illness	X
Assistance in changing behaviors to minimize disease impact	X
Material and logistic resources	
Help in managing disruptions in work, school, and family	X
Financial advice and/or assistance	

as psychosocial deal with the generic self-management challenges discussed above. For these reasons, we believe that the quality of patient self-management is just as important in cancer care as with other chronic illnesses, and should be a critical component of every cancer patient's care.

There is now considerable evidence in other chronic diseases that interventions directed at improving patient knowledge, skills, and confidence in managing their illnesses improves outcomes.[22] These interventions share with self-management supportive interventions for other chronic conditions the common premise that patients (and their families) have a major role in addressing or managing these challenges, and their ability to manage competently can be improved by information, empowerment and other support. Interventions have been designed to assist patients' coping with the various challenges presented by cancer and its treatment: physical symptoms such as fatigue or nausea, psychological distress, sexual dysfunction, interacting with multiple providers, and so forth.

Such interventions, most often provided by nurses in the cancer care setting, have been variously termed psychoeducational, self-care, self-management support, and, more recently, cognitive-behavioral interventions. They have been administered to patients before therapy or the onset of symptoms as prevention, or to patients experiencing symptoms or distress, or to patients following therapy. They have involved nurse counseling alone, or have been complemented by computer programs, video presentations, and other tools. In the oncology nursing literature, the term self-care[9] has often been used to describe patient behaviors to manage symptoms and other challenges and is therefore indistinguishable from self-management. To illustrate the interchangeability of all these terms, Givens and colleagues recently stated that the goal of their cognitive-behavioral intervention for patients undergoing chemotherapy "was to assist patients to acquire self-management knowledge, skills, and behaviors to address symptom problems."[23] While there may be differences in the underlying theory, the interventions described under the four rubrics share much in common. However, intervention elements are often mixed, which has contributed to confusion about what works and what does not.

In general, self-management support interventions include basic information about the illness and its treatment; information and coaching about skills needed to manage the illness (e.g., use a pillbox), control symptoms (e.g., exercise for fatigue, mouth care for mucositis) and interact with health care (e.g., communicate unrelieved pain to providers), and efforts to increase patient self-efficacy.[24] The education and coaching are generally tailored to the needs and learning styles of individual patients, encourage active patient participation in care, and involve some form of problem-solving assistance. These basic elements of self-management support have often been combined with specific psychological or physical modalities such as relaxation response or exercise. Tested self-management interventions in conditions other than cancer have more often been conducted in groups, while self-care interventions in cancer have generally been individually administered by nurses.

In addition to variation in nomenclature, cancer self-management interventions also vary with respect to the nature and breadth of the primary intervention target(s). Many primarily target symptoms associated with the cancer or with the therapy. Others target emotional distress, while others primarily focus on changing behavior—for example, increasing physical activity to prevent or ameliorate fatigue. Although most cancer support interventions have such a primary focus, they will also mention other components aimed at providing information, improving coping, and reducing stress or distress.

THE EFFECTIVENESS OF SELF-MANAGEMENT SUPPORT INTERVENTIONS

Conditions other than cancer. A number of review articles and meta-analyses have consistently shown that disease-specific self-management programs produce clinically important benefits in patients with diabetes, hypertension, and asthma.[25-28] Somewhat less consistent impacts were noted for patients with arthritis.[25] Efforts to disentangle the multiple components of these interventions to find the active ingredient(s) have been largely unsuccessful,[25] but self-management interventions may be less successful with respect to symptom control than with other outcomes.[26] The studied interventions vary widely in primary target (physiologic measures, symptoms, behaviors), setting, duration, group versus individual, intervention personnel, and other characteristics. However, most programs transmitted information and applied elements of social learning theory, especially goal setting, problem solving, and action planning. The magnitude of the effects of self-management programs on outcomes often compares favorably with medication effects. For example, participation of patients/families in self-management supports interventions:

1. reduced average HbA1c 0.8% among diabetic patients in several different meta-analyses[25,27,28]
2. reduced average systolic blood pressure 5 mm Hg and diastolic BP 4.3 mm Hg among hypertensive patients in one review[25]; and
3. improved quality of life and medication behaviors in the majority of asthma and arthritis interventions studied.[26]

The programs described above, while often efficacious, have limitations that have made them less attractive to real-world healthcare delivery systems. Disease-specific programs may be less relevant to individuals with multiple chronic conditions or other conditions, and would require the availability of a suite of disease-specific programs to serve a population. Since patients with any chronic condition face a common set of self-management tasks, Lorig, Holman and colleagues postulated that a generic self-management program focused on these common

tasks could meet the needs of any chronically ill patient.[7] Although their CDSMP, a lay person-led workshop given in community settings can positively impact important health outcomes, there is concern as to the duration of their effect. Norris and colleagues in their review of diabetes self-management programs observed that about two-thirds of the reduction in HbA1c noted at the end of the interventions were lost when measured a few months after the end of the intervention.[28] This observation suggests that self-management support needs ongoing reinforcement and renewal, which should not be unexpected given the undulating nature of most chronic illnesses and the changeability of medical treatment and life circumstances. This has led to a growing interest in making self-management support a routine part of medical care for the chronically ill.[2] Efforts to integrate self-management support into clinical practice tend to address the following:

- making the identification, review, and documentation (e.g., in a patient registry) of self-management goals a part of every visit;
- adapting or developing a standard set of educational materials that emphasize the patient's role;
- identifying (and often training) someone, generally a nurse or medical assistant, in the practice to provide ongoing collaborative goal-setting, problem-solving, and action-planning support;
- implementing structured individual or group visits with time committed to self-management support; and
- identifying and making links with relevant community programs and resources that would help patients meet self-management goals.

While there have been very few rigorous evaluations of practice-based self-management support, a few randomized controlled trials (RCT) and studies of practices with the best chronic disease performance measures generally support the importance of integral self-management support programs.[29-31]

Cancer interventions. Peer support programs are supportive interventions that involve interaction with others with the same condition. Such programs for cancer patients are available in most communities. Although mostly provided in group settings, peer support can also be provided one to one (e.g., the American Cancer Society's Reach to Recovery Program), and through the internet.[32] Despite the widespread availability of peer support programs, rigorous evidence of their effectiveness is relatively sparse but suggests positive impacts on knowledge and emotional distress. For example, Campbell and colleagues found little evidence of a positive impact of peer support programs on quality of life.[33] Whether cancer peer support programs with more emphasis on self-management, for example, modeled on CDSMP, would increase their effectiveness on outcomes such as symptoms or quality of life needs further research.

Nurse counseling or care management is the most frequently studied approach to delivering information and support to cancer patients. Earlier meta-analyses of randomized trials suggest that these counseling interventions are effective in reducing symptoms of cancer or its treatment,[34,35] as well as symptoms of anxiety, depression and psychological distress.[36] However, because of the admixture of different intervention components, these meta-analyses are of limited help in identifying the intervention elements that contribute to their effectiveness. The PRO-SELF Program, the most extensively tested strategy, targets various symptoms of cancer and its treatment, and has been evaluated in multiple randomized trials.[37-39] The intervention involves nurse coaching with patients and their families. The content includes information to assist patients "in managing the cancer treatment experience" including basic information about the disease and its treatment, symptoms, and approaches to symptom management. In addition to information, patients receive coaching in the skills necessary to manage symptoms—for example, mouth care for mucositis[40] or opioid use for pain[41]—and problem-solving assistance.

McCorkle and colleagues have developed and studied nurse interventions to help cancer patients and their family caregivers manage the impacts of the illness and its treatment. Delivered in the home by advanced practice nurses, the interventions generally involved assessment of physical, psychosocial, and functional health status; teaching, support, and counseling; the provision of direct care if needed; assistance in accessing community resources; and coordination with other healthcare providers and settings. In a series of randomized trials, the home nurse intervention helped lung cancer patients maintain independence longer and reduced rehospitalizations,[42] improved mental health status among solid tumor patients[43]; reduced distress among the spouses of dying lung cancer patients[44]; and improved survival among older postsurgical cancer patients.[45]

More recent randomized trials have helped further clarify the potential of nurse coaching interventions to benefit cancer patients. A recent study of the impact of the PRO-SELF program on pain among cancer patients with bone metastases showed significantly reduced pain intensity and increased appropriate use of opioids. Givens and colleagues tested a cognitive-behavioral intervention among solid tumor patients undergoing chemotherapy that began with collaborative problem identification by patient and nurse.[46,47] The nurse would then propose interventions that would be collaboratively evaluated and an action plan developed. These were supported by classes focused on self-management, problem solving and communication with providers. Those receiving the experimental intervention reported significantly less severe symptoms at 10 and 20 weeks follow-up. Related interventions have been shown in RCTs to improve mood and vigor among patients with malignant melanoma,[48] reduce psychological distress after radiotherapy,[49] reduce fatigue and improve functional status among cancer survivors,[50] and improve sexual function and reduce worry among patients with prostate cancer.[51]

Although the interventions described above vary in theoretical underpinnings, target problem, patient population, counseling strategy employed, and outcomes measured, they provide convincing evidence that assessment, monitoring, and teaching by a trained oncology nurse is valued by patients and their families, and impacts both physical and psychological critical outcomes such as symptoms, psychosocial distress, and functional status.

DELIVERING SELF-MANAGEMENT SUPPORT TO CANCER PATIENTS

Since self-management begins the moment a person has to deal with an illness, support for self-management ideally should be available at the point of diagnosis or even before and continue as long as the condition impacts a patient's life. In early cancer care, patients usually are shifting from provider to provider, or institution to institution as the diagnosis is confirmed, the tumor is staged, and treatment decisions are being made. The multiplicity of providers in cancer care complicates the delivery of self-management support (SMS) in the period before definitive treatment begins.

Every cancer care provider should help patients receive self-management support by integrating it into their treatment plan, and/or by linking patients with effective programs in the community. One useful framework for planning SMS service delivery in the practice is 5 A's to behavior change. This strategy, derived from smoking cessation research, has recently been applied to self-management support in general.[52] Table 63–3 defines and describes the 5 A's for self-management support.

While all 5 A's could be delivered by the same individual, for example, an Oncology nurse educator or even a physician, it has often proven more effective and efficient in noncancer settings for a practice or healthcare system to divide the five functions among different individuals or service programs. A receptionist, medical assistant or even a computer in the waiting room could administer a standardized *assessment* questionnaire to patients, and then summarize the results. Many such instruments have been developed and are nicely summarized in the recent Institute of Medicine report.[21] The clinician provides *advice* or information but may want help from individuals or resources with greater expertise in modern cancer treatment. The responsibility for assuring that patient perspectives are heard and *agreement* is truly bilateral rests primarily with the clinician as it may be difficult for many patients to challenge strong physician recommendations. The clinician should begin the agreement process by actively eliciting patient questions, concerns, and preferences. It may be useful to follow the clinician

Table 63–3. The 5 A's of self-management support[52]

Assess	Assessing patients for their information needs and learning preferences, behaviors, psychosocial distress and problems, progress toward self-management goals, and self-efficacy
Advise	Providing patients with relevant, scientifically grounded information delivered in accord with their learning preferences, culture, and literacy
Agree	Finding common ground between the patient's perspective and professional advice
Assist	The collaborative process of defining problems, setting goals to deal with problems, developing action plans to achieve goals, and revising over time
Arrange	Helping patients identify and link with needed services

interaction with conversation with a nurse or other clinical staff member trained in motivational interviewing or a related counseling strategy who could review the agreements made with the clinician to be certain that both patient and clinician are understood, and that the patient does in fact agree. This clinical team member would then "*assist*" the patient by collaborating with them on the establishment of goals and an action plan. This person or a social worker or community health worker, if available, might help patients identify and *arrange* referrals to resources that might help patients achieve their goals—for example, an exercise or smoking cessation program, a peer support program, or a financial counselor.

The particular challenges of delivering self-management support to cancer patients stem from the multiple handoffs involved in early cancer care, the complexity and rapidly changing nature of the information necessary to respond to patient questions, and the high levels of psychosocial distress. A well-trained oncology nurse with training in self-management and emotional support counseling techniques and ready access to additional expertise in cancer care has been shown to be effective in providing information, supporting self-management, and alleviating emotional distress in the treatment setting. On the basis of the nurse intervention literature, linking cancer patients with a trained cancer nurse specialist to provide support early in their course would be well worth testing. However, given the current organization of and reimbursement for cancer care, early oncology nurse self-management support may not be sustainable outside of integrated, multispecialty practice organizations or comprehensive cancer centers. An alternative strategy would be concerted efforts by primary care physicians, surgeons, and others involved in early cancer care to encourage their patients to participate in community-based cancer-specific group self-management courses or peer support programs that provide peer support, specific cancer information and skills, as well as self-management training and support (goal setting and problem solving). These have been proven to be effective in conditions such as diabetes and asthma and show promise for adapting with patients with cancer and their families.

In this chapter, we have reviewed the evolution of self-management support and its natural fit with chronic illnesses such as diabetes, asthma, and arthritis. The common usage and recognition of self-management has been slow to emerge in cancer care. There have been multiple studies with interventions that reflect the key components of self-management but few have been described explicitly. Future studies need to explore what patients do to help themselves, what enables patients to act for themselves, and how our healthcare system can support patients and families in their efforts. For self-management to be effective and sustaining, multiple levels of interventions are needed that target the patient, family, and system of care. The essential component of successful self-management is open and ongoing communication between patients and healthcare professionals so a partnership is formed and they can collaborate and negotiate the healthcare system. There is a growing demand by consumers and professionals which emphasizes the patients' central role in managing their cancer and the treatment effects. Self-management will become even more common practice as more patients are surviving longer and assuming increasing responsibility for managing their illness and becoming more proactive in decisions affecting their treatment choices and how they live.

REFERENCES

1. Parsons T. *The social system*. New York: the Free Press; 1951.

2. Anderson RM, Funnell MM. Patient empowerment: reflections on the challenge of fostering the adoption of a new paradigm. *Patient Educ Couns*. 2005 May;57(2):153–157.

3. Freidson E. *A study of the sociology of applied knowledge*. New York: Dodd-Mead; 1970.

4. Clark NM. Management of chronic disease by patients. *Annu Rev Public Health*. 2003;24:289–313.

5. Barlow J, Wright C, Sheasby J, Turner A, Hainsworth J. Self-management approaches for people with chronic conditions: a review. *Patient Educ Couns*. 2002 Oct-Nov;48(2):177–187.

6. Corbin JM, Strauss A. A nursing model for chronic illness management based upon the Trajectory Framework. *Sch Inq Nurs Pract*. 1991 Fall;5(3):155–174.

7. Lorig K, Holman HR, Sobel D, Laurent D, González V, Minor M. *Living a healthy life with chronic conditions*. 2nd ed. Boulder, CO: Bull Publishing; 2000.

8. Lorig KR, Holman H. Self-management education: history, definition, outcomes, and mechanisms. *Ann Behav Med*. 2003 Aug;26(1):1–7.

9. Lorig KR, Sobel DS, Stewart AL, et al. Evidence suggesting that a chronic disease self-management program can improve health status while reducing utilization and costs: a randomized trial. *Medical Care*. 1999;37(1):5–14.

10. Lorig KR, Ritter P, Stewart AL, et al. Chronic disease self-management program: 2-year health status and health care utilization outcomes. *Medical Care*. 2001;39(11):1217–1223.

11. Lorig KR, Sobel DS, Ritter PL, Laurent D, Hobbs M. Effect of a self-management program on patients with chronic disease. *Eff Clin Pract*. 2001;4(6):256–262.

12. Glasgow RE, Osteen VL. Evaluating diabetes education. Are we measuring the most important outcomes? *Diabetes Care*. 1992 Oct;15(10):1423–1432.

13. Orem DE. The utility of self-care theory as a theoretical basis for self-neglect. *J Adv Nurs*. 2001 May;34(4):545–551, 552–553.

14. Clark NM. Asthma self-management education. Research and implications for clinical practice. *Chest*. 1989 May;95(5):1110–1113.

15. Anderson RM. Patient empowerment and the traditional medical model. A case of irreconcilable differences? *Diabetes Care*. 1995 Mar;18(3):412–415.

16. VonKorff M, Gruman J, Schaefer J, Curry SJ, Wagner EH. Collaborative management of chronic illness. *Ann Inter Med*. 1997 Dec 15;127(12):1097–1102.

17. Heisler M, Smith DM, Hayward RA, Krein SL, Kerr EA. How well do patients' assessments of their diabetes self-management correlate with actual glycemic control and receipt of recommended diabetes services? *Diabetes Care*. 2003 Mar;26(3):738–743.

18. Funnell MM, Anderson RM. Patient empowerment: a look back, a look ahead. *Diabetes Educ*. 2003 May-Jun;29(3):454–458.

19. Bodenheimer T, Lorig K, Holman H, Grumback K. Patient self-management of chronic disease in primary care. *JAMA*. 2002 Nov 20;228(19):2469–2475.

20. MacVicar MG, Winningham ML, Nickel JL. Effects of aerobic interval training on cancer patients' functional capacity. *Nurs Res*. 1989;38:348–351.

21. Institute of Medicine (IOM). 2008. Cancer care for the whole patient: meeting psychosocial health needs: Adler NE, Page AE, (eds). Washington, DC: The National Academies Press.

22. Chodosh J, Morton SC, Mojica W, et al. Meta-analysis: chronic disease self-management programs for older adults. *Ann Intern Med*. 2005 Sep 20;143(6):427–438.

23. Given C, Given B, Rahbar M, Jeon S, et al. Effect of a cognitive behavioral intervention on reducing symptom severity during chemotherapy. *J Clin Oncol*. 2004 Feb 1;22(3):507–516.

24. Lev EL, Daley KM, Conner NE, Reith M, Fernandez C. An intervention to increase quality of life and self-care self-efficacy and decrease symptoms in breast cancer patients. *Sch Inq Nurs Pract*. 2001;15(3):277–294.

25. Newman S, Steed L, Mulligan K. Self-management interventions for chronic illness. *Lancet*. 2004 Oct 23–29;364(9444):1523–1537. Review.

26. Barlow J, Wright C, Sheasby J, Turner A, Hainsworth J. Self-management approaches for people with chronic conditions: a review. *Patient Educ Couns*. 2002 Oct-Nov;48(2):177–187.

27. Shojania KG, Ranji SR, McDonald KM, et al. Effects of quality improvement strategies for type 2 diabetes on glycemic control: a meta-regression analysis. *JAMA*. 2006 Jul 26;296(4):427–440.

28. Norris SL, Lau J, Smith SJ, Schmid CH, Engelgau MM. Self-management education for adults with type 2 diabetes: a meta-analysis of the effect on glycemic control. *Diabetes Care*. 2002 Jul;25(7):1159–1171.

29. Fleming B, Silver A, Ocepek-Welikson K, Keller D. The relationship between organizational systems and clinical quality in diabetes care. *Am J Manag Care*. 2004 Dec;10(12):934–944.

30. Nutting PA, Dickinson WP, Dickinson LM, et al. Use of chronic care model elements is associated with higher-quality care for diabetes. *Ann Fam Med*. 2007 Jan-Feb;5(1):14–20.

31. Piatt GA, Orchard TJ, Emerson S, et al. Translating the chronic care model into the community: results from a randomized controlled trial of a multifaceted diabetes care intervention. *Diabetes Care*. 2006 Apr;29(4):811–817.

32. McTavish FM, Gustafson DH, Owens BH, et al. CHESS: an interactive computer system for women with breast cancer piloted with an under-served population. *Proc Annu Symp Comput Appl Med Care*. 1994;599–603.

33. Campbell HS, Phaneuf MR, Deane K. Cancer peer support programs-do they work? *Patient Educ Couns*. 2004 Oct;55(1):3–15.

34. Meyer TJ, Mark MM. Effects of psychosocial interventions with adult cancer patients: a meta-analysis of randomized experiments. *Health Psychol*. 1995 Mar;14(2):101–108.

35. Devine EC, Westlake SK. The effects of psychoeducational care provided to adults with cancer: meta-analysis of 116 studies. *Oncol Nurs Forum*. 1995 Oct;22(9):1369–1381.

36. Sheard T, Maguire P. The effect of psychological interventions on anxiety and depression in cancer patients: results of two meta-analyses. *Br J Cancer*. 1999 Aug;80(11):1770–1780.

37. West CM, Dodd MJ, Paul SM, et al. The PRO-SELF(c): Pain Control Program—an effective approach for cancer pain management. *Oncol Nurs Forum*. 2003 Jan-Feb;30(1):65–73.

38. Kim JE, Dodd M, West C, et al. The PRO-SELF pain control program improves patients' knowledge of cancer pain management. *Oncol Nurs Forum*. 2004 Nov 16;31(6):1137–1143.

39. Dodd MJ, Miaskowski C. The PRO-SELF Program: a self-care intervention program for patients receiving cancer treatment. *Semin Oncol Nurs*. 2000 Nov;16(4):300–308. Discussion 308–316.

40. Larson PJ, Miaskowski C, MacPhail L, et al. The PRO-SELF Mouth Aware program: an effective approach for reducing chemotherapy-induced mucositis. *Cancer Nurs*. 1998 Aug;21(4):263–268.

41. Miaskowski C, Dodd M, West C, et al. Randomized clinical trial of the effectiveness of a self-care intervention to improve cancer pain management. *J Clin Oncol*. 2004 May 1;22(9):1713–1720.

42. McCorkle R, Benoliel JQ, Donaldson G, Georgiadou F, Moinpour C, Goodell B. A randomized clinical trial of home nursing care of lung cancer patients. *Cancer*. 1989;4:199–206.

43. McCorkle R, Jepson C, Yost L, et al. The impact of post-hospital home care on patients with cancer. *Res Nurs Health*. 1994;17:243–251.

44. McCorkle R, Robinson L, Nuamah I, Lev E, Benoliel J. The effects of home nursing care for patients during terminal illness on the bereaved's psychological distress. *Nursing Research*. 1998;47(1):2–10.

45. McCorkle R, Strumpf N, Nuamah I, et al. A randomized clinical trial of a specialized home care intervention on survival among elderly post-surgical cancer patients. *J Am Geriatr Soc*. 2000;48:1707–1713.

46. Doorenbos A, Given B, Given C, Verbitsky N, Cimprich B, McCorkle R. Reducing symptom limitations: a cognitive behavioral intervention randomized trial. *Psychooncology*. 2005 Jul;14(7):574–584.

47. Sherwood P, Given BA, Given CW, et al. A cognitive behavioral intervention for symptom management in patients with advanced cancer. *Oncol Nurs Forum*. 2005 Nov;32(6):1190–1198.

48. Boesen EH, Ross L, Frederiksen K, et al. Psychoeducational intervention for patients with cutaneous malignant melanoma: a replication study. *J Clin Oncol*. 2005 Feb;23(6):1270–1277.

49. Stiegelis HE, Hagedoorn M, Sanderman R, et al. The impact of an informational self-management intervention on the association between control and illness uncertainty before and psychological distress after radiotherapy. *Psychooncology*. 2004 Apr;13(4):248–259.

50. Gielissen MF, Verhagen S, Witjes F, Bleijenberg G. Effects of cognitive behavior therapy in severely fatigued disease-free cancer patients compared with patients waiting for cognitive behavior therapy: a randomized controlled trial. *J Clin Oncol*. 2006 Oct 20;24(30):4882–4887.

51. Giesler RB, Given B, Given CW, et al. Improving the quality of life of patients with prostate carcinoma: a randomized trial testing the efficacy of a nurse-driven intervention. *Cancer*. 2005 Aug 15;104(4):752–762.

52. Glasgow RE, Emont S, Miller DC. Assessing delivery of the five 'As' for patient-centered counseling. *Health Promot Int*. 2006 Sep;21(3):245–255. Epub 2006 Jun 2.

CHAPTER 64

Building Problem-Solving Skills through COPE Education of Family Caregivers

Julia A. Bucher and James R. Zabora

Coping with cancer remains a daunting challenge that families are not thoroughly equipped to tackle. For several decades, clinicians and researchers have described stress, demands, burdens, needs, and reactions among people with cancer and their caregivers. However, less is known about the effect of interventions focused on giving families information and support that moderates their distress and least is known about the effect or likelihood of improving family caregiver skills through the cancer experience. This chapter will summarize the conceptual framework for problem solving education (PSE), describe COPE skill building education for people with cancer and their families, and describe the effects on problem-solving skills among family caregivers when COPE education is modified.

CONCEPTUAL FRAMEWORK FOR PSE

Problem solving education for family caregivers is based on problem solving therapy (PST), which is well known to be effective for people with anxiety-related disorders, suicidal ideation, substance abuse, mental retardation, and schizophrenia.[1] In addition, many research reports suggest a strong positive treatment effect of PST on depression among adults,[2] among people with cancer (Nezu, Nezu, Freidman, Faddis, Houts, 1999),[3] and among distressed adults with cancer and their family caregivers reported in Project Genesis (Nezu, Nezu, Felgoise, McClure, Houts, 1993).[4]

In an informative meta-analysis by Cuijpers, van Straten, and Warmerdam (2007)[5] conclude that "Although there is no doubt that PST can be an effective treatment for depression, more research is needed to ascertain the conditions and subjects in which these positive effects are realized."

Although quite flexible in implementation, PST usually is offered in 10 therapy sessions or less, wherein the therapist teaches basic steps in planning and evaluating approaches to specific problems. Five key concepts undergird PST: orientation, problem definition, generating alternatives, decision making, and implementation (see Table 64–1). The first, *orientation*, refers to one's understanding of and reactions to problems encountered with living in general. Education about orientation provides people with a rational, constructive, and positive outlook about most problems and emphasizes a step-by-step problem-solving process as an effective means of approaching and coping with problems as challenges. Activities that help people adopt a positive outlook or orientation overlap with many cognitive therapy techniques used for depression including stopping negative thoughts, role playing, and challenging distorted thinking.

The *problem definition* concept helps people learn ways to view their problems objectively by differentiating objective facts from their own inferences, assumptions, and problem interpretations. It also encourages people to collect facts about the problem such as how often does it happen, how common is it, and how long might it take to solve. By defining a problem more specifically, people learn to set realistic problem-solving goals.

In *generating alternatives*, people learn to break out of their restricted views of their problems by using brainstorming. Brainstorming involves freeing the imagination and thinking of new ideas without criticism. Brainstorming also allows others to get involved and create a list of possible solutions. This also allows for the possibility of combining ideas to create solutions previously unknown. This activity expands people's views of what is possible and can almost be a fun activity.

Decision making refers to selecting those brainstormed ideas that are feasible and also likely to be helpful. People learn to do a "cost benefit" analysis of their options and decide which strategies they want to try. The problem plan is fashioned around these specific ideas.

Implementation includes carrying out the problem plan, monitoring progress with implementation steps as well as outcomes, reinforcing steps that lead to solutions, and troubleshooting steps that do not lead t solutions and thus lead to the development of a new plan.

A form of brief therapy, the five concepts behind PST are explored in far more detail in the book by Nezu, Nezu, and Perri[2] in relation to the role of the counselor. The conceptual framework that supports their effectiveness is described next.

Problem solving therapy and PSE are undergirded by stress model theory (SMT), which suggests that any individual must experience a series of cognitive appraisals related to a crisis event or level of distress in their lives (Lazarus and Folkman, 1984).[6] In other words, before one can act and respond to a crisis, to reduce the distress associated with it, the person must develop a personal meaning of the specific crisis or event. Primary appraisal describes this process as defining what the crisis event means to people at this point in their lives. To define the crisis event, people use all of their available resources.

The SMT postulates that people possess a number of internal and external resources. Examples of internal resources include some specifically focused upon by PST counselors, such as *level of optimism* and the *ability to solve problems*. The level of distress can serve as an "appropriate marker" to identify high-risk patients and families and, if they lack internal resources such as these, then the delivery of PST would be a priority intervention to strengthen problem-solving skills and reduce distress levels.

Table 64–1. PST concepts and examples of skills focused upon in therapy

PST concepts	Examples of problem-solving skills
1. Orientation	Identifying attitude toward action
2. Problem definition	Defining a clear problem that can be influenced or changed in some way
	Parsing a problem situation into smaller problems
	Understanding when the problem happens
	Identifying underlying issues
3. Generating alternatives	Brainstorming options
	Listing strategies
	Weighing pros and cons of strategies
4. Decision making	Selecting actions
	Enlisting help with actions if needed
	Designing a plan with a timeline
5. Implementation	Carrying out a plan of action
	Monitoring progress
	Reinforcing actions that work
	Troubleshooting obstacles
	Evaluating what worked and to what degree
	Adjusting the plan of action

Table 64–2. Comparison of PST concepts and COPE adaptation of problem solving education (PSE) with example skills taught in COPE education

Problem-solving therapy concepts	PSE components	PSE skills taught with COPE model
1. Orientation 2. Problem Definition	1. Optimism	Making the conscious decision to try to actively solve problems to the best of one's ability Trying on a "can do" attitude Seeing problems as a normal part of life Setting reasonable goals that can be achieved with reasonable effort
3. Generating alternatives	2. Creativity	Freeing oneself from the constraints of stressful thinking Committing to learning how to think differently Brainstorming options with others while withholding any judgments Combining options and strategies generated by brainstorming Listing all potential actions
4. Decision making	3. Planning	Deciding on actions from the brainstorming list Committing to a reasonable goal
5. Implementation		Taking action Reflecting on results of actions Revising actions based on experience
	4. Expert Information Understand the problem Know when to get professional help, what information to present, and what questions to ask Deal with or prevent the problem Confront obstacles to carrying out the problem plan Carry out and adjust your plan	Using accurate expert information Being open to being honest about different perspectives Learning about the context of the problem from different perspectives Encouraging inquisitiveness by oneself and others Listing questions Pursuing answers Enlisting help from professionals such as oncology nurses, cancer information hotlines, or community agencies

Stress model theory also identifies external resources, such as social supports and the "family." If social supports are adequate and available then individuals possess a greater likelihood to define a crisis event in a positive or "can-do" manner rather than a negative manner. PST can zero in on and guide people to try to strengthen social support resources.

The presence or absence of internal and external resources not only facilitates people's definition of crisis but also promotes the development of a secondary appraisal, which is related directly to initiating effective strategies or actions to respond to crisis events (Lazarus, 1991).[7] Failure to respond to the demands of a crisis event and to solve the related and complex problems that follow may result in significant levels of emotional distress that can cause disruptions in daily functioning.

Extending the benefits of PST to PSE capitalizes on promoting specific problem-solving skills, helping families plan and use expert information, and strengthen internal resources through the cancer crisis. In addition, the COPE educational intervention in particular seeks to create a more effective "problem-solving team" by integrating family caregivers into skill development and action planning and thus improve the strength of external resources for people with cancer.

In essence, the relevance of boosting problem-solving skills for people with cancer and family caregivers lies in the moderating role that problem-solving skills serve to enhance coping in the general stress-distress relationship (Houts, Nezu, Nezu, Bucher, 1999).[8] The more effectively that people resolve or cope with stressful problems, the more probable it is that they will experience a higher level of QOL and less distress as compared with those people facing similar problems who have difficulty in coping. Families naturally require guidance and support to manage the multiple problems associated with cancer, its related treatments, their adverse reactions, the uncertain prognosis, rehabilitation issue, distressing symptoms, or even decline and death. Teaching and reinforcing problem-solving skills has become an accepted intervention for families with cancer as listed in the recent report of the Institute of Medicine (Adler and Page, 2007).[9] Although counseling therapy sessions permit

education, the challenge is to move what is taught within PST to the purely educational session or opportunity.

ADAPTATION OF PSE FROM PST

COPE as an educational model. Ten years ago, the skills education and development used in PST were translated into an education model that could be offered easily to family caregivers of people with cancer to improve problem-solving skills (Houts, Nezu, Nezu, Bucher, 1999).[8] PST as an intervention serves families well but may not be as widely available as PSE because of the cost and stigma of therapy as opposed to less expensive and possibly more acceptable and accessible community education sessions.

The educational adaptation of PST for family members of people with cancer is labeled "COPE" to stand for four components that summarize PST skills in lay language for teaching purposes: Creativity, Optimism, Planning, and Expert Information. Table 64–2 illustrates the fit of the four PSE components with the five PST concepts and also lists example exercises that participants are reminded of and practice within COPE education. These exercises demand cognitive, attitudinal, and behavioral skills that are familiar to many adults in day-to-day life; however, the skills are not automatically resurrected or deliberately practiced in the face of unfamiliar events and stressors such as the cancer experience.

The component of Expert Information ("E") was added to components of PST because people with cancer and family caregivers uniformly report information and understanding information as their number one need across the different stages of the disease and its effects. Coping with physical illness requires accurate information not just about the disease as a biological phenomenon but also about management of the illness itself, such as how to get information from medical staff, learn about community resources, manage symptoms, prevent depression, or coordinate care across settings (also called transition care). Literature for family caregivers had not been organized before to coach specific problem-solving skills or list clearly stated actions to take with the reasons to take the actions. Therefore, to round off the education model adapted from PST, the developers created a collection of information, first known as the "Cancer Home Care Plan" (Houts, Nezu, Nezu, Bucher, 1993)[10] and eventually the *Homecare guide for cancer* (Houts, Nezu, Nezu, Bucher, Lipton, 1994; Houts, Nezu, Nezu, Bucher, Lipton, 1995).[11,12]

The collection of Expert ("E") Information about common problems experienced by people with cancer—and helpful actions to cope with or prevent these problems—was well known to experienced oncology professionals about cancer home care—and cancer care in general—but not well known to people with cancer or their family caregivers. The information was presented per specific problem, such as nausea or finding help, chapter by chapter, to support problem-solving behavior according to a step-by-step action plan similar to the planning part of PST and similar to how healthcare professionals approach clinical care with Expert Information:

Understand the problem. Know when to get professional help, what information to present, and what questions to ask to get help and answers

Deal with or prevent the problem
Confront obstacles to carrying out the problem plan
Carry out and adjust your plan

The guides were written for caregivers of people under cancer treatment (Houts, Nezu, Nezu, Bucher, Lipton, 1994; Houts, Nezu, Nezu, Bucher, 1999),[11–13] for children (Houts, Neeley, Kandsberger, Bucher, Nezu, Nezu, 1998),[14] for people with HIV/AIDS (Houts, Bucher, Damianos, Ehmann, Jacik, Johnston, Kreher, Nezu, Nezu, Zulo,1997),[15] and for caregivers of people with late stage cancer (Houts, Bucher, Mount, Britton, Nezu, Nezu, Harvey, 1997).[16] The versions for families of people under treatment were translated into Spanish,[17] Italian,[18] (Pannuti, Tannenberger, Houts, Bucher, 1995), and German[19] (Tannenberger, Pannuti, Houts, Bucher, 1995).

A great deal of clinical field testing further refined the guides and their format. The current comprehensive written reference designed to support COPE is titled: *The American Cancer Society complete guide to family caregiving* (Bucher and Houts, In print).[19] The manual instructs readers on how to manage a variety of problems and each chapter follows the above action-oriented subheadings.

The other components of COPE are directly adapted from PST and renamed for the public. See Table 64–1.

1. *Creativity* helps participants select types of people to brainstorm with, practice brainstorming solutions to a problem, and combine ideas to create new ideas.
2. Participants practice *Optimism* and parse a problem into its smaller parts, select a part amenable to alteration, and improve one's attitude that, indeed, something can be done about a part of a problem through actions that will have a positive effect.
3. Participants learn and practice *Planning* just as it is taught to and used by nurses, social workers, physicians, and other professionals and they learn how to evaluate the outcomes of implementing the plans. If the plan did not work, they are encouraged to try something again that worked a little, think about what made that action work, strengthen that part of the plan, and perhaps set smaller goals.
4. Finally, caregivers are oriented to key sources of *Expert Information* explained earlier. Examples are *The American Cancer Society complete guide to family caregiving* (In print),[19] other written sources; internet sources for caregivers and people with cancer; and of course other people such as peers in cancer support groups, oncology nurses, and social workers.

The structure, scenario scripts, flip chart material, and facilitators of the COPE Education Program teach people to use basic skills with short explanations, discussion, and application to family caregiver scenarios. The program can be held in three 2-hour educational sessions or within one-on-one sessions of varying lengths with a COPE coach. Participants are encouraged to get as much Expert Information as possible that is focused on the specific problems that they are attacking and use the skills that they practiced. Column 3 in Table 64–2 lists example exercises practiced in COPE sessions.

APPLIED RESEARCH THAT SUPPORTS COPE PSE

Tests of the COPE education model initially used process measures and later added outcome measures as test designs steady progressed from descriptive to comparative designs.

Development and initial field testing. The COPE education model was offered first as community education for cancer family caregivers. Over 3000 caregivers attended three in-person small group sessions to build skills in structured problem solving. Sessions were 2 hours in length with a break. The course was offered by nurses and social workers at medical clinics, senior centers, churches, and home healthcare agencies under the cosponsorship of community organizations and funded by the PA Department of Health for 5 years. Descriptive outcomes revealed that a majority of attendees felt more confident with their problem-solving skills and would recommend the course to others (Bucher and Houts, 1999).[20] In addition, they agreed that using the *Home care guide* to help solve problems was very helpful.

Modifications COPE education for varied groups. In the next attempt to explore the effectiveness of PSE among diverse cancer populations, a series of pilot studies were designed to test the efficacy of PSE under specific conditions. In the first initiative, COPE education was beneficial when delivered to people with cancer and their families in a busy oncology clinic (Bucher, Loscalzo, Zabora, Houts, and BrintzenhofeSzoc, 2001).[21,22] Sixty people with cancer with advanced disease along with a family caregiver participated in one 90-minute educational session. After the session, 83% of caregivers stated that having and using the *Home care guide* made a great deal of difference to them and 65% reported improved problem-solving skills. Most importantly, problem-solving scores were significantly higher at posteducation evaluation. Only 6% of caregivers did not feel confident to provide care. However, 30% of patients and caregivers did not derive any benefit from the education and further subanalyses revealed that these families tended to be more "extreme" in their level of family functioning, such as highly enmeshed or highly disconnected. Consequently, one 90-minute session simply was insufficient to improve the response of these families to the stresses coping with a cancer diagnosis, related treatments, and uncertain future.

For these investigators, the next logical step was to increase the "dose of the intervention" for extreme families from one to three PSE sessions in comparison to what was delivered to "balanced families with higher levels of family functioning" who would receive only one longer educational session. Results from this pilot dosing study (n = 30) indicated that "extreme families" experienced an increase in problem-solving skills and a modest decrease in distress after 3 sessions; however, the decrease in distress was not sustained at 6 months. Consideration has been given to designing a larger dose-escalation study to attempt to identify the number of sessions of PSE that are necessary to benefit highly problematic families especially with advanced cancer (Zabora, 2008).

In a third pilot study, these same investigators explored the effectiveness of PSE in relation to a specific problem, that is, depression among African-American cancer survivors. In this study, eligibility was based on a minimum score of 16 on the CES-D8 and the intervention consisted of four sessions that were targeted for the problem of depression. The cancer survivors' (n = 12) depression scores decreased by 2.5 points on the Brief Symptom Inventory (BSI)-18 while QOL scores increased by nearly 6 points at 30 days after intervention. Unfortunately, the small sample size did not allow for significance according to Dr. Zabora who communicated this from Johns Hopkins University at the time. In the qualitative comments, these African-American cancer survivors indicated a lower level of stigma associated with the intervention, a positive response to the educational format, and greater confidence to manage problems associated with their illness.

The results from these three pilot studies led to the development of two larger funded research projects. In the first, a collaborative cross-national research team conducted a randomized clinical trial entitled "Simultaneous Care: Linking Palliation to Phase I and II Clinical Trials." PSE offered a theoretically-driven, well-defined, and systematic intervention for use in palliative care. More than 500 patients enrolled in this study that now has concluded with final data analyses are underway according to Dr. Zabora at the time of this writing.

In the second research project, funded by the Centers for Disease Control, Men Against Breast Cancer (MABC) investigators partnered with leading survivorship experts to develop a psychoeducational program for men entitled *Partners in Survival*. Its intent is to bring critical problem-solving skills to spouses or partners of medically underserved groups of women with breast cancer who frequently report a perceived lack of support from a gamut of external resources: the healthcare team, spouses, family, and friends. *Partners in Survival* seeks to shore up skills and support for these women through all the stages of illness by strengthening the skills of a key external resource: the men in their lives. To date, over 200 spouses and partners have enrolled in this intervention that provides PSE in varying formats including 3-hour workshops as well as a 2 day male caregiver conference for men helping women. In essence, improved "problem-solving skills" for men, such as developing plans for certain challenges such as relationship strains, may enable families to effectively resolve some of the many difficulties associated with treatment and recovery (Loscalzo, 2008).[23]

Comparison group research design. Finally, McMillan and colleagues (2006)[24] conducted a randomized clinical trial to test the effects of COPE education. They divided 354 family caregivers of community dwelling hospice patients with advanced cancer into three groups. One group received standard hospice care. The second group received standard care and three supportive visits, and the third group received standard care plus three visits to learn COPE problem-solving coping skills. These home visits were at least an hour in length with education, practice exercises, and discussion led in a standardized format.

The COPE group showed significantly greater improvement in three key variables: caregiver quality of life (QOL), caregiver burden from patient symptoms, and caregiver task burden. Clearly, guided PSE and reinforcement of the use of these skills assisted these families to cope with the multiple and complex challenges that may not be addressed by healthcare or even hospice teams who (1) are not on site 24 hours/day and (2) do not delve into all levels of family challenges or distress. The problem-solving skills guided families to create plans of action and follow these plans, an intervention itself known to reduce anxiety about problems and concerns.

To boost the likelihood of translating these findings into practice, this research team has made a How To manual available at http://health.usf.edu/nocms/nursing/CaregiverInterventionManualB.pdf. Their results not only underscore the flexibility of the intervention but also suggest that this type of skill development could be incorporated into clinical practice.

SUMMARY

Certainly nurses, social workers, physicians, counselors, ministers, other support staff, and volunteers support problem solving by providing information and support. However, their interactions and interventions typically, and appropriately, are focused on providing expert advice and giving answers rather than on stepping back and taking steps to coach and improve problem-solving skills. Families can be helped in the long run by learning and using basic step-by-step approaches, developing plans, and evaluating the results of carrying out these plans no matter what challenge they confront.[25,26] In the face of cancer, such skills even may reduce distress and boost an invaluable sense of being able to cope.

ACKNOWLEDGEMENT

Peter S. Houts PhD, Professor Emeritus, Penn State University

REFERENCES

1. Chang EC, D'Zurilla EJ, Sanna LJ (eds). *Social problem solving: Theory, research, and training.* New York: Oxford University Press; 2004.

2. Nezu AM, Nezu CM, Perri MG. *Problem-solving therapy for depression: Theory, research, and clinical and guidelines.* New York, NY: John Wiley and Sons; 1989.

3. Nezu AM, Nezu AM, Freidman SH, Faddis S, Houts PS. *Helping cancer patients cope: A problem-solving approach.* Washington DC: American Psychological Association; 1999.

4. Nezu AM, Nezu CM, Felgoise SH, McClure HS, Houts PS. Project Genesis: assessing the efficacy of problem solving therapy for distressed adult cancer patients. *J Consult Clin Psychol.* 1993;71(6):1036–1048.

5. Cuijpers P, van Straten A, Warmerdam L. Problem solving therapies for depression: a meta-analysis. *Euro Psychiatry.* 2007;22(1):9–15.

6. Lazarus RS, Folkman S. *Stress, appraisal, and coping.* New York: Springer Publishing Co.; 1984.

7. Lazarus RS. *Emotion and adaptation.* New York: Oxford University Press; 1991.

8. Houts PS, Nezu AM, Nezu CM, Bucher JA. The prepared family caregiver: a problem-solving approach to family caregiver education. *Patient Educ Couns.* 1999;27:63–73.

9. Adler NE, Page EK, eds. *Cancer care for the whole patient: Meeting psychosocial health needs.* Bethesda, MD: Institute of Medicine; 2007.

10. Houts PS, Nezu AM, Nezu CM, Bucher JA (eds). *Cancer home care plan.* Hershey, PA: Pennsylvania State University College of Medicine; 1993.

11. Houts PS, Nezu AM, Nezu CM, Bucher J, et al. (eds). *Homecare guide for cancer.* Philadelphia, PA: American College of Physicians; 1994.

12. Houts PS, Nezu AM, Nezu CM, Bucher J (eds). *Caregiving: A step by step resource for families of persons with cancer.* Atlanta, GA: American Cancer Society; 1999.

13. Houts PS, Neeley JA, Kandsberger D, et al. (eds). *Homecare guide for younger persons with cancer.* Hershey, PA: Penn State College of Medicine; 1998.

14. Houts PS, Bucher JA, Damianos FP, et al. (eds). *Homecare guide for HIV/AIDS.* Philadelphia, PA: American College of Physicians; 1997.

15. Houts PS, Bucher JA, Mount B, et al. (eds). *Homecare guide for advanced cancer.* Philadelphia, PA: American College of Physicians; 1997. www.acponline.org. Accessed August 13, 2009.

16. Houts PS, Nezu AM, Nezu CM, Bucher JA, et al. (eds). *Guia para el cuidado del paciente con cancer en al hogar.* Philadelphia, PA: American College of Physicians; 1994.

17. Pannuti F, Tannenberger S, Houts PS, Bucher JA. *Consigli alla famiglia per la migliore assistenza ai sofferenti presso il loro domicilio.* Bologna, Italy: ANT; 1995.

18. Tannenberger S, Pannuti F, Houts PS, Bucher JA. *Jeman in meiner familie hat krebs - Was kann ich tun?* Bern, Germany: W. Zuckschwerdt Verlag; 1995.

19. Bucher J, Houts PS, eds. *The American Cancer Society complete guide to family caregiving.* Atlanta, GA: American Cancer Society; In print.

20. Bucher JA, Houts PS, Nezu AM, Nezu CM. Improving problem-solving skills of family caregivers through group education. *J Psychosoc Oncol.* 1999;16(3/4):73–84.

21. Bucher JA, Loscalzo M, Zabora J, Houts PS, Hooker C, BrintzenhofeSzoc K. Problem-solving cancer care education for patients and caregivers. *Cancer Pract.* 2001;9(2):66–70.

22. Loscalzo MJ, Bucher J. Teaching patients with cancer and their families to solve problems: the COPE model. *J Psychosoc Oncol.* 1999;16(3/4):93–117.

23. Loscalzo MJ, Hayison M. *We love: A breast cancer action plan and caregivers guide for men.* Savage MD: Bartleby Press; 2007.

24. McMillan SC, Small BJ, Weitzner M, Schonwetter R, Moody L, Haley WE. Impact of coping skills intervention with family caregivers of hospice patients with cancer a randomized clinical trial. *Cancer.* 2006.106:214–222.

25. Sorensen S, Pinquart M, Duberstein P. How effective are interventions with caregivers? An updated meta-analysis. *Gerontologist.* 2002;42:356–372.

26. Bucher J, ed. The Application of problem-solving therapy to psychosocial oncology care. *J Psychosoc Oncol.* 1999;16(3/4):27–40, 73–84.

CHAPTER 65

The Wellness Community's Integrative Model of Evidence-Based Psychosocial Programs, Services, and Interventions

Mitch Golant and Kim Thiboldeaux

Globally, more than 11 million people are diagnosed with cancer annually, and it is estimated that 16 million new cases will be diagnosed each year by 2020. Cancer causes 7 million deaths annually—or 12.5% of deaths worldwide. However, over the last twenty years, cancer is no longer viewed as a death sentence. Of course, people are still dying of cancer, but increasingly it is being treated as a chronic illness. Consider this hopeful statistic: there are more than 12 million cancer survivors in the United States compared to 5.8 million in 1982.[1] Encouraged by earlier detection and better treatments, many people live with this disease for years. Patients may go through treatment, some may experience recurrence, and others may undergo a second course of treatment or even a third. According to the National Coalition for Cancer Survivorship, a cancer survivor is *a person living with, through, and beyond cancer*.

Through this lengthy and ever-extending pattern of diagnosis, recurrence, and treatment, it is evident that survivorship is an integral part of cancer care. As The Wellness Community (TWC) faces the reality of longer survival periods and increased numbers of cancer survivors, it is imperative to recognize that the needs of cancer survivors are evolving. TWC's very notion of cancer survivorship is changing as well. Therefore, a comprehensive model of care needs to be adopted which casts a net across time that is wide enough to capture the broad spectrum of needs cancer survivors and caregivers will encounter during the cancer continuum. These are not only medical and treatment needs but also psychological and emotional supportive care needs. The November 2007 Institute of Medicine report entitled *Cancer care for the whole patient*[2] says it best:

- "Health is determined not just by biological processes but by people's emotions, behaviors, and social relationships."
- "Good quality health care must attend to patients' psychosocial problems and provide services to enable them to better manage their illnesses and underlying health."

A fundamental shift in patient care and survivorship is emerging linked to the fact that people will live longer and have multiple cancers or other co-morbidities that may directly or indirectly impact treatment and recovery. Treatments for cancer have become increasingly complex and multimodal. Cancer is a disease that affects the entire family and often a community. The needs of families will only grow. The National Cancer Institute (NCI) estimates the number of Americans diagnosed annually will double in the next 50 years—from 1.3 to 2.6 million. Yet, according to the International Union against Cancer (UICC), 5-year survival rates are increasing. In fact, the majority of those diagnosed (approaching 70%) can expect to be alive in 5 years.

All of these factors taken together underscore that the role of community-based support services and interventions has become critically important in total cancer patient care. Again, the 2007 IOM report, seizing this key idea outlines the essential role that community-based organizations play in cancer care and survivorship. As the report confirms, nearly 85% of patients are being treated in community cancer centers, hospitals, and practices rather than in large comprehensive cancer centers. Community-based services provide the psychosocial support essential to a survivor's well-being. In fact, since joining forces with Gilda's Club in July 2009, TWC is the largest provider of cancer support worldwide. In the United States, the combined organization is now comprised of nearly 50 affiliates, 12 affiliates in development, and over 100 satellite locations. The Wellness Community/Gilda's Club has several international facilities and affiliates as well as a Web presence through TWC Online. Taken together all of these facilities reach over 300,000 people with cancer each year. In this context, the community is one key to the cancer patient's long-term survival. Creating a seamless delivery system of care for all patients is essential to improving quality care and survivorship (see Fig. 65–1).

This chapter provides background about TWC programs, philosophy and services, and its Community-Initiated Research Collaboration (CIRC) model of evidence-based research in partnership with academic and scientific partners.

TWC VISION

The Wellness Community is an international nonprofit organization dedicated to providing support, education and hope for people with cancer and their loved ones. TWC's Vision is to be the Gold Standard in community-based support for all people affected by cancer.

Not only are all of its program's services provided without charge to patients and families, but also are led by licensed healthcare professionals—psychologists, social workers, and marriage and family therapists. Most importantly, professionals are trained to deliver these programs in a similar manner across the United States, so that they are uniform throughout multiple sites.

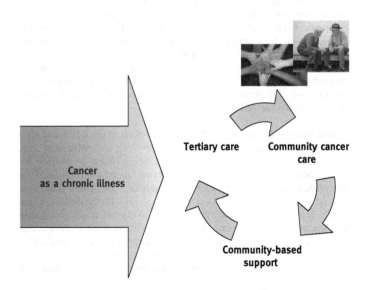

Fig. 65–1. An integrative model of care.
SOURCE: Reprinted with permission from the Wellness Community.

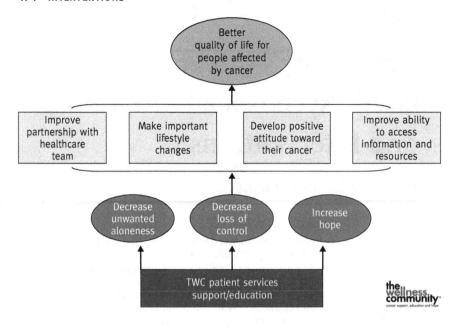

Fig. 65–2. Patient active concept.

THE PATIENT ACTIVE CONCEPT

The three most significant psychosocial stressors for people with cancer are: unwanted aloneness, loss of control, and loss of hope.[3-5] The central organizing principal of TWC's program is the patient active concept (see Fig. 65–2), which seeks to alleviate these stressors. The concept states that *People with cancer who participate in their fight for recovery, along with their healthcare team, rather than acting as helpless and hopeless passive victims of the illness, will improve their quality of life and may enhance the possibility of their recovery.* This concept combines the will of the patient with the skill of the physician, and it has a particularly positive effect on outcomes.[6,7] TWC's programs provide a range of activities aimed at improving one's ability to become Patient Active.

PATIENT ACTIVE SUPPORT GROUPS

At TWC, ongoing, weekly cancer support groups are provided for men and women with mixed diagnoses. Typically, participants stay in these groups between 12 and 18 months. TWC also offers diagnosis-specific support groups for people with brain tumors, breast cancer, prostate cancer, lung cancer, and some other cancers. TWC includes the entire family, not just the patient, so weekly 2-hour family/caregiver and bereavement support groups provide support to these populations. In addition, there are many similar support groups at The Wellness Community Online (TWCO) (www.thewellnesscommunity.org).[8]

The importance of support groups. Professionally facilitated support groups can play a crucial role in augmenting and enhancing care. This is especially true if families and friends are unable to provide the much-needed emotional support for the cancer patient or if the family is providing support but the patient needs more or if the patient is satisfied with family support but still wants to meet others with the disease. These groups provide patients a safe environment to express emotions because they are with those who can identify with what they are experiencing. Support groups encourage confronting, contemplating, and reevaluating traumatic events and may counter the social constraints that can exist in other relationships, thereby facilitating emotional assimilation and accommodation.

One can broaden these safe environments for emotional expression to many different situations including individual therapy, psychoeducational programs, online support groups, and face-to-face support

groups. Community-based support programs like those at TWC offer survivors a place where they can join together with other survivors to reduce the distress associated with the disease.

Why we facilitate groups at TWC. TWC offers many support groups because research consistently shows that they help to decrease distress, depression, anxiety, and pain. Indeed, research makes it clear that professionally facilitated support groups improve quality of life, positively impact treatment adherence, and diminish distress, depression, and anxiety.[3,9–16]

Why support groups? In particular, professionally-led support groups help patients to order their experience or trauma. They also detoxify the traumatic experience and replace it with more hopeful words, thoughts or images. The patient becomes accustomed to talking about cancer and witnesses others who are going on with their lives. The combination of cognitive completion and detoxification provides the framework upon which the support groups actually help. In a cross-sectional study of 289 participants in TWC's support groups, we looked at whether length of time in these support groups was linked to improved quality of life (FACT–G) and decreases in depression (CES–D). We found that patients who had spent more time in the TWC groups (over 6 months) had lower scores on the CES–D, $F(1, 286) = 4.06$, $p = 0.05$, and reported less severe physical symptoms, $F(1, 286) = 14.99$, $p = 0.00$; a better relationship with their doctor, $F(1, 286) = 6.02$, $p = 0.02$; higher well-being, $F(1, 286) = 2.91$, $p = 0.09$; and better functional performance, $F(1, 286) = 6.64$, $p = 0.01$. Interestingly, there was no difference in the quality of social relationships.[17]

Support groups offer nonjudgmental support for patients who may not receive it from family and friends. Confronting, contemplating, and reevaluating the experience of the diagnosis and treatment helps manage and facilitate the emotional adaptation to cancer. In a randomized clinical trial comparing TWC's Patient Active Support Group with Stanford University's Supportive-Expressive Therapy, TWC's participants reported significant improvements in developing a new attitude toward the illness ($t(40) =1.72$, $p = 0.05$), making changes in their lives that they thought were important ($t(40) =1.72$, $p = 0.05$), better communicating with their physician ($t(40) =1.72$, $p = 0.05$), and better accessing cancer-related information and resources ($t(40) =2.84$, $p = 0.01$).[9]

Two other models and methodologies have proven quite useful in helping cancer patients enrolled in support groups at TWC: Psychoeducational programs that combine emotional support with information on coping with the illness, and techniques to create a synergetic environment for reducing distress, improving quality of life, and enhancing the possibility of recovery. They are described below.

PSYCHO-EDUCATIONAL PROGRAMS

TWC's psycho-educational programs are comprised of state-of-the-science information about managing cancer and its treatment coupled with interventions that improve quality of life and enhance learning. TWC National Patient Educational Programs are delivered across the United States and around the world. Topics include treatment options, side-effect management, proper nutrition during and after treatment, stress-reduction exercises and problem-solving exercises in several formats:

- *Ask The Doctor/Professional.* Discussion group where patients and caregivers can interact directly with healthcare professional on cancer-specific topics or better managing treatment.
- *Frankly Speaking Series.* These workshops include interactive lectures, stress-reduction exercises, and a take-home patient workbook on topics such as side effect management, new discoveries in treatment and disease-specific information (e.g., lung cancer, lymphoma, and colorectal cancer). For a list of downloadable *Frankly speaking* booklets go to: www.thewellnesscommunity.org/education
- *Patient Active Guides.* This series of disease-specific handbooks incorporates the latest medical information, Patient Active strategies to better cope with the illness, and tips to communicate with professionals in making treatment decisions (e.g., *Patient Active Guide to Living with Ovarian Cancer* and the *Patient Active Guide to Living with Advanced Breast Cancer*). These programs are downloadable at www.thewellnesscommunity.org/education

The rationale behind psycho-educational programs at TWC. Although managing emotions and distress is a *process* that takes time and varies depending on the course of treatment and the disease itself, the literature shows that psycho-educational programs provide a safe haven for cancer patients to express emotions and learn more adaptive ways of coping, all of which decrease the emotional burden of cancer.[10,18-20]

How patients think about their distress can worsen it. Often we hear the comment: "I know my doctor is giving up on me. He didn't tell me how I was doing, and I know that means things are bad." When a patient is distressed, it is challenging for him or her to consider that doctors are seeing patients every 5–10 minutes, and without a scheduled consultation meeting, the physician may have no time to accurately convey what is happening with the disease. Psycho-educational programs provide a roadmap for patients on how to better communicate with their healthcare team.[8]

Similarly, validation and empathy are key factors that enable patients to absorb new information. Psycho-educational programs provide a safe place to learn new information in an environment where others are asking the same questions and expressing the same concerns. This give-and-take—information and support—helps normalize the cancer experience and bolsters the patient through the many unknowns of treatment and recovery, providing direction in face of cancer's ambiguity. Participating in psycho-educational programs also gives patients an opportunity to model positive interactions with their medical team.

The Wellness Community elicits input and feedback on these programs from medical professionals, patients, and caregivers. In addition, the materials are updated regularly and are available in hard copy and on the Web. Many of the materials are also available in Spanish.

MIND/BODY AND STRESS-REDUCTION PROGRAMS

Stress-reduction exercises (including strength training, tai chi, or yoga) and mind-body programs like meditation, relaxation, and visualization are offered at local Wellness Communities and are incorporated in to many of the Frankly Speaking programs. Similar stress-reduction programs have been shown to reduce anxiety, and diminish pain and fatigue.[21-24] They are downloadable at http://www.thewellnesscommunity.org/mm/Learn-About/Additional-Resource

ONLINE SUPPORT GROUPS

The Wellness Community Online is a web site that mirrors the programs provided in a brick-and-mortar center. The site focuses on three elements: education, support, and hope. It includes downloadable educational programs, a nutrition guide, relaxation and visualization exercises, moderated public discussion boards, and professionally facilitated support groups. TWCO is based on research in partnership with Stanford University and the University of California in San Francisco. Findings from the research showed that women with breast cancer in professionally led online support groups experienced significant reductions in depression and in negative reaction to pain. They also experienced significant increases in life fulfillment, finding new possibilities or meaning after cancer, as well as deepened spirituality.[25]

PROGRAM REACH

In 2007, TWC held more than 13,486 support group sessions. Nearly 9000 of those support groups were for patients, and more than 4400 were for caregivers. In addition, more than 2300 educational workshops and nearly 6400 stress-reduction programs were offered in the same timeframe.

The Wellness Community Online was officially launched in February, 2002, on Good Morning America. By 2008, it offered 14 online support groups, four caregiver groups, and one teen support group—part of *Group Loop. Teens. Talk. Cancer. Online.* (www.grouploop.org). There is also a Spanish Language Group and a Bereavement Group. TWCO has served more than 1600 participants in these online support groups; on average, patients and caregivers spend between 12 and 18 months in them. In 2007, over a quarter of a million unique visitors entered the site.

In addition, TWC has partnered with many other patient, private, and governmental agencies including the Lance Armstrong Foundation, the National Coalition for Cancer Survivorship, the NCI, the Leukemia and Lymphoma Society, and the British Columbia Cancer Agency in Canada. These partnerships have helped TWC design innovative programs to reach more cancer patients and their families. They've also provided opportunities for research and clinical staff training.

TWC IS COMMITTED TO QUALITY ASSURANCE

In 2004, TWC launched a national Quality Assurance Program designed to provide a framework for assessing quality of leadership, governance, and programs at all local Wellness Communities. The Quality Assurance Program consists of an intensive self-assessment by each local community, followed by a site visit from a multidisciplinary team, led by TWC's headquarters office.

The Quality Assurance Program consists of 116 quality measures organized under five key areas of focus: (1) Governance, (2) Operations and Administration, (3) Fund Development, (4) Marketing and Outreach, and (5) Program. All local Wellness Communities are subject to the quality assurance (QA) process every 3 years to ensure ongoing quality performance and consistency in the delivery of clinical and educational programs. In addition, the program allows for the identification and sharing of best practices across TWC's system, a critical element to learning and improving service delivery organization-wide.

All programs are based on evidence. Dr. Lee Jong-Wook, former Director-General of the World Health Organization (WHO) laments the "gap between today's scientific advances and their application—between what we know and what is actually being done."[26] The role of TWC is to step into this gap and translate evidence-based research into practice to better serve people with cancer and their families. Since 1982 TWC has been a service delivery organization. However, in 1996 TWC implemented into its strategic plan a four-fold commitment to evidence-based practice and research. The goals of TWC's research agenda are to:

- develop programs and services based upon research;
- utilize research data to improve training and program delivery;
- answer questions important to TWC and psychosocial-oncology community;
- become the Gold Standard in psychosocial-oncology support services.

Research collaborations. TWC either integrates research into its programs and services that it conducts in collaboration with its academic or hospital partners or applies psychosocial research that has already been completed by others. TWC's research model is called Community-Initiated Research Colloborations (CIRC), and refers to research collaborations between community-based nonprofits and medical or academic centers.[27] There are several key elements to this collaborative research model:

Power is equal. A critical feature of shared power is CIRC is shared equity in the resources and budget allocation among the partners. To conduct a study with the proper support requires that the funding be shared so that the community partner has the opportunity to hire new staff to oversee the study but also so that staff time typically allocated for program delivery can be reapportioned to allow for research demands. Most importantly, the research questions and project aims are guided by the needs of the community as well as those of the academic or scientific partner. It is important for the research to truly answer questions that are important to the community organizations and that the researchers share in these interests equally.

Mediation integrated into the model. In the CIRC model, mediation is included as an essential and expected component of the discussions and not only during a crisis. In essence, effective collaborations include effective conflict resolution. By way of example, in TWC's randomized clinical trial with Stanford University, it took the research team and the community group 1 year to determine how randomization would occur—without a wait-listed control!

The goal is to further science not just evaluate programs. Any research study with an academic or scientific partner requires a *rigorous system* of investigation to determine the effectiveness of the intervention or area of inquiry. In this system, it is incumbent upon the researchers to educate the community partner of the potential benefits and risks of the study through staff in-service training.

Results are disseminated through professional and public forums. All papers and presentations are shared jointly—and where applicable—the community partner may be first author on research articles. This includes the opportunity to present findings at scientific or professional meetings and conferences.

CIRC is a win-win for researchers and community partners.

Benefits for the researcher. Researchers often find they have done excellent work which has been published in an outstanding journal only to have their important findings sit on a shelf or in a library. TWC has heard from its research partners that the most exciting aspect of the CIRC model is that it provides an opportunity for scientists to test whether their research is effective in the real world. The CIRC model creates a vehicle whereby academic scholars are able to participate in innovative research and bring scientific clarity to an issue which is of great value to people in need. Also, researchers receive real help with recruitment thereby impacting more people with evidence-based interventions. Taken together, these elements provide an opportunity for true professional growth. This is especially true since the National Institute of Health is focused on *translational or effectiveness* research that can be disseminated widely into the community.

Benefits for the community. The research partnership creates an opportunity to test a community's innovative ideas and programs in a structured and focused manner. However, most importantly, the community partner wants to know that their programs and services are helping their target population. Evidence-based research is a significant method for guaranteeing quality not only for people in the community but also for the funders. Evidence is a key to assessing true value. Moreover, research data can reveal strengths and weaknesses and thus provide opportunities for growth and productive change. In particular, the research findings can illuminate hidden issues—like identifying unmet needs or better methods of delivering program services. It also provides the opportunity to focus on underserved populations to design effective interventions that can have a larger impact beyond a small community. Moreover, it is rare for community groups to have Institutional Review Board sanction for programs or interventions. Joining with a research partner lends increased credibility and safety monitoring to the organization and the program services.

Ultimately, because the research is taking place in the community—in what is called a "translational setting"—there is a real opportunity for positive findings to be disseminated widely.

CASE STUDIES: EXAMPLES OF TWC'S COMMUNITY-INITIATED RESEARCH

COLLABORATION

Case study #1: Frankly speaking about cancer series. To test the efficacy of psycho-educational programs in the community, TWC studied the *Frankly speaking about cancer treatment: take control of side effects through medicine, mind, and body,* program. The findings from the study were published in *Cancer nursing*: "Managing Cancer Side Effects to Improve Quality of Life: A Cancer Psychoeducational Program."[17]

The program goals were to educate people with cancer and their caregivers about the major side effects of cancer and cancer treatment and to empower them to proactively integrate medicine with mind and body techniques to prevent and/or limit the impact of specific cancer treatment side effects. Results from this pilot study are encouraging.

The Wellness Community found a significant decrease among participants in anxiety from baseline to 30-day follow-up. This is particularly noteworthy because increased anxiety interferes with a patient's ability to integrate and process new information. Under those circumstances, a patient is likely to be less effective in preventing or limiting cancer treatment side effects. TWC believes that the mind/body exercise aspect of the program may have played a significant role in decreasing patients' anxiety levels, thereby helping them to remain focused, integrate the information presented, and better manage side effects.

In addition, the 30-day follow-up evaluation revealed that feelings of increased ability to manage side effects were associated with greater improvements on the SF-36 Mental Health Scale. This finding underscores that people in the study not only benefited from the information in the program, but also may have been empowered to improve their emotional attitudes toward managing cancer treatment side effects thereby improving their quality of life and overall mental health.

Findings also revealed that participants without children show a greater decrease in work interference because of emotional problems than do participants with children. This warrants adding a component to the program that helps participants better cope with their children.

In 2006 TWC updated *Frankly Speaking About Cancer Treatment: Take Control of Side Effects through Medicine, Mind, and Body,* the patient journal, and workshop to include additional management tools for fatigue, hair loss, infection, anemia, skin problems, pain, gastrointestinal issues, and emotional stressors. We are investing adding a unique program to help parents cope with their children's issues. The patient journal now includes new tools for health and wellness including a side effect tracking log, an exercise log, and tips for good nutrition and stress management. These improvements were made in response to the ongoing demand for this program, and to address feedback learned from thousands of people surveyed.

DISSEMINATION. The Wellness Community introduced the updated program in 2006 and held 15 *Frankly speaking about cancer treatment* education workshops for survivors and caregivers at local Wellness Communities around the country, Gilda's Clubs, and at The Eisenhower Lucy Curci Cancer Center in Rancho Mirage, CA. The program was held in markets including Newton MA, Shorewood WI, St. Louis MO, Sarasota FL, several locations in California, and Toronto, Ontario, Canada.

In 2007, TWC received an educational grant from the Amgen Foundation to create TWC's International Network Program which was designed to test the feasibility of delivering the *Frankly speaking about cancer treatment: take control of side effects through medicine, mind, and body* in four countries—Canada, the UK, Ireland, and Italy—through partnerships with British Columbia Cancer Agency and Hope and Cope in Canada; Maggie's Centre in England and Scotland; ARC Cancer Support Centre in Ireland, and the University of Ferrara and Associazione Italiana Malati di Cancro (AiMAC) in Italy. Moreover, the program materials are translated into Italian and will be translated into French. The program was delivered in all of these countries in fall 2008 and Spring 2009. Each of the sites replicated the pilot study findings originally published in the *Cancer Nursing* journal article in 2003.[17]

Case study #2: Effectiveness of electronic support groups for women with breast carcinoma: a pilot study of effectiveness (2003). In this study done in partnership with Stanford University and the University of California at San Francisco, TWC found that women with breast cancer in professionally facilitated online support groups experienced significant increases in posttraumatic growth in three areas: Seeing new possibilities, zest for life, and spirituality. These women also experienced decreases in depression. This study was significant because it suggested that even support received in a nontraditional setting such as in an online support group was associated with reductions in depression and also the ability to "see the silver lining" in the traumatic experience.[28]

Case study #3: Do cancer support groups reduce physiological stress: a randomized clinical trial.[9,3,10] In this on going randomized clinical trial in partnership with Stanford University, TWC has identified many positive outcomes. When compared to those in supportive-expressive therapy (the Stanford Model), women in TWC support groups show significant reductions in posttraumatic stress symptoms, significant increases in making important life changes, an increasingly positive attitude toward their illness, better access to cancer-related information/resources, and better communication with their physicians.

Case study #4: Cancer transitions: moving beyond treatment. Cancer transition is an evidence-based posttreatment survivorship program developed by TWC in partnership with the Lance Armstrong Foundation. The six week program for survivors (less than 2 years posttreatment) was piloted at ten TWC affiliates across the United States in 2007 (phase I) and 2008 (phase II). A total of 151 survivors of breast (n=76), blood (n=16), gynecologic (n=22), lung (n=8), colorectal (n=9), prostate (n=4), and other (n=15) cancers participated in the program. The intervention included education and support on medical issues, exercise, nutrition and emotional needs that survivors face after treatment. Pre- and posttest questionnaires were completed on site and included the SF-12 health survey, an impact of cancer scale, the International Physical Activity Questionnaire, and a fat- and fiber-related dietary behavior questionnaire. Three and 6-month follow-up questionnaires were mailed. Participation

rates at the six sessions ranged from 75–94%. Following the intervention, there was a significant increase (mean±SE) in the mental component summary score of the SF-12 (2.4±0.8, p=0.002), and the increase was maintained at 3 months (2.7±1.0, p=0.01) and 6 months (2.9±1.2, p=0.023). There were significant increases over time in the role physical (F=7.49, p<0.001), vitality (F=4.26, p=0.0058), social function (F=3.94, p=0.0090) and the role emotional (F=5.54, p=0.0010). There was a reduction in the negative impact of cancer; the greatest impact was on health-related worry with a significant (p<0.01) decrease at all time points. Participants also reported less negative changes to their body, lower life interference, and a reduction in their negative outlook on life. There was a significant increase in physical activity, and, during Phase II, a significant improvement in fat- and fiber-related dietary behavior. Results from the pilot study showed that participants experienced positive changes following the 6-week intervention in health-related quality of life and lifestyle change and at 3- and 6-month follow-up. Cancer survivors participating in the program felt a significant decrease in health worry as well as a significant increase in quality of life around physical, mental and social functioning. Participants increased physical activity and improved fat- and fiber-related dietary habits.

NEW DIRECTIONS

When Harold Benjamin founded TWC in 1982 there were only 5.8 million cancer survivors. In 2008, there are over 12 million. This profound change in the cancer survivorship landscape requires TWC to continue to develop innovative programs and partnerships to better meet the growing needs of patients and families. To that end, TWC has embarked on several innovative programs that are geared toward addressing some of these needs.

In 2009 TWC opened the nation's first *community-based* Cancer Survivorship Research and Training Institute in Philadelphia, Pennsylvania. The Research and Training Institute (RTI) will work closely with our academic and scientific partners to translate research into practice as well as train the next generation of psychosocial oncologists in delivering state-of-the-science care. Moreover, the RTI will provide the research expertise to help our local TWC's develop and grow innovative evidence-based programs as well as fulfill the IOM's call for integrative care across the cancer continuum.

REFERENCES

1. Cordova M, Giese-Davis J, Golant M, et al. Mood disturbance in community cancer support groups: the role of emotional suppression and fighting spirit. *J Psychiatr Res.* 2003;55:461–467.

2. Lieberman M, Golant M. Therapeutic norms and patient benefit; cancer patients. Professionally directed support groups. *Group Dynamic: Theory, Research and Practice.* 2004:8(4):265–276.

3. Giese-Davis J, Kronenwetter C, Golant M, et al. Cancer support groups: Different models, different participant experiences. *Group Dynamics: Theory, Research and Practice (in revision).*

4. Cordova MJ, Giese-Davis J, Golant, M, Kronenwetter M, Chang V, Spiegel D. Breast cancer as trauma: Posttraumatic Stress and Posttraumatic Growth. *J Clini Psychol Med Setting.* 2007;14:308–319.

5. Lieberman M, Golant M, Giese-Davis J, et al. Electronic support groups for breast carcinoma: a clinical trial of effectiveness. *Cancer.* 2003 Feb;97(4): 920–925.

6. Golant M, Altman T, Martin C. Managing cancer side effects to improve quality of life: a cancer psychoeducation program, *Cancer Nursing.* 2003 Feb;26(1): 37–46.

7. Jong-Wook L. Keynote address. *Health Promo Int.* 2006;21(Suppl 1):5–6.

8. Institute of Medicine. (IOM). Cancer care for the whole patient. In: Adler NE, Page AK (eds). *Meeting psychosocial health needs.* Washington, DC: The National Academies Press; 2007.

9. Giese-Davis J, Golant M, Angell K, Rowland J. Community/research collaborations, how to reach more people more of the time with evidence-based interventions. *Ann Behav Med.* 2002;(Suppl)24:19p.

10. Thiboldeaux K, Golant M. *The total cancer wellness guide: Reclaiming your life after diagnosis.* BenBella, Dallas, Texas; 2007:306.

11. Rowland J, Mariotto A, Aziz N, et al. Cancer survivorship—United States, 1971–2001. *MMWR*. 2004;53:526–529.

12. Watson M, Greer S, Rowden L, et al. Relationships between emotional control, adjustment to cancer and depression and anxiety in breast cancer patients. *Psychol Med*. 1991;21:51–57.

13. Watson M, Haviland JS, Greer S, Davidson J, Bliss JM. Influence of psychological response on survival in breast cancer: a population-based cohort study. *Lancet*. 1999 Oct 16;354(9187):1331–1336.

14. Han WT, Collie K, Koopman C, et al. Breast cancer and problems with medical interactions: relationships with traumatic stress, emotional self-efficacy, and social support. *Psychooncology*. 2005 Apr;14(4):318–330.

15. Loscalzo MJ, Zabora JR. Care of the cancer patient: response of family and staff. In: Bruera E, Portenoy RK (eds). *Topics in palliative care*. New York: Oxford University Press; 1998:1–4

16. Goodwin PJ, Ennis M, Bordeleau LJ, et al. Health-related quality of life and psychosocial status in breast cancer prognosis: analysis of multiple variables. *J Clin Oncol*. 2004 Oct 15;22(20):4184–4192.

17. Kissane DW, Love A, Hatton A, et al. Effect of cognitive-existential group therapy on survival in early-stage breast cancer. *J Clin Oncol*. 2004 Nov 1;22(21):4255–4260. Epub 2004 Sep 27.

18. Spiegel D, Giese-Davis, JE. Depression and cancer: mechanisms and disease progression. *Biol Psychiatr*. 2003 Aug 1;54(3):269–282.

19. Goodwin PJ, Ennis M, Pritchard KI, Koo J, Trudeau ME, Hood N. Diet and breast cancer: evidence that extremes in diet are associated with poor survival. *J Clin Oncol*. 2003 Jul 1;21(13):2500–2507.

20. Spiegel D, Butler LD, Giese-Davis J, et al. Supportive-expressive group therapy and survival in patients with metastatic breast cancer: a randomized clinical intervention trial. *Cancer*. 2007;110(5):1130–1138.

21. Raison CL, Giese-Davis J, Miller AH, Spiegel D. Depression in cancer: mechanisms, consequences and treatment. In: Evans DL, Charney DS, Lewis L (eds). *The physician's guide to depression and bipolar disorders*. New York: McGraw-Hill; 2006:377–410.

22. Daugherty C, Ratain MJ, Grochowski E, et al. Perceptions of cancer patients and their physicians involved in phase I trials [*J Clin Oncol*. 1995 Sep;13(9):2476]. *J Clin Oncol*. 1995;13(5):1062–1072.

23. Houts PS, Nezu AM, Nezu CM, Bucher JA. The prepared family caregiver: a problem-solving approach to family caregiver education. *Pat Edu Counseling*. 1996;27(1):63–73.

24. Nezu AM, Nezu CM, Houts PS, Friedman SH, Faddis S. Relevance of problem-solving therapy to psychosocial oncology. *J Psychoso Oncol*. 1999;16(3–4):5–26.

25. Carlson LE, Speca M, Patel KD, Goodey E. Mindfulness-based stress reduction in relation to quality of life, mood, symptoms of stress and levels of cortisol, dehydroepiandrosterone sulfate (DHEAS) and melatonin in breast and prostate cancer outpatients. *Psychoneuroendocrinology*. 2004 May;29(4):448–474.

26. Antoni MH, Lehman JM, Kilbourn KM, et al. Cognitive—behavioral stress management intervention decreases the prevalence of depression and enhances benefit finding among women under treatment for early-stage breast cancer. *Health Psychol*. 2001;20:20–32.

27. Spiegel D, Bloom J. Group therapy and hypnosis reduce metastatic breast carcinoma pain. *Psychosom Med*. 1983;45:333–339.

28. Carlson LE, Bultz B. Mind-body interventions in oncology current treatment options in oncology. August 13 epublication; 2008.

Survival Following Psychotherapy Interventions

David W. Kissane

Life is not a process of mere predictable cause and effect. Both cause and effect are aspects of something greater than either.-Laurens van der Post, in *Jung and the story of our time*, 1975

INTRODUCTION

How does psychological wellness impact upon the course and outcome of cancer? Does living better mean living longer? Such questions were posed after the publication in 1989 of a survival advantage from participation in group therapy for women with metastatic breast cancer.[1] A flurry of studies blossomed as a result to examine the effect of psychotherapy interventions on length of survival with cancer. The outcome of such trials is reviewed in this chapter, together with consideration of some moderators of change.

INFLUENTIAL EARLY SURVIVAL STUDIES

Yalom led group therapy trials at Stanford during the 1970s, culminating in a group intervention that became known as supportive-expressive group therapy (SEGT).[2,3] Although the cohort in Spiegel et al.'s initial study was small at 86 subjects, after 10 years, the patients in the group intervention survived nearly 18 months longer.[1] Fox pointed out that the control arm had very poor survival times (2.8% alive at 5 years) compared to SEER data (32% alive at 5 years)—SEER data is drawn from the National Cancer Institute (NCI)'s Surveillance, Epidemiology and End Results (or SEER) data.[4] An inadvertent sampling bias seemed to have occurred, which may have influenced the outcome finding by Spiegel and colleagues of extended survival.[5,6]

Shortly thereafter, a psycho-educational group intervention to promote coping in patients with early stage melanoma (N = 68) further raised hopes that psychotherapeutic interventions can extend survival.[7] However, when compared again with SEER data, the control subjects in this study by Fawzy and colleagues had done more poorly (72% alive at 5 years compared to 92% in the SEER data).[8] Reclassification of a single subject in this trial would have rendered the survival findings nonsignificant.[8]

There were also mixed results from other studies. For instance, one study of supportive counseling delivered individually to male patients with stage IV cancer (N = 120) failed to reveal any survival advantage,[9] as did another using supportive group therapy in mixed cancers (N = 127).[10] Yet a different individual intervention that promoted adherence to treatments for hematologic malignancies (N = 94) achieved a survival benefit.[11] There were methodological weaknesses in some of these studies, such as selection biases, nonuse of randomization and no attention to treatment integrity, which made replication studies necessary to examine more carefully the impact of psychotherapy on survival.

MECHANISMS OF EFFECT

There has been much investigation of immune mechanisms that might be altered by stress reduction, such as natural killer cell activity,[7,12,13] flattened diurnal cortisol rhythms,[14] circadian dysregulation,[15] and the hypothalamic-pituitary-adrenal axis altered by depression.[16,17] One noteworthy coping intervention for women with early stage breast cancer showed benefits in reducing anxiety, promoting adherence to anticancer treatments and improving immune function.[18] For example, T-cell proliferation did increase with a blastogenic response to phytohemagglutinin and concanavalin A for group therapy subjects. However, a path analysis for health outcomes at 12 months showed that the reduction in emotional distress mediated good health outcomes, but not immune mechanisms.[13] Science has, thus, not been able to close the loop in terms of psychoneuroimmunological mechanisms. Is there a key psychoneuroimmunological pathway or ingredient, or is the percentage of variance attributable to these mechanisms quite small?

Alternative mechanisms of effect include behavioral ones, like adherence to anticancer treatments, improved diets, and increased physical activity, or social support mechanisms.[19-21] The latter have been studied through group interventions,[22,23] with Bloom recently arguing for greater focus on the supportive milieu[21] but relatively less attention has been applied to biobehavioral mechanisms.[24] Recent studies, for instance, have shown the ability of group therapy to improve anticancer treatment adherence.[18,25]

REPLICATION STUDIES OF SEGT IN BREAST CANCER

Better powered, randomized controlled trials (RCTs) that carefully utilized the manualized SEGT intervention for women with metastatic breast cancer were conducted in Canada (N = 235), the United States (N = 125) and Australia (N = 227).[26-28] Although significant psychological benefits were achieved as a result of SEGT in each study, no extension of survival was found.[25,29,30] Taken together, these studies cast doubt about the ability of SEGT to prolong survival.

COGNITIVELY ORIENTED GROUP THERAPY IN BREAST CANCER

Other studies made use of cognitive-behavioral group therapy in both advanced[31-33] and early stage breast cancer.[18,34,35] Cognitive-existential group therapy highlighted a novel adaptation to reduce the fear of cancer recurrence among women with primary breast cancer.[34] Again, although quality of life benefits were evident as a result of these interventions, survival has not thus far been improved.[31,33,36]

PSYCHO-EDUCATIONAL GROUP THERAPY IN MELANOMA

A meticulous replication of Fawzy's psycho-educational intervention in patients with primary melanoma was undertaken in Denmark.[37] No survival advantage was obtained, although poorer survival was seen in the socioeconomically disadvantaged study refusers.[38]

DOES PSYCHOTHERAPY EXTEND SURVIVAL?

The characteristics of RCTs reporting survival outcomes are summarized in Table 66–1. Recent trials of group therapy with improved methodology have failed to demonstrate any survival benefit. Other studies have methodological concerns, such as the study by Kuchler et al., where randomization assignment was not adhered to, with 34 patients in the control arm transferring to receive the psychotherapy intervention and 10 patients in the intervention arm swapping across into the controls.[39,40] After the individual supportive intervention was delivered, patients in the intervention arm received twice as much chemotherapy as control arm subjects,[8] creating a clear explanation for the apparent survival gain.

Table 66–1. Randomized controlled trials of psychosocial interventions on survival (nonrandomized studies excluded)

Study year and authors	Type of intervention	N in treatment group	N in control group	Follow-up period	Hazard ratio (95% CI)	p-value (Univariate analysis)
Spiegel et al. 1989	Supportive-expressive group therapy in metastatic breast cancer	50	36	10 yrs	0.51 (0.31, 0.82)	p <0.0001
Fawzy et al. 1993	Psycho-educational group intervention in primary melanoma	34	34	6 yrs and 10 yrs	Not available 0.35 (0.12, 0.99)	p = 0.0066
Fawzy et al. 2003						
Ilnyckyj et al. 1994	Supportive-group therapy in mixed cancers	96	31	11 yrs	1.18 (0.77, 1.83)	p >0.1
Cunningham et al. 1998	Cognitive-behavioral group therapy in metastatic breast cancer	30	36	5 yrs	0.76 (0.43, 1.35)	p = 0.35
Edelman et al. 1999	Cognitive-behavioral group therapy in metastatic breast cancer	60	61	5 yrs	0.77 (0.56, 1.06)	p >0.10
Kuchler et al. 1999	Supportive-individual therapy in gastrointestinal cancers at initial surgery (47% proved metastatic)	136	135	2 yrs and 10 yrs	0.61 (0.45, 0.84) 0.65 (0.49, 0.86)	p = 0.002 p = 0.003
Kuchler et al. 2007						
McCorkle et al. 2000	Supportive nursing postsurgical home care in mixed cancers	190	185	3.66 yrs	0.49 (0.32, 0.75)	p = 0.001
Goodwin et al. 2001	Supportive-expressive group therapy in metastatic breast cancer	158	77	7 yrs	1.06 (0.78, 1.45)	p = 0.72
Kissane et al. 2004	Cognitive-existential group therapy in primary breast cancer	154	149	7 yrs	1.35 (0.76, 2.39)	p = 0.31
Kissane et al. 2007	Supportive-expressive group therapy in metastatic breast cancer	147	80	8.3 yrs	0.92 (0.69, 1.24)	p = 0.60
Spiegel et al. 2007	Supportive-expressive group therapy in metastatic breast cancer	64	61	14 yrs	0.93 (0.62, 1.40)	p = 0.73
Boesen et al. 2007	Psycho-educational group intervention in primary melanoma	128	130	6 yrs	1.30 (0.50, 3.50)	p = 0.61
Andersen et al. 2008	Stress-reducing group therapy in regional breast cancer	114	113	11 yrs	0.51 (0.28, 0.93)	p = 0.028[a]

[a] Based only on the less conservative multivariate statistic, rather than a Kaplan Meier univariate statistic.

A recent, stress-reduction, psychologic group intervention for regional breast cancer made consistent use of relaxation therapy and treatment adherence principles.[13,18] A longer model of therapy offered 26 sessions in weekly groups for 4 months and monthly groups for the next eight. Using multivariate analysis, survival was significantly increased by the intervention.[41]

An impressive, supportive intervention by nurses delivering home care to the elderly after surgery showed a significant survival benefit among these cancer patients, but important physical treatments were combined with this mode of care delivery.[42] Three meta-analyses and one systematic review failed to find an effect of psychotherapy on survival.[43–46]

SOCIAL DISADVANTAGE AND SURVIVAL

Social disparity and poorer cancer outcome has been an important finding seen in Denmark,[38] the United Kingdom,[47,48] Sweden,[49,50] and the United States.[51] In the United States, the 5-year relative survival rate for all cancers combined is lower for African-Americans (57%) than it is for whites (68%), while the death rate for African Americans is 38% higher than for white males and 17% higher than for white females.[51] Attention to factors such as access to preventive screening, early diagnosis, and adherence to treatment are crucial to correct this social inequality. Andersen and colleagues found reduced-chemotherapy dose intensity and more drop outs from chemotherapy for controls compared to group therapy,[18] a finding similar to Richardson et al.[11] and Kissane et al.[25] but dissimilar to Kogon et al.[52]

Psychotherapeutic and psycho-educational interventions that promote understanding of the benefits of anticancer therapies alongside risks may help eliminate the social disparities seen currently in oncology through the behavioral mechanism of enhanced treatment adherence. Meta-analyses show that adherence reduces the risk of a poor treatment outcome by 26%.[53] Health beliefs may influence treatment adherence[54] and the odds of nonadherence is three times higher if co-morbid depression exists.[53]

DEPRESSION AND SURVIVAL

Several studies have highlighted the association between helpless/hopeless and depressed mental states and shorter survival.[55–58] The linkage of prospective data about depression from the New Haven Epidemiologic Catchment Area Study with the Connecticut Tumor Registry showed that women with major depression were at increased risk for late-stage breast cancer diagnosis compared to their nondepressed counterparts.[59]

In Australia's RCT of SEGT, depression prophylaxis held up as a key finding across all time points, and in posthoc analyses, remaining in a depressed state after 6 months showed a trend to shorter survival.[25] Depressed patients received significantly less anticancer treatment than nondepressed patients.[25] These are intriguing findings. Indeed, DiMatteo and colleagues showed in meta-analyses of adherence to treatment that depression makes the odds of nonadherence three times higher.[53] Conversely, social support and cohesive family relations improve the odds of adherence.[60] Active treatment of depression to improve compliance with anticancer therapies is an important behavioral pathway.

Recently, Gallo and colleagues reported that older patients with major depression in primary care practices that had implemented a "depression care management algorithm" were less likely to die from cancer over a 5-year period than comparable patients in usual care practices.[61] This was seen in the so-called PROSPECT study (Prevention of Suicide in Primary Care Elderly: Collaborative Trial), where the effectiveness of care management on reducing risk factors for late-life suicide was examined.[62] Randomization was conducted at the practice level and contrasted an algorithm for management of depression coordinated by a care manager with usual care within control arm practices. Twenty primary care practices in New York, Philadelphia and Pittsburgh took part and over 1200 randomly sampled patients were identified through age-stratified depression screening with the CES-D. Major depression at baseline was confirmed with the SCID and Hamilton Depression Rating Scale. The PROSPECT algorithm included citalopram 30 mg daily, plus or minus augmentation with interpersonal psychotherapy. Patients with depression in the intervention arm practices were 45% less likely to have died at 5 years than patients with depression in the usual care practices. The benefit appeared attributable to a reduction in death from cancer.

Given that depression influences adherence to treatment, it can be hypothesized that treatment adherence mediates the poorer survival outcome for those who remain depressed. This important outcome from the PROSPECT study is in keeping with findings from the Marsden prospective cohort of cancer patients followed by Watson and colleagues,[55,56] in which depression has been associated with poorer survival.

CONCLUSION—THE TRANSFORMATIVE BENEFITS OF GROUP THERAPY

In meta-analyses, group therapy has been more effective than individual therapy, perhaps because of the additive influence of the group-as-a-whole.[63] When groups coalesce around constructive rather than restrictive solutions for the group-as-a-whole, the creative potential that is harnessed has the ability to enrich quality of life. Groups transform existential ambivalence into an appreciation of deeper meaning and value in life.[28] Although group therapy may not directly prolong survival, the psychosocial gains make these clinical programs very worthwhile.

Shorter survival in oncology has been associated with social deprivation and depression, while treatment adherence is one important behavioral pathway that could explain this. Interventions that promote adherence to anticancer treatments and treat depression remain important in future studies. Group therapy can prophylactically prevent the onset of depression[25] and do much to ameliorate the suffering of patients with cancer.

REFERENCES

1. Spiegel D, Bloom JR, Kraemer HC, et al. Effect of psychosocial treatment on survival of patients with metastatic breast cancer. *Lancet*. 1989;2(8668): 888–891.

2. Spiegel D, Spira J. *Supportive-expressive group therapy: a treatment manual of psychosocial intervention for women with metastatic breast cancer*. Stanford, CA: School of Medicine, Stanford University; 1991.

3. Spiegel D, Classen C. *Group therapy for cancer patients: a research-based handbook of psychosocial care*. New York: Basic Books; 2000.

4. Fox BH. A hypothesis about Spiegel et al 1989 paper on psychosocial intervention and breast cancer survival. *Psychooncology*. 1998;7:361–370.

5. Fox BH. Rejoinder to Spiegel et al. *Psychooncology*. 1998;7:518–519.

6. Fox BH. Clarification regarding comments about a hypothesis. *Psychooncology*. 1999;8:366–367.

7. Fawzy FI, Fawzy NW, Hyun CS, et al. Malignant melanoma: effects of an early structured psychiatric intervention, coping, and affective state on recurrence and survival 6 years later. *Arch Gen Psychiatry*. 1993;50(9):681–689.

8. Coyne J, Stefanek M, Palmer S. Psychotherapy and survival in cancer: the conflict between hope and evidence. *Psychol Bull*. 2007;133:367–394.

9. Linn M, Linn B, Harris R. Effects of counseling for late stage cancer. *Cancer*. 1982;49:1048–1055.

10. Ilnyckyj A, Farber J, Cheang M, Weinerman BH. A randomized controlled trial of psychotherapeutic intervention in cancer patients. *Ann Royal Coll Phy Sur Canada*. 1994;27:93–96.

11. Richardson JL, Shelton DR, Krailo M, Levine AM. The effect of compliance with treatment on survival among patients with hematologic malignancies. *J Clin Oncol*. 1990;8(2):356–364.

12. Miller G, Cohen S. Psychological interventions and immune mechanisms: a meta-analytic review and critique. *Health Psychol*. 2001;20:47–63.

13. Andersen B, Farrar W, Golden-Kreutz D, et al. Distress reduction from a psychological intervention contributes to improved health for cancer patients. *Brain Behav Immun*. 2007;21:953–961.

14. Sephton S, Sapolsky R, Kraemer H, Spiegel D. Diurnal cortisol rhythm as a predictor of breast cancer survival. *J Natl Cancer Inst*. 2000;92:994–1000.

15. Sephton S, Spiegel D. Circadian disruption in cancer: a neuroendocrine-immune pathway from stress to disease? *Brain Behav Immun*. 2003;17:321–328.

16. Spiegel D, Giese-Davis J, Taylor CB, Kraemer H. Stress sensitivity in metastatic breast cancer: analysis of hypothalamic-pituitary-adrenal axis function. *Psychoneuroendocrinology*. 2006;31:1231–1244.

17. Giese-Davis J, Wilhelm F, Conrad A, et al. Depression and stress reactivity in metastatic breast cancer. *Psychosom Med*. 2006;68:675–683.

18. Andersen B, Farrar W, Golden-Kreutz D, et al. Psychological, behavioral, and immune changes after a psychological intervention: a clinical trial. *J Clin Oncol.* 2004;22:3570–580.

19. Andersen BL. Psychological interventions for cancer patients to enhance the quality of life. *J Consult Clin Psychol.* 1992;60(4):552–568.

20. Andersen BL. A biobehavioural model of cancer stress and disease course. *Am Psychol.* 1994;49(5):389–404.

21. Bloom J. Improving the health and well-being of cancer survivors: past as prologue. *Psychooncology.* 2008;17(6):525–532.

22. Spiegel D, Bloom JR, Yalom I. Group support for patients with metastatic cancer: a randomized prospective outcome study. *Arch Gen Psychiatry.* 1981;38:527–533.

23. Cain E, Kohorn E, Quinlan D, Latimer K, Schwartz PE. Psychosocial benefits of a cancer support group. *Cancer.* 1986;57:183–189.

24. Andersen B. Biobehavioral outcomes following psychological interventions for cancer patients. *J Consult Clin Psychol.* 2002;70:590–610.

25. Kissane D, Grabsch B, Clarke D, et al. Supportive-expressive group therapy for women with metastatic breast cancer: survival and psychosocial outcome from a randomized controlled trial. *Psychooncology.* 2007;16:277–286.

26. Goodwin PJ, Leszcz M, Quirt G, et al. Lessons learned from enrollment in the BEST study—a multicenter, randomized trial of group psychosocial support in metastatic breast cancer. *J Clin Epidemiol.* 2000;53(1):47–55.

27. Classen C, Butler LD, Koopman C, et al. Supportive-expressive group therapy and distress in patients with metastatic breast cancer. *Arch Gen Psychiatry.* 2001;58:494–501.

28. Kissane DW, Grabsch B, Clarke DM, et al. Supportive-expressive group therapy: the transformation of existential ambivalence into creative living while enhancing adherence to anti-cancer therapies. *Psychooncology.* 2004;13(11):755–768.

29. Goodwin PJ, Leszcz M, Ennis M, et al. The effect of group psychosocial support on survival in metastatic breast cancer. *N Engl J Med.* 2001;345(24): 1719–1726.

30. Spiegel D, Butler L, Giese-Davis J, et al. Effects of supportive-expressive group therapy on survival of patients with metastatic breast cancer. *Cancer.* 2007;110:1130–1138.

31. Cunningham AJ, Edmonds CV, Jenkins GP, et al. A randomized controlled trial of the effects of group psychological therapy on survival in women with metastatic breast cancer. *Psychooncology.* 1998;7:508–517.

32. Edelman S, Bell DR, Kidman AD. A group cognitive behaviour therapy programme with metastatic breast cancer patients. *Psychooncology.* 1999;8: 295–305.

33. Edelman S, Lemon J, Bell DR, Kidman AD. Effects of group cognitive behaviour therapy on the survival time of patients with metastatic breast cancer. *Psychooncology.* 1999;8:474–481.

34. Kissane DW, Bloch S, Miach P, Smith GC, Seddon A, Keks N. Cognitive-existential group therapy for patients with primary breast cancer—techniques and themes. *Psychooncology.* 1997;6:25–33.

35. Kissane DW, Bloch S, Smith GC, et al. Cognitive-existential group psychotherapy for women with primary breast cancer: a randomised controlled trial. *Psychooncology.* 2003;12:532–546.

36. Kissane DW, Love A, Hatton A, et al. Effect of cognitive-existential group therapy on survival in early-stage breast cancer. *J Clin Oncol.* 2004;22(21): 4255–4260.

37. Boesen E, Ross L, Frederiksen K, et al. Psychoeducational intervention for patients with cutaneous malignant melanoma: a replication study. *J Clin Oncol.* 2005;23:1270–1277.

38. Boesen E, Boesen S, Frederiksen K, et al. Survival after a psycho-educational intervention for patients with cutaneous malignant melanoma: a replication study. *J Clin Oncol.* 2007;25:5698–5703.

39. Kuchler T, Henne-Bruns D, Rappat S, et al. Impact of psychotherapeutic support on gastrointestinal cancer patients undergoing surgery: survival results of a trial. *Hepatogastroenterology.* 1999;46:322–335.

40. Kuchler T, Bestmann B, Rappat S, Henne-Bruns D, Wood-Dauphinee S. Impact of psychotherapeutic support for patients with gastrointestinal cancer undergoing surgery: 10-year survival results of a randomized trial. *J Clin Oncol.* 2007; 25:2702–2708.

41. Andersen BL, Yang HC, Farrar WB, et al. Psychologic intervention improves survival for breast cancer patients: a randomized clinical trial. *Cancer.* 2008;113(12): 3450–3458.

42. McCorkle R, Stumpf N, Nuamah I, et al. A specialized home care intervention improves survival among older post-surgical cancer patients. *J Am Geriatr Soc.* 2000;48:1707–1713.

43. Newell SA, Sanson-Fisher RW, Savolainen NJ. Systematic review of psychological therapies for cancer patients: overview and recommendations for future research. *J Natl Cancer Inst.* 2002;94(8):558–584.

44. Chow E, Tsao M, Harth T. Does psychosocial intervention improve survival in cancer? A meta-analysis. *Palliat Med.* 2004;18:25–31.

45. Smedslund G, Ringdal G. Meta-analysis of the effects of psychological interventions on survival time in cancer patients. *J Psychiatr Res.* 2004;57:123–131.

46. Edwards AGK, Hailey S, Maxwell M. Psychological interventions for women with metastatic breast cancer. *Cochrane Database Syst Rev.* 2004;2(CD004253).

47. Coleman M, Rachet B, Woods L, et al. Trends and socioeconomic inequalities in cancer survival in England and Wales up to 2001. *Br J Cancer.* April 5, 2004;90: 1367–1373.

48. Leigh Y, Seagroatt V, Goldacre M, McCulloch P. Impact of socio-economic deprivation on death rates after surgery for upper gastrointestinal tract cancer. *Br J Cancer.* 2006;95:940–943.

49. Lagerlund M, Bellocco R, Karlsson P, Tejler G, Lambe M. Socio-economic factors and breast cancer survival—a population based cohort study. *Cancer Causes Control.* 2005;16:419–430.

50. Halmin M, Bellocco R, Lagerlund M, Karlsson P, Tejler G, Lambe M. Long-term inequalities in breast cancer survival—a ten year follow-up study of patients managed within a National Health Care System (Sweden). *Acta Oncol.* 2008;47(2):216–224.

51. American Cancer Society. *Cancer facts and figures 2007.* Atlanta: American Cancer Society; 2007.

52. Kogon MM, Biswas A, Pearl D, Carlson RW, Spiegel D. Effects of medical and psychotherapeutic treatment on the survival of women with metastatic breast cancer. *Cancer.* 1997;80(2):225–230.

53. DiMatteo M, Giordani P, Lepper H, Croghan TW. Patient adherence and medial treatment outcomes: a meta-analysis. *Med Care.* 2002;40(9):794–811.

54. DiMatteo MR, Haskard KB, Williams SL. Health beliefs, disease severity, and patient adherence: a meta-analysis. *Med Care.* 2007;45(6):521–528.

55. Watson M, Haviland JS, Greer S, Davidson J, Bliss JM. Influence of psychological response on survival in breast cancer: a population-based cohort study. *Lancet.* 1999;354:1331–1336.

56. Watson M, Homewood J, Haviland J, Bliss JM. Influence of psychological response on breast cancer survival: 10-year follow-up of a population-based cohort. *Eur J Cardiol.* 2005;41:1710–1714.

57. Hjerl K, Andersen E, Keiding N, Mouridsen HT, Mortensen PB, Jørgensen T. Depression as a prognostic factor for breast cancer mortality. *Psychosomatics.* 2003;44:24–30.

58. Spiegel D, Giese-Davis J. Depression and cancer: mechanisms and disease progression. *Biol Psychiatr.* 2003;54:269–282.

59. Desai M, Bruce M, Kasl S. The effects of major depression and phobia on stage at diagnosis of breast cancer. *Int J Psychiatry Med.* 1999;29:29–45.

60. DiMatteo MR. Social support and patient adherence to medical treatment: a meta-analysis. *Health Psychol.* 2004;23(2):207–218.

61. Gallo J, Bogner H, Morales K, Post EP, Lin JY, Bruce ML. The effect of a primary care practice-based depression intervention on mortality in older adults. *Ann Intern Med.* 2007;146:689–698.

62. Bruce M, Have TT, Reynolds C, et al. Reducing suicidal ideation and depressive symptoms in depressed older primary care patients: a randomized controlled trial. *JAMA.* 2004;291:1081–1091.

63. Sheard T, Maguire P. The effect of psychological interventions on anxiety and depression in cancer patients: results of two meta-analyses. *Br J Cancer.* 1999;80:1770–1780.

Psychosocial Interventions for Couples and Families Coping with Cancer

Talia Irit Zaider and David W. Kissane

For most adults, the mutuality of a close relationship empowers the expression of psychosocial needs. Author and family therapist Esther Perel observed that today, "we turn to one person to provide what an entire village once did: a sense of grounding, meaning, and continuity."[1] We now know that the quality of a person's relationships with significant others is highly consequential for his or her physical and mental health.[2] Mounting evidence also suggests that proximity to a loved one has a regulatory effect on emotional functioning, helping to modulate emotional and physiological responses to life stressors.[3] When an illness such as cancer strikes, the supportive potential of family relationships will powerfully shape the psychosocial course of disease.[4]

A cancer diagnosis marks a major transition in a family's life, described by Rolland as an "uninvited guest"[5] that must be accommodated by the couple or family.[6] At every stage of illness, families are faced with challenges that threaten to disrupt the stability of their relationships and their quality of life. These include the rearrangement of roles and responsibilities around patient care, the renegotiation of future plans and shifting of priorities, adjustment to losses in functioning, the management of uncertainty, the fear of recurrence or, in advanced stages of illness, the burden of care, and prospect of death. Researchers and practitioners alike have argued that the psychosocial impact of cancer should be construed in relational terms.[7,8] Although medically, cancer happens to the individual patient, psychosocially, illness is shared problem. Families affected by cancer function as interdependent emotional units, such that the needs, goals, and emotional responses of patients and their close partners are highly correlated and mutually influencing.[9] For this reason, there has been increased interest in approaching the psychosocial care of the cancer patient with a family-centered lens. In this chapter, we begin with an overview of supportive therapies designed for the intimate couple, and follow this with a description of psychosocial care of the family as a whole.

COUPLE-BASED PSYCHOSOCIAL INTERVENTIONS

Over the last two decades, there has been a proliferation of supportive interventions tested for couples coping with cancer. The predominant therapeutic approach has been aimed at promoting relationship enhancement (RE) and/or preventing relationship distress, especially for couples at the early stages of disease. RE/prevention models emphasize the instruction of relationship skills that are intended to prevent adverse outcomes and maximize the couple's capacity for mutual support. For couples facing advanced-stage cancer, alternative intervention approaches focus more on the exploration of existential, emotional, and attachment-based themes. The content and efficacy of these couple-based intervention models are described below.

Early-stage cancers. Here the aim is to prophylactically strengthen relational competencies (e.g., communication, decision making, problem solving) so that patients and their partners are well equipped to metabolize the chronic strain associated with illness. These RE/prevention models share several characteristics: first, they are delivered normatively—that is, they are designed to benefit all couples affected by a cancer diagnosis regardless of how much distress exists individually or relationally. Second, these therapies lean heavily on didactic methods, using psycho-educational material and homework exercises to teach skills. Finally, they are typically oriented toward the reduction

of individual-level distress. Thus, aspects of the couple's relationship are construed as either facilitating or aggravating each individual partner's own adjustment. This is reflected in the outcomes used to evaluate the efficacy of the intervention (e.g., patient and partner symptoms of depression, anxiety or cancer-related distress), as well as in the theoretical underpinnings that underlie most early stage couples interventions.

The social-cognitive processing model[10] serves as a basis for involving the partner or spouse in psychosocial interventions. Open communication with the significant other helps the patient make sense of and integrate their cancer experience, which ultimately enables better adaptation and lower distress for the patient (or partner). Because this perspective construes the relationship as empowering to the individual members of the couple, Manne and Badr[11] referred to this as a "resource theory" of couples adaptation to cancer. Though many of the interventions we describe below are informed by this theoretical framework (i.e., relationship-as-resource), and therefore have as their endpoint the goal of improving individual adaptation, the interventions focus on relational processes within the couple as a means toward this end. Below we describe specific RE/prevention interventions for couples affected by early stage breast and prostate cancers.

Breast cancer. The CanCOPE intervention was designed for couples facing early stage breast or gynecological cancers.[12] Its major premise is that a mutually supportive and communicative relationship is a necessary condition for promoting effective coping responses. Across seven sessions, CanCOPE educates couples about psychological and medical ramifications of their cancer diagnosis and its treatment. Couples are trained to use active, problem solving coping and to monitor mutually and challenge each other's negative thoughts about cancer-related experiences. Couples are taught effective communication strategies, and are encouraged to practice empathic listening, validation of each other's perspectives and self-disclosure about cancer-related concerns. Finally, CanCOPE includes a module for discussing treatment-related changes in sexual responsiveness, sexual satisfaction, and body image concerns that arise for women diagnosed with breast and gynecological cancers. Couples are given relevant educational material and are instructed in strategies to help restore their sexual intimacy (e.g., sensate focus exercises).

In a randomized controlled trial comparing CanCOPE to the delivery of medical information only or a coping-training intervention for the patient alone, CanCOPE reduced the effort needed by the couple to cope, reduced women's psychological distress marginally, and enhanced sexual intimacy. Furthermore, CanCOPE couples were more likely to engage in communal and mutually supportive coping when observed discussing cancer-related stress. CanCOPE was delivered in the home, making it highly accepted by couples (94% participation). Couples reported high marital satisfaction and little conflict before the intervention, but more distressed couples were more likely to drop out. It remains unclear whether the content and format of CanCOPE would meet the needs of a high-risk population.

Manne and colleagues[13] developed an active coping group intervention for couples couple-focused group intervention (CG) affected by early stage breast cancer. Guided by cognitive-social processing theory, the overarching goal of CG is patient-centered in aiming to reduce the breast cancer patient's distress and improve her well-being by harnessing resources within her relationship. Weekly group sessions focus on increasing emotional expression, teaching stress management strategies within the couple (e.g., relaxation exercises), practicing effective coping and communication skills, enhancing mutual support, and recognizing the impact of cancer-related changes, both currently and in the future. A randomized controlled trial comparing CG to usual care showed a relative impact of CG in reducing women's depressive symptoms up to 6 months after treatment. Like CanCOPE, this intervention does not specifically target a distressed group, but demonstrated benefit regardless of how psychologically distressed women were before enrollment. The group format makes CG more cost-effective than the home-based CanCOPE, but also more difficult to customize to the particular needs of a couple.

Kayser[14] developed the Partners in Coping Program (PICP) based on a model of dyadic coping which recognizes the mutual influence of one partner's coping style on the other partner's distress. PICP is a delivered on an outpatient basis, across nine sessions that occur during the first year after diagnosis. Although guided by a different theoretical model, the content of the intervention is similar to the two prior therapies in its focus on helping both patient and partner identify and improve individual coping styles and communication skills to promote supportive exchanges. Although there were trends toward improved outcomes, a randomized controlled trial showed few differences between PCIP and standard care.

More recently, couple-based interventions have focused on the adaptation and growth of the couple as a unit. Promising preliminary results were obtained for Baucom and colleagues'[15] Relationship enhancement couples therapy for early stage breast cancer. Sessions of RE-incorporated elements similar to those previously described (e.g., communication skills training, enhancement of problem-solving skills, psycho-education regarding the psychological, physical, and sexual changes associated with breast cancer treatment), but targeted the growth and well-being of the couples' relationship rather than either the patient's or the partner's own adjustment per se. Couples receiving RE showed significant improvements relative to usual care, not only in the individual functioning, but also in the perceived quality of their mutual relationship. These results were sustained 1 year after intervention.

Intimacy enhancing couples' therapy (IECT) is again based on a relationship model that directly focuses on promoting behaviors (e.g., disclosure and responsiveness) that enhance closeness.[11] An uncontrolled pilot in women with early stage breast cancer showed preliminary efficacy in increasing responsiveness and intimacy, reducing individual distress and increasing general relationship closeness.

Prostate cancer. Treatment-related changes in the prostate cancer patient's quality of life and sexual functioning (e.g., incontinence, loss of libido, erectile dysfunction) can compromise his sense of masculinity, and disrupt communication and sexual intimacy for the couple. Qualitative accounts from men with early stage prostate cancer highlight the tendency to hold back from expressing concerns or fears, particularly with regard to the loss of sexual functioning.[16,17] High-distress levels are evident among the partners of men with prostate cancer, with accompanying changes in the couples' relationship.[18]

An early source of stress from prostate cancer is the decision-making process that unfolds as the couple is presented with numerous treatment options. Davison and colleagues[19] included significant others in the delivery of a customized information and decision-making support tool for early stage prostate cancer. This computer-based program was developed to help healthcare providers tailor the provision of information to the specific priorities and decision-making styles of patients and their partners. This decision-aide reduced distress for both patients and their partners. Interestingly, over half of men expressed a preference to share decision making collaboratively, whereas the majority of partners preferred a more passive role. Within-couple differences in decision-making preferences may contribute to the degree of relational strain experienced during this process.

A couple-focused sexual rehabilitation intervention for patients with localized prostate cancer and their partners[20] educated them about the sexual impact of surgery or radiation therapy. Couples were instructed in strategies to improve sexual communication, address negative beliefs

about cancer and sexuality, and increase the expression of affection in the relationship. In-session and home exercises (e.g., touching exercises) reinforced the skills learned in sessions. Distress was relieved and sexual functioning improved, although these gains were not maintained 6 months later. Interestingly, a substantial portion of couples (nearly 40%) withdrew from the therapy, 21% citing high marital distress, and 9% the explicit discussion of sexual topics. Perhaps because of its relatively brief and didactic nature, a sexual rehabilitation intervention may be most suitable for couples who are already functioning well in their relationship and are therefore able to assimilate educational material readily. Moreover, couples who share a trusting, communicative, and cohesive relationship may be better able to incorporate new ways of enjoying sexual intimacy (e.g., without a firm erection). Couples, however, with high levels of distress or longstanding marital conflict may need an intervention that more broadly addresses their relational constraints (e.g., poor communication).

The FOCUS intervention, developed by Northouse and colleagues,[21] is couple based and designed to impact a broader array of relational concerns relevant to prostate cancer. The intervention is named after the five core areas targeted: *F*amily involvement, *O*ptimistic attitude, *C*oping effectiveness, *U*ncertainty reduction, *S*ymptom management. FOCUS is similar to other RE/prevention programs in that it uses a supportive-educative approach to enhance communication, coping, the management of uncertainty and self-care strategies. A randomized controlled trial of this intervention showed numerous benefits to the spouses of men with prostate cancer. Spouses demonstrated improved quality of life, a greater sense of self-efficacy in coping and managing symptoms, improved communication about the illness, a reduction in hopelessness, and a less negative view of their caregiving role. Benefits to the spouse's quality of life were sustained 12 months after intervention. Interestingly, patient characteristics, such as his level of initial distress, or his phase of illness, did not appear to influence outcomes.

Advanced-stage cancers. Disease progression presents distinct challenges for families and is associated with an increase in distress among patients and their significant others.[22] Couples coping with advanced illness experience a more pronounced loss of reciprocity in the relationship, as partners are called upon to serve as caregivers and patients become more dependent and less functional. As the threat of loss insinuates itself into the couple's life, open and responsive communication becomes essential to sustaining connection, and addressing salient end-of-life concerns while both partners are able to do so (e.g., identifying palliative care needs, planning for the future, managing uncertainty and existential distress). When asked what constitutes quality of life at the end of life, family caregivers, patients, and healthcare professionals alike agreed on a common set of needs that included symptom management, decision making, preparation for death, sense of life completion, support, and affirmation of the whole person.[23,24] Relational processes, such as saying goodbye, spending time with family, resolving conflicts, and confiding in loved ones, predominate. Couple's therapy is well suited to help achieve these goals. The emphasis on themes of caregiving, anticipated loss, and existential concerns differentiates the support of advanced-stage couples from early stage interventions.[22] The evidence base for the utility of couple-based interventions is more limited in palliative care, where family-centered models have predominated. Theoretical models guiding couple's therapy include attachment theory, equity theory, and coping and stress-appraisal theory. The controlled trials discussed below provide promising evidence for the value of a couple-based approach, but also raise important questions about the needs of this population.

Northouse adapted the FOCUS program described earlier[25] to aim to change aspects of patient and caregiver coping. Guided by the stress-appraisal model of Lazarus and colleagues, appraisal of caregiving, and feelings of uncertainty and hopelessness are examined. Home-based sessions delivered by trained nurses focused on promoting an optimistic attitude, reducing feelings of uncertainty, promoting mutual support and communication among family members, and practicing active coping strategies. FOCUS was associated with improved immediate outcomes for patients, who showed a decrease in hopelessness and in negative appraisal of the illness. However, these benefits were not sustained at follow-up 6 months later. Family caregivers showed a reduction in negative appraisal of caregiving, although this effect was also not sustained. The intervention showed no effect on patient or partner's quality of life, coping, or feelings of uncertainty.

This intervention is brief, home based, and confers immediate psychosocial benefits, especially to the patient. A larger dosage of the intervention may be needed to sustain its effects over time. However, the applicability of some aspects of the model encouraging optimistic thinking and reducing uncertainty may be limited in the face of more imminent death. Nearly 20% of the patients died during this trial, one-third experienced disease progression, and over half required a change in treatment. Patients who dropped out were more symptomatic and had a more persistent illness course. Given that the goals of palliative care include achieving comfort, saying goodbye, confiding wishes and fears to loved ones and planning for the future, the intervention may not have tapped the relational processes most salient at this phase.

Kuijer and colleagues[26] adopted a more relational approach to supporting couples with advanced illness. They addressed inequities in the caregiving relationship, a process shown to generate distress, relationship dissatisfaction, and perceived burden. This five-session intervention aims to restore a realistic balance of supportive exchange so that caregivers perceive more benefit relative to their investment and patients also perceive more gains. Sessions focused on creating more mutually supportive interactions, targeting both instrumental needs (e.g., patients taking on manageable self-care tasks) and psychological processes (revising the patient and partner's own standards about how much investment is possible).

A randomized controlled trial showed an improvement in relationship quality and reduction in perceptions of inequity for both parties who received this intervention.[26] A greater mitigating effect on psychological distress emerged for the patient than the partner. Furthermore, changes in the patient's perceptions of equity following the intervention did predict relationship quality 3 months later.

The advantage of this approach is that it makes use of conjoint sessions to address a relational source of distress (i.e., loss of reciprocity in the relationship) that would not be as easily addressed in an individualized format. The intervention may need to address additional existential *content* that couples face at the end of life (e.g., saying goodbye, resolving old conflicts). The facilitation of open communication about these concerns may prove especially important.

Challenges at the end of life. Couples facing advanced illness may experience not only a shift in the distribution of tasks, but also a skew in the exchange of emotional support. A challenge is how to continue leaning on, and drawing comfort from one's partner when the threat of separation is imminent. This can be particularly distressing for couples with limited capacity to comfort each other to begin with. As noted by McWilliams, "It is very painful to say goodbye when you are vaguely aware of not having said a satisfactory 'hello' to the other person."[27]

Attachment theory provides a useful frame for understanding how couples manage perceived or threatened loss. Application of this theory to couples dealing with advanced illness has yielded promising results. According to attachment theory,[28,29] seeking proximity with a close other is protective under conditions of danger or threat. The goal of proximity-seeking behaviors is to ultimately restore emotional stability and safety. Temporary separation from a loved one is associated with physiological and affective dysregulation, evidenced by changes in sleeping patterns, increases in physical symptoms and cortisol levels, in addition to subjective reports of distress.[3] The regulatory effects of close proximity to an attachment figure is more pronounced for individuals with high "attachment anxiety," a classification that refers to a person's stable tendency to feel uncertain about the availability and responsiveness of an intimate partner.[3]

When faced with the existential threat posed by illness, couples with a secure attachment process will draw support effectively from one another, remaining responsive to each other's needs whether in the role of caregiver or care receiver. Attachment theory proposes that when proximity is not achievable in a time of need, partners enact a kind of "separation protest" (e.g., clinging, following, blaming, coercive, or controlling behavior). This behavior can easily shape a pattern of demand-withdraw, which is associated with high distress in couples coping with cancer.[30] An alternative response to a perceived breach in attachment security is to deny the need for contact altogether, and avoid engagement or shut down emotionally, behavior that unfortunately amplifies disconnection and diminishes the sense of safety.

Guided by attachment theory, McLean and Nissim[31] adapted an empirically supported intervention for relationship distress called emotion-focused couples therapy (EFCT) to address the disruptions in emotional engagement that occur for some facing advanced cancer. The goal of EFT is to strengthen a couple's capacity to shore up safety and connectedness, particularly during periods of vulnerability. Rather than instructing couples to use communication or problem-solving skills per se, the EFT therapist assumes that these skills already exist and will emerge spontaneously in a context of safe connection. Sessions help couples to recognize destructive or distancing interaction cycles, choreographing new ways of interacting that restore closeness and open emotional expression. McLean and her colleagues piloted this intervention and showed improved marital functioning, decreased depression, and subjective reports of benefit and satisfaction.

This model targets couples who present with high relationship distress. EFT is a fully relational model in that its focus is on the functioning of the couple as a pair, and relies on conjoint sessions to facilitate growth and reparation. A disadvantage of this approach is that it requires more sessions than the psycho-educational interventions described above, and needs more experienced therapists trained in systems and experientially based couple techniques.

FAMILY-CENTERED PSYCHOSOCIAL INTERVENTIONS

Meta-analyses on family-centered care. Higginson and colleagues contrasted the small but positive effect size in their meta-analyses of palliative care on patient outcomes (26 studies, d = 0.33, 95% confidence intervals 0.10–0.56) with the negligible effect on caregivers and families (13 studies, d = 0.17, 95% confidence intervals −0.14–0.48).[32] Harding and Higginson[33] suggested adroitly that support for caregivers and families needed to focus on high-risk caregivers, in the process respecting the resilience present in many families, and targeting our limited resources to those most in need. Bereavement researchers have similarly advocated focusing interventions on high-risk populations following a loss.[34] Continuity of care for the family from palliative care through to bereavement is an admirable goal for any psychosocial care team. Indeed, bereavement care should not be an add-on after the fact.

Resilience and family strengths. In the past decade, the field of family therapy has matured toward strength-based models of intervention—a family resilience approach. This counterbalances the usual mental health tendency to characterize families on the basis of deficit and pathology. This resilience model strives to harness areas of competence, affirm skills, and identify capacities for growth. Viewing any family through a resilience lens helps to humanize their experience and to find hope for mastery and reintegration at a time when families may feel challenged or potentially overwhelmed.

Resilience has been defined as a "dynamic process encompassing positive adaptation within the context of significant adversity."[35] Within this concept, we do not include those who destabilize temporarily under stress before returning to their prior level of functioning.[36] Walsh has usefully identified three overarching domains of family resilience, embracing their belief systems, organization patterns and communication processes.[37] The Family Focused Grief Therapy Model considers these dimensions through its exploration of family functioning and helps clinicians to specifically recognize resilient families. These families accept whatever the level of threat and form a belief in their ability to respond.[38] The affirmation of strengths allows services to then focus scarce resources on those "at risk" or in greater need.

Table 67–1. Guideline to conducting a basic family meeting

1. Round of introductions, welcome, and putting people at ease
2. Leaders declare their goal of meeting together
   A. To review the status of the patient's illness
   B. To consider the family's needs in care provision
   C. To understand more about how the family gets on
   D. To aim at optimizing the journey ahead
3. Identify and explore any other agendas that the family might have; agree on agenda and timetable accordingly
4. Check each family member's understanding of the seriousness of illness
5. Check each family member's understanding of the current goals of medical care
6. Are there symptoms that are a worry to the patient or family?
   A. Pain or other physical symptoms and related treatment concerns?
   B. Any concerns about nursing or hospice visits? Hygiene?
   C. Any concerns about walking, moving, transferring? Resources?
   D. Any concerns about coping? If so, who?
   E. Any needs for respite?
7. Clarify the patient's and family's view of what the future holds:
   A. If relevant, has the place of death been discussed?
   B. If at home, who from the family will be providing care?
   C. If in hospital, who will accompany? Help? Support?
8. How is the family managing emotionally: Is anyone a concern or do you expect family members to manage satisfactorily? Is there anything we can do to help?
9. Affirm family strengths: commitment, willingness, caring and concern for one another. If concerns exist and are agreed to, discuss referral for ongoing family therapy
10. Offer written educational material in accordance with institutional norms or issues raised at the meeting
11. "Before concluding are there any questions that you have as a family?"
12. Arrange follow-up care plan and ensure consensus

The routine family meeting. We recognize two tiers of intervention, the first of which is a brief and focused single family meeting, in which the key dimensions of family competence and coping are assessed as care needs are reviewed. Table 67–1 presents guidelines to this basic family meeting. As is often the case, the assessment of the family during this meeting is itself a form of intervention, as family members are invited to take notice of, and make explicit, their ways relating with each other and dealing with the illness. This first meeting has certain general purposes that are undoubtedly part of routine practice (e.g., introducing the family to the oncology or palliative care team, reviewing the goals of care and engaging caretakers in helping deliver this). Additional strategies can be introduced as appropriate to aid in planning for care of the family-as-a-whole.

This family meeting is an opportunity for the healthcare team to gain information from the family, but also for the family to openly acknowledge how they interact and communicate with one another, what values are prioritized, and which members, if any, are suffering significant distress. In this way, the meeting itself models and fosters the very processes that contribute to resilience.

For all families, regardless of how well they are functioning, a critical component of this meeting is the affirmation of family strengths and resources. The healthcare team can use this time to reassure well-functioning families that their cohesion, communication, and conflict resolution (the three C's of relational life) will prove to be a great source of mutual support. Likewise, families who struggle to cope and have greater difficulty working together may be reminded of aspects of family life that are valued, unique, and genuinely positive (e.g., caring concern for each other, commitment to the patient). Written material can be offered to summarize issues raised during this meeting.

Screening families to identify those at risk of morbid outcome. We advocate for the use of routine screening as a tool to gauge the predominant "family environment," and determine any level of risk facing each family.[7] The Family Relationships Index (FRI)[39] has proven to be a reliable and informative screening device that is minimally intrusive and can be easily administered to patients and their relatives in the clinical setting. In our most recent sample of palliative care families, the FRI was found to be extremely sensitive to detecting maladaptive family patterns (86% sensitivity), although some risk for false positives was evident.[40] Its sensitivity and specificity in detecting families at risk have been confirmed by other groups.[41] The FRI is a feasible and acceptable method of screening, although some training and facilitation may be needed to integrate screening into existing practices.

The scale is best used at the time of new admission to the service, when family members are likely to be accompanying the patient. Each family member completes the scale independently and without consulting with one another to ensure honest and confidential responses. Additionally, a comment to normalize the divergence in views among members may help clarify the importance of obtaining each member's perspective. The FRI can be used to derive scores on three key dimensions of family competence—cohesiveness, communication, and conflict resolution. Families are considered to be at risk if one or more respondents score 9 or less out of 12 on the FRI, or less than 4 on cohesiveness, a particularly sensitive predictor of family outcomes.[42] Families in which at least one member indicates difficulties in family functioning could be offered the option of additional family meetings as part of an ongoing program of support. The following is a sample script used by the practitioner in this scenario:

We notice in your questionnaire responses that some of you feel that an aspect of family life—communication, teamwork, or conflict—can be a challenge at times. We'd like to tell you about some options for services that try to help families as they strive to support a sick relative. These services use ongoing meetings like this to support the family…

The screening should supplement, but not replace, a broader discussion with the family that aims to elicit family members' perceptions of family functioning and coping. Should maladaptive patterns (e.g., high conflict, fractured relationships) emerge during this discussion or from the FRI, the task for psycho-oncology is not to try to solve these issues there and then, but rather to help synthesize the information so that a plan for further support can be established.

Engaging the family in focused family therapy. Preventive family therapy can be commenced in the setting of advanced cancer for those families deemed at greater risk and continued by the clinician into bereavement if the patient dies subsequently. The Family Focused Grief Therapy (FFGT) model was developed empirically to optimize coping and mutual family support during palliative care, and support the sharing of grief systemically in bereavement. Its efficacy has been demonstrated in a randomized controlled trial[43]; the greater any relational dysfunction in the family, the more sessions will likely be needed over the subsequent year to 18 months. In general, mild family dysfunction will be aided by 4–6 sessions over as many months, while 10–12 sessions will prove necessary for those at greatest risk.

Using this model, therapists make use of circular questions and summaries to engage and guide the family toward optimal functioning and mutual support.[44] Openness to discussion of death and dying and early containment of conflict prove beneficial until improved communication and closeness help family members to tolerate differences of opinion.

CONCLUSION

Relationship-focused interventions delivered at both the early and advanced stages of cancer do effectively enhance the quality of family relationships, strengthen their capacity to maintain functioning amid illness-related changes and reduce the risk for psychiatric morbidity. Implicit in this is the concept that maladaptive relational processes can constrain the full coping potential of the patient and the family-as-a-whole.

The existing evidence base for couple- and family-based psychosocial interventions within oncology leans heavily on preventive, psychoeducational approaches. This RE/prevention approach to supporting couples and families can be delivered normatively, across relatively few sessions, and administered by trained healthcare practitioners of medical and psychosocial disciplines (e.g., nurse practitioners, psychologists, social workers). Few interventions target groups at risk for poor adjustment, whether through high levels of relationship discord or elevated distress. Although many couples and families describe having supportive relationships, the substantial minority who experience these as fractured or conflictual are also at higher risk for psychological morbidity.[7] As described above, a routine family meeting in which relational functioning is assessed along with the adjustment of each individual provides an opportunity to identify couples and families in greater need of supportive services.

A large meta-analytic review of trials comparing family-based psychosocial interventions for various chronic illnesses with usual medical care found that there were clear benefits to including a family member in the psychosocial support of medically ill patients.[45] Benefits to the patient were particularly strong when the intervention focused on couples and addressed relationship issues. Given the centrality of the intimate relationship in the patient's journey with cancer, future research must strive for a more integrated, and evidence-based model that will guide how to best help families sustain their essential functions in the face of adversity and anticipated loss.

REFERENCES

1. Perel E. *Mating in captivity.* New York, HarperCollins; 2007:XIV.

2. Kiecolt-Glaser JK, Newton TL. Marriage and health: his and hers. *Psychol Bull.* 2001;127(4):472–503.

3. Diamond LM, Hicks AM, Otter-Henderson KD. Every time you go away: changes in affect, behavior, and physiology associated with travel-related separations from romantic partners. *J Pers Soc Psychol.* 2001;95(2):385–403.

4. Manne S. Cancer in the marital context: a review of the literature. *Cancer Invest.* 1998;16(3):188–202.

5. Rolland J. In sickness and in health: the impace of illness on couples' relationships. *J Marital Fam Ther.* 1994;20(4):327.

6. Rolland JS. *Families, illness, & disability: an integrative treatment model.* New York, Basic Books; 1994:235.

7. Kissane DW, Bloch S, Burns W, McKenzie DP, Posterino M. Psychological morbidity in the families of patients with cancer. *Psychooncology.* 1994;3:47–56.

8. Zaider T, Kissane DW. Resilient families. In: Monroe B, Oliviere D (eds). *Resilience in palliative care.* Oxford, Oxford University Press; 2007.

9. Hagedoorn M, Sanderman R, Bolks HN, Tuinstra J, Coyne JC. Distress in couples coping with cancer: a meta-analysis and critical review of role and gender effects. *Psychol Bull.* 2008;134(1):1–30.

10. Lepore SJ, Ragan JD, Jones S. Talking facilitates cognitive-emotional processes of adaptation to an acute stressor. *J Pers Soc Psychol.* 2000;78(3):499–508.

11. Manne S, Badr H. Intimacy and relationship processes in couples' psychosocial adaptation to cancer. *Cancer.* 2008;112(Suppl 11):2541–2555.

12. Scott JL, Halford WK, Ward BG. United we stand? The effects of a couple-coping intervention on adjustment to early stage breast or gynecological cancer. *J Consult Clin Psychol.* 2004;72(6):1122–1135.

13. Manne SL, Ostroff JS, Winkel G, et al. Couple-focused group intervention for women with early stage breast cancer. *J Consult Clin Psychol.* 2005;73(4):634–646.

14. Kayser K. Enhancing dyadic coping during a time of crisis: a theory-based intervention with breast cancer patients and their partners. In: Revenson TA, Kayser K, Bodenmann G (eds). *Couples coping with stress: Emerging perspectives on dyadic coping.* Washington, DC: American Psychological Association; 2005:175–194.

15. Baucom DH, Porter LS, Kirby JS, et al. A couple-based intervention for female breast cancer. *Psychooncology.*2008;18(3):276–283.

16. Boehmer U, Clark JA. Communication about prostate cancer between men and their wives. *J Fam Pract.* 2001;50(3):226–231.

17. Maliski SL, Heilemann MV, McCorkle R. From "death sentence" to "good cancer": couples' transformation of a prostate cancer diagnosis. *Nurs Res.* 2002;51(6):391–397.

18. Couper J, Bloch S, Love A, Macvean M, Duchesne GM, Kissane D. Psychosocial adjustment of female partners of men with prostate cancer: a review of the literature. *Psychooncology.* 2006;15(11):937–953.

19. Davison BJ, Goldenberg SL, Gleave ME, Degner LF. Provision of individualized information to men and their partners to facilitate treatment decision making in prostate cancer. *Oncol Nurs Forum.* 2009;30(1):107–114.

20. Canada AL, Neese LE, Sui D, Schover LR. Pilot intervention to enhance sexual rehabilitation for couples after treatment for localized prostate carcinoma. *Cancer.* 2005;104(12):2689–2700.

21. Northouse LL, Mood DW, Schafenacker A, et al. Randomized clinical trial of a family intervention for prostate cancer patients and their spouses. *Cancer.* 2007;110(12):2809–2818.

22. McLean LM, Jones JM. A review of distress and its management in couples facing end-of-life cancer. *Psychooncology.* 2007;16(7):603–616.

23. Steinhauser KE, Christakis NA, Clipp EC, McNeilly M, McIntyre L, Tulsky JA. Factors considered important at the end of life by patients, family, physicians, and other care providers. *JAMA.* 2000;284(19):2476–2482.

24. Steinhauser KE, Clipp EC, McNeilly M, Christakis NA, McIntyre LM, Tulsky JA. In search of a good death: observations of patients, families, and providers. *Ann Intern Med.* 2000;132(10):825–832.

25. Northouse L, Kershaw T, Mood D, Schafenacker A. Effects of a family intervention on the quality of life of women with recurrent breast cancer and their family caregivers. *Psychooncology.* 2005;14(6):478–491.

26. Kuijer RG, Buunk BP, De Jong GM, Ybema JF, Sanderman R. Effects of a brief intervention program for patients with cancer and their partners on feelings of inequity, relationship quality and psychological distress. *Psychooncology.* 2004;13(5):321–334.

27. McWilliams AE. Couple psychotherapy from an attachment theory perspective: a case study approach to challenging the dual nihilism of being an older person and someone with a terminal illness. *Eur J Cancer Care (Engl.).* 2004;13(5):464–472.

28. Bowlby J. *Attachment and loss: Attachment.* Vol. 1. New York, Basic Books; 1969.

29. Bowlby J. *Attachment and loss: Separation.* Vol. 2. New York, Basic Books; 1973.

30. Manne SL, Taylor KL, Dougherty J, Kemeny N. Supportive and negative responses in the partner relationship: their association with psychological adjustment among individuals with cancer. *J Behav Med.* 1997;20(2):101–125.

31. McLean LM, Nissim R. Marital therapy for couples facing advanced cancer: case review. *Palliat Support Care.* 2007;5(3):303–313.

32. Higginson IJ, Finlay IG, Goodwin DM, et al. Is there evidence that palliative care teams alter end-of-life experiences of patients and their caregivers? *J Pain Symptom Manage.* 2003;25(2):150–168.

33. Harding R, Higginson IJ, Donaldson N. The relationship between patient characteristics and carer psychological status in home palliative cancer care. *Support Care Cancer.* 2003;11(10):638–643.

34. Stroebe M, Hansson RO, Schut H, Stroebe W. Bereavement research 21st century prospects. In: eds. *Handbook of bereavement research and practice,* pp. 577–603. Washington, DC: American Psychological Association; 2008.

35. Luthar SS, Cicchetti D, Becker B. The construct of resilience: a critical evaluation and guidelines for future work. *Child Dev.* 2000;71(3):543–562.

36. Bonanno GA. Loss, trauma, and human resilience: have we underestimated the human capacity to thrive after extremely aversive events? *Am Psychol.* 2004;59(1):20–28.

37. Walsh F. Family resilience: a framework for clinical practice. *Fam Process.* 2003;42(1):1–18.

38. Patterson JM. Integrating family resilience and family stress theory. *J Marriage Fam.* 2001;64:349–360.

39. Moos RH, Moos BS. *Family environment scale manual.* StanfordConsulting Psychologists Press; 1981.

40. Kissane DW, McKenzie M, McKenzie DP, Forbes A, O'Neill I, Bloch S. Psychosocial morbidity associated with patterns of family functioning in palliative care: baseline data from the Family Focused Grief Therapy controlled trial. *Palliat Med.* 2003;17(6):527–537.

41. Edwards B, Clarke V. The psychological impact of a cancer diagnosis on families: the influence of family functioning and patients' illness characteristics on depression and anxiety. *Psychooncology.* 2004;13(8):562–576.

42. Kissane DW, Bloch S. *Family focused grief therapy: A model of family-centred care during palliative care and bereavement.* Buckingham and Philadelphia, Open University Press; 2002.

43. Kissane DW, McKenzie M, Bloch S, Moskowitz C, McKenzie DP, O'Neill I. Family focused grief therapy: a randomized, controlled trial in palliative care and bereavement. *Am J Psychiatry.* 2006;163(7):1208–1218.

44. Dumont I, Kissane DW. Techniques for framing questions in conducting family meetings in palliative care. *Palliat Support Care.* 2009;7(2):163–170.

45. Martire LM, Lustig AP, Schulz R, Miller GE, Helgeson VS. Is it beneficial to involve a family member? A meta-analysis of psychosocial interventions for chronic illness. *Health Psychol.* 2004;23(6):599–611.

PART X

Special Considerations

Matthew J. Loscalzo, ED

CHAPTER 68

The Older Patient

Barbara A. Given and Charles W. Given

AGING AND CANCER

The fastest growing segment of the population comprises persons 65 and older. Individuals aged 85 and older will double by 2030. More than 8 million cancer survivors are over 65, and by 2030, 60%–70% of all malignancies and approximately 80% of cancer deaths will occur to this age group.[1] The median age of patients at the point of diagnosis is over 65 for those with colon, lung, pancreas, stomach, and urinary bladder cancers. Analyzing factors relevant to aging and cancer points to the importance of understanding cancer in the older person.

When diagnosed with cancer, older individuals are already dealing with multiple medical problems often resulting in co-morbidities. Aging involves progressive decline in functional reserve of multiple organs and body systems, reduced tolerance of stress and greater physical impairments. The prevalence of co-morbid conditions and decreasing social and economic resources compounds the repercussions for the older cancer patient. These factors exacerbate tolerance of the cancer and cancer treatment.

Given the increased life expectancy resulting from improved treatment of cancer and cancer control, cancer and aging will be an important area of concern for the future healthcare system. We delineate information-relevant psychosocial areas relevant to cancer treatment in the older adult patient. Chronological age is not the focus; we consider how the biological, psychological, and social factors add to the complexity of care of the older cancer patient. Older cancer patients face the challenge of finding individualized, patient-oriented care. We will not examine specific sites of cancer; these topics are addressed in other chapters (see Chapters 38 and 39 on palliative care).

Impact of aging and psychosocial aspects for cancer. Aging is associated with a number of molecular, cellular, and physiological changes that influence the incidence of, biology of, and progression of treatment response to cancer. Lower maximal heart rate and cardiac output occur in addition to decreased perfusion to the kidney, and subsequently to reduced renal excretion of drugs.[2] There is a decreased response to catacholamines resulting in hypoxemia. The aging lung has lower vital capacity and decreased elasticity in the lung tissue. There is lower gastric emptying. A combination of reduced digestion of proteins and lowered absorption often occurs and results in reduced absorption of amino acids, decreased protein synthesis, increased concentration of catabolic cytokines in the circulation, and reduced production of anabolic hormones.[3-5] Malnutrition may be present in those over 65 and is an independent factor for toxicity from cancer treatment and an important predictor of survival and platelet counts.[6,7] Decreased bone marrow reserve results in hematopoietic suppression. Myelosuppression and the risk of febrile neutropenia becomes a main dose-limiting toxicity among older cancer patients.[8] With aging, there is a decrease in total body water in hepatic mass and blood flow and an increase in body fat. The older adult is vulnerable to mucositis and the other gastrointestinal side effects of cancer therapy; in addition, these physiological changes may accentuate cognitive and physical functional decline. Taken together, the molecular and physiological factors may compromise the ability of the older adult to tolerate cancer treatment.

We focus on psychosocial aspects of care during cancer treatment. The physiological and biological changes that occur during cancer treatment, as well as the altered physical, cognitive, and social function, may affect how the patient, family, and healthcare professionals including primary care face treatment decisions and respond to the side effect and responses to cancer treatment; thus, it is essential to focus on the psychosocial aspects of care.

The age group "over 65" is not homogeneous; age alone is not an independent consideration for cancer care. Older patients are physiologically, psychologically, socially, economically, and culturally diverse. Chronological, biological, and functional age are not the same; each has to be considered individually within the consideration of cancer treatment methods. To ensure a comprehensive approach to care, an assessment such as the comprehensive geriatric assessment (CGA) is to be completed.[9]

Cancer care professionals in collaboration with primary care professionals need to rely on a comprehensive assessment, such as the CGA,[10,11] that provides information regarding an older individual's physiological, functional, and cognitive age rather than "chronological age" as a standard for determining treatment and psychosocial care.[12] Older patients may not present with typical signs and symptoms either to the original disease or to the treatment; thus, the entire area of symptom management becomes an additional element to be added to the plan of care. A coordinated effort is needed between primary care provider and cancer specialist (Table 68–1).

A CGA may be used to anticipate and plan for complications that may arise in older cancer patients to reduce treatment interruptions and their late effects and to make cancer care, both, more effective and efficient.[10,11,13] Using such a tool that distinguishes among older adults with or without health status problems, or physiological or psychosocial conditions is important in the development and implementation of treatment plans (Table 68–2).

On the basis of an assessment, the cancer treatment decisions and plan should reflect consideration of physical, cognitive, social and emotional factors. Even poor vision and limited hearing may alter aspects of treatment decisions and must also play a vital role in the care plan. Older persons place high value on the ability to function in their social roles and the ability to participate in daily activities. Many of the cancer-specific performance status assessments do not fully recognize cognitive factors, activities of daily life (ADL), and instrumental activities of daily life (IADL) or quality of life. Quality of life is a critical concern to the treatment decisions and treatment plan. Optimal outcomes for the patient must extend beyond disease free survival and include continued function and quality of life with a minimum of late effects.[14]

If health care professionals' understanding of prognosis (expected survival) and of the potential outcomes of therapy is ignored, patients may receive treatments inconsistent with their preferences.[15]

Co-morbidity. Co-morbid conditions increase with age and can complicate treatment based on how they may impact cardiac, renal, pulmonary, and hepatic function, possibly reducing life expectancy and increasing resource requirements for older patients with cancer.[16-19] Co-morbidity, disability, frailty, and geriatric syndromes may overlap or occur independently and are integral assessments in the plan of care.[20] Completion of the CGA at diagnosis can document co-morbidity, frailty, and ability together by the clinical variables to organize treatment and can provide markers for observation and follow-up. Consideration of co-morbidity in the plans of care are critical variables for older patients.

Table 68–1. Examples of CGA and potential clinical applications for psychosocial care

Area	Assessment	Measure
Functional Status Activities of daily life(ADL) and Instrumental activities of daily living (IADL)	Relation to life expectancy, functional dependence symptom distress such as weakness, fatigue, pain, vomiting, eating, dressing	ADL, IADL, performance status, use of cane
Co-morbidity Co-morbid conditions	Number of conditions, relation to functional dependence, complexity of care, polypharmacy	Co-morbid indices, e.g., Charleston
Mental status Mental cognitive status	Relation of adherence, decisions, communication, understanding, participation in interventions, delirium	Mini-Mental Status, Folstein Mental Status
Emotional conditions Depression, anxiety	Relation to survival; adherence, participate in interventions, symptom	Geriatric Depression Scale (GDS)
Nutritional status Nutritional assessment	Weight loss, symptom, weakness, functioning, anorexia, vomiting	Weight, Mini-Nutritional Assessment
Geriatric syndromes Delirium, dementia, depression, falls, incontinence	Physical functional dependence, mental health, cognitive status, osteoporosis	Falls, Geriatric Depression Scale

Table 68–2. Assessment areas for older patients

Physical functional status
Psychological health
Polypharmacy
Symptom experience
Social health status and support (income, access to transportation and presence of a caregiver)
Cognitive status
Quality of life
Co-morbidity
Loss
Geriatric syndromes
Patient preferences
Nutritional status
Financial status

THE TREATMENT COURSE

Many of the oncology treatment guidelines are based on clinical trials in which older adults are either underrepresented or absent; thus, we know little about the overall response of the older adult to treatment. The trial data are especially sparse for individuals aged 75 and older. Patients diagnosed with cancer at 70 years and older do not always receive the same cancer treatment as their younger counterparts because of physicians' concerns regarding co-morbidity, toxicity, adverse events, limited life expectancy, and functional status.[15] Treatment recommendations for the older adult range from the standards recommended to younger patients to less intensive variations of standard regimens, to best supportive or palliative care; therefore careful attention and detailed individualized assessment related to cognitive, emotional, physical, and social status is paramount. The usual study endpoints of efficacy and toxicity do not fully address the risks and benefits of therapy for an older adult: Quality of life, psychosocial functioning, and subjective responses may be important outcome considerations.[21] Older cancer patients may view the consequences associated with treatment differently than younger patients.

Because the older individual who is physically, socially, and cognitively fit has a life expectancy exceeding 5 years, consideration for cancer treatment should be given to adjuvant therapy for fit individuals the same as younger patients.[22,23]

Adjuvant chemotherapy has led to improvements in relapse-free and overall survival in older patients with breast, colon, and nonsmall-cell lung cancer and a therapeutic plan of care must be emphasized.[23]

Careful assessments balancing older patients' willingness to tolerate symptoms and late effects of treatment against their current health should be made explicit to patients and families. Aggressive symptom management interventions and treatment of adverse effects need to be introduced promptly. Anemia resulting from treatment has negative effects that may alter the psychosocial functioning. Careful monitoring of hematologic indicators is critical because they can have significant impacts on cognition, fatigue, and functional dependence that compromise health-related quality of life. Compromised function leads to an increased need for family care and hinders support systems to keep patients functioning, moving, and carrying out their daily activities.[24,25]

Psychosocial assessments for the older cancer patient. Psychosocial assessment of patients and their caregivers should include determining the psychological, social, and financial resources. Healthcare professionals should determine the preferences of older cancer patients and respond to their wishes for treatment. Patients deserve to know the probable immediate impact during treatment on their resources as well as possible late effects on their quality of life. Once patients, families, and the health team have established these parameters, progress may begin.

Given that co-morbidity often exists in the older adults and quality of life is a priority, it is important that patients are allowed to make treatment decisions after having received explanations of all reasonable treatment options, including forgoing cancer-specific treatment. Patient and family participation in treatment plan decision making is a necessary consideration; however, the presence of frailty and geriatric syndromes may affect its benefits. Topics important to older cancer patients include symptom management, respite care, discharge planning, survivor issues, and involvement of older children in their care.[26] Each of these areas warrants consideration for the treatment decision, the establishment of the plan of care throughout the care trajectory. To make fully informed decisions, patients require information regarding outcomes, adverse effects, and a description of the usual experience of treatment participation (e.g., frequency and length of procedures, recovery period).[12]

The main elements of the assessment for the older adult with cancer include physical functional status, activities of daily living (ADL), instrumental activities of daily living (IADL), customary roles, gait, balance and risk for falls, co-morbidity, mental status (depression, anxiety), and cognitive status. In addition, screening assessment should include questions relevant to older adults, such as quality of life, self-rated health, sleep, pain, social resources, financial stability, caregivers' availability, and social support systems.[11,27] The prevention of poor nutritional status, weight loss, and sarcopenia should be assured for those in treatment, especially with chemotherapy in which mucositis or anorexia may occur.[28] Asking questions about oral and dental status may point out problems. These assessments can detect unaddressed problems so professionals may recommend interventions to make treatment decisions, provide guidance for clinical evaluation to improve care management, and facilitate survival.[29,30] Providers then catalogue the person's resources and strengths, assess the need for services, and develop a coordinate care plan.[12,31,32]

PLAN OF CARE

An interdisciplinary team of health professionals versed in primary care, gerontology, and oncology should be involved in designing and implementing care plans. From the assessment summary, the cancer patient may be classified as healthy, vulnerable, or frail. It is important to determine which older patients can benefit from cancer treatment and which patients may benefit more from supportive or palliative care.

Cancer care and primary care professionals must listen, discuss, and realize what individuals are feeling about their decisions and what is happening during treatment, rather than simply provide information about medications or other treatments.[33] Older patients wish to receive more individualized, or caring communication, instead of cold facts about treatment plans or about medications for their side effects, making the shared-care plan optimal for a positive patient–provider relationship.

Older patients may assume a *passive* role in the treatment decision making, while some may favor an *active* role or collaborative role.[34,35] They may want to discuss their options with their primary care providers. Preference for a passive role in treatment decisions may be more common among older female patients who have less education, poorer performance status, or more co-morbid illness.[15,34] Care demands concordance of physician perception of patient preference for prognostic information.[15] Active communication and interaction about preferences may help healthcare professionals identify which patients will benefit most from shared decision making and may assist patients in achieving their desired roles in the process. Patients must be encouraged to actively participate in communication about their care as higher physical functioning and social functioning has been documented with those who are actively involved.[35–37] We next identify major areas of concern for care, including physical function, psychological health and loss, polypharmacy, symptom experience, social health, cognitive status, and quality of life. Following these sections, intervention strategies will be presented.

Physical function. Older cancer survivors may suffer from greater impairment in physical function and health-related quality of life than their younger counterparts may.[11,38,39] Older patients are more likely to require assistance with function, and professionals must identify and assess existing physical function before treatment.

The effects of cancer on physical function, especially with advanced age, may be due to age-related co-morbid illness.[40] *Karnofsky* performance status (KPS) and *Eastern Cooperative Oncology Group* (ECOG) Performance Status, which are common performance status measures for cancer treatment, do not specifically address ADL or IADL, the independent predictors of morbidity and mortality in the older patient, and function assessment should go beyond the traditional cancer-specific performance measures.[12,41,42] The need for functional assistance may persist in older cancer survivors for years after a cancer diagnosis due to lack of return to previous functional state as a result of fatigue, weakness, pain, or peripheral neuropathy.[43] In addition, osteoarthritis, neuropathy, and osteoporosis, common in older patients, may aggravate functionality. Rehabilitation to return to precancer functional status is an integral consideration as part of the treatment and care plan. Poor physical functioning becomes increasingly important because of its association with negative therapeutic outcomes.[44]

When clinicians are aware of the functional performance change, potential or existing, they can collaborate with the older adult to identify preferences and select appropriate treatment plans, rehabilitation, and home care to reduce the impact of negative functional performance. Patients with physical function disability need environmental support.

Psychological health and loss. Several psychological health problems may occur in the older adult with cancer. The most frequent are anxiety, depression, and loss.[45,46] Depression is not automatic with growing old, but the multiple losses older adults endure in physical, emotional, social, and family areas may worsen with a cancer diagnosis. Premorbid depression history should be assessed upon the cancer diagnosis and established treatment plan. Risks for depression among older adults include severe co-morbidity, lack of financial resources, loss of spouse, functional disability, inadequate emotional support, uncontrolled pain, poor physical condition, medications, advanced disease, previous depression, and other previous life losses. Healthcare professionals must ensure the availability of resources and support for those at risk for depression. Higher levels of symptom severity, lower levels of prior physical functioning, and greater physical functioning deficits that occur with treatment have predicted higher levels of depressive symptoms (depression is a treatable condition and is an essential component of a plan of care).[47] Depression in older adults is associated with increased risk for postoperative morbidity, posttreatment disability, mortality, increased resource requirements, and needs for family caregivers during the treatment phase.[11,48,49]

Although not all cancer patients are depressed, most patients have periods of distress at the crisis points of illness, such as diagnosis, recurrence, treatment failure, and transition from curative to palliative care, and healthcare professionals must identify and manage these periods.

Anxiety is another mental health condition common among older cancer patients. The diagnosis, medication side effects, and unmanaged symptoms, especially pain, can result in anxiety. Patients with situational anxiety may overreact, be unable to comprehend information, and may have physical symptoms such as agitation, diarrhea, or tachycardia. Professionals need to determine the presence of anxiety, explore patients' fears and concerns, and prescribe needed medications. Strategies to reduce uncertainty and to acknowledge patient concerns are necessities; supportive expressive therapy is a preferred approach to lessening anxiety symptoms and improving overall patient coping.

Losses, including functional control, relationship, and energy loss, often affect quality of life for the older cancer patient and are crucial issues possibly exacerbating depression and anxiety.[50] During treatment, restrictions may impose functional loss from the limitations in activity due to risks of neutropenia, or limited household chores that result from fatigue. The loss of favorite activities and independence, and the perceived burden of care resulting from those losses, are common areas of concern. Functional decline, or losses in function due to cancer or cancer treatment, may be associated with decreased independence and a challenge to effective coping with the treatment.[51] The issue of being a burden to family members may also be an important concern; for some individuals, the perception and fear of being a burden is more significant than the loss of the activity or function itself.

Among older cancer patients, diagnoses generate fears of death, dependency, disfigurement, pain, disability, and loss of relationships.[52] Each of these has particular meaning in the context of retirement, widowhood, and other medical disabilities and losses.[53]

Polypharmacy. Polypharmacy is present often in the older patient and can ultimately affect treatment tolerance and outcomes. There is a three-fold more use of medication in the older person compared to younger patients because co-morbid illnesses exist. A review of the patient's medication list must be a part of the assessment and recognition of situations can lead to prevention. Some recommend the " brown bag" approach where patients bring in all their medications for health professionals to review so that polypharmacy can be prevented. Older patients are more vulnerable to adverse drug events and an adverse reaction can lead to polypharmacy when it is misinterpreted as a new medical condition. Off protocol dietary supplements or minerals need to be reviewed with the patients as well. In addition to adverse events, the high rate of side effects may lead to poor quality of life. Risk rises with number of drugs. Contributing to the risk of adverse events are the changes in pharmacokinetics and pharmacodynamics that occur with aging. These factors have to be considered for patients receiving chemotherapy.[54]

Symptom experience. Older patients experience cancer-related symptoms from the disease, from its treatment, and from co-morbid conditions. Often, older adults may underreport symptoms and side effects from cancer treatment or may report them after they become more severe. Studies about older cancer patients have indicated a high prevalence of pain, fatigue, weakness, dry skin, pruritus, dyspnea, delirium, cough, nausea, vomiting, depression, and anxiety.[55] Symptom management in the older adult requires an interdisciplinary approach to optimize planning, management, and outcomes.[56]

Older adults may be less likely to report pain, resulting in undertreated ailments.[57,58] The ability of the patient to express pain may be impaired by cognitive decline. Uncontrolled pain in the older adult can lead to anorexia, nausea, insomnia, and fatigue. Compounding the under treatment of pain, the pharmacokinetics analgesics, including opioids may be a problem for the patient, causing adverse events such as constipation, neurotoxicity, or respiratory depression. The careful assessment of need and response to pain management is essential to quality care.

Clinicians need to understand the complexity involved in vulnerability, immobility, confusion, and bowel and bladder elimination among the older patient being treated for cancer. Patient perception declines with age, and co-morbidity interferes with treatment. Symptom expression may not be a reliable factor; but symptom distress has been identified as the strongest predictor of poor physical and mental functions in older cancer patients.[59] Using strategies to try to discern accurately the symptoms and the etiology of the symptoms so that they can be controlled and managed appropriately.

Social health (personal and social resources). Social support resources are integral to an older cancer patient's life, often acting as a buffer against the psychological impacts of cancer treatment. Living alone, for example, may pose challenges to effective cancer treatment.[60] Older adults may have fewer social resources, less resilience, loss of social relationships such as widowhood, and declining adaptability. Many older adults are on a fixed income with limited financial resources.[30,61] Professionals must assess the availability of support resources as part of the care plan's development. More psychosocial resources including optimism, mastery, and spirituality may result in better patient outcomes.[30,62] Social isolation can impact overall psychological well-being and may limit favorite activities of older adults. Providers also need to assess socioeconomic environment, familial context, social network, patient preference, organization of care—including the family.[63] Older cancer adults may need home care during or following treatment and during the immediate postrecovery period.

Cognitive status. Determining cognitive status in an older patient with cancer is an important element of a care plan. Cognitive dysfunction affects the ability of patients to determine the risks and benefits of cancer therapy and may affect decision making. Cognitive and communicative changes alter interactive ability, understanding as they confront a cancer diagnosis and treatment, and the ability to make decisions.[37] Cognitive changes may affect the ability to adhere to the treatment plan and recognize the signs of chemotoxicity. Toxic effects such as dehydration, malnutrition, and electrolyte imbalance can increase the risk of delirium or cognitive decline in the older patient. With the frequent use of oral chemotherapy agents, cognitive assessment will determine whether the patient has the capacity for decision making and judgment to consent and subsequently follow oral medication instructions. Oral agents require patients to follow complex dosing, recognize signs of toxicity, and seek help in response to early complications. If the patient takes an incorrect number of pills, the treatment could result in serious adverse events or be ineffective and nontherapeutic.

New cognitive deficits could imply metastatic brain disease. Length of survival of cognitively impaired patients even with similar treatments was about a third of that of nonimpaired patients.[11] Coping with cognitive decline, therefore, must be a priority[64] consideration for assessment and planning interventions.

Quality of life. Cancer-related variables, for example, treatment, including duration of survival and type of cancer treatment, may not be significantly associated with survivors' well-being and predictors of self-rated health.[65–67] The ability to function, to do what is important to

Table 68–3. NCCN senior adult oncology practice guidelines

Screening and assessment		
Specific issues related to age		
Neurotoxicity	Bone Marrow	Renal
Cardiac	Diarrhea	Mucositis
	Anorexia	
Comprehensive geriatric assessment		
Criteria to define frailty (weight, exhaustion, physical activity, work time, grip strength)		
Procedure for functional assessment		
Vulnerable elderly survey		
Disease specific issues related to age		

NCCN Clinical Practice Guidelines In Oncology. *Senior Adult Oncology.* Fort Washington, PA: National Comprehensive Cancer Network; 2007.

them daily, and to cope with changes and symptom control may be more significant.

Perkins[30] indicates that psychosocial coping variables will be associated with higher levels of life satisfaction and general health perception and lower levels of depression, after controlling for demographic, cancer-related, and health status variables. Lower fatigue and higher physical functioning predict higher life satisfaction and high levels of mastery, spirituality, and optimism also predict high levels of life satisfaction. Lower levels of social support, optimism, and spirituality predict higher levels of depression. Intervention studies enhancing optimism and mastery must be developed and implemented to assess evidence-based outcomes for future psychological adjustment and treatment outcomes for older adults.[30]

Intervention strategies. Recognizing older adults who appear stable and functional but have limited ability to recover due to limited resources and from the stressors associated with cancer treatment may be extremely helpful in tailoring treatment plans.[12,17] The assessment information collected by an interdisciplinary team should establish goals of care and direct cancer-specific and symptom-specific treatment in light of co-morbidities, functional status, and psychological and social resources.

There are numerous successful psychosocial interventions for symptom management.[68–71] For the older adult, this includes the coordination and follow-up care with supportive resources, and these needs should be shared with primary care providers from the beginning. An interdisciplinary assessment approach such as the CGA is essential through the diagnostic, treatment, follow-up, and survival period.[10]

Lack of systematic referral of older persons to major cancer treatment centers may lead to inadequate diagnosis and treatment but when cancer-specific treatment ends it is critical to include the primary care provider.

National Comprehensive Cancer Network (NCCN) guidelines exist for the older adult and represent an attempt to formalize an approach specific to those with cancer. See Table 68–3 for items from the NCCN Guidelines.

We need to determine for which patients these treatment protocols are acceptable and for which patients they are not. Under these circumstances, older patients and their families need to be informed of the risks and potential benefits from treatment. Patients need to be actively engaged in making treatment decisions. When treatment is not recommended, patients and their families should be provided with the best guidance and support to receive maximum benefit from palliation. Primary care professionals should be participants in the plan of care. Supportive interventions are important for those needing palliative care but that focus is beyond the scope of this paper. (See Chapters 38 and 39.)

Managing the cancer care of older patients and their families will enable more patients to participate in active treatment and maintain their quality of life. As cancer therapy becomes more effective and as the number of older persons who participate in cancer treatment—outcomes such as quality will become even more important. We need to be ready to provide this care.

REFERENCES

1. Yancik R, Ries LA. Cancer in older persons: an international issue in an aging world. *Semin Oncol.* 2004;3:128–136.

2. Cova D, Balducci L. Cancer chemotherapy in the older patient. In: Balducci L, Ershler WB, Layman Newark GH, (eds). *Comprehensive geriatric oncology.* London and New York: Taylor & Francis; 2004:463–488.

3. Hamerman D. Frailty, cancer cachexia and near death. In: Balducci L, Ershler WB, Layman Newark GH, (eds). *Comprehensive geriatric oncology.* London and New York: Taylor & Francis; 2004:223–235.

4. Kinney JM. Nutritional frailty, sarcopenia and falls in the elderly. *Curr Opin Clin Nutr Metabol Care.* 2004;7:15–20.

5. Vantallia TB. Frailty in the elderly: contribution of sarcopenia and visceral protein depletion. *Metabolism.* 2003;52(10, Suppl 2):22–26.

6. DiFiore F, Lecleire S, Rigal O, et al. Predictive factors of survival in patients treated with definitive chemoradiotherapy for squamous cell esophageal carcinoma. *World J Gastroenterol.* 2006;12:4185–4190.

7. Kastritis E, Bamias A, Bozas G, et al. The impact of age in the outcome of patients with advanced or recurrent cervical cancer after platinum-based chemotherapy. *Gynecol Oncol.* 2007;104:372–376.

8. Gomez H, Mas L, Casanova L, et al. Elderly patients with aggressive non-Hodgkin's lymphoma treated with CHOP chemotherapy plus granulocyte-macrophage colony-stimulating factor: identification of two age subgroups with differing hematologic toxicity. *J Clin Oncol.* 1998;16:2352–2358.

9. Cohen HJ. The cancer aging interface: a research agenda. *J Clin Oncol.* 2007;25:1945–1948.

10. Extermann M, Hurria A. Comprehensive geriatric assessment for older patients with cancer. *J Clin Oncol.* 2007;25:1824–1831.

11. White HK, Cohen HJ. The older cancer patient. *Med Clin N Am.* 2006;90:967–982.

12. Bernabei R, Venturiero V, Tarsitani P, Gambassi G. The comprehensive geriatric assessment: when, where, how. *Crit Rev Oncol Hematol.* 2000;33:45–56.

13. Azziz N. Late effects of cancer treatments. In P Ganz, (ed). *Cancer survivorship today and tomorrow.* New York: Springer; 2007:54–76.

14. Elkin EB, Kim SHM, Casper ES, Kissane DW, Schrag D. Desire for information and involvement in treatment decisions: elderly cancer patients' preferences and their physicians' perceptions. *J Clin Oncol.* 2007;25:5275–5280.

15. Extermann M, Balducci L, Lyman GH. What threshold for adjuvant therapy in older breast cancer patients? *J Clin Oncol.* 2000;18:1709–1717.

16. Ferrucci L, Guralnik JM, Cavazzini C, et al. The frailty syndrome: a critical issue in geriatric oncology. *Crit Rev Oncol Hematol.* 2003;46:127–137.

17. Firat S, Bousamra M, Gore E, Byhardt RW. Comorbidity and KPS are independent prognostic factors in stage I non-small-cell-lung cancer. *Int J Radiat Oncol Biol Phys.* 2002;52:1047–1057.

18. Piccirillo JF, Tierney RM, Costas I, Grove L, Spitznagel EL Jr. Prognostic importance of comorbidity in a hospital-based cancer registry. *JAMA.* 2004;291:2441–2447.

19. Koroukian SM, Murray P, Madigan E. Comorbidity, disability, and geriatric syndromes in elderly cancer patients receiving home health care. *J Clin Oncol.* 2006;24:2304–2310.

20. Hurria A, Lichtman SM, Gardes J, et al. Identifying vulnerable older adults with cancer: integrating geriatric assessment into oncology practice. *J Am Geriatr Soc.* 2007;55:1604–1608.

21. Gridelli C, Maione P, Rossi A. Treatment of stage I-III non-small-cell lung cancer in the elderly. *Oncology (Williston Park).* 2006;20:373–380.

22. Muss HB, Biganzoli L, Sargent DJ, Aapro M. Adjuvant therapy in the elderly: making the right decision. *J Clin Oncol.* 2007;25:1870–1875.

23. Denny SD, Kuchibhatla MN, Cohen HJ. Impact of anemia on mortality, cognition, and function in community-dwelling elderly. *Am J Med.* 2006;119:327–334.

24. Inzitari M, Carlo A, Baldereschi M, et al. ILSA Working Group. Risk and predictors of motor-performance decline in a normally functioning population-based sample of elderly subjects: the Italian longitudinal study on aging. *J Am Geriatr Soc.* 2006;54:318–324.

25. Penninx PW, Pahor M, Cesari M, et al. Anemia is associated with disability and decreased physical performance and muscle strength in the elderly. *J Am Geriatr Soc.* 2004;52:719–724.

26. Lewis M, Pearson V, Corcoran-Perry S, Narayan S. Decision making by elderly patients with cancer and their caregivers. *Cancer Nurs.* 1997;20:389–397.

27. Extermann M. Approach to the newly diagnosed colorectal cancer patient: special considerations-colorectal cancer in the elderly patient: assessment and treatment. In: S Lichtman, (ed). *CMP healthcare media.* New York: Oncology Publisher Group; 2005:1–10.

28. Bozzetti F. Nutritional issues in the care of the elderly patient. *Crit Rev Oncol Hematol.* 2003;48:113–121.

29. Extermann M, Aapro M, Bernabei R, et al. Task Force on CGA of the International Society of Geriatric Oncology. Use of comprehensive geriatric assessment in older cancer patients: recommendations from the task force on CGA of the International Society of Geriatric Oncology (SIOG). *Crit Rev Oncol Hematol.* 2005;55:241–252.

30. Perkins EA, Small BJ, Balducci L, Extermann M, Robb C, Haley WE. Individual differences in well-being in older breast cancer survivors. *Crit Rev Oncol Hematol.* 2007;62:74–83.

31. Fried LP, Tangen CM, Walston J, et al. Cardiovascular Health Study Collaborative Research Group. Frailty in older adults: evidence for a phenotype. *J Gerontol A Biol Sci Med Sci.* 2001;56:M146-M156.

32. Solomon D, Brown AD, Brummel-Smith K, et al. National Institutes of Health Consensus Development Conference Development Conference Statement: geriatric assessment methods for clinical decision-making. *J Am Geriatr Soc.* 1988;36:342–347.

33. Skalla KA, Bakitas M, Furstenberg CT, Ahles T, Henderson JV. Patients' need for information about cancer therapy. *Oncol Nurs Forum.* 2004;31:313–319.

34. Hack TF, Degner LF, Parker PA, SCRN Communication Team. The communication goals and needs of cancer patients: a review. *Psychooncology.* 2005;14:831–845.

35. Hack TF, Degner LF, Watson P, Sinha L. Do patients benefit from participating in medical decision making? Longitudinal follow-up of women with breast cancer. *Psychooncology.* 2006;15:9–19.

36. Davison BJ, Goldenberg SL, Gleave ME, Degner LF. Provision of individualized information to men and their partners to facilitate treatment decision making in prostate cancer. *Oncol Nurs Forum.* 2003;30:107–114.

37. Sparks L, Nussbaum JF. Health literacy and cancer communication with older adults. *Patient Educ Couns.* 2008;71:345–350.

38. Arndt V, Merx H, Sturmer T, Stegmaier C, Ziegler H, Brenner H. Age-specific detriments to quality of life among breast cancer patients one year after diagnosis. *Eur J Cancer.* 2004;40:673–680.

39. Cimprich B, Ronis DL, Martinez-Rasmos G. Age at diagnosis and quality of life in breast cancer survivors. *Cancer Pract.* 2002;10:85–93.

40. Robb C, Haley WE, Balducci L, et al. Impact of breast cancer survivorship on quality of life in older women. *Crit Rev Oncol Hematol.* 2007;62:84–91.

41. Extermann M, Overcash J, Lyman GH, Parr J, Balducci L. Comorbidity and functional status are independent in older cancer patients. *J Clin Oncol.* 1998;16:1582–1587.

42. Repetto L, Fratino L, Audisio RA, et al. Comprehensive geriatric assessment adds information to Eastern Cooperative Oncology Group performance status in elderly cancer patients: an Italian group for geriatric oncology study. *J Clin Oncol,* 2002;20:494–502.

43. Keating NL, Norredam M, Landrum MB, Huskamp HA, Meara E. Physical and mental health status of older long-term cancer survivors. *J Am Geriatr Soc.* 2005;53:2145–2152.

44. Chen H, Cantor A, Meyer J, et al. Can older cancer patients tolerate chemotherapy? A prospective pilot study. *Cancer.* 2003;97:1107–1114.

45. Miovic M, Block S. Psychiatric disorders in advanced cancer. *Cancer.* 2007;110:1665–1676.

46. Roth AJ, Modi R. Psychiatric issues in older cancer patients. *Crit Rev Oncol Hematol.* 2003;48:185–197.

47. Kurtz ME, Kurtz JC, Stommel M, Given CW, Given B. Physical functioning and depression among older persons with cancer. *Cancer Pract.* 2001;9:11–18.

48. Audisio RA, Ramesh H, Longo WE, Zbar AB, Pope D. Preoperative assessment of surgical risk on oncogeriatric patients. *Oncologist.* 2005;10:262–268.

49. Langa KM, Valenstein MA, Fendrick AM, Kabeto MU, Vijan S. Extent and cost of informal caregiving for older Americans with symptoms of depression. *Am J Psychiatry.* 2004;161:857–863.

50. Wallberg B, Michelson H, Nystedt M. The meaning of breast cancer. *Acta Oncol.* 2003;42:30–35.

51. Gignac MA, Cott C, Badley EM. Adaptation to chronic illness and disability and its relationship to perceptions of independence and dependence. *J Gerontol B Psychol Sci Soc Sci.* 2000;55B:362–372.

52. Holland JC, Rowland J, Lebovits A, Rusalem R. Reactions to cancer treatment: assessment of emotional response to adjunct radiotherapy. *Psychiatr Clin North Am.* 1979;2:347–358.

53. Holland JC. Psychological aspects of cancer. In: Holland JF, Frei E, (eds). *Cancer medicine.* 2nd ed. Philadelphia, PA: Lea & Febiger; 1982:1175–1203.

54. Tam-McDevitt J. Polypharmacy, aging, and cancer. *Oncology (Williston Park).* 2008;22:1052–1060.

55. Rao A, Cohen HJ. Symptom management in the elderly cancer patient: fatigue, pain, and depression. *J Natl Cancer Inst Monogr.* 2004;32:150–157.

56. Bernabei R, Gambassi G, Lapane K, et al. Management of pain in elderly patients with cancer. SAGE Study Group. Systematic assessment of geriatric drug use via epidemiology. *JAMA.* 1998;279:1877–1882.

57. Balducci L. Management of cancer pain in geriatric patients. *J Support Oncol.* 2003;1:175–191.

58. Carreca I, Balducci L, Extermann M. Cancer in the older person. *Cancer Treat Rev.* 2005;31:380–402.

59. Kurtz, ME, Kurtz JC, Stommel M, Given CW, Given B. The influence of symptoms, age, comorbidity and cancer site on physical functioning and mental health of geriatric women patients. *Women Health.* 1999;29:1–12.

60. Bouchardy C, Rapiti E, Fioretta G, et al. Undertreatment strongly decreases prognosis of breast cancer in elderly women. *J Clin Oncol.* 2003;21:3580–3587.

61. Sammarco A. Quality of life among older survivors of breast cancer. *Cancer Nurs.* 2003;26:431–438.

62. Zeiss AM, Lewinsohn PM, Rohde P, Seeley JR. Relationship of physical disease and functional impairment to depression in older people. *Psychol Aging.* 1996;11:572–581.

63. Bouchardy C, Rapiti E, Blagojevic S, Vlastos AT, Vlastos G. Older female cancer patients: importance, causes, and consequences of undertreatment. *J Clin Oncol.* 2007;25:1858–1869.

64. Hurria A, Goldfarb S, Rosen C, et al. Effect of adjuvant breast cancer chemotherapy on cognitive function from the older patient's perspective. *Breast Cancer Res Treat.* 2006;98:343–348.

65. Dorval M, Maunsell E, Deschenes L, Brisson J. Type of mastectomy and quality of life for long term breast carcinoma survivors. *Cancer.* 1998;83:2130–2138.

66. Ganz PA, Guadagnoli E, Landrum MB, Lash TL, Rakowski W, Silliman RA. Breast cancer in older women: quality of life and psychosocial adjustment in the 15 months after diagnosis. *J Clin Oncol.* 2003;21:4027–4033.

67. Mandelblatt JS, Edge SB, Meropol NJ, et al. Predictors of long-term outcomes in older breast cancer survivors: perceptions versus patterns of care. *J Clin Oncol.* 2003;21:855–863.

68. Sikorskii A, Given C, Given B, Jeon S, McCorkle R. Testing the effects of treatment complications on a cognitive-behavioral intervention for reducing symptom severity. *J Pain Symptom Manage.* 2006;32:129–139.

69. Sikorskii A, Given CW, Given B, et al. Symptom management for cancer patients: a trial comparing two multimodal interventions. *J Pain Symptom Manage.* 2007;34:253–264.

70. McCorkle R, Strumpf NE, Nuamah IF, et al. A specialized home care intervention improves survival among older post-surgical cancer patients. *J Am Geriatr Soc.* 2000;48:1707–1713.

71. McCorkle R, Dowd M, Ercolano E, et al. Effects of a nursing intervention on quality of life outcomes in post-surgical women with gynecological cancers. *Psychooncology.* 2009;18:62–70.

Adolescent and Young Adult Patients

Sheila J. Santacroce and Brad J. Zebrack

Adolescent and young adult (AYA) patients have characteristics that distinguish them from children and youth, and also from more mature adults, most notably in the psychosocial sphere. Not only can usual psychological and social trajectories and their outcomes be adversely affected by cancer and its treatment, but also usual development has the potential to unfavorably affect cancer therapy. Thus, AYA patients merit special attention from psycho-oncologists as a potential means to support medical treatment, psychosocial adaptation, and best possible outcomes in all domains. In this chapter, firstly we define the AYA population and describe its prominent developmental characteristics and inherent challenges. Second, we summarize trends in the epidemiology, etiology, and prognosis of cancer in this population. Third, we discuss issues specific to AYA patients. Fourth, we tell about prevalent psychosocial effects of cancer for AYA patients and provide guidance about assessment, information, and intervention. Throughout, lacking a body of evidence, we offer recommendations about what we see as constituting reasonable psycho-oncology care for this special population.

DEFINING AND DESCRIBING THE POPULATION

Most investigations of AYAs and cancer have focused on survivors of pediatric malignancy. While these studies variably define the AYA population, developmental theories can provide a rationale for assigning an age range. The late teenage years to mid-20s represent a period of "emerging adulthood,"[1] with the transition from adolescence to adulthood occurring by age 20.[2] In some instances, age 30 years serves as an upper boundary for "young adult."[2] The National Cancer Institute (NCI)[3] recently extended the range to include 15–39 year olds, based on the Surveillance, Epidemiology, and End Results (SEER) program data showing that people in this age range have not shared in the improvements in cancer mortality and survival that have been experienced by other patients.[4] For this review, the AYA age range was considered to be 15–39 years, excepting some epidemiological data which is reported in the literature.

According to Arnett: "Having left the dependency of childhood and adolescence, and having not yet entered the enduring responsibilities that are normative in adulthood, emerging adults often explore a variety of possible life directions in love, work, and worldview" (p.469).[1] In reviewing developmental tasks of young adults, Rowland[2] suggests that the transition from adolescence to young adulthood is marked by maturation. Intellectually AYAs can be egocentric about the origin of ideas, believing that they are the first to experience profound feelings or see the world's complexities. One task of this period is to curb egocentric tendencies. Communication skills peak by the end of the phase. Most individuals complete their formal education, undertake jobs consonant with goals, and map plans for advancement. Meanwhile, large numbers of young adults delay marriage and child bearing and some return to the parental home while exploring careers.[5] Postponements can be more likely when cancer occurs.

EPIDEMIOLOGY OF ADOLESCENT AND YOUNG ADULT CANCER

Cancer is the leading cause of death from disease for AYAs in the United States.[4] For females 20–39 years of age, cancer occurs nearly twice as often as death from heart disease which is the second leading cause of disease-related death for this group.[6] Overall, cancer incidence increases

with age and, thus, cancer is considered a disease of aging and the aged. Cancer incidence, however, peaks during the first 5 years of life. A second peak occurs during adolescence and early adulthood, most prominently in males.[7] About five times as many people are diagnosed with cancer during the second 20 years of life as are during the first 20. Approximately two-thirds of these individuals are diagnosed between ages 30–39 years, which is consistent with an increase in incidence as a function of age. Non-Hispanic whites have the highest incidence of cancer between ages 15–29 years.[4]

The types of malignancies that occur in AYA differ from those occurring in pediatric and older adult populations. In 15–29 year olds, lymphomas predominate with Hodgkin's lymphoma accounting for 12% of all cases in the age group.[8] Other prevalent cancers include melanoma, testes and female genital tract malignancies, thyroid cancer, soft tissue sarcomas, leukemia, central nervous system (CNS) malignancy, and breast cancer.[4]

For AYAs, cancer mortality is higher in males than for females even when accounting for incidence. Generally, cancer death rates follow incidence by ethnicity and race, except for 15–40 year old African-Americans/Blacks who have the highest death rate relative to incidence by race/ethnicity.[4] Although between 1975 and 2000 cancer mortality rates declined overall, 20–44 year olds had less improvement in mortality than younger and older people with cancer; the least improvement in mortality was seen in AYA African-American/Blacks.[4]

Development of cancer in AYAs seems unpredictable. Less than 5% of cancers in 15–29 year olds have been attributed to a family cancer syndrome.[9] In contrast to older adults, substantial exposures to known carcinogens by 15–29 years of age are rare. Notable exceptions include exposures to chemotherapy and/or radiotherapy during treatment for childhood cancer as a factor in the development of subsequent malignancy,[10] and exposure to human papilloma virus (HPV) as a factor in the development of uterine and cervical carcinoma.[11] However, not everyone with these exposures develops malignancy. As knowledge of genetics develops, we may better understand individual and environmental factors, and the interplay between them, that can lead to the development of cancer in AYAs.

SPECIAL ISSUES AND CONSIDERATIONS

Accessing care and obtaining a diagnosis. Cancer symptoms in AYAs can be nonspecific. Heightened patient and provider awareness of the peak in cancer incidence in this age group and information about the cancers that tend to occur is essential to timely medical care, appropriate evaluation, and accurate diagnosis. Delay in diagnosis and treatment may adversely affect survival and undermine trust in health professionals. On the basis of data about children with cancer,[12] diagnosis delays for AYAs may be related to person and healthcare factors.

Characteristic developmental features can lead AYAs to view themselves as invulnerable to cancer or the consequences of risky health behaviors that include lack of regular healthcare and/or not following medical recommendations. With normative increases in cognitive abilities, a central task for AYAs is becoming independent in functioning, including in health self-management. In pursuing independence, AYAs may not consult parents about symptoms of a change in their health yet be unclear how to access care on their own or clearly present their symptoms and concerns to health professionals. More so than children, AYAs are likely to lack a regular primary care provider and also have the lowest rates of primary care of any age group perhaps because they have the highest lifetime rates of being under- or uninsured.[13]

When AYAs seek healthcare, physicians tend to spend significantly less time with them than with older adults.[13] Noteworthy symptoms may not resonate with protem health professionals who are unfamiliar with the patient's usual state and may not have access to an established medical record. Nononcology health professionals can lack awareness of the prevalence of cancer in AYAs and assign symptoms to stress or fatigue/depression without considering the possibility of cancer. When cancer does come to mind, fear and misinformation or lack of information about prognosis, possible treatments and treatment centers, including centers that can offer access to clinical trials, can impede diagnosis-referral and initiation of therapy.

Treatment. The goal of treatment for cancer in AYAs is long-term cure with minimal adverse effects.[14] Two core issues exist with regards to achieving this goal: (1) what treatment approach and care setting should be used, and (2) enrollment in clinical trials.

Approach and setting. Common AYA malignancies like the lymphomas also occur during childhood[7] and are within the scope of pediatric oncology. Pediatric oncologists tend to use intensive multimodal treatment regimens. This treatment is typically centralized at tertiary care centers, uses a multidisciplinary approach and includes supportive care that aims to address developmental, psychosocial, and quality of life aspects of the cancer experience. Parents are key team members and communications about their child's condition and treatment are conducted mainly with them. Visiting hours are unrestricted and sleeping accommodations and other provisions are made for parents in or near the child's hospital room. Conversely, some AYA malignancies are more typically seen in adults and fall within the scope of adult oncology. Much adult cancer care is delivered in the community and while community oncologists can have expertise with particular malignancies, their practice isn't usually conducted in the context of a multidisciplinary team. Further, adult oncology care is directed at the patient who is deemed autonomous in decision making and ongoing care.

While each approach has valuable features, neither is ideal for AYAs. The developmental perspective that characterizes pediatrics focuses on infant, child, and younger adolescents. Environments and policies created with the 0–14 year old in mind are not suited to AYAs. Because pediatric providers usually communicate with parents, AYAs may be sidelined in decision making and become dependent in ongoing care. Adolescents can be appalled at the idea of sleeping in a room with their parent, preferring the company of friends. In contrast, adult health professionals may treat 15–39 year olds exclusive of parents or other potential sources of tangible assistance and emotional support. Clinical experience suggests that AYAs can be upset by hospitalization among older adults especially those with dementia. In Australia and the United Kingdom, specialized units for AYAs have instituted developmentally-based policies such as late morning wake-ups, open visiting hours, and recreation space geared toward AYA interests, and opportunities to interact with same-age peers.[15,16]

Lacking other evidence about where AYAs are best treated, treatment approach and setting decisions should be guided by what will likely provide the patient with the best outcomes.[17] On the basis of data that shows better treatment outcomes for pediatric versus adult protocols in terms of complete remission and event-free survival for AYAs with acute lymphoblastic leukemia, some suggest that treatment should be guided by disease biology, not patient age, and rigorously managed by experienced oncology health professionals at major cancer centers according to collaborative clinical trials to maximize individual outcomes and establish efficacious cancer treatments for AYAs.[18]

Enrollment in clinical trials. Pediatric and adult settings can each lack opportunities for AYA enrollment in clinical trials. In the United States, approximately 71% of 0–14 year olds with cancer are enrolled with the national clinical trials group,[19] and much of the improvement that has been made in survival rates for children has been attributed to

clinical trials. In contrast, 10%–15% of 15–19 year olds and approximately 2% of 20–29 year olds with cancer are enrolled in such trials.[20] While disparities in clinical trial participation for 20–29 year olds are similar across racial and ethnic groups, disparity in male participation stands out.[21] One assumption is that the absence of improvement in survival for AYAs relates to the low rate of participation in trials.[21,22]

Clinical trials can indirectly and directly benefit participants. Trials can offer opportunities to be in research that may improve medical care and outcomes for future patients, and entail close clinical monitoring which may improve the participants' cancer experience. Generally, potential improvements on standard treatment can only be accessed via clinical trial and, thus, some participants may directly experience better outcomes as a result of being assigned to the innovative treatment condition.[23]

The same factors that can delay diagnosis can be potential barriers to enrolling AYAs in clinical trials.[22] Moreover, community primary care and specialty professionals may not know about opportunities for participation in clinical trials or prefer to retain AYA patients rather than refer them to a clinical trials group member institution. Some health professionals may view cancer as challenging enough for AYAs and not want to add the responsibilities entailed in clinical trial participation. Given their developmental characteristics AYAs can be assumed to be at risk for suboptimal adherence. Health professionals can hesitate to commit the time and effort needed to assure that AYAs understand what a trial involves and then support ongoing adherence.[23,24]

Communication and decision making. Communication and decision making for AYA patients can be sensitive issues. Some AYAs prefer to be shielded from communication about their cancer and potential late effects and/or to assume a dependent position. Others want a prominent or fully independent role. Because wide variability in cognitive capacity normally exists within the AYA population and because cancer, treatments, and associated stressors can impair cognition, the individual's capabilities are important to assess throughout the illness course. In terms of style, AYA patients typically prefer face-to-face healthcare communications that are honest, non-judgmental, respectful, and inclusive of them.[25,26] Given their task of identity formation, AYAs also value talking with health professionals about non-illness aspects of life; such talk can convey recognition that their identity comprises more than patient.[27] Engaging AYAs in communications and decision making lays groundwork for supportive future communications, thus enhancing the likelihood for informed decisions and treatment adherence.[28]

Patients age 18 years or more are considered adults who can provide informed consent. Their parents are deemed to have no rights to their child's health information without specific patient agreement. Patients between 15 and 18 years of age should also be engaged in healthcare communications and decision making, and give assent. The assent process includes helping the patient understand the condition; explaining what tests, treatments, and side effects are anticipated; assessing the patient's understanding of what has been explained; and asking the patient to go along with the plan.[29] Most AYAs lack experience to guide communications and decision making regarding cancer and rely heavily on parental support throughout their illness, but some AYAs are completely independent from their parents in healthcare communications, decision making and other functions. In general, parents feel responsible to protect and advocate for their child, no matter their child's age or level of independence, and can struggle with their child and their child's health professionals over information and control of care.[30] Health professionals must determine, as early as feasible, the extent to which AYAs wishes to involve parents in communications and decision making. Health professionals can help AYA patients realize that parental involvement is currently needed at a level that may have been unacceptable under usual conditions, and help parents by offering structured guidance about how to promote individual and family development in the setting of cancer.[27,30] One approach is for the health professional, with patient permission, to give information to the patient first and then, to the extent specified, to parents and patient together.[27] This way offers AYAs repetition of complex and significant information plus opportunities to learn from parent questions, and may also promote development of an open, trusting healthcare relationship between all parties.

Adherence. Treatment adherence is another significant issue for AYAs and their health professionals. Some researchers have proposed that a person must take at least 95% of a prescribed regimen to be considered adherent.[31] The level of adherence necessary to inhibit disease recurrence or progression is unknown.[32] Studies suggest that 10%–59% of AYAs with cancer have suboptimal adherence at some point during treatment,[33] and suboptimal adherence in adolescents with chronic conditions other than cancer has been estimated at about 50%.[34] Factors contributing to suboptimal adherence include cultural and linguistic differences, and poor communications between patients, families and health professionals.[35,36] Adherence can also be adversely affected by AYA developmental features including urges to be like peers and one's former self, concern about side effects that could interfere with normalcy, feeling exempt from the consequences of suboptimal adherence, regression to concrete thinking under stress, and lack of parental involvement.[37]

Health professionals should expect that AYAs will have difficulties with adherence and regularly assess adherence using a non-judgmental, understanding, and hopeful approach.[38] In potentially life-threatening illness, AYAs' prospects for disease control and long-term survival may be enhanced through parental help with obtaining and organizing medications and other treatment aspects, and establishing systems to maximize adherence.[37] However, given their drive for independence, AYAs can be irritated by parental involvement. Health professionals can help AYAs establish acceptable and supportive roles for parents and other concerned individuals with regards to supporting adherence. At diagnosis, AYAs and their parents should be encouraged to discuss their understandings of the disease and its prognosis, treatment goals and beliefs about treatment efficacy, and to define their roles and responsibilities in adherence considering developmental stage and daily routines.[38] Patients should be provided routinely with precise written information about treatment and copies of treatment calendars and road maps; regular reminders via cell phone and other electronic means may also help promote adherence for AYAs.[39,40] Open communications that offer AYAs opportunities to address questions, explore treatment options and feel that they are listened to can also promote treatment adherence.[5,36]

DEVELOPMENTALLY-SPECIFIC EFFECTS OF CANCER ON AYA PATIENTS

Five universal areas of stress and disruption exist for people with cancer: (1) interpersonal relationships, (2) dependence–independence, (3) achievement, (4) body-sexual image and integrity, and (5) existential issues.[2] Nature and extent of stress and disruption people experience in each domain are affected by developmental themes, AYAs being no exception.

Interpersonal relationships. The stress associated with cancer can heighten AYA patients' needs for support from friends.[41] Diagnosis of a friend's cancer can be a source of stress for healthy young people who may respond by avoiding interactions with AYA patients. Isolation and alienation are commonly reported among AYA patients as they miss out on life experiences common to non-ill peers.[42] Self-view is shaped in part by the person's social roles such as student, athlete, or employee. When these roles are lost or changed or attainment delayed due to cancer, alienation from role- and age-peers can occur.[43] In adolescents with cancer, those with low levels of social support and high levels of uncertainty have been shown to have the highest levels of psychological distress.[41] Cancer can deprive AYAs from regular participation in activities normal for the age, including experimentation with sex and other forms of intimacy. AYA adult patients can be challenged in sexual and intimate relationships.[44,45] Some AYAs adjust to cancer-related changes in sexual desire and function without distress. Others feel increased distress including symptoms of depression or anxiety, which in turn can further influence sexual desire and function. The AYA patient may be confused or embarrassed about sexual problems, unaware they may relate to cancer, and hesitate to raise these concerns with health professionals. A main worry for AYA patients is deciding if, when, and how to disclose medical history,[46] struggling with what and how much to say particularly to those with whom long-term intimacy may be desired.

Faced with varied potential reactions, AYAs can lack confidence because they doubt acceptance. Severe loss of opportunities for peer interaction can be experienced as major deprivations that multiply other illness stressors. Affirming peer interactions can ease illness-related stress and renew adaptive capacities. Quality friendships can promote AYAs' social reintegration, deflect criticism and stigma, and reduce feelings of isolation.[47]

Dependence–independence. Seriously ill people can become dependent, at least temporarily. For AYAs, this may involve recommencing dependency on parents. As they negotiate cancer, AYAs can discover that generations within the family use different coping strategies. An important factor in spousal interaction, coping symmetry can also affect child–parent interaction. For example, parents may want to discuss issues that AYAs do not wish to discuss, or vice-versa, perhaps because doing so may evoke long buried feelings. Some AYAs can desire to protect parents from worry and upset, perhaps out of guilt for what their parents are going through or because they perceive that parental distress is already high.[48,49] While AYA patients identify parents as their primary source of support, the relationship is tenuous as young people attempt to balance desire for independence with forced dependence on parents to accompany them to healthcare, to help them understand the cancer experience, to care for and love them.[50]

Achievement. Rowland[2] has also identified milestone achievements of young adulthood that include career planning, maturing perspective on parents, and committing to another person; AYA patients can face disruptions in affecting these achievements. School attendance can be sporadic, leading to social functioning disruption and sometimes limiting educational attainment, thereby work and career options. Overall, when employed, AYAs most often work at jobs that do not offer benefits including health insurance or, given their sense of immortality and/or competing expenses, may opt out of available benefits. Even when they have health insurance AYA patients can lose coverage when they miss work for extended periods of time, leave school, or age out of eligibility under parental employment benefits. To be eligible for supplemental security income (SSI), social security disability insurance (SSDI) or Medicaid, AYAs must be unemployed, or if working, earn below "substantial gainful employment." Meeting eligibility requirements can require AYAs to return to work prematurely, or remain under- or unemployed. Neither means to insurance supports successful developmental achievements for AYAs.

Body-sexual image and integrity. Altered appearances, including weight changes, hair loss, and scarring can cause AYAs to feel different from peers with an adverse impact on self-esteem. Fears that the body will never return to normal, of being unrecognizable to others or mistaken for the opposite sex can lead to shame, isolation, and regressive behaviors.[51] Patients can perceive physical changes as threats to their well-being, which can generate anxiety. Self-image and life outlook seem worse among AYAs who perceive treatment-related physical changes as moderate to severe versus those who perceive them as mild or not at all limiting.[52]

The effects of cancer and it treatment on fertility are widely reported. Yet many AYAs do not recall adequate discussion with a health professional before treatment initiation about risk of infertility or available means to decrease the risk,[53] possibly because they were more concerned about threats to current function and survival than potential late effects.[28] For males fertility preservation (FP) options include semen cryopreservation. For females FP methods are more invasive and experimental[54] and can include in vitro fertilization (IVF), ovarian tissue cryopreservation, ovarian transposition, and pharmacological protection.[55] Options for FP vary by acuity, treatment, gender, age, and resources. Health professionals' assessments of these factors influence the extent to which FP options are presented to patients.[56] Less than 50% of age-appropriate males bank sperm and less than 50% receive suitable education, counseling, and resources.[56] Primary barriers to FP include lack of available information and difficulty in communicating about fertility.[57] Physician factors that impede discussion about FP include lack of knowledge about resources or referrals; duration of practice; specialty; lack of training to discuss FP; and lack of knowledge about national guidelines. Once informed, conditions that preclude patients from taking advantage of FP include parental refusal, patient inability to produce a viable sample, time constraints related to treatment and/or acuity, lack of adequate counseling, anxiety, perception of FP as low priority, gender, and parity.[56,58,59] Fertility concerns are prevalent, can effect treatment decisions and heighten distress, and may impact adherence for AYA patients.[60,61] All AYA patients should be thoroughly informed about the potential effects of their treatment on fertility as well as FP.[28]

A related area of stress and disruption concerns sexual identity. During the transition from adolescence to adulthood individuals realize that they are sexual beings, develop sexual identity, and conceptualize reproductive capacity. Adolescents display concern about attractiveness to peers and explore intimate relationships. Not surprising, cancer and its treatment can affect sexuality regardless of age, race, sexual orientation, gender, or socioeconomic background.[62–65] Effects on sexuality and intimacy are experienced not only by AYAs during treatment and long-term survivorship, but also by their current and future partners.[66] Cancer, its treatment, and their effects such as early menopause, osteoporosis, altered cognition, infertility, and fatigue can affect AYAs' sexual behaviors, attitudes, and identity.[67–69] Altered body image and self-esteem, changed relationships and other social challenges can take a toll on AYAs, for whom exploring and developing sexual and intimate relations is normative. Addressing AYAs' sexuality and intimacy concerns acknowledges the importance of developing a sense of self as a sexual being, and the formation of safe and healthy intimate relationships. Emergence of a favorable sexual identity depends upon acquiring accurate sexual knowledge, developing favorable interpersonal relationships, and addressing body image concerns.[68]

Existential issues. Uncertainty, that is, difficulty knowing the meaning of illness-related events[70] has been identified as the single greatest psychosocial stressor for people affected by potentially fatal illnesses like cancer.[71] The concept has four aspects: ambiguity about the state of one's health and meaning of symptoms and test results; lack of information about the illness, its treatment and treatment side effects; complexity of available information; healthcare relationships and the system of care; and unpredictability of one's future.[70] While it can ease uncertainty in the area of ambiguity, a cancer diagnosis is widely associated with death and so is also a potentially traumatic event that can generate fear and helplessness,[72] and expand uncertainty into every facet of life.[73] Uncertainty may be especially intense for AYAs who typically can grasp the nature of cancer but can lack that social support, experience with and expectancy of personal vulnerability to cancer that can promote the formation of an illness schema and reduce uncertainty.[70] Patients can develop three kinds of characteristic posttrauma symptoms (PTS) in response to the intense fear, helplessness, and uncertainty that is initially concerned with not getting well: (1) reexperiencing, (2) avoidance of reminders/numbing of cognition and emotion, and (3) hyperarousal exhibited as irritability, insomnia, and hypervigilance to one's bodily state and provider communications/behaviors.[72] Characteristic PTS for AYAs further include a sense of biological fragility, narrowing interests and social withdrawal, and/or resolve to live fully in the moment with heightened risk taking such as substance abuse.[74] Overall, AYAs are more likely to develop PTS than children.[74] Across age groups, females are more likely to develop PTS than males.[75] People with inadequate social support and those with a history of exposure to other traumatic stressors are also at heightened risk for developing PTS.[76] Four to six weeks following diagnosis, PTS can represent normative self-protective efforts against perceived threat and intense uncertainty. Most patients do not go on to have a clinically significant level of persistent PTS in all three clusters with impaired function, that is, full-blown posttraumatic stress disorder (PTSD).[72] However, PTS in one or two clusters can impede AYAs' development and general health, treatment adherence and healthcare use, and expansion of cancer-related knowledge.[77] At diagnosis, AYAs may benefit from concrete communications that highlight what will be done immediately to manage the situation and protect their well-being. Over the longer term, efforts to booster social support,

cognitive schema for the illness, and coping skills including skills for communicating about cancer with healthcare professionals, family and friends are potential means for managing uncertainty and maximizing medical and quality of life outcomes. Adolescent patients appreciate health care communications that convey hope, defined as a reality-based sense of positive expectations for health and normalcy in future,[78] which may be a means to lessen uncertainty in the area of unpredictability and also support optimal treatment adherence.[79] Some AYA patients, especially females, may find religiosity and spirituality helpful in promoting hopefulness and thus managing uncertainty.[80] Adolescent patients at the completion of 1 year of treatment[81] and young adult long-term survivors[82] have been shown to have perspective on the cancer experience and ongoing uncertainty that encompasses benefit. These beneficial aspects, termed posttraumatic growth, generally include changed perceptions of the self and improved personal relationships, new directions for one's life, greater appreciation of life, greater sense of personal strength, and enhanced spirituality.[83] Posttraumatic growth does not seem to occur exclusive of PTS nor is it consistently associated with reduced emotional distress. Posttraumatic growth does seem to indicate the development of a resultant fuller and perhaps wiser life perspective following cancer.[84]

CARE OF AYA PATIENTS

Along with the psychosocial outcomes previously described, AYA patients have supportive care needs, many of which are not being met.[85] In general, distinctive outcomes and needs of AYAs have not been described due to the regular inclusion of AYAs in studies of children or older adults.[86]

Psycho-oncology providers should start by evaluating the extent to which cancer is having effects on the AYA patient's developmental tasks. Given their age-based risk, AYAs should be evaluated for characteristic PTS as well as risk factors that can heighten an individual's risk for developing PTSD and/or additional chronic psychological conditions. Other high priority areas to address include physical concerns, treatment effects, personal changes, and school and social life.[47,87] Assessment should also include evaluation of identity formation including sexual identity, social and developmental histories, plus personal history and feelings about past coping strategies[68]; overall AYAs prefer to use the strategies of humor, religious beliefs, cognitive reframing, and imagination.[88]

Jacobs and Hobbie[89] suggest that long-term follow-up care for adults who have been treated for cancer should include assessment and information regarding late effects emphasizing quality of life and health maintenance/promotion. At diagnosis and throughout treatment, AYA patients could also benefit from a quality of life/health maintenance and promotion perspective. An age-appropriate environment that conveys hope and offers age-relevant information that can empower AYA patients to take steps starting at diagnosis to manage potential late effects, for example, access FP to manage risk of infertility, may be means to reduce uncertainty and maximize treatment outcomes.[90–92] Information needs assessment should include evaluating readiness for information as ill-timed discussions may increase distress,[67] and appraisal of cognitive capacity for absorbing information and potential effects on emotions and behavior.[68]

The main topics AYA patients want information about are their cancer and its treatment, the decision-making process, the healthcare system, and survivorship issues such as what can be done about late effects.[85,93,94] A sizeable proportion also want information about healthy diet, exercise, infertility, complementary and alternative approaches, and insurance. Addressing AYAs' information needs requires health professionals to (1) use a caring manner and understandable language, (2) allow time for AYAs to process information, (3) not assume AYAs are confident to ask questions, and (4) expect AYAs' and parental concerns to differ.[94] Many AYAs independently access cancer-related information.[84] The extent to which extant information is understandable to people of varied ages and education levels is a concern. With usage prevalent in the age group,[95] development of developmentally-appropriate web-based information for AYA patients has great potential.

Developmental theory can guide intervening with AYAs. Health professionals should be educated about developmental influences on AYA behavior and to intervene in fitting ways.[94,96] Also guided by developmental theory, supportive care interventions for AYA should target favorable body image, economic and emotional independence, social involvement, identity formation, and career direction.[90] Primary intervention goals are to promote functional coping and quality of life.[97] Interventions that aim to enhance social support and involvement seem to have great potential to enhance quality of life since quality of life in AYA patients has been shown to be largely a function of social support,[61,98] and social support may mitigate adverse psychosocial outcomes.[98] While parents are identified as a primary source of support, peers who have experienced cancer can also play important roles.[99,100] Interventions that aim to enhance peer support can offer safety and encouragement not usually available to AYA[67] and promote their psychological adjustment.[90] Peer support provides AYA patients with opportunities to address mutual concerns, and can also decrease feelings of social isolation, depression, and anxiety.[101] Participation in oncology camps, adventure programs, and day picnics offers experiences that can promote successful achievement of AYA developmental tasks. Wilderness adventure and advocacy skills training programs can provide AYA patients with experiences that boost self-image, raise confidence, and improve independence.[88,102,103] For AYA survivors it is not inconsequential that they make friends through peer programs as this is a critical task for the age and relevant to AYA patients.

CONCLUSION

AYA patients face distinct developmental tasks that can be challenged by cancer. Psycho-oncology healthcare professionals must cultivate awareness and sensitivity to the tasks for this age so they can best assist AYA patients to achieve normalcy and healthy maturation throughout the cancer experience.

REFERENCES

1. Arnett JJ. Emerging adulthood: a theory of development from late teens through the twenties. *Am Psychol.* 2000;55:469–480.

2. Rowland JH. Developmental stage and adaptation: adult model. In: JC Holland, JH Rowland, (eds). *Handbook of psycho-oncology.* New York, NY: Oxford University Press; 1990:29–33.

3. Adolescent and Young Adult Oncology Progress Review Group. *Closing the gap: Research and care imperatives for adolescents and young adults with cancer.* National Cancer Institute, NIH Pub No. 06-6067. Bethesda MD 2006.

4. O'Leary M, Barr R, Ries LAG, eds. *Cancer epidemiology in older adolescents and young adults 15 to 29 Years of Age, including SEER incidence and survival: 1975–2000.* National Cancer Institute, NIH Pub No. 06-5767. Bethesda, MD 2006.

5. Arnett JJ. Emerging adulthood: understanding the new way of coming of age. In: JJ Arnett, JL Tanner (eds). *Emerging adults in America: Coming of age in the 21st century.* Washington DC: American Psychological Association Press; 2006:3–20.

6. Jemal A, Siegel R, Ward E, Murray T, Xu J, Thun MJ. Cancer statistics 2007. *CA: Cancer J Clin.* 2007;57:43–66.

7. Birch JM, Bleyer A. Epidemiology and etiology of cancer in adolescents and young adults. In: A Bleyer, R Barr (eds). *Cancer in adolescents and young adults.* New York: Springer; 2007:39–59.

8. Bleyer A, Albritton K, Ries L, Barr R. Introduction. In: A Bleyer, R Barr (eds). *Cancer in adolescents and young adults.* New York: Springer; 2007:4–5.

9. Bhatia S, Sklar C. Second cancers in survivors of childhood cancer. *Cancer.* 2002;2:124–132.

10. Oeffinger KC, Mertens AC, Sklar CA, et al. for the Childhood Cancer Survivor Study. Chronic health conditions in adult survivors of childhood cancer. *N Engl J Med.* 2006;355:1572–1582.

11. Franco EL, Schlecht NF, Saslow D. The epidemiology of cervical cancer. *Cancer J.* 2003;9:348–359.

12. Dang-Tan T, Franco EL. Diagnosis delays in childhood cancer. *Cancer.* 2007;110:703–713.

13. Ziv A, Boulet JR, Slap GB. Utilization of physician offices by adolescents in the United States. *Pediatrics.* 1999;104:35–42.

14. Albritton K, Eden T. Access to care before and during therapy. In: A Bleyer, R Barr (eds). *Cancer in adolescents and young adults.* New York: Springer; 2007:61–69.

15. Mulhall A, Kelly D, Pearce S. A qualitative evaluation of an adolescent cancer unit. *Eur J Cancer.* 2004;3:16–22.

16. Reynolds BC, Windebank KP, Leonard RC, Wallace WH. A comparison of self-reported satisfaction between adolescents treated in a "teenage" unit with those treated in adult or pediatric units. *Pediatr Blood Cancer.* 2005;44:259–263.

17. Bleyer A. Young adult oncology: the patients and their survival challenges. *CA: Cancer J Clin.* 2007;57:242–255.

18. Jeha S. Who should be treating adolescents and young adults with acute lymphoblastic leukemia? *Eur J Cancer.* 2003;39:2579–2583.

19. Liu L, Krailo M. Reaman GH. Bernstein L. Surveillance, Epidemiology and End Results Childhood Cancer Linkage Group. Childhood cancer patients' access to cooperative group cancer programs: a population-based study. *Cancer.* 2003;97:1339–1345.

20. Bleyer A, Budd T, Montello M. Adolescents and young adults with cancer: the scope of the problem and criticality of clinical trials. *Cancer.* 2006;107:1645–1655.

21. Bleyer A, Montello M, Budd T, Saxman S. National survival trends of young adults with sarcomas: lack of progress is associated with lack of clinical trial participation. *Cancer.* 2005;103:1891–1897.

22. Bleyer A, Budd T, Montello M. Older adolescents and young adults with cancer, and clinical trials: lack of participation and progress in North America. In: A Bleyer, R Barr (eds). *Cancer in adolescents and young adults.* New York: Springer; 2007:71–81.

23. Burke ME, Albritton K, Marina N. Challenges in the recruitment of adolescents and young adults to cancer clinical trials. *Cancer.* 2007;110:2385–2393.

24. Ferrari A, Bleyer A. Participation of adolescents with cancer in clinical trials. *Cancer Treatment Rev.* 2007;33:603–608.

25. Decker CL, Haase JE, Bell C. Uncertainty in adolescents and young adults with cancer. *Oncol Nurs Forum.* 2007;34:681–688.

26. Ljungman G, Mcgrath PJ, Cooper E, et al. Psychosocial needs of families with a child with cancer. *J Pediatr Hematol Oncol.* 2003;25:223–231.

27. Grinyer A. Young adults with cancer: parent interactions with health care providers. *Eur J Cancer Care.* 2003;13:88–95.

28. Abrams AN, Hazen EP, Penson RT. Psychosocial issues in adolescents with cancer. *Cancer Treatment Rev.* 2007;33:622–630.

29. Kools S, Tong EM, Hughes R, et al. Hospital experiences of young adults with congenital heart disease: divergence in expectations and dissonance in care. *Amer J Critical Care.* 2002;11:115–127.

30. American Academy of Pediatrics, Committee on Bioethics. Informed consent, parental permission, and assent in pediatric practice. *Pediatrics.* 1995;95:314–317.

31. Davies HA, Lennard L, Lilleyman JS. Variable mercaptopurine metabolism in children with leukemia: a problem of noncompliance? *Br Med J.* 1993;306:1239–1240.

32. Lau RCW, Matsui D, Greeburg M, Koren G. Electronic measurement of compliance with mercaptopurine in pediatric patients with acute lymphoblastic leukemia. *Med Ped Oncol.* 1998;30:85–90.

33. Simon C, Zyanski SJ, Eder M, Raiz P, Kodish ED, Simonoff LA. Groups potentially at risk for making poorly informed decisions about entry into clinical trials for childhood cancer. *J Clin Oncol.* 2003;21:2173–2178.

34. Shaw RJ. Treatment adherence in adolescents: development and psychopathology. *Clin Child Psych.* 2001;6:137–150.

35. Lancaster D, Lennard L, Lilleymoan JS. Profile of non-compliance in lymphoblastic leukemia. *Arch Dis Child.* 2006;76:365–366.

36. Spinetta JJ, Masera G, Eden T, et al. Refusal, non-compliance, and abandonment of treatment in children and adolescents with cancer: a report of the SIOP working committee on psychosocial issues in pediatric oncology. *Med Pediatr Oncol.* 2002;39:114–117.

37. Malbasa T, Kodish E, Santacroce SJ. Adolescent adherence to oral therapy for leukemia: a focus group study. *J Pediatr Onc Nurs.* 2007;24:139–151.

38. Williams AB. Adherence to HIV regimens: 10 vital lessons. *Amer J Nurs.* 2001;101:37–44.

39. Gesundheit B, Greenberg M, Or R, Gideon K. Drug compliance by adolescent and young adult patients: challenges for the physician. In: A Bleyer, R Barr (eds). *Cancer in adolescents and young adults.* New York, NY: Springer; 2007:353–363.

40. Puccio JA, Belzer M, Olson J, et al. The use of cell phone reminder calls for assisting HIV-infected adolescents and young adults to adhere to highly active antiretroviral therapy: a pilot study. *AIDS Pat Care STDs.* 2006;20:438–444.

41. Neville K. The relationships among uncertainty, social support, and psychological distress in adolescents recently diagnosed with cancer. *J Pediatr Onc Nurs.* 1998;15:37–46.

42. Levin Newby W, Brown RT, Pawletko TM, Gold SH, Whitt JK. Social skills and psychological adjustment of child and adolescent cancer survivors. *Psychooncology.* 2000;9:113–126.

43. Hughes J, Sharrock W, Martin PJ. *Understanding classical sociological theory.* London, England: Sage Publications Ltd.; 2003.

44. Fobair P, Stewart SL, Chang S, D'Onofrio C, Banks PJ, Bloom JR. Body image and sexual problems in young women with breast cancer. *Psychooncology.* 2006;15:579–594.

45. Jonker-Pool G, Hoekstra JJ, van Imhoff GW, et al. Male sexuality after cancer treatment- needs for information and support: testicular cancer compared to malignant lymphoma. *Patient Educ Counc.* 2004;52:143–150.

46. Thaler-Demers D. Intimacy issues: sexuality, fertility, and relationships. *Semin Oncol Nurs.* 2001;17:255–262.

47. Larouche SS, Chin-Peuckert L. Changes in body image experienced by adolescents with cancer. *J Pediatr Oncol Nurs.* 2006;23:200–209.

48. Chesler M, Barbarin O (eds). *Childhood cancer and the family.* New York: Bruner/Mazel; 1987.

49. Zebrack B, Chesler M, Orbuch T, Parry C. Mothers of survivors of childhood cancer: their worries and concerns. *J Psychosoc Oncol.* 2002;20:1–26.

50. Woodgate RL. The importance of being there: perspectives of social support by adolescents with cancer. *J Pediatr Onc Nurs.* 2006;23:122–134.

51. Die-Trill M, Stuber ML. Psychological problems of curative cancer treatment. In: J Holland (ed). *Psycho-Oncology.* New York: Oxford University Press; 1998.

52. Zebrack BJ, Chesler MA. Health-related worries, self-image and life outlooks of survivors of childhood cancer. *Health Soc Work.* 2001;26:245–256.

53. Schover LR, Brey K, Lichtin A, Lipshultz LI, Jeha S. Knowledge and experience regarding cancer, infertility, and sperm banking in younger male survivors. *J Clin Oncol.* 2002;20:1880–1889.

54. Weintraub M, Gross E, Kadari A, et al. Should ovarian cryopreservation be offered to girls with cancer. *Pediatr Blood Cancer.* 2007;48:4–9.

55. Grady MC. Preconception and the young cancer survivor. *Maternal Child Health J.* 2006;10S:165–168.

56. Quinn GP, Vadaparampil ST, Gwede CK, et al. Discussion of fertility preservation with newly diagnosed patients: oncologists' views. *J Cancer Survivorship.* 2007;1:146–155.

57. Edge B, Holmes D, Makin G. Sperm banking in adolescent cancer patients. *Arch Dis Child.* 2006;91:149–152.

58. Bashore L. Semen preservation in male adolescents and young adults with cancer: one institution's experience. *Clin J Oncol Nurs.* 2007;11:381–386.

59. Goodwin T, Oosterhuis EB, Kiernan J, Hudson MM, Dahl GV. Attitudes and practices of pediatric oncology providers regarding fertility issues. *Pediatr Blood Cancer.* 2006;48:80–85.

60. Partridge AH, Gelber S, Peppercorn J, et al. Web based survey of fertility issues in young women with breast cancer. *J Clin Oncol.* 2004;22:4174–4183.

61. Wenzel L, Dogan-Ates A, Habbal R, et al. Defining and measuring reproductive concerns of female cancer survivors. *J NCI.* 2005;34:94–98.

62. Katz A. The sounds of silence: sexuality information for cancer patients. *J Clin Oncol.* 2005;1:238–241.

63. Pelusi J. Sexuality and body image: research on breast cancer survivors documents altered body image and sexuality. *Cancer Nurs.* 2006;29S:32–38.

64. Zabora J. Psychosocial consequences of breast cancer. In: K Bland, E Copland (eds). *The breast: Comprehensive management of benign and malignant disorders.* 3rd ed. St. Louis, MO: Saunders; 2004:1569.

65. Svetlik D, Dooley K, Weiner M, Williamson G, Walter A. Declines in satisfaction with physical intimacy predict caregiver perceptions of overall relationship loss: a study of elderly caregiving spousal dyads. *Sex Disability.* 2005;23:65–79.

66. Evan E, Kaufman M, Cook A, Zeltzer LK. Sexual health and self-esteem in adolescents and young adults with cancer. *Cancer.* 2006;107S:1672–1679.

67. Evan E, Zeltzer LK. Psychosocial dimensions of cancer in adolescents and young adults. *Cancer.* 2006;107:1663–1671.

68. Hampton T. Cancer treatment's trade-off: years of added life can have long-term costs. *JAMA.* 2005;294:167–168.

69. Zebrack BJ, Casillas J, Nohr L, Adams H, Zeltzer LK. Fertility issues for young adult survivors of childhood cancer. *Psychooncology.* 2004;13:689–699.

70. Mishel MH. Uncertainty in illness. *Image: J Nurs Scholarship.* 1988;20:225–232.

71. Santacroce SJ. Parental uncertainty and posttraumatic stress in serious childhood illness. *Image: J Nurs Scholarship.* 2003;35:45–51.

72. American Psychological Association. *Diagnostic and statistical manual of mental disorders: DSM-IV-TR.* 4th ed. Washington, DC: Author; 2000.

73. Cohen MH. Diagnostic closure and the spread of uncertainty. *Issues Compr Pediatr Nurs.* 1993;16:135–146.

74. Shaw JA. Children, adolescents and trauma. *Psychiatric Q.* 2000;71:227–243.

75. Kessler R, Sonnega A, Bromet E, Hughes M, Nelson C. Posttraumatic stress disorder in the National Comorbidity Survey. *Arch Gen Psychiatry.* 1995;52:1048–1060.

76. Bisson J. *Posttraumatic stress disorder.* In: D Tovey (ed). *Clinical evidence.* 13th ed. London: BMJ Publishing; 2005:306–309.

77. Santacroce SJ, Lee Y-L. Uncertainty, posttraumatic stress, and health behavior in young adult childhood cancer survivors. *Nurs Res.* 2006; 55:259–266.

78. Hinds PS. The hopes and wishes of adolescents with cancer and the nursing care that helps. *Oncol Nurs Forum.* 2004;31:925–934.

79. Hinds PS, Quargenenti A, Fairclough D, et al. Hopefulness and its characteristics in adolescents with cancer. *West J Nurs Res.* 1999;21:600–616.

80. Hendricks-Ferguson V. Relationships of age and gender to hope and spiritual well-being among adolescents with cancer. *J Pediatr Oncol Nurs.* 2006;23:189–199.

81. Jorngarden A, Mattsson E, von Essen L. Health-related quality of life, anxiety and depression among adolescents and young adults with cancer: a prospective longitudinal study. *Eur J Cancer.* 2007;43:1952–1958.

82. Parry C. Embracing uncertainty: an exploration of the experiences of childhood cancer survivors. *Qual Health Res.* 2003;13:227–248.

83. Tedeschi RG, Calhoun LG. The Posttraumatic Growth Inventory: measuring the positive legacy of trauma. *J Trauma Stress.* 1996;9:455–471.

84. Tedeschi RG, Calhoun LG. Posttraumatic growth: a new perspective on psychotraumatology. *Psychiatr Times.* 2004;21:58, 60.

85. Zebrack B. Information and service needs for young adult cancer patients. *Support Care Cancer.* 2008;16:1353–1360.

86. Haase JE, Phillips CR. The adolescent/young adult experience. *J Pediatr Oncol Nurs.* 2004;21:145–149.

87. Hedstrom M, Kreuger A, Ljungman G, Nygren P, vonEssen L. Accuracy of assessment of distress, anxiety, and depression by physicians and nurses in adolescents recently diagnosed with cancer. *Pediatr Blood Cancer.* 2006;46:773–779.

88. Elad P, Yagil Y, Cohen LH, Meller I. A jeep trip with young adult cancer survivors: lessons to be learned. *Support Care Cancer.* 2003;11:201–206.

89. Jacobs LA. Hobbie WL. Leadership & professional development. The living well after cancer program: an advanced practice model of care. *Oncol Nurs Forum.* 2002;29:637–638.

90. Eiser C, Kuperberg A. Psychological support for adolescents and young adults. In: A Bleyer, D Barr (eds). *Cancer in adolescents and young adults.* Berlin Heidelberg, FRG: Springer-Verlag; 2007:365–374.

91. Greving D. Santacroce S. Cardiovascular late effects. *J Pediatr Oncol Nurs.* 2005;22:38–47.

92. Pagano-Therrien J, Santacroce SJ. Bone mineral density decrements and children diagnosed with cancer. *J Pediatr Oncol Nurs.* 2005;22:328–38.

93. Zebrack, B, Mills J, Weitzman, T. Health and supportive care needs of young adult cancer patients and survivors. *J Cancer Survivorship.* 2007;1:137–145.

94. Palmer S, Mitchell A, Thompson, K. Unmet needs among adolescent cancer patients: a pilot study. *Palliat Support Care.* 2007;5:127–134.

95. Rideout V. *Generation Rx.com: How young people use the internet for health information.* Menlo Park, CA: Henry J. Kaiser Family Foundation; 2001:12–11

96. Craig F. Adolescents and young adults. In: A Goldman, R Hain, S Liben (eds). *Oxford textbook of palliative care for children.* New York: Oxford University Press; 2006:108–118.

97. Kyngas H, Mikkonen R, Nousiainen EM, et al. Coping with the onset of cancer: coping strategies and resources of young people with cancer. *Eur J Cancer Care.* 2001;10:6–11.

98. Sammarco A. Perceived social support, uncertainty, and quality of life of younger breast cancer survivors. *Cancer Nurs.* 2001;24:212–219.

99. Ritchie MA. Sources of emotional support for adolescents with cancer. *J Pediatr Oncol Nurs.* 2001;18:105–110.

100. Zebrack B, Bleyer A, Albritton K, Medearis S, Tang J. Assessing the health care needs of adolescent and young adult (AYA) cancer patients and survivors. *Cancer.* 2006;107:2915–2923.

101. Shannon C, Smith IE. Breast cancer in adolescents and young women. *Eur J Cancer.* 2003;39:2632–2642.

102. Stevens B, Kagan S, Yamada J, et al. Adventure therapy for adolescents with cancer. *Pediatr Blood Cancer.* 2004;43:278–284.

103. Zebrack B, Oeffinger K, Hou P, Kaplan S. Advocacy skills training for young adult cancer survivors: the Young Adult Survivors Conference (YASC) at Camp Make-a-Dream. *Support Care Cancer.* 2006;14:779–782.

Disparities in the Impact of Cancer

Carolyn C. Gotay

INTRODUCTION

What are health disparities? As defined by the (U.S.) Minority Health and Health Disparities Research and Education Act, "A population is a health disparity population if there is a significant disparity in the overall rate of disease incidence, prevalence, morbidity, mortality or survival rates in the population as compared to the health status of the general population."[1]

Cancer illustrates a health condition with multiple disparate outcomes. This chapter discusses how cancer's effects differ among different populations, and possible explanations for these disparities. Part I focuses on disparities in the cancer care continuum, including incidence and mortality rates, cancer risk factors, screening, and cancer treatment. These factors all contribute to how individual cancer patients deal with cancer (Part II) and psychosocial support that is required (Part III). While much current data and research are based on populations in the developed world, a global perspective on the "world population" will be included where possible.

PART I: DISPARITIES ACROSS THE SPECTRUM OF CANCER CONTROL

The global cancer burden. Cancer is the second leading cause of death worldwide, accounting for 7.9 million deaths (13% of all deaths) in 2007. Lung, stomach, liver, colon, and breast cancers cause the most deaths, with lung cancer the most common cause of cancer death in both developed and developing countries. Global cancer deaths are projected to increase by 45% between 2007 and 2030, with 12 million annual deaths estimated by 2030.[2]

Even within countries or regions, cancer rates can vary markedly. Consider the state of Hawaii, with a highly ethnically diverse population. Breast cancer incidence rates vary from 93.1 (per 100,000 population) for Filipinos to 162.4 for Native Hawaiians, colon cancer rates in men go from 33.4 in Chinese to 52.0 in Japanese, and prostate cancer rates vary from 100.5 in Native Hawaiians to 155.7 in Caucasians.[3]

Cancer prevention. At least 30% of cancers could be prevented, based on current knowledge of risk factors and effective interventions.[2] According to the World Health Organization (WHO), tobacco is the single largest preventable cause of cancer in the world today, causing 80%–90% of all lung cancer deaths. While comprehensive cancer control programs have been effective in reducing tobacco use in many developed countries, tobacco use is increasing in the developing world, implying greater future disparities in lung cancer rates and the associated death and suffering. Initiating and sustaining comprehensive tobacco control programs are a high priority globally, and the WHO has an active program in this area.[2] Given different roles that tobacco plays in various cultures (e.g., ceremonial, religious, and medicinal use in Native American and First Nations communities), tobacco control strategies need to be tailored to the values and attitudes of the particular group.

Infectious agents account for nearly 22% of cancer deaths in the developing world and 6% in industrialized countries.[4] These include viral hepatitis B and C in liver cancer, human papilloma virus (HPV) in cervical cancer, and the bacterium *Helicobacter pylori* in stomach cancer. Newly developed HPV vaccines hold considerable promise for eradicating cervical cancer, as do hepatitis vaccinations and antibiotics to eliminate *H pylori*. Preventing these cancers will go a long way toward eliminating some cancer disparities, particularly since no effective treatments are available for liver, stomach, and advanced cervical cancer.

Other major modifiable risk factors for cancer include nutrition (particularly, low intake of plant-based nutrients and excessive alcohol use), obesity, inactivity, and exposure to carcinogenic environmental agents (e.g., ultraviolet radiation, chemical carcinogens).[4] These factors may disproportionately affect different groups: for example, exposure to chemical carcinogens is more prevalent in the developing world and among lower-paid factory workers in some developed countries. Other risk factors appear to have global applicability. For example, the WHO states that "Obesity has reached epidemic proportions globally, with approximately 1.6 billion adults and at least 20 million children under the age of 5 being overweight…and more than 75% of obese children live in low- and middle- income countries."[3] While approaches to prevent and reduce obesity require cultural tailoring, given group differences in preferences for foods, forms of physical activity, and other factors, the need to reduce the risk for obesity transcends group boundaries.

Cancer screening and early detection. If a cancer cannot be prevented, the next best step is catching it early when it is much more likely to be successfully treated and controlled. Screening modalities have been shown to reduce cancer mortality and are recommended for use in the population at specified intervals, and for particular age groups. These include Pap testing for cervical cancer, mammography for breast cancer, and several strategies for colorectal screening (e.g., fecal occult blood testing, sigmoidoscopy, colonoscopy).

Challenges arise because these screening tests require access to healthcare services and trained professionals to interpret the results and provide follow-up care. As such, they are not available in most developing countries, with the consequence that "for a long time to come, as many as 80%-90% of cancer patients in the developing countries will probably continue to be diagnosed with far-advanced, incurable cancer, if they are diagnosed at all."[5] Even in developed countries, screening tests are often not covered by heathcare insurance, despite the availability of population-based healthcare.

While insurance coverage and having a usual source of medical care are significant predictors of use of cancer screening tests, a number of other factors contribute to disparities in use of screening. Most research on barriers to cancer screening has focused on mammography in the United States. Two recent comprehensive reviews have concluded that lower breast cancer screening rates are associated with older age, lower socioeconomic status (SES), rural residence, and racial and ethnic minority status.[6,7] Patient barriers include access and logistical challenges; knowledge, attitudes, and cultural beliefs; language and acculturation; and literacy, whereas a strong predictor of receiving screening is physician recommendations. Vulnerable groups are less likely to receive provider recommendation for breast cancer screening, possibly due to poor communication, provider assumption about patient age and financial resources, and discrimination.[6]

Much less is known about barriers to screening tests other than mammography and about disparities in populations outside the United States, although some evidence indicates that similar barriers to mammography, such as educational and financial concerns[8] and incentives such as a physician recommendation[9] are important in European populations.

Table 70–1. Mean FACT-G scores in different patient groups compared to norms

Study		FACT-G	PW	SW	EW	FW
Brucker et al. (Norm)		80.9	21.3	22.1	18.7	18.9
Ell et al. (U.S.)[a]		n/a[e]	20.9	17.9	15.7	14.3
Dapueto et al. (Uruguay)[b]		63.7	15.7	16.6	18.6	13.5
Ashing-Giwa et al. (U.S.)[c]	Total sample	62.8	21.7	18.9	17.0	20.0
	African-American	64.8	21.2	20.1	18.1	20.0
	European-American	63.0	22.0	18.9	17.1	20.3
	Latina	59.0	20.6	16.7	15.8	18.6
	Asian-American	64.5	22.6	20.1	17.4	21.1
Wong et al (China)[d]	Liver	71.2[f]	n/a	n/a	n/a	n/a
	Lung	71.3	n/a	n/a	n/a	n/a

[a] Sample was 79% Hispanic.
[b] Study used the FACT-G S4 (Spanish version 4).
[c] Study used the FACT-G; data in Table 70–1 reflect the chapter author's weighting of the mean scores in the original paper (which went 0–100) to generate the same scale metric as that used in the other studies.
[d] Study used the FACT-G Ch (Chinese version).
[e] Mean data were not reported.
[f] Mean data reflect baseline scores.
ABBREVIATIONS: EW, emotional well-being; FACT-G, *functional assessment of cancer therapy-general*; FW, functional well-being; n/a, not available; PW, physical well-being; SW, social well-being.

Treatment. Effective cancer therapies can determine whether patients live or die, how long they survive, how long they live without evidence of disease, and control of symptoms. In this area, as well, there is considerable evidence of disparities. These disparities have been explored most extensively in the United States, and the Institute of Medicine (IOM) commissioned a comprehensive assessment of this issue. The title of the report summarizing the findings—"Unequal Treatment: Confronting Racial and Ethnic Disparities in Health Care"—indicates the conclusions. Considerable evidence indicated that members of certain groups—particularly poor people, the elderly and racial/ethnic minorities—were less likely to receive less effective treatment and supportive care. This finding did not emerge in every study, and sometimes it disappeared when correlates such as stage of disease, having healthcare insurance, income, and co-morbidity were controlled. Nonetheless, the consistency of findings led the IOM to develop a series of recommendations directed at policy, the healthcare system, providers, surveillance, and research to eliminate disparities in healthcare.[10]

Disparities in cancer treatment are not limited to the United States. Molassiotis[11] points out that European countries differ considerably in the availability of pharmaceutical agents and access to specialty care, both within and between countries. As well, many countries in the developing world have virtually no access to cancer treatment technologies and skilled personnel at all, reflecting considerable disparity between the potential for successful treatment in patients diagnosed in the developing compared to developed world.

PART II: DISPARITIES IN PSYCHOSOCIAL IMPACT OF CANCER

In groups and countries where cancer is generally associated with late diagnosis, inadequate treatment and symptom control, and often death, it seems reasonable to expect that the distress associated with a cancer diagnosis is likely to be considerable and greater than in an environment where cancer is found early, pain can be controlled, nausea can be prevented, and hope for a cure can be provided.

We will examine the evidence available that assesses the psychosocial impact of cancer in defined groups. Empirical research using three different methodologies will be reviewed: studies of individual groups, comparisons with normative data, and comparative studies.

Studies of specified cultural groups. Pandey and colleagues[12] studied 50 breast cancer patients in India. While the sample included

patients with both early and advanced disease, most had advanced disease. This reflects the most common disease presentation in India, which does not have active breast cancer screening programs in effect. Results indicated that patients reported problems in a number of areas, particularly recreation, social life, mobility, physical activity, and sleep and attitude. The study concluded that until there is a change in healthcare in India, such that early detection of breast cancer is a reality for most of the population, women will be diagnosed with advanced disease that needs intensive treatment, and psychosocial well-being will be impacted accordingly.

Baider et al.[13] studied psychological functioning in two groups of breast cancer patients: those who were second-generation Holocaust survivors: that is, at least one parent had survived the Holocaust (n = 106); and Israeli breast cancer patients who were not (n = 102). Results indicated that the women from Holocaust families were much more distressed by their cancer experience and reported clinically significant levels of psychopathology. The authors propose that the family experience of trauma may extend beyond the person who experiences the trauma and affect the adjustment of a family member who subsequently experiences a different kind of stressor. While this study focused on a historically and culturally distinct experience, Baider and colleagues suggest that similar findings may emerge when families experience other kinds of traumatic situations.

Studies in a single culture can provide a rich picture of the nuances in a given group. Methods can be tailored to the understanding and communication style of the target group, and a common language can be used. However, interpretation of results in these studies needs to be carefully considered, in order not to attribute findings to culture, when other variables, such as socioeconomic factors or lack of medical care, may be explanatory; or to attribute universal cultural values—such as the importance of the family—to a single group.

Comparisons with normative data. Another approach to understanding differences across ethnic and cultural groups is to compare outcomes of a specific group to normative data.

Table 70–1 provides an example of the comparative approach to quality of life (QOL) assessment using one questionnaire: the Functional Assessment of Cancer Therapy—General (FACT-G). The FACT-G assesses health-related QOL and provides an overall rating and four subscales—Physical Well-being (PW), Social/Family Well-being (SFW), Emotional Well-being (EW), and Functional Well-being (FW).

Normative data have been developed based on a large (N = 2,236) sample of mostly White U.S. cancer patients.

Table 70–1 provides a comparison of FACT overall and subscale scores (as available) for a normative cancer patient sample,[14] a predominantly Hispanic-American sample,[15] a Uruguayan sample,[16] a multiethnic sample from California,[17] and a Chinese sample.[18] Regarding subscale comparisons, a few findings stand out: the Uruguayan cancer patients had the lowest, or almost lowest, overall and subscale scores, except for EW; all groups scored lower than the normative sample for SW and EW; and Hispanics/Latinos across two studies reported the lowest subscale scores of any United States group. Regarding overall FACT-G scores, all of the ethnic subgroups of California residents (including European Americans) reported lower scores than both the cancer norms and Chinese, as did Uruguayans. These data imply that the norms are based on healthier cancer patients and are more likely to provide useful comparative information for higher functioning patient groups. The differences between the U.S. Asians and the Chinese sample may suggest interesting hypotheses for further study.

While comparisons using normative data can be quite informative, there are limitations to such approaches. For example, differences between countries, and across specific samples (e.g., cancer site, treatment, time since diagnosis, age), should also be considered in comparisons. Information on SES would be particularly useful, although equivalent indicators of SES can be difficult to define cross-culturally. In addition, cancer treatments may change over time, with different QOL impacts, and normative data may become outdated.

Comparative studies. Advantages of comparing groups within a single study include the use of a standard approach to recruiting and enrolling study participants, collection of data at the same time, use of common metrics, and being able to identify areas of both similarity and difference among groups. Three different comparative approaches are discussed below.

Patient census comparisons. Carlson et al.[19] examined psychological functioning in consecutive patients during a 1-month period at a regional cancer center in Alberta, Canada. 2776 patients (90% of the total possible) completed questionnaires. Most (78%) reported European, Canadian, or British ancestry, with the remaining patients reflecting a number of other groups. Findings indicated that minority group patients, and those with lower incomes, reported more distress. They were also significantly more likely to use cancer center psychological support services. Similarly, Moadel et al.[20] assessed psychosocial needs in oncology outpatient waiting rooms; 248 patients (70% of the total eligible) completed questionnaires. The sample was almost half Whites, with the remainder African-Americans (AA), Hispanics, and patients of other ethnicities. Results indicated that ethnicity was the most important predictor of unmet psychosocial needs in all areas, even controlling for SES. Among minority groups, Hispanics identified the highest number of needs.

Subgroup comparisons. Regions including large numbers of minority subgroups offer the opportunity to examine differences in psychosocial functioning in a single research study. Gotay et al.[21] assessed QOL in newly-diagnosed breast and prostate cancer patients (N = 227) from the four main ethnic groups in Hawaii (Filipino, Native Hawaiian, Japanese, White). Scores for a number of psychosocial outcomes varied significantly according to ethnicity, with ethnicity remaining a significant predictor in multivariate analyses. In all instances, the Filipino women reported worse outcomes than the other groups, which did not differ, pointing out the need for follow-up studies to understand more about needs in Filipinas.

Fobair and colleagues[22] investigated the impact of breast cancer in young women (N = 549); 71% were White and the remainder Asian (16%), Latina (8%) or Black (5%). Results indicated no differences in body image across ethnic groups, but lower prevalence of sexual activity in Asian women, and fewer sexual problems in Latinas. The investigators suggest that cultural factors may affect both of these findings. They also raise the possibility that the study methodology—in this case, face-

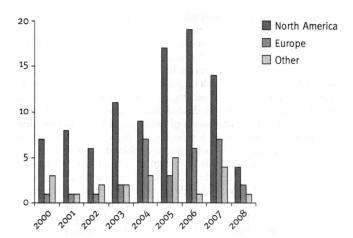

Fig. 70–1. Numbers of psychotherapy studies in cancer patients across time and location.

to-face interviews—may have affected results, since openly discussing sexual matters with a stranger may be uncomfortable and result in less complete responses in Asian and Latina women.

International comparisons. Studies comparing psychological well-being across different countries offer the opportunity to examine the impacts of culture, region, and healthcare systems, among other factors. Shim et al.[23] conducted a survey of QOL in breast cancer patients in Germany, Japan, and South Korea (N = 413). A number of similarities in patterns of results were found across the countries, although the specific effects differed. For example, social support, particularly negative support, was an important correlate of QOL in all three groups. However, social support was a more powerful correlate of PW in Japanese and of mental well-being in Germans. The authors speculate that this may reflect social support's traditional expression in Japanese culture less through emotions and more through instrumental support.

Psychometric properties of assessment tools in different groups are also important to consider. Scott et al.[24] reported on a pooled analysis of 103 studies comprising 27,891 patients from 22 countries that used one of 14 language versions of the same well-validated assessment tool: the European Organization for Research and Treatment of Cancer Quality of Life Questionnaire (EORTC QLQ-C30). Analyses were conducted to identify differential item functioning (DIF); DIF indicates when individuals from one group give systematically different responses as compared to comparable individuals in another group. Results showed that DIF was present on at least one subscale in all translations. This implies the need for continued validation and refinement of questionnaires, and care in interpreting results that go across countries and different translations, even for well-validated instruments.

PART III. DISPARITIES IN THE RECEIPT AND IMPACT OF PSYCHOSOCIAL INTERVENTIONS IN CANCER PATIENTS

Given cultural differences in values and attitudes toward cancer, and the different cancer-related outcomes experienced by subgroups of cancer patients, it would seem reasonable to expect that (1) some subgroups would be less likely to receive psychosocial care than others; (2) psychosocial interventions would have different effects on different subgroups; and (3) interventions available should be tailored to be culturally appropriate to specific subgroups.

Regarding whether there are disparities in the receipt of psychosocial care, the IOM report on health disparities stated that minority patients were less likely to receive supportive care in general. It is likely that the same is true for psychosocial oncology support, although no study investigating this issue could be identified. It is well-recognized that psychological support is underutilized and unavailable to the majority of cancer patients in the United States, across all subgroups.[25]

To explore whether psychosocial interventions have different effects in different subgroups, we undertook a literature search of empirically based psychosocial intervention studies listed on Medline. It should be noted that this analysis provides a perspective on only a portion of the much broader psychosocial oncology literature. Preliminary searches using alternate search terms indicated that the descriptor "psychotherapy" yielded the most inclusive set of psychosocial interventions. Thus, the search terms used were psychotherapy, clinical trial or randomized-controlled trial (RCT), and cancer, published 2000 or later (The 2008 data reflect only citations up to 8/01/08.). A total of 297 abstracts emerged from the initial search; all abstracts were reviewed and excluded from further consideration if they did not meet analytic criteria (empirical study of psychosocial outcomes in adult cancer patients written in English). While omitting non-English papers could interject bias, only 11 papers were excluded on this basis. One hundred and forty-six papers met inclusion criteria and were examined in greater detail.

As illustrated in Fig. 70–1, the volume of literature in this area has increased markedly over time, particularly in North America. European studies come from many countries (the United Kingdom and the Netherlands being the most frequent), and the "other" countries include those in Asia (China, Japan, South Korea), as well as Australia, Brazil, and Israel. The most common type of intervention in this review (N = 28) was studies focusing specifically on relaxation: for example, visualization and guided imagery, mindfulness meditation, progressive muscle relaxation, hypnosis, or massage. Eleven of these studies were based in North America, eight in Europe, and nine elsewhere (five from Asia, and two each from Australia and Israel). The next largest number (N = 25) was described as "cognitive behavioral:" such interventions generally included multiple techniques for stress reduction, problem solving, accessing information, and learning coping skills. Most of these studies were conducted in North America. Fourteen studies (11 from North America) used "expressive therapies:" the therapeutic application of music (n = 8), art (n = 4), dance (n = 1), or writing (n = 1). Numerous other interventions were reported: for example, education, symptom management, supportive-expressive group therapy, and couples therapy. The largest numbers in all cases were from North America, with one exception: there were seven trials of aromatherapy reported (sometimes combined with massage or reflexology), five conducted in the United Kingdom and one each in Japan and Australia.

It should be noted that ethnic or cultural differences were almost never reported, with a few exceptions. Some studies applied intervention approaches originally developed in Anglo North American populations (e.g., support groups) to different populations (e.g., Latinas, Europeans, Chinese, and Japanese); most studies found evidence suggesting efficacy in these new populations.

On the basis of this review, there is currently insufficient information to judge whether different populations experience disparate psychosocial outcomes based on the interventions received. Most research is based on North American samples, with little emphasis on subgroup differences within these studies. The large differences in the relative frequencies of the different kinds of psychosocial support in this analysis do imply international and cultural differences in preferences for types of care. Relaxation therapies are relatively more popular outside North America. Cognitive behavior therapy is dominant in North America, where problem solving and patient self-efficacy is highly emphasized; it should be noted that most of these interventions also included relaxation/stress reduction as one component. Expressive therapies, particularly music therapy, are receiving considerable attention in North America, whereas aromatherapy appears to be widely studied in the United Kingdom (and elsewhere in the world) and not at all in North America.

Psychosocial interventions for specified cancer patient populations.
Although psychosocial interventions aimed at populations that experience disparate cancer outcomes were not common in this literature, a few studies did address this issue, with examples discussed below.

Differential intervention impacts in specified groups. Patient characteristics may affect intervention effectiveness, as explored in studies reported by Mishel, Gil, and colleagues.[26,27] Their intervention was designed to reduce uncertainty and fear of recurrence in breast cancer survivors. A four-session, nurse-directed program was delivered by telephone, manual, and audiotapes. Participants were 509 recurrence-free breast cancer survivors (360 White (W), 149 AA), 5–9 years after diagnosis. Primary outcomes—uncertainty management and coping—were assessed 10 months after enrolment on the study, with follow-up at 20 months.

Results indicated that the intervention benefited both W and AA women, but through different coping strategies: AAs improved in cognitive reframing (especially regarding catastrophizing) and sharing additional information with the nurse, while Ws improved in satisfaction with social support and ability to distract themselves. A number of positive effects persisted 20 months later. The authors believe that some culturally linked factors may have influenced which coping strategies were most effective in the specific group: for example, high levels of fatalism has been noted in other studies of AAs, and the intervention's emphasis on reducing catastrophic thoughts may have directly affected this aspect of cognitive reframing.

Modifying interventions to enhance effectiveness in disparate groups.
Interventions demonstrated as effective in some groups may require modifications for different kinds of patients. Dwight-Johnson, Ell, and colleagues[28,29] focused on depression, widely recognized as a frequent, troubling, and underdiagnosed problem in cancer patients within a public health system. Fifty-five patients were randomly assigned to a Multifaceted Oncology Depression Program that provided a specialized team to track the patient's treatment for depression or usual care. Results indicated that this program resulted in significant improvements in depression and emotional functioning.

Despite these positive indications, the investigators identified a number of features requiring modification for future programs for low-income populations, especially Latinos. These include logistical features (e.g., using the telephone for contact and data collection; coordinating depression and cancer treatment appointments; reimbursing patients for time, transportation, and out-of-pocket medical costs) and culturally based modifications (e.g., further adapting Spanish language materials for literacy and idiomatic content; including patient navigation/case management as part of the protocol; attending to the needs and roles of family members; providing support groups in English and Spanish; and providing formal staff training in cultural competence). The effectiveness of this intervention is currently being tested in a randomized clinical trial.

Developing a group-specific intervention.
Another approach to providing psychosocial support is starting from the values and preferences of a particular group and developing an intervention that is based on these values. Mokuau et al.[30] describe this kind of intervention developed for Native Hawaiians. Focus groups in Native Hawaiian cancer survivors underlined the primary importance of the family (`ohana`), rather than the individual, in healthcare. Based on this finding, a `ohana`-focused supportive intervention was developed that also incorporated other aspects of Hawaiian culture, including an emphasis on spirituality. Intervention sessions began and ended with a *pule* (prayer) asking for ancestral and contemporary spiritual guidance, often delivered by a *kupuna* (elder) in the `ohana`. Cultural values were invoked throughout the intervention, illustrations in written materials depicted Hawaiian scenes and symbols, and the intervention was delivered by individuals who were of Native Hawaiian ancestry or who were long time Hawaii residents. The intervention itself included "modern" technologies, such as teaching the family members how to use the internet to access cancer information, but it was delivered in a traditional context.

This study was a randomized pilot study with a limited number of participants (six patients and 10 family members in the intervention and four patients and eight family members in the control group). Despite the small sample size, intervention group participants experienced significant positive changes on a number of measures, suggesting that a more extensive test of this intervention is warranted.

CONCLUSIONS AND RECOMMENDATIONS

Although the specific types of cancer differ regionally, cancer is a major health challenge across the globe. Considerable evidence shows that individuals who have fewer resources experience higher cancer rates, less screening, less adequate treatment, higher death rates, and more negative sequelae of the disease and its therapy. These disparities are found across countries, and in subgroups within countries and regions such as members of different ethnic populations.

While it is likely that similar disparities are found in psychosocial consequences of cancer, considerably fewer data are available to support or refute this claim. Most research has been conducted in developed countries, particularly the United States. Further, within the ethnically heterogeneous United States, few studies have focused on possible variations in psychosocial outcomes among individuals in different ethnic groups. The vast majority of studies do not report outcomes according to ethnicity and do not have the statistical power to detect differences.

Nonetheless, a body of evidence is beginning to be developed in both assessment of psychosocial outcomes and development and testing of interventions in population subgroups and international populations. Regarding outcomes, current information indicates that minority groups are likely to experience worse effects of cancer. The review of intervention studies conducted for this chapter indicates an increasing volume of intervention trials and international research, although most in North American samples. Specific kinds of interventions seem to be of more interest in different parts of the world. Selected studies have shown that interventions may work in different ways in different populations. Approaches may need to be tailored to match the needs and preferences of particular groups, and new approaches building on cultural values and practices of a specific group are also warranted.

To move this field forward, the following are needed:

More studies that include enough individuals in disparate groups to allow for adequate statistical power to detect possible group differences. For this kind of research to be successful, additional resources for recruitment of individuals from underrepresented groups are needed, including attention to activities such as translation and validation of assessment tools in the preferred language of the target group, approaches to intervention and measurement that are feasible in individuals who have low levels of literacy, and community participation to build support for the research and trust between researchers and patients. The most important first step is the acknowledgement that identifying possible differences among population subgroups is an important goal for more psychosocial oncology research.

More attention to understand the meaning of cancer in the context of culture, and the appropriateness of different assessment tools and intervention approaches in disparate groups. There are benefits to using common metrics and intervention approaches across subgroups and internationally. However, explanatory models for health and illness, values and preferences, roles of the family, and many other aspects of day-to-day life vary enormously from one group to another. More attention is needed to modifying interventions or developing new approaches that are consistent with cultural traditions, and to developing assessment tools that reflect the differences that distinguish groups, as well as the common threads that go across them all.

More attention to a comprehensive model of assessing and reducing health disparities. The causes of health disparities, as well as solutions to reduce them are complex and multifaceted. The covariation of ethnicity, race, and SES poses a particular challenge to understanding disparities. In addition, historical factors, the social context of health and illness, and many other variables go together to determine the outcomes individuals experience. In a comprehensive review of descriptions, causes, and mechanisms for health disparities in the United States, Adler and Rehkopf[31] propose research studies based on multiple sources of data, including natural experiments, and analytic methods, such as structural equation modeling, as ways to untangle causal influences on health disparities. Such approaches could aid in understanding the relationships between social factors, biological processes, and changes over time and across locations. Another consideration should be the identification of strengths, not only weaknesses and limitations, in groups that experience disparate cancer outcomes. Recognized cultural strengths provide building blocks for developing supportive interventions, with the ultimate goal to ensure that all cancer patients receive the care they need delivered in a manner that is comfortable to them, so that their psychosocial well-being is the highest possible.

ACKNOWLEDGMENT

Thanks to Nicole Bartley for editorial assistance in the preparation of this chapter.

REFERENCES

1. Minority Health and Health Disparities Research and Education Act. United States Public Law 106–525. 2000;2498.
2. Cancer. World Health Organization Website. http://www.who.int/topics/cancer/en. Accessed August 2008.
3. American Cancer Society/Cancer Research Center of Hawai'i/Hawai'i Department of Health. *Hawai'i: cancer facts & figures 2003-2004.* Honolulu, Hawaii: American Cancer Society; 2003.
4. World Cancer Research Fund/American Institute for Cancer Research. *Food, nutrition, physical activity, and the prevention of cancer: a global perspective.* Washington, DC: AICR; 2007
5. Stjernsward J, Teoh N. Current status of the global cancer control problem of the World Health Organization. *J Pain Symptom Manage.* 1993;8:340–347.
6. Peek ME, Han JH. Disparities in screening mammography: current status, interventions, and implications. *J Gen Intern Med.* 2004;19:184–194.
7. Masi CM, Blackman DJ, Peek, ME. Interventions to enhance breast cancer screening, diagnosis, and treatment among racial and ethnic minority women. *Med Care Res Rev.* 2007;64;S195–S242.
8. Borras JM, Guillen M, Sanchez V, Junca S, Vicente R. Educational level, voluntary private health insurance and opportunistic cancer screening among women in Catalonia. *Eur J Cancer Prev.* 1999;8:427–434.
9. Pivot X, Rixe O, Morere JF. Breast cancer screening in France: results of the EDIFICE survey. *Int J Med Sci.* 2008;5:106–112.
10. Institute of Medicine of the National Academies. *Unequal treatment: Confronting racial and ethnic disparities in health care.* Washington, DC: National Academy of Sciences; 2003.
11. Molassiotis A. Disparities in cancer care in Europe. *Eur J Oncol Nurs.* 2006;10:167–168.
12. Pandey M, Singh SP, Behere BP, Roy SK, Singh S, Shukla VK. Quality of Life in patients with early and advanced carcinoma of the breast. *Eur J Surg Oncol.* 2000;26:20–24.
13. Baider L, Peretz T, Ever Hadani P, Perry S, Avramov R, Kaplan De-Nour, A. Transmission of response to trauma? Second-generation Holocaust survivors' reaction to cancer. *Am J Psychiatry.* 2000;157:904–910.
14. Brucker PS, Yost K, Cashy J, Webster K, Cella D. General population and cancer patient norms for the Functional Assessment of Cancer Therapy—General (FACT-G). *Eval Health Prof.* 2005;28:192–211.
15. Ell K, Sanchez K, Vourlekis B, et al. Depression, correlates of depression, and receipt of depression care among low-income women with breast or gynecological cancer. *J Clin Oncol.* 2005;23:3052–3060.
16. Dapueto JJ, Francolino C, Servente L, et al. Evaluation of the Functional Assessment of Cancer Therapy—General (FACT-G) Spanish version 4 in South America: classic psychometric and item response theory analyses. *Health Qual Life Outcomes.* 2003;1:32.
17. Ashing-Giwa K, Tejero JS, Kim J, Padilla GV, Hellemann G. Examining predictive models of HRQOL in a population-based, multiethnic sample of women with breast carcinoma. *Qual Life Res.* 2007;16:413–428.
18. Wong WS, Fielding R. The association between patient satisfaction and quality of life in Chinese lung and liver cancer patients. *Med Care.* 2008;46:293–302.
19. Carlson LE, Angen M, Cullum J, et al. High levels of untreated distress and fatigue in cancer patients. *Br J Cancer.* 2004;90:2297–2304.
20. Moadel AB, Morgan C, Dutcher J. Psychosocial needs assessment among an underserved, ethnically diverse cancer patient population. *Cancer.* 2007;109(Suppl 2):446–454.
21. Gotay C, Holup J, Pagano I. Ethnic differences in quality of life among early breast and prostate cancer survivors. *Psychooncol.* 2002;11:103–113.
22. Fobair P, Stewart SL, Chang S, D'Onofrio C, Banks PJ, Bloom JR. Body image and sexual problems in young women with breast cancer. *Psychooncol.* 2006;15:579–594.

23. Shim E, Mehnert A, Koyama A, et al. Health-related quality of life in breast cancer: a cross-cultural survey of German, Japanese, and South Korean patients. *Breast Cancer Res Treat.* 2006;99:341–350.

24. Scott NW, Fayers PM, Bottomley A, et al. Comparing translations of the EORTC QLQ-C30 using differential item functioning analyses. *Qual Life Res.* 2006;15:1103–1115.

25. Institute of Medicine (IOM). 2008. *Cancer care for the whole patient: Meeting psychosocial health needs.* Adler NE, Page AEK, (eds). Washington, DC: The National Academies Press.

26. Mishel MH, Germino BB, Gil KM, et al. Benefits from an uncertainty management intervention for African-American and Caucasian older long-term breast cancer survivors. *Psychooncology.* 2005;14:962–978.

27. Gil KM, Mishel MH, Belyea M, Germino B, Porter LS, Clayton M. Benefits of the uncertainty management intervention for African American and White older breast cancer survivor: 20 month outcomes. *Intern J Behav Med.* 2006;13:286–294.

28. Dwight-Johnson M, Ell K, Lee P. Can collaborative care address the needs of low-income Latinas with comorbid depression and cancer? Results from a randomized pilot study. *Psychosomatics.* 2005;46:224–232.

29. Ell K, Quon B, Quinn DI, et al. Improving treatment of depression among low-income patients with cancer: the design of the ADAPt-C study. *Gen Hosp Psychiatry.* 2007;29:223–231.

30. Mokuau N, Braun KL, Wong LK, Higuchi P, Gotay CC. Development of a family intervention for Native Hawaiian women with cancer: a pilot study. *Soc Work.* 2008;53:9–19.

31. Adler NE, Rehkopf DH. U.S. disparities in health: descriptions, causes and mechanisms. *Annu Rev Public Health.* 2008;29:235–252.

PART XI

Psychological Issues for the Family

Matthew J. Loscalzo, ED

CHAPTER 71

The Family's "Stuck Points" in Adjusting to Cancer

Frances Marcus Lewis

Cancer invades and causes ripple effects in the family.[1]

Families matter. They matter because they form the first line of support to the patient with cancer. They also matter because they are directly impacted by cancer-related pressures and are often on their own to understand the disease and treatment, how to help the patient manage, how to correctly interpret the patient's symptoms, and how to maintain some semblance of balance between family life and life with the cancer. Increasingly we have come to learn that cancer threatens the core functions of a household family, even high functioning families.[2] Cancer can take over the family's life at the expense of maintaining nurturing and caring interpersonal communication, quality parenting, and supportive marital communication.[2-4]

Families suffer unnecessarily when cancer is diagnosed, when it recurs, or when it moves to an advanced stage. General advice or broad-stroke help from professionals is not sufficient to help. Targeted, planned, systematic professional services are needed to help families deal with their "stuck points," the cross-cutting issues that are known from research to affect how a family experiences, adjusts, and functions when a family member has cancer.

There are 4 purposes to this chapter (1) to conceptualize cancer as a family illness, not a patient's disease; (2) to describe "stuck points" family members experience in adjusting to and managing cancer; (3) to describe four levels of service for family-focused psycho-oncology that can be responsive to the "stuck points"; and (4) to propose future needed directions for programs in family-focused psycho-oncology.

CANCER AS A FAMILY'S ILLNESS, NOT A PATIENT'S DISEASE

In the past 20 years, there has been a growing awareness that cancer is a family's illness, not patient's diagnosis. Initial awareness grew out of seminal papers by healthcare providers and behavioral scientists in the 1960s and 1970s.[1,5,6] However, it was not until the 1980s and 1990s that family-focused psycho-oncology came to fruition in the research programs of a small but now growing number of teams, including Compas[7]; Given[8]; Hilton[9]; Hoskins[10]; Lewis[11-14]; Northouse[15]; and Wellisch.[16]

In the 2000s, the diagnosis of cancer still represents a major threat to family members and their functioning as a household, despite the success of early diagnosis and increasingly successful medical treatment for the disease. Even when diagnosed early, family members, including children, adolescents, adult children, and spouses, worry about the patient dying or suffering from the cancer.[14,17,18] The cancer causes "ripple effects" in the family by creating fears, uncertainty, disrupted life plans, rearranged schedules and routines, changed interpersonal communication, existential worries, alterations in household members' functioning, and heightened household tension, among other ripples.

Cancer is not a single stressor event for families but is better characterized as a series of multiple, interwoven, and layered psychosocial transitions.[19] The threat and tension generated by the cancer recycles when the cancer recurs, causing heightened concern by both patients and family members.[20-22] Cancer also challenges the assumptive world of the family, not just the patient, including the family's values, orientation, and self-formulation.[19] During psychosocial transitions, family members search for answers to questions like, Why me? Why has this happened to our family? Why us? Why now?[17] These internal reflections are invisible to others, including other members of the same family.

From a family systems perspective, a family experiencing cancer attempts to reconfigure itself around the cancer and, in the process, there is destabilization, even in high resource and well-adjusted households. This destabilization occurs in both patient–spouse dyads and in the parent–child dyad.[3,11,12,23] Destabilization is accompanied by distress. Both distress and destabilization are normative processes, not pathological ones. From a family systems perspective, destabilization eventually gets worked out and there is restabilization. In the ideal, restabilization is reflected in new arrangements families make to take care of the patient, changes in the ways family members communicate and support each other, new goals it generates for itself as a family, and a new self-reformulation. Families experience "stuck points" in the process of restabilization.

"STUCK POINTS" EXPERIENCED BY FAMILY MEMBERS

Families, regardless of type or stage of cancer, experience "stuck points," that is, cross-cutting issues on which they get "stuck," and with which they struggle, often with few or no resources. These issues are known from research to affect how a family experiences and restabilizes, that is, adjusts, and functions when a family member has cancer. Knowledge of these "stuck points" can enable psycho-oncology clinicians to help families.

Stuck point 1. Families do not know how to support the dependent child who is experiencing parental cancer. The report card is mixed on the family's ability to support the child whose parent has cancer. During treatment or repeated cycles of treatment, parents are in "survival mode."[13] Although family members claim they want to help their child, they are often too distressed, too symptomatic, or too emotionally exhausted to support their child in the ways they want. Diagnosed mothers of children claim they do not know what to say or how to help their child deal with the impact of her breast cancer in ways that care, not scare.[23] Parents are especially concerned about their ability to respond to their child's *emotional* needs, particularly when those needs compete with the diagnosed parent's abilities in the moment.[13] As one mother stated, "I was aware…that the kids' emotional needs had to take second place to mine and that was hard. With the fatigue, I just didn't have enough energy to listen."[13]

A large proportion of school-age and adolescent children are likely on their own to interpret and manage the impact of parental cancer. In an interview study of 81 children of mothers diagnosed with cancer, the majority of both young and older children said they did not talk with their mother about her cancer.[24] When asked *who helped them cope with the mother's cancer*, 11% of the younger children and 37% of the older children did not report that anyone helped them deal with their mother's breast cancer.[24] When asked what *the family did that helped the children cope*, 25% of the younger and 15% of the older children said that the family did nothing to help them.

Even when diagnosed parents interact with their child about the cancer, the content and form of the discussion is more like a biology class than a nurturing, interactive conversation.[25] In a study of mothers of 30 school-age children, mothers used a biomedical-talk-teach-tell model to talk with their child about their cancer and did not report attending to the child's thoughts and feelings.[25] The language the ill mothers use may include frightening images, words, or experiences, as illustrated in this mother's statements to her 8-year-old son about her cancer. "It (cancer) was a group of bad cells that if allowed to grow could cause...well, I think I did mention that it could be fatal."[25] A mother of two boys, ages 12 and 9, said, "I told them I didn't plan to (die)...but that some people did."

Single parents may be at particular risk for challenges in assisting their child with the cancer. In a comparative study of 22 single compared to 104 married mothers with breast cancer, single mothers with breast cancer scored significantly lower on parenting quality on a standardized measure of parenting.[14] Analyses also revealed that single women overly relied on their children for support, even when the single women's network size and quality of support were comparable to those of married mothers.[14] Single mothers viewed their children as a major source of the ill mother feeling like or loved. Single mothers confided in their children about their cancer and also turned to their children as a major source of help.[13] Note this single mother's statements.

I just want her to be there for me...if I had a rough day. Maybe I do expect her to be the other adult. I think I expect some emotional support for me...I want her to feel what I'm going through...it's hard as a single mom.

The challenge for families to support the child is made more complex because children do not always share their questions, worries, or concerns about the parent's cancer. Confidential interviews with children reveal that children see both the ill parent and household members as overly burdened by the cancer and do not want to add to that burden. Some children conceal their thoughts, fears, and feelings to protect their ill parent or not cause more tension in their relationship with the ill parent.[24] Children who were 8–12 years old at the time of their mother's diagnosis were asked to describe what it was like for them to talk with their mother or other parent about the mother's breast cancer.[18] Here is what one 12-year old child said, "*I didn't want to upset her. I didn't want to, you know, like make her cry or anything.*" A child who was 8 years old at the time of his mother's diagnosis worried that talking would cause a permanent disconnection between him and his mother.[18] Here are his words.

It'd be like you'd lost contact. It's like you...like...they built moon base, and then they lost contact with earth. It's like you can see it so close, yet so far? I was just afraid that I would upset her so bad or something that she'd just would never talk to me again.

Stuck point 2. Spouses do not know how to respond supportively to the patient's expressed thoughts and feelings about the cancer. Cancer is known to cause communication difficulties and marital tension in the diagnosed patient and spouse, the largest evidence of which has been documented in couples experiencing breast cancer.[26] These communication challenges can affect couples' martial adjustment.[10,22,27–30]

In a recently completed interview study involving 77 couples dealing with early stage breast cancer, the majority (65%) of their top-ranked concerns related to interpersonal tension, relationship issues, or communication problems that both spouses explicitly attributed to the cancer.[3] In that same study, 22% of couples said they wanted help in developing new ways of being together as a couple that emphasized their relationship, not the cancer. Couples said the cancer had taken precedence over everything, including their time alone as a couple and they wanted to find a way to instead focus on their relationship again.

Couples experiencing the acute phase of breast cancer treatment have treatment-related demands that distract them from attending to and supporting each other's thoughts, feelings, and needs for support about the cancer. Some scientists interpret this form of interaction as aversive communication; others view it as the spouse's absence of skills and confidence.[31]

Tension in the patient–spouse dyad can be heightened when the ill and non-ill spouse experience different disease trajectories or hold different views about how to help the patient heal from the cancer.[15,32,33] These different views cause an interpersonal disconnection between them. For example, wives with breast cancer are known to want their spouse to be a good listener for them at a time when the spouse thinks he should support her by doing the dishes or cleaning the house. Such spouse behavior can be viewed as nonsupportive by the patient. In another example, spouses commonly attempt to cheer up their ill wife by telling her she will be okay. The diagnosed wife, in contrast, views such behavior as uncaring or as the spouse's not fully understanding the seriousness of her experience.[30]

Nonresponsiveness to patients' thoughts and feelings can be influenced by gender-related issues. Husbands of wives with breast cancer are known to protect themselves from their own feelings,[34] to ride out their feelings, or to attempt to forget them.[30]

Stuck point 3. Family members struggle with the effects of the patient's and spouse's depressed mood on the household. The patient's depressed mood has diffuse negative effects on other members of the household, on interpersonal relationships, and on the quality with which the diagnosed patient is able to support other family members. Rates and duration of depressed mood and anxiety vary by stage of disease, by recurrence, by type of treatment, and by type of measurement, among other factors. See Fann and others for a recent review of the evidence.[35]

Women with breast cancer experience high rates of depressed mood and affective problems for up to or longer than 2 years after diagnosis.[36–38] Depressed mood in mothers with breast cancer is known to be disruptive to routines in the home and to negatively affect overall tension in the household.[11,12] Even in the absence of depressed mood, treatment demands or preoccupation with the cancer can make the diagnosed woman physically or emotionally unavailable for other family members. Side effects caused by polychemotherapy, hormonal therapy and surgical and radiation treatment can result in months of symptoms.

Psychosocial morbidity in spouses of women with breast cancer has been demonstrated in both cross sectional and longitudinal studies with significantly elevated levels documented up to 3 years after diagnosis. In some studies, spouse distress exceeds levels in the diagnosed woman.[10,15,39]

Depressed mood in the spouse has known negative consequences for the diagnosed patient who is attempting to heal from the cancer. Greater mood disturbance in the spouse has been associated with higher distress in cancer patients.[40] Spouses' depressed mood can constrain their support to the patient and their ability to listen to, respond to, or work collaboratively with the patient to manage the cancer. Studies reveal that the diagnosed wife interprets this inaccessibility as rejection or abandonment.[41] Depressed mood can also cause distancing or criticism and negatively affect the ways in which couples cope with their problems and challenges.[42] Marital tension or conflict have high potential to distract from the couple's processes of appraising, reconfiguring around, and adjusting to the demands of the cancer.[43]

There is beginning evidence that the effects of depressed mood in the diagnosed parent of dependent children may affect the child. Admittedly, the evidence is mixed. Short-term depressed mood is situational depressed mood, not clinical depression, and there is no study that definitively documents the effects of parental situational depression on dependent children when a parent has cancer. Short-term depressed mood in an ill parent may be partially compensated by quality parenting by the non-ill parent or by the other yet-to-be studied factors.[44]

The largest body of evidence of the effects of parental depressed mood on children's adjustment comes from studies of mothers with breast cancer. Depressed mothers have impaired parenting characterized by less psychological availability, communicativeness, as well as increased irritability. When parent–child relations are characterized by parental withdrawal, indifference, or unreliability, children show impaired functioning in the form of behavioral, social, and self-esteem problems.[44,45] In a seminal study of children whose mother had breast cancer or diabetes, children of mothers with serious illness tended to have lower self-esteem scores than children of well mothers (F 1,46 = 3.01, p =0.09).[45] In that same study, children of mothers with breast cancer scored lower on a standardized measure of self-esteem on more occasions than did children of well mothers (F 1, 27 = 5.71, p =0.02).[45] The authors of that study speculated that children of mothers with cancer may internalize self-deprecating views compared to children of non-ill parents.

In a more recently completed study of 87 adolescents and 174 ill and non-ill parents, results revealed that mothers' depressed mood was significantly associated with three measures of adolescent functioning: total behavior problems ($t_{85} = -2.97$; $p < 0.01$); externalizing problems ($t_{85} = -2.34$; $p < 0.05$); and internalizing problems ($t_{85} = -2.98$; $p < 0.01$).[44] In contrast, fathers' (non-ill parents) mood was not related to any measure of adolescent functioning.

Stuck point 4. Tension in the marriage from the cancer has significant negative consequences for the household's functioning. Tension in the marriage that is attributed to the cancer has negative effects on the household. As such, marital tension from the cancer is a family matter, not a private matter between the diagnosed patient and spouse. The earliest evidence of the deleterious effects of marital tension on the household came from a study of 80 diagnosed women with breast cancer, their 8–12 year old school-age children, and spouses.[12] Heightened marital tension negatively affected the quality of the parent–child relationship, the family member's coping behavior, and the overall functioning of the household.[12] It appeared that an escalating positive or deviation amplifying feedback loop was operating in which worsening conditions in the marriage resulted in diminished coping, poorer parenting quality, lower child functioning, and less well-adjusted functioning in the household.[12]

Stuck point 5. Families use coping behavior that may be nonresponsive to pressures on the household from the cancer. "Coping" is a popular term in psycho-oncology and although the concept has relevance to studies of an individual patient's adaptation to bounded and delimited stressors, its validity in depicting a family system's response to cancer in a member is less clear. In two studies of families impacted by maternal breast cancer, the illness-related demands reported by either the patient or the spouse-caregiver never significantly predicted family member coping behavior.[11,12] In another study of 111 families of women with breast cancer, data obtained on three occasions at 4-month intervals revealed that family members did not change their coping behavior over time, even when the number of illness-related demands changed (Multivariate $F = 6.70$, $p < 0.01$). Instead of modifying how they coped with the changing demands from the cancer, family members' coping behavior remained unchanged. Furthermore, in cross-lagged analyses involving these same households, family members' coping behavior did not reduce the cancer-related pressures they experienced at the next occasion in which they were assessed. This suggests that families may continue to use coping behavior that is ineffective in reducing the cancer-related issues families experience. It is as if the families as households put the cancer "under the table, not on top of it." If family members are not coping with the illness-related demands, with what are they coping? Evidence from hundreds of patients and spouse-caregivers reveal that family members are attempting to manage tension in the family system, especially heightened tension in the patient–spouse relationship that is accentuated or caused by the cancer.[11,12]

FOUR LEVELS OF SERVICE FOR FAMILY-FOCUSED PSYCHO-ONCOLOGY PROGRAMS

This chapter has described five "stuck points" family members are likely to experience when a member has cancer. Four levels of family-focused psycho-oncology services are needed to help families manage their "stuck points." When a patient is put on a chemotherapy protocol, there are certain minimums the patient will receive, including instructions about the drugs, symptoms to expect, how to manage side effects, symptoms to report to the medical provider, among others. This information creates a cognitive map for the patient. There are no such minimums and no such cognitive map for the family of a patient with cancer. The future of family-focused services in psycho-oncology needs to include four levels of service: Level 1, minimum; Level 2, programmatic; Level 3, personalized, and Level 4, case-intensive.

Level 1 is the minimum service all families need to be offered. Contact involves minimum contact by a professional or specially trained assistant who offers the family member access to predeveloped printed, auditory, web based, or audio-visual (AV) materials to help them manage the impact of the cancer on the family, including symptom interpretation, among other things. There are exemplary models of this Level 1 service at agencies like the Princess Margaret Hospital in Toronto, among others. Princess Margaret Hospital has a major learning center that is called the "Patient & Family Library" in which trained volunteers are positioned to assist family members access materials that are relevant to their situation. The agency also has 22 "Resource Centres of the Patient & Family Library" in clinic waiting areas throughout the hospital. The goal of the family encounter in Level 1 service is to guarantee the family's access to materials as informed consumers.

Level 2 service is programmatic service. It involves enrolling, not merely offering families, entry into predeveloped programs that are available from the agency or in collaboration with other agencies. Ideally, these predeveloped programs are evidence-based programs that have been previously and formally evaluated for short-term impact or efficacy. At minimum the programs have been well described and evaluated in the published literature. Examples of well described programs include the FOCUS Program[46] and the Enhancing Connections Program,[47] among others. Provider agencies will need to create a systematic process by which previously tested programs are identified and then brought to the agency for further dissemination.

Level 3 or personalized service, includes all that is offered in Level 1, plus personalized services from a specially trained professional who assists the family members interpret and integrate the information they obtained from Level 1 materials. The focus of the professional in Level 3 service is to systematically coach the family on ways to gain and implement new cognitive, behavioral, and emotional methods to manage the family's "stuck points." Such coaching is targeted self-management and focuses on skills to maintain and protect the family's core functions as well as better manage the illness.[2] Trained professionals can include nurses, clinical psychologists, social workers, masters prepared patient educators, certified masters prepared counselors, and chaplains, among others. Level 3 services are not informal or conversational but are instead services that add to the competencies and self-confidence of the family to manage the impact of cancer. Families are not receiving therapy; they are being assisted to manage the impact of cancer on their lives as a family.

Level 4 service is case-intensive service for highly distressed families that are too challenged to communicate among family members, too distressed to read and plan ways to carry out the recommendations in Level 1 materials, or too unclear on what they need to work on to manage, as would be the case in Level 2 services. In Levels 1, 2, and 3, family members are communicating with each other, even if they are depressed, anxious, grieving, or otherwise distressed. In Level 4, communication between family members is essentially nonexistent or extremely challenged. Families needing Level 4 service include severely disrupted families who require more intensive therapy and some may benefit from pharmacologic support.

FUTURE DIRECTIONS FOR FAMILY-FOCUSED SERVICES AND PROGRAMS

All families experience "stuck points" when a member has cancer. Our goal in psycho-oncology is to help them get "un-stuck" or to prevent the intensity, duration, or level of destabilization that is caused by the "stuck point." When cancer is cast as a long term, chronic illness, there is an even greater imperative to help families add to their competencies to manage the impact of the cancer while they protect and nurture their lives as families.

Family members with cancer have been treated with benign neglect by clinicians because we have confused valuing the family with programs and service.[2] The reality is that families are primarily on their own to manage the transitions and contingencies of a patient's cancer, even as the cancer causes ripple effects in family members' lives and families' core functions.

When agencies commit to systematizing family-focused psycho-oncology services like those described in Levels 1, 2, and 3, new structures will be developed. For example, new methods of record keeping will be needed. The medical record in most agencies does not include data on parenting status and very few agencies systematically document the patient's marital or partnership status. How can we offer family-focused psycho-oncology services if we do not know the composition of the patient's household family. If we are to outreach them with programs to help them support their dependent child about the cancer, then we need to know about parenting status. The child-rearing status of the patient is absent from the medical record. It is as if patients were hermetically isolated individuals, not members of a family.

Level 1 and 2 services will require specific structures and personnel in the agency to identify psycho-educational programs that have been developed and tested that meet the agency's standards for evidence-based programs. This will require on-going annual monitoring of new programs, replacing out-dated programs, and maintaining a library of updated materials. The director of "libraries" needs to be in close contact with professional staff so that they are apprised of the current offerings.

Future programs and services need to develop creative ways to channel families into Levels 1, 2, and 3 services and programs. Merely having a resource library or center is not enough; getting the materials into the hands of family members is the minimum goal. Caution is also in order. It is not normative for many families to ask or receive help from outsiders, and it will not be a simple matter to tell families about these services. Many families choose to handle things on their own, even as they struggle and suffer unnecessarily with their "stuck points." We will need creative ways to offer families these services.

A prescription for healing families is needed. Healing involves helping the family stabilize its core functions, including relationships between members that have been altered or challenged by the cancer. Healing also involves helping family members add to their competencies to manage the illness, including reorganizing routines around treatment, symptom management, long-term care, and survivorship while concurrently protecting time to be a family, not just a family with cancer.

Providers ideally could identify and note the programs and services they want a specific family or, alternatively all families of their patients, to receive, inclusive of Level 1, 2, and 3 services. By making these referrals in writing, the provider is normalizing the provision of family-focused services in the same way a provider would normalize and prescribe physical therapy when a patient fractures a bone.

Future programs with families need to include the use of new channels, including the World Wide Web and telephone-delivered interventions, including recently evolved telehealth methods like the videophone, among others. Telephone-delivered psycho-educational programs hold great promise; see the efficacy-tested telephone intervention by Mishel,[48] among others.

The family's "stuck points" are part of the natural history of the family's experience with cancer; they are not signs of pathology. Although we have well-developed programs to assist individual patients to better adjust to cancer, we need comparable programs to assist *families qua families* better self-manage, self-regulate, and thrive. A little intervention can go a long way to help families adapt and more is not always better. Level 1 and 2 services may be sufficient to help most families.

Healing from cancer is much more than surgical wound healing, cancer remission, or cure. Healing needs to involve family members, all of whom have been impacted by the patient's cancer. It is not enough to only help the patient; our work in helping families heal is a social and professional imperative. Psycho-oncology clinicians are ideally positioned to be the stewards of family-focused services.

ACKNOWLEDGMENTS

Research reported in this chapter was made possible through grants from the National Institutes of Health: R01 NR 01000, R01 CA 78424, R01-CA-55347, R01 NR 04135; the Department of Defense, Breast Cancer Research Program, U.S. Army Medical and Materiel Command; American Cancer Society; Oncology Nursing Foundation; Lance Armstrong Foundation; Tennis Fund, University of Washington, School of Medicine; Nesholm Family Foundation; Dorothy S. O'Brien Special Projects Fund, Cancer Lifeline; and Susan G. Komen Breast Cancer Foundation, Puget Sound Affiliate.

REFERENCES

1. Parkes CM. The emotional impact of cancer on patients and their families. *J Laryng Otol.* 1975;89(12):1271–1279.
2. Lewis FM. Family-focused oncology nursing research. *Oncol Nurs Forum.* 2004;31(2):288–292.
3. Shands ME, Lewis FM, Sinsheimer J, Cochrane BB. Core concerns of couples living with early stage breast cancer. *Psychooncology.* 2006 Dec;15(12):1055–1064.
4. Manne S, Sherman M, Ross S, Ostroff J, Heyman RE, Fox K. Couples' support-related communication, psychological distress, and relationship satisfaction among women with early stage breast cancer. *J Consult Clin Psychol.* 2004 Aug;72(4):660–670.
5. Barckley V. The crisis in cancer. *Am J Nurs.* 1967 Feb;67(2):278–280.
6. Litman TJ. The family as a basic unit in health and medical care: a social-behavioral overview. *Soc Sci Med.* 1974 Sep;8(9–10):495–519.
7. Compas BE, Ey S, Worsham NL, Howell DC. When mom or dad has cancer: II. Coping, cognitive appraisals, and psychological distress in children of cancer patients. *Health Psychol.* 1996;15(3):167–175.
8. Given B, Given CW. Patient and family caregiver reaction to new and recurrent breast cancer. *J Am Med Womens Assoc.* 1992 Sep-Oct;47(5):201–206, 212.
9. Hilton BA. A study of couple communication patterns when coping with early stage breast cancer. *Can Oncol Nurs J.* 1993;3(4):159–166.
10. Hoskins CN. Adjustment to breast cancer in couples. *Psychol Rep.* 1995;77(2):435–454.
11. Lewis FM, Hammond MA. The father's, mother's, and adolescent's functioning with breast cancer. *Fam Relat.* 1996;45:456–465.
12. Lewis FM, Hammond MA, Woods NF. The family's functioning with newly diagnosed breast cancer in the mother: the development of an explanatory model. *J Behav Med.* 1993;16(4):351–370.
13. Lewis FM, Zahlis EH, Shands ME, Sinsheimer JA, Hammond MA. The functioning of single women with breast cancer and their school-aged children. *Cancer Pract.* 1996;4(1):15–24.
14. Lewis FM, Fletcher KA, Cochrane BB, Fann JR. Predictors of depressed mood in spouses of women with breast cancer. *J Clin Oncol.* 2008 Mar 10;26(8):1289–1295.
15. Northouse LL, Swain MA. Adjustment of patients and husbands to the initial impact of breast cancer. *Nurs Res.* 1987;36(4):221–225.
16. Wellisch DK, Gritz ER, Schain W, Wang HJ, Siau J. Psychological functioning of daughters of breast cancer patients. Part I: daughters and comparison subjects. *Psychosomatics.* 1991 Summer;32(3):324–336.
17. Houldin A, Lewis FM. Salvaging their normal lives: a qualitative study of patients with recently diagnosed advanced colorectal cancer. *Oncol Nurs Forum.* 2006 Jul;33(4):719–725.
18. Zahlis EH. The child's worries about the mother's breast cancer: sources of distress in school-age children. *Oncol Nurs Forum.* 2001;28(6):1019–1025.
19. Lewis FM. Psychosocial transitions and the family's work in adjusting to cancer. *Semin Oncol Nurs.* 1993;9(2):127–129.
20. Northouse LL, Dorris G, Charron-Moore C. Factors affecting couples' adjustment to recurrent breast cancer. *Soc Sci Med.* 1995;41(1):69–76.
21. Cella DF, Mahon SM, Donovan MI. Cancer recurrence as a traumatic event. *Behav Med.* 1990 Spring;16(1):15–22.
22. Lewis FM, Deal LW. Balancing our lives: a study of the married couple's experience with breast cancer recurrence. *Oncol Nurs Forum.* 1995;22(6):943–953.
23. Zahlis E, Lewis FM. Mothers' stories of the school-age child's experience with the mother's breast cancer. *J Psychosoc Oncol.* 1998;16(2):25–43.
24. Issel LM, Ersek M, Lewis FM. How children cope with mother's breast cancer. *Oncol Nurs Forum.* 1990;17(3):5–13.
25. Shands ME, Lewis FM, Zahlis EH. Mother and child interactions about the mother's breast cancer: an interview study. *Oncol Nurs Forum.* 2000;27(1):77–85.
26. Wimberly SR, Carver CS, Laurenceau J-P, Harris SD, Antoni MH. Perceived partner reactions to diagnosis and treatment of breast cancer: Impact on psychosocial and psychosexual adjustment. *J Consult Clinical Psychol.* 2005;73(2):300–311.
27. Hilton BA. Issues, problems, and challenges for families coping with breast cancer. *Semin Oncol Nurs.* 1993;9(2):88–100.
28. Hilton BA. Family communication patterns in coping with early breast cancer. *West J Nurs Res.* 1994 Aug;16(4):366–388. Discussion 388–391.
29. Lichtman RR, Taylor SE, Wood JV. Social support and marital adjustment after breast cancer. *J Psychosoc Oncol.* 1987;5(3):47–74.
30. Samms MC. The husband's untold account of his wife's breast cancer: a chronologic analysis. *Oncol Nurs Forum.* 1999;26(8):1351–1358.
31. Lewis FM, Cochrane BB, Fletcher KA, et al. Helping her heal: a pilot study of an educational counseling intervention for spouses of women with breast cancer. *Psychooncology.* 2007;17(2):131–137.

32. Baider L, Kaplan De-Nour A. Couples' reactions and adjustment to mastectomy: a preliminary report. *Int J Psychiatry Med.* 1984;14(3):265–276.

33. Quint JC. The impact of mastectomy. *Am J Nurs.* 1963;63(11):88–92.

34. Sabo D, Brown J, Smith C. The male role and mastectomy: support groups and men's adjustment. *J Psychosoc Oncol.* 1986;4(1/2):19–31.

35. Fann J, Thomas-Rich A, Katon W, et al. Major depression after breast cancer: a review of epidemiology and treatment. *Gen Hosp Psychiatry.* 2008 30(2):112–126.

36. Bloom JR, Cook M, Fotopoulis S, et al. Psychological response to mastectomy: a prospective comparison study. *Cancer.* 1987;59(1):189–196.

37. Fallowfield LJ, Hall A, Maguire GP, Baum M. Psychological outcomes of different treatment policies in women with early breast cancer outside a clinical trial. *BMJ.* 1990 Sep 22;301(6752):575–580.

38. Goldberg JA, Scott RN, Davidson PM, et al. Psychological morbidity in the first year after breast surgery. *Eur J Surg Oncol.* 1992;18:327–331.

39. Hoskins CN, Baker S, Budin W, et al. Adjustment among husbands of women with breast cancer. *J Psychosoc Oncol.* 1996;4(1):41–69.

40. Ben-Zur H, Gilbar O, Lev S. Coping with breast cancer: patient, spouse, and dyad models. *Psychosom Med.* 2001;63:32–39.

41. Hagedoorn M, Kuijer RG, Buunk BP, DeJong GM, Wobbes T, Sanderman R. Marital satisfaction in patients with cancer: does support from intimate partners benefit those who need it most? *Health Psychol.* 2000;19(3):274–282.

42. Manne SL. Intrusive thoughts and psychological distress among cancer patients: the role of spouse avoidance and criticism. *J Consult Clin Psychol.* 1999;67(4):539–546.

43. Weihs K, Enright T, Howe G, Simmens SJ. Marital satisfaction and emotional adjustment after breast cancer. *J Psychosoc Oncol.* 1999;17(1):33–49.

44. Lewis FM, Darby EL. Adolescent adjustment and maternal breast cancer: a test of the "faucet hypothesis". *J Psychosoc Oncol.* 2004;21(4):83–106.

45. Armsden GC, Lewis FM. Behavioral adjustment and self-esteem of school-age children of women with breast cancer. *Oncol Nurs Forum.* 1994;21(1):39–45.

46. Northouse LL, Mood DW, Schafenacker A, et al. Randomized clinical trial of a family intervention for prostate cancer patients and their spouses. *Cancer.* 2007 Dec 15;110(12):2809–2818.

47. Lewis FM, Casey SM, Brandt PA, Shands ME, Zahlis EH. The enhancing connections program: pilot study of a cognitive-behavioral intervention for mothers and children affected by breast cancer. *Psychooncology.* 2006 Jun;15(6):486–497.

48. Mishel MH, Belyea M, Germino BB, et al. Helping patients with localized prostate carcinoma manage uncertainty and treatment side effects: nurse-delivered psychoeducational intervention over the telephone. *Cancer.* 2002 Mar 15;94(6):1854–1866.

CHAPTER 72

Spouse Caregivers of Cancer Patients

Laurel L. Northouse and Ruth McCorkle

Over the past two decades, the role of family caregivers has become essential as treatment for adults with cancer has shifted to outpatient facilities and as patients survive longer with active disease.[1] Spouses are most often the primary caregivers to people with cancer,[2] and although they received little or no preparation, spouses are consumed with patient responsibilities such as assistance with activities of daily living, medication administration, physical care, emotional support, transportation, and household management. Historically, spouse caregivers have played a major role in providing care; however, the level of technical, psychological, and physical support currently demanded of caregivers is unprecedented.[1,3] Too often the responsibility for complex care resides with spouse caregivers without regard for their resources or skills to provide the care.

As the demands of caregiving increase, spouses experience a myriad of physical, mental, and social consequences, which may exceed those of their ill partners.[2,4-6] There is concern not only for the mental and physical well-being of spouse caregivers, but also for their ability to provide complex care when their own health is compromised. Studies indicate that when spouse caregivers are highly distressed, cancer patients report more problems adjusting to the illness over time.[7] In light of the essential role of spouses and the multiple care demands they face, it is important to understand their experiences and identify ways to help them.

This chapter focuses on spouses as primary caregivers to people with cancer. The chapter begins with a discussion of the interdependence of patients and spouses and the reciprocal effect they have on one another. We discuss the common needs of spouse caregivers, as well intervention studies that have been conducted to address their needs. The chapter concludes with directions for future research.

INTERDEPENDENCE OF PATIENTS AND SPOUSES

One of the unique aspects of the patient–spouse relationship is the partners' interdependence on one another as they cope with the demands of cancer. Patients and spouses share the same household, same resources, and rely on one another for emotional and instrumental support. When one partner is diagnosed with cancer, both partners experience stress associated with the illness. In a recent meta-analysis, Hagedoorn and colleagues[8] examined 46 studies of cancer patients and their spouses to determine to what extent they influence one another during the cancer experience. They found a moderate significant relationship ($r = .29$) between the emotional distress of patients and their spouses. On the basis of these findings, the researchers concluded that couples react to cancer as an emotional system; each partner affects the other (see Fig. 72–1). This reciprocal relationship was evident across various types of cancer and stages of cancer. They also found that couples who are coping with cancer reported moderate levels of distress, and that their distress was significantly higher than couples without cancer or community samples.

The interdependence of cancer patients and their spouses is evident in many other aspects of the illness, such as dealing with changing family roles,[9] managing symptoms, and maintaining the family's quality of life.[2] Spouses often assume the responsibilities of ill partners, which can help to maintain family function, but it can also lead to spouses' role overload. Research indicates that as the number of illness-related demands increase, spouses are at greater risk of developing depression.[10]

The concept of caregiver burden (i.e., the distress that caregivers feel as a result of providing care) is closely related to the interdependence that exists between patients and their spouses. Caregiver burden increases when patients report more symptom distress or have trouble meeting their basic needs.[4,11,12] It also increases when spouses need to provide more hours of care or a higher intensity of care. In a national study of caregivers of patients with chronic disease five levels of caregiver burden have been identified[13] (see Table 72–1). The level of burden was based on an index derived from the number and types of care provided, as well as the number of hours of care provided. The levels of burden increased as the intensity and the hours of care increased. At the highest level of burden (Level 5), the majority of caregivers were women (71%), many of the caregivers rated their own health as fair or poor, and they were likely to say that caregiving made their health worse.[13] These findings underscore the interrelationship between caregiver burden and caregiver well-being. Spouses of cancer patients are vulnerable to caregiver burden because of their primary caregiving role, and because their lives are so intertwined with the lives of their ill partners.

COMMON NEEDS OF SPOUSE CAREGIVERS

There have been a number of systematic reviews identifying the needs of caregivers beginning in the 1980s[14-17]; the majority of respondents in these reports were spouses. In the mid-1990s, participants were expanded to include a broader base of caregivers, including siblings, parents, and other relatives or friends.[18] As the field has grown, these reviews targeted caregivers of patients with specific sites of cancer.[19,20] Out of these reviews came consistent documentation of the needs associated with caring for a member with cancer.

Information. Spouses consistently report the need for information. Spouses search for information can be extensive, as they use many sources for obtaining information, including the internet. Spouses may be more active than patients in seeking information,[21] and often initiate a search for information to supplement the information provided by health professionals.[22] Spouses want information about specific treatments, the expected course of care, about traditional as well as alterative approaches to treatment, the ways to manage symptoms, and which community resources are available.[20,23] Spouses also need information on the emotional aspects of the illness, and patients' expected course of emotional recovery.[24] Table 72–2 indicates that spouses' needs for information extend over the course of illness and can vary from one phase to another.

Spouses report *more* uncertainty about the cancer patient's illness than patients themselves[25]; this may be due in part to spouses' limited information and lack of regular contact with health professionals. There are barriers, however, that can make it difficult for spouses to obtain information from professionals. For example, the Health Insurance Portability and Accountability Act (HIPAA), which mandates confidentiality of patient information, has created a "HIPAA scare" and created some confusion about information that can be provided to family caregivers.[26] In addition, child care or work responsibilities can limit spouses' availability to attend clinic appointments and get first-hand information. Spouses who are able to attend clinic appointments often find that the appointments are brief or rushed, with little time for questions. Furthermore, some providers direct their comments primarily to

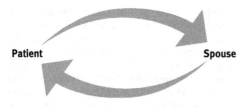

Fig. 72-1. Reciprocal relationship between cancer patient's and spouse's emotional distress.

Table 72-1. Caregiver burden and hours of care in United States

Levels of caregiver burden	Hours of caregiving per week	Percent of caregivers at each level[a]
1	3.5	33
2	9.8	17
3	12.0	15
4	33.1	21
5	87.2	10

[a]Missing data accounted for 4%
SOURCE: National Alliance for Caregiving and AARP, Caregiving in the U.S.[13]

Table 72-2. Information needs of cancer patients and spouses over the course of illness

Diagnostic phase	Hospital phase	Treatment phase	Survivorship phase	Recurrent phase
• Type and purpose of diagnostic procedures that will be performed • When test results can be expected • The person who is coordinating the care • Common emotions that develop while awaiting diagnosis (e.g., anxiety, uncertainty) • How to talk to people about the diagnosis • Making treatment decisions, pros/cons of options	• Type of surgery planned • When pathology report will be available • Expected length of hospitalization and time to recover • Role limitations to anticipate when patient is discharged • The effects of illness on other family members • Concerns about pain and other common symptoms	• Type and length of treatments planned • Anticipated side effects and when they may occur • Ways to reduce side effects • Likelihood of temporary role changes • Availability of education, support groups, and community resources • How and who to talk with about the patient's or spouse's unresolved concerns	• When follow-up examinations or tests are necessary • Common concerns during this phase (e.g., fear of recurrence) • Importance of balancing needs of patient and family • Availability of education, support groups, and community resources • Adjusting to a new self-image • Working after cancer treatment, financial issues	• Type of treatment planned • Anticipated side effects, when they may occur, and ways to manage them • Common feelings during this phase (e.g., uncertainty, sadness, fear, growth) • Ways to maintain hope regardless of recurrence • Availability of support groups and community resources

patients, which leaves little opportunity for spouses to get their questions asked.

A number of strategies have been identified to help spouses to obtain information. These include encouraging spouses to attend clinic appointments or consultation sessions, bringing a list of questions to clinic visits, and telephoning office nurses with additional questions. There are also web sites available through major organizations such as the American Cancer Society or the National Cancer Institute. In the future, web-based programs are likely to increase because they will be able to reach more patients and their spouses at a lower cost; web sites may provide information tailored to specific needs of each person.[27]

Support. Spouse caregivers also need support. In early descriptive studies, spouses' needs for support were overlooked as professionals and others focused solely on the support needs of patients. Spouses were perceived to be immune to the effects of cancer since they were "well" and patients were sick. To some extent, this perception was reinforced by early descriptive studies in which spouses ranked their own needs as less important than patients' needs.

Several studies compared the support perceived by patients and spouses and found that spouses consistently perceived less support from friends and professionals,[28,29] even though their own levels of emotional distress were similar to or even higher than patients' distress.[25] Spouses report less support than patients across all phases of illness,[9] including

the advanced phase where the demands of illness are especially high.[25] Some spouses report anger at professionals because of their lack of support.[30] This is not surprising since the spouses' needs for support have been documented for many years, and there is still a lack of routine strategies for professionals to identify the needs of spouse caregivers and provide support.[1]

There is evidence across numerous studies that spouses of cancer patients benefit from both emotional and instrumental support from others. Spouses with more support report a higher quality of life,[2] less emotional distress,[31] less fear of cancer recurrence,[2] and greater posttraumatic growth.[32] In light of the positive benefits of support, the challenge for health professionals is to find systematic ways to provide support to spouses, as well as to patients, in busy healthcare settings.

Communication. Effective communication, especially with their ill partners, is another need of spouse caregivers. Cancer patients often consider spouses to be their primary confidantes; this is especially the case for male patients.[33] However, communicating about cancer can be difficult for several reasons. Partners may have different styles of communication or preferences for disclosure[34] or partners may hold erroneous beliefs that discussing fears about cancer can hinder the patient's adjustment.[34,35] Some partners engage in protective buffering to hide feelings from one another.[36] Other couples may respond to one another in a critical or an insensitive manner that hinders open communication about the illness.[37]

Although communicating about the illness can be difficult, effective communication has been associated with a number of benefits for cancer patients and their spouses. More open communication has been associated with higher relationship satisfaction,[34,38] greater intimacy,[38] less use of cancer-related avoidance,[38] and less emotional distress.[39] Open communication also enables couples to process the cancer experience and enhance partners' ability to support one another.[36] Health professionals can facilitate effective communication among couples by providing information to both partners at the same time, and by offering them opportunities to discuss difficult issues in the presence of a health professional.[34] Professionals also can be role models to couples by demonstrating open, honest, respectful, and supportive communication as patients and spouses discuss their feelings. Also, including spouses in interventions offered to patients, and educating them about the negative consequence of criticism may help to reduce negative interactions among patients and spouses.[40] Encouraging spouses to use support groups, telephone support services such as Cancer Care, or talk with friends who are also dealing with cancer also may facilitate more open communication.

Effective coping. Spouses as well as patients need effective strategies for coping with the stress of cancer. In general, the use of active coping strategies such as problem solving, positive reframing, planning, and acceptance have been associated with higher quality of life in caregivers,[41,42] while avoidant strategies such as denial, behavioral disengagement, and uses of drugs and alcohol have been related to poorer quality of life or higher emotional distress.[43]

A recent longitudinal analysis indicated that spouses of cancer patients used avoidant rather than active coping to deal with their own symptom distress (e.g., fatigue, pain).[44] In this study, spouses of prostate cancer patients, who had higher symptom distress of their own, had a tendency to deny or minimize their own symptoms over time. This pattern of coping was associated with lower mental quality of life in spouses at 8-months follow-up, and could eventually lead to spouses' poorer physical quality of life over time. Other studies have reported that spouses in demanding caregiving situations tend to exercise less, get less sleep, forget to take prescription medications, and have less time to recuperate from their own illnesses than do noncaregivers.[45] These studies indicate that spouses need active strategies to deal with their own symptom distress and to maintain their health.

Spouses also need more active coping strategies to manage the tension that cancer creates in marital relationships.[46] In a qualitative study, couples coping with breast cancer said they needed better ways to be together as a couple instead of just being "a couple with cancer". These couples wanted relief from the cancer and needed help to learn new ways to enjoy one another.[46] Maliski and colleagues described couples' experiences with incontinence and impotence after prostate cancer surgery.[47] Couples described their work in managing their lives as individuals and then as a couple. Their findings lend support for the development of specific interventions targeted to the patient and spouse separately, and to the couple together.

Self-efficacy. Spouses also need self-efficacy or confidence in their ability to provide care for their ill partner with cancer. Spouses are often expected to provide complex care without skills to do so. Too often skill-enhancement programs focus on building patients' skills rather than spouses' skills.[48] Spouses need confidence in their ability to provide emotional support as well as physical care.[49] Husbands of breast cancer patients reported no confidence in their ability to support their wives. They struggled on their own to understand and respond to their wives' emotions.[50] Keefe and colleagues found that three-fourths of the caregivers (most were spouses) reported low or moderate efficacy to manage patients' cancer pain.[51]

Research indicates that caregivers who report more self-efficacy have less strain, have more positive moods, and their ill family members have higher physical[51] and mental well-being.[52] In a longitudinal study, Kershaw and colleagues found that self-efficacy had far reaching effects on patients and their spouse caregivers. Spouses with higher caregiver self-efficacy at baseline reported less negative appraisal of caregiving,

hopelessness, and uncertainty at 4-months follow-up, and those spouses had better mental quality of life at 8-months follow-up.[44]

Closely related to the concept of self-efficacy is the concept of preparedness or perceived readiness to provide care. Over 50% of spouse caregivers of prostate cancer patients in one study reported feeling unprepared for their caregiving role.[49] Schumacher and colleagues examined preparedness and mutuality (e.g., positive relationship quality) among adult caregivers (mostly spouses) of cancer patients. They found that caregivers who felt more prepared for their caregiving role had more vigor, less fatigue, and higher overall mood scores.[53] Mutuality between caregivers and patients was related to less caregiver strain, tension, depression, and anger. They contend that two factors may be needed to protect caregivers' well-being: a personal resource (preparedness) and an interpersonal resource (mutuality). The researchers recommend assessing those two factors, and tailoring interventions to meet caregivers' need.[54]

INTERVENTIONS TO HELP SPOUSE CAREGIVERS

Even though spouse caregivers have many needs, the number of interventions designed to help them has been relatively small. There are several literature reviews of interventions conducted with caregivers of patients with cancer which provide an overview of intervention research in this area.[55,56] These reviews tend to cover a relatively small number of studies that offer various types of interventions, including stress and activity management programs, problem-solving interventions, and telephone counseling. However, most of these studies involved small sample sizes, and measured a variety of outcomes. The reviews indicate that positive results were most likely for self-reported improvement in caregivers' coping skills and knowledge. Studies that focused on education for palliative and hospice care had a tendency to show decreases in caregiver stress.

Although not cancer specific, Martire and colleagues conducted a meta-analysis of psychosocial interventions in chronic illness to determine if it was beneficial to include a family member in the intervention.[57] They analyzed 70 randomized clinical trials (five in cancer) that assessed both patient and family member outcomes. The strongest evidence for the efficacy of family interventions was in reducing the caregiver's burden. Family interventions also reduced depression in family caregivers, and reduced caregiver anxiety when relationship issues were addressed. Depression in patients was also reduced—but only when the intervention was offered to spouses of patients or to couples, possibly because of the greater proximity or intimacy of couples. This meta-analysis indicated that interventions offered to spouse-spouse dyads, to patient-caregiver dyads (e.g., daughter or sister), or to spouses or other caregivers alone can have positive effects on both patients and caregivers. However, the outcomes varied depending on the content addressed in the intervention and in the types of caregivers (e.g., spousal vs. nonspousal) who participated in them.

Interventions with cancer patients and caregivers: single studies. A review of individual studies in the cancer literature revealed varied results and an array of outcomes. Intervention studies have been conducted with cancer patients and their caregivers, or with caregivers only. The studies have been categorized into four broad intervention areas: (1) supportive-educative, (2) caregiving skills/symptom management, (3) coping skills, and (4) relationship-focused interventions. These are not necessarily discrete categories because some interventions address more than one area.

Supportive-educative interventions. In view of patients' and spouses' common needs for support and information, it is no surprise that the majority of interventions are supportive-educative or psycho-educational interventions. These interventions have produced a variety of positive outcomes whether offered to patients and spouses jointly, or to spouses alone. Most commonly reported outcomes of these interventions are less emotional distress or improved quality of life in patients and/or partners,[58–62] increased caregiver self-efficacy,[60,62,63] increased rewards of caregiving,[64,65] and better caregiver coping.[65,66] Other positive outcomes but reported less often are improved caregiver physical well-being or health,[58,59,63] less negative appraisal of the illness or less uncertainty,[62,67] better communication between partners,[62] and greater caregiver knowledge about community resources.[66] The outcomes associated with supportive-educative interventions indicate that they are effective in providing patients and spouses with support and information, but can also produce many other positive outcomes.

Caregiver skills/symptom management interventions. Since spouses benefit when they feel confident in providing care, several studies have focused on improving caregivers' skills. These programs have been offered to patients and caregivers together or to caregivers alone. Interestingly, when a symptom management intervention was offered *jointly* to patients and caregivers, patients' own symptom management improved, caregivers spent less time helping patients to manage symptoms, and caregivers reported less negative reactions to caregiving.[68] Interventions to increase caregivers' skills or preparedness have increased caregivers' information about caregiving,[49] their knowledge and attitude toward pain management,[69] and decreased caregivers' depressive symptoms.[70]

Robinson and colleagues offered a family caregiver education program to over 700 caregivers in the state of Pennsylvania to enhance caregivers' knowledge and skill. One of the unique aspects of the program was that researchers educated not only the caregivers, but also the health professionals from across the state so they could bring the program back to their local communities. The caregivers who participated in the program were more knowledgeable about their role and about community resources, were less overwhelmed, were better able to cope with the caregiving experience, and were more prepared to communicate with health professionals.[66] This study points out the importance of educating both caregivers and professionals on ways to build caregiving skills in both groups.

Coping skills interventions. Since the use of active coping strategies has been associated with higher quality of life, some intervention programs have included coping skills in their program content. Two studies focused primarily on ways to improve the coping skills of patients and/or caregivers.[71,72] The CanCope Program was developed by researchers in Australia to help breast cancer patients and their partners *jointly* to cope with cancer and support each other. In a randomized clinical trial they compared outcomes for couples in (1) a couple-based program; (2) an individually-based, patient-only program; and (3) a control condition. The couple-based coping program produced more positive outcomes than the patient-only program or control condition. The couple-based program increased partners' supportive communication with one another, increased their intimacy as a couple, and decreased their coping effort. It also lessened patients' use of avoidant coping, and also decreased patients' distress.[72] In another study, caregivers of hospice patients were offered (1) a standard hospice program only, (2) hospice plus supportive visits, or (3) hospice with a coping skills intervention. Caregivers in coping skills intervention reported less caregiver burden and greater quality of life than caregivers in the other two conditions.[71] These studies document the value of teaching coping skills to couples and/or caregivers who are trying to manage the demands of cancer.

Relationship-focused interventions. Since cancer can cause stress in couples' relationships, a few studies have focused on relationship issues. Kuijer and colleagues from New Zealand and the Netherlands developed an intervention to help couples reduce inequity (e.g., over-investment or underbenefit) in their relationships as they coped with cancer. The intervention focused on ways partners support one another, maintain "give and take" in their relationships, and change their expectations of one another over the course of illness. Couples who participated in the intervention reported greater equity in their relationships and higher marital satisfaction than couples in the control condition.[73] To improve relationships, some investigators contend that it may be necessary to include both partners in the intervention. For example, Manne et al.[65] offered an intervention to wives of men with prostate cancer to lessen wives' distress, increase their personal growth, and facilitate

marital communication. Although wives benefited from the intervention on some variables, the intervention did not improve communication with their husbands. The researchers suggest that the intervention might not have been able to improve marital communication because husbands were not included in the intervention.

From the four categories of interventions above (supportive-educative, caregiving skills/symptom management, coping skills, and relationship-focused interventions), it is clear that interventions offered to couples or to spouses alone can have many positive effects. These interventions have addressed spouses' needs for support, information, communication, effective coping skills, and caregiver self-efficacy—the common needs of spouses that were identified earlier in the chapter. Even though the majority of intervention programs were helpful, few of them have been disseminated into clinical practice settings where they could be available to others. Translating and disseminating effective interventions into standard clinical care still remains a challenge for both researchers and clinicians.

Delivery of interventions to patients and family caregivers. A report by the Institute of Medicine (IOM), titled "Cancer Care for the Whole Person: Meeting Psychosocial Health Needs," addresses the importance of finding ways to provide psychosocial care to cancer patients and their families.[74] According to the report, current cancer care provides state-of-the-science biomedical treatment, but fails to provide adequate psychosocial care. The report states that there should be a standard of care that all patients with cancer and their families should receive high-quality cancer care that includes appropriate psychosocial health services.

On the basis of extensive review of the scientific literature, the committee for the IOM report developed a model for effective delivery of psychosocial services. Key aspects of the model include (1) identifying psychosocial health needs, (2) linking patients and families to psychosocial services they need, (3) supporting patients and families as they manage the illness, (4) coordinating psychosocial and biomedical care, and (5) following up on the delivery of care to determine its effectiveness, and making modifications as needed. The report contends that a combination of activities rather than a single activity only, is needed to deliver appropriate psychosocial healthcare.

DIRECTIONS FOR FUTURE RESEARCH

On the basis of the review of literature and on the recommendations of the IOM report, several directions for future research are listed below.

1. There is a need for comprehensive screening tools that can address a range of psychosocial stressors that interfere with patients' and spouses' ability to manage cancer.[74] In a classic study with widowers of formerly ill patients, Parkes[75] identified a number of factors that predict negative outcomes: age, socio-economic status, gender, culture, previous mental illness, prior life crises, strength of the relationship, and social support. Screening tools that incorporate a range of key factors will be valuable for identifying patients and caregivers at risk of poorer outcomes.
2. Targeted interventions are needed. Not all patients and spouses need intensive programs. Determining what program is optimal for which patients and their caregivers will produce better outcomes and use fewer healthcare resources.
3. There is a need for studies with caregivers who have been overlooked in prior studies, or who are underserved in clinical settings. This includes caregivers from different ethnic backgrounds, those with few socio-economic resources, and those with same gender partners.[8]
4. Interventions are needed that can effectively link patients and caregivers with various healthcare services that they need, using a variety of services such as case management and patient navigators.[74]
5. Finally, programs are needed to educate health professionals so they are more prepared to meet the psychosocial needs of cancer patients and their caregivers.[74]

In summary, spouses' lives are interdependent with patients' lives; each partner affects the other. Spouses have a number of needs that must be addressed for them to maintain their own emotional well-being and to provide effective care to patients. A variety of different intervention programs have been developed and tested to meet spouses' needs, but considerably more research is essential. Attending to the psychosocial needs of cancer patients and their spouses is an integral part of quality cancer care.[74]

REFERENCES

1. Given BA, Given CW, Kozachik S. Family support in advanced cancer. *CA Cancer J Clin.* 2001;51:213–231.

2. Mellon S, Northouse LL, Weiss LK. A population-based study of the quality of life of cancer survivors and their family caregivers. *Cancer Nurs.* 2006;29:120–131.

3. Hudson P. Positive aspects and challenges associated with caring for a dying relative at home. *Int J Palliat Nurs.* 2004;10:58–65.

4. Given B, Wyatt G, Given C, et al. Burden and depression among caregivers of patients with cancer at the end of life. *Oncol Nurs Forum.* 2004;31(6):1105–1115.

5. McCorkle R, Siefert ML, Dowd MF, Robinson JP, Pickett M. Effects of advanced practice nursing on patient and spouse depressive symptoms, sexual function, and marital interaction after radical prostatectomy. *Urol Nurs.* 2007;27:65–77.

6. Northouse LL, Mood D, Kershaw T, et al. Quality of life of women with recurrent breast cancer and their family members. *J Clin Oncol.* 2002;20(19):4050–4064.

7. Northouse LL, Templin T, Mood D. Couples' adjustment to breast disease during the first year following diagnosis. *J Behav Med.* 2001;24(2):115–136.

8. Hagedoorn M, Sanderman R, Bolks HN, Tuinstra J, Coyne JC. Distress in couples coping with cancer: a meta-analysis and critical review of role and gender effects. *Psychol Bull.* 2008;134(1):1–30.

9. Northouse LL, Mood D, Templin T, Mellon S, George T. Couples' patterns of adjustment to colon cancer. *Soc Sci Med.* 2000;50(2):271–284.

10. Lewis FM, Woods NF, Hough EE, Bensley LS. The family's functioning with chronic illness in the mother: the spouse's perspective. *Soc Sci Med.* 1989;29(11):1261–1269.

11. McCorkle R, Yost LS, Jepson C, Malone D, Baird S, Lusk E. A cancer experience: relationship of patient psychosocial responses to caregiver burden over time. *Psychooncology.* 1993;2:21–32.

12. Stetz K. Caregiving demands during advanced cancer: the spouse's needs. *Cancer Nurs.* 1987;10:260–268.

13. National Alliance of Caregiving, AARP. *Caregiving in the U.S.* 2004.

14. Hull MM. Family needs and supportive nursing behaviors during terminal cancer: a review. *Oncol Nurs Forum.* 1989;16:787–792.

15. Kristjanson JL, Norby PA. The family's cancer journey: a literature review. *Cancer Nurs.* 1994;17:1–17.

16. Lewis FM. The impact of cancer on the family: a critical review of the literature. *Patient Educ Couns.* 1986;8:269–289.

17. Northouse LL. The impact of cancer on family: overview of the literature. *Int J Psychiatr Med.* 1984;14(3):87–113.

18. Laizner A, Shedga L, Barg F, McCorkle R. Needs of family caregivers of persons with cancer: a review. *Semin Oncol Nurs.* 1993;9:114–120.

19. Couper J, Bloch S, Love A, Macvean M, Duchesne GM, Kissane D. Psychosocial adjustment of female partners of men with prostate cancer: a review of the literature. *Psychooncology.* 2006;15:937–953.

20. Resendes LA, McCorkle R. Spousal responses to prostate cancer: an integrative review. *Cancer Invest.* 2006;24:192–198.

21. Echlin KN, Rees CE. Information needs and information-seeking behaviors of men with prostate cancer and their partners: a review of literature. *Cancer Nurs.* 2002;25:35–41.

22. Lavery JF, Clarke VA. Prostate cancer: patients' and spouses' coping and marital adjustment. *Psychol Health Med.* 1999;4(3):289–302.

23. Hilton BA, Crawford JA, Tarko MA. Men's perspectives on individual and family coping with their wives' breast cancer and chemotherapy. *West J Nurs Res.* 2000;22:438–459.

24. Oberst MT, Scott DW. Postdischarge distress in surgically treated cancer patients and their spouses. *Res Nurs Health.* 1988;11(4):223–233.

25. Northouse LL, Mood DW, Montie JE, et al. Living with prostate cancer: Patients' and spouses' psychosocial status and quality of life. *J Clin Oncol.* 2007;25:4171–4177.

26. Levine C. HIPAA and talking with family caregivers: what does the law really say? *Am J Nurs.* 2006;106:51–53.

27. Strecher VJ. Internet methods for delivering behavioral and health-related interventions (eHealth). *Ann Rev Clin Psychol.* 2007;3:53–76.

28. Davis-Ali S, Chesler M, Chesney BK. Recognizing cancer as a family disease: worries and support related by patients and spouses. *Soc Work Health Care.* 1993;19(2):45–65.

29. Northouse LL. Social support in patients' and husbands' adjustment to breast cancer. *Nurs Res.* 1988;37(2):91–95.

30. Hilton BA, Crawford JA, Tarko MA. Men's perspectives on individual and family coping with their wives' breast cancer and chemotherapy. *West J Nurs Res.* 2000;22(4):438–459.

31. Eton DT, Lepore SJ, Helgeson VS. Psychological distress in spouses of men treated for early-stage prostate carcinoma. *Cancer.* 2005;103:2412–2418.

32. Weiss T. Correlates of posttraumatic growth in husbands of breast cancer survivors. *Psychooncology.* 2004;13:260–268.

33. Harrison J, Maguire GP, Pitceathy C. Confiding in crisis: gender differences in pattern of confiding among cancer patients. *Soc Sci Med.* 1995;41:1255–1260.

34. Hilton BA. Family communication patterns in coping with early breast cancer. *West J Nurs Res.* 1994;16(4):366–388.

35. Zhang AY, Siminoff LA. Silence and cancer: why do families and patients fail to communicate? *Health Commun.* 2003;15:415–429.

36. Manne SL, Dougherty J, Veach S, Kless R. Hiding worries from one's spouse: protective buffering among cancer patients and their spouses. *Cancer Res Ther Control.* 1999;8:175–188.

37. Manne SL, Alfieri T, Taylor KL, Dougherty J. Spousal negative responses to cancer patients: the role of social restriction, spouse mood, and relationship satisfaction. *J Consult Clin Psychol.* 1999;67(3):352–361.

38. Porter LR, Keefe FJ, Hurwitz H, Faber M. Disclosure between patients with gastrointestinal cancer and their spouses. *Psychooncology.* 2005;14:1030–1042.

39. Manne SL, Ostroff JS, Norton TR, Fox K, Goldstein L, Grana G. Cancer-related relationship communication in couples coping with early stage breast cancer. *Psychooncology.* 2006;15:234–247.

40. Manne SL, Pape SJ, Taylor KL, Dougherty J. Spouse support, coping, and mood among individuals with cancer. *Ann Behav Med.* 1999;21(2):111–121.

41. Kershaw T, Northouse L, Kritpracha C, Schafenacker A, Mood D. Coping strategies and quality of life in women with advanced breast cancer and their family caregivers. *Psychol Health.* 2004;19:139–155.

42. Malcarne VL, Banthia R, Varni JW, Sadler GR, Greenbergs HJ, Ko CM. Problem-solving skills and emotional distress in spouses of men with prostate cancer. *J Cancer Educ.* 2002;17:150–154.

43. Banthia R, Malcarne VL, Varni JW, Ko CM, Sadler GR, Greenbergs HL. The effects of dyadic strength and coping styles on psychological distress in couples faced with prostate cancer. *J Behav Med.* 2003;26(1):31–52.

44. Kershaw T, Mood DW, Newth G, et al. Longitudinal analysis of a model to predict quality of life in prostate cancer patients and their spouses. *Ann Behav Med.* 2008;36(2):117–128.

45. Burton LC, Newsom JT, Schultz D, Hirsch CH, German PS. Preventive health behaviors among spousal caregivers. *Prev Med.* 1997;26:162–169.

46. Shands ME, Lewis FM, Sinsheimer J, Cochrane BB. Core concerns of couples living with early stage breast cancer. *Psychooncology.* 2006;15:1055–1064.

47. Maliski S, Heilemann M, McCorkle R. Mastery of postprostatectomy incontinence and impotence: his work, her work, our work. *Oncol Nurs Forum.* 2001;28:985–991.

48. Lewis FM, Fletcher KA, Cochrane BB, Fann JR. Predictors of depressed mood in spouses of women with breast cancer. *J Clin Oncol.* 2008;26:1289–1295.

49. Giarelli E, McCorkle R, Monturo C. Caring for a spouse after prostate surgery: the preparedness needs of wives. *J Fam Nurs.* 2003;9(4):453–485.

50. Zahlis EH, Shands ME. Breast cancer: demands of the illness on patient's partner. *J Psychosoc Oncol.* 1991;9(1):75–93.

51. Keefe FJ, Ahles TA, Porter LS, et al. The self-efficacy of family caregivers for helping cancer patients manage pain at end-of-life. *Pain.* 2003;103:157–162.

52. Campbell LC, Keefe FJ, McKee DC, et al. Prostate cancer in African Americans: relationship of patient and partner self-efficacy to quality of life. *J Pain Symp Manage.* 2004;28(5):433–444.

53. Schumacher KL, Stewart BJ, Archbold PG, Caparro M, Mutale F, Agrawal S. Effects of caregiving demand, mutuality, and preparedness on family caregiver outcomes during cancer treatment. *Oncol Nurs Forum.* 2008;35:49–56.

54. Schumacher KL, Stewart BJ, Archbold PG. Mutuality and preparedness moderate the effects of caregiving demand on cancer family caregiving outcomes. *Nurs Research.* 2007;56:425–433.

55. Harding R, Higginson I. What is the best way to help caregivers in cancer and palliative care? A systematic literature review of interventions and their effectiveness. *Palliat Med.* 2003;17:63–74.

56. Pasacreta JV, McCorkle R. Cancer care: impact of interventions on caregiver outcomes. *Annu Rev Nurs Res.* 2000;18:127–148.

57. Martire LM, Lustig AP, Schulz R, Miller GE, Helgeson VS. Is it beneficial to involve a family member? A meta-analysis of psychosocial interventions for chronic illness. *Health Psychol.* 2004;23(6):599–611.

58. Budin WC, Hoskins CN, Haber J, et al. Breast cancer: education, counseling, and adjustment among patients and partners: a randomized clinical trial. *Nurs Res.* 2008;57:199–213.

59. Jepson C, McCorkle R, Adler D, Nuamah I, Lusk E. Effects of home care on caregivers' psychosocial status. *Image J Nurs Sch.* 1999;31(2):115–120.

60. Lewis FM, Cochrane BB, Fletcher KA, et al. Helping her heal: a pilot study of an educational counseling intervention for spouses of women with breast cancer. *Psychooncology.* 2008;17:131–137.

61. McCorkle R, Robinson L, Nuamah I, Lev E, Benoliel JQ. The effects of home nursing care for patients during terminal illness on the bereaved's psychological distress. *Nurs Res.* 1998;47:2–10.

62. Northouse LL, Mood DW, Schafenacker A, et al. Randomized clinical trial of a family intervention for prostate cancer patients and their spouses. *Cancer.* 2007;110:2809–2818.

63. Pasacreta JV, Barg F, Nuamah I, McCorkle R. Participant characteristics before and 4 months after attendance at a family caregiver cancer education program. *Cancer Nurs.* 2000;23(4):295–303.

64. Hudson P, Aranda S, Hayman-White K. A psycho-educational intervention for family caregivers of patients receiving palliative care: a randomized controlled trial. *J Pain Symp Manage.* 2005;30:329–341.

65. Manne S, Babb J, Pinover W, Horwitz E, Ebbert J. Psychoeducational group intervention for wives of men with prostate cancer. *Psychooncology.* 2004;13:37–46.

66. Robinson KD, Angeletti KA, Barg FK, Pasacreta JV, McCorkle R, Yasko J. The development of a family caregiver cancer education program. *J Cancer Educ.* 1998;13:116–121.

67. Northouse L, Kershaw T, Mood D, Schafenacker A. Effects of a family intervention on the quality of life of women with recurrent breast cancer and their family caregivers. *Psychooncology.* 2005;14:478–491.

68. Given BA, Given CW, Sikorskii A, Jeon S, Sherwood P, Rahbar M. The impact of providing symptom management assistance on caregiver reaction: results of a randomized trial. *J Pain Symp Manage.* 2006;32:433–443.

69. Ferrell BR, Grant M, Chan J, Ahn C, Ferrell BA. The impact of cancer pain education on family caregivers of elderly patients. *Oncol Nurs Forum.* 1995;22:1211–1218.

70. Kozachik SL, Given CW, Given BA, et al. Improving depressive symptoms among caregivers of patients with cancer: results of a randomized clinical trial. *Oncol Nurs Forum.* 2001;28(7):1149–1157.

71. McMillan SC, Small BJ, Weitzner M, et al. Impact of coping skills intervention with family caregivers of hospice patients with cancer. *Cancer.* 2006;106:214–222.

72. Scott JL, Halford WK, Ward BG. United we stand? The effects of a couple-coping intervention on adjustment to early stage breast or gynecological cancer. *J Consult Clin Psychol.* 2004;72:1122–1135.

73. Kuijer RG, Buunk BP, DeJong GM, Ybema JF, Sanderman R. Effects of a brief intervention program for patients with cancer and their partners on feelings of inequity, relationship quality and psychological distress. *Psychooncology.* 2004;13:321–334.

74. IOM. *Cancer care for the whole patient: Meeting psychosocial needs.* Washington, DC: National Academy of Science; 2008.

75. Parkes M. Determinants of outcome following bereavement. *Omega.* 1975;6:303–323.

Gender and Caregiving

Matthew J. Loscalzo, Youngmee Kim, and Karen L. Clark

CHANGING ROLES OF WOMEN AND MEN IN SOCIETY

Very little can be said about women or men that will fit into clearly defined categories. The two genders have more intrasexual variation than between the sexes. The inclinations of women and men are important in how they manage and cope with stress and the expectations they have on their social support systems.

The changing social demands on women and men in western society have never been as dramatic as in the last 50 years. Both women and men have been confronted with expectations and opportunities that have put particular stress on their ability to adapt to rapid social changes that may outstrip the organisms' psychophysiological ability to adapt. Advances in the scientific study of gender have legitimized and to some degree lessened the political angst that once plagued the ability to better understand the complex influences of sex and gender. The groundbreaking 2001 Institute of Medicine Report (IOM), *Exploring the biological contributions to human health: does sex matter?* documented the gaps in knowledge and potential benefit of being able to develop a reliable body of scientific information that better informs how we treat illness and promote wellness in women and men.[1]

Approximately 65% of women (ages 25–64) now work outside of the home.[2] Within the context of the demanding workplace, these are primarily competitive rather than the collaborative relationships that have comprised women's relationships for many millennia. This has been a double stressor for women as they no longer can depend on the support and feedback from other women on a consistent basis to manage their stress. This may leave women feeling emotionally unfulfilled, isolated, diluted, and frustrated. Within the context of cancer, women may turn to men to provide the kind of support which they have historically received from their sisters, mothers, grandmothers, aunts, and female friends. Men are seldom equipped to intuitively respond in a helpful way or to comprehend what women need from them. One of the well-documented gender differences found in the literature is on the stress response. When under stress, women have been shown to reach out to others and to "tend and befriend,"[3] as an initial response to control their sense of danger and fear. Women feel secure in reaching out to others when trying to manage the stress associated to their vulnerability and do not experience any diminution of self-esteem by asking for help. For women, their level of self-efficacy (i.e., confidence that she can be a good caregiver) has been shown to be an indicator of how they manage stress related to chronic illness.[4]

For men, who have traditionally gained their sense of purpose and direction in a highly competitive action oriented environments, such as work, recent social demands focusing on high levels of verbal communication, collaborative team work, and sensitivity to their emotional impact on others has created stress and confusion. Within the context of cancer, both as care recipients and caregivers, many men are confronted with demands from their loved ones that do not come naturally to them and which leads to a sense of shame and guilt that encourages their natural inclination to withdraw. When men experience stress, there is an innate tendency to react with the fight-or-flight response. When confronted with stressors that are not manageable by immediate action there is a strong inclination to turn inward to access internal resources and for reflection related to problem solving. Unlike women, men may experience a sense of diminished self-esteem by sharing their vulnerabilities with others. Although women are adept at prospectively sharing their emotional concerns to reduce their immediate sense of threat, it is only in retrospect that men are generally comfortable sharing their fears and concerns with others, once the sense of threat is reduced to manageable levels. The ways in which many women and men manage their vulnerabilities (women seeking emotional connection and men seeking space and time to think) has significant implications within the context of caregiving. Although female caregivers report higher levels of emotional distress,[5] male caregivers may express their distress by becoming rebellious or aggressive, or by smoking and drinking more.[4]

At first impression, it would appear that the mismatches of women and men in regulating stress are misaligned and maladaptive. For women, reaching out to a variety of others, verbally processing, sharing detailed internal vulnerabilities, and not expecting resolutions or fixes are natural inclinations for managing stress. For men, turning inward, self-reliance, taking action, outcome orientation and problem resolution are natural inclinations for managing stress. The changing social demands on women and men when confronted with serious life-threatening illness are different than the more predatory obvious and external dangers for which men and women have had to adapt together throughout history. Research has clearly demonstrated that the intellectual differences between women and men are very small compared to their many similarities.[1] But when it comes to coping with cancer, sometimes small differences can have a big impact.

DEARTH OF RESEARCH IN GENDER AND CAREGIVING

There is a dearth of research on gender as a primary variable in cancer studies and there is even a greater lack of research on the influence of gender in caregiving of care recipients with cancer. The majority of caregiver research has focused on Alzheimer's disease. In the few studies that do exist on cancer caregiving and gender; women generally report higher levels of distress than men.[5] Most of the few existing studies focus on women's caregiver roles and even less studies have looked at men as caregivers. The first meta-analysis[6] that studied gender differences in caregiving in 1992, concluded that more research was needed on gender roles and finding meaning in the caregiving experience. Since then very little has changed. Fromme et al. (2005) stated, "In the last three decades of family caregiving research, only a few studies have provided insight into the roles that men play."[7] Overall, most of the studies have been descriptive in nature or have investigated gender effects as a secondary rather than a primary variable.

In research focused on the biological mechanisms of illness, there has been a significant interest in the role of gender; however, psychosocial research has not adequately addressed or accepted the importance and implications of gender. This is especially problematic given the importance placed on interpersonal relationships of the psychosocial model. There may be a number of reasons why gender has been underappreciated as a primary focus of psychosocial research: lack of funding, political sensitivities, misperceptions about the quality and presence of existing data; it is so obvious that people do not see it or that gender is too complex to study. Gender is always an essential component of people and their relationships. It will not be possible to understand the complex interpersonal relationships in the caregiver context without first some fundamental understanding of the influence of gender in these highly stressful, emotionally charged environments. This gap in knowledge may deprive women and men in receiving psychosocial services in a manner that is consistent with their psychological, social, and biological requirements. Although it is widely accepted that women and men access psychosocial services differently, there has been a virtual collusion of silence in addressing these unique needs.

CAREGIVERS ARE PREDOMINANTLY FEMALE BUT THE NUMBERS OF MALE CAREGIVERS ARE INCREASING

The family's involvement in cancer care continues to expand in response to an increased number of older individuals with chronic illness and disabilities, and changes in healthcare delivery; such as, earlier discharge of hospitalized patients.[8] The number of people diagnosed and living with cancer is also increasing. Approximately 10.8 million Americans with a history of cancer are alive today[9] and their family members are the primary source of support for various aspects of care.[10] According to a recent national survey, caregivers of individuals with cancer were predominantly middle aged, middle-class individuals with some college education, married, employed full- or part-time, and more female. Caregivers are more likely to care for parents or parents-in-law rather than other family members. Care recipients are predominately in their late 60s. Socio-demographic variables for caregivers and care recipients are equivalent between the genders and similar with those of caregivers for individuals with other types of diseases.[11]

Although traditional socialization practices in many cultures reinforce men to be protectors and providers and women to be nurturers and caregivers,[12] increased egalitarian perspectives on both work and family responsibilities have been reflected in a recent social trend. Namely, an increasing number of men have assumed caregiving responsibilities: 25% of the caregivers surveyed were male in 1987, 28% in 1997, and 39% in 2004.[13,14] This trend has also been the case with cancer caregivers, pinpointing that male caregivers are a fast growing population. We have little reliable information about the specific strains placed on cancer caregivers by gender, many of whom may be ill prepared for these tasks. Even though over time more men are becoming caregivers, there are still more women in the caregiving role.

GENDER IS SIGNIFICANT IN REPORTING DISTRESS

Despite the fact that gender as a primary research variable has been understudied, the most widely used validated measures of psychological distress are not gender normed. The Brief Symptom Inventory is the only widely known distress measure that is gender normed.[15] There is general recognition that women report higher levels of distress than men; further highlighting the ambiguity that gender studies creates in the psycho-social scientific community. Conversely, Hagedoorn et al. (2000) found that male and female patients reported equal levels of distress.[16] This ambiguity raises the question of whether distress is the same experience for men and women; an important question yet to be addressed. Recent studies documenting that women and men respond differently to stress; "tend and befriend" for women and "fight or flight" for men are providing cues as to some of the important influences that relate to how men and women frustrate or support each other during stress; for example, caregiving.

Distress in caregivers. A recent review[10] documented the detrimental impact of cancer on various aspects of family caregivers' quality of life, physical health, and emotional well-being. Levels of physical strain and emotional stress resulting from cancer caregiving were equivalent to that of dementia caregiving, both of which were higher than caregiving for individuals with diabetes or frailty. Even after adjusting for socio-demographic characteristics, level of burden, duration of caregiving, hours of care per week, and the care recipient's disease group, the levels of physical strain and emotional stress were still higher for cancer and dementia caregivers than for diabetes or frailty caregivers.[11] Matthews (2003) found that the caregivers' assessment of their global cancer-related distress was higher than reported by survivors.[17] On the other hand, Hodges et al. (2005)[18] reported that cancer survivors and their family caregivers often report similar levels of psychological distress. As the conclusion of a meta-analysis suggested, caregivers' subjective appraisal of the caregiving situation (perceived the situation as stressful and/or as an experience of personal growth) plays a significant role in their mental and physical quality of life outcomes.[19] A more recent study[20] looking at 101 patients with advanced gastrointestinal (GI) or lung cancer and their spouses, found that spousal caregivers of patients with advanced cancer are a high-risk population for depression and that subjective caregiving burden and relational variables, such as caregivers' attachment orientations and marital dissatisfaction, are important predictors of caregiver depression.

The burden of cancer caregiving may weigh more heavily on caregivers of some socio-demographic groups than others. For example, carrying out multiple social roles has an influence on the extent to which the caregivers psychologically adjusted to cancer in their family. More specifically, cancer caregivers who were employed and took care of children reported the highest levels of emotional distress.[21] Overall, the quality of the caregivers' emotional attachments, marital satisfaction, and support in managing children and work influence the ability to cope with the emotional demands of caregiving. Although societal expectations of these demands are changing, there is still an unequal burden placed on women.[22]

Women still perceive themselves as being primarily responsible for the physical and emotional care of their loved ones. This expectation is strongly reinforced by social norms of almost every society throughout the world. Because self-efficacy relates to self-perceptions and role expectations, it is an important construct for understanding how effective people feel in any given situation. For example, when female caregivers reported high self-efficacy and felt they took good care of the recipients, caregiver distress was lower and equal to the distress reported by male caregivers.[4] In a large study of 263 patient and spouse dyads, Northouse et al. (2007) found that female caregivers of prostate cancer patients had less confidence in their ability to manage the illness.[23] These studies support the importance of self-efficacy for females in managing caregiver distress.

Caregiver distress in females and males. Psychological distress may have a different influence on each person's quality of life, depending on their gender, rather than role as a survivor or caregiver.[24] Specifically, women appeared to perceive lack of emotional mutuality or reciprocity with an ill spouse as the result of neglecting the spouse's emotional concerns and her own deficiencies in interpersonal sensitivity. For female caregivers this led to feelings of isolation and social inadequacy, and thus poorer mental health. On the other hand, male caregivers who are emotionally disconnected from their ill spouses are less likely to suffer from the emotional abandonment and more likely to have their time and energy freed up, which results in better physical functioning. Men tend to be less emotionally sensitive to their social environment, use more emotional distancing, and compartmentalizing, problem solving may seem to be a more natural and comforting way for them to communicate their commitment and to manage their distress. Although these behaviors may not be soothing to the female care recipients on an emotional level, women do say that in some circumstances these are the very same traits that they value highly in men.

The male defense is to withdraw emotionally to keep functioning and has negative implications for greater stress in women. Women's distress is the strongest predictor of men's physical health over and above the men's distress, couple (dis)similarity in distress, survivor's age, and cancer stage. This effect occurred regardless of whether the men were the care recipients or the caregivers. This is consistent with findings that men are profoundly impacted by the emotional state of the women in their lives.[24] In a study looking at men as caregivers at end of life, the strongest predictor of high end-of-life caregiver distress was the perceived female decedent's emotional distress.[7]

It is noteworthy that the adverse effect of having a male partner who is less emotionally resourceful or has distanced himself psychologically is limited to men's physical health, but not vice versa.[24] This finding on the unequal influence of gender on the partner's distress is consistent with findings in some studies[25,26] although other studies have found no gender differences[27,28] and the effects of social support on physical health have not been consistent.[29,30]

Table 73–1. Predicators and outcomes of high distress in cancer care-givers by gender

Female	Male
Predictors of high distress	
Younger age[1]	Older, less educated, recently married, uncertain of the future, less adjusted marriages[40]
Lower income[1]	More frequent use of denial[41]
Working outside the home[42]	Confusion over behavioral expectations[43]
Receiving care from men[5]	No one to speak with honestly[43]
Providing care to men[5]	Sharing struggles less[7]
Lower confidence[23]/self-efficacy[4]	Demands of emotional support from spouse[22]
	Emotional state of spouse[24]
	Spouse's distress[24]
Outcomes of high distress	
Report greater distress overall[17]	Increased complaining of physical symptoms[4]
Report clinically meaningful levels of depression, anxiety, pain, fatigue and sleep problems[14]	Increased smoking and drinking[4]
Feeling insecure and incompetent[4]	More likely to become rebellious and aggressive[4]
Feeling isolated[24]	Negligence at work[43]
Feeling socially inadequate[24]	

Table 73–2. Characteristics of caregivers by gender

Female caregiver	Male caregiver
Regardless of roles, more reported distress[5]	Report less distress overall[5,22]
When in role of patient, highest level of distress[5]	Use more denial and distancing, less active engagement coping strategies[4]
When caregiving is perceived as central to identity, experience more distress[4]	Higher caregiver esteem[22]
More likely to care for sicker dependents[34]	Engage less in caregiver role[6]
Provide more burdensome tasks[34]	More likely to hire caregivers[46]
Information gathering and emotional roles most important[47]	Provide occasional, informational or tangible support[34]
Provide more personal care[34]	Provide less personal care[6]
Provide more frequent, tangible and medical and symptom care[34]	Provide hands on care equal to female caregivers[7]

As displayed in Table 73–1, female and male caregivers differ in the causes of distress and in the negative consequences of not managing that distress. For example, female caregivers express more distress overall[17]; however, male caregivers appear to have more severe consequences as a result of caregiver distress. These trends are consistent with women's inclinations to openly express their vulnerabilities through verbal communication. While men tend to minimize and somatize their vulnerabilities through nonverbal and sometimes harmful behaviors (e.g., substance use[4]).

GENDER AND CAREGIVER ROLES MATTER

Examining the effect of gender on appraisal and caregiving outcomes may provide useful information. As a recent meta-analysis demonstrated, gender played a key role in emotional distress: women reported greater levels of distress than men, regardless of a person's role as a care recipient or caregiver.[5] Specifically, male caregivers reported higher caregiver's esteem, which refers to a sense of value and worth as a caregiver, resulting in less stress from providing care to their wives with cancer.[22,31] On the other hand, female caregivers often reported greater burden and lower self-esteem as a caregiver due in part to the fact that women are often expected to be the family caregivers, and therefore they perceive providing care as doing what they are supposed to do.[32] When women cannot meet these social expectations they feel they have failed. By internalizing this social expectation and not utilizing paid external support (as men more frequently do) women experience greater caregiver distress.[6]

The intensive nature of cancer caregiving may require the involvement of both men and women in diverse and unfamiliar tasks to meet the multidimensional needs of the care recipients. These complex, demanding, and novel tasks need to be balanced with the caregivers' own personal needs. Among spousal or adult offspring caregivers of

lung cancer patients,[33] providing emotional support, transportation, and monitoring symptoms were reported as the most time-consuming. The most difficult care tasks were emotional support, behavioral management, monitoring symptoms, and household duties.

Kim et al. (2007) found that the levels and types of involvement differed between genders.[34] For example, female, compared with male caregivers provided more frequent tangible, medical and symptom management. Since the unique challenges associated with cancer caregiving involve various acute side effects as a result of surgery, chemotherapy, radiation therapy, or a combination of all of these (e.g., catheter care, emesis, dyspnea, fatigue, pain), requiring the caregiver to deliver complex medical care. Since female caregivers are more frequently involved in medical and symptom management tasks, they assume a disproportionate burden and a diminution of their own quality of life. It is interesting to note that there were no differences found between male and female caregivers in perceived levels of difficulty providing various types of care[34] and in the total number of duties related to assistance provided for symptom management.[35]

Another aspect related to caregivers' gender and caregiving stress is the care recipient's functional status. Women are more likely to be involved in caring for sicker dependents with poor mental or physical functioning status. They are also more likely to provide personal care and perform household tasks that require a more constant and burdensome commitment than the occasional tasks of providing informational or tangible support, that are more likely to be performed by male caregivers.[19] For a summary of caregiver characteristics by gender see Table 73–2.

Within the context of seriously ill male care recipients and the ongoing demands on women from multiple perspectives, it is easy to understand how women can become socially isolated, emotionally deprived, and physically exhausted. At the same time, the now dependent male who may have perceived his role as provider and protector may be inclined to withdraw and to feel demoralized and depressed. So while women are deprived of the emotional support, communication, and connection that are so important to them, men may increasingly avoid the very contact and connection that women are missing because men perceive the requests for support as a criticism of their ability to be an adequate protector and provider. Since taking care of others is at the core of many women's self-identity,[4] when women do not feel effective as caregivers there are direct and powerful implications for their sense of self-worth. Therefore, it is important to create programs to support and reinforce women's effectiveness and self-efficacy as caregivers as this is central to their role-identity. It is also essential to help women redefine and to expand the limits of their role-identity in the face of a serious illness which may cause significant changes in the care recipient for which they may have little control. The opportunities for education and mental health consultation in these situations are as obvious as if they are essential.

GENDER-BASED CAREGIVER INTERVENTIONS

Gender has been shown to be an important component in caregivers' self-efficacy, role-identity, and stress interventions. Yet programs targeting these critical areas are nearly nonexistent. One exemplar program that has received national attention and Centers for Disease Control and Prevention funding is Men Against Breast Cancer (MABC). MABC is the first national nonprofit organization designed to provide targeted support services to educate and empower men to be effective caregivers for women with breast cancer. MABC partners with community-based organizations, health educators, and cancer centers to bring the Partners' In Survival (PIS) workshops to primarily minority and underserved populations throughout the United States. The PIS program is a strengths-based psycho-educational intervention that focuses on maximizing the inherent synergies of women and men to solve cancer-related problems together. Men are trained in the C.O.P.E. (Creativity, Optimism, Planning, and Expert information) model[36,37] of problem solving for problems common in women receiving treatment for cancer (e.g., depression, fatigue, pain, anxiety, menopausal symptoms). The men learn how to communicate more effectively and to understand the underlying intentions of women in a respectful and honest environment, while becoming proficient in the C.O.P.E problem-solving model. The men then work with the women in their lives to solve mutually agreed upon cancer-related problems. The goal is to provide men with an opportunity to do something meaningful (their "mission") and to provide the women with the collaboration that enables them to feel a sense of emotional connection and self-efficacy.

Although the data from this 5-year study are still being analyzed, the feasibility of implementing this program has been clearly demonstrated. Men will attend and enthusiastically participate in programs that are male-friendly and focus on their specific interests and motivations. To date, 202 men have participated in the PIS workshops: 41.0% African-American, 39.0% Caucasian, 12.0% Latino, and 8% other or unidentified. These findings are important because we know so little about men as caregivers. There is reluctance in the field to study or to fund research on this underserved population. The data from MABC show male caregivers with poor problem-solving skills at baseline are significantly more likely to report higher levels of distress. Similar finding were seen in spouses of prostate cancer patients.[38] Those women with poor problem-solving skills (avoidance, impulsivity, negative problem orientation) reported more distress. Poor problem-solving skills in the spousal caregivers predicted distress in patients. These findings demonstrate that coping difficulties by the caregiver have a significant impact on how prostate cancer patients manage their illness-related stress. The results from Ko et al. (2005) and MABC support the need for specific problem-solving gender-based caregiver interventions.

An additional example of a caregiver gender-based intervention is Men and Women Getting the Best out of Each Other, problem-solving group. The four week 2-hour sessions are manualized courses that are interactive and based on the C.O.P.E problem-solving model. Any man or woman who is coping with illness is encouraged to participate. This problem-solving group takes a strengths-based approach maximizing the ability of women and men to work together through the challenges of cancer. They build-off of each others' strengths through the identification of differences in the way men and women cope with and manage stress. This problem-solving group is an opportunity for men and women to speak honestly, openly, and respectfully to encourage communication, problem solving, and teamwork. The goal of the group is to help men and women empathically understand the motivations underlying potentially alienating gender-based behaviors. For example, participants learn how to solve problems together and integrate mutual support into their lives, rather than responding emotionally. This group also helps to maximize the potential that the caregivers and care recipients' expectations and demands are aligned through enhanced understanding, knowledge

Table 73–3. Benefit finding of caregiving for both men and women

Benefit finding
Accepting things[39]
Couples getting closer[48]
Empathy for all human beings[39]
Getting closer to family members[39]
Increased spirituality[49]
Positive self-view[39]
Reprioritization[39]

about gender-based perceptions, and responses. Care recipients and their family members or caregivers report being extremely satisfied with this problem-solving group (N = 57). The participants stated that the group was meaningful to them (100%) and personally helpful to them (98%), that they learned at least one thing to help themselves or a loved one cope better (100%). They reported that the group was a good place to discuss and resolve problems (98%). The implications of these preliminary findings are that healthcare providers should encourage partners to actively engage in activities that teach them to enhance their own feelings of self-efficacy, which appears to be the case more among female caregivers.

CAREGIVING AS AN OPPORTUNITY FOR GROWTH

Although the findings of many of these studies have focused on the negative secondary impact of cancer on the family, such as caregiving stress and heightened levels of psychological distress, recent studies report that family caregivers are also able to find benefit in the challenges associated with cancer in the family.[39] Those individuals with greater levels of perceived caregiving stress and lower education were related to greater benefit finding in the cancer caregiving experience. Men and women reported equivalent levels of benefit-finding experiences from caregiving, such as accepting things, empathy for all human beings, getting closer to family members, positive self-view, and reprioritization, with an exception where women were less likely to report changes in appreciation in life due to cancer caregiving (see Table 73–3).

CONCLUSIONS/FUTURE DIRECTIONS

There has also been extremely limited funding available for the essential research that will inform interventions and programs to understand how to best support women and men in their caregiver roles. Hopefully, the changing demographics relating to age and increased budgetary implications for the healthcare system and consumer demand will motivate increases in support for such basic and essential information.

Since gender is one of the most basic biological and psycho-social characteristics of individuals, knowledge of caregivers' gender can be the first step toward understanding the complexities of cancer caregiving. Once intergender variations are more fully and objectively understood, additional components of the caregiver should be studied, such as; intragender differences, culture, age, race/ethnicity, relationship characteristics, stage in life span, and other demographics. Another important factor to be considered is the alignment of expectations and demands of the caregiver and the care recipient. This "fit" is essential for both the caregiver and care recipient's quality of life and can be gained through honest and open communication, education, and a deep understanding of the innate differences between men and women and how these differences are magnified in times of stress. For example, female caregivers report more emotional distress overall; however, male caregivers suffer more physically. In female caregivers, her self-efficacy is highly related to how well she copes as a caregiver. For male caregivers, the emotional state of the care recipient is an important component in how he will cope as a caregiver.

The areas of interdependence in the caregiver experience are more common than there are differences. However, to benefit from the unique contributions of women and men, there need to be honest, open, and respectful negotiations over higher levels of reciprocity and conscious choices made about what each individual is capable and willing to provide. The self-awareness afforded to modern women and men through the development of the cerebral frontal cortex, communication skills, education, understanding, social values of equality, and an inherent belief in the worth of all human life creates, an environment where men and women can make conscious decisions about what it means to reach their full potential, independently and interdependently.

Never before have women and men been able to use history, science, and technology in a society that increasingly values the equality of the sexes to make conscious and deliberate decisions about how to benefit from our shared values while fully exploiting the synergies of our individual biological, psychological, social, and spiritual inclinations. The caregiver experience is a microcosm of how men and women continue to evolve together and how we are recreating each other through our increasing respect and commitment to enhancing the humanity of both.

REFERENCES

1. Institute of Medicine. *Exploring the biological contributions of human health: Does sex matter?* Washington, DC: National Academy Press; 2001.

2. Bureau of Labor Statistics. *Women in the labor force*. Available at URL: http://www.bls.gov/cps/wlf-databook2007.html. Accessed July 30, 2008.

3. Taylor SE, Klein LC, Lewis BP, Greunewald TL, Gurung RA, Updegraff JA. Biobehavioral responses in stress in females: tend-and-befriend, not fight-or-flight. *Psychol Rev*. 2000;107(3):411–429.

4. Hagedoorn M, Sanderman R, Buunk BP, Wobbes T, Sanderman, R. Failing in spousal caregiving: the 'identity-relevant stress' hypothesis to explain sex differences in caregiver distress. *Br J Health Psychol*. 2002;7:481–494.

5. Hagedoorn M, Sanderman R, Bolks HN, Tuinstra J, Coyne JC. Distress in couples coping with cancer: a meta-analysis and critical review of role and gender effects. *Psychol Bull*. 2008;134(1):1–30.

6. Miller B, Cafasso L. Gender differences in caregiving: fact or artifact. *Gerontologist*. 1992;32(4):498–507.

7. Fromme EK, Drach LL, Tolle SW, et al. Men as caregivers at the end of life. *J Palliat Med*. 2005;8:1167–1175.

8. Edwards BK, Howe HL, Ries LAG, et al. Annual report to the nation on the status of cancer, 1973–1999, featuring implications of age and aging on U.S. cancer burden. *Cancer*. 2002;94(10):2766–2792.

9. National Cancer Institute—Cancer Control and Population Sciences. Estimated Cancer Prevalence. *SEER* 2008; Ries LAG, Melbert D, Krapcho M, et al. (eds). SEER Cancer Statistics Review, 1975–2004, National Cancer Institute. Bethesda, MD, http://seer.cancer.gov/csr/1975_2004/, based on November 2006 SEER data submission, posted to the SEER web site, 2007. Available at: URL: http://cancercontrol.cancer.gov/ocs/prevalence/prevalence.html. Accessed June 18, 2008.

10. Kim Y, Given BA. Quality of life of family caregivers of cancer survivors across the trajectory of the illness. *Cancer*. 2008;11(Suppl 112):2556–2568.

11. Kim Y, Schulz R. Family caregivers' strains: comparative analysis of cancer caregiving with dementia, diabetes, and frail elderly caregiving. *J Aging Health*. 2008;20(5):483–503.

12. Gilligan C. *In a different voice: Psychological theory and women's development*. Cambridge, MA: Harvard University Press; 1982.

13. National Alliance for Caregiving, American Association of Retired Persons. *Family caregiving in the U.S.: Findings from a national survey*. Washington, DC: National Alliance for Caregiving; 1997.

14. National Alliance for Caregiving and AARP. *Caregiving in the U.S.* Washington, DC: National Alliance for Caregiving and AARP; 2004. Available at http://www.caregiving.org/data/04finalreport.pdf.

15. Derogatis LR, Morrow GR, Fetting J, et al. The prevalence of psychiatric disorders among cancer patients. *JAMA*. 1983;249:751–757.

16. Hagendoorn M, Buunk, BP, Kuijer RG, Wobbest T, Sanderman R. Couples dealing with cancer: role and gender differences regarding psychological distress and quality of life. *Psychooncology*. 2000;9:232–242.

17. Matthews BA. Role and gender differences in cancer-related distress: a comparison of survivor and caregiver self-reports. *Oncol Nurs Forum*. 2003;30(3):493–499.

18. Hodges LJ, Humphris GM, Macfarlane G. A meta-analytic investigation of the relationship between the psychological distress of cancer patients and their carers. *Soc Sci Med*. 2005;60:1–12.

19. Pinquart M, Sörensen S. Differences between caregivers and noncaregivers in psychological health and physical health: a meta-analysis. *Psychol Aging*. 2003;18(2):250–267.

20. Braun M, Mikulincer M, Rydall A, Walsh A, Rodin G. Hidden morbidity in cancer: spouse caregivers. *J Clin Oncol*. 2007;25:4829–4834.

21. Kim Y, Baker F, Spillers RL. Cancer caregivers' quality of life: effects of gender, relationship, and appraisal. *J Pain Symp Manage*. 2007;34(3):294–304.

22. Kim Y, Loscalzo MJ, Wellisch DK, Spillers RL. Gender differences in caregiving stress among caregivers of cancer survivors. *Psychooncology*. 2006;15(12):1086–1092.

23. Northouse LL, Mood DW, Montie JE, et al. Living with prostate cancer: patients' and spouses' psychosocial status and quality of life. *J Clin Oncol*. 2007;27:4171–4177.

24. Kim Y, Kashy DA, Wellisch DK, Spillers RL, Kaw CK, Smith TG. Quality of life of couples dealing with cancer: dyadic and individual adjustment among breast and prostate cancer survivors and their spousal caregivers. *Ann Behav Med*. 2008;35:230–238.

25. Baider L, Ever-Hadani P, Goldzweig G, Wygoda MR, Peretz T. Is perceived family support a relevant variable in psychological distress? A sample of prostate and breast cancer couples. *J Psychos Res*. 2003;55(5):453–460.

26. Kiecolt-Glaser JK, Newton T, Cacioppo JT, MacCallum RC, Glaser R, Malarkey WB. Marital conflict and endocrine function: are men really more physiologically affected than women? *J Consult Clin Psychol*. 1996;64(2):324–332.

27. Baider L, Koch U, Esacson R, De Nour AK. Prospective study of cancer patients and their spouses: the weakness of marital strength. *Psychooncology*. 1998;7(1):49–56.

28. Burman B, Margolin G. Analysis of the association between marital relationships and health problems: an interactional perspective. *Psychol Bull*. 1992;112(1):39–63.

29. Kiecolt-Glaser JK, Newton TL. Marriage and health: his and hers. *Psychol Bull*. 2001;127(4):472–503.

30. Shumaker SA, Hill DR. Gender differences in social support and physical health. *Health Psychology*. 1991;10(2):102–111.

31. Baider L, Koch U, Esacson R, De Nour AK. Prospective study of cancer patients and their spouses: the weakness of marital strength. *Psychooncology*. 1998;7(1):49–56.

32. Kim Y, Loscalzo MJ, Wellisch DK, Spillers RL. Gender differences in caregiving stress among caregivers of cancer survivors. *Psychooncology*. 2006;15(12):1086–1092.

33. Bakas T, Lewis RR, Parsons JE. Caregiving tasks among family caregivers of patients with lung cancer. *Oncol Nurs Forum*. 2001;28(5):847–854.

34. Kim Y, Carver CS. Frequency and difficulty in caregiving among spouses of individuals with cancer: effects of adult attachment and gender. *Psychooncology*. 2007;16(8):714–723.

35. Given B, Given CW, Sikorskii A, Jeon S, Sherwood P, Rahbar M. The impact of providing symptom management assistance on caregiver reaction: results of a randomized trial. *J Pain Symptom Manage*. 2006;32(5):433–443.

36. Houts PS, Nezu AM, Nezu CM, Bucher JA. The prepared family caregiver: a problem-solving approach to family caregiver education. *Patient Educ Couns*. 1996;27(1):63–73.

37. Nezu AM, Nezu CM, Felgoise SH, McClure KS, Houts PS. Project Genesis: assessing the efficacy of problem-solving therapy for distressed adult cancer patients. *J Consul Clin Psychol*. 2003;71(6):1036–1048.

38. Ko CM, Malcarne VL, Varni JW, et al. Problem-solving and distress in prostate cancer patients and their spousal caregivers. *Support Care Cancer*. 2005;13:367–374.

39. Kim Y, Schulz R, Carver CS. Benefit finding in the cancer caregiving experience. *Psychosom Med*. 2007;69:283–291.

40. Lewis FM, Fletcher KA, Cochrane BB, Fann JR. Predictors of depressed mood in spouses of women with breast cancer. *J Clin Oncol*. 2008;8:1289–1294.

41. Sabo D, Brown J, Smith C. The male role and mastectomy: support groups and men's adjustment. *J Psychos Oncol*. 1986;4(1/2):19–31.

42. Gaugler JE, Given WC, Linder J, Kataria R, Tucker G, Regine W. Work, gender and stress in family cancer caregiving. *Support Care Cancer*. 2008;16:347–357.

43. Lalos A, Jacobson L, Lalos O, Stendahl U. Male experience of gynecological cancer. *J Psychosom Obstet Gynaecol*. 1995;16:153–165.

44. Fletcher BS, Paul SM, Dodd MJ, et al. Prevalence, severity, and impact of symptoms on female family caregivers of patients at the initiation of radiation therapy for prostate cancer. *J Clin Oncol*. 2008;26:599–604.

45. Kim Y, Loscalzo MJ, Wellisch DK, Spillers RL. Gender differences in caregiving stress among caregivers of cancer survivors. *Psychooncology*. 2006;15(12):1086–1092.

46. Emanuel EJ, Fairclough DL, Slutsman J, Alpert H, Baldwin D, Emanuel LL. Assistance from family members, friends, paid care givers, and volunteers in the care of terminally ill patients. *N Engl J Med*. 1999;341:956–963.

47. Srirangam SJ, Pearson E, Grose C, Brown SC, Collins GN, O'Reilly PH. Partner's influence on patient preference for treatment in early prostate cancer. *Br J Urol Sur Int*. 2003;92:365–369.

48. Dorval M, Guay S, Mondor M, et al. Couples who get closer after breast cancer: frequency and predictors in a prospective investigation. *J Clin Oncol*. 2005;23:3588–3596.

49. Kim Y, Wellisch DK, Spillers RL, Crammer C. Psychological distress of female cancer caregivers: effects of type of cancer and caregivers' spirituality. *Support Care Cancer*. 2007;15(12):1367–1374.

CHAPTER 74

Addressing the Needs of Children When a Parent Has Cancer

Cynthia W. Moore and Paula K. Rauch

INTRODUCTION

For many parents, the thought, "What will I tell my children?" follows a cancer diagnosis with lightning speed. Parents wonder whether to tell children about the diagnosis, how to share the news in an age-appropriate manner, what reactions to anticipate, and when to be worried. There may be one child they have particular concerns about due to temperament or preexisting challenges, or there may be family circumstances such as a recent death that elevate concern about all the children.

Both the existing research and the clinical experience of the authors in providing guidance to parents with cancer underscore the need for members of the psycho-oncology team to understand how children cope with parental cancer. This chapter provides an overview of key issues of concern to parents and recommendations to support children's emotional health, so that clinicians can respond to these concerns with informed sensitivity.

REVIEW OF THE LITERATURE

Studies of parental cancer's effects on children focus particularly on two areas: first, the prevalence of negative psychological outcomes, and second, the factors associated with risk and resilience[1-3] Parents may be encouraged to learn that children and adolescents who have a parent with cancer seem not to experience serious psychological difficulties, such as a diagnosable depression or anxiety disorder, more frequently than their peers. However, these children are at increased risk for internalizing problems. Approximately 20%–25% of children coping with parental illness experience depressed and anxious mood, poor concentration, intrusive thoughts, school difficulty, sleep problems, or somatic complaints.[3-8] When asked about their reactions to a parent being ill, children report a variety of worries. Latency age (6–12 years) children fear, among other things, that the parent will die or stay sick for a long time, have significant changes in their appearance, or require hospitalizations and therefore separations from the child.[9] Adolescents worry about the possibility of the parent's dying, and also express pity for the parent, try to comfort the parent, feel angry, and struggle to find meaning in the situation.[1,9]

Efforts to identify risk and protective factors for psychosocial outcomes in these children have the potential to guide clinical interventions. A number of parent and family characteristics are related to children's functioning, though medical variables, such as stage of illness and type of cancer, are generally not.[2] Maternal depression increases children's distress[10,11] Children from families with both a depressed mother and poorly defined family roles may be at particular risk for internalizing problems, with girls more at-risk than boys. Family style may also affect children's functioning. For example, adolescents from families with open communication tend to be less anxious and distressed and have fewer externalizing problems.[3,12] Less cohesive families are likelier to have adolescents with more anxiety, depression and externalizing behaviors.[2,3,12] While many aspects of family functioning tend to be good for most children, the hope over time is to identify which aspects are particularly critical in families facing cancer so that more general family interventions can be fine-tuned to address medical illness. A family's ability to solve problems flexibly may be one such target area. Flexible problem solving predicted less adolescent psychological distress in families dealing with parental cancer, but not in families without illness.[12]

Importance of communication. Many parents worry that sharing information about their cancer will cause unnecessary distress to children. Yet in one recent qualitative study, 8–15-year-olds clearly expressed the importance of having a "precise knowledge" of the parent's illness, even though being included in these conversations could be difficult.[9] A number of studies have suggested that open communication is valuable in ultimately reducing children's anxiety.[13-16] While parents are aware that they should use "age appropriate" explanations, they are often uncertain about how those explanations should actually sound. Both parents and oncology nurses have voiced a need for more developmentally based information about children's understanding of illness and characteristic responses to a parent's cancer.[17,18] Research also demonstrates that families avoid communication about the emotional aspects of illness, suggesting that education about the importance of talking about feelings may also be beneficial.[9,19]

A DEVELOPMENTAL PERSPECTIVE ON CHILDREN'S AND ADOLESCENTS' UNDERSTANDING OF ILLNESS

The nuts and bolts of *how* to talk with children openly and honestly varies according to the child's developmental stage. Parents can benefit from guidance around how their children are likely to understand the cancer diagnosis, and how to respond to their needs.

Infants and toddlers. Children this young do not have the verbal capacity to comprehend the idea of "cancer." They are most affected by changes in caregivers and routines necessitated by the parent's treatment, and may react to such disruptions by being more difficult to feed or soothe. Organizing a small number of caregivers who can maintain consistency in the details of the child's daily routine such as naptime, meals, baths, and bedtime, will minimize the stress on these children.

Preschoolers. Preschoolers benefit from hearing simple explanations of a parent's illness and treatment that make clear that nothing they thought or did caused the cancer. In the absence of such information, they are capable of creating their own, often egocentric, explanations for the parent's illness or changes in behavior, such as, "I kicked Daddy when we were wrestling and made him get sick," or, "Mommy is mad at me and that's why she's not playing." Talking to a preschooler about the name of the illness, basics of treatment, and the expected changes to the child's routine or experience within the family, will help the child adapt. For example, a 4-year-old might be told: "Daddy is sick with something called colon cancer. He will be going to the doctor for a special medicine called chemotherapy, and Mom will go with him to keep him company. The medicine will help make the cancer better, but Dad will feel pretty tired for a few days after he takes it. On the days he has doctor's appointments, you'll have a play date with Brian after preschool, until we get home."

School-age children. Six- to twelve-year-olds may have heard of cancer, and may be curious, but have erroneous beliefs, about its causes and course. They generally expect illness to "follow the rules," for example, if you follow your doctor's recommendations then your cancer will be cured. Most school-age children are familiar with the idea that germs transmit illness, and may be confused thinking that cancer is also contagious. As with younger children, it can be helpful to ask the child what ideas they have about how the parent got cancer, so that misperceptions can be corrected. A 10-year-old girl whose father was dying of esophageal cancer shared that she understood that "stress can cause illnesses, and I know he was upset that I wasn't doing all my homework."

Somatic complaints such as headaches and stomachaches are a common manifestation of stress in children this age, so monitoring visits to the school nurse may provide an indication of how the child is coping. Maintaining a normal routine as much as possible will help the child to feel secure, but this can get complicated when there are multiple children heading in multiple directions after school. Families willing to ask for help with rides, shopping for school supplies, and so on, will have an easier time preserving their children's consistent participation in activities.

Adolescents. A new capacity for abstract thinking allows adolescents to comprehend both the current and potential impact of a parent's illness as well as uncertainty about prognosis. Thus, they are susceptible to a variety of worries, for example, about family finances (Will there be money for college?), the well-being of other family members (How will my younger siblings handle this?), and concerns about justice and meaning (How could this happen to MY family?). In addition to a clear description of the illness and treatment, teens may need to hear that because cancer treatment is so individual, reading about it on the internet or talking to friends about their experiences with cancer is likely to give them misinformation.

Adolescents need a say in how information about the illness is disseminated to their school. Many are intensely private, and some worry that they will be treated differently, or pitied, if others learn of the parent's cancer. However, given the pressure on adolescents to perform, informing a trusted teacher or guidance counselor about the illness can facilitate the creation of a safety net of support quickly, should the need arise.

Parents frequently impose new responsibilities on adolescents, particularly girls, in response to feeling overwhelmed by the demands of the illness and treatment. For instance, teens may be expected to provide care to the ill parent or younger siblings, to shop for groceries, cook, or clean. It is easy to sympathize with parents wanting their older children to "step up to the plate" and help out. However, some adolescents are asked to take on responsibilities for which they have not been well prepared, or roles—such as "man of the house"—that are unrealistic. An adolescent may react by trying overly hard to fulfill a parent's needs, and thereby miss out on spending time with peers or on other age-appropriate pursuits. Alternatively, adolescents may react by spending less time at home and avoiding the parent's declining health and increasing requests. Frustration on both sides may be minimized when parents offer choices about how teens might most comfortably help, and explicitly recognize the critical importance of their child's peer relationships and outside interests.

FACILITATING PARENT–CHILD AND CHILD–PARENT COMMUNICATION

In addition to the developmental considerations outlined above, some general guidelines can help relieve parents' anxiety about initiating conversations about illness. First, choosing a specific time and place to begin talking can concretize the task for parents. Children usually feel more comfortable talking at home or somewhere private, where they will not feel self-conscious about an emotional reaction to difficult news. While family meetings with everyone together are often preferred for significant updates, one-on-one, unstructured conversations at times the child tends to be most talkative (e.g., driving in the car, or at bedtime) are a good opportunity for parents to respond individually to each child's questions. Parents who communicate with adolescents living away from home via cell phone calls and email may want to discuss with them in advance how they prefer to be updated. Given the variety of settings in which a cell phone may be answered, parents may also need to check whether the adolescent is in a comfortable place for a conversation, before sharing difficult news.

Parents will want to share enough about the current situation that children are not caught unawares by significant events, but not say so much that children feel anxious for too long about events that may or may not occur in the future. They may start by asking the child what he or she has noticed about the parent lately, then acknowledging those observations, elaborating on them, providing an explanation, and discussing solutions to problems that have arisen. For example, in response to a 7 year old's comment that her mother hasn't been getting up in the morning to help her prepare for school, parents might say, "You're right, Mom has been staying in bed later than usual. Remember how she went to the doctor's for her special medicine a few days ago? That medicine makes her extra tired for a few days. We hope she'll start feeling better soon, hopefully by the weekend. Is there anything that would make the morning times easier for you?" In addition to providing information and facilitating problem solving, it is crucial for parents to inquire about and validate children's feelings and reactions to the illness, whether positive or negative, and to model that emotions change at different times.

SPECIFIC ISSUES IN COMMUNICATION

Symptoms. Children usually feel curious and concerned about the physical symptoms they observe in their parents, including hair loss, fatigue, and nausea. Even once they understand that these are related to cancer treatment, they may need reassurance that a parent who seems sicker due to treatment side effects is actually getting better. The impossibility of hiding hair loss sometimes encourages otherwise reluctant parents to discuss a cancer diagnosis. Elementary school-age children, in particular, may express concern about the parent being scrutinized by peers. It may help for the parent to plan with the child how to explain physical changes to peers, and also to discuss the types of camouflage (wigs, scarves) the parent will utilize, and in what settings. Fatigue is exasperating to children in part because it is invisible, and manifests mainly in the parent's inactivity. Younger children may feel that the parent just doesn't want to play with them, while adolescents become impatient with a parent who "always lies around...she doesn't even *try* to stay busy." Mood changes and irritability, which can be caused by steroid medications or depression, are similarly challenging. Children may believe that they are the cause of the parent's short fuse, and feel guilty, withdraw, act out, or take on too much responsibility for cheering up the parent.

Children who prefer not to talk. Some children, usually school-age and older, make it clear that they want to hear only the most minimal updates. They tend not to ask questions or share feelings, and parents frequently worry about their adjustment to the illness. Although parents may accurately sense that the child is protecting him or herself from unwanted bad news, it is important even for these children to receive brief, factual updates about the treatment plan and significant changes in the parent's functioning. It may help to identify another adult that the child knows well, with whom he or she can speak about the parent's cancer, since children may feel they need to protect parents from their distress.

Anxious children. Parents also worry about conversations with children who ask "a million questions about things that even *I* haven't thought about yet!" When parents think in advance about the kinds of questions their children are likely to have, based on their developmental stage, and history, they can then plan how to be both reassuring and honest. Parents seem particularly afraid of the question, "Are you going to die?" no matter what stage of illness they have. When they feel prepared even for this very difficult question, conversations can proceed more freely. A child may be reassured with a response like, "Yes, sometimes people die of cancer, like Aunt Holly. But my cancer is a very different kind than hers. None of my doctors are worried about my dying, and neither am I. I'm planning to do everything I can to get better. If anything changes, I will let you know." Or, if a parent is more sick, "Yes, people can die from my type of cancer, but I'm still really confident that this new treatment will help slow down the cancer."

Though parents may worry about burdening their children with bad news, they frequently find that their children feel trusted, reassured and included in the family team by knowing more and having an opportunity to share their particular concerns.

SUPPORTING FAMILY FUNCTIONING IN WAYS THAT BENEFIT THE CHILDREN

Cancer can be enormously disruptive to a family's typical routines. For example, an ill parent may not feel well enough to help children get ready for school every morning, to coach baseball, or shop for a prom dress. The well parent may work longer hours, finances may be tight, and activities may be cut or vacation plans curtailed. Families may benefit from meals and practical help from friends and extended family members, but harnessing so much good will can prove exhausting, and the help can at times feel intrusive. When there are many disruptions in family life, and when they last for a long time, children's adjustment can suffer.

Consistent routines and rules, and continued enjoyment of family time help children flourish, despite parental illness. For example, frequent visitors, telephone calls, or repeated inquiries from well-wishers about the parent's health while the child and parent are together can lead children to feel that their whole world is about cancer. Concrete adjustments often help, like limiting visitors and calls to times of day when children are not present, updating many people at once by using an email distribution list or phone tree, or designating a "Minister of Information" who will keep family and friends up-to-date on developments.

Having a trusted friend or relative coordinate offers of help and communicate the details of what would truly feel helpful to the family can also make it easier for the family to protect their time. Because it can be difficult to call to mind exactly what sort of help might be needed at exactly the moment help is offered, some families designate a "Captain of Kindness," to orchestrate who will help, when, doing what. For instance, materials needed by a child for their historical figure costume and book report can be purchased by a willing parent of a classmate when they are shopping for their own child. Parents with limited energy can be reminded that it makes sense to spend time and energy doing things that will give both they and their child the most satisfaction.

PREPARATION FOR SPECIFIC EVENTS

Though much about cancer is unpredictable, hospitalizations may be scheduled far enough in advance that families can discuss the reason for the treatment and separation, whether visits will be possible, and practical concerns such as who will care for children while a parent is away. It may help to frame longer separations as a short-term challenge important for the family's long-term benefit. Table 74–1 summarizes strategies to prepare for separations that can help maintain connections between an absent parent and the children.

COMMON CHALLENGES

In asking "what-if" sorts of questions, clinicians must raise anxiety enough to facilitate planning, but not so much that the parent becomes overwhelmed and withdrawn. To start, parents can be asked, "What are your concerns about your children if treatment doesn't go as well as we hope?" or, "A lot of parents have a hard time thinking about who would care for their children if they couldn't for any reason…but find it enormously reassuring once plans are made. Is that something we could talk about together?" Parents need to be aware that although they are quite optimistic, their children may still conceal worries about a variety of frightening possibilities, such as where they would live and who would care for them if anything happened to the parent.

Table 74–1. Managing separations and hospital visits

Preparation for separations
Infants/toddlers
Minimize number of different caregivers when possible
Leave caregivers detailed notes about feeding and nap times, strategies for soothing, favorite ways to play

School-age children and teens
Describe the reason for the treatment and expected length of separation
Invite children's help in choosing caregivers, planning rides to school, and activities
Discuss preferences about who will provide updates on parent's condition, when and how

Keeping in touch
Phone calls, email, instant messaging, video conferencing help keep parents in touch with caregivers and older children
Both children and parents appreciate receiving cards, drawings
Display family photos at home and in hospital
Have a trusted adult available to assist children processing news updates about the ill parent

Preparation for children's visits to the hospital
Describe how ill parent will look and behave, what the child may hear or see (e.g., medical equipment, roommates)
Encourage but do not force a reluctant child to visit; elicit questions and concerns, problem-solve, and correct misperceptions
Pack activities—quiet games, art supplies, homework
Consider delaying visit if the parent is agitated, delirious, or at high risk of infection

Helping children cope with parental cancer is made more complicated when parents experience frequent conflict, are estranged, or are divorced. These parents often insist they cannot safely share medical or financial information. However, for both parents to be able to answer children's questions and respond sensitively to a variety of reactions, both require basic information about the practical impact of the diagnosis and treatment plan on the children. If too much conflict exists, another adult may serve as an intermediary. Children should not be asked to convey this information to the other parent.

Ill parents may worry that if they don't survive, their children will have no choice but to live with a clearly inadequate parent, or alternatively, may be unaware that even a long-absent parent can have legal rights to a child. A referral to a family lawyer can be invaluable in many of these complicated situations. It is critical that extended family members are not left to fight for custody of a child without having a record of the parent's wishes.

Even when both parents are actively raising children, frequently an ill parent will verbalize the sense that should they die, the children's practical needs will be met, but they won't be as lovingly nurtured. With ample empathy for the painfulness of the situation, clinicians may be able to encourage parents to consider who else in their children's lives share some of the qualities they most value in their own parenting. Relationships between children and these adults can often be deepened in advance of a parent's death, in ways that the surviving parent is able to tolerate and even appreciate.

WHEN TO RECOMMEND PSYCHOLOGICAL ASSESSMENT OF A CHILD BEYOND PARENT GUIDANCE

Having cancer seems to elicit advice—both welcome and unwelcome—from all corners. Commonly, parents are advised to get children into therapy right away by well-meaning friends or relatives, yet experience

Table 74-2. Guidelines to identify children who may require psychological assessment and treatment

Child verbalizes a wish to speak to a therapist
Child verbalizes thoughts of self-harm
Child has preexisting mental health issues (e.g., anxiety, depression) and experiences an increase in symptoms
Child's functioning at school, with peers or at home is noticeably different for more than several weeks, or in two or more arenas

suggests that not all children need, or will benefit from, seeing a therapist. Parents appreciate guidance in determining when this added support is critical enough to warrant the sacrifices involved. Table 74-2 provides guidelines to help determine which children may need psychological assessment and treatment. School counselors and pediatricians may be helpful in referring parents to an appropriate resource for the child.

END OF LIFE ISSUES

Informing a child that a parent probably won't survive much longer is fraught with sadness and worry. Parents express concern about when to share this news, what to say, and how their children might react. Very young children are unlikely to understand or benefit from advance warning that a parent's death is imminent. Children around age 4 and older, however, may regret missing the opportunity to say good-bye in whatever way is meaningful, and may perceive adults' protectiveness as being excluded.

In deciding when to inform children about an impending death, parents must balance speaking soon enough so that the child has time to process the news and say good-bye, with waiting long enough so that the child isn't made too anxious for too long, confused by a "dying" parent who still seems to function relatively well, or pressured to keep the relationship happy, and conflict free over an impossibly long period. Ideally, the conversation will occur before the ill parent experiences irreversible changes in mental status or cognitive function, preventing a two-way conversation between parent and child. If there is hope that the parent may be alert for a number of days, but concern that a sudden change in function is possible, it is generally better to err on the side of informing children sooner than later. Children can be told that time with the parent is precious, and that it is important for them to say anything that needs to be said soon.

Some children quite willingly visit a dying parent, while others balk due to concerns that can be alleviated fairly easily once they are discovered and discussed. For example, a child may feel embarrassed to cry in front of other people, or fear being alone with the parent at the time of death. A plan to clear the room of other visitors while the child is there, or to ensure the presence of an adult at all times, may help the child feel safe enough to visit. Some worries are harder to address; for example, an adolescent's concern that he will not be able to remember his mother as healthy if he sees her at the very end of life. If a visit will not be possible, the child may be encouraged to send a note for another adult to read to the parent, to say something over the telephone, or to simply send hugs.

Sharing news of a parent's death is one of the hardest conversations an adult can have with a child. Euphemisms for death—being called to be with God, being taken by the angels, gone to Heaven—keep us at arm's length from the painfulness of a loss, but are confusing to preschoolers and even some 6–12 year olds because they lack a clear understanding of biological death. Death should be explained to young children in simple, concrete terms: "Death is when the body completely stops working…the heart stops, breathing stops, so it's *not* like just being asleep." Parents should be prepared for questions like, "Can we give him more medicine and make him better?" or, repeatedly, "When is Mommy coming home?" as children struggle to come to terms with the irreversibility and permanence of this separation.

Attending a parent's funeral or memorial can help all but the youngest children to process the loss, if they are well prepared. A description of what children will see and hear during the rituals, and the ways emotions may be expressed by different people is a good start. If a child expresses a strong desire to stay home, even after discussions about what would allow him to attend, it is usually best to honor this. Having an adult attend the funeral with a younger child will allow her to leave if needed during the service, without pulling away the other parent who will likely need to stay. Children can be invited, but not required, to participate in the service in a number of ways—sharing some favorite memories, playing an instrument, choosing photographs for a collage, even arranging napkins. Older children should be given choices about which photographs that include them will be on display, and which of their peers are invited. Finally, the presence of many friends and relatives at the funeral provides a rare opportunity to collect written stories and memories about the parent, which enrich that parent's legacy.

CHALLENGES AND RECOMMENDATIONS FOR PROVIDING A RANGE OF CLINICAL SERVICES

A growing emphasis on family-centered care has resulted in the creation of a variety of programs to meet the needs of children with ill parents. Hospitals may provide family friendly visiting areas, equipped with art supplies and home-like furnishings.[20] Informational brochures to facilitate conversations between children and parent exist, and resource rooms often have books on parenting with cancer on hand (see examples in reference list).[21,22] Organizations such as the Wellness Community and Cancer Care offer support groups for children who have a parent with cancer, sometimes along with a concurrent parent group. A structured intervention that educates parents with cancer about talking with their children is being developed and evaluated.[23] The Parenting at a Challenging Time program (PACT) at Massachusetts General Hospital offers free parent guidance consultations with a child psychiatrist or psychologist to patients with cancer, and has created a web site to provide information to parents who do not have direct access to the program (www.mghpact.org).

The range of programs being developed suggests a growing appreciation of the importance of meeting the needs of children affected by parental cancer. However, the lack of availability of services at many treatment centers underscores the importance of better understanding the obstacles to addressing children's needs as a matter of course in a parent's treatment for cancer. Clearly, constraints on funding and staff time are significant obstacles, as are a lack of child development expertise in staff trained to work primarily with adults, and a lack of formal structure for support or supervision.[18] The intensity of parents' distress about their children may be a less obvious impediment, as staff can be wary about opening a "Pandora's box" of parents' concerns that seems difficult to close.

CONCLUSIONS

Cancer centers, like families, are unique, and there is no "one size fits all" approach to offering parenting support in every possible setting. At a minimum, patients need the importance of their role as parents acknowledged by their medical team, and their concerns about children heard and validated. In addition, some basic resources should be offered, such as a written list of books and web sites that address children's needs around parental cancer, as well as a list of local therapists and nonprofit agencies that work with cancer patients and their families. Many treatment settings could go further, and support one or two staff members in developing expertise in this area. Ideally, these providers would already have a background in mental health to which they could add a solid working knowledge of child development gleaned from formal classes or supervision.

The field of psycho-oncology has begun to fill a critical gap in services for parents with cancer, with research and the development of new interventions. Our hope is that before long, information and support for these parents in caring for their children will be so readily accessible that "What will I tell my children?" will not even need to be spoken before help is offered.

REFERENCES

1. Grabiak BR, Bender CM, Puskar KR. The impact of parental cancer on the adolescent: an analysis of the literature. *Psychooncology.* 2007;16(2):127–137.

2. Osborn T. The psychosocial impact of parental cancer on children and adolescents: a systematic review. *Psychooncology.* 2007;16(2):101–126.

3. Watson M, St. James-Roberts I, Ashley S, et al. Factors associated with emotional and behavioural problems among school age children of breast cancer patients. *Br J Cancer.* 2006;94:43–50.

4. Welch AS, Wadsworth ME, Compas BE. Adjustment of children and adolescents to parental cancer: Parents' and childrens' perspectives. *Cancer.* 1996;77(7):1409–1418.

5. Siegel K, Karus D, Raveis VH. Adjustment of children facing the death of a parent due to cancer. *J Am Acad Child Adolesc Psychiatry.* 1996;35(4):442–450.

6. Birenbaum LK, Yancey DZ, Phillips DS, Chand N, Huster G. School-age children's and adolescents' adjustment when a parent has cancer. *Oncol Nurs For.* 1999;26(10):1639–1645.

7. Nelson E, While D. Children's adjustment during the first year of a parent's cancer diagnosis. *J Psychosoc Onc.* 2002;20(1):15–36.

8. Visser A, Huizinga GA, Hoekstra HJ, et al. Emotional and behavioural functioning of children of a parent diagnosed with cancer: a cross-informant perspective. *Psychooncology.* 2005;14:746–758.

9. Thastum M, Johansen MB, Gubba L. Coping, social relations, and communication: a qualitative exploratory study of children of parents with cancer. *Clin Child Psychol Psychiatry.* 2008;13(1):123–138.

10. Heiney SP, Bryant LH, Walker S, Parrish RS, Provenzano FJ, Kelly KE. Impact of parental anxiety on child emotional adjustment when a parent has cancer. *Oncol Nurs Forum.* 1997;24:655–661.

11. Lewis FM, Darby EL. Adolescent adjustment and maternal breast cancer: a test of the faucet hypothesis. *J Psychosoc Oncol.* 2003;21(4):81–104.

12. Lindqvist B, Schmitt F, Santalahti P, Romer G, Piha J. Factors associated with the mental health of adolescents when a parent has cancer. *Scand J Psychol.* 2007;48(4):345–351.

13. Rosenheim E, Reicher R. Informing children about a parent's terminal illness. *J Child Psychol Psychiatry.* 1985;26(6):995–998.

14. Nelson E, Sloper P, Charlton A, While D. Children who have a parent with cancer: a pilot study. *J Cancer Educ.* 1994;9(1):30–36.

15. Grant KE, Compas BE. Stress and symptoms of anxiety/depression among adolescents: searching for mechanisms of risk. *J Consult Clin Psychol.* 1995;63:1015–1021.

16. Issel LM, Ersek M, Lewis FM. How children cope with mother's breast cancer. *Oncol Nurs Forum.* 1990;17(Suppl 3):5–12.

17. Barnes J, Kroll L, Lee J, Burke O, Jones A, Stein A. Factors predicting communication about the diagnosis of maternal breast cancer to children. *J Psychosom Res.* 2002;52(4):209–215.

18. Turner J, Clavarino A, Yates P, Hargraves M, Connors V, Hausmann S. Oncology nurses, perceptions of their supportive care for parents with advanced cancer: challenges and educational needs. *Psychooncology.* 2007;16(2):149–157.

19. Shands ME, Lewis FM, Zahlis EH. Mother and child interactions about the mother's breast cancer: an interview study. *Oncol Nurs Forum.* 2000;27(1):77–85.

20. Pengelly M. Family matters in acute oncology. *Cancer Nurs.* 2006;5(3):20–23.

21. Rauch P, Muriel A. *Raising an emotionally healthy child when a parent is sick.* New York: McGraw-Hill; 2006.

22. McCue K, Bonn R. *How to help children through a parent's serious illness.* New York: St. Martin's Griffin; 1994.

23. Lewis FM, Casey SM, Brandt PA, Shands ME, Zahlis EH. The Enhancing Connections Program: pilot study of a cognitive-behavioral intervention for mothers and children affected by breast cancer. *Psychooncology.* 2006;15(6):486–497.

CHAPTER 75

Psychosocial Research and Practice with Adult Children of Cancer Patients

Catherine E. Mosher and Talia R. Weiss

Even though I know we all have to die, at some point… it's just *impossible* for me to really think that my mother is not going to be there… and I think that I have to get maybe a little bit—stronger.…adult daughter of a breast cancer patient[1, p. 54-55]

As this quotation illustrates the psychosocial and existential implications of parental cancer in adulthood can be profound. Adults' heightened awareness of their parent's mortality as well as their own cancer risk may precipitate distress.[1] In addition, many of these adults experience psychological strain associated with multiple role demands, such as balancing responsibilities related to caring for parents, caring for children, and employment.[2] Conversely, having a parent with cancer may lead to a positive shift in priorities and closer relationships with others.[3,4] The number of adult children of cancer patients is substantial, as 60% of cancer survivors are 65 years of age and older.[5] For years, this diverse group was neglected in the psychosocial literature because the impact of parental cancer was assumed to be minimal. Today, due in large part to greater awareness of breast cancer risk, mainly first-degree female relatives (FDRs) (i.e., mother, sister, or daughter) of breast cancer patients are assessed for symptoms of psychological distress.[6]

This chapter first reviews the literature on emotional distress and post-traumatic stress responses to parental cancer. We refer the reader to Part IV of this book for information on emotional responses to testing for genetic susceptibility to cancer. Second, the challenges associated with caring for a parent with cancer are discussed. Third, research on coping efforts and personal growth related to parental cancer is reviewed. Finally, directions for future research and implications for clinical practice are presented.

PSYCHOLOGICAL ADJUSTMENT TO PARENTAL CANCER

Emotional distress. Most studies of psychological adjustment to parental cancer have focused on daughters of breast cancer patients, with a few studies examining daughters of ovarian cancer patients.[7] Wellisch and colleagues[8,9] pioneered studies that examined the distress and quality of life of daughters of breast cancer patients. No differences between women with and without maternal histories of breast cancer were found in psychological symptoms or body image ratings.[8] However, daughters of breast cancer patients reported significantly less frequent sexual intercourse, lower sexual satisfaction, and greater feelings of vulnerability to breast cancer.

A number of studies have examined FDRs of breast cancer patients, but the percentage of participants with a maternal history of the disease is rarely reported. However, when that information is included, 45%–100% of the participants have a maternal history of the disease.[10-12] FDRs of breast cancer patients have been found to have higher levels of general distress, anxiety, somatization, and depression on the Brief Symptom Inventory (BSI)[13] compared to women without familial histories of the disease.[6] In a study of self-referred women at a cancer prevention center in the U.S.,

Kash and colleagues[14] found that 27% of FDRs of breast cancer patients endorsed levels of distress on the BSI consistent with a need for psychological counseling. This figure increased to 53% in another study of FDRs attending a one-day educational program about breast cancer.[11]

A few studies have suggested that FDRs may experience levels of emotional distress comparable to that of patients recently diagnosed with breast cancer.[11,15,16] One study examined women attending a high-risk clinic for FDRs of breast cancer patients in the U.S.[15] Almost one-third (28.8%) of this sample scored above 16 on the Center for Epidemiologic Studies Depression Scale (CES-D),[17] which is considered a cutoff point for clinically significant depressive symptoms. In addition, 51.9% scored above the clinical cutoff point for the State-Trait Anxiety Inventory (STAI)[18] trait measure, indicating significant symptoms of anxiety. Similar results were obtained in a sample of Australian women, with 29% reporting significant general distress before attending a familial cancer clinic.[19]

Although accumulating evidence documents the distress felt by women at risk for breast or ovarian cancer, some studies have revealed low levels of general psychological morbidity among these samples.[20-23] Indeed, some studies have found no differences between the levels of depression experienced by these women and members of the general population.[20,21,23] Similarly, Zakowski et al.[22] found that FDRs of breast cancer patients recruited through mammography screening programs in the U.S. did not report higher general distress on the BSI than women without family histories of this disease. These null BSI results were replicated in samples of predominantly racial and ethnic minority women (75% African American, 10% Hispanic) at three U.S. medical centers.[10] Other studies in Scotland and Australia have not found higher rates of general distress among FDRs recruited through familial cancer clinics relative to a number of comparison groups (e.g., general practitioner attendees, members of a twin registry).[10,24,25] Thus, rates of distress among FDRs have not consistently varied as a function of recruitment strategies (e.g., recruitment via high-risk clinics vs. general medical centers).

Compas and colleagues[26,27] examined U.S. samples that included both daughters and sons of cancer patients. For young adults (mean age = 23 years) whose parents had cancer, mean BSI scores were approximately one-half standard deviation above the normative mean, suggesting moderate levels of symptoms of anxiety and depression.[26] Participant sex was not significantly related to young adults' symptoms of anxiety and depression, which points to the importance of assessing sons' psychological adjustment to parental cancer.

Researchers have assessed predictors of psychological distress among female FDRs of breast cancer patients. Similar levels of mood disturbance and depression have been found among younger and older FDRs, although a few studies have found younger age to be a predictor of distress.[21,28] In addition, mixed evidence has been obtained regarding the relationship between the timing of the illness, including age at the time of the relative's cancer diagnosis and the recency of the event, and subsequent

Portions of this chapter are reprinted from Mosher, C. E., & Danoff-Burg, S. (2005). Psychosocial impact of parental cancer in adulthood: A conceptual and empirical review. *Clinical Psychology Review*, 25, 365–382, with permission from Elsevier.

psychological distress.[9,22] Research also has found inconsistent associations between the mental health status of women with cancer and that of their adult daughters.[29,30] Past cancer stressors (i.e., cancer-related caregiving and death), current caregiving burden, and perceptions of future risk for developing cancer have been found to predict distress among FDRs.[10,19,29] FDRs whose experiences included both maternal caregiving and maternal death from breast cancer were reported to have the highest levels of both breast cancer-specific distress and general depressive symptoms.[10] However, women who had one of these experiences without the other did not report higher distress than was observed in the comparison group of women without family histories of breast cancer.[10] Reduced distress among FDRs has been associated with greater optimism and social support.[10,12,31] Future research should explore other potential predictors of distress, including both objective and perceived illness severity, types of medical treatments received, and the types of caregiving provided. It is also important to assess whether the active treatment phase of the mother's illness is most distressing relative to the pre- and posttreatment phases.

Posttraumatic stress symptoms. With the advent of the fourth edition of the *Diagnostic and Statistical Manual of Mental Disorders* (DSM-IV),[32] cancer and other life-threatening illnesses have been conceptualized as possible precipitants of posttraumatic stress disorder (PTSD) symptoms (i.e., intrusive thoughts, avoidance, and hyperarousal). The majority of studies on this topic have examined women diagnosed with early- to middle-stage breast cancer and their female FDRs. For example, using the PTSD Reaction Index (RI),[33,34] Boyer and colleagues[35] found that 21% of American breast cancer patients and 13% of their daughters reported symptoms consistent with PTSD. The prevalence of PTSD symptoms in the daughters was comparable to that found in previous studies of women with breast cancer, and mothers with PTSD symptoms were more likely to have daughters with these symptoms.

To date, most studies of PTSD responses in adult children of cancer patients have used the Impact of Event Scale[36] or the Impact of Event Scale—Revised (IES-R).[37] As discussed earlier in this chapter, Compas and colleagues[26] studied male and female young adult children of American patients with various cancers. The mean IES score for this sample ($M = 11.82$) was well below the cutoff point of 26, above which a moderate or severe impact is indicated.[36] Young adults' stress response symptoms on the IES were significantly correlated with the perceived seriousness and stressfulness of the parent's cancer. In a Dutch study of adolescent and young adult children of cancer patients (ages 11 to 23 years), 21% of sons and 35% of daughters reported clinically elevated stress response symptoms on the IES.[38]

The remaining studies of stress reactions to parental cancer have primarily focused on FDRs of breast cancer patients, a subset of whom are daughters. With one exception,[10] findings suggest that FDRs of breast cancer patients have significantly higher levels of cancer-related intrusive thoughts and avoidance compared to women without such family histories.[6,22] Using the IES-R, one study found that 4% of FDRs of breast cancer patients in the U.S. reported symptoms consistent with a diagnosis of probable PTSD related to familial breast cancer.[15] Other researchers administered the IES to Australian FDRs of breast cancer patients and found that 8% merited a probable PTSD diagnosis related to their personal risk of developing breast cancer.[19] A third U.S. study[20] found that 53% of FDRs experienced intrusive thoughts related to their familial history of breast cancer, and that levels in these women were comparable to those found in studies of individuals exposed to other types of trauma.[36] In addition, 30% of these women reported breast cancer-related worries that interfered with their daily lives.[20] Finally, using diagnostic interviews, a U.S. study found that 15.8% of FDRs reported current threshold or subthreshold PTSD related to familial breast cancer, whereas another 23.7% endorsed past-only levels of threshold or subthreshold PTSD.[39]

Given the marked variability in levels of distress among FDRs of cancer patients,[10,20] it is important to assess predictors of their stress responses. For example, age has been inversely associated with stress response severity among FDRs of breast cancer patients,[12,21] whereas other research has not found this association.[19] In a study of FDRs of ovarian cancer patients, Schwartz et al.[40] found a positive relationship between perceived risk for ovarian cancer and intrusive thoughts, as well

as direct and indirect (via perceived risk) positive relations between the dispositional attentional style of monitoring (i.e., scanning for threat-relevant information) and intrusive thoughts. Overestimating personal breast cancer risk also has been associated with greater stress response symptoms in FDRs.[19] Another study found that avoidance partially mediated the relation between social constraints and two types of distress (i.e., breast cancer-related intrusions and general distress) among FDRs of breast cancer patients.[41] From a social cognitive processing perspective, the findings suggest that unsupportive or negative reactions from others during disclosure of stressor-related thoughts and feelings may result in attempts to avoid such thoughts and feelings; this inadequate exposure to the stressor may prevent its cognitive processing and prolong distress.

Researchers have begun to identify particular aspects of women's experiences with familial cancer that may influence their current levels of stress response symptoms. Compared to women who had either a mother or a sister with breast cancer, women who had a history of breast cancer in both of these relatives were found to experience greater intrusive thoughts.[11] Another potential predictor of posttraumatic stress is a parent's death from cancer, which may be preceded by a lengthy and painful decline in the parent's health and long-term caregiving by close family members. Among FDRs of breast cancer patients, those whose parent(s) had died of cancer were found to have the highest levels of intrusive thoughts, avoidance, and perceived risk.[22] Results suggested that perceived personal risk of breast cancer mediated the effect of parental death on intrusive thoughts and avoidance regarding breast cancer. Caring for a parent or other relative with breast cancer also has been associated with higher levels of cancer-specific stress responses.[10,12]

ADULT OFFSPRING CAREGIVERS

Approximately 20% of primary family caregivers for cancer patients are their children, many of whom are women employed outside the home (see Chapter 74 for a review of gender issues in caregiving).[42] Although there is limited research focusing exclusively on the caregiving process for cancer patients and their caregivers, it is clear that cancer may change the family's identity, roles, and daily functioning and that the disease's effects may be profound and long-lasting, regardless of the medical outcome.[43] The psychosocial literature also documents the distress that caregivers may experience as they provide physical and emotional support for the patient.[44,45] The multiple demands of caregiving, such as monitoring the patient's symptoms around the clock, administering medications, and coping with treatment side effects, may be physically and emotionally exhausting for caregivers.[43,46]

The caregiving literature in general indicates that adult daughters are heavily involved in the informal support and care of dependent older people.[2,47] In fact, adult daughters who care for their parents have been referred to as the "sandwich generation" or "women in the middle" because of the strain involved in balancing multiple role demands.[48] For example, a study of young to middle-aged (18–64 years) caregivers of cancer patients in the United States found that employed caregivers with children reported a higher level of caregiving stress than employed or unemployed caregivers with no children.[2] Research also indicates that employed caregiving daughters managing competing demands do not reduce their caregiving.[49] Instead, they eliminate their leisure time,[50] decrease their work hours, or leave the workforce.[49,51] Despite the recognition that these women provide critical parental support, most research on caring for adult cancer patients has studied samples comprised primarily or entirely of spouses.[52]

It is important to separately examine the caregiving experiences of spouses and adult children because research has documented differential perceptions of burden and adaptational outcomes for these groups.[53,54] Investigations of caregivers for older adults have yielded mixed findings; some research has found more strain and lower well-being among spouse caregivers as compared to grown offspring caregivers,[54] whereas another study found that offspring experienced more strain in their caregiving role than spouse caregivers.[53] Studies of adult children and spouse caregiving teams support the notion that children experience less physical and financial problems than spouses but are equally likely to experience psychological distress.[54,55] Finally, the American Cancer Society survey of spouse and offspring caregivers of cancer survivors found that adult daughters reported the highest levels of caregiving stress, whereas sons reported the lowest levels of caregiving stress.[56] Thus, gender and relationship type may be important to consider when examining cancer caregiving burden.

Raveis and colleagues[49,52] examined predictors of anxiety and depression symptoms among American women caring for a parent with cancer. These researchers found that caregivers' mean state anxiety score on the STAI was only slightly above the normative mean for working women,[18] although 31% of the caregivers scored at or above the 80th percentile of the normative sample scores.[52] Likewise, although the average depression score for caregivers was not exceptionally elevated, 30% of the sample reported scores that met the criteria for probable caseness of depression.[49] Caregivers with medical conditions, a greater sense of filial duty, and greater caregiving burden were found to have higher state anxiety and depressive symptoms.[49,52] Correlates of lower state anxiety and fewer depressive symptoms included having a positive outlook on the caregiving experience and performing a greater variety of caregiving tasks.[52]

Cultural differences in perceptions of the caregiving experience have yet to be elucidated because the vast majority of studies on caregiving have been conducted in Western cultures. In general, Western cultures place a greater emphasis on individualism, whereas Eastern cultures place greater emphasis on collectivism, such as the welfare of one's family (familism). One qualitative study of women who cared for relatives with cancer in India (30% daughters) found that religious beliefs and practices were associated with positive views of caregiving tasks and hope.[57] In addition, the family was frequently characterized as a source of emotional and instrumental support. A study of Korean caregivers of cancer patients (32% children) found that the majority of caregivers experienced severe financial difficulties and many made major life changes (e.g., altered educational plans).[58] Income loss and major life changes were associated with decrements in caregivers' quality of life. Taken together, research suggests that cultural and economic factors deserve further attention in the cancer caregiving literature.

COPING AND PERSONAL GROWTH

Parental cancer provides an important model for examining coping and adaptation to stressful circumstances. To date, research on parental cancer has yielded equivocal findings regarding the relation of coping strategies to adjustment outcomes. For example, both avoidance and engaged coping were associated with higher distress among American FDRs of breast cancer patients (45% daughters).[31] Another study found that problem-focused coping strategies were positively associated with anxiety among Norwegian women with *BRCA1* carrier status.[59] Conversely, emotion-focused strategies were positively associated with anxiety among Norwegian women who had a family history of breast/ovarian cancer in the absence of demonstrated mutations. A third study found that passive coping strategies (i.e., acceptance or denial of stressors) were positively correlated with cancer-related intrusive thoughts and avoidance among American women with family histories of breast cancer.[60] This relationship was not found among women without such family histories. Finally, a U.S. study of preadolescent, adolescent, and young adult children of cancer patients found that increasing age was related to higher levels of symptoms of anxiety and depression and the greater use of emotion-focused coping and avoidance.[27] Further research is needed to clarify the relations between coping and psychological adjustment to parental cancer within specific medical, cultural, and relational contexts.

Studies of coping and adaptation to parental cancer have rarely assessed personal growth and existential issues, despite their central importance when faced with suffering and potential loss. Indeed, the most commonly cited personal concern of adult children of newly diagnosed cancer patients was the search for life's meaning.[61] In studies of American female college students with parental cancer histories,[3] the vast majority (93.3%) indicated that cancer had caused at least one positive change in their lives, particularly in the interpersonal and existential domains. The majority (75%) of female caregivers of relatives with cancer in India also spontaneously reported positive personal changes related to their caregiving experience (e.g., acceptance, reprioritization of life issues).[57] A U.S. study found that the posttraumatic growth or positive

life changes of daughters of breast cancer survivors was comparable to that reported for breast cancer patients.[4] Posttraumatic growth was positively associated with social support, active and problem-focused coping and emotional processing strategies, and life satisfaction. In addition, caring for one's mother following her breast cancer diagnosis was associated with greater posttraumatic growth. The American Cancer Society Quality of Life Survey for Caregivers identified six domains of benefit finding in caregiving (i.e., acceptance, empathy, appreciation, family, positive self-view, and reprioritization).[62] Acceptance of circumstances and appreciating new relationships with others were associated with better adjustment, whereas becoming more empathic toward others and reprioritizing values was related to greater depressive symptoms. Clearly, further research is needed to identify aspects of benefit finding that promote or hinder adjustment to parental cancer.

DIRECTIONS FOR FUTURE RESEARCH

Methodological directions. Most investigations regarding adult children of cancer patients have been limited by a lack of comparison groups as well as a lack of longitudinal designs. In studies of adjustment without control groups, one cannot presume that the source of participants' emotional distress was their experiences related to parental cancer. Cross-sectional approaches do not firmly establish predictors of adjustment throughout the cancer experience. True prospective designs are needed to evaluate changes in the relations between contextual and individual difference variables and psychosocial outcomes from the time of the parent's cancer diagnosis, during adjuvant treatment, and during recovery. Adult children's responses to parental cancer relapse and their involvement in end-of-life caregiving and treatment decision-making also deserve further study.

The enormous diversity in adjustment to parental cancer has yet to be fully explored due to primarily homogeneous samples with regard to gender, race/ethnicity, and socioeconomic status. Researchers have mainly studied convenience samples of middle- and upper-class White women coping with maternal breast cancer. Indeed, the focus on female FDRs of cancer patients parallels the focus on female cancer patients in the psycho-oncological literature.[63] Meyerowitz and Hart[63] contend that the implicit assumption that "women feel and men act" (p. 67) still guides the research agenda. Although women's emotions are fully explored, the degree to which caring for a parent with cancer disrupts their educational and career development is largely unknown. Conversely, the feelings of men facing parental cancer are rarely studied; indeed, the unique experience of sons has been neglected in the psycho-oncological literature.

Few psychosocial interventions have been developed for adult daughters and sons of cancer patients. However, initial results of group interventions with FDRs of breast cancer patients[16,64] and information regarding their support needs[65] may guide the development of future interventions. To date, intervention trials with FDRs of breast cancer patients have primarily focused on coping skills for dealing with personal cancer risk.[16,64] Descriptive studies indicate that many FDRs of breast cancer patients want personalized information regarding their own breast cancer risk as well as measures to reduce this risk.[65] Thus, further development of lifestyle interventions and genetic counseling interventions for this population is warranted (see Parts II and IV of this book). In addition, many FDRs have expressed the need for information regarding methods of communicating with their children and other family members about their own breast cancer risk and their relative's experience with breast cancer.[65] The development of communication skills interventions would directly address this need. Finally, many FDRs want further information about ways to support their relative during her experience with breast cancer.[65] Examining the unmet needs of sons and daughters of patients with different types of cancer would inform intervention development.

Few psychosocial and behavioral interventions for cancer patients' caregivers have been developed and evaluated.[47] European group programs are primarily directed toward cancer patients and rarely include their relatives.[66] In Australia, the "Living with Cancer Education Programme" provides information and support to cancer patients and their family members and friends in eight weekly 2-hour sessions.[67,68] Participants reported high satisfaction with the program and significant improvement in coping abilities, knowledge, and communication. In the

U.S. literature, few interventions for family caregivers of cancer patients have been reported.[47] Intervention trials have primarily focused on spouse caregivers, and, thus, there is a need to develop interventions that are tailored to the needs and preferences of adult children caregivers.

Conceptual directions. Although research on adult children of cancer patients has generated useful descriptive data, a theoretical framework often has been lacking in the literature. Precipitants of psychological distress may be subsumed under conceptual frameworks, such as the stress, appraisal, and coping model.[69] In addition, an ecological or contextual perspective would provide a broader framework for elucidating the mechanisms underlying individual differences in adjustment.[70] Reciprocal and interdependent relationships between attributes of individuals and their social systems account for the marked variability in adaptational outcomes.[70] Contextual variables include the sociocultural context (e.g., age, gender, socioeconomic status), the interpersonal context (e.g., social networks), the situational context (e.g., stress), and the temporal context (e.g., disease stage).[70] Given the seemingly endless array of contextual factors, researchers may have to restrict their analysis to theoretically significant variables, such as the degree of social support provided by friends and family or interactions with the health care system.

A final conceptual issue to consider is that the majority of studies focus on symptoms of psychopathology without examining adult children's concomitant psychological strength in the face of a parent's life-threatening illness. Indeed, most individuals and their families achieve positive psychosocial outcomes as reflected in measures of affective distress, quality of life, and role competence.[71] Family members often report feeling closer to one another after gathering resources to fight cancer.[72,73] Furthermore, evidence suggests that the majority of mother–child relationships stay strong or grow stronger following breast cancer.[74] The strength and interdependency of the parent–child relationship during all phases of cancer merits greater research attention.

IMPLICATIONS FOR CLINICAL PRACTICE

Although adult children of cancer patients are an understudied population, results of descriptive studies and intervention trials provide some guidance with regard to their clinical care. First, when conducting a clinical interview, the extent to which parental cancer contributes to distress, lifestyle changes, or existential concerns should be assessed. Risk factors for distress should be noted during the interview, such as a parent's functional disability, cognitive impairment, or other unrelieved symptoms (e.g., pain, fatigue, depressive symptoms).[75] The duration and course of the parent's illness and the adult child's degree of involvement in emotional and instrumental caregiving tasks also should be noted. Multiple roles (e.g., employment, childcare, and parental care) may contribute to caregiving burden and distress.[2]

In addition to assessing the degree to which the parent's suffering and caregiving demands are affecting the adult child, it is important to evaluate whether feelings of personal vulnerability to cancer are heightened. These feelings may be associated with an extensive family history of cancer or a personal genetic predisposition to cancer. The extent to which the adult child engages in cancer screening and self-care (e.g., plant-based diet, exercise) and has a supportive social network should be assessed. Finally, cultural sensitivity will enhance the assessment and therapy process, especially if the adult child raises existential or spiritual concerns associated with parental cancer. A culturally competent clinician has an understanding of general cultural differences in spiritual beliefs, conceptualizations of illness and caregiving, doctor–patient communication, and health-related coping strategies while simultaneously recognizing the great diversity of experiences within each culture.

A comprehensive needs assessment and an understanding of the individual's cultural context should inform intervention strategies. First, practical concerns may need to be addressed, such as financial needs related to the parent's medical care, respite care, or finding time for exercise and other self-care. Training in assertive communication with professionals and/or family members may be necessary to address practical needs. Second, some individuals may need to cultivate relationships that allow for discussion of thoughts and feelings regarding parental cancer.

For young adults in particular, few of their peers may have experienced parental cancer, and, thus, different avenues for obtaining support may be needed (e.g., computer-based support). Emotional and existential concerns may be processed during counseling, and skills for communicating with others about the parent's cancer or personal cancer risk may be practiced during the sessions. Finally, some individuals may benefit from discussion of ways to reduce their parent's suffering. For example, individuals may delineate their role in the parent's symptom management or activities that they can continue to enjoy with the parent. Throughout the therapeutic process, the strengths of individuals coping with parental cancer (e.g., optimism, spiritual beliefs, bond with the ill parent) may be mobilized to effectively address existential and psychosocial challenges.

REFERENCES

1. Raveis VH, Pretter S. Existential plight of adult daughters following their mother's breast cancer diagnosis. *Psychooncology*. 2005;14(1):49–60.

2. Kim Y, Baker F, Spillers RL, Wellisch DK. Psychological adjustment of cancer caregivers with multiple roles. *Psychooncology*. 2006;15(9):795–804.

3. Leedham B, Meyerowitz BE. Responses to parental cancer: a clinical perspective. *J Clin Psychol Med Settings*. 1999;6(4):441–461.

4. Mosher CE, Danoff-Burg S, Brunker B. Post-traumatic growth and psychosocial adjustment of daughters of breast cancer survivors. *Oncol Nurs Forum*. 2006;33(3):543–551.

5. Office of Cancer Survivorship. *Estimated US cancer prevalence counts: who are our cancer survivors in the US?* National Cancer Institute; 2007. http://cancercontrol.cancer.gov/ocs/prevalence. Accessed September 22, 2008.

6. Valdimarsdottir H, Bovbjerg DH, Kash K, Holland JC, Osborne MP, Miller DG. Psychological distress in women with a familial risk of breast cancer. *Psychooncology*. 1995;4(2):133–141.

7. Mosher CE, Danoff-Burg S. Psychosocial impact of parental cancer in adulthood: a conceptual and empirical review. *Clin Psychol Rev*. 2005;25:365–382.

8. Wellisch DK, Gritz ER, Schain W, Wang H-J, Siau J. Psychological functioning of daughters of breast cancer patients. Part I: daughters and comparison subjects. *Psychosomatics*. 1991;32:324–336.

9. Wellisch DK, Gritz ER, Schain W, Wang H-J, Siau J. Psychological functioning of daughters of breast cancer patients. Part II: characterizing the distressed daughter of the breast cancer patient. *Psychosomatics*. 1992;33(2):171–179.

10. Erblich J, Bovbjerg DH, Valdimarsdottir HB. Looking forward and back: distress among women at familial risk for breast cancer. *Ann Behav Med*. 2000;22(1):53–59.

11. Baider L, Ever-Hadani P, Kaplan De-Nour A. Psychological distress in healthy women with familial breast cancer: like mother, like daughter? *Int J Psychiatry Med*. 1999;29(4):411–420.

12. Zapka J, Fisher G, Lemon S, Clemow L, Fletcher K. Relationship and distress in relatives of breast cancer patients. *Fam Syst Health*. 2006;24(2):198–212.

13. Derogatis LL, Spencer PM. *Administration and procedures: BSI manual: I*. Baltimore, MD: Clinical Psychometric Research; 1982.

14. Kash K, Holland JC, Halper MS, Miller DG. Psychological distress and surveillance behaviors of women with a family history of breast cancer. *J Natl Cancer Inst*. 1992;84:24–30.

15. Lindberg NM, Wellisch DK. Identification of traumatic stress reactions in women at increased risk for breast cancer. *Psychosomatics*. 2004;45(1):7–16.

16. Schwartz MD, Lerman C, Audrain J, et al. The impact of a brief problem-solving training intervention for relatives of recently diagnosed breast cancer patients. *Ann Behav Med*. 1998;20(1):7–12.

17. Radloff LS. The CES-D scale: A self-report depression scale for research in the general population. *Appl Psychol Meas*. 1977;1:385–401.

18. Spielberger CD. *State-trait anxiety inventory: STAI (Form Y)*. Redwood City, CA: Mind Garden; 1983.

19. Meiser B, Butow P, Schnieden V, et al. Psychological adjustment of women at increased risk of developing hereditary breast cancer. *Psychol Health Med*. 2000;5(4):377–388.

20. Lerman C, Daly M, Sands C, et al. Mammography adherence and psychological distress among women at risk for breast cancer. *J Natl Cancer Inst*. 1993;85(13):1074–1080.

21. Lerman C, Kash K, Stefanek M. Younger women at increased risk for breast cancer: perceived risk, psychological well-being, and surveillance behavior. *J Natl Cancer Inst Monogr*. 1994(16):171–176.

22. Zakowski SG, Valdimarsdottir HB, Bovbjerg DH, et al. Predictors of intrusive thoughts and avoidance in women with family histories of breast cancer. *Ann Behav Med*. 1997;19(4):362–369.

23. Coyne JC, Benazon NR, Gaba CG, Calzone K, Weber BL. Distress and psychiatric morbidity among women from high-risk breast and ovarian cancer families. *J Consult Clin Psychol.* 2000;68(5):864–874.

24. Butow P, Meiser B, Price M, et al. Psychological morbidity in women at increased risk of developing breast cancer: a controlled study. *Psychooncology.* 2005;14(3):196–203.

25. Rees G, Fry A, Cull A, Sutton S. Illness perceptions and distress in women at increased risk of breast cancer. *Psychol Health.* 2004;19(6):749–765.

26. Compas BE, Worsham NL, Epping-Jordan JE, et al. When mom or dad has cancer: Markers of psychological distress in cancer patients, spouses, and children. *Health Psychol.* 1994;13(6):507–515.

27. Compas BE, Worsham NL, Ey S, Howell DC. When mom or dad has cancer: II. Coping, cognitive appraisals, and psychological distress in children of cancer patients. *Health Psychol.* 1996;15(3):167–175.

28. Wellisch DK, Lindberg NM. A psychological profile of depressed and nondepressed women at high risk for breast cancer. *Psychosomatics.* 2001;42(4):330–336.

29. Cohen M, Pollack S. Mothers with breast cancer and their adult daughters: the relationship between mothers' reaction to breast cancer and their daughters' emotional and neuroimmune status. *Psychosom Med.* 2005;67(1):64–71.

30. Kim Y, Wellisch DK, Spillers RL. Effects of psychological distress on quality of life of adult daughters and their mothers with cancer. *Psychooncology.* 2008;17(11):1129–1136.

31. Fletcher KE, Clemow L, Peterson BA, Lemon SC, Estabrook B, Zapka JG. A path analysis of factors associated with distress among first-degree female relatives of women with breast cancer diagnosis. *Health Psychol.* 2006;25(3):413–424.

32. American Psychiatric Association. *Diagnostic and statistical manual of mental disorders.* 4th ed. Washington, DC: Author; 1994.

33. Frederick C. Psychic trauma in victims of crime and terrorism. In: Van den Bos GR, Bryant BK, (eds). *Cataclysms, crises, and catastrophes.* Washington, DC: American Psychological Association; 1987:65–68.

34. Pynoos RS, Frederick C, Nader K, Arroyo W, et al. Life threat and posttraumatic stress in school-age children. *Arch Gen Psychiatry.* 1987;44(12):1057–1063.

35. Boyer BA, Bubel D, Jacobs SR, Knolls, ML, Harwell, VD, Goscicka M. Posttraumatic stress in women with breast cancer and their daughters. *Am J Fam Ther.* 2002;30(4):323–338.

36. Horowitz M, Wilner N, Alvarez W. Impact of Event Scale: a measure of subjective stress. *Psychosom Med.* 1979;41(3):209–218.

37. Weiss D, Marmar CR. The impact of event scale—revised. In: Wilson JP, Keane TM, (eds). *Assessing psychological trauma and PTSD: A practitioner's handbook.* New York: Guilford; 1997:399–411.

38. Huizinga GA, Visser A, van der Graaf WTA, et al. Stress response symptoms in adolescent and young adult children of parents diagnosed with cancer. *Eur J Cancer.* 2005;41(2):288–295.

39. Hamann HA, Somers TJ, Smith AW, Inslicht SS, Baum A. Posttraumatic stress associated with cancer history and BRCA1/2 genetic testing. *Psychosom Med.* 2005;67(5):766–772.

40. Schwartz M, Lerman C, Daly M, Audrain J, Masny A, Griffith K. Utilization of ovarian cancer screening by women at increased risk. *Cancer Epidemiol Biomarkers Prev.* 1995;4(3):269–273.

41. Schnur JB, Valdimarsdottir HB, Montgomery GH, Nevid JS, Bovbjerg DH. Social constraints and distress among women at familial risk for breast cancer. *Ann Behav Med.* 2004;28(2):142–148.

42. Ferrell BR. The family. In: Doyle D, Hanks GWC, MacDonald N, (eds). *Oxford textbook of palliative medicine.* 2nd ed. New York: Oxford University Press; 1998:909–917.

43. Blanchard CG, Albrecht TL, Ruckdeschel JC. The crisis of cancer: psychological impact on family caregivers. *Oncology.* 1997;11:189–194.

44. Kurtz ME, Kurtz JC, Given CW, Given B. Relationship of caregiver reactions and depression to cancer patients' symptoms, functional states and depression—a longitudinal view. *Soc Sci Med.* 1995;40(6):837–846.

45. Given CW, Stommel M, Given B, Osuch J, Kurtz ME, Kurtz JC. The influence of cancer patients' symptoms and functional states on patients' depression and family caregivers' reaction and depression. *Health Psychol.* 1993;12(4):277–285.

46. Porter LS, Keefe FJ, McBride CM, Pollak K, Fish L, Garst J. Perceptions of patients' self-efficacy for managing pain and lung cancer symptoms: correspondence between patients and family caregivers. *Pain.* 2002;98:169–178.

47. Kim Y, Given BA. Quality of life of family caregivers of cancer survivors. *Cancer.* 2008;112(Suppl 11):2556–2568.

48. Brody EM. "Women in the middle" and family help to older people. *Gerontologist.* 1981;21:471–480.

49. Raveis VH, Karus DG, Siegel K. Correlates of depressive symptomatology among adult daughter caregivers of a parent with cancer. *Cancer.* 1998;83:1652–1663.

50. Stephens MAP, Townsend AL, Martire LM, Druley JA. Balancing parent care with other roles: interrole conflict of adult daughter caregivers. *J Gerontol B Psychol Sci Soc Sci.* 2001;56(1):P24-P34.

51. Enright RB, Friss L. *Employed caregivers of brain-impaired adults: An assessment of the dual role.* San Francisco: Gerontological Society of America; 1987.

52. Raveis VH, Karus D, Pretter S. Correlates of anxiety among adult daughter caregivers to a parent with cancer. *J Psychsoc Oncol.* 1999;17(3–4):1–26.

53. Johnson CL, Catalano DJ. A longitudinal study of family supports to impaired elderly. *Gerontologist.* 1983;23:612–618.

54. Lowenstein A, Gilbar O. The perception of caregiving burden on the part of elderly cancer patients, spouses and adult children. *Fam Syst Health.* 2000;18(3):337–346.

55. Hoyert DL, Seltzer MM. Factors related to the well-being and life activities of family caregivers. *Fam Relat.* 1992;41(1):74–81.

56. Kim Y, Baker F, Spillers RL. Cancer caregivers' quality of life: effects of gender, relationship, and appraisal. *J Pain Symptom Manage.* 2007;34(3):294–304.

57. Mehrotra S, Sukumar P. Sources of strength perceived by females caring for relatives diagnosed with cancer: an exploratory study from India. *Support Care Cancer.* 2007;15:1357–1366.

58. Yun YH, Rhee YS, Kang IO, et al. Economic burdens and quality of life of family caregivers of cancer patients. *Oncology.* 2005;68:107–114.

59. Geirdal AO, Dahl AA. The relationship between coping strategies and anxiety in women from families with familial breast-ovarian cancer in the absence of demonstrated mutations. *Psychooncology.* 2008;17(1):49–57.

60. Kim Y, Valdimarsdottir HB, Bovbjerg DH. Family histories of breast cancer, coping styles, and psychological adjustment. *J Behav Med.* 2003;26(3):225–243.

61. Germino BB. Family members' concerns after cancer diagnosis. Unpublished doctoral dissertation. Seattle, WA: University of Washington; 1984.

62. Kim Y, Schulz R, Carver CS. Benefit finding in the cancer caregiving experience. *Psychosom Med.* 2007;69(3):283–291.

63. Meyerowitz BE, Hart S. Women and cancer: have assumptions about women limited our research agenda? In: Stanton AL, Gallant SJ, (eds). *The psychology of women's health: Progress and challenges in research and application.* 1st ed. Washington, DC: American Psychological Association; 1995:51–84.

64. Wellisch DK, Hoffman A, Goldman S, Hammerstein J, Klein K, Bell M. Depression and anxiety symptoms in women at high risk for breast cancer: pilot study of a group intervention. *Am J Psychiatry.* 1999;156(10):1644–1645.

65. Chalmers K, Marles S, Tataryn D, Scott-Findlay S, Serfas K. Reports of information and support needs of daughters and sisters of women with breast cancer. *Eur J Cancer Care (Engl).* 2003;12(1):81–90.

66. Kotkamp-Mothes N, Slawinsky D, Hindermann S, Strauss B. Coping and psychological well being in families of elderly cancer patients. *Crit Rev Oncol Hematol.* 2005;55(3):213–229.

67. Todd K, Roberts S, Black C. The Living with Cancer Education Programme. I. Development of an Australian education and support programme for cancer patients and their family and friends. *Eur J Cancer Care (Engl).* 2002;11(4):271–279.

68. Roberts S, Black C, Todd K. The living with cancer education programme. II. Evaluation of an Australian education and support programme for cancer patients and their family and friends. *Eur J Cancer Care (Engl).* 2002;11(4):280–289.

69. Lazarus RS, Folkman S. *Stress, appraisal, and coping.* New York: Springer; 1984.

70. Revenson TA. All other things are not equal: an ecological approach to personality and disease. In: Friedman HS, (ed). *Personality and disease.* New York: John Wiley & Sons; 1990:65–94.

71. Compas BE, Harding A. Competence across the lifespan: lessons from coping with cancer. In: Pushkar D, Bukowski WM, Schwartzman AE, Stack DM, White DR, (eds). *Improving competence across the lifespan: building interventions based on theory and research.* New York: Plenum Press; 1998:9–26.

72. Lewis FM, Woods NF, Hough EE, Bensley LS. The family's functioning with chronic illness in the mother: the spouse's perspective. *Soc Sci Med.* 1989;29(11):1261–1269.

73. Taylor SE, Brown JD. Illusion and well-being: a social psychological perspective on mental health. *Psychol Bull.* 1988;103(2):193–210.

74. Lichtman RR, Taylor SE, Wood JV, Bluming AZ, Dosik GM, Leibowitz RL. Relations with children after breast cancer: the mother-daughter relationship at risk. *J Psychsoc Oncol.* 1985;2:1–19.

75. Given B, Sherwood P. Family care for the older person with cancer. *Semin Oncol Nurs.* 2006;22(1):43–50.

CHAPTER 76

Bereavement: A Special Issue in Oncology

Wendy G. Lichtenthal, Holly G. Prigerson, and David W. Kissane

INTRODUCTION

According to the World Health Organization (WHO),[1] 7.6 million patients died of cancer in 2005. On the basis of the estimate that each patient leaves four survivors behind,[2] approximately 30.4 million individuals were bereaved because of cancer that year. Professionals in psycho-oncology witness grief that begins with the many losses cancer patients suffer before their death, including loss of physical capacity, important personal roles and activities, significant relationships, and some future plans. Providers are also able to provide continuity of care from pre- to postbereavement because of the trusting relationships they form with the patient and family during the illness.

Practitioners who take a family-centered approach can enhance the quality of life of the patient and the family during palliative care and position themselves to facilitate bereavement care.[3] Specifically, clinicians can help the family understand the dying process, which may provide comfort and some sense of predictability. Psycho-oncology clinicians need to understand risk factors for morbid outcomes, be comfortable with the multiple presentations of grief, and be able to manage such expressions or to make appropriate referrals when risk factors are apparent or clinical intervention seems necessary.

Many terms are used, often interchangeably, to indicate reactions to loss. The following are definitions that grief theorists maintain in the literature:

- *Bereavement* is an event; the **state** of loss resulting from death.[4,5]
- *Grief* is the distressing **emotional response** to any loss, including related feelings, cognitions, and behaviors.[4]
- *Mourning* is the **process of adaptation**, which includes culturally, religious, and socially influenced behaviors, such as grieving rituals.[6]
- *Anticipatory grief* is the **distress** and related emotions, cognitions, and behaviors, that occur before an expected loss.[6]
- *Pathological grief* is a severely distressing and disabling **abnormal emotional response** to loss that involves mental and/or physical dysfunction.[2,7,8]
- *Disenfranchised grief* is kept hidden, typically among individuals who have less social permission to express their response.[9]

We begin this chapter with a brief overview of influential theoretical models of grief that have contributed to our understanding of the ways in which grief presents clinically. Descriptions of grief phenomena follow, organized chronologically from palliative care to bereavement, including the impact of loss on children. We then discuss pathological reactions to bereavement, such as prolonged grief disorder (PGD), and related risk factors. Finally, various grief interventions are discussed, including broad descriptions, indications, and, when available, research examining their efficacy.

THEORETICAL MODELS OF GRIEF

An understanding of general bereavement theories can assist staff with comprehending observed behaviors and with making appropriate referrals when necessary. These models suggest adaptive tasks as well as potential preventive strategies and interventions (see references 4 and 7 for summaries).

Initiatives to develop a neurobiopsychosocial model of grief have been advanced through use of technology such as functional magnetic resonance imaging (fMRI).[10] For example, a recent fMRI study found increased activity in the posterior cingulate cortex, a brain region believed to be involved in retrieval of emotion-laden episodic memories, during a grief arousal task.[11]

Attachment theory has been among the most influential frameworks in the bereavement field. With a focus on interpersonal bonding, this theory posits that children instinctually attach to their caregivers, seeking safety and security to promote their survival, and internalize working models of these early attachments.[12] Researchers distinguish secure from insecure attachment styles, which may be anxious, avoidant, or disorganized/hostile, among infants.[13] Those with more insecure attachment styles are at increased risk for separation distress and prolonged grief reactions.[2,14]

Psychodynamic theories also consider the influence of early relationships.[7] For example, object relations theorists view these relationships, beginning with the initial separation between infant and mother, as models that influence emotional reactions to separations. Yearning for the lost object is considered an adaptive response to the initial and subsequent separations, including bereavement. Freud argued that adaptation to bereavement occurs via "grief work," which involves processing one's emotions to sever the bond to the deceased.[4,7] He proposed that pathological mourning occurred when individuals were ambivalent about their loss.[15]

Interpersonal theories focus on the way interaction patterns and roles shape identity and self schemas, influencing how individuals grieve.[15] For example, in his treatment for stress-response syndromes, Horowitz[16] described how person schemas related to deceased individuals (e.g., an "ambivalent" schema) can be identified and modified as they emerge in current relationships.

Several models consider the cognitive processes involved in adaptation to loss.[5,17] Parkes[5] proposed that alteration of one's assumptions about the way in which the world works was key to adjustment (e.g., accommodating the inevitability of death into one's "assumptive world"[5,18]). Neimeyer[19] described a related adaptive task, "meaning reconstruction," which involves individuals making sense of and finding meaning in the loss by developing a coherent narrative about how the loss fits into their lives. In cognitive stress theory, cognitive appraisals of a situation determine how stressful an event is perceived to be, influencing coping strategies and the related physiological impact.[7,20] Making meaning of adverse life events such as bereavement can result in positive emotions, which can improve or maintain physical health and, according to a social-functional viewpoint, yield interpersonal benefits.[4,7,20]

Sociological models consider the influence of society on individual mourning, including culture-specific rituals (e.g., self-mutilation). Some cultures support continuing rather than severing bonds through speaking to the deceased or seeking spiritual guidance from deceased ancestors.[21] Social constructionists propose that culture and social norms powerfully shape the content of expressions of grief as well as the extent to which public and private grieving practices are sanctioned.[22] Social support of the bereaved serves to reduce isolation and buffer additional stressors. Family systems theory considers the reciprocal influences individual members of a bereaved family have on one another.[3] Grief responses often greatly depend on the role of the deceased individual and the family's level of functioning before the loss.[3]

Cognitive-behavioral theory focuses on the relationship between emotions, thoughts, and behaviors related to grieving, particularly those that are maladaptive and play a role in prolonged or severe grief responses.[7,23,24] Distorted cognitions (e.g., unrealistic thoughts that one should have done more to care for the deceased) and associated feelings (e.g., guilt) can result in unhelpful ruminations about the deceased. Avoidance becomes negatively reinforcing, and may prolong the course of grief by reducing opportunities for processing the loss as well as for pleasurable, corrective experiences.[24]

A widely accepted contemporary theory is Stroebe and Schut's[25] dual process model of coping, which posits that adaptive coping involves engagement in both loss-orientation and restoration-orientation tasks.[7] Loss-oriented thoughts, emotions, and behaviors focus on the deceased and confronting the reality of the loss. Restoration-oriented activities reflect assimilation in the world in the absence of the deceased. Central to this model is the hypothesis that oscillation between loss-oriented and restoration-oriented phases permits the person to actively confront their grief for a time and then take respite as they make efforts to reengage in life.[4,7] The dual process model suggests clear prescriptions for adaptive coping, and psychotherapeutic grief interventions have incorporated it into their theoretical rationales.[23,26]

CLINICAL PRESENTATIONS OF GRIEF

Clinicians in oncology may witness grieving in numerous contexts, including anticipatory grieving as illness progresses, acute grief at the time of death, and in some cases, prolonged grieving that does not abate with time.

Anticipatory grief. A feature of grief among survivors of deceased cancer patients is that it begins well before the death. From the time of diagnosis, the patient and family often recognize that the malignancy may be fatal.[6] Cognitive and emotional acceptance is a dynamic process, waxing and waning as acknowledgment of the prognostic reality competes with a desire to maintain hope for a cure. Loved ones may present with unrealistic optimism, protest, anger, or heightened protectiveness of the patient.

More intense anticipatory grieving may be observed when bad news or serious disease progression is communicated to the patient. Sensitive communication can assist the family in processing this information and in coping. Families may grow closer and more cohesive as they adapt to the multiple losses associated with advanced illness. They have the opportunity to express their attachment through acts of caregiving and may make attempts to resolve relationship issues. However, members in more dysfunctional families may react with denial, hostility, avoidance, or other maladaptive behaviors, resulting in tension and conflict.

While some theorists have suggested that the presence of anticipatory grief diminishes the intensity of postloss grief, studies in this area have yielded inconsistent findings. In fact, intense anticipatory grief may be a risk factor for morbid outcome.[27] As illness progresses, providers can encourage open communication and opportunities to say goodbye, allowing patients and families to address unfinished business and express appreciation for one another.[28]

Grief around the time of death. When the family is at the patient's bedside at the time of death, they are often emotional and exceptionally attentive to details related to the patient's well-being. Vivid memories of these moments can remain with survivors long after the patient's death, necessitating that clinicians exhibit the utmost respect and sensitivity. Practitioners are key providers of reassurance about the patient's comfort and of information about the dying process, including the meaning of sounds, secretions, and changes in breathing patterns and levels of consciousness.

Family members who are not present should be contacted by staff when the patient's condition begins to deteriorate and death appears imminent. If the death occurs before the family can be reached, relatives should be offered an opportunity to view the body, and given information about the sequence of events leading up to the death. Staff should respect and honor cultural and religious practices, including those related to autopsy, time alone with the patient, and pastoral counseling. Culture may influence expressions of acute grief, and clinicians could consult with a cultural intermediary to ensure they respond sensitively to a family's practices and needs. Efforts should be made to prevent

disenfranchised grief,[9] and so expected deaths should not be minimized. Families greatly appreciate clinicians communicating their sympathy through a phone call or other personal means. Other types of support include prescription of anxiolytics or sleep aids, referrals for psychosocial services, and direction about making funeral arrangements.

Acute grief following the death. The course of grief is variable and may be expressed in very different ways, even within a given family system. Emotions are often intensely distressing following the loss, making it difficult to distinguish between "normal" and pathological responses during the first months of bereavement. The course of adaptive grief has characteristic emotions, cognitions, behaviors, and physical symptoms. Emotions that come and go in waves include sadness, guilt, anger, despair, and anxiety.[5,7] Individuals often initially experience a profound sense of yearning for the lost individual. Survivors of patients who were intensely suffering may experience a sense of relief in parallel with their sadness. Thoughts during the acute phase of grief range from deliberate reminiscing about the deceased to unbidden, intrusive images and memories. Behaviors include searching for the deceased, social withdrawal, or alternatively seeking support and comfort. Physical symptoms include difficulty sleeping, fatigue, anorexia, mild weight loss, numbness, restlessness, tension, tremors, and sometimes pain.

Early theorists proposed that there were consecutive stages of "normal" or adaptive grief that individuals need to pass through to achieve acceptance of the loss, including shock, yearning, angry protest, sad or depressed mood, and finally, recovery from the loss.[29,30] This trajectory, widely accepted in the field for years, is illustrated in the top panel

Hypothesized grief resolution (as illustrated in Jacobs, 1993)*

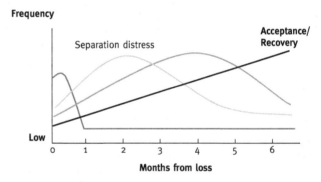

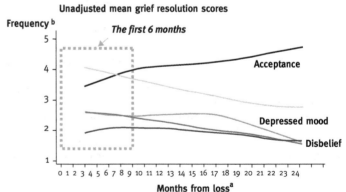

a: All of the lines start from 2 months after loss and end at 24 months
b: 1= Less than once a month; 2= Monthly; 3= Weekly; 4=Daily;
    5= Several times a day except for indicator of "depressed mood"

Fig. 76–1. Proposed grief resolution model and observed grief symptoms over time.

SOURCE: Reprinted from Jacobs SC, "Diagram of the dimensions of grief." *Pathologic grief: maladaptation to loss*, 1993. With permission from the American Psychiatric Association.

of Fig. 76–1. While the stage theory has not been subjected to explicit empirical testing, grief indicators among bereaved community-based participants in the Yale Bereavement Study demonstrated that yearning was the predominant initial reaction, rather than shock and disbelief, as previously conjectured.[31] See the bottom panel of Fig. 76–1. Participants were assessed between 2 and 24 months from their loss, and it is possible that shock or other symptoms were elevated during the first 2 months, but not captured. Declines in shock, yearning, and sad mood and an increase in acceptance were observed over the 22-month study period, while anger generally remained low and relatively stable.[31] Rescaling these grief indicators and comparing their respective peak frequencies during the first 6 months of loss revealed a sequence similar to the order of stages proposed by past bereavement theorists.[5,30]

The commonly held contemporary perspective is that stages of grief overlap, intense emotions may wax and wane in the early phases of bereavement, bonds to the deceased individual may continue, and grief may be experienced intermittently throughout one's life.[7] Adaptive coping is widely believed to follow the dual process model of coping, with an oscillation between confrontation of the loss, including processing related emotions, and reengagement in life without the deceased.[25] The intensity and duration of grieving is largely related to the strength and degree of security of the attachment. No firm timelines for adaptation have been established, but cultural sanctions may influence the duration of expressions of grief.[9]

While grieving may not completely "resolve," 80%–90% of bereaved individuals have come to accept the death of their loved one by 6 months postdeath.[2] In other words, the majority of individuals are able to *adapt* to the loss as indicated by their ability to acknowledge the loss and transform their relationship to the deceased; to reengage in work, leisure, and creative activities; to maintain and develop personal relationships; and to consider their lives and the future as potentially meaningful and satisfying.[2] They may continue to grieve throughout their lives, when activated by reminders of the deceased or anniversaries, but their reactions will gradually become less intense and will be briefer in duration. Recent investigations have demonstrated that resilience following bereavement is common.[4,7,32]

Pathological responses to bereavement

Bereavement-related psychopathology. In the acute phase of grief, intense distress, and waves of sadness and anxiety are typical and expected. For a subset of individuals, however, the stress of bereavement interacts with existing vulnerabilities, resulting in pervasive, persistent depressed mood, or the exacerbation of premorbid psychiatric conditions. Given that sadness is so common during the first 2 months of bereavement, the diagnosis of a clinical depression is dependent on features such as profound loss of interest, pervasive sadness, psychomotor retardation, deep guilt, worthlessness, hopelessness/helplessness, loss of meaning, and suicidal ideation. Neurovegetative features of depression are less discriminatory.

Bereaved individuals may also meet criteria for anxiety disorders, presenting with symptoms of separation anxiety, panic disorder, generalized anxiety, phobias, and/or somatization disorders. They may exhibit symptoms of post-traumatic stress disorder (PTSD) when circumstances of the death are perceived as traumatic, involving, for example, gross disfigurement, weeping bedsores, foul odors, or agitated delirium. In addition, those who have a history of substance, bipolar, or psychotic disorders are at heightened risk of relapse. According to the rules of *DSM-IV-TR*,[33] adjustment disorder diagnoses should be deferred if the clinical symptoms are due to the stress of bereavement.

Prolonged grief disorder. While grief diminishes in its intensity among the majority of bereaved individuals, approximately 10%–20% exhibit a more prolonged and severe grief response.[2] These people may appear "stuck" in their grief, experiencing intense pining and yearning for the lost individual, with distressing ruminations and intrusive thoughts about the absence of the deceased, a struggle to find meaning in their lives without their loved one, and difficulty accepting the

reality of the loss and moving forward.[2] To help clinically recognize these individuals, researchers have empirically identified a cluster of characteristic symptoms. PGD is distinct from bereavement-related depression and anxiety.[2] Although PGD may be co-morbid with depression or anxiety, symptoms of PGD, such as intense longing for the deceased, disbelief about the death, and feeling that life lacks meaning without the deceased, can be clinically distinguished from symptoms of depression, such as depressed mood, psychomotor retardation, and changes in appetite or weight.[2,34] In a study of PGD, PTSD, and major depressive disorder among recent widows, PGD was identified as the most prevalent disorder with the lowest co-morbidity rate.[35] Formerly referred to as both complicated grief and traumatic grief, PGD may emerge in response to losses involving either traumatic or nontraumatic circumstances. It has been associated with increased risk of negative mental and physical health outcomes, including cancer, hypertension, cardiac events, adverse health behaviors, hospitalization, depressive symptoms, functional impairment, and suicidal ideation.[2]

Several terms and subtypes have been used to describe grief pathology in the bereavement literature, such as *chronic grief, inhibited grief,* and *delayed grief.*[5,7] While bereavement experts have historically acknowledged and described pathological grief responses, there continues to be debate about whether symptoms of PGD constitute a distinct mental disorder.[2] "Normal" and abnormal grief responses are believed to fall on the same continuum. Pathological symptoms are intensified and prolonged manifestations of acute grief symptoms. On the basis of the growing empirical evidence suggesting the clinical and research utility of standardizing diagnostic criteria, bereavement experts have proposed that PGD be established as a distinct mental disorder in the next edition of *Diagnostic and statistical manual of mental disorders*[36] (i.e., *DSM-V*).[2,4,34] The proposed diagnostic criteria[2] are presented in Fig. 76–2. The criterion stating that the diagnosis should not be made until at least 6 months have elapsed since the death was developed to clinically identify those individuals whose grief appears to be persisting and who might benefit from intervention, while remaining conservative and not being overly inclusive of those individuals whose grief will resolve naturally with time.[2] The onset of symptoms typically occurs at the time of death, but delayed and chronic grief can also meet the 6-month timing criterion.

Risk factors. Most individuals who suffer a loss gradually adapt without need for psychosocial interventions. Because resources are limited, it is important to triage those at heightened risk to clinical service. Staff should hold a regular multidisciplinary death review to identify family members at risk for psychopathology.[3,7] Individuals at risk for psychiatric disorders in general are also vulnerable to onset or recurrence during bereavement. Risk factors for negative bereavement outcomes are shown in Table 76–1. Studies of the etiology of PGD have demonstrated the key role of early disturbances in secure attachment, including insecure attachment styles; high-marital dependency and close, security-enhancing relationships; close kinship relationship to the deceased; and childhood separation anxiety.[2,14,37] Heightened risk for PGD has also been observed among African-Americans, those who perceived themselves as less prepared for the loss, and those with reduced social support.[2,38]

SPECIFIC CIRCUMSTANCES

Sudden death. Even when the course of illness is protracted, deaths may be perceived as unexpected and sudden by the family. This may be due to expectations about the amount of time they had left with the patient based on the prognosis given. Unexpected deaths can be due to secondary conditions, including sepsis, pulmonary emboli, cardiac events, or hemorrhage. Individuals who perceive themselves as psychologically unprepared for the loss are at greater risk for PGD and depression, particularly when the death is perceived as violent.[2,4,38] Clinicians should assess family members' understanding of the circumstances surrounding the death and help the bereaved make sense of any aspects that were perplexing.

A: Event Criterion: Bereavement (loss of a significant other)

B: Separation Distress: The bereaved person experiences yearning (e.g., craving, pining, or longing for the deceased; physical or emotional suffering as a result of the desired, but unfulfilled, reunion with the deceased) daily or to a disabling degree.

C: Cognitive, Emotional, and Behavioral Symptoms: The bereaved person must have 5 (or more) of the following symptoms experienced daily or to a disabling degree:

1. Confusion about one's role in life or diminished sense of self (i.e., feeling that a part of oneself has died)
2. Difficulty accepting the loss
3. Avoidance of reminders of the reality of the loss
4. Inability to trust others since the loss
5. Bitterness or anger related to the loss
6. Difficulty moving on with life (e.g., making new friends, pursuing interests)
7. Numbness (absence of emotion) since the loss
8. Feeling that life is unfulfilling, empty, and meaningless since the loss
9. Feeling stunned, dazed, or shocked by loss

D: Timing: Diagnosis should not be made until at least six months have elapsed since the death.

E: Impairment: The disturbance causes clinically significant impairment in social, occupational, or other important areas of functioning (e.g., domestic responsibilities).

F: Relation to Other Mental Disorders: The disturbance is not better accounted for by major depressive disorder, generalized anxiety disorder, or posttraumatic stress disorder.

NOTE: Proposed diagnostic criteria for PGD outlined by Prigerson et al.[2]

Fig. 76-2. Proposed diagnostic criteria for prolonged grief disorder.

Table 76-1. Risk factors for pathological grief outcomes

Category	Description
Circumstances of death	Perceived preparedness for loss
	Untimely within the life cycle (e.g., death of child)
	Sudden and unexpected (e.g., death from septic neutropenia during chemotherapy)
	Traumatic (e.g., shocking cachexia and debility)
	Stigmatized (e.g., AIDS or suicide)
Personal vulnerability	History of psychiatric disorder (e.g., clinical depression, separation anxiety)
	Childhood adversity (e.g., abuse, neglect, controlling parenting)
	Personality and coping style (e.g., intense worrier, low self-esteem)
	Attachment style (e.g., insecure)
	Cumulative experience of losses
Nature of the relationship with the deceased	Overly dependent (e.g., security-enhancing relationship)
	Ambivalent (e.g., angry and insecure with alcohol abuse, infidelity, gambling)
Family and social support	Family dysfunction (e.g., poor cohesion and communication, high conflict)
	Isolated (e.g., new migrant, new residential move)
	Alienated (e.g., perception of low social support)

ABBREVIATION: AIDS, acquired immunodeficiency syndrome.

Grief during childhood. A child's ability to understand the permanency of death and to express their grief varies according to developmental stage.[6,7] The capacity for abstract thinking develops around ages 8–10. Open, age-appropriate discussion of the loss and support from surviving family and caregivers promotes adaptive grieving. Other strategies that clinicians may suggest include participation in mourning rituals, facilitation of emotional expression through, for example, physical activities, and construction of a memory book to preserve the child's bond to the deceased.[6,7]

Loss of a child. Parents who suffer the loss of a child have potentially the most profound grief reactions.[7,37] Losing a child to cancer often occurs after a lengthy battle with the illness. When caregiving for the child has long been the priority, parents may become disconnected from relationships and roles that were previously meaningful. The intense pain of acute grief often deepens the sense of isolation. Parents may find solace in connecting with other bereaved parents through support groups. They may need additional assistance coping with guilt related to concerns that they could have done more to prevent the death. Finding ways to honor and memorialize their child's life may help parents to move forward, and so staff should facilitate this when possible.

INTERVENTIONS

Grief intervention research in recent decades has yielded inconsistent findings, likely due to variations in the populations targeted and other aspects of methodology. To determine which individuals might benefit from psychotherapy and counseling, several systematic reviews and meta-analyses of grief interventions have been conducted.[39–42] These studies are summarized in Table 76-2. Grief interventions have not generally been effective, yielding small to moderate effects (as compared to the larger effects observed in meta-analyses of psychotherapy in general). A debate about how these findings should be interpreted has risen in the field, with some proposing that the majority of individuals do not require interventions because their symptoms dissipate naturally,[42,43] whereas others advocate cautious optimism about the utility of grief counseling.[44] Amid the variable findings, the result that is consistent is that treatments targeting high risk or symptomatic individuals demonstrate stronger effects.[42]

Staff support. Families have expressed that continuity of care is greatly appreciated. Efforts to follow-up with bereaved families after the patient's death, by offering condolences over the telephone, through a sympathy card or personal visits, by attending the funeral, or by conducting annual commemoration services are generally welcome when close relationships have been formed.

Individual psychotherapy

Supportive counseling. Interventions in which support is offered generally facilitate an adaptive grieving process.[17] They permit a venue for emotional expression and discussion of the loss, as well as a safe place to consider actions related to moving forward with life. Counselors help to promote adaptive coping.

Psychodynamic and interpersonal psychotherapies. Psychodynamic interventions are typically longer term and focus on events from childhood and internalized object relations that may be influencing the patient's unconscious conflicts and current related grief response. Empirical studies of this type of approach are generally lacking, although supportive-expressive approaches have been examined in a variety of populations, including individuals with depression.[45] Individuals who struggle with unresolved issues influenced by early relationships and conflicts, including those related to attachment security, might benefit from a psychodynamic approach.

Interpersonal psychotherapy (IPT) is a short-term (12–16 weeks) manualized treatment that is based in part on psychodynamic theory.

Table 76-2. Systematic reviews and meta-analyses of bereavement interventions

Authors	No. of studies	Study selection	Effect size	Possible conclusions
Currier, Neimeyer and Berman[42]	61	Randomized and non-randomized studies No-intervention control group Participants did not choose study condition 48 peer-reviewed articles and 16 dissertations	0.16[a]	Generally all participants (intervention and control) improved over time Clinical and self-referrals associated with better outcomes, though differences diminished at follow-up Age/sex of participants and timing of intervention did not appear to impact effects
Currier, Holland and Neimeyer[41]	13	Controlled studies of interventions for children	0.14	Lack of support for efficacy of interventions Earlier intervention yielded stronger effects Targeting distress associated with better outcomes
Allumbaugh and Hoyt[39]	35	Controlled and noncontrolled	0.43	Effects stronger for self-identified participants Low statistical power Moderating variables impact effects
Kato and Mann[40]	13	Randomized controlled trials Treatment and control groups recruited similarly Postloss interventions	0.11	Interventions may be ineffective Control groups also improve May need stronger dose of interventions Methodological problems common
Fortner and Neimeyer[46,b]	23	Randomized controlled trials	0.13	Greater effects with high-risk populations
Schut, Stroebe, van den Bout, and Terheggen[47]	16 primary; 7 secondary; 7 tertiary[c]	Organized help Focused on treating grief Methodologically sound	Low to modest effects	Strongest effects with individuals exhibiting psychopathology/pathological grief Greater effects with self-referred
Jordan and Neimeyer[43]	4	Reviews and meta-analyses	N/A	Generally low efficacy of interventions Intervention may not be necessary for most bereaved Need to develop new approaches Need to improve methodology of studies

[a]The effect size of $d = 0.16$ for randomized studies at posttreatment; for nonrandomized studies ($n = 12$), the effect size was $d = 0.51$ at posttreatment. Tests of both effect size estimates were statistically significant.

[b]From unpublished work of Fortner and Neimeyer (1999) described by Neimeyer.[46]

[c]Primary preventive interventions were open to all bereaved individuals. Secondary preventive interventions were open to high-risk individuals. Tertiary preventive interventions were open to individuals with complicated grief or other psychopathology.

Its efficacy in treating a variety of disorders has been demonstrated.[48] IPT was designed to treat depression by focusing on relationship problems theorized to maintain depressive symptoms. Therapists use strategies such as communication skill building to help resolve complicated grief. It is indicated for bereaved individuals who would benefit from improvement in current interpersonal functioning.

Cognitive-behavioral therapy. Cognitive-behavioral therapy (CBT) approaches with bereaved individuals focus on identifying and challenging maladaptive thoughts and behaviors. Specifically, the goals are to modify dysfunctional thinking that prevents adaptive processing of the loss, exposure to avoided thoughts and situations, and engagement in restorative tasks.[24] It is indicated when individuals are struggling with excessive guilt and anger, for those who are avoiding reminders of the loss, and for those avoiding resuming functional activities.

Group psychotherapy. One of the primary benefits of groups for the bereaved is the mutual support offered by those who have experienced similar losses. These individuals offer validation to one another, while reducing the isolation that may occur during bereavement. Groups also permit emotional expression and processing. Bereaved individuals can share effective coping strategies with one another. Piper and colleagues[49] examined short-term group psychotherapy for complicated grief and

found that individuals who have more social support; a history of mature relationships; and high scores on measures of extraversion, openness, and conscientiousness responded more positively than their counterparts.

Family therapy. Using a family-centered approach throughout the course of cancer treatment and palliative care permits providers to identify those who might be at risk for poor psychological outcomes after death. Kissane et al.[3,26] developed Family Focused Grief Therapy (FFGT), a 6–10 session preventive intervention for high-risk families that begins during palliative care with the patient and continues with surviving members after the patient's death. This approach fosters continuity of care, permitting clinicians a better understanding of the patient's and family's journey of illness that may impact their grief. Families are screened to identify those exhibiting risk factors previously associated with negative bereavement outcomes, including high conflict, low cohesion, and/or communication deficits.[3,26] Dysfunctional families and "Intermediate" families, who display moderate levels of disturbance, are targeted.[3,26] The goals of FFGT are to address families' risk factors by facilitating mutual support and the sharing of grief. In a randomized controlled trial (RCT) of FFGT, significant decreases in distress 13 months after death were observed.[26,50] The use of routine screening of family functioning and implementation of this type of family-centered intervention may assist high-risk families in oncology settings.

Combined psychopharmacological approaches. Bereavement-related mental disorders are treated using standard psychopharmacological and psychotherapeutic approaches.[4,7] Anxiolytics and sleep aids may be particularly useful during the acute phase of bereavement. Selective serotonin and noradrenergic reuptake inhibitors may be used to reduce depressive symptoms.

Treatments for PGD. Symptoms of PGD do not appear to respond as well to traditional treatments for bereavement-related depression (e.g., interpersonal therapy or antidepressants).[2] Efforts are underway to develop specific interventions for PGD. Shear and colleagues[23] developed complicated grief treatment (CGT), a 16-session manualized treatment using CBT principles that involved psychoeducation about the dual process model of coping, exposure to avoided loss-related thoughts, retelling the story of the death, imaginal conversations with the deceased, and development of personal goals to assist with restorative behaviors. In a RCT comparing CGT to IPT, a greater percentage of patients responded to CGT (51%) than to IPT (28%), and time to response was more rapid.[23]

Boelen et al.[24] found that 12 sessions of CBT was more efficacious in reducing PGD and other psychopathological symptoms than 12 sessions of supportive counseling. They also found that exposure was more potent than cognitive restructuring, and greater benefits were observed when treatment began with exposure followed by cognitive restructuring than when the order was reversed.[24]

CONCLUSIONS

Several disciplines have contributed to our understanding of bereavement, but theoretical models are not mutually exclusive. Integration of empirically-supported models of intervention within a biopsychosocial framework is desirable. To this end, efforts to bridge the substantial divide between clinicians and researchers should continue.[4,51] However, ethical concerns about the vulnerabilities of bereaved individuals make it difficult to recruit and design methodologically sound treatment outcome studies.

Clinically relevant controversies remain in the bereavement field, including whether a distinction between normal and pathological grief can be made and, moreover, whether PGD should be established as a mental disorder in *DSM-V*. Psychotherapy for grief should target those individuals who are at greatest risk and would likely benefit the most. Recognition of resilience among the bereaved underscores adaptive pathways that can be promoted.[2,34]

The importance of continuity of care of families from end of life to bereavement is gaining increasing recognition in palliative care. Unfortunately, there is still a great need to establish infrastructures within these settings to facilitate support for the bereaved. Establishing routine screening of patients, caregivers, and families is critical to identifying those at risk and applying evidence-based approaches to reducing the suffering of those in greatest need.

REFERENCES

1. WHO. *Cancer control: Knowledge into action, WHO guide for effective programmes.* Switzerland: Palliative Care Geneva; 2007.

2. Prigerson HG, Horowitz MJ, Jacobs SC, et al. Prolonged grief disorder: psychometric validation of criteria proposed for DSM-V and ICD-11. *PLoS Med.* 2009 Aug;6(8):e1000121.

3. Kissane DW, Bloch S. *Family focused grief therapy. A model of family-centered care during palliative care and bereavement.* Buckingham: Open University Press; 2002.

4. Genevro J, Marshall T, Miller T. Report on bereavement and grief research. *Death Studies.* 2004;28:491–575.

5. Parkes C. *Bereavement studies of grief in adult life.* 3rd ed. Madison, CT: International Universities Press; 1998.

6. Raphael B. *The anatomy of bereavement.* London: Hutchinson; 1983.

7. Stroebe M, Hansson R, Stroebe W, Schut H. (eds). *Handbook of bereavement research: consequences, coping, and care.* Washington: APA Books; 2001.

8. Jacobs S. *Pathologic grief: Maladaptation to loss.* Washington, DC: American Psychiatric Press; 1993.

9. Doka K. Disenfranchised grief. In: Doka K, (ed). *Disenfranchised grief: Recognizing hidden sorrow.* Lexington, MA: Lexington Books; 1989:3–11.

10. Freed PJ, Mann JJ. Sadness and loss: toward a neurobiopsychosocial model. *Am J Psychiatry.* 2007 Jan;164(1):28–34.

11. O'Connor MF, Gundel H, McRae K, Lane RD. Baseline vagal tone predicts BOLD response during elicitation of grief. *Neuropsychopharmacology.* 2007 Oct;32(10):2184–2189.

12. Bowlby J. The making and breaking of affectional bonds I & II. *Br J Psychiatry.* 1977;130:201–210.

13. Ainsworth M, Blehar M, Waters E, Wall S. *Patterns of attachment: A psychological study of the strange situation.* Hillsdale, NJ.: Erlbaum; 1978.

14. Vanderwerker LC, Jacobs SC, Parkes CM, Prigerson HG. An exploration of associations between separation anxiety in childhood and complicated grief in later life. *J Nerv Ment Dis.* 2006 Feb;194(2):121–123.

15. Shapiro ER. Grief in interpersonal perspective: theories and their implications. In: Stroebe M, Hansson R, Stroebe W, Schut H, (eds). *Handbook of bereavement research: Consequences, coping, and care.* Washington, DC: American Psychological Association; 2001:301–327.

16. Horowitz MJ. A model of mourning: change in schemas of self and other. *J Am Psychoanal Assoc.* 1990;38(2):297–324.

17. Worden JW. *Grief counseling and grief therapy: A handbook for the mental health practitioner.* 4th ed. New York: Springer Pub.; 2008.

18. Janoff-Bulman R. *Shattered assumptions: Towards a new psychology of trauma.* New York: Free Press; 1992.

19. Neimeyer R. *Meaning reconstruction and the experience of loss.* Washington, DC: American Psychological Association; 2001.

20. Bonanno GA, Kaltman S. Toward an integrative perspective on bereavement. *Psychol Bull.* 1999 Nov;125(6):760–776.

21. Klass D, Walter T. Processes of grieving: how bonds are continued. In: Stroebe MS, Hansson RO, Stroebe W, Schut H, (eds). *Handbook of bereavement research: Consequences, coping, and care.* Washington, DC: American Psychological Association; 2001.

22. Rosenblatt PC. A social constructionist perspective on cultural differences in grief. In: Stroebe MS, Hansson RO, Stroebe W, Schut H, (eds). *Handbook of bereavement research: Consequences, coping, and care.* Washington, DC: American Psychological Association; 2001:298–300.

23. Shear K, Frank E, Houck PR, Reynolds III CF. Treatment of complicated grief: a randomized controlled trial. *JAMA.* 2005;293:2601–2068.

24. Boelen PA, de Keijser J, van den Hout MA, van den Bout J. Treatment of complicated grief: a comparison between cognitive-behavioral therapy and supportive counseling. *J Consult Clin Psychol.* 2007 Apr;75(2):277–284.

25. Stroebe M, Schut H. The dual process model of coping with bereavement: rationale and description. *Death Stud.* 1999 Apr-May;23(3):197–224.

26. Kissane D, Bloch S, McKenzie M, et al. Family focused grief therapy: a randomized controlled trial in palliative care and bereavement. *Am J Psychiatry.* 2006;163:1208–1218.

27. Levy LH. Anticipatory grief: its measurement and proposed reconceptualization. *Hosp J.* 1991;7(4):1–28.

28. Prigerson HG, Maciejewski PK. Grief and acceptance as opposite sides of the same coin: setting a research agenda to study peaceful acceptance of loss. *Br J Psychiatry.* 2008 Dec;193:435–437.

29. Kübler-Ross E. *On death and dying.* New York: Macmillan; 1969.

30. Bowlby J. Processes of mourning. *Int J Psychoanal.* 1961 Jul-Oct;42:317–340.

31. Maciejewski PK, Zhang B, Block SD, Prigerson HG. An empirical examination of the stage theory of grief. *JAMA.* 2007 Feb 21;297(7):716–723.

32. Bonanno GA. Loss, trauma, and human resilience: have we underestimated the human capacity to thrive after extremely aversive events? *Am Psychol.* 2004 Jan;59(1):20–28.

33. APA. *Diagnostic and statistical manual of mental disorders,* 4th ed. Text Revision (DSM-IV-TR). Washington, DC: American Psychiatric Association; 2000.

34. Lichtenthal WG, Cruess DG, Prigerson HG. A case for establishing complicated grief as a distinct mental disorder in DSM-V. *Clin Psychol Rev.* 2004 Oct;24(6):637–662.

35. Silverman GK, Johnson JG, Prigerson HG. Preliminary explorations of the effects of prior trauma and loss on risk for psychiatric disorders in recently widowed people. *Isr J Psychiatry Relat Sci.* 2001;38(3–4):202–215.

36. American Psychiatric Association. *Diagnostic and statistical manual of mental disorders,* 4th ed. Washington, DC: Author; 1994.

37. Wijngaards-de Meij L, Stroebe M, Schut H, et al. Patterns of attachment and parents' adjustment to the death of their child. *Pers Soc Psychol Bull.* 2007 Apr;33(4):537–548.

38. Barry LC, Kasl SV, Prigerson HG. Psychiatric disorders among bereaved persons: the role of perceived circumstances of death and preparedness for death. *Am J Geriatr Psychiatry.* 2002 Jul-Aug;10(4):447–457.

39. Allumbaugh D, Hoyt W. Effectiveness of grief therapy: a meta-analysis. *J Community Psychol.* 1999;46:370–380.

40. Kato PM, Mann T. A synthesis of psychological interventions for the bereaved. *Clin Psychol Rev.* 1999 Apr;19(3):275–296.

41. Currier JM, Holland JM, Neimeyer RA. The effectiveness of bereavement interventions with children: a meta-analytic review of controlled outcome research. *J Clin Child Adolesc Psychol.* 2007 Apr-Jun;36(2):253–259.

42. Currier JM, Neimeyer RA, Berman JS. The effectiveness of psychotherapeutic interventions for the bereaved: a comprehensive quantitative review. *Psychol Bull.* 2008 Sep;134(5):648–661.

43. Jordan JR, Neimeyer RA. Does grief counseling work? *Death Stud.* 2003 Nov;27(9):765–786.

44. Larson DG, Hoyt WT. What has become of grief counselling? An evaluation of the empirical foundations of the new pessimism. *Prof Psychol: Res Prac.* 2007;38:347–355.

45. Crits-Christoph P, Connolly MB. Empirical basis of supportive-expressive psychodynamic psychotherapy. In: Bornstein RF, Masling JM, (eds). *Empirical studies of the therapeutic hour.* Washington, DC: American Psychological Association; 1998:109–151.

46. Neimeyer RA. Searching for the meaning of meaning: grief therapy and the process of reconstruction. *Death Stud.* 2000 Sep;24(6):541–558.

47. Schut H, Stroebe M, van den Bout J, Terheggen M. The efficacy of bereavement interventions: determining who benefits. In: Stroebe M, Hansson R, Stroebe W, Schut H, (eds). *Handbook of bereavement research: Consequences, coping, and care.* Washington, DC: American Psychological Association; 2001:705–738.

48. Markowitz JC, Weissman MM. Interpersonal psychotherapy: principles and applications. *World Psych.* 2004 Oct;3(3):136–139.

49. Piper WE, Ogrodniczuk JS, Joyce AS, Weideman R, Rosie JS. Group composition and group therapy for complicated grief. *J Consult Clin Psychol.* 2007 Feb;75(1):116–125.

50. Kissane D, Lichtenthal WG, Zaider T. Family care before and after bereavement. *Omega (Westport).* 2007;56(1):21–32.

51. Stroebe M, Hansson R, Schut H, Stroebe W. (eds). *Handbook of bereavement research and practice: 21st century perspectives.* Washington, DC: American Psychological Association; 2008.

PART XII

Survivorship

Ruth McCorkle, ED

Positive Consequences of the Experience of Cancer: Perceptions of Growth and Meaning

Annette L. Stanton

I have learned to be more patient and take some time for people and things. I still find myself getting hurried and upset at things. Then I stop to realize, "This is not important, slow down, focus on the important things in life." It is great to have this new perspective on life in general. It makes you focus on friends and family, happiness, quality of life, and your true feelings.-Research participant diagnosed with breast cancer[1]

In their conversations with individuals diagnosed with cancer, researchers and clinicians in psycho-oncology are likely to hear statements such as the one above offered by a woman living with breast cancer. Indeed, it seems impossible to interact intensively with individuals affected by cancer without becoming aware of the benefits some extract as they struggle with the demands of the experience. This chapter begins with a consideration of the prevalence and meaning of finding benefit in the experience of cancer, followed by a summary of findings on the conditions that promote benefit finding as well as the role of benefit finding in adjustment to cancer. The chapter closes with thoughts on clinical implications of the research on finding benefit in cancer.

FINDING BENEFIT IN THE EXPERIENCE OF CANCER: PREVALENCE AND SIGNIFICANCE

Reviewing the empirical literature on finding benefit in the experience of cancer, Stanton, Bower, and Low[2] found that positive life changes are reported by the majority of individuals diagnosed with a variety of cancers, including cancers of the breast, lung, colon, prostate, and others. Most adolescent and adult survivors of childhood cancers also report finding benefit. There also is some evidence that finding benefit in the experience of cancer increases over time, as documented by Manne et al.[3] in both breast cancer patients and their partners from approximately 4 months after diagnosis through 18 months later (also see reference 4). In addition, cancer patients are more likely to report growth through their experience than are comparison adults reflecting on change over similar time frames. Cordova, Cunningham, Carlson, and Andrykowski[5] compared the responses on the Posttraumatic Growth Inventory (PTGI[6]), a commonly used measure of perceived benefit arising from a designated stressor, of women with breast cancer to responses of age- and education-matched women with no cancer history who completed the PTGI to refer to the extent of change perceived on each item since the cancer diagnosis of their matched counterpart (e.g., in the last 2 years). Women diagnosed with cancer reported significantly more posttraumatic growth than did the comparison sample, and they reported more growth in the specific domains of relating to others, spirituality, and appreciation of life (but not personal strength or new possibilities in life) (see also reference 7).

Several domains of benefit are reported by individuals diagnosed with cancer. A primary perceived benefit involves the interpersonal realm, including heightened intimacy, awareness of one's importance to significant others, and compassion. Both Petrie and colleagues[8] and Sears, Stanton, and Danoff-Burg[9] found enhanced relationships to be the most commonly cited category of benefit in cancer patients responding to an open-ended question on cancer-related positive consequences (33% and 46% of the respective samples). A second benefit involves sharpened appreciation for life, endorsed by 85% of Hodgkin disease survivors in a study by Cella and Tross,[10] for example. A bolstered sense of personal strength and skills, deepened spirituality, and valued change in life priorities and goals also are commonly cited. Such benefits also are evident in the broader literature on perceived positive change from traumatic experiences (i.e., posttraumatic growth, Tedeschi and Calhoun[6,11]), although distinct stressful or traumatic events catalyze the report of benefit to different degrees (e.g., reference 12). A unique category of benefit spontaneously offered by individuals with cancer (and other medical stressors) regards improvement in health-related behaviors (e.g., reference 9).

What does it mean to report benefit from the experience of a life-threatening disease? In part, benefit finding might represent a natural propensity to maintain a positive self-view, such that perceptions of growth might be achieved by derogating one's precancer status (e.g., reference 13) or by comparing oneself to others who are worse off. Individuals can seek benefit as an intentional strategy to cope with mortality threat and illness-related demands (e.g., coping through positive reappraisal), or they can report benefits that already have accrued through their experience with the disease.[14] In a sample of breast cancer patients who recently had completed primary medical treatments, Sears et al.[9] found that these constructs had different predictors. Further, actively coping through positive appraisal of the cancer experience (e.g., "I look for something good in what is happening"[15]) predicted perceived cancer-related growth, as well as improved positive mood and perceived physical health, 1 year later. In contrast, simply reporting having found benefit in the cancer experience at study entry did not predict improved adjustment at 1 year, leading the authors to suggest that it is those individuals who make active use of their perceptions of benefit through cognitive reminders or behavioral instantiation (e.g., spending more time with close friends) that are most likely to experience salutary outcomes.

It is quite possible that reports of benefit serve distinct functions for different individuals. For some survivors, reporting cancer-related benefits might be akin to wishful thinking, whereas citing benefits might signify important and sustained positive shifts in cognitions, emotions, or behaviors for others. Evidence for these distinct motivational functions comes from two longitudinal studies, one of women with breast cancer[16] and the other of mothers caring for children undergoing stem cell transplantation.[17] In both cases, finding benefit in the cancer-related experience (or positive reappraisal coping in[16]) predicted improved adjustment over time for women with high personal resources (i.e., high dispositional hope or optimism) and declining adjustment for those with lower personal resources (i.e., personality × benefit-finding interaction). Stanton et al.[16] also found that women with high hope who reported coping through positive reappraisal were unlikely to engage in avoidant coping, whereas the relation between positive reappraisal coping and avoidance-oriented coping was positive for women low in hope. They suggested that benefit finding might serve an avoidant function for those with low personal resources and an approach-oriented function for those with greater resources, with distinct consequences for adjustment. If expression of the sentiment that "Cancer is the best thing that ever happened to me" or "I appreciate every day so much more now" carries distinct motivational significance for different individuals, then researchers might need to assess potentially moderating variables carefully to elucidate the nature of the relationship between benefit finding and adjustment.

WHAT CONDITIONS PROMOTE BENEFIT FINDING?

Over the past several decades, researchers and clinicians have attempted to understand how individuals are able to extract benefit in the face of experiences that also carry the potential for disability, psychosocial disruption, and loss of life. Theories of finding meaning and growth through adversity suggest that life disruption sufficient to prompt a search for meaning is necessary for growth to occur (e.g., references 11, 18, and 19). Through the search for meaning and associated cognitive processes, life threat can prompt enhanced appreciation for life and a commitment to live according to one's fundamental priorities, considerate reactions of others can take on special meaning and motivate deepened relationships, and the recognition that one can surmount major difficulties can bring a sense of pride and self-regard. The intrapersonal and interpersonal contexts influence the ultimate adaptive consequences of the process of making meaning in stressful or traumatic experiences (e.g., reference 20).

In a review of 29 independent, quantitative studies, and seven additional substudies based on those samples, Stanton and colleagues[2] examined correlates of finding benefit in the experience of cancer. Potential correlates included a number of sociodemographic factors, stressor characteristics, personality attributes, social context variables, and coping processes. Concordant with theory, Stanton et al. concluded that significant cancer impact and personal engagement are the most consistent precursors of finding benefit. That is, although the evidence is not entirely consistent and comes primarily from cross-sectional studies, more life disruption and perceived threat are associated with more perceived growth from the experience of cancer. Further, intentional engagement with the experience of cancer, as evidenced through dispositional approach tendencies and approach-oriented coping strategies such as problem-focused coping, active acceptance of the cancer diagnosis, and intentional positive reappraisal, is related to more perceived growth. Amid numerous null or inconsistent findings, there also was some evidence that greater cancer-related benefit finding is related to younger age (perhaps owing to higher perceived threat and life disruption in younger adults with cancer), being of ethnic minority status (mediated by religious coping in[21]), higher dispositional optimism and other positive personality attributes, and greater social support regarding the cancer experience.

The relations documented by Stanton et al.[2] with regard to benefit finding in the cancer experience are similar to those found in a meta-analysis of 87 cross-sectional studies of benefit finding across a variety of stressors, including cancer.[22] The meta-analysis revealed significant associations of benefit finding with objective event severity and subjective threat, coping through positive reappraisal and acceptance, younger age, ethnic minority status, female gender, optimism, and religiosity. The one inconsistent association is that the meta-analysis[22] suggested a relation between benefit finding and coping through denial, whereas most studies reviewed by Stanton et al.[2] found no significant relation with avoidance-oriented coping.

Progress is evident in delineating the factors that promote perceptions of growth through the cancer experience, and most empirical findings are consistent with theories that finding benefit is catalyzed by significant perceived event impact and intentional approach toward the stressor through cognitive processing and other active coping strategies. A supportive social context and positive personal attributes also might facilitate finding benefit. However, the preponderance of cross-sectional studies and heterogeneous effects limit the conclusions that can be drawn regarding determinants of finding benefit.

WHAT IS THE ROLE OF BENEFIT FINDING IN ADJUSTMENT TO CANCER?

A common belief in the lay community is that positive thinking can affect not only adjustment to cancer but also disease outcome, and the adaptive consequences of finding benefit in the experience of cancer have received study. Of course, perceiving growth as a result of one's experience might be valuable in its own right, representing the maintenance or enhancement of a sense of mastery and meaning in the face of life-threatening disease. Whether benefit finding bodes well for other domains of adjustment is less clear. Certainly, notable positive findings exist, such that perceived positive meaning in the cancer experience at 1–5 years after diagnosis predicted an increase in positive affect 5 years later in a sample of 763 breast cancer patients,[23] and finding benefit in the year after surgery predicted lower distress and depressive symptoms 4–7 years later in another sample of women diagnosed with breast cancer.[24] However, reviews of the literature reveal a mixed picture. The Stanton et al.[2] review revealed mixed evidence that cancer-related benefit finding is associated with lower distress or more positive mood, and the authors suggested that relations between benefit finding and adjustment might be conditioned by individual differences in motivational functions of benefit finding, the timing of finding benefit relative to cancer diagnosis and treatment, and other factors. The Helgeson et al.[22] meta-analysis of cross-sectional research on various stressors demonstrated that benefit finding was not related to anxiety, global distress, and quality of life. Benefit finding was related significantly to lower depressive symptoms, more positive well-being, and greater cancer-related intrusive/avoidant thoughts. However, there was significant variability in effect sizes across studies, and relations varied as a function of duration of the stressor, how benefit finding was assessed, and the racial composition of the sample. A more focused review by Algoe and Stanton,[25] which targeted only longitudinal studies of individuals who had experienced serious physical illness (including cancer), demonstrated inconsistent relations between benefit finding and psychological adjustment, but somewhat more consistent evidence of a relationship between finding benefit and subjective or objective markers of better physical health (see also reference 26). The reviews were consistent in their conclusion that additional research to identify moderators of the relation of benefit finding with psychological and physical health is warranted, in light of emerging evidence that the association is dependent on characteristics of the stressful context and the person.

In addition to having a direct relationship with particular adaptive outcomes or having effects dependent on other variables, finding benefit in the cancer experience might have additional, complex relations with physical and psychological health. First, benefit finding might serve as a mechanism for the relations of more stable individual difference factors with outcomes. For example, Tallman, Altmaier, and Garcia[27] found that high optimism before bone marrow transplant predicted benefit finding at 1 year after transplant, which in turn predicted lower depressive symptoms and better physical functioning 3 years after transplant (see also reference 28 in a noncancer sample). Second, finding benefit might serve a stress-buffering function. For example, in a cross-sectional study, the relation of posttraumatic stress symptoms with higher depressive symptoms and lower quality of life was attenuated in women who endorsed more posttraumatic growth.[29] Siegel and Schrimshaw[30] reported a similar finding in women living with human immunodeficiency virus/acquired immunodeficiency syndrome (HIV/AIDS), as did McMillen et al.[12] in three types of disaster. Third, benefit finding that is sustained or increases over time might promote adjustment. Schwarzer et al.[4] found that finding benefit in cancer was not associated with well-being at any point in a longitudinal study, but that an increase in finding benefit from the week before surgery through 1 year predicted increased well-being in a sample of patients with various cancers.

The mechanisms through which finding benefit in the experience of cancer might promote positive outcomes also are receiving study (see reference 26 for a review). Dunigan, Carr, and Steel,[31] who found that posttraumatic growth was associated with longer survival in hepatocellular carcinoma, suggested that finding benefit promotes biological homeostasis through hypothalamic modulation of glucocorticoids (note that the relation was reduced to a trend when gender was controlled in analyses). This hypothesis is consistent with the finding of Cruess et al.[32] that an increase in benefit finding after participation in a cognitive-behavioral stress management (CBSM) intervention[33] was associated with a reduction in cortisol in breast cancer patients; moreover, benefit finding mediated the effect of the intervention on cortisol. Altered immune function also might result from finding benefit or meaning.[34,35] The nature and significance of neuroendocrine and immune changes associated with finding benefit requires continued investigation.

Clearly, the relation of benefit finding with adaptive outcomes is not straightforward. Rather, the impact of finding benefit in the experience of cancer likely is dependent on a number of characteristics of the person, the disease context, and the social milieu. Accordingly, any clinical implications of findings must be advanced with caution.

CLINICAL IMPLICATIONS OF BENEFIT FINDING IN CANCER

In the past decade, researchers have examined the effect of psychosocial interventions on benefit finding in cancer and other stressors. Although not originally designed to promote benefit finding, Antoni's CBSM intervention has been demonstrated to increase cancer-related benefit finding in two trials of women with breast cancer[33,36] and a trial of men with prostate cancer.[37] The development of perceived ability to relax[36] and broader stress management skills[37] mediated the effects of CBSM on benefit finding.

Research also has explicitly prompted the consideration of cancer-related benefits. Stanton and colleagues[1] randomly assigned women who had completed primary treatments for breast cancer to write over four sessions about their deepest thoughts and feelings about their experience with breast cancer (EXP), positive thoughts and feelings about their experience (POS), or the facts of the experience (CTL). Compared with the CTL condition, both EXP and POS produced significantly fewer medical appointments for cancer-related morbidities over the next 3 months, and EXP participants reported significantly fewer physical symptoms, with a similar trend evident for POS (see also references 38 and 39 for comparable findings in noncancer samples). The writing interventions did not have direct effects on psychological outcomes, but EXP was more effective in reducing distress for participants low in cancer-related avoidance, and POS appeared somewhat more effective for more highly avoidant participants.

Such controlled, experimental evidence promotes confidence in the results of longitudinal, naturalistic research that finding benefit in the experience of cancer can carry salutary health consequences. However, few trials are available, and much is left to learn about whether, when, and how to prompt consideration of benefits during clinical encounters. Certainly, discussing positive consequences gleaned during the cancer experience is not the same as an insistence on positive thinking. A sole focus on positive thinking, accompanied by a suppression of negative thoughts and feelings, is clinically contraindicated[40–42] and is likely to exact a psychological and physiological toll (e.g., reference 43). Indeed, it is possible that inducing women to consider the positive consequences of their experience with breast cancer was effective in part because the trial was conducted after the completion of primary medical treatments,[1] when women likely already had had considerable time to process and express negative emotions surrounding cancer. An instruction to generate benefits shortly after diagnosis might have induced suppression of negative emotions, with very different outcomes. It also is important to note that none of the trials that prompted benefit finding suggested that women should identify any particular benefit, but rather encouraged self-generation of positive consequences. One woman wrote, "The first time I was asked to write about the positive aspects for 20 minutes, I thought, 'Are you kidding?!' Then as I started thinking about it I was amazed at all of the things that came to mind!"[1]

The empirical literature on benefit finding has not matured sufficiently to offer definitive procedural guidance for clinicians. Certainly, the direct suggestion that one should experience any specific benefit can be perceived as minimizing the impact of the cancer experience; however, spontaneous reports of illness-related benefits offer a potentially useful entrée into a cancer patient's efforts to adapt to the disease. Further, a sensitively timed query about any positive consequences that might have occurred amid the negative aspects could prompt productive cognitive and emotional processing. Helping individuals make active use of benefits found, for example, through changing health behaviors, making the most of time with loved ones, and living according to deeply held values and priorities, also can be productive. In tandem, the next decade of basic research and clinical trials promise to illuminate further what it means to find benefit in the face of life-threatening disease, the conditions under which finding benefit promotes positive adaptive outcomes, and the place of benefit finding in clinical interventions for individuals diagnosed with cancer.

REFERENCES

1. Stanton AL, Danoff-Burg S, Sworowski LA, et al. Randomized, controlled trial of written emotional expression and benefit-finding in breast cancer patients. *J Clin Oncol.* 2002;20:4160–4168.

2. Stanton AL, Bower JE, Low CA. Posttraumatic growth after cancer. In: Calhoun LG, Tedeschi RG, (eds). *Handbook of posttraumatic growth: Research and practice.* Mahwah, NJ: Erlbaum; 2006:138–175.

3. Manne S, Ostroff J, Winkel G, Goldstein L, Fox K, Grana G. Posttraumatic growth after breast cancer: patient, partner, and couple perspectives. *Psychosom Med.* 2004;66:442–454.

4. Schwarzer R, Luszczynska A, Boehmer S, Taubert S, Knoll N. Changes in finding benefit after cancer surgery and the prediction of well-being one year later. *Soc Sci Med.* 2006;63:1614–1624.

5. Cordova MJ, Cunningham LLC, Carlson CR, Andrykowski MA. Posttraumatic growth following breast cancer: a controlled comparison study. *Health Psychol.* 2001;20:176–185.

6. Tedeschi RG, Calhoun LG. The posttraumatic growth inventory: measuring the positive legacy of trauma. *J Traumatic Stress.* 1996;9:455–471.

7. Bishop MM, Beaumont JL, Hahn EA, et al. Late effects of cancer and hematopoietic stem-cell transplantation on spouses or partners compared with survivors and survivor-matched controls. *J Clin Oncol.* 2007;25:1403–1411.

8. Petrie KJ, Buick DL, Weinman J, Booth RJ. Positive effects of illness reported by myocardial infarction and breast cancer patients. *J Psychosom Res.* 1999;47:537–543.

9. Sears SR, Stanton AL, Danoff-Burg S. The yellow brick road and the emerald city: benefit finding, positive reappraisal coping, and posttraumatic growth in women with early-stage breast cancer. *Health Psychol.* 2003;22:487–497.

10. Cella DF, Tross S. Psychological adjustment to survival from Hodgkin's disease. *J Consult Clin Psychol.* 1986;54:616–622.

11. Tedeschi RG, Calhoun LG. Posttraumatic growth: conceptual foundations and empirical evidence. *Psychol Inq.* 2004;15:1–18.

12. McMillen JC, Smith EM, Fisher RH. Perceived benefit and mental health after three types of disaster. *J Consult Clin Psychol.* 1997;65:733–739.

13. Widows MR, Jacobsen PB, Booth-Jones M, Fields KK. Predictors of posttraumatic growth following bone marrow transplantation for cancer. *Health Psychol.* 2005;24:266–273.

14. Tennen H, Affleck G. Benefit-finding and benefit-reminding. In: Snyder CR, (ed). *Handbook of positive psychology.* New York: Oxford University Press; 2002:584–597.

15. Carver CS, Scheier MF, Weintraub JK. Assessing coping strategies: a theoretically-based approach. *J Pers Soc Psychol.* 1989;56:267–283.

16. Stanton AL, Danoff-Burg S, Huggins ME. The first year after breast cancer diagnosis: hope and coping strategies as predictors of adjustment. *Psychooncology.* 2002;11:93–102.

17. Rini C, Manne S, DuHamel KN, et al. Mothers' perceptions of benefit following pediatric stem cell transplantation: a longitudinal investigation of the roles of optimism, medical risk, and sociodemographic resources. *Ann Behav Med.* 2004;28:132–141.

18. Janoff-Bulman R, Frantz, CM. The impact of trauma on meaning: from meaningless world to meaningful life. In: Power M, Brewin CR, (eds). *The transformation of meaning in psychological therapies.* New York: Wiley; 1997:91–106.

19. Janoff-Bulman R, Berger A. The other side of trauma: towards a psychology of appreciation. In: Harvey JH, Miller ED, (eds). *Loss and trauma: General and close relationship perspectives.* Philadelphia, PA: Brunner/Mazel; 2000:29–44.

20. Calhoun LG, Tedeschi RG. (eds). *Handbook of posttraumatic growth: Research and practice.* Mahwah, NJ: Erlbaum; 2006.

21. Urcuyo KR, Boyers AE, Carver CS, Antoni MH. Finding benefit in breast cancer: relations with personality, coping, and concurrent well-being. *Psychol Health.* 2005;20:175–192.

22. Helgeson VS, Reynolds KA, Tomich PL. A meta-analytic review of benefit finding and growth. *J Consult Clin Psychol.* 2006;74:797–816.

23. Bower, JE, Meyerowitz BE, Desmond KA, Bernaards CA, Rowland JH, Ganz PA. Perceptions of positive meaning and vulnerability following breast cancer: predictors and outcomes among long-term breast cancer survivors. *Ann Behav Med.* 2005;29:236–245.

24. Carver CS, Antoni MH. Finding benefit in breast cancer during the year after diagnosis predicts better adjustment 5 to 8 years after diagnosis. *Health Psychol.* 2004;23:595–598.

25. Algoe SB, Stanton AL. Is benefit finding good for individuals with chronic disease? In: Park CL, Lechner SC, Antoni MH, Stanton AL, (eds). *Medical illness and positive life change: Can crisis lead to personal transformation?* Washington, DC: American Psychological Association. 2009:173–193.

26. Bower JE, Epel E, Moskowitz JT. Biological correlates: How psychological components of benefit finding may lead to physiological benefits. In: Park CL, Lechner SC, Antoni MH, Stanton AL, (eds). *Medical illness and positive life change: Can crisis lead to personal transformation?* Washington, DC: American Psychological Association. 2009:155–172.

27. Tallman BA, Altmaier E, Garcia C. Finding benefit from cancer. *J Counseling Psychol.* 2007;54:481–487.

28. Davis CG, Nolen-Hoeksema S, Larson J. Making sense of loss and benefiting from the experience: two construals of meaning. *J Pers Soc Psychol.* 1998;75:561–574.

29. Morrill EF, Brewer NT, O'Neill SC, et al. The interaction of post-traumatic growth and post-traumatic stress symptoms in predicting depressive symptoms and quality of life. *Psychooncology.* 2008;17:948–953.

30. Siegel K, Schrimshaw EW. The stress moderating role of benefit finding on psychological distress and well-being among women living with HIV/AIDS. *AIDS Behavior.* 2007;11:421–433.

31. Dunigan JT, Carr BI, Steel JL. Posttraumatic growth, immunity and survival in patients with hepatoma. *Dig Dis Sci.* 2007;52:2452–2459.

32. Cruess DG, Antoni MH, McGregor BA, et al. Cognitive-behavioral stress management reduces serum cortisol by enhancing benefit finding among women being treated for early stage breast cancer. *Psychosom Med.* 2000;62:304–308.

33. Antoni MH, Lehman JM, Kilbourn KM, et al. Cognitive-behavioral stress management intervention decreases the prevalence of depression and enhances benefit finding among women under treatment for early-stage breast cancer. *Health Psychol.* 2001;20:20–32.

34. Bower JE, Kemeny ME, Taylor SE, Fahey JL. Cognitive processing, discovery of meaning, CD4 decline, and AIDS-related mortality among bereaved HIV-seropositive men. *J Consult Clin Psychol.* 1998;66:979–986.

35. McGregor BA, Antoni MH, Boyers A, Alferi SM, Blomberg BB, Carver CS. Cognitive-behavioral stress management increases benefit finding and immune function among women with early-stage breast cancer. *J Psychosom Res.* 2004;56:1–8.

36. Antoni MH, Lechner SC, Kazi A, et al. How stress management improves quality of life after treatment for breast cancer. *J Consult Clin Psychol.* 2006;74:1143–1152.

37. Penedo FJ, Molton I, Dahn JR, et al. A randomized clinical trial of group-based cognitive-behavioral stress management in localized prostate cancer: development of stress management skills improves quality of life and benefit finding. *Ann Behavioral Med.* 2006;31:261–270.

38. Danoff-Burg S, Agee JD, Romanoff NR, Kremer JM, Strosberg JM. Benefit finding and expressive writing in adults with lupus or rheumatoid arthritis. *Psychol Health.* 2006;21:651–665.

39. King LA, Miner KN. Writing about the perceived benefits of traumatic events: implications for physical health. *Pers Soc Psychol Bull.* 2000;26:220–230.

40. Holland JC, Lewis S. *The human side of cancer: Living with hope, coping with uncertainty.* New York: Harper Collins; 2000.

41. Rittenberg CN. Positive thinking: an unfair burden for cancer patients? *Supp Care Cancer.* 1995;3:37–39.

42. Stanton AL, Tennen H, Affleck G, Mendola R. Coping and adjustment to infertility. *J Soc Clin Psychol.* 1992;11:1-13.

43. Gross JJ. Emotion regulation: affective, cognitive, and social consequences. *Psychophysiology.* 2002;39:281–291.

Changing Health Behaviors after Treatment

Wendy Demark-Wahnefried

A conceptual framework for the care of older adults over the trajectory of the cancer experience has been provided by Rose and O'Toole (Fig. 78–1).[1] This simple, yet elegant framework can be applied to old and young alike. This chapter will focus primarily on the three final stages of the right-hand pathway associated with early stage disease, that is, adjuvant therapy and follow-up, long-term survivorship, and health maintenance. Given advances in early detection and treatment, this is the path that will mark the footsteps of 66% of patients who are newly diagnosed with cancer.[2] Indeed, it is good news and we must celebrate the fact that the clear majority of cancer patients go onto "cure." However, the bad news is that a substantial proportion of these survivors will return to the point of diagnosis, either via recurrence or the discovery of second cancers.[3,4] In addition, many more will run head-long into other co-morbid conditions, such as cardiovascular disease, diabetes, or osteoporosis.[3,5–7] As the number of cancer survivors increase, and more and more data gather on the late effects associated with cancer and its treatment, the significance of health promotion within this high-risk population becomes ever more important, not only to improve quality of life (QOL) and reduce the burden of suffering, but also in terms of sheer economics.[3,8] For example within the United States in 2007, the indirect costs of cancer far outweighed the direct costs by a factor of two-to-one, with estimates of 131 billion dollars.[8] Therefore as the number of cancer survivors increase with each passing year, it is imperative that we turn our attention to the long-term health issues of cancer survivors and begin to deliver care that prevents adverse sequelae and that can preserve or improve functional status and overall health[5,9]; we can not afford otherwise.

Advances in the development of therapeutic agents with fewer side effects, and the institution of survivorship care plans (next chapter) are likely to make a large impact on survivors' health and well-being.[6] Included within this effort, but sometimes overlooked are the health or lifestyle practices of cancer survivors. As addressed in previous chapters, evidence exists that lifestyle factors, such as diet, physical activity, and the use of tobacco, alcohol, sun-protective strategies, or complementary therapies may make a difference, not only in preventing the primary risk of cancer (as addressed in Chapters 2–5), but also in improving QOL and ameliorating symptoms during treatment (as addressed in Chapters 31, 36, and 58–61).[5,9] Such factors may be even more relevant after the flurry of primary treatment ends and the long-term futures of most survivors begin to unfold.

Data clearly show that cancer survivors are at increased risk for second cancers, thus the lifestyle factors addressed in Chapters 2–5 become even more important.[4] Diet, physical activity, and alcohol and tobacco-use also are well-recognized factors that are associated with prevalent forms of co-morbidity among cancer survivors, and which often kill or cripple survivors at much higher rates than the cancer itself.[3,10,11] Furthermore, studies among patients diagnosed with tobacco- or alcohol-induced cancers show that continued smoking and/or drinking leads to increased rates of complications and decreased survival.[10,12] Data also are beginning to accumulate suggesting that physical activity and weight control may be just as important as chemotherapy for enhancing disease-free survival.[13–16]

The potential benefits of physical activity, as well as exercise interventions targeting cancer survivors were already covered in a previous chapter by Courneya (see Chapter 61). Likewise, complementary therapies and related interventions also were addressed in forerunning chapters (see Part IX). To avoid redundancy, this chapter will "fill-in-the-gaps" and address other important lifestyle behaviors in cancer survivors, that is, diet and weight control, tobacco- and alcohol-use, and sun exposure. It also will address overarching issues, such as the need for interventions and what is currently known (or not known) about how best to deliver them.

DIET AND WEIGHT CONTROL

The first nutrition guidelines that specifically addressed cancer survivors were established by the American Cancer Society (ACS) in 2003.[17] Three years later, these guidelines were updated.[18] In 2007, the American Institute for Cancer Research (AICR) in collaboration with the World Cancer Fund (WCF) also addressed dietary guidelines for cancer survivors.[19] Because the risk of co-morbid disease, including second cancers is a significant concern for cancer survivors, these guidelines are based heavily upon those used for primary cancer prevention, as well as those used for the prevention of other prevalent chronic diseases, such as cardiovascular disease and diabetes.[17–19] These guidelines also include recommendations for physical activity. Table 78–1 summarizes the ACS *"Nutrition and physical activity during and after cancer treatment: An American Cancer Society guide to informed choices,"* and the WCF/AICR *"Recommendations for cancer prevention after treatment"* according to common themes.

Weight management. It should be noted that weight management is the lead item in both sets of recommendations. This recommendation takes into account that although anorexia and cachexia may be of concern in select subsets of cancer patients (i.e., those diagnosed with specific gastro-intestinal, respiratory, or head and neck cancers, or those diagnosed with later stage disease) for the majority of cancer survivors, obesity and overweight are problems that are far more prevalent.[5,9,17,18,20] Indeed, data suggest that in the two largest segments of cancer survivors, that is, survivors of breast and prostate cancer, the prevalence of overweight and obesity (body mass index [BMI] >24.9) exceeds 70%, whereas the prevalence of underweight (BMI <18.5) is nil.[21] These data are not surprising given that obesity is a well-established risk factor for cancers of the breast (postmenopausal), colon, kidney (renal cell), esophagus (adenocarcinoma), and endometrium.[7,19] Increased premorbid body weight and/or body weight at the time of diagnosis also has been associated with increased mortality (overall and cancer-specific) for all cancers combined and specifically for non-Hodgkin lymphoma and multiple myeloma, and cancers of the breast, esophagus, colon and rectum, cervix, uterus, liver, gallbladder, stomach, pancreas, prostate, and kidney.[22] Finally, additional weight gain is common during or after treatment for a variety of cancers.[17,18,20,23] Such weight gain has been found to reduce QOL and exacerbate risk for functional decline, co-morbidity, and perhaps even cancer recurrence and cancer-related death.[15,20] While studies exploring the relationship between postdiagnosis weight gain and disease-free survival have been somewhat inconsistent,[15,17,18,23] one of the largest studies (n = 5204) by Kroenke et al.[15] found that breast cancer survivors who experienced increases in BMI after diagnosis of at least 0.5 units had a significantly higher relative risk (RR) of recurrence and all-cause mortality. This accumulating evidence of adverse effects of obesity in cancer survivors, plus evidence indicating that obesity has negative consequences for overall health and physical function make weight management a priority for cancer survivors.[5,9,13,18–20] While

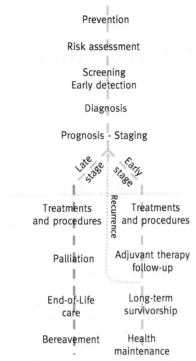

Fig. 78–1. Conceptual framework for care along the cancer continuum. Modified from Rose et al.[1]

Table 78–1. Nutrition guidelines for cancer survivors

Diet or nutrition factor	American Cancer Society (2006)[18]	World Cancer Fund/ American Institute for Cancer Research (2007)[19]
Weight	Achieve and maintain a healthy weight	Be as lean as possible without becoming underweight
Dietary pattern	*Consume a healthy diet with an emphasis on plant sources* Choose foods and beverages in amounts that achieve and maintain a healthy weight Eat five or more servings of a variety of fruits and vegetables/day Choose whole grains in preference to refined grains Limit consumption of processed and red meat	Avoid sugary drinks, limit energy-dense foods (foods high in sugar and fat, and low in fiber) Eat more of a variety of vegetables, fruits, whole grains, and legumes Limit consumption of processed and red meat
Other		Limit consumption of salty foods
Alcohol	If drink limit to 1–2 drinks/day	If drink limit to 1–2 drinks/day
Supplements	Don't use supplements to protect against cancer	Don't use supplements to protect against cancer

the pursuit of a desirable weight can be postponed until primary treatment is complete, among patients who are overweight or obese there are no contraindications to a modest rate of weight loss (no more than two pounds per week) during treatment as long as the oncologist approves and it does not interfere with treatment.[17,18]

To date, there have been a handful of studies that have tested weight-loss interventions among cancer survivors, with one of these studies aimed at endometrial cancer survivors,[24] and the remainder targeting breast cancer survivors.[5,9,20,25] By-in-large these studies have been feasibility trials, with the largest enrolling 107 participants. While the earliest of these trials experienced difficulty with recruitment due to reported disbelief that obesity is a problem for cancer patients, more recent trials have found high levels of interest for weight-loss interventions among cancer survivors.[20] In general, larger weight losses have been observed with interventions that utilize theory-driven models and group support.

While energy restriction can be achieved by portion control and reducing the energy density of the diet via the substitution of low-energy density foods (e.g., water-rich vegetables, fruits, whole grains, and soups) for foods that are higher in calories,[26] more intensive programs that promote energy deficits of up to 1000 calories/day may yield better results.[27] Therefore, overweight survivors may benefit from set reductions in energy intake, in combination with increased energy expenditure (via exercise), since previous studies have found exercise to be a strong predictor of weight loss among cancer survivors.[20] In addition, given evidence that sarcopenic obesity (gain of adipose tissue at the expense of lean body mass) is a documented side effect of both chemotherapy and hormonal therapy,[20,28] exercise, especially resistance exercise, may be especially important for cancer survivors since it is considered the cornerstone of treatment for this condition (see Chapter 61 for further detail). Until more is known, guidelines established for weight management in the general population should be applied to cancer survivors, and include not only dietary and exercise components, but also behavior therapy.[17,18,29]

Dietary pattern. The choice of foods and their proportions within an overall diet (dietary pattern) may be more important than absolute amounts.[18–20] Given that cancer survivors are at high risk for other chronic diseases, guidelines suggest prudent diets that rely heavily on unrefined plant foods such as fruits, vegetables and whole grains, and which contain limited amounts of fat, simple sugars, and red or processed meats.[7,17–19] Observational studies of breast cancer survivors (n = 2619) and colorectal cancer survivors (n = 1009) within the Nurse's Health Study cohort suggest that as compared to those who reported a Western-type diet (e.g., high proportional intakes of meat, refined grains, high-fat dairy products, and desserts), those who reported a prudent diet (e.g., high proportional intakes of fruits, vegetables, whole grains, and low-fat dairy products) had significantly better outcomes, for example, improved overall survival and reduced rates of colorectal recurrence and mortality, respectively.[30,31] Furthermore, cross-sectional data from 714 breast cancer survivors participating in the Health, Eating, Activity and Lifestyle (HEAL) study, as well as 688 elderly breast and prostate cancer survivors, suggest that diet quality during survivorship is significantly and positively associated with mental and/or physical functioning.[32,33] A recent randomized controlled trial among 641 overweight elderly breast, colorectal and prostate cancer survivors indeed found significantly improved physical functioning with a multicomponent intervention that promoted improvements in diet quality and physical activity with concomitant weight loss.[34]

In contrast, no differences were observed in either disease-free or overall survival in the recently completed Women's Healthy Eating and Living (WHEL) trial, which tested a low fat, high fiber, and high fruit and vegetable (i.e., three fruit servings, five vegetable servings plus 16 oz. of vegetable juice per day) diet against usual care among 3088 pre- and postmenopausal women followed over 7 years.[35] Null findings have been attributed to high baseline fruit and vegetable intakes in both study arms (mean of 7.4 servings/day), as well as an absence of weight loss, despite the low-energy density diet.[36] Indeed, findings of WHEL differ markedly from the Women's Intervention Nutrition Study (WINS), in which the dietary intervention was solely focused on dietary fat restriction (<15% of total energy) and tested against a healthy diet.[37] In this trial of 2437 post-menopausal women followed for 5 years, a significantly reduced risk of recurrence was observed (Hazards Ratio: 0.76; 95% Confidence Interval: 0.60, 0.98) among women assigned to the low-fat diet, an effect which was even stronger among participants with estrogen-receptor negative disease. These findings, however, may have been confounded by the six pound weight loss observed with the low-fat diet over the course of the study period (data which reinforce the importance of weight control as a key lifestyle factor in cancer survivors).

Thus, in summary, dietary pattern may be important for QOL and the prevention of various co-morbid conditions among survivors. Furthermore, diet pattern also may play a role in energy regulation and weight maintenance, which appears to be a key issue, not only for survivors, but also for the population-at-large (pun intended). Other recommendations that pertain to the avoidance of red and processed meats, as well as limiting the consumption of salty foods are based more on the prevention of select cancers (i.e., colorectal and other aero-digestive cancers),[17-19] and for which survivors may be at greater risk given their increased susceptibility for second primaries.[4]

Alcohol use. National data from the United States and Australia suggest that while moderate-to-heavy drinking is noted more frequently among select groups of cancer survivors (i.e., survivors of head, neck, lung, and prostate cancers), alcohol consumption among cancer survivors overall is similar to that of the general population.[38,39] Furthermore, alcohol-use diminishes significantly with age, and "risky-use" (>2 drinks per day for men and >1 drink/day in women) is noted among only 4.1% of cancer survivors who are age 65 and older.[38] The low prevalence of risky drinking among the majority of cancer survivors, plus the proven cardio-protective benefit of light alcohol consumption form the basis of the recommendations established by both the ACS and the WCF/AICR.[18,19] However, continued alcohol-use is strongly discouraged among survivors of renal and head and neck cancers due to significantly higher rates of treatment complications, co-morbidity, and second cancers.[12] Currently, the "jury is still out" regarding alcohol-use among breast cancer survivors.[18] On one hand, alcohol is associated with increased primary risk of breast cancer in a population where risk is already high; however, balancing that are data which show no increase in risk of recurrence or all-cause mortality among breast cancer survivors.[18,20] Furthermore, recent findings suggest a 55% reduction in rates of ovarian cancer (95% confidence interval: 0.2–1.0) among breast survivors who continue to imbibe.[40]

SMOKING CESSATION

As noted in the Institute of Medicine (IOM) report, "*From cancer patient to cancer survivor – lost in translation*," nearly one-third of all cancers are caused by smoking, thus there is a high likelihood of tobacco-use among survivors, especially those who have been diagnosed with smoking-related malignancies, that is, lung, head and neck, cervix, bladder, kidney, pancreas, and myeloid leukemia.[7] Persistent tobacco-use after diagnosis also is associated with poorer outcomes, including increased complications of treatment, progressive disease, second primaries, and increased co-morbidity.[10] Thus, while smoking cessation plays a substantial role in prevention and primary care, this need is heightened among cancer survivors,[10] and may be even more critical among survivors of heritable cancers who may be particularly sensitive to the carcinogenic effects of tobacco.[41] Fortunately, the cancer diagnosis, especially if it is a tobacco-related cancer, often prompts many patients to stop smoking, as evidenced by quit rates that exceed 50%.[10,42] Unfortunately these early successes are often short-lived, as evidenced by substantial rates of relapse, which are unsurprising given that most institutions fail to offer their survivors smoking prevention (61%) or cessation (75%) programs, and many even lack a referral system (42%).[10] Recent data from the National Health Interview Survey also suggest that current smoking rates may be especially high in younger cancer survivors (ages 18–40) than in the general population, though subsequent controlled analyses on data with longer follow-up suggest that these differences may not be as discrepant as previously thought.[38]

Given evidence that combined interventions that utilize behavioral counseling along with pharmacotherapy are effective, definitive guidelines exist for providing care as it relates to smoking cessation. The 5-A approach endorsed by the U.S. Preventive Services Task Force provides a concrete framework for healthcare providers to deliver appropriate care regarding smoking cessation, and is a featured element within the IOM report.[7] Despite this extant framework, the barriers to long-standing smoking cessation success are substantial, and findings from intervention trials have been mixed. The IOM report provides a solid overview of studies conducted up until 2005 and notes the significance of smoking cessation within the survivor population and the numerous barriers that exist.[7] In an important study which appeared after this report, Emmons et al. found that a peer telephone counseling intervention with tailored materials was effective in promoting higher quit rates in 796 currently smoking adult childhood cancer survivors both at 8-month (16.8% vs. 8.5%; *p* <0.01) and 12-month follow-up (15% vs. 9%; *p* <0.01).[43] This home-based intervention also was found to be cost effective. This recent positive trial not only is important for it's contribution to smoking cessation research, but also paves the way more generally for future health promotion programs by testing innovative strategies that are well-accepted and more readily disseminable to survivor populations who often are hard to reach. As with other lifestyle interventions, more research is necessary to determine approaches that are optimally effective and that promote permanent smoking cessation in what is likely to be a particularly resistant population. Furthermore, since smokers are likely to practice other unhealthful behaviors (i.e., sedentary behavior, high-red meat consumption, and excessive alcohol-use) they also may be prime candidates for multiple risk factor interventions.[5,7,42] As noted in the IOM report, as well as in other studies, smokers may benefit especially from interventions that incorporate social or familial support.[7]

SUN-PROTECTIVE BEHAVIORS AND SKIN CANCER SCREENING

While recent findings suggest that vitamin D and modest sunlight exposure may be protective, not only for the primary risk of some solid tumors, but also for survival of select cancers,[44,45] it also is well-known that for many cancer survivors, especially those who received locoregional radiotherapy and hematopoietic cell transplantation, the risk for melanoma and basal cell skin cancers is high and may be exacerbated by exposure to the sun.[46,47] Thus, at a minimum all cancer survivors should be closely monitored for skin cancers, and sun-protective behaviors should be endorsed for those who are know to be at increased risk for melanoma (survivors of melanoma and survivors who received locoregional radiotherapy and hematopoietic stem cell radiation). A recent study by Manne and Lessin of 229 melanoma survivors; however, suggests only moderate adherence to such guidelines, and suggests a need for interventions.[48] To date, only one trial has been reported which addressed sun exposure in 200 survivor-caregiver dyads. This study, although effective, is more than decade old.[49]

HEALTH BEHAVIOR CHANGE AND PREFERENCES FOR DELIVERY AMONG CANCER SURVIVORS

Levels of interest in lifestyle interventions among cancer survivors. A recent review by Stull et al.[50] suggests that while most survivors attribute their cancer diagnosis to factors beyond their control (with the exception of tobacco use), they often become interested in modifying their diet and exercise behaviors after diagnosis in hopes of "preventing recurrence." Surveys among adult survivor populations suggest "extremely high to very high" levels of interest in diet (54%) and exercise (51%) interventions, as well as comparable levels of interest in smoking cessation programs (60%), among adult cancer survivors who currently smoke.[21] These findings are remarkably similar in pediatric cancer survivor populations, with even higher levels of interest noted among their parents.[51] Van Weert et al.[52] recently reported even higher levels of interest (80%) in multiple behavior interventions. Thus, the cancer diagnosis may signal an opportune time or a "teachable moment" for undertaking health behavior change.[5,10,42] While some reviews and recent studies suggest that cancer survivors may begin to adopt healthier lifestyle practices on their own,[5,53,54] large population-based studies in the United States and Australia suggest that, for the most part, cancer survivors' health behaviors parallel those of the general population—a population marked by inactivity; overweight or obesity; suboptimal fruit, vegetable, and fiber consumption; and high intakes of fat.[38,39] Similar results were found in another study that tracked lifestyle behaviors longitudinally over time in a cohort of women (n = 2321) with early stage breast cancer.[23] These studies suggest that although many cancer patients report healthful lifestyle changes after diagnosis, these changes may not generalize to all populations of cancer survivors, may be temporary, or may indicate that even after undertaking behavior change, cancer survivors' behaviors are similar to the general population.[9] Given higher rates of co-morbidity among survivors and evidence that diet, exercise, and tobacco-use affect risk for other cancers and other chronic diseases, these recent data support a tremendous need for lifestyle interventions that target the vulnerable population of cancer survivors.

Preferences, barriers, and other considerations in delivering lifestyle interventions to cancer survivors. While cancer survivors may have high levels of interest in lifestyle interventions, they may have special needs (i.e., fatigue, incontinence, lymphedema, food intolerances or digestive disorders, long-term addictions to tobacco or alcohol, etc.) that must be considered if attempts to promote healthful lifestyle practices are to succeed.[50] Timing of interventions also may be of critical importance, since readiness to pursue various lifestyle changes may wax and wane along the survivorship continuum. Findings from a survey study of 978 breast and prostate cancer survivors suggest that while most survivors prefer lifestyle interventions that are initiated at the "time of diagnosis or soon thereafter"; interventions offered "anytime" also garner high levels of interest.[21] Given evidence that levels of psychological distress after diagnosis differ in males (low initial levels which decrease significantly over time) versus females (high initial levels that decrease less precipitously), it is postulated that optimal intervention timing may differ between the sexes.[55] Thus, interventions that capitalize on moderate levels of distress (not too overwhelming, but enough to motivate behavior change) may yield the best results; however, this statement is speculative at best, and there are no firm data yet to support it. Other factors, such as concurrent demands of treatment and rehabilitation are likely to play key roles influencing distress and readiness to pursue lifestyle change.[6] The targeted behavior, the patients' self-efficacy in pursuing behavior change, and various patient characteristics also are likely to influence uptake.[11,50] For example, in a recent study that tested the feasibility of a home-based diet and exercise intervention to prevent adverse body composition change among 90 breast cancer patients during active treatment, Demark-Wahnefried and colleagues found that while participants demonstrated excellent adherence to a low-fat, high-fruit, and vegetable and calcium-rich diet, their adherence to strength training and aerobic exercise was much poorer.[56] These results differed remarkably from a smaller pilot study (n = 10) that tested the feasibility of a clinic-based diet and exercise program conducted by the same investigators which found excellent adherence to both the diet and exercise components.[57] Of note, however, there was a much higher refusal rate for the clinic-based study (55% vs. 19%), and the subjects who agreed to participate in the clinic-based program also appeared much more fit, as indicated by a BMI mean of 24.1 versus 25.8. This comparison provides an overarching example of the biases that are inherent in conducting intervention research among cancer survivors or for that matter any population, that is, the individuals who enroll are likely to be much different than the population for which you hope to generalize findings—bias that is accentuated with increasing demands placed on the study population (e.g., travel, time) and in accruing self-referrals versus Population-based samples (i.e., those ascertained from cancer registries).[58,59]

As reviewed by Stull et al.[50] the preponderance of reported health behavior interventions among cancer survivors have been conducted in self-referred or clinic-recruited samples and have utilized clinic-based interventions. Although the potential acceptability and reach for home-based interventions is notably greater than for clinic-based programs, to date relatively few studies have employed this approach. Indeed, more research is necessary in this arena, especially since time and travel are well-recognized and significant barriers to participation.[59] Telephone counseling has offered traditional means of addressing the barrier of distance and has been used with varying levels of success among cancer survivors, as well as in other high-risk populations.[11,35,43,50] Web-based formats offer future promise; however, access issues may serve as barriers among cancer survivors who tend to be elderly.[11] Indeed, interventions that are delivered via mailed print materials receive the highest levels of interest, not only in a sample of 978 breast and prostate cancer survivors (mean age of 63 years), but also among 209 childhood cancer survivors (mean age of 19).[21,51] Similarly, Rutten et al.[60] reported that cancer survivors were twice as likely to report reliance on print materials as sources of health information rather than the internet or other media sources. It is currently unknown whether these results are apt to change over time or whether there is a definite hard-set preference for print materials over computer-based venues. The salience of distance-medicine based approaches, whether they are delivered via the telephone, the mail, the web, or via other home-based approaches is especially important for interventions that target highly mobile or geographically-dispersed survivor populations (e.g., childhood cancer survivors) or those needing long-term follow-up.

While the mode of intervention delivery is important, the use of behavioral theory to guide intervention development and evaluation is perhaps even more critical. Recent reviews however, of dietary, exercise, and smoking cessation intervention trials suggest that less than one-third are theoretically based.[50] This is unfortunate since a solidly designed intervention that "fits" behavioral theory to the targeted behavior and the needs of the study sample not only has an increased probability of success, but also has the advantage of being perceived by participants as "a well-conceived" study, and more likely to reduce attrition. To date and among cancer survivors, the most frequently-used theories for behavioral interventions have been Social Cognitive Theory, the Theory of Planned Behavior, and the Transtheoretical Model.[50,61–63] Multibehavior interventions can particularly benefit from a solid and unified theoretical framework, which can enhance the organization and presentation of key components, and allow a systematic approach for testing issues such as behavioral sequencing.

BRIDGING THE GAP—HOW CAN WE LINK CANCER SURVIVORS TO THE INTERVENTIONS THAT THEY NEED AND/OR WANT?

While the preceding sections of this chapter were devoted to reviewing some of the important health behaviors for cancer survivors, and then reviewed some of the "what," "where," "when," and "how's" of intervening to improve health behaviors, the last topic remaining is "who." "Who" should receive the intervention? and "who" should deliver it? In the realm of cancer survivorship, such interventions could benefit not only survivors (as a means of tertiary or quaternary prevention), but also family members who might be at increased risk and who may derive primary preventive benefit. In addition, family members, especially if they receive appropriate training, could serve as a source of support for interventions that target the cancer survivor. Indeed, much more research is needed in both of these areas. Likewise, "who" delivers the intervention also can make an impact, and also is an area where more research is needed. That being said, what is known is that the recommendation of the healthcare provider is a critical first step in motivating patients to consider lifestyle change. Jones et al.[64] found that the oncologist's recommendation directly influenced perceived behavioral control and was associated with increased physical activity in a randomized controlled trial of 450 breast cancer survivors. Unfortunately, data suggest that only a minority of oncology care physicians appear to offer guidance regarding healthful lifestyle change, and report barriers, such as competing treatment or health concerns, time constraints, or uncertainty regarding the delivery of appropriate health behavior messages.[21,65] Therefore, strategies are needed to efficiently and effectively bring to bear the motivational power of the physician.

SUMMARY

As the number of cancer survivors continues to grow world-wide, so too does the need for effective health promotion interventions. While research has begun on crafting interventions aimed at improving the lifestyle behaviors of this vulnerable population, more research is needed to develop innovative approaches that can most effectively accomplish the following: (1) promote behavior change in content areas that are most likely to contribute to the overall health and well-being of cancer survivors; (2) provide delivery at a point in time most likely to ensure uptake; (3) combine or sequence messages to facilitate change in multiple arenas; (4) use delivery channels and formats that are well understood, well accepted, and cost effective; (5) provide guidance to overcome common barriers; and (6) target cancer populations that are currently underserved, and/or most in need (i.e., survivors diagnosed with underrepresented cancers, minorities, and the elderly), as well as to extend interventions to other survivorship populations (i.e., caretakers or other family members).

REFERENCES

1. Rose JH, O'Toole E, Koroukian S, Berger N. Geriatric oncology and primary care: promoting partnerships in practice and research. *J Am Geriatr Soc.* In press.

2. Ries LAG MD, Krapcho M, et al. (eds.) *SEER cancer statistics review, 1975–2004.* www.seer.cancer.gov/csr/1975_2004. Accessed July 14, 2008.

3. Aziz NM. Cancer survivorship research: state of knowledge, challenges and opportunities. *Acta Oncol.* 2007;46:417–432.

4. Ng AK, Travis LB. Second primary cancers: an overview. *Hematol Oncol Clin North Am.* 2008;22(2):271–289.

5. Demark-Wahnefried W, Aziz NM, Rowland JH, Pinto BM. Riding the crest of the teachable moment: promoting long-term health after the diagnosis of cancer. *J Clin Oncol.* 2005;23(24):5814–5830.

6. Ganz PA. Psychological and social aspects of breast cancer. *Oncol (Williston Park).* 2008;22(6):642–646, 650–653.

7. Hewitt M, Greenfield S, Stovall EL. *Institute of medicine and national research council: From cancer patient to cancer survivors: Lost in transition.* Washington, DC: National Academies Press; 2005.

8. American Cancer Society. Cancer Facts & Figures – 2008. American Cancer Society, 2008. http://www.cancer.org/docroot/MIT/content/MIT_3_2X_Costs_of_Cancer.asp

9. Jones LW, Demark-Wahnefried W. Diet, exercise, and complementary therapies after primary treatment for cancer. *Lancet Oncol.* 2006;7(12):1017–1026.

10. Gritz ER, Fingeret MC, Vidrine DJ, Lazev AB, Mehta NV, Reece GP. Successes and failures of the teachable moment: smoking cessation in cancer patients. *Cancer.* 2006;106(1):17–27.

11. Pinto BM, Trunzo JJ. Health behaviors during and after a cancer diagnosis. *Cancer.* 2005;104(Suppl 11):2614–2623.

12. Deleyiannis FW, Thomas DB, Vaughan TL, Davis S. Alcoholism: independent predictor of survival in patients with head and neck cancer. *J Natl Cancer Inst.* 1996;88(8):542–549.

13. Chlebowski RT, Aiello E, McTiernan A. Weight loss in breast cancer patient management. *J Clin Oncol.* 2002;20(4):1128–1143.

14. Holmes MD, Chen WY, Feskanich D, Kroenke CH, Colditz GA. Physical activity and survival after breast cancer diagnosis. *JAMA.* 2005;293(20):2479–2486.

15. Kroenke CH, Chen WY, Rosner B, Holmes MD. Weight, weight gain, and survival after breast cancer diagnosis. *J Clin Oncol.* 2005;23(7):1370–1378.

16. Meyerhardt JA, Heseltine D, Niedzwiecki D, et al. Impact of physical activity on cancer recurrence and survival in patients with stage III colon cancer: findings from CALGB 89803. *J Clin Oncol.* 2006;24(22):3535–3541.

17. Brown JK, Byers T, Doyle C, et al. Nutrition and physical activity during and after cancer treatment: an American Cancer Society guide for informed choices. *CA Cancer J Clin.* 2003;53(5):268–291.

18. Doyle C, Kushi LH, Byers T, et al. Nutrition and physical activity during and after cancer treatment: an American Cancer Society guide for informed choices. *CA Cancer J Clin.* 2006;56(6):323–353.

19. World Cancer Fund—American Institute for Cancer Research. *Food, nutrition, physical activity and the prevention of cancer: A global perspective.* http://www.dietandcancerreport.org/. Accessed July 14, 2008.

20. Rock CL, Demark-Wahnefried W. Nutrition and survival after the diagnosis of breast cancer: a review of the evidence. *J Clin Oncol.* 2002;20(15):3302–3316.

21. Demark-Wahnefried W, Peterson B, McBride C, Lipkus I, Clipp E. Current health behaviors and readiness to pursue life-style changes among men and women diagnosed with early stage prostate and breast carcinomas. *Cancer.* 2000;88(3):674–684.

22. Calle EE, Rodriguez C, Walker-Thurmond K, Thun MJ. Overweight, obesity, and mortality from cancer in a prospectively studied cohort of U.S. adults. *N Engl J Med.* 2003;348(17):1625–1638.

23. Caan B, Sternfeld B, Gunderson E, Coates A, Quesenberry C, Slattery ML. Life After Cancer Epidemiology (LACE) Study: a cohort of early stage breast cancer survivors (United States). *Cancer Causes Control.* 2005;16(5):545–556.

24. von Gruenigen VE, Courneya KS, Gibbons HE, Kavanagh MB, Waggoner SE, Lerner E. Feasibility and effectiveness of a lifestyle intervention program in obese endometrial cancer patients: a randomized trial. *Gynecol Oncol.* 2008;109(1):19–26.

25. Mefferd K, Nichols JF, Pakiz B, Rock CL. A cognitive behavioral therapy intervention to promote weight loss improves body composition and blood lipid profiles among overweight breast cancer survivors. *Breast Cancer Res Treat.* 2007;104(2):145–152.

26. Rolls BJ, Roe LS, Meengs JS. Reductions in portion size and energy density of foods are additive and lead to sustained decreases in energy intake. *Am J Clin Nutr.* 2006;83(1):11–17.

27. Saquib N, Natarajan L, Rock CL, et al. The impact of a long-term reduction in dietary energy density on body weight within a randomized diet trial. *Nutr Cancer.* 2008;60(1):31–38.

28. Demark-Wahnefried W, Peterson BL, Winer EP, et al. Changes in weight, body composition, and factors influencing energy balance among premenopausal breast cancer patients receiving adjuvant chemotherapy. *J Clin Oncol.* 2001;19(9):2381–2389.

29. National Heart Lung and Blood Institute. *The practical guide: Identification, evaluation, and treatment of overweight and obesity in adults.* Vol NIH Pub No. 00–4084; 2000.

30. Kroenke CH, Fung TT, Hu FB, Holmes MD. Dietary patterns and survival after breast cancer diagnosis. *J Clin Oncol.* 2005;23(36):9295–9303.

31. Meyerhardt JA, Niedzwiecki D, Hollis D, et al. Association of dietary patterns with cancer recurrence and survival in patients with stage III colon cancer. *JAMA.* 2007;298(7):754–764.

32. Demark-Wahnefried W, Clipp EC, Morey MC, et al. Physical function and associations with diet and exercise: results of a cross-sectional survey among elders with breast or prostate cancer. *Int J Behav Nutr Phys Act.* 2004;1(1):16.

33. Wayne SJ, Baumgartner K, Baumgartner RN, Bernstein L, Bowen DJ, Ballard-Barbash R. Diet quality is directly associated with quality of life in breast cancer survivors. *Breast Cancer Res Treat.* 2006;96(3):227–232.

34. Morey MC, Snyder DC, Sloane R, et al. Effects of home-based diet and exercise on functional outcomes among older, overweight long-term cancer survivors. RENEW: A randomized controlled trial. *JAMA.* 2009;301:1883–1891.

35. Pierce JP, Natarajan L, Caan BJ, et al. Influence of a diet very high in vegetables, fruit, and fiber and low in fat on prognosis following treatment for breast cancer: the Women's Healthy Eating and Living (WHEL) randomized trial. *JAMA.* 2007;298(3):289–298.

36. Gapstur SM, Khan S. Fat, fruits, vegetables, and breast cancer survivorship. *JAMA.* 2007;298(3):335–336.

37. Chlebowski RT, Blackburn GL, Thomson CA, et al. Dietary fat reduction and breast cancer outcome: interim efficacy results from the Women's Intervention Nutrition Study. *J Natl Cancer Inst.* 2006;98(24):1767–76.

38. Bellizzi KM, Rowland JH, Jeffery DD, McNeel T. Health behaviors of cancer survivors: examining opportunities for cancer control intervention. *J Clin Oncol.* 2005;23(34):8884–8893.

39. Eakin EG, Youlden DR, Baade PD, et al. Health behaviors of cancer survivors: data from an Australian population-based survey. *Cancer Causes Control.* 2007;18(8):881–894.

40. Trentham-Dietz A, Newcomb PA, Nichols HB, Hampton JM. Breast cancer risk factors and second primary malignancies among women with breast cancer. *Breast Cancer Res Treat.* 2007;105(2):195–207.

41. Foster MC, Kleinerman RA, Abramson DH, Seddon JM, Tarone RE, Tucker MA. Tobacco use in adult long-term survivors of retinoblastoma. *Cancer Epidemiol Biomarkers Prev.* 2006;15(8):1464–1468.

42. McBride CM, Ostroff JS. Teachable moments for promoting smoking cessation: the context of cancer care and survivorship. *Cancer Control.* 2003;10(4):325–333.

43. Emmons KM, Puleo E, Park E, et al. Peer-delivered smoking counseling for childhood cancer survivors increases rate of cessation: the partnership for health study. *J Clin Oncol.* 2005;23(27):6516–6523.

44. Giovannucci E, Liu Y, Rimm EB, et al. Prospective study of predictors of vitamin D status and cancer incidence and mortality in men. *J Natl Cancer Inst.* 2006;98(7):451–459.

45. Zhou W, Suk R, Liu G, et al. Vitamin D is associated with improved survival in early-stage non-small cell lung cancer patients. *Cancer Epidemiol Biomarkers Prev.* 2005;14(10):2303–2309.

46. Leisenring W, Friedman DL, Flowers ME, Schwartz JL, Deeg HJ. Nonmelanoma skin and mucosal cancers after hematopoietic cell transplantation. *J Clin Oncol.* 2006;24(7):1119–1126.

47. Maule M, Scelo G, Pastore G, et al. Risk of second malignant neoplasms after childhood leukemia and lymphoma: an international study. *J Natl Cancer Inst.* 2007;99(10):790–800.

48. Manne S, Lessin S. Prevalence and correlates of sun protection and skin self-examination practices among cutaneous malignant melanoma survivors. *J Behav Med.* 2006;29(5):419–434.

49. Robinson JK, Rademaker AW. Skin cancer risk and sun protection learning by helpers of patients with nonmelanoma skin cancer. *Prev Med.* 1995;24(4):333–341.

50. Stull VB, Snyder DC, Demark-Wahnefried W. Lifestyle interventions in cancer survivors: designing programs that meet the needs of this vulnerable and growing population. *J Nutr.* 2007;137:243S–248S.

51. Demark-Wahnefried W, Werner C, Clipp EC, et al. Survivors of childhood cancer and their guardians. *Cancer.* 2005;103(10):2171–2180.

52. van Weert E, Hoekstra-Weebers J, Grol B, et al. A multidimensional cancer rehabilitation program for cancer survivors: effectiveness on health-related quality of life. *J Psychosom Res.* 2005;58(6):485–496.

53. Alfano CM, Day JM, Katz ML, et al. Exercise and dietary change after diagnosis and cancer-related symptoms in long-term survivors of breast cancer: CALGB 79804. *Psycho Oncology.* 2008; http://www3.interscience.wiley.com/cgi-bin/fulltext/119815598/PDFSTART. Accessed July 21, 2008.

54. Humpel N, Magee C, Jones SC. The impact of a cancer diagnosis on the health behaviors of cancer survivors and their family and friends. *Support Care Cancer.* 2007;15(6):621–630.

55. McBride CM, Clipp E, Peterson BL, Lipkus IM, Demark-Wahnefried W. Psychological impact of diagnosis and risk reduction among cancer survivors. *Psychooncol.* 2000;9(5):418–427.

56. Demark-Wahnefried W, Case LD, Blackwell K, et al. Results of a diet/exercise feasibility trial to prevent adverse body composition change in breast cancer patients on adjuvant chemotherapy. *Clin Breast Cancer.* 2008;8(1):70–79.

57. Demark-Wahnefried W, Kenyon AJ, Eberle P, Skye A, Kraus WE. Preventing sarcopenic obesity among breast cancer patients who receive adjuvant chemotherapy: results of a feasibility study. *Clin Exerc Physiol.* 2002;4(1):44–49.

58. Snyder DC, Sloane R, Lobach D, et al. Differences in baseline characteristics and outcomes at 1- and 2-year follow-up of cancer survivors accrued via self-referral versus cancer registry in the FRESH START diet and exercise trial. *Cancer Epidemiol Biomarkers Prev.* 2008;17(5):1288–1294.

59. Watson JM, Torgerson DJ. Increasing recruitment to randomised trials: a review of randomised controlled trials. *BMC Med Res Methodol.* 2006;6:34–46.

60. Rutten LJ, Arora NK, Bakos AD, Aziz N, Rowland J. Information needs and sources of information among cancer patients: a systematic review of research (1980–2003). *Patient Educ Couns.* 2005;57(3):250–261.

61. Ajzen I. From intentions to actions: a theory of planned behavior. In: J Kuhl, J Beckman, (eds). *Action-control: From cognition to behavior.* Heidelberg: Springer; 1985:11–39.

62. Bandura A. *Social learning theory.* Englewood Cliffs, NJ: Prentice Hall; 1977.

63. Prochaska JO, DiClemente CC. Stages and processes of self-change of smoking: toward an integrative model of change. *J Consult Clin Psychol.* 1983;51(3):390–395.

64. Jones LW, Courneya KS, Fairey AS, Mackey JR. Effects of an oncologist's recommendation to exercise on self-reported exercise behavior in newly diagnosed breast cancer survivors: a single-blind, randomized controlled trial. *Ann Behav Med.* 2004;28(2):105–113.

65. Sabatino SA, Coates RJ, Uhler RJ, Pollack LA, Alley LG, Zauderer LJ. Provider counseling about health behaviors among cancer survivors in the United States. *J Clin Oncol.* 2007;25(15):2100–2106.

CHAPTER 79

Implementing the Survivorship Care Plan: A Strategy for Improving the Quality of Care for Cancer Survivors

Patricia A. Ganz and Erin E. Hahn

INTRODUCTION AND BACKGROUND

Looming before us is a major expansion of the number of individuals diagnosed with cancer, simply by virtue of the aging of the population and the high incidence of cancer as part of the aging process. Maintaining the quality of care for these new cancer survivors will be challenged by an anticipated shortage of health professionals—medical oncologists and nurses—to care for the increased number of newly diagnosed and surviving cancer patients.[1] Although the National Coalition for Cancer Survivorship and the National Cancer Institute's Office of Cancer Survivorship define survivorship as beginning at the time of diagnosis and extending through death, a recent Institute of Medicine (IOM) report on adult cancer survivors (described below) focused on the posttreatment phase of the cancer survivorship continuum.[2] This phase was described as needing specific attention, especially with regard to coordination and quality of care. Thus, in this chapter, we focus on posttreatment cancer survivors, and the survivorship care plan.

Over the past decade, the IOM has been engaged in a concerted effort to examine the quality of health care in the United States, and to identify critical issues that are central to improving the delivery of healthcare to the population. The IOM definition of quality is "the degree to which health services for individuals and populations increase the likelihood of desired outcomes and are consistent with current professional knowledge."[3] In its investigations of quality of care, various IOM committees have identified overuse, misuse, and underuse of healthcare services, as well as poor coordination of care, especially for those individuals with chronic illness. In particular, one of the first IOM investigations of quality of care focused on the disparities in cancer care service delivery in the 1999 report Ensuring Quality Cancer Care[4] in which a wide gulf was found between ideal cancer care and that received by most Americans. Subsequently, the IOM Committee on Quality of Health Care in America issued two key reports: *To err is human: Building a safer health system*[5] and *Crossing the quality chasm: a new health system for the 21st century,*[6] that laid the foundation and created the vision for the transformation that is necessary to improve the quality of healthcare. The former high-profile report brought to public attention the high human and fiscal cost of medical errors and the critical issue of patient safety, while the latter identified six key dimensions of quality healthcare (safety, effectiveness, patient centered, timely, efficient, equitable) that should be the focus of improvement efforts within the healthcare system.

With this background in mind, in 2004 the National Cancer Policy Board and the IOM established a committee on cancer survivorship to examine issues related to improving care and quality of life.[2] Early in its deliberations, the committee decided to focus its efforts on describing the quality of care needs for patients with cancer who were beyond the acute phase of treatment and living with cancer—and its aftermath—as a chronic disease. The resulting IOM report, *From cancer patient to cancer survivor: Lost in transition*, outlines the key issues facing cancer survivors and makes concrete recommendations as to how to address these problems. Fig. 79–1 describes the cancer care trajectory and highlights the enlarging time/phase/place in which patients live free of cancer, but often with burdens of long-term and late effects.

Why is cancer survivor care special? Shouldn't coordination of care between specialist and generalists be expected? Cancer patients often require treatment by multiple specialists (surgeons, radiation oncologists, medical oncologists) due the use of multimodal therapies and the frequent use of organ sparing treatments. Chemotherapy administration may require both inpatient and outpatient visits, and radiation therapy may not be given in the same facility where surgery and chemotherapy are received. As a result, there is seldom a single integrated medical record and there may be limited formal (written) communication between the specialists. Primary care providers are often not included in the management of the patient during this time, and it may be months to years after the completion of treatment that the patient returns for regular check-ups with the primary care provider. In addition, patients may become so focused on the cancer and the potential risk of its recurrence that they may neglect other aspects of their health and have limited follow-up with their regular provider. Adding to this situation is the failure of the oncology care system to provide education and guidance to patients at the end of active cancer treatment—something that is very effective at diagnosis and during treatment—and as a result, the patient often feels "lost in transition." Although treatments may be completed, often patients are left with many physical symptoms, which for the most part gradually resolve. Oncology specialists are not always able to predict the time course of recovery, and many patients need a lot of psychological support during this time—something that is not always forthcoming. Thus, it is the intensity, complexity, and length of cancer treatment that magnifies the need for coordination of care during the phase of extended survival off cancer treatment.

Cancer survivors face some unique challenges. In the short-term, many survivors need to have an understanding of what treatments they received and what kind of follow-up is necessary. This is for their own information, so that they can understand how they can recover effectively, but also so they can tell others (family, friends, employer, other health professionals) what to expect. Often, they have put many activities on hold and they are looking forward to resuming a normal life. They need guidance during this early posttreatment time which is often lacking in the current healthcare delivery system. They are also eager to have a better understanding of whether there are any long-term effects of the treatments that need monitoring (e.g., cardiac or pulmonary toxicity, second cancers, etc.) and whether other specialists are required. There is a tendency to worry about every ache and pain, and during this time, many scans, and tests are likely to be done to look for cancer recurrence, and many additional specialists may be consulted.

There are some special populations that are worthy of mention, as their care coordination needs are more substantial. These include the

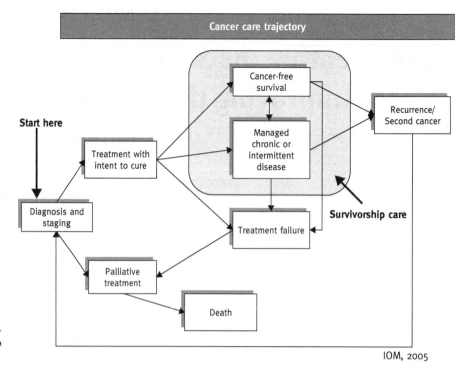

Fig. 79–1. The cancer treatment trajectory with special identification of the posttreatment survivorship care phase.

adult survivors of childhood cancer, who often suffer from an increased number of chronic conditions[7] as well as a substantial risk for second malignancies.[8,9] Bone marrow transplant patients (both children and adults) also sustain considerable toxicities from the conditioning regimens and risk for graft versus host disease. There are high rates of physical and psychological complications in this patient population.[10–12] Finally, older individuals make up the majority of cancer patients and survivors, and in the context of their follow-up care, co-morbid conditions may add to the specific toxicities of cancer treatment, especially cardiac, pulmonary, and renal toxicities.

As can be seen, there are many challenges associated with ensuring quality care for cancer survivors. One of the proposed first steps in accomplishing this is the widespread implementation of treatment summaries and survivorship care planning. This key recommendation of the IOM report has been embraced by a number of leading organizations, including the American Society of Clinical Oncology (ASCO). The Lance Armstrong Foundation LIVESTRONG Survivorship Centers of Excellence and others are also working hard to incorporate treatment summaries and care plans into their work. The *treatment summary and care plan* is seen as the roadmap and communication vehicle for quality care, and thus we will use this chapter to describe it in some detail. We will also provide some perspective on the health policy impact of survivorship care plans as they relate to current legislation, accountability, and quality improvement activities that are underway.

WHAT IS THE SURVIVORSHIP CARE PLAN?

The IOM report recommends the development and utilization of a treatment summary and survivorship care plan, a synoptic document that describes the patient's cancer treatment experience and provides guidance for the patient's future care. Per the recommendations from the IOM Workshop Summary *Implementing survivorship care planning,* [13] survivorship care plans should always contain certain core elements: a cancer treatment history, the potential long-term and late effects of treatment, recommended surveillance for long-term and late effects, and recommended surveillance for recurrence and new cancers.[13] Additionally, links to resources that provide psychosocial support for survivors should be included in the care plan, as well as information on general health and wellness for cancer survivors. The plan should also contain a clear timeline for the patient's follow-up care, and ideally will

identify the appropriate physician to provide it. These core items will allow for improved communication between the treating oncologist(s) and the primary care provider as well as educating and empowering the patient (see Tables 79–1 and 79–2 for examples of the content).

It is critical for the survivorship care plan to have a comprehensive cancer treatment history that includes information on surgeries, chemotherapy, radiation, blood transfusions and/or bone marrow transplant, and any continuing medical therapies such as endocrine therapy. Complications the patient experienced during treatment should also be noted, such as chemotherapy toxicities. This section should also include provider contact information for the medical oncologist, surgeon, radiation oncologist, and other treating clinicians. Accurate treatment records and a clear understanding of the patient's cancer treatment experience are essential to create the most effective and informative plan for the patient's future care.

On the basis of the patient's cancer treatment history, the known potential long-term and late effects of each treatment should be described along with recommendations for surveillance and evaluation of these effects. Long-term and late effects can include fatigue, pain, sexual dysfunction, cardiac problems, psychological distress, and many other conditions.[14] It is essential to provide the patient with guidance on what symptoms require an immediate visit with a clinician, such as chest pain, shortness of breath, or localized limb swelling, and what does not. This vital information must be provided to the patient in a clear, easy to read written format so that the patient is not struggling to remember verbal information given during a visit that may not be accurately recalled. This section will also assist primary care providers to identify long-term and late effects that present in their survivor patient population.

The psychosocial needs of the survivor are frequently neglected both during and after treatment. The treatment summary and care plan can fill this gap by including recommendations and/or referrals for depression, anxiety, and relationship issues. Information on organizations that provide support and resources, such as The Wellness Community or the Lance Armstrong Foundation, should be included in the care plan. Also important are resources and tools for general health and wellness, such as the nutrition guidelines for survivors from the American Cancer Society (ACS), as maintaining a healthy weight and effectively managing co-morbid conditions is essential for cancer survivors and may help reduce the risk of early morbidity in this population. (see Table 79–3 for list of resources). Support for the need of these physical and emotional

Table 79–1. Example of treatment summary content

Name:
Date of birth:
Current age:

Cancer diagnosis
Date of Tissue Diagnosis:
Age at Diagnosis:
Cancer Detection:
Stage of Cancer:
Site of Cancer:

Pathological findings
Cancer Type:
Tumor Size:

Treatment history
Surgical Procedures and Dates:
Radiation Treatments:
- Fields treated
- Toxicities
Chemotherapy regimen:
Dates:
- Number of cycles received:
- Total dose in mg/meters^2 of those with cumulative late effects:
- Other oncologic medical therapies
- Chemotherapy toxicities

Treating physicians and contact information
Surgeon:
Medical Oncologist:
Radiation Oncologist:
Primary Care Provider:
Other:

SOURCE: Adapted from Hewitt M, Greenfield S, Stovall E. "From Cancer Patient to Cancer Survivor: Lost in Transition," 2005. With permission from the National Academy of Sciences, Courtesy of the National Academies Press, Washington, D.C.

Table 79–2. Example of survivorship care plan description of long term and late effects

Surgical
- Numbness
- Weakness
- Pain
- Loss of range of motion
- Lymphedema
Chemotherapy
- Fatigue
- Neuropathy
- Cognitive dysfunction
- Weight gain
- Sexual dysfunction
- Psychological distress
- Ovarian failure with associated menopausal symptoms
- Osteoporosis from premature ovarian failure
- Increased risk of leukemia after anthracycline-based chemotherapy
- Increased risk of cardiac dysfunction after anthracycline-based chemotherapy and/or Herceptin
Radiation
- Fibrosis
- Breast pain
- Telangectasia
- Atrophy
- Poor cosmetic outcome
- Cardiac late effects
Hormone therapies
- Tamoxifen
  - Hot flashes
  - Increased risk of stroke
  - Increased risk of uterine cancer
  - Increased risk of blood clots
- Aromatase inhibitors
  - Increased risk of osteoporosis
  - Increased risk of fractures
  - Vaginal dryness
  - Arthralgias

services among survivors can be found in a large scale Internet based survey (N = 1020) conducted by the Lance Armstrong Foundation in 2004, which demonstrated that 54% reported chronic pain, 70% reported depression due to cancer, 49% had unmet nonmedical needs, and that 53% found emotional needs harder than physical needs.[15] Additionally, a recent report from the IOM, *Cancer care for the whole patient: Meeting psychosocial health needs,* underlines the importance of coordinating medical care with psychosocial serves and linking survivors to appropriate psychosocial care providers.[16]

Obstacles and challenges to completing the treatment summary and survivorship care plan. The creation of an effective and informative survivorship care plan depends upon obtaining primary-source treatment records. Without accurate pathology reports, chemotherapy records, operative reports, radiation summaries, and other treatment records, the survivorship care plan could be greatly compromised. However, depending on where the patient was treated, getting timely access to patient records can be a struggle, and all records are not equal in clarity and content.

Radiation oncologists often provide a treatment plan and concluding summary note, both of which are particularly helpful in identifying the extent of the patient's radiation treatment. These notes typically include an introductory note at the beginning of treatment outlining the planned radiation therapy course and a concluding note summarizing the total radiation received, areas radiated, and details of any changes or problems encountered during the treatment. In addition, surgeons routinely provide a detailed operative report with the pre- and postoperative diagnosis clearly stated along with the details of the procedure. However, medical oncologists seldom provide a detailed treatment plan at the beginning of treatment or a summary of care received upon completion of treatment, making determination of chemotherapy treatment actually received a problem. Medical records may contain a brief letter dictated to the primary care provider outlining the proposed treatment course, but there is rarely an organized summary of what treatment the patient actually received. It is extremely important to include the chemotherapy medications given during treatment as they can have significant long-term and late effects; for example, doxorubicin and cyclophosphamide can potentially have cardiac late effects.[17] If the medical oncologist has not summarized the chemotherapy and/or ongoing endocrine treatment that a patient has received, it may be necessary to search for a chemotherapy treatment flow sheet or nursing notes to help determine the prescribed treatments and the total dose received.

It can be time-consuming to request and collect treatment records from the surgical, radiation, and medical oncologist offices, but it is absolutely essential to creating an accurate treatment summary and care plan document. Collecting records from large academic institutions and cancer centers can be much simpler than collecting records from individual physician offices scattered throughout the community, but both can be accomplished. Record retrieval can be carried out by administrative, research, or clinical staff; staff can also be trained to abstract records to begin populating the treatment summary and care plan with these data before the patient's visit.

Table 79–3. Online resources for cancer survivors

Organization and description	Web site
American Cancer Society Survivors Network: ACS is a nation-wide voluntary health organization that provides cancer resources online and in the community; ACS has developed this site specifically for survivors	http://www.cancer.org http://www.acscsn.org
CancerCare: CancerCare is a nonprofit organization that provides free professional support services online and by telephone for anyone affected by cancer	www.cancercare.org
Lance Armstrong Foundation (LAF): The LAF provides information and survivorship resources online and in the community	www.livestrong.org
NCI Office of Cancer Survivorship: OCS provides current information on survivorship research, resources, and publications	http://cancercontrol.cancer.gov/ocs/
The IOM report *"From Cancer Patient to Cancer Survivor: Lost in Transition"* can be accessed online at no charge	www.iom.edu/
The Wellness Community (TWC): TWC provides support groups, activities, and other resources online and in their many community sites	www.thewellnesscommunity.org
The National Coalition for Cancer Survivors (NCCS): NCCS is the oldest survivor-led cancer advocacy organization in the country, advocating for quality cancer care for all Americans and empowering cancer survivors	http://www.canceradvocacynow.org/
People Living With Cancer (PLWC): PLWC provides expert up-to-date information on cancer and survivorship; it is the patient site of ASCO	http://www.cancer.net/

Prospective preparation of the treatment summary and care plan is preferred to retrospective reconstruction of past treatments. The ASCO recently created sample templates for a combined treatment plan/treatment summary for breast and colon cancer patients that are designed to be used prospectively; there is also an associated one-page survivorship care plan that outlines the recommended follow-up care and surveillance for these patients (see Table 79–4 for web site URL). ASCO has also developed a generic template that can be used for any cancer site, and has in preparation other disease-specific templates, which can be quickly completed before or during a patient visit by the treating physician or other staff. These templates cover all of the core elements of the treatment

Table 79–4. Links and online resources for preparing treatment summaries and survivorship care plans

Links to web-based survivorship tools:
ASCO treatment summary and care plan templates for breast and colon cancer: www.asco.org/treatmentsummary
LIVESTRONG care plan, powered by Penn Medicine OncoLink:http://www.livestrongcareplan.org
A Prescription for Living treatment summary and care plan from the American Journal of Nursing: http://www.cc.nih.gov/nursing/nursingresearch/Rx_for_Living.pdf
Journey Forward, guiding survivors as they move ahead. NCCS, Wellpoint, UCLA, Genentech, www.journeyforward.org

summary and survivorship care plan as recommended in the IOM report on cancer survivorship care.

A more comprehensive approach to the survivorship care plan may include information on the patient's co-morbid conditions from primary care as well as specialist care such as cardiology, endocrinology, or pulmonology. This more holistic approach is much more resource intensive and may be easier to carry out in specialized survivorship clinical practices or in large healthcare institutions with access to multiple areas of care. The comprehensive plan will provide a broader picture of the patient's overall health along with the core elements of the survivorship care plan and may assist with providing well-coordinated care for cancer survivors.

Emerging trends. There is currently a national effort underway to educate both the healthcare community and the general public about survivorship issues and to encourage the use of survivorship care plans (Table 79–4). Organizations such as ASCO, the Lance Armstrong Foundation, the National Coalition for Cancer Survivorship (NCCS) and various health plans are interested invested in educating oncologists, oncology nurses, primary care providers, and patients about the importance of survivorship care and the use of survivorship care plans. These efforts include providing practical information on provider billing, access to publicly available care plan templates and survivorship guidelines, and survivorship care plan tool kits with resources for patients and providers. There is also momentum to include treatment plans and care summaries as a reportable quality of care measure. As part of many of these efforts, programmatic evaluation is planned to determine patient and provide satisfaction with the care plans, and downstream examination of adherence to guideline care for cancer surveillance and health promotion. This is an area that is ripe for further research to support implementation and the most effective models of care.

There are excellent publicly available resources and guidelines that can be used to create or supplement survivorship care plans in clinical practice. ASCO has templates for breast and colon cancer treatment summary and care plans, as well as a generic chemotherapy treatment plan and treatment summary and general background materials for care plans. ASCO is also currently promoting integration of the treatment plan and summaries into oncology electronic health records by hosting symposia and workshops with electronic health record system vendors.

The National Comprehensive Cancer Network (NCCN) and the ACS also have resources and materials focused on survivorship issues, guidelines, and survivorship care plans. Other e-resources such as the Oncolink survivorship care plan tool, Oncolife, and Prescription for Living, a care planning tool developed for use in nursing are providing web-based survivorship tools specifically for patients to use with their healthcare team (see Table 79–1). All of these resources are dedicated to assisting clinicians in providing high-quality survivorship care and empowering and informing cancer survivors.

Implementing the survivorship care plan. Each practice setting needs to decide on a strategy that will permit the implementation of survivorship care plans: prevalent or incident cases? Cover all disease types or begin with one? A focus on incident cases may simply mean adding the survivorship care plan and discussion into the first follow-up visit after active treatment ends; focusing on prevalent cases may require doing outreach to patients who are no longer being seen in regular follow-up care. Concentrating on one common cancer, such as breast, may ease the transition to using the care plans in a clinical practice. In addition, decisions must be made on the format of the plan and the communication with other treating physicians. Using uniform templates with drop down menus, check boxes, and prepopulated data fields will reduce the amount of time needed to complete the plan. A consistent approach across the practice is the most efficient method for implementing survivorship care plans for your survivor population.

The key goal of survivorship care planning is better communication between the oncology team, primary care providers, and the patient, which will lead to better coordinated care for the survivor. A well-prepared survivorship care plan will empower the patient and inform clinicians involved in their care and can provide a framework for a shared-care model. Primary care providers who have received a treatment summary and survivorship care plan are extremely appreciative and have reported greater self-efficacy in the follow-up care of cancer patients in their practice. In addition, for busy medical oncologists, having this single note in the chart can simplify follow-up care for patients who are only seen periodically after treatment ends.

HEALTH POLICY IMPLICATIONS OF THE SURVIVORSHIP CARE PLAN

The need for coordination of care for cancer survivors is emblematic of the challenges faced by many patients with chronic diseases, where complex care is often delivered by specialists in the absence of primary care involvement. In addition, the real or perceived shortage of primary care providers in the United States leads patients to rely heavily on their subspecialty physicians. Unfortunately, as a result, many important healthcare processes are often ignored or overlooked in specialty only care. Indeed, several studies in the Medicare population have shown that optimal cancer care occurs when adult cancer patients are treated by both cancer specialists and primary care providers.[18-20] No doubt similar findings would occur in other chronic diseases. The important role of preventive health services for noncancer conditions, as well as management of co-morbid conditions, cannot be overlooked in the cancer survivor. The implementation of treatment summaries and survivorship care plans may be a first step in enhancing better care for cancer survivors, and may serve as a model testable in other chronic diseases. Two recent efforts call for the implementation of treatment summaries into the standard care of cancer patients and survivors: Legislation pending in Congress ("Comprehensive Cancer Care Improvement Act" HR 1078 and S. 2790), and the recently developed Oncology Physician Performance Measurement Set developed by ASCO and the American Society of Therapeutic Radiation Oncology (ASTRO) with the American Medical Association Physician Consortium for Performance Improvement.

CONCLUSION

Medical oncology is a relatively young specialty, compared to surgery and radiation oncology. It has been traditional for surgeons to describe their cancer treatment (surgery) with a detailed operative note. Similarly, it is customary for radiation oncologists to provide a treatment summary of the amount of radiation given and the specific ports involved, including a short-term description of local tissue tolerance and complications. Until the last half of the twentieth century pharmacological treatments for cancer were primarily palliative. With the advent of combination chemotherapy and multimodality therapies, many pediatric and adult cancers are now curable. However, treatment is administered over a prolonged period of time, largely in the outpatient setting. The tradition of preparing a treatment summary is largely absent from the culture of medical oncology practice.

Documentation of drug type and dosages received will ultimately be important, as more information is gathered about the late toxicities of various treatments. Since cancer in older adults frequently co-occurs with other co-morbid conditions, communication about known potential organ toxicities (e.g., heart, lung, kidney) to the patient and their primary care providers are likely to be critical in prevention of secondary late and long-term effects. Furthermore, the development of a treatment summary and care plan is essential for improving the quality and coordination of care for the growing population of cancer survivors. The time has come for this to occur, and we predict that we are at the tipping point for widespread adoption of the cancer treatment summary and survivorship care plan. As these efforts roll out in the coming years, through both natural and planned experiments, there will be ample opportunity for formal research and informal evaluative projects. Examination of patient and provider satisfaction are key measures, but reduction in duplication/unnecessary testing and better coordination care will be important outcomes to measure.

REFERENCES

1. Erikson C, Salsberg E, Forte G, Bruinooge S, Goldstein M. Future supply and demand for oncologists: challenges to assuring access to oncology services. *J Oncol Pract.* 2007;3:79–86.

2. Hewitt M, Greenfield S, Stovall E. *From cancer patient to cancer survivor: Lost in transition.* Washington, DC: The National Academies Press; 2006.

3. Chassin MR, Galvin RW; National Roundtable on Health Care Quality. The urgent need to improve health care quality: Institute of Medicine National Roundtable on Health Care Quality. *JAMA.* 1998;280:1000–1005.

4. Hewitt M, Simone JV. *Ensuring quality cancer care.* Washington, DC: National Academy Press; 1999.

5. Kohn LT, Corrigan J, Donaldson M. *To err is human: Building a safer health system.* Washington, DC: National Academy Press; 2000.

6. Kohn LT, Corrigan JM, Donaldson MS. *Crossing the quality chasm: A new health system for the 21st Century.* Washington, DC: National Academy Press; 2001.

7. Oeffinger KC, Mertens AC, Sklar CA, et al. Chronic health conditions in adult survivors of childhood cancer. *N Engl J Med.* 2006;355:1572–1582.

8. Kenney LB, Yasui Y, Inskip PD, et al. Breast cancer after childhood cancer: a report from the Childhood Cancer Survivor Study. *Ann Intern Med.* 2004;141:590–597.

9. Mertens AC, Yasui Y, Neglia JP, et al. Late mortality experience in five-year survivors of childhood and adolescent cancer: the childhood cancer survivor study. *J Clin Oncol.* 2001;19:3163–3172.

10. Syrjala KL, Roth-Roemer SL, Abrams JR, et al. Prevalence and predictors of sexual dysfunction in long-term survivors of marrow transplantation. *J Clin Oncol.* 1998;16:3148–3157.

11. Shankar SM, Carter A, Sun CL, et al. Health care utilization by adult long-term survivors of hematopoietic cell transplant: report from the bone marrow transplant survivor study. *Cancer Epidemiol Biomarkers Prev.* 2007;16:834–839.

12. Fraser CJ, Bhatia S, Ness K, et al. Impact of chronic graft-versus-host disease on the health status of hematopoietic cell transplantation survivors: a report from the Bone Marrow Transplant Survivor Study. *Blood.* 2006; 108:2867–2873.

13. Hewitt M, Ganz PA. *Implementing cancer survivorship care planning: Workshop summary.* Washington, DC: National Academies Press; 2007.

14. Ganz PA. Monitoring the physical health of cancer survivors: a survivorship-focused medical history. *J Clin Oncol.* 2006;24:5105–5111.

15. Wolff SN, Nichols C, Ulman D, et al. Survivorship: an unmet need of the patient with cancer-implications of a survey of the lance armstrong foundation (LAF). *J Clin Oncol.* 2005 ASCO Annual Meeting Proceedings 23, 16S, Part I or II (June 1 Suppl). 2005;6032.

16. Adler NE, Page AEK. *Cancer care for the whole patient: Meeting psychosocial health needs.* Washington, DC: Institute of Medicine, National Academies Press; 2007.

17. Carver JR, Shapiro CL, Ng A, et al. American Society of Clinical Oncology Clinical Evidence Review on the ongoing care of adult cancer survivors: cardiac and pulmonary late effects. *J Clin Oncol.* 2007;25:3991–4008.

18. Earle CC, Neville BA. Under use of necessary care among cancer survivors. *Cancer.* 2004;101:1712–1719.

19. Earle CC, Burstein HJ, Winer EP, Weeks JC. Quality of non-breast cancer health maintenance among elderly breast cancer survivors. *J Clin Oncol.* 2003;21:1447–1451.

20. Earle CC. Failing to plan is planning to fail: improving the quality of care with survivorship care plans. *J Clin Oncol.* 2006;24:5112–5116.

Adult Survivors of Childhood Cancer

Lisa A. Schwartz, Branlyn E. Werba, and Anne E. Kazak

The survival rate of pediatric cancer has increased dramatically in recent decades, with approximately 80% of childhood cancer survivors reaching 5-year survival. Young adults who are survivors of childhood cancer are no longer unusual; one out of every 640 adults between the ages of 20 and 39 is now a survivor of childhood cancer.[1] For these adults, the impact of the intensive treatment responsible for their survival may also result in life-long morbidities related to medical problems, risk for future medical problems or second cancer diagnosis, and cognitive difficulties. Moreover, because of the cancer experience and long-term effects, survivors also face psychosocial challenges as adults. The goals of this chapter are to (1) provide rationale for the unique health and psychosocial issues of adult childhood cancer survivors, (2) describe the potential physical, neurocognitive, and psychosocial issues relevant to this population and factors that may contribute to risk and resiliency, (3) describe the impact of these issues on developmental outcomes, and (4) discuss future directions and clinical implications for healthcare providers and research.

RATIONALE FOR ATTENTION TO THE NEEDS OF ADULT CHILDHOOD CANCER SURVIVORS

The long-term problems and risks of childhood cancer survivors, known as late effects, coupled with the burgeoning population of childhood cancer survivors have resulted in critical national attention to the issues facing this population. As an example, childhood cancer survivorship issues were the focus of a report from the Institute of Medicine[1] and care guidelines have been developed (e.g., Children's Oncology Group (COG) guidelines).[2] In addition, the Childhood Cancer Survivorship Study (CCSS) was formed as a multiinstitutional consortium to study long-term outcomes of childhood cancer survivors. Using epidemiological methods, the CCSS has assessed the physical functioning and quality of life over 14,000 survivors treated between the years 1970 and 1986 who were under age 21 at diagnosis. A second cohort, treated between the 1987 and 1999, is being recruited. The CCSS and the many single site and smaller collaborative research reports in this field are significant and comprehensive sources of current understanding of long-term outcomes of childhood cancer survivors.

It is critical to examine the needs of adult childhood cancer survivors as potentially unique from cancer survivors who were adults when ill. First, these survivors experienced treatment during critical developmental periods when they had not reached full physical, emotional, or cognitive maturation. Therefore, their long-term medical, psychological, and cognitive late effects may differ as a function of their stage of development at diagnosis and treatment. Similarly, in addition to the general trauma of cancer, these patients may have not yet fully developed coping skills, emotional regulation, and cognition to help them through the experience. In fact, some who were infants or young children at the time of treatment remember very little, if anything, of the treatment experience. Their risk for long-term difficulties may increase when entering adulthood, as these survivors gain the cognitive ability to process and comprehend the implications of the cancer experience in terms of physical and psychosocial vulnerabilities. Furthermore, the cancer experience may have interrupted education or time with family and friends. Subsequently, adult identity formation and attainment of young adult developmental milestones may be delayed or difficult to achieve. Further discussion of the long-term sequelae of childhood cancer survivorship as it relates to adults is presented below.

LONG-TERM HEALTH VULNERABILITY

Childhood cancer survivors may be burdened with life-long medical problems and risks that require attention to health-promoting behaviors and medical follow-up.

Physical late effects. Many childhood cancers and related treatments put survivors at increased risk for long-term medical morbidities and early death, though the impact of treatment is often not apparent until adulthood. In fact, morbidities seem to increase with age rather than plateau.[3] Some treatments (e.g., radiation and certain chemotherapies) cause irreversible tissue and organ damage or may be carcinogenic. Subsequent physical late effects may impact major organ systems (e.g., heart, lungs, vision, endocrine, and immune systems). The CCSS found that 62% of survivors have at least one chronic condition and 28% had a severe or life-threatening condition.[3] High-risk chronic health conditions that occur at a rate eight times higher than siblings, include second cancers, cardiovascular disease, renal dysfunction, severe musculoskeletal problems, and endocrinopathies.[3] A significant minority also are at risk for infertility as a result of treatment. This late effect often causes distress in adulthood and serves as a reminder of cancer's long-term impact.[4] Other nonspecific outcomes have been reported such as increased frequency of fatigue and pain.[5,6] Furthermore, because of such physical late effects, survivors have also reported more functional limitations compared to siblings.[7] These include less ability to attend work or school, and engage in self-care and routine activities. Not surprisingly, brain tumor and bone cancer survivors are often most at risk for such limitations. Unfortunately, as described next, survivors' often demonstrate suboptimal health-promoting behaviors and lack sufficient knowledge to enhance medical outcomes.

Health promotion and knowledge. Health promotion and long-term medical surveillance are critical given the risk for second cancers and later chronic health conditions such as cardiac and pulmonary disease, diabetes, and osteoporosis. Therefore, the optimal health of survivors is not only dependent on medical surveillance, but also dependent on patients, providers, and other supportive people having accurate knowledge, and survivors following-through with important health-promoting behaviors.

Health-promoting practices are similar to those recommended for the general public. However, health-promoting behaviors are more critical for survivors because of their vulnerable health status. For example, smoking and other tobacco use may exacerbate risk of cardiac and pulmonary disease, including lung cancer; alcohol may exacerbate liver and cardiac damage resulting from various therapies; and ultraviolet exposure may increase risk of skin cancer heightened by radiation.[8] Modifiable behaviors that are especially important for survivors include eating a balanced diet, exercising regularly, avoidance of tobacco, minimizing alcohol intake, sunscreen use, and safe sex practices to avoid sexually transmitted diseases. As summarized in a review,[8] many studies have demonstrated that survivors engage in health-risk behaviors at equal or lower rates as same-age peers. However, survivors still engaged in smoking, drinking, and marijuana use at a rate that should be concerning based on their increased risk for new cancer diagnoses and other diseases. Furthermore, health-risk behaviors among survivors have been found to be qualitatively different from controls. As an example, survivors who smoke are less likely to attempt to or successfully quit smoking.[9] Risk factors for these unhealthy behaviors seem to be similar to that of the general population. However, because mood difficulties have been found to be a significant risk factor, survivors are at increased risk for health-harming behaviors given their potential for anxiety and distress related to late effects and cancer history.[8]

Exercise and diet practices are also not at optimal levels for most survivors. The CCSS found that survivors were less likely to meet recommendations for physical activity and to report fewer leisure activities than siblings.[10] Higher levels of worry and more barriers to physical activity have been identified as important predictors of inactivity among survivors.[11] In another study of over 200 adolescent and young adult survivors, 79% did not meet guidelines for fruits and vegetables, 68% did not meet guidelines for calcium intake, 52% did not meet guidelines for exercise, and 42% were overweight or obese.[12] Those over 18 years of age, compared to adolescents, were more likely to smoke (17% vs. 1%), be obese (22% vs. 15%), and to have suboptimal calcium intake (76% vs. 58%).[12]

Furthermore, screening practices are not optimal for survivors, despite being essential to monitor risk for future cancers. Examples of important screening practices include breast and testicular self-examinations, mammograms, skin examinations, Pap smears, and colonoscopies. Data from the CCSS showed that, although screening practices related to self-examinations and imaging tended to be higher than siblings, screening practices remained below optimal levels given survivors' risk for health problems, including a new cancer diagnosis.[13]

Clearly, appropriate medical follow-up and disease knowledge is also essential for health promotion, disease management, and monitoring for future problems. To facilitate optimal care, survivors should have a complete record of cancer-related details including date of diagnosis; cancer histology and stage; and treatment history including surgery, chemotherapy, and radiation. Unfortunately, previous studies evaluating health knowledge of childhood cancer survivors demonstrate survivors' suboptimal knowledge about their cancer diagnosis, treatment, and cancer-related health risks. For example, CCSS findings showed that although survivors knew about their diagnosis and treatment in general, they did not know specifics such as the names of chemotherapy, even when prompted with the name.[14] In addition, only 35% thought their cancer treatment could cause long-term effects on their health.[14] Thus, despite best efforts to educate patients, they may still lack all the knowledge they need to actively manage their health and navigate the medical system. Furthermore, many healthcare providers lack familiarity with cancer-related health risks and risk-reduction methods relevant for this population.

Taken together, long-term physical late effects and need for continued care may heighten the risk for psychological late effects as described later. This is especially true for survivors transitioning to adulthood as they realize the impact of their disease and face the potential for worsening late effects. Furthermore, as described below, childhood cancer survivors often experience neurocognitive late effects that have long-term implications for educational and vocational attainment.

NEUROCOGNITIVE LATE EFFECTS AND IMPACT ON EDUCATIONAL AND VOCATIONAL ATTAINMENT

Cancers, related treatments involving the central nervous system (CNS), and the cumulative negative impact of cancer on school attendance and achievement have all been associated with ongoing long-term cognitive effects. Specific neurocognitive effects have been documented with magnetic resonance imaging, computerized tomography scans, and neuropsychological testing. In addition to evidence of decreased intelligence quotient (IQ), especially in those survivors of brain tumors and acute lymphoblastic leukemia (ALL), evidence suggests impairments in the following: attention and concentration, processing speed (e.g., more time required to complete work, slower to understand), visual perceptual skills (e.g., difficulty with writing, interpretation of visual information such as maps or puzzles), executive functioning (e.g., problems with planning, insight, organization), memory, and cognitive fatigue (difficulty with concentrating for long periods of time and more tired than

expected after a day at work or school).[15] In general, the acquisition of new information and skills may occur at lower rates than healthy peers and, ultimately, result in poorer academic achievement.

The specific pattern of neurocognitive deficits seen in childhood cancer survivors depends in part on age at diagnosis, type of cancer, type of cancer treatment, and tumor site.[15] Risk is highest for CNS malignancies, cranial radiation therapy, intrathecal therapy for those treated for ALL, and those who received a blood/stem cell transplant. In terms of age, the degree of brain maturation at the time of therapy has been directly correlated with the potential for CNS insult, with children under the age of 3 are at greatest risk.[15] Finally, the effects of cancer and cancer treatment on neurocognitive functioning are often delayed, with most deficits not evident until 1 or more years posttreatment.[16,17]

The impact of cancer survivorship on educational and vocational attainment beyond high school is only beginning to be understood. Some survivors may successfully compensate for cognitive limitations until they reach high school or college, when coursework requires more complex abstract reasoning, attention, and organization. Some studies have found that young adult survivors are less likely than controls to have educational plans beyond high school,[18] are less likely to go on to attend college than when compared to the general population or siblings,[18,19] and less often hold an advanced degree.[20] Furthermore, evidence suggests that survivors are less likely to be employed than peers and experience more job discrimination.[20] In contrast, a recent qualitative study found several ways in which cancer may have had a positive impact on survivors, including increased motivation and determination to succeed in educational and career pursuits and a tendency to choose careers that help others.[21] As survivors live longer and potentially experience less treatment related toxicities with treatment advances, it will be important to continue to examine the impact of physical (e.g., neurocognitive status) and environmental (e.g., missed school and experiences) factors that influence outcomes among subgroups of survivors at different points of development.

PSYCHOLOGICAL LATE EFFECTS AND IMPACT ON ADJUSTMENT

Attention to psychological late effects and overall psychosocial adjustment is important given the health and neurocognitive vulnerabilities associated with childhood cancer survival. Findings are generally supportive of the positive adaptation made by the majority of survivors. Most cancer survivors are found to be well adjusted relative to healthy control participants, nonill siblings, and standardized norms. However, it is important to note that some studies suggest that young adult survivors exhibit a tendency to deny or minimize problems.[22,23] Survivors may also experience response shift whereby judgments of well-being may be made relative to expectations for someone having had cancer as opposed to comparing themselves to healthy never-ill individuals.[22] Thus, many survivors may be functioning well compared to peers, others may have adapted a coping style that minimizes or reframes outcomes, and a select few may acknowledge difficulties as survivors.

Psychological vulnerability. Despite generally positive outcomes, some areas of potential concern exist, especially as survivors enter adulthood. Young adulthood is a potentially stressful developmental period that includes setting and pursuing goals related to employment, living arrangements, spouse selection, and parenthood. For survivors, this may be an especially distressing period due to the potential for increased awareness of, and reflection on, the impact of cancer on their health, education, and relationships. Specific ways in which survivors may experience continued impact of their cancer on their development and experience of distress are discussed below.

Studies show more negative moods, tension, and depression in young adult survivors than in their siblings[19] and report suicidal symptoms and global psychological distress.[24] Also, the presence of pain, fatigue, and other somatic symptoms may be partially related to anxiety and worry. In addition, up to 50% of young adult survivors experience posttraumatic stress (PTS) in the form of intrusive, avoidant, and arousal symptoms.[25-27] In fact, research has shown that up to 20% of young adult survivors meet criteria for the psychiatric diagnosis of posttraumatic stress disorder (PTSD).[25,27,28]

Attention has also focused on understanding how PTS may be relevant to the experience of distress for cancer survivors and their family members during young adulthood. Cancer can be an ongoing trauma in terms of threat of future cancers or late effects, current late effects, reminders of the cancer, and losses such as diminished social, cognitive, and reproductive capacity. Young adult survivors' cognitive maturity and enhanced awareness of the implications of their cancer, in conjunction with newly identified late effects in early adulthood, may "re-expose" them to the trauma of cancer. Symptoms of PTS for these young adults may include rumination, intrusive thoughts, frequent nightmares about cancer or related experiences, increased arousal when thinking or talking about cancer, avoidance of thinking or talking about cancer, avoidance of healthcare settings or doing things to take care of health, hypervigilance of body and symptoms, and feeling life is prematurely shortened. Such symptoms have been shown to relate to distress and impairment in this population[28] as well as health behaviors.[29]

There are several factors that have been associated with distress of childhood cancer survivors during young adulthood. Survivors' perception that their cancer treatment was intense[27] and that their perceptions of current health and life threat[27] have been associated with both PTS and more general distress. Demographic factors including female gender, lower socioeconomic status, lack of employment, lower educational achievement, and single status have also been associated with increased distress.[27,30] Objective medical data related to the cancer, treatment, age at diagnosis, or time since treatment has rarely been shown to predict distress. Thus, it is important to assess the patient's perceptions of their experience, in addition to demographic and disease factors, when assessing risk for poor psychosocial outcomes.

Because of increasing cognitive maturity, young adult survivors are also likely to experience positive benefits as a result of their cancer experience. Research has shown that survivors have enhanced coping abilities and motivation in various life domains[31] and experience posttraumatic growth (PTG).[32] PTG is the process of applying positive interpretations and finding meaning in a traumatic event. By doing so, the experience of trauma may facilitate positive changes related to self-concept, relationships, and life philosophy. While not yet widely studied in adult childhood cancer survivors, one study with adolescent survivors found that the majority of them and their parents identified positive consequences as a result of their cancer in the domains of self, relationships, and future plans.[32] Thus, interventions to enhance PTG, and reduce the negative impact of PTS and other forms of distress are indicated.

SOCIAL RELATIONSHIPS AND RELATED DEVELOPMENTAL OUTCOMES

Social and romantic development may also be impacted for survivors. In contrast with evidence that childhood and adolescent survivors' social skills are similar to their peers,[33] young adult survivors are more likely to report difficulty forming relationships with same-sex peers and romantic relationships, and are less satisfied with both types of relationships.[34,35] In addition, these survivors evidence lower marriage rates and/or marry later than peers,[20] and may have a higher rate of divorce than the general population.[36] Although the specific factors that may lead to these developmental outcomes have not been well-studied, young adult survivors may experience unique challenges that impact relationships into adulthood, such as how and when to disclose information related to their health and fertility, a past history of relationship disruptions or less opportunity to develop relationships, and potential changes in appearance that become more salient to a survivor with age.

The experience of childhood cancer may also impact family relationships and autonomy development into adulthood. Developmentally, parents are critical in the transition to young adulthood. Childhood cancer survivors are no exception, particularly given the central role that parents continue to play in monitoring their offspring's health. Whereas parents of never-ill individuals in this age group are not likely to be aware of healthcare visits made by their offspring, parents of survivors were three times more likely to attend medical appointments than parents of controls.[37] Further, young adult survivors live longer with their parents and are less independent from their parents than peers.[18,35] Therefore,

facilitating the transfer of responsibility for healthcare from the parent to the child is critical in this adult population.

One potential factor that may continue to impact a young adult survivors' autonomy development and parent–child relationship may be the ongoing impact of cancer on parental adjustment. Although most studies have not found an increase in psychiatric symptoms such as depression and anxiety in parents of long-term survivors of childhood cancer,[38] studies support the enduring experience of PTS among parents. Parents may retain traumatic memories of caring for their sick children and continue to fear for their child's life. Levels of PTS have been shown to be higher for parents of survivors compared to control groups,[39] and specifically among parents of adult survivors.[38] Parents of adult survivors also reported significantly greater unresolved anger and sorrow than parents of child patients on active treatment, which may, in part, explain why accompanying their adult children to medical visits may be comforting or decrease anxiety related to their child's health.[38]

Along with increased parental experience of PTS, it is not surprising that parents of young adult survivors also report PTG, which may also influence their young adults' development. In the previously mentioned study of PTG, almost all mothers and fathers identified at least one positive outcome of cancer; the most reported change was in how parents thought about their life.[32] Parents also report that a unique bond was created with their now adult childhood cancer survivor through experiencing a potentially traumatic event together.[37] A unique relationship between mothers and survivors may also develop due to the "polarization" of roles for parents during cancer treatment (i.e., mothers become more likely to be the main caregiver, whereas the father may focus on continuing to work and other family responsibilities).[40] In fact, survivors report closer relationships with mothers than fathers,[40] though this may not necessarily lead to better outcomes in all domains. For example, the combination of lower encouragement from fathers and greater involvement with mothers was associated with impaired close relationships outside the family, especially for female survivors.[40]

Finally, a survivor's relationship with their sibling may also be impacted by cancer. During treatment, siblings may experience less time with their parents, interruptions in their routines, and worry that their sibling will die. Unfortunately, it is unknown if distress and/or positive growth occurs long term for siblings, and how this may impact the adult survivor–sibling relationship. Not surprisingly, in a study of adolescent siblings of survivors, one-third of the sample reported moderate to severe levels of PTS.[41] Taken together, there is ample evidence to support PTS as a salient model of long-term adjustment for the entire family and the need for family-centered assessment and interventions in the context of long-term survivorship care.

LONG-TERM CARE FOR SURVIVORS

Adult survivors of childhood cancer require long-term surveillance to monitor for future cancer risk and morbidities and manage current physical and psychological problems. Care should be risk-based and comprehensive (COG guidelines).[2] Risk-based care incorporates assessment and knowledge of the previous cancer, cancer therapy, genetic predispositions, lifestyle behaviors, and co-morbid health conditions. Because of the long-term morbidities, life-time health promotion, and health navigation skills are critical for optimal outcomes.

Furthermore, survivors will inevitably require transfer to adult-oriented care. The transfer of care has proven to be a considerable challenge for survivors and their providers.[42] Many patients and families are reluctant to leave their pediatric oncologists and the associated comprehensive care. Providers are also apprehensive to transfer given the paucity of adult providers with expertise in caring for pediatric cancer survivors. While many models of transition focus on the acquisition of disease skills and knowledge, many other factors may contribute to the successful transition of survivors to adult care. A recently developed model of transition, the Socio-ecological Model of Adolescent/Young Adult Readiness for Transition (SMART) emphasizes the importance of understanding the socio-ecology of the transition process with regards to the relationships, goals, beliefs, and feelings (in addition to patient disease skills and knowledge) of the patient, parent, and provider.[43]

Given the increased risk for PTS among adult survivors, the transition process to adult care may serve as an additional cancer-related traumatic event, and warrants further research and clinical attention.

FUTURE DIRECTIONS AND CLINICAL IMPLICATIONS

Existing research supports the overall promise of healthy survival for many childhood cancer survivors as they enter adulthood. In particular, ongoing epidemiological research has been instrumental in describing this growing population while science has also progressed in terms of understanding ongoing medical risks associated with cancer and its treatment during childhood. There has also been a substantive increase in the number of studies investigating psychosocial outcomes in the past decade.

Most results support the resiliency and quality of life of long-term survivors. However, a significant minority experience distress, including PTS. In addition, some adult survivors are achieving young adult developmental milestones at slower rates, or with more difficulty, than their peers. These developmental tasks include becoming increasingly independent from one's family, pursuing educational and vocational goals, and establishing intimate relationships with friends and romantic partners. Poor psychosocial outcomes are more prevalent with neurocognitive difficulties and/or increased likelihood of restrictive health problems that impair the ability to attain goals of adulthood. However, outcomes are most often predicted by subjective appraisal of the cancer experience and related coping abilities, and can be influenced by family narratives of, and reactions to, the cancer experience. Such difficulties can be exacerbated by the already difficult developmental period of transition to adulthood.

Unfortunately, for survivors, little is known about approaches to facilitate an optimal transition to adulthood in terms of psychosocial outcomes, engagement in medical care, and health-promoting behaviors. While treatments that are effective with younger survivors and/or their parents (e.g., cognitive remediation, cognitive behavioral/family therapy approaches, problem-solving therapies) may be helpful, they have not been tested with this age group. Many adult survivors, like their never-ill peers, are difficult to reach and engage in intervention programs or medical follow-up. That is, they are engaged in busy lives and may be less connected with the healthcare system. Some are also on less-adaptive trajectories, engaging in risky behaviors, facing difficult personal challenges, and learning how to cope and adapt to life stressors more generally.

Thus, engaging young adult survivors in follow-up care remains a significant challenge. Such care in early adulthood is particularly important to promote successful transition to adulthood, in addition to providing the necessary medical care to manage problems and promote long-term physical and psychological health. Annual follow-up appointments provide an ideal setting for monitoring medical risks as well as broaching concerns about overall psychological adjustment and worries about well-being. Social relationships are also an area of importance, as well as having the skills necessary to navigate the healthcare system (this being a nonnormative experience for young adults in general). Beyond describing psychological symptoms, identifying the beliefs of young adult survivors about their health, psychological well-being, and ability to stay well is also critical, as they are modifiable targets of intervention to improve outcomes. Furthermore, the artificial divide between the study of psychological outcomes and health outcomes should be diminished given burgeoning research showing that one influences the other (e.g., relationship between PTS and health behaviors). In summary, significant next steps in adult childhood cancer survivorship care are to engage young adult survivors in long-term care, extend assessment of them beyond typical psychological and medical outcomes (e.g., assess developmental goals, beliefs, health care utilization), and to better understand the influence of such outcomes on long-term well-being and health-promoting behaviors.

REFERENCES

1. Hewitt M, Weiner SL, Simone JV. (eds). *Childhood cancer survivorship: Improving care and quality of life*. Washington DC: National Academies Press; 2003.

2. Children's Oncology Group. *Long-term follow-up guidelines for survivors of childhood, adolescent, and young adult cancers*. Version 2.0; 2006. Available at www.survivorshipguidelines.org. Accessed July 31, 2008.

3. Oeffinger KC, Mertens AC, Sklar CA, et al. Chronic health conditions in adult survivors of childhood cancer. *N Engl J Med*. 2006;355(15):1572–1582.

4. Zebrack BJ, Casillas J, Nohr L, Adams H, Zeltzer LK. Fertility issues for young adult survivors of childhood cancer. *Psychooncology*. 2004;13(10):689–699.

5. Hudson MM, Mertens AC, Yasui Y, et al. Health status of adult long-term survivors of childhood cancer: a report from the Childhood Cancer Survivor Study. *JAMA*. 2003;290(12):1583–1592.

6. Mulrooney DA, Ness KK, Neglia JP, et al. Fatigue and sleep disturbance in adult survivors of childhood cancer: a report from the childhood cancer survivor study (CCSS). *Sleep*. 2008;31(2):271–281.

7. Ness KK, Gurney JG, Zeltzer LK, et al. The impact of limitations in physical, executive, and emotional function on health-related quality of life among adult survivors of childhood cancer: a report from the Childhood Cancer Survivor Study. *Arch Phys Med Rehabil*. 2008;89(1):128–136.

8. Clarke SA, Eiser C. Health behaviours in childhood cancer survivors: a systematic review. *Eur J Cancer*. 2007;43(9):1373–1384.

9. Emmons K, Li FP, Whitton J, et al. Predictors of smoking initiation and cessation among childhood cancer survivors: a report from the childhood cancer survivor study. *J Clin Oncol*. 2002;20(6):1608–1616.

10. Florin TA, Fryer GE, Miyoshi T, et al. Physical inactivity in adult survivors of childhood acute lymphoblastic leukemia: a report from the childhood cancer survivor study. *Cancer Epidemiol Biomarkers Prev*. 2007;16(7):1356–1363.

11. Finnegan L, Wilkie DJ, Wilbur J, Campbell RT, Zong S, Katula S. Correlates of physical activity in young adult survivors of childhood cancers. *Oncol Nurs Forum*. 2007;34(5):E60–E69.

12. Demark-Wahnefried W, Werner C, et al. Survivors of childhood cancer and their guardians. *Cancer*. 2005;103(10):2171–2180.

13. Yeazel MW, Oeffinger KC, Gurney JG, et al. The cancer screening practices of adult survivors of childhood cancer: a report from the Childhood Cancer Survivor Study. *Cancer*. 2004;100(3):631–640.

14. Kadan-Lottick NS, Robison LL, Gurney JG, et al. Childhood cancer survivors' knowledge about their past diagnosis and treatment: Childhood Cancer Survivor Study. *JAMA*. 2002;287(14):1832–1839.

15. Nathan PC, Patel SK, Dilley K, et al. Guidelines for identification of, advocacy for, and intervention in neurocognitive problems in survivors of childhood cancer: a report from the Children's Oncology Group. *Arch Pediatr Adolesc Med*. 2007;161(8):798–806.

16. Mulhern RK, Palmer SL, Reddick WE, et al. Risks of young age for selected neurocognitive deficits in medulloblastoma are associated with white matter loss. *J Clin Oncol*. 2001;19(2):472–479.

17. Langer T, Martus P, Ottensmeier H, Hertzberg H, Beck JD, Meier W. CNS late-effects after ALL therapy in childhood. Part III: neuropsychological performance in long-term survivors of childhood ALL: impairments of concentration, attention, and memory. *Med Pediatr Oncol*. 2002;38(5):320–328.

18. Boman KK, Bodegard G. Life after cancer in childhood: social adjustment and educational and vocational status of young-adult survivors. *J Pediatr Hematol Oncol*. 2004;26(6):354–362.

19. Zeltzer LK, Chen E, Weiss R, et al. Comparison of psychologic outcome in adult survivors of childhood acute lymphoblastic leukemia versus sibling controls: a cooperative Children's Cancer Group and National Institutes of Health study. *J Clin Oncol*. 1997;15(2):547–556.

20. Langeveld NE, Ubbink MC, Last BF, Grootenhuis MA, Voute PA, De Haan RJ. Educational achievement, employment and living situation in long-term young adult survivors of childhood cancer in the Netherlands. *Psychooncology*. 2003;12(3):213–225.

21. Brown C, Pikler VI, Lavish LA, Keune KM, Hutto CJ. Surviving childhood leukemia: career, family, and future expectations. *Qual Health Res*. 2008;18(1):19–30.

22. O'Leary TE, Diller L, Recklitis CJ. The effects of response bias on self-reported quality of life among childhood cancer survivors. *Qual Life Res*. 2007;16(7):1211–1220.

23. Phipps S, Larson S, Long A, Rai SN. Adaptive style and symptoms of posttraumatic stress in children with cancer and their parents. *J Pediatr Psychol*. 2006;31(3):298–309.

24. Recklitis C, O'Leary T, Diller L. Utility of routine psychological screening in the childhood cancer survivor clinic. *J Clin Oncol*. 2003;21(5):787–792.

25. Hobbie WL, Stuber M, Meeske K, et al. Symptoms of posttraumatic stress in young adult survivors of childhood cancer. *J Clin Oncol*. 2000;18(24):4060–4066.

26. Langeveld NE, Grootenhuis MA, Voute PA, de Haan RJ. Posttraumatic stress symptoms in adult survivors of childhood cancer. *Pediatr Blood Cancer*. 2004;42(7):604–610.

27. Rourke MT, Hobbie WL, Schwartz L, Kazak AE. Posttraumatic stress disorder (PTSD) in young adult survivors of childhood cancer. *Pediatr Blood Cancer*. 2007;49(2):177–182.

28. Schwartz L, Drotar D. Posttraumatic stress and related impairment in survivors of childhood cancer in early adulthood compared to healthy peers. *J Pediatr Psychol.* 2006;31(4):356–366.

29. Lee YL, Santacroce SJ, Sadler L. Predictors of healthy behaviour in long-term survivors of childhood cancer. *J Clin Nurs.* 2007;16(11C):285–295.

30. Zebrack BJ, Zevon MA, Turk N, et al. Psychological distress in long-term survivors of solid tumors diagnosed in childhood: a report from the childhood cancer survivor study. *Pediatr Blood Cancer.* 2007;49(1):47–51.

31. Gray RE, Doan BD, Shermer P, et al. Psychologic adaptation of survivors of childhood cancer. *Cancer.* 1992;70(11):2713–2721.

32. Barakat LP, Alderfer MA, Kazak AE. Posttraumatic growth in adolescent survivors of cancer and their mothers and fathers. *J Pediatr Psychol.* 2006;31(4):413–419.

33. Noll RB, Bukowski WM, Davies WH, Koontz K, Kulkarni R. Adjustment in the peer system of adolescents with cancer: a two-year study. *J Pediatr Psychol.* 1993;18(3):351–364.

34. Mackie E, Hill J, Kondryn H, McNally R. Adult psychosocial outcomes in long-term survivors of acute lymphoblastic leukaemia and Wilms' tumour: a controlled study. *Lancet.* 2000;355(9212):1310–1314.

35. Stam H, Grootenhuis MA, Last BF. The course of life of survivors of childhood cancer. *Psychooncology* 2005;14(3):227–238.

36. Green DM, Zevon MA, Hall B. Achievement of life goals by adult survivors of modern treatment for childhood cancer. *Cancer.* 1991;67(1):206–213.

37. Ressler IB, Cash J, McNeill D, Joy S, Rosoff PM. Continued parental attendance at a clinic for adult survivors of childhood cancer. *J Pediatr Hematol Oncol.* 2003;25(11):868–873.

38. Hardy KK, Bonner MJ, Masi R, Hutchinson KC, Willard VW, Rosoff PM. Psychosocial functioning in parents of adult survivors of childhood cancer. *J Pediatr Hematol Oncol.* 2008;30(2):153–159.

39. Barakat LP, Kazak AE, Meadows AT, Casey R, Meeske K, Stuber ML. Families surviving childhood cancer: a comparison of posttraumatic stress symptoms with families of healthy children. *J Pediatr Psychol.* 1997;22(6):843–859.

40. Hill J, Kondryn H, Mackie E, McNally R, Eden T. Adult psychosocial functioning following childhood cancer: the different roles of sons' and daughters' relationships with their fathers and mothers. *J Child Psychol Psychiatry.* 2003;44(5):752–762.

41. Alderfer MA, Labay LE, Kazak AE. Brief report: does posttraumatic stress apply to siblings of childhood cancer survivors? *J Pediatr Psychol.* 2003;28(4):281–286.

42. Freyer DR, Brugieres L. Adolescent and young adult oncology: transition of care. *Pediatr Blood Cancer.* 2008;50(Suppl 5):1116–1119.

43. Schwartz LA, Tuchman LK, Ginsberg J, Hobbie W. Addressing the challenge of transition to adult-oriented care for childhood cancer survivors: a pilot study of a new assessment tool to assess transition readiness. In the Cancer Survivorship Conference of the National Cancer Institute, Lance Armstrong Foundation, and the American Cancer Society. Atlanta, GA; 2008.

PART XIII

Building Psychosocial Programs

Marguerite S. Lederberg and Ruth McCorkle, EDS

CHAPTER 81

Building Psychosocial Programs: A Roadmap to Excellence

Matthew J. Loscalzo, Barry D. Bultz, and Paul B. Jacobsen

INTRODUCTION

Programs that focus on the psychosocial aspects of cancer have never before received the amount of funding or recognition than in the present. The convergence of aging populations, increasing numbers of cancer survivors and their caregivers, the emergence of many cancer-centric advocacy groups, the growth of professional organizations, and increases in funding have created a momentous time for a specialty (psychosocial oncology) that impacts cancer patients from time of diagnosis to palliative care, their caregivers and our communities. There is the potential for new alliances of patients and caregivers, advocacy groups, professionals and community-based organizations. All stakeholders working together can create a more informed, comprehensive, and compassionate approach to caring for people with chronic life-threatening diseases which transcends any single disease and has the potential to revolutionize healthcare internationally.

Psychosocial oncology has become recognized as an essential component of comprehensive cancer care.[1,2] Internationally, psychosocial programs have dramatically increased in scope, practice, and influence over the past 25 years. Where there were once isolated, individual biobehavioral clinicians and researchers within larger medical and surgical departments, there are now free standing psychosocial programs and departments. With the exception of a few large academic institutions, psychosocial services and behavioral research have reflected the funding sources and have not been well integrated. With the increasing complexity of medical and psychosocial care and raised expectations for evidence-based practice, investigators, clinicians, and educators are expected to work much more closely together and to demonstrate quality and effectiveness. This is an important shift of the zeitgeist of professionals who are highly committed to their professional identities and to their special areas of expertise and interests.

Integrated psychosocial departments did not come from large established programs but rather from smaller and newer cancer centers where there were less established boundaries and scarcer resources so efficiency was essential. Separate profession-based departments providing parallel services and programs are a luxury that few cancer centers can afford and perhaps in context of the patient requirements for psychosocial support, may be seen as redundant. Simultaneously, many professionals are finally catching up with the realities of the clinical setting and the benefits of an integrated interdisciplinary psychosocial department.

Although funding for biobehavioral research in cancer has traditionally been minuscule, when compared to overall governmental and foundation funding for bio-medical research, there have been incremental gains in recent years reflecting the growing respect for the importance and quality of psychosocial oncology and all its facets. In addition, the increase in the number of cancer survivors and their caregivers has given rise to a dramatic number of cancer-centric advocacy groups that have lobbied for greater investment in providing for the minimal psychosocial requirements for service and research with a focus to improve the quality of life for those affected by cancer. The growth and evolution of cancer-specific professional organizations focused on psychosocial oncology such as the Canadian Association of Psychosocial Oncology, the American Psychosocial Oncology Society, the International Psychosocial Oncology Society, the Association of Oncology Social Work, the Association of Pediatric Oncology Social Work, the Oncology Nursing Society and others have all matured to a point where there is informational cross over, mutual support, and enough interorganizational competitiveness to encourage individual excellence. In many ways, the professional organizations and established hospital-based departments of psychiatry, psychology, social work, pastoral care, and other counselors were following and not leading the obvious reality that cancer care is a team effort.

To better facilitate patient adjustment and to integrate with the cancer care service delivery system psychosocial departments were encouraged to focus on meaningful research that could ultimately inform and influence practice. These same skills were also essential to evaluate the effectiveness of the services provided. While intuitive wisdom acknowledged patient challenges accompanying each step of aspect of care, it seemed that it was really the large sample distress prevalence studies[3-5] that drove physicians, insurers, and administrators to acknowledge that a supportive patient care area was required. But as this chapter will explain, although reliable, objective information is the foundation of any quality program, data alone is never enough.[6] The personal human element is influential in all relationships and institutions are no different. Having insight, deciphering latent motivation, and engaging others under stress is at the core of any mental health team. Institutions can be seen as large personalities, each with its own language and priorities. Once mental health professionals apply their clinical acumen to treat each institutional encounter as the engagement phase of treatment, they start to *think like a program*. By having every member of the team, from the secretary to the psychiatrist, thinking like an integrated program creates a transformative experience for the department and for the institution. (For a discussion of creation of the model team see Loscalzo and von Gunten.)[7] The synergy of quality data, understanding what motivates your constituents, and processes that demonstrate value all support the nurturing of programs. The true worth of psychosocial values was and is how well patients and families are able to maximize the benefit of medical care, navigate the illness process, and manage distress.

With the use of standardized measures, prevalence of distress was consistently being pegged at the 40% range for a general population of cancer patients. The challenge for researchers and psychosocial directors was to identify and treat those patients in the most immediate need in a timely way and to systematically triage to the appropriate professional or resource. Given that screening for pain and biological indicators had already been conceptualized as standard practice for cancer patients and given the prevalence of distress was objectively established it seems logical and necessary to routinely screen for distress. While the *National Comprehensive Cancer Network* (NCCN) has supported this position, of the 18 NCCN member affiliates, it is surprising to learn that only three programs screen routinely as of 2007.[8] None the less, Bultz and Carlson (2006)[9] and Holland and Bultz (2007)[10] believe that with the current science, timing is ripe for a shift to routinely Screen Distress as the 6th vital sign in cancer care. All cancer centers and psychosocial programs should embrace screening as a core and necessary component of comprehensive cancer program delivery. While insurers may argue about the costs associated with screening and added expense for additional patient resources, ignoring the evidence has its own costs both in terms of patient satisfaction and patient desire to be treated in for-profit institutions. Despite any argument against screening, the Institute of Medicine[1] is strongly recommending screening in its publication of *Cancer care for the whole patient: Meeting psychosocial heath needs* (2007).[1] Unquestionably, screening for distress will provide the method to identify and directly support the patient in need. In the authors' experience, screening has also been a powerful and successful instrument to increase and tailor staffing levels based on the resulting data.

The application of systematic screening processes to identify and address biopsychosocial problems elevates the psychosocial domains as the standard of care.[9,11] Advances in, and ready access to, technology has made real-time electronic transfer of information possible resulting in innovative touch-screen programs that identify, address and triage patient and family problems, and support interprofessional commitment to excellence.[12] Cancer, while both an acute and chronic disease, has the potential to serve as a roadmap to excellence in the care of many patients facing the challenges of a life-threatening disease.

Technology must be used to bring people together. The introduction of electronic medical records is only the beginning, web-based screening will be the next step. The shifts from inpatient to outpatient treatments and now to chemotherapy at home also has major implications for the increased need for psychosocial support to maximize adherence and to minimize the great potential for social isolation in these populations. Paradoxically, the increasing encroachment of technology into all aspects of patient care only highlights the need for the partnership with a team of trained professionals who can make assessments, communicate with team members, coordinate care, provide timely interventions, and follow through with referrals. Some existing psychosocial screening and triage programs have the technology and potential to humanize the illness experience by identifying which patients need what services and at what point in time. Technology integration is not an option but an enormous opportunity for integrated programs that seize the opportunity to create a future based on the very humanistic values on which all healing is based.

Although progress has been steady but variable, there has been very little information or guidance, resources, or support available to assist leaders in creating psychosocial programs of excellence. Almost all of the early formal programs work in profession silos rather than as integrated indisciplinary teams did not have a focus. Therefore, it is not surprising that integrated psychosocial programs that are patient and family-centered, rather than guild-centered, are still extremely few in number. Although the importance of teamwork and integrated programs may be extolled as having virtuous attributes, in reality, it takes relentless perseverance in building psychosocial programs: for example, educating key administrative institutional leaders about the vision, benefits, and goals of the psychosocial program. Team building; leadership among professionals; and maximizing the synergies of research, clinical care, and education are the base upon which psychosocial programs are built.

Psychosocial programs are relatively new developments in medicine and there are no models which have been systematically evaluated. In many ways, evaluating extant psychosocial programs is irrelevant as there is already a trend to integrate palliative care and psychosocial programs. Whole-person; patient-centered care; biopsychosocial screening; and the resulting triage, program evaluation, and the demand for resource-wise integrated departments, makes the synergy of professionals and their diverse perspectives apparent.

This chapter addresses a void at a time when many new programs are being created and others reconsidering the structure, limits, and opportunities for their departments. The authors admit to having the viewpoint that patient-family-community centered programs that are founded on humanistic values naturally lead to the integration of professionals toward the actualization of evidence-based programs that include research, clinical care, education, and advocacy.

INTEGRATED PROGRAMS OF PSYCHOSOCIAL CARE

The international interest in creating programs that integrate all psychosocial providers, researchers, and educators into one clearly defined department or program stems from a variety of converging sources.

Regulatory bodies and funding sources have long called for increased teamwork and integration of professional efforts to maximize efficiency, quality, and safety,[13] as well as the need to reduce administrative costs associated with like-focused departments. Funders of research in particular have demanded that professionals demonstrate the ability to test models and to discover new knowledge that has relevance across the continuum. Institutions see integrated programs for the benefit they can bring by using resources most efficiently, enhancing their profile in the market place and mitigating the endless destructive interprofessional politics endemic to complex emotionally charged health systems. Forward-looking professionals realize that there are many enhanced opportunities by working closely with individuals who bring divergent skills to the program but who share similar interests and values. Without question, the exponential growth in the number of cancer survivors and their caregivers world-wide is one of the most robust drivers of the need for efficient, patient and family-centered programs of integrated biopsychosocial care.[14]

Patients and their caregivers almost always come to the cancer setting with inadequate information, knowledge, and skills in how to best manage the cancer experience. The disease, treatment, temporary and permanent physical and mental side effects, possibility of disability and death, and potential financial devastation are superimposed on overwhelmed health systems that create unintended iatrogenic distress. It must be noted that the distress that cancer patients and their families experience is communicated to the healthcare staff who seldom have an opportunity to process the challenges of caring for so many individuals affected by life-threatening illness. In some ways, the stress and isolation experienced by patients and their families is similar to that of healthcare professionals trying to humanize the healthcare system. For the committed professionals who function daily in highly emotionally charged environments where simple errors can have dire consequences for all involved, staff can become traumatized. Being able to readily access an organized and effective program of psychosocial services for their patients and families may significantly reduce the likelihood of burn-out. The possibilities that integrated programs offer are still being explored. Table 81–1 outlines key characteristics of model programs.

Truly integrated programs look well beyond the multidisciplinary professional perspective by including all constituents and potential allies in the pursuit of creating natural synergies toward programs of excellence at every level. Physicians, nurses, and other healthcare professionals all benefit, directly and indirectly, when there are systems in place to identify and manage psychosocial problems through clinical services, staff support, consultation on patient and family management, education about common psychosocial problems, and collaborative research to discover new knowledge.

LEVERAGING FOR GROWTH AND MAXIMIZING INFLUENCE

Research and education as the foundation for credibility. Many psychosocial oncology programs were started for the purpose of meeting the demand for psychosocial care among patients and families. Most of the literature relates to clinical care. While clinical care remains the core activity, the more successful programs have expanded their mission to include research and education. There are many reasons why research and education contribute to a program's success and should be an essential part of its mission.

All of the major cancer centers are actively engaged in basic, clinical, and population science research aimed at preventing, curing, and controlling cancer. By also engaging in research, psychosocial programs link to these larger efforts to advance the science of cancer care. The benefits of engaging in research may include greater resources in the form of intramural and extramural funds available for research and greater opportunities for collaboration with other cancer professionals through joint projects and publications. Engagement in research also signals that a psychosocial oncology program and its members value scientific evidence and are part of the growing movement within oncology and other fields of medicine toward evidence-based clinical practice. Finally,

Table 81–1. What do the best integrated programs look like?

Biopsychosocial programs and services as the foundation and connective tissue of medical care
Psychosocial programs seen as seamless with institutional vision, mission, strategic plan
Institution can clearly identify the benefits of the program:
Quality care
Safety
Patient satisfaction
Services provided supporting the mission
Efficient services
Resource preservation
Staff and faculty morale
Innovative programs
Minimize disruptions to system by helping complex patients and families
Affiliations with clinical training and research programs
Marketing and institutional profile
Community values the program
Media exposure
Humanitarian mission
Guidance and support to senior leadership
Teams who do not waste time focusing on turf and conflict
Attractive to students, interns, postdocs and other trainees
Evidenced-based processes carefully integrated into the very fabric of all programs and services
Comfortable taking risks and learning from failures
Compassionate team (from secretaries to scientists) of diverse experts all sharing humanistic values
Horizontal hierarchy based on individual expertise, specific skill required, and the encouragement of role-blurring
Relentless honesty, direct, open, and timely communication, and profound respect for colleagues and other constituents
Maximizing technology to bring people closer together
Systematic universal prospective ongoing screening
Tailored to the unique needs of the individual patient, family, community
Creates healthy dependence at all levels of the institution on services

engagement in research is likely to earn a program and its members recognition in the larger scientific community through publications in peer-reviewed journals and presentations at professional meetings.

Professional education activities, in the form of training and continuing education programs can also yield multiple dividends. The presence of trainees encourages program members to remain abreast of recent developments in their fields of expertise so they can communicate this wisdom to the next generation of clinicians and researchers. The questions posed by trainees may challenge program members to examine and advance current clinical practices rather than maintain the status quo. Likewise, the fresh perspectives of trainees may stimulate new lines of scientific investigation and or new approaches to old questions. Given the scarcity of individuals trained in psychosocial oncology, many programs also find their own trainees to be among the best-qualified candidates for open positions. Conducting continuing professional education for established professionals is another activity that encourages program members to remain abreast of recent developments and to examine their current practices. These activities also have the potential to establish a program's reputation as a center of excellence in psychosocial oncology through presentations that showcase innovative and thoughtful approaches to care delivery.

Ultimately, research and education informs and drives the development of new knowledge and innovative ways to expand the boundaries and perceptions of what psychosocial programs have to contribute to the patient, family, clinical staff, and greater community. It is only through the meticulous application of scientific principles to whole patient and family care that psychosocial programs will be able to truly develop the discipline of a "science of caring" that connects the illusory chiasm in cancer medicine.

Marketing and public affairs. Departments of Marketing and Public Affairs are focused on showing the institution in the best light possible. This leads to community recognition of the institution as a benefit and to being competitive in the market place. Marketing and public affairs are both essential functions for the survival of a quality institution. Within these departments are highly creative individuals who are able to translate and carefully craft the language of psychosocial care for the specific targeted audience. Historically, the major barrier to utilization of Marketing and Public Affairs Departments has been the reluctance of psychosocial professionals to actively orient and educate these professionals who focus on getting the message of the institution into the public domain. It is the responsibility of the psychosocial department to continually feed stories, information, and ideas to these two departments. It is only within the context of ongoing relationships that the information can be understood and as having value to the institution. Patient and family stories, new research, innovative interventions, creative and artistic therapies, tailored programs to specific constituents, practical things people can do to support others, and new program models are all examples of topics that are of particular interest to the public and enhance the competitiveness of the institution in the market place. More importantly, these are areas that are the primary focus of psychosocial programs (see Table 81–2).

Table 81–2. How to know what your institution values?

Ask them
Peruse strategic plan, annual report, marketing materials
Peruse the home page web site
Read press releases
Know the financial metrics used by the institution
Get as high up in the hierarchy as you can, then go higher
Know what the senior leadership values
Understand where the bulk of the resources go
Research information and interests about new faculty and employees
Know what buildings are being built and why
Talk to the Board of Directors whenever possible

Development matters: but you have to ask. It was once considered "common wisdom" that it was difficult or impossible to raise money for psychosocial and palliative care programs from external sources. The etiology of this attitude (*large donations only go to medicine or bench-science*) and resulting disinclination to mount fund-raising efforts for psychosocial programs are now moot. Many psychosocial programs have raised large sums of money to support and to enhance the size and depth of their programs. Experience consistently demonstrates that one of the barriers to raising money is the lack of a relationship between the psychosocial program and the Development Office of institutions. You have to ask, many times!

The other barrier to maximizing your relationship with the Development Office is creating "products" for which individuals, foundations, and corporations can see as having great value. Examples of successful fundable projects are Chairs or Professorships, multiuse buildings that provide psychosocial services, touch-screen screening programs, professional and community educational series, community outreach, patient navigation programs, research for specific patient populations or problems, integrative medicine education or research, indigent care, pet therapy, creative arts, musical instruments, salary support as seed money for new programs.

Working with the Development Office is a relationship, not a single event: it is necessary to create opportunities for ongoing communication and coordination based on reliable and trusting relationships. If you make your institution look good, your program will be valued and the Development Office will want to help support your program. If there is reluctance from the Development Office to actively support your program it is essential that you go as high up in the administrative system to advocate for support. This is a time when the Patient and Family Advisory Council (to be discussed later) can be a potent (and hard to ignore) advocate for the program.

People who have the financial or resource capability and who are philanthropic (you need both) want to create meaning in their lives by giving. They are also people who are highly selective about quality and value. Value in these situations is measured by inherent worth of the services, what the donor sees as important and how the donor benefits. Although motivations vary greatly, no people or entities will give money unless they are sure that the money will be used wisely, that there is a deliverable product or service that can be clearly described in understandable language and that the effort will be carefully evaluated. Psychosocial programs are well positioned to receive such funding because outcomes can be measured.

Basic demographics predict that philanthropic giving will grow exponentially over the next 20 years in line with the baby boom generation. Since cancer most commonly affects the elderly there is an opportunity for psychosocial programs to offer potentials for giving that can dramatically further research, education, and clinical care by partnering with donors. Most donors will come through the Development Office; it is, therefore, essential to have an ongoing relationship with the Development Office and to understand how the individual fund-raisers are incentivized. Having this insight will help to frame your approach to engaging the Development Office—but, remember, you have to ask!

The patient and family advisory council. Until recently, the primary interactions professionals had with patients and their families were within the clinical setting and within clearly defined hierarchical boundaries, with the professionals being in the one-up positions. This reflection of the medical model is limiting and is increasingly inconsistent in an age of consumer rights and regulations relating to informed consent. In addition, the medical model also resulted in the psychosocial concerns of patients and families, and the professionals providing these services, being relegated to a lower level on the hierarchy for funding. Funding, whether for clinical, educational, or research programs is still the most accurate reflection of the values of the institution or the healthcare system. Until recently, psychosocial programs have not had the strong relationships with the full spectrum of constituents that other medical specialties have enjoyed. This is changing, quickly. In fact, psychosocial programs can and should have a central and highly visible role to play in leading the transition in the changing relationships with patients, families, and healthcare

professionals. Enhancing communication, interpreting motivations and behaviors, psychosocial screening and tailored triage, problem solving, providing emotional support, alchemizing distress into meaningful activity, counseling, education, mediation, and advocacy are all areas of expertise for psychosocial providers. The Patient and Family Advisory Council is one important way to manifest this contribution.

A number of forward-looking medical institutions have created variances of highly organized programs where patients, their families, healthcare staff, hospital administrators, and community leaders meet to discuss ways to maximize the benefits of medical care and psychosocial services to patients, families, and community.[15] Although the structure and operations of the Councils are beyond the scope of this manuscript, the benefits are not. Patients and family members can and will always speak in a voice that will have higher emotional authority than professionals with an "agenda." Hospital administrators specifically, hear the concerns of patients and families as being much more objective than requests from their colleagues who from their perspective are always asking for more: more money, more space, more resources, more recognition, more respect, more appreciation, and more of everything.

Because psychosocial services, education, and research will never be reliable or robust revenue streams (with the exception of philanthropy), it is essential for successful programs to leverage their influence to assure that in the competition for resources their strategies are focused and effective. Having patients and families advocating for additional resources for psychosocial services, education, and research has a powerful impact. It is highly recommended that whenever possible a high-ranking member of the Board of Directors be a member of the Council. It is also suggested that the Council make periodic progress reports to the institution's leadership. Whether the problem is parking, uncommunicative physicians, talking to children about cancer, fatigue, depression, anxiety or spiritual crisis; patient and families, along with healthcare professionals need to use many voices to communicate the same consistent messages. Although these tailored messages will differ by institution and situation, the mantra must be the same—*the biopsychosocial perspective is the foundation for maximizing the benefits of medical care and to promote quality of life. This can only be achieved with psychosocial services that are at least as good as the medical care provided.*

The Council can be a robust and powerful resource for the psychosocial program with implications that can reverberate at all levels of the institution and community. By having many voices with one focused message, the psychosocial program can clarify the inseparable and dynamic connection between psychosocial wellness and physical health. The Council is increasingly an essential voice toward program excellence.

Hospital administrators. Although mental health professionals tend to be astute as it relates to the needs of patients and families, this wisdom and training has not been applied to encounters with the goals of the institution in general and to hospital administrators specifically. Being able to demonstrate the contributions of psychosocial services at every opportunity is essential for a successful program. Institutions and administrators deserve the same amount of respect, assessment, and insight as do clinical situations. It has long been recognized that the best clinicians are also superb administrators. Individual psychosocial providers must apply their understanding of motivation and skills of engagement to all of their constituents, in other words—*Think like a clinician but act like a program at all times!*

For too many hospital administrators psychosocial services are seen as ancillary and are not perceived as contributing to the core financial mission of the institution. However, hospital administrators do value safety, cost avoidance and reduction, quality, patient satisfaction, resource efficiency, staff retention, and minimizing disruption to hospital systems and processes. Psychosocial services can make major contributions in all of these areas. Mental health services, as with most of the services provided in medical institutions, do not result in a profit. Although third party reimbursement for mental health services are significantly less than payment for medical care there is significant political action toward reconciling this stigmatizing disparity.

Social work	Psychology	Psychiatry	Palliative care
• Does not require consult request form	• Fax consult request • Doctor-doctor contact needed for urgent consult	• Fax consult request • Doctor-doctor contact needed for urgent consult	• Fax consult request • Doctor-doctor contact needed for urgent consult
Phone:			
Fax:			
• Urgent assessment of suicidal, homicidal or upset patients • Adjustment to illness • Coping skills • Stress management • Family counseling • Advanced directives • Suicide assessment • Community referrals • Bereavement • End-of-life counseling • Compliance enhancement • Gate keeper for psychosocial services	• Assessment & stabilization of *illness-related distress* including: ~Adjustment to illness ~Psychological stability for treatment ~Medical compliance ~Stress & coping ~Body image & sexual functioning ~Neuropsychological functioning • Inpatient & outpatient consultation available	• Assessment & treatment of altered mental state • Pharmacologic treatment of depression, anxiety & agitation • Substance dependence • Psychiatric stability for treatment	• Pain and symptom assessment & management • End-of-life communications • Goals of care discussions • Diarrhea/Constipation • Nausea/Vomiting • Sedation • Substance abuse consultation

Fig. 81–1. Supportive care medicine triage.

But even with medical parity, it is extremely unlikely that psychosocial services will ever be seen as a meaningful revenue stream for hospitals. Therefore, other ways to demonstrate value must be developed and cogently communicated, preferably through scripted mantras, to administrators at every opportunity and by every member of the department.

Another key area for psychosocial departments relates to the major contribution made to the institution in times of crisis, either through natural disaster or due to human tragedy, such as the death of a beloved colleague, unanticipated death of a patient, violence in the work place, or a major medical error resulting in serious injury or death. The importance of a proactive approach by the psychosocial leader, resulting in clearly defined steps to communicate and implement a plan of action to stabilize the situation is essential and will result in recognition for the value of psychosocial services that cannot be accomplished in any other manner. It is in the best interest for psychosocial providers to have team-centered protocols in place for mental health support and for the practical resources needed in times of crises. Psychiatry, psychology, social work, chaplaincy, administrative support staff, and others should all have clearly defined roles and procedures in the event of a crisis (Fig. 81–1). No single event will more potently imprint on administrators the value (and gratitude) of psychosocial services as an integrated and highly organized program deftly implemented in a time of crisis. Ultimately, psychosocial programs must be perceived as part of the essential fabric and connective tissue of the institution where there is a sense of profound healthy interdependence and respect.

MAINTAINING AND DEVELOPING PROFESSIONAL IDENTITY

The integration of multiple disciplines into a unified psychosocial department or program creates a number of opportunities. The benefit to the hospital is the elimination of duplication of the financial costs to the institution and the clarity of messaging to other healthcare providers (nurses and physicians) and patients that a psychosocial department is the "one stop-shop" to refer patients for emotional, financial, spiritual,

practical, and other concerns. For too long, professional rivalries and the primitive "need" for separate departments have created confusion about where to refer and who would be the best provider to care for the multiple and complex supportive care needs of the patient.

With the opportunity of building a unified interdisciplinary psychosocial department, there will be clear challenges as well as benefits to the professionals. Resistance to integration will likely focus on fear of change, sense of loss of familiar ways of doing things, ostensible dilution of professional identity, shift in the hierarchy, and the impact on staffing levels (jobs). Keeping in mind the unique value of each profession may not be enough to build a commitment to a blended department, but working together and collaborating in areas of clinical service, teaching, and research will create opportunities to learn from each other and develop trust. Irrespective of profession, a leader committed to the value of providing excellence in service, education, and research will help an integrated program overcome the political rivalries that inevitably occur. Striving for excellence at ever opportunity and at every level must be the departmental mantra. Respect for, and learning from, discipline differences must become the only acceptable behavior of all departmental members. Not all professionals are suited for such high demands and interpersonal expectations. Ultimately, there needs to be space within integrated programs for the strengthening of a sense of professional identify based on the universal humanistic and patient-centered values of Hippocrates, Galen, Maimonides, while more recently Cicely Saunders, Elisabeth Kubler-Ross, and perhaps you.

CREATING THE FUTURE OF BIOPSYCHOSOCIAL PROGRAMS

Changing demographics and economics will always influence healthcare change. It is how these powerful political forces drive healthcare policies that are most important to patients, families, healthcare professionals, and community. Healthcare is always a highly politicized charged process, both nationally and within institutions. It is essential that new and meaningful partnerships with patients, families, and especially among healthcare professionals are forged. Integrated departments of psychosocial and palliative care are at the vanguard of new models for the provision of psychosocial care. But as it relates to state of the art medical care overall, almost all psychosocial programs around the world are anachronisms that are so focused on ostensible turf and boundary struggles, that they are not able to see beyond the reflexive fear that blinds them to the promise of what can be ultimately achieved by working as a integrated team.

Bringing together compassionate expertise of highly skilled teams of mental and medical health professionals, researchers, and educators, holds the most promise to advance the humanistic vision of psychosocial care, while fully appreciating the other powerful economic and political forces that are endemic to healthcare systems everywhere. The different perspectives of physicians, psychologists, social workers, nurses, spiritual counselors, educators, and others, all within one clearly defined department, results in creative tension that when focused on one common vision has the greatest probability to result in a superior program that inculcates patient-centered whole-patient care; that is the challenge before us.

REFERENCES

1. Institute of Medicine (IOM). Adler NE, Page AEK (eds). *Cancer care for the whole patient: Meeting psychosocial health needs*. Washington DC: National Academy Press; 2008.

2. Institute of Medicine. *Meeting psychosocial needs of women with breast cancer*. Washington DC: National Academy Press; 2001.

3. Zabora J, BrintzenhofeSzoc K, Curbow B, Hooker C, Piantadosi S. The prevalence of psychological distress by cancer site. *Psychooncology. 2001;*10:19–28.

4. Cella DF, Tulsky DS, Gray G, et al. The functional assessment of cancer therapy scale: development and validation of the general measure. *J Clin Oncol.* 1993;11:570–579.

5. Carlson LE, Angen M, Cullum J, et al. High levels of untreated distress and fatigue in cancer patients. *Br J Cancer.* 2004;90:2297–2304.

6. Ariely D. *Predictably irrational: The hidden forces that shape our decisions.* London, UK: HarperCollins; 2008.

7. Loscalzo MJ, von Gunten C. The palliative care team. In: Chochinov H, Breitbart W (eds). *Handbook of psychiatry in palliative medicine*, 2nd ed. Oxford University Press. 2009.

8. Jacobsen PB. Screening for psychological distress in cancer patients: challenges and opportunities. *J Clin Oncol.* 2007;25:4526–4527.

9. Bultz BD, Carlson LE. Emotional distress: the sixth vital sign—future directions in cancer care. *Psychooncology.* 2006;15:93–95.

10. Holland JC, Bultz BD, National comprehensive Cancer Network (NCCN). The NCCN guideline for distress management: a case for making distress the sixth vital sign. *J Natl Compr Canc Netw.* 2007;1:3–7.

11. Jacobsen PB, Donovan KA, Trask PC, et al. Screening for psychologic distress in ambulatory cancer patients: a multicenter evaluation of the distress thermometer. *Cancer.* 2005;103:1494–1502.

12. Loscalzo MJ, Clark KL. Problem-related distress in cancer patients drives requests for help: a prospective study. *Oncology.* 2007;21:1133–1138.

13. Institute of Medicine. *To err is human: Building a safer health system.* Washington DC: National Academy Press; 1999.

14. President's Cancer Panel. *Living beyond cancer: A European dialogue.* Bethesda, MD: National Cancer Institute; 2004.

15. Medical News Today. *Many hospitals establish patient advisory councils.* Available at URL: http://www.medicalnewstoday.com/articles/79199.php. Accessed September 12, 2008.

CHAPTER 82

Oncology Staff Stress and Related Interventions

Mary L. S. Vachon

Working in oncology has been both stressful and rewarding from its inception to the present. This chapter focuses primarily on recent research from 2000 on, in occupational stress and its relevance for understanding stressors, coping mechanisms, and programs of intervention relevant to oncology.

OCCUPATIONAL STRESS

The concepts of stress, burnout, compassion fatigue, and moral distress are relevant in a discussion of stress in oncology. Of these, the issues of stress and burnout are most studied.

Burnout. Table 82–1 shows the symptoms of burnout which include physical, emotional, occupational, and social symptoms. Burnout is a form of mental distress manifested in "normal" people who did not suffer from prior psychopathology and who experience decreased work performance resulting from negative attitudes and behaviors.[3]

Components of burnout. Burnout is a psychological syndrome in response to chronic interpersonal stressors on the job. The three key dimensions are as follows[4]:

Overwhelming **emotional exhaustion** (EE)—the basic *individual stress dimension* of burnout refers to feelings of being overextended and depleted of one's emotional and physical resources Exhaustion is the most widely and most thoroughly analyzed and studied aspect of burnout. Exhaustion prompts action to distance oneself emotionally and cognitively from work, as a way to cope with work overload.[3]

Feelings of **cynicism** and detachment from the job (**depersonalization**) (DP)—the *interpersonal context* dimension of burnout, refers to a negative, callous, or excessively detached response to various aspects of the job. It is an attempt to put distance between oneself and various aspects of the job. Research shows a consistent and strong relationship between exhaustion and cynicism both of which emerge in the presence of work overload and social conflict.[3] Sense of **ineffectiveness** and **lack of personal accomplishment** (PA)—the *self-evaluation dimension* of burnout refers to feelings of incompetence and a lack of achievement and productivity at work. PA arises more clearly from a lack of resources to get the work done (e.g., lack of critical information, lack of necessary tools, or insufficient time). It may be directly related to EE and DP, or be more independent.[5]

Demographic characteristics related to burnout include being single and younger; males score slightly higher on cynicism than females. Personality characteristics associated with burnout include neuroticism, lower levels of hardiness and self-esteem.[3,5] Supportive spouses or partners are helpful in preventing burnout[6,7]; work-home interference is associated with burnout.[8] Research is much stronger for the association between burnout and a wide range of job characteristics including the following: chronically difficult job demands, an imbalance between high demands and low resources, and the presence of conflict (whether between people, between role demands, or between important values.[5]

The impact of burnout. Highly motivated health professionals with intense investment in their profession are at a greater risk for the development of burnout.[9] Burnout is associated with suboptimal patient care practices and medical errors on the part of physicians.[10] DP in physicians was associated with lower patient satisfaction and longer postdischarge

recovery.[11] Burnout was associated with a lower satisfaction with career choice; it was a stronger predictor of low career satisfaction than screening positive for depression in all models. It was also associated with poorer health.[12]

BURNOUT IN ONCOLOGY

Stress and burnout in oncology. This review focuses on five studies from before 2000[13–17] and 18 from 2000 onward.[8,12,18–33] One-third of the studies were from the United States. Studies were primarily of oncologists and oncology nurses, but some also included psychosocial staff, and support staff.

Burnout scores. In Maslach and Jackson's[34] normative sample of U.S. physicians and registered nurses, 33% had high EE, 33% high DP and 33% low PA. Most of the reviewed studies did not report an overall score on the Maslach Burnout Inventory (MBI) but 28% of surgical oncologists (31% of those under 50 vs. 22% over 50) and women (37% vs. 26%) had overall high-burnout scores.[12] Using a similar population and instrument, burnout in a large sample of oncologists decreased overtime from 56%[15] to 34%.[33] In another large sample of American oncologists,[18] 61.7% reported feeling burned out.

Emotional exhaustion. Emotional exhaustion is the scale that is most responsive to the organizational environment and social interactions that characterize human service work.[20] The lowest rate of EE reported in the studies reviewed was 15% in Japanese palliative care physicians.[19] Approximately one-quarter of oncologists in Japan[19]; the United Kingdom[16]; Italy, Spain and Portugal,[32] and surgical oncologists in the United States reported high EE.[12] One-third of Italian haemato-oncology doctors and nurses[20] and Canadian gynecologic oncologists[8] reported high EE, as did 40% of oncology and transplant staff in Greece.[29] The highest rate of EE (53.3%) was found in physicians working in Cancer Care Ontario which compared with 37.1% of allied staff.[23]

Kash et al.[27] used mean scores. The total sample mean for burnout was 29.22. The normative score for U.S. physicians and nurses was >17.[34] House staff had significantly higher EE (34.03) than nurses (29.2) and medical oncologists (25.1).

EE and anger. Oncologists and ophthalmologists were assessed using the MBI and the State-Trait Anger Expression Inventory.[31] Oncology staff showed higher mean scores on the MBI, EE, and DP scales. Increasing burnout was associated with higher anger expressed toward the environment and loss of anger control. Higher scores on State Anger were associated with a pathological state of EE. Anger, as a response to frustration, appears to be a constant clinical feature of burnout and it should not be underestimated in theoretical and preventive contexts. Previously, Vachon[14] reported that in a study of 581 international caregivers to the critically ill, dying, and bereaved, the 110 caregivers in oncology were more likely to report problems with anger, irritability, and frustration than were the caregivers in other specialties. The burned out oncologists in Allegra et al.'s[18] sample reported feeling frustrated (78%), emotionally exhausted (69%) and had a lack of satisfaction with work (50%).

DP (diminished empathy). Depersonalization "may be interpreted as an attitude of 'patient refusal' in the oncology staff actuated

Table 82–1. Signs and symptoms of burnout

Physical
Fatigue
Physical and emotional exhaustion
Headaches
Gastrointestinal disturbances
Weight loss
Sleeplessness
Hypertension
Myocardial infarction

Psychological
Anxiety
Depression
Boredom
Frustration
Low morale
Irritability
May contribute to alcoholism and drug addiction

Occupational
Depersonalization in relationships with colleagues, patients, or both
Emotional exhaustion, cynicism, perceived ineffectiveness
Job turnover
Impaired job performance
Deterioration in the physician–patient relationship and a decrease in the quantity and quality of care

Social
Marital difficulties

SOURCE: The table is adapted from information in references 1 and 2.

as a defense mechanism toward the bewildering and frightening experiences that come with the daily assistance of oncology patients."[31' p. 648] In Greece, DP was higher in those in pediatric oncology without children and with fewer years of practice.[29]

The lowest report of DP was 4% of the allied health staff in the Ontario study.[23] Nurses in the Kash et al.[27] study had lower rates than house staff or oncologists. Physicians in oncology more commonly reported rates of DP from 10% to 15%.[8,12,16,19] Approximately one-quarter of physicians in oncology in Ontario[23]; Italy, Spain and Portugal,[32] and Italian oncologists and nurses reported DP.[20] The house staff in Kash et al.'s[27] study scored significantly higher than oncologists. High emotional empathy has been found to be associated with mental well-being in internal medicine residents.[35]

Low PA. American surgical oncologists were least likely to report low feelings of PA (9.6%).[12] One-third of Canadian gynecologic oncologists[8]; about half of Ontario oncologists and allied health professionals[23]; about half of Japanese palliative care physicians and 65% of oncologists reported low PA.[19] In the Kash et al. study[27] the group was almost identical to the mean of 36.53 reported by Maslach and Jackson,[34] but nurses' had a significantly lower sense of accomplishment (34.94) than oncologists (38.03).

Psychiatric disturbance. Psychiatric disturbance in oncology staff ranged from a low of 12% of palliative care physicians[19] to between a quarter and one-third of the sample in the other studies.[8,20,23] Kash et al.[27] found women had more psychological distress/demoralization (30% vs. 24.5%) and house staff had more than oncologists (30% vs. 21.6%).

Demographic variables and burnout in oncology. Younger caregivers report more stressors, exhibit more manifestations of stress and fewer coping strategies[14] and are more prone to burnout and stress reactions.[12,16,27,36] Emotional sensitivity and the ability to connect with

patients rose after the age of 35.[37] Those with more years of experience were less likely to report stress-related symptoms and burnout.[14,33] Surgeons with fewer years of experience had a lower sense of P A.[12]

Those with more responsibility for dependents, either children or elderly parents, reported more stress.[27] Being single was an independent risk factor for burnout.[36] Females may be more at risk of mental health problems and burnout.[12,17,27] However, in a large, recent study of U.K. National Health Service physicians, male and midaged consultants were particularly at risk.[38]

Personality factors relevant to burnout in oncology. The profession of medicine with its delay of satisfactions may lead people to experience burnout.[2,39] The compulsive triad in physicians of doubt, guilt feelings, and an exaggerated sense of responsibility can have an enormous impact on professional, personal, and family lives.[2,39] A diminishing awareness of one's physical and emotional needs leads to a self-destructive pattern of overwork. A psychology of postponement takes root in which physicians habitually delay in attending to their significant relationships and other sources of renewal until all the work is done or the next professional hurdle is achieved.[2,40]

The personality characteristic of hardiness—a sense of commitment, control, and challenge,[41,42] helped to alleviate burnout in oncology staff and was associated with a greater sense of PA.[27]

Religiosity, spirituality, and meaning making. Being religious has been associated with a decreased risk of burnout.[27] Current work tends to speak of spirituality in contrast to religiosity. Kearney and Mount[43] define spirituality as "of, or pertaining to, affecting or concerning the spirit or higher moral questions" and speak of the need for the caregiver to experience his or her own inner depths as he or she is with a patient experiencing spiritual pain.

A MODEL FOR UNDERSTANDING OCCUPATIONAL STRESS

Recent research on burnout has focused on the degree of match or mismatch between the person and six domains of the job environment. The greater the gap or mismatch between the person and the environment, the greater the likelihood of burnout. The greater the match or fit the greater the likelihood of engagement with work. Six areas of work life encompass the major organizational antecedents of burnout. These include workload, control, reward, community, fairness, and values.[4]

Burnout arises from chronic mismatches between people and their work settings in some or all of these areas. The area of values may play a central mediating role for the other areas[4] although, for individuals at risk of burnout, fairness in the work environment may be the tipping point determining whether people develop job engagement or burnout.[3]

Emotion-work variables (e.g., requirement to display or suppress emotions on the job, requirements to be emotionally empathic) account for additional variance in burnout scores over and above job stressors.[4]

Workload. Excessive workload exhausts the individual to the extent that recovery becomes impossible. Workload has long been a major issue in oncology.[8,13,14,17,18,20,23–27]

Whippen and Cannelos[15] and Whippen et al.[33] report insufficient personal time and or vacation time as two of the three most commonly reported stressors leading to burnout. In their replication study in 2004, over one-third said that their burnout affected patient care. A lack of confidence in having sufficient time to communicate with patients was associated with burnout in Japanese oncologists,[19] while French oncology nurses felt time pressure which did not allow them to deal with the psychological components of care and to face suffering and death.[25]

Burnout was also associated with being overloaded and its effect on home life.[16,26] Performing more than 11 surgical cases a week, was associated with burnout and surgical oncologists who worked longer hours (24% worked more than 70 hours a week) were more likely to have EE.[12] In gynecologic oncologists, low PA was associated with having fewer partners, a high number of follow-ups and culposcopy patients and spending a high percentage of time with gynecologic oncology patients.[8]

Control. Control is related to inefficacy or reduced PA. Mismatches often indicate that individuals have insufficient control over the resources necessary to do their work or insufficient authority to pursue the work in what they believe is the most effective manner. Stress results from a lack of knowledge in interpersonal skills and a lack of communication skills and/or management skills.[13,16,17,24] There are issues when patients become more demanding consumers.[13,14,23]

In gynecologic oncologists, high EE, and a negative association with job satisfaction was associated with a loss of ability to bring about positive change in the organization. High EE and high stress was associated with "insufficient input into my unit" and inadequate facilities.[8]

Consistently, caregivers report having difficulty performing in their jobs because of a lack of organizational resources.[8,13,16,17,20,23] In addition, they report feeling disenfranchised[27] and having an imbalance between their job and their authority.[26]

Reward. Lack of reward may be financial when one doesn't receive a salary or benefits commensurate with achievements, or lack of social rewards when one's hard work is ignored and not appreciated by others. The lack of intrinsic rewards (e.g., doing something of importance and doing it well) can also be a critical part of this mismatch. Issues with the financial reward for work was noted by physicians.[17-20] Almost half of Italian oncology nurses, compared with one-third of oncologists reported low salaries.[20] Low PA and high stress was reported when pay was inequitable.[8] There are frequent complaints of a lack of resources to do one's work.[8,17]

Reports of communication problems with administration often reflect a lack of social rewards.[14,26] In the Ramirez et al. study[16] deriving little satisfaction from work was associated with burnout for oncologists. There were concerns about the future funding of units and feeling that skills were being underutilized.[22] Oncology support staff reported feeling a lack of value and recognition. Their lowest satisfaction score was with job recognition.[21]

Community. This mismatch arises when people lose a sense of personal connection with others in the workplace. Social support from people with whom one shares praise, comfort, happiness, and humor affirms membership in a group with a shared sense of values. Problems with colleagues were reported in many studies.[13,14,16,17,20,21,26] In the Kash study[27] oncologists reported less support from their colleagues than did nurses or fellows. A lack of support from administration was found in Italian nurses[20] as well as support staff at Massachusetts General Hospital (MGH).[21] In Greek staff, a lack of role clarity was associated with burnout.[29] French nurses reported that the absence of a doctor at the time of a patient's death was associated with distress lasting for a week after the patient's death.[25] Gynecologic-oncologists had high DP and high-job stress if they had difficult relations with colleagues.[8] High EE and high-job stress were associated with taking on managerial responsibilities and relationships with colleagues.[8]

Fairness. This mismatch arises when there is perceived unfairness in the workplace. Fairness communicates respect and confirms people's self-worth. Mutual respect between people is central to a shared sense of community. There are concerns about funding[17]; nurses not feeling supported in meeting patients' emotional needs[27]; and having inadequate resources to do the job properly.[23,24] In Turkey, oncology nurses and oncologists experienced an imbalance between their jobs and responsibilities, unfairness in job promotion, inadequacy of equipment, and high cost of drugs.[26]

Values. People might feel constrained by their job to do something unethical and not in accord with their own values. Alternatively, there may be a mismatch between their personal career goals and the values of the organization. People can also be caught in conflicting values of the organization, as when there is a discrepancy between a lofty mission statement and actual practice, or when the values are in conflict (e.g., high-quality service and cost containment do not always coexist). Staffing problems can lead to not being able to do the job properly, a decrease in quality patient care and decreased staff morale.[23,24]

Gynecologic-oncologists had high EE and high-job stress if their expertise was not being put to good use.[8] Burned out oncology surgeons[12] were less satisfied with their career choice. Surgeons in private practice were less likely to say they would become a physician again, and less likely to say they would become a surgical oncologist again. Devoting less that 25% of one's time to research was associated with burnout in that study.

Emotion/work variables. Emotion/work variables require the individual to display or suppress emotions on the job and involve the requirement to be emotionally empathic. Staff report difficulty in various aspects of communicating with sick, suffering, and dying patients and their family members,[14,15,18,20,23,24,26,32] particularly if they are young.[14,20]

A recent study of academic oncologists[44] found that those who viewed their roles as encompassing both biomedical and psychosocial aspects of care reported a clear method of communicating with patients and families about end-of life issues, an ability to positively influence patient and family coping with and acceptance of the dying process. They described communication as a process, made recommendations to the patient using an individualized approach, and viewed the provision of effective EOL care as very satisfying. In contrast, oncologists who described primarily a biomedical role reported a more distant relationship with the patient, a sense of failure at not being able to alter the course of the disease, and an absence of collegial support. In their descriptions of communication encounters with patients and families, these physicians did not seem to feel they could impact patients' coping with and acceptance of death and made few recommendations about EOL treatment options. Physicians who viewed EOL care as an important role reported increased job satisfaction.

In a Southern European study, low psychosocial orientation and burnout symptoms were associated with lower confidence in communication skills and higher expectations of a negative outcome following physician-patient communication.[32] Confidence in communication was not related to age or years in practice. Physicians who scored high on DP considered it very unlikely that a positive outcome would be achieved as a result of communicating with their patients. Japanese oncologists and palliative care physicians who were less confident in dealing with psychologic care and demonstrated higher levels of EE were more likely to choose continuous-deep sedation for patients with refractory physical and psychologic distress.[30] Insufficient confidence in the psychological care of patients was associated with physician burnout rather than involvement in EOL care.[19]

In the original burnout study by Whippen and Cannelos[15] administering palliative or terminal care was a contributing factor to burnout in 53% of respondents. In the later study[33] this dropped to 31%. Frustration with limited therapeutic success dropped to 22% versus 45%.

Kash et al.[27] found that nurses and house staff most often see patients, rather than the patient when they are most ill with symptoms, or in the terminal stage of disease. The stressors contributing most to burnout and demoralization were dealing with a high number of deaths, or struggling over a Do Not Resuscitate (DNR) decision with another colleague or family member. Ethical issues also contributed to burnout in Italy where oncologists reported more difficulty with ethical and moral problems than did nurses but seemed to have better judgment on the communication training received.[20] Cohen and Erickson[45] suggest that students and novice nurses in oncology may experience more uncertainty and distress related to ethical issues, evolving from conflicting values or beliefs about what is the right or best course of action.

Oncology nurses[25] reported feeling impotent if patients didn't improve and over one-third reported disgust with preparing dead bodies for the mortuary, especially with stuffing orifices.

Rural nurses working in Australia with oncology patients found that a key issue in providing psychosocial care was their own "emotional toil." They are multiskilled generalists providing care to patients with cancer without necessarily having specialist knowledge or skill. This results in fatigue and EE that impact on their own well-being.[28]

JOB ENGAGEMENT AND COMPASSION SATISFACTION

Job engagement[5] and compassion satisfaction (CS)[46] are two frameworks to understand what keeps workers functioning and enjoying their work in challenging situations.

JOB ENGAGEMENT

Job engagement is conceptualized as being the opposite of burnout. Engagement is defined as a persistent, positive-affective-motivational state of fulfillment in employees that is characterized by vigor, dedication, and absorption.[5] Engagement is associated with a sustainable workload, feelings of choice and control, appropriate recognition and reward, a supportive work community, fairness and justice, and meaningful and valued work.

Maslach and Leiter[3] describe the continuum between the negative experience of burnout and the positive experience of engagement. There are three interrelated dimensions to this continuum: exhaustion-energy, cynicism-involvement, and inefficacy-efficacy. Exhaustion and cynicism are the two primary measures of burnout. They "go together," both appearing strongly in people experiencing burnout and they both fade away in people experiencing engagement with their work. A potential early warning sign of burnout is the appearance of one, but not the other of these signs. They suggest there is a push to move from an inconsistent pattern to a consistent one. A predictor of whether an inconsistent pattern will evolve toward burnout or engagement will be the presence of a negative incongruence between the person and the job. For someone who is experiencing one of the burnout dimensions, this level of incongruity can be the tipping point into burnout. In a university setting the workplace incongruity (tipping point) that determined whether people changed was their perception of fairness in the workplace.

Compassion satisfaction. Compassion satisfaction[46] is satisfaction derived from the work of helping others. It may be the portrayal of efficacy. Caregivers with CS derive pleasure from helping others, like their colleagues, feel good about their ability to help and make a contribution. There may be a balance between compassion fatigue and CS. Caregivers may experience compassion fatigue, yet they like their work because they feel positive benefits from it. They believe what they are doing is helping others and may even be redemptive. When a person's belief system is well maintained with positive material, a person's resiliency may be enhanced.[47] What seems to count most for resilience is the opportunity to encounter pain within a context of meaning and to find that one's compassion (one's suffering with) has power. These sustain an underlying belief that the world is good and in order.[48]

COPING

Job satisfaction and meaning making. When caregivers to the critically ill, dying, and bereaved were asked what enabled them to continue working in the field, the top coping mechanism identified was as follows: a sense of competence, control, or pleasure in one's work.[14] One-third of Italian oncologists and nurses[20] were very satisfied with their jobs and 60% were quite satisfied. More than 80% would repeat their choice to work with oncology patients.

Sources of satisfaction for oncology staff include the following:

- dealing well with patients and relatives[16,24]
- patient care or patient contact[20,24]
- having professional status and esteem, deriving intellectual satisfaction, and having adequate resources to perform one's role[16]
- being perceived to do one's job well[24]
- having good relationships with colleagues[8,14,20,24]
- personal ideals[24]

Oncology was perceived to be a special environment, often because of longstanding relationships with patients.[24] Attachment to work and patients hardly declines, even in burnout. Stress may be "double-edged" in the sense that a task done badly was a source of stress, but the same job done well was a source of satisfaction.[16,20]

Hamilton,[49] a neurosurgeon, writes of coming to recognize how we are all connected "…as a physician, you have unparalleled entry into the lives of others. Every patient is an existential conduit to seeing your own struggle" [p.63]. Taylor,[50] a neuro-anatomist had a left brain stroke at age 37. In *My stroke of insight* she says the experience made her aware that …"I am part of a greater structure-an eternal flow of energy and molecules

from which I cannot be separated" [p.160]. "My left hemisphere had been trained to perceive myself as a solid, separate from others. Now, released from that restrictive circuitry my right hemisphere relished in its attachment to the eternal flow. I was no longer isolated and alone [p.69]. She speaks of being sensitive to the energies of her caregivers.

I experienced people as concentrated packages of energy. Doctors and nurses were massive conglomerations of powerful beams of energy that came and went…With this shift onto my right hemisphere, I became empathic to what others felt. Although I could not understand the words they spoke, I could read volumes from their facial expressions and body language. I paid very close attention to how energy dynamics affected me. I realized that some people brought me energy, while others took it away [p.74-75].

Hamilton[49] says "Medicine was not meant to be a mechanical transaction. It's a spiritual quest, putting your own soul on the line, along with the patient's" [p.123].

Katz[51] redefines counter-transference and speaks of the alchemical reaction which occurs when two individuals engage together at the most vulnerable time in human existence-the EOL. Alchemy is "that space" that takes its own place in the poignant relationship between helper and patient. Through the experience both can be transformed.

PERSONAL WELLNESS

A number of recent documents[52-54] have addressed the concept of wellness for cancer survivors, but caregivers also need to address their personal wellness. We cannot continue to give if we are empty vessels. Meier, Back, and Morrison[55] propose a model for increasing physician self-awareness, which includes identifying and working with emotions that may affect patient care. Kearney, Weininger, Vachon, Mount, and Harrison[56] have written of the need for physicians to be "connected" to continue to practice end-of-life care.

Elit et al.[8] found that three areas must be addressed to decrease stress and burnout in physicians–physician well-being, job description, and environment. Physician well-being seems to be inversely correlated to number of hours on call, number of hours in direct patient contact, and lack of vacation time. The Joint Committee on Accreditation has mandated that all hospitals have a program to address physician well-being, separate from disciplinary processes.[57]

Spickard et al.,[2] note the best prevention for physician burnout is to promote personal and professional well-being on all levels: physical, emotional, psychological, and spiritual. This must occur throughout the professional life-cycle of physicians, from medical school through retirement. It is a challenge not only for individual physicians in their own lives but also for the profession of medicine and the organizations in which physicians work. Of course this concept applies equally well to all other professional caregivers. Shanafelt and his colleagues have done a series of articles on wellness in residents,[10] oncologists[35,39] and surgical oncologists.[12,58] The well-being and personal wellness strategies of medical oncologists in the North Central Cancer Treatment Group were assessed.[35] Half reported high overall well-being. Being age 50 or younger, male, and working 60 hours or less per week were associated with increased overall well-being.

Ratings of the importance of a number of personal wellness promotion strategies differed for oncologists with high-well-being compared with those without high well-being. Developing an approach/philosophy to dealing with death and end-of-life care, using recreation/hobbies/exercise, taking a positive outlook and incorporating a philosophy of balance between personal and professional life were all rated as substantially more important wellness strategies by oncologists with high well-being…Oncologists with high overall well-being also reported greater career satisfaction [p.23].

These coping strategies are similar to the top five coping strategies identified two decades ago[14]: a sense of competence, control or pleasure in one's work; team philosophy, building and support; control over aspects of practice; lifestyle management; and a personal philosophy of illness, death and one's role in life.

Oncologists can shape their career and increase their likelihood of achieving personal and professional satisfaction through: identifying professional goals, optimizing career fit, identifying and managing stressors specific to practice type, and achieving optimum work-life balance.[39] Shanafelt suggests that surgical oncologists[58] can find meaning, balance, and personal satisfaction in their career through asking oneself and reflecting on a series of questions related to: one's greatest priority in life and whether one has been living life in a way that demonstrates that; asking where one is most irreplaceable; looking at adequate balance between home and personal life; how much professional achievement one is willing to sacrifice to have more time with family; checking if one is asking more of a spouse than one should; asking what type of legacy one wishes to leave one's children; inquiring what person or activity one might have been neglecting; how one would relive the past year; asking one's self what one would like life to be like in 10 years and asking one's self what do I fear? Shanafelt[58] also suggests looking at relationships, taking time for personal reflection, spiritual practices, self-care and hobbies, and personal interests. Caring for one's self, cultivating personal relationships, and nurturing personal interests is what makes time away from work meaningful and provides individuals with opportunity for achievement and personal growth outside of work.

A study of 549 surgical oncologists[12] found that devoting less than 25% of time to research was associated with greater burnout and there was a lower physical quality of life associated with a low sense of PA. Factors associated with problematic alcohol use include screening positive for depression and devoting at least 25% of time to research. Kuerer

et al. concluded that there was a need to encourage faculty to be attentive to their physical health (e.g., maintaining fitness, establishing a primary care physician, staying current with recommended health maintenance measures).

STUDIES OF INTERVENTION

While new findings regarding the interpersonal dynamics between the worker and other people in the workplace have yielded new insights into the sources of stress, effective interventions to prevent burnout have yet to be developed.[5] The model proposed by Maslach and her colleagues suggests that effective interventions to deal with burnout should be framed in terms of the three dimensions of exhaustion, cynicism, and sense of inefficacy. Currently their interventions are focusing on building job engagement, rather than reducing burnout.[3] Programs of intervention in oncology could focus on one or more of the issues addressed above in the section on *A model for understanding occupational stress*.

A Cochrane Review assessed the prevention of occupational stress in healthcare workers,[59] concluding there was limited evidence for the effectiveness of person- and work-directed interventions to reduce stress levels in healthcare settings. Only two trials, one in oncology[60] were rated as being of high quality, based on receiving 75% on the internal validity subscales.

One of the reviewed studies that could have relevance for oncology is an 8 week Mindfulness-Based Stress Reduction (MBSR) program for nurses in a hospital system.[61] Work had already been done to improve

Table 82–2. Intervention: communication studies

Authors	Sample	Design	Results
Fallowfield et al.[63,64]	160 U.K. oncologists from 34 cancer centers	Allocated to written feedback plus course; course alone; written feedback alone on control Each clinician had 6–10 interviews with patients videotaped at baseline and three months postintervention	Improved communication skills in oncologists assigned to training Twelve month follow-up—no demonstrable attrition in communication behaviors in those who had shown improvement previously, including fewer leading questions, appropriate use of focused and open-ended questions and responses to patient cues Additional skills not apparent at 3 months included fewer interruptions and increased summarizing of information Expressions of empathy declined Twelve–fifteen months after intervention, clinicians had integrated key communication skills into practice and were applying others
Razavi et al.[65]	72 oncology nurses	Randomly assigned to 24-hours psychological training program or wait-list period	Significant training effect on attitudes, especially those related to self-concept, and occupational stress related to inadequate preparation Limited changes found regarding posttraining skills Trained staff were significantly more in control of the interview Consolidation of the skills through posttraining sessions is needed
Razavi et al.[66]	63 Belgian physicians	Basic training program, randomly assigned to consolidation workshops	Communication skills improved more in the consolidation-workshop group than in the waiting-list group Simulated interviews—significant increases in open and open-directive questions and utterances alerting patients to reality, and significant decrease in premature reassurance Actual patient interviews—significant increase in acknowledgements and empathic statements, educated guesses, and negotiations Patients interacting with physicians who benefited from consolidation workshops reported higher scores concerning their physicians' understanding of their disease
Wilkinson et al.[67]	U.K. nurses	Randomized to 3-day communication skills training program, or control group	Communication skills scores for the intervention group increased significantly Control scores decreased Confidence scores increased significantly for experimental group and decreased in control group
Butow et al.[68]	35 oncologists from six teaching hospitals in six Australian cities	Participated in a 1.5-day intensive communication skills training program	Videotaped simulated patient interviews Intervention group displayed nonsignificantly more creating environment and fewer blocking behaviors after completion and 12 months later The intervention doctors valued the training highly but there was not a significant change in stress or burnout Baseline stress and burnout scores were, somewhat less than those reported elsewhere

employee satisfaction and retention; a nursing advisory council was set up; there was work to enhance the model of self governance and increased opportunity for education and professional development. Mindfulness: being fully present to one's experience without judgment or resistance; emphasis on self-care, compassion and healing makes it relevant as an intervention for helping caregivers. The treatment group had decreased scores on the MBI which lasted 3 months. These included decreased EE and DP and a trend toward significance in PA.

INTERVENTION TO IMPROVE THE ONCOLOGY WORKPLACE

Communication training. Fellowes, Wilkinson, and Moore[62] did a Cochrane Review of communication skills training for healthcare professionals in oncology. Three trials, involving 347 health professionals met the criteria.[63-66] At the time of that review the work of Wilkinson, Perry, and Blanchard [67] was noted as being ongoing and has been reported. Table 82-2 briefly describes these studies, as well as the Delvaux, Razavi et al.[60] study and a recent Australian study.[68]

Team intervention. LeBlanc et al.[69] did a quasi experimental study of a team-based burnout intervention on 29 oncology units in the Netherlands. Nine wards were randomly selected to participate in the Take Care! intervention. The program consists of six monthly 3-hour sessions including education about the mechanisms of stress and feedback about the participants' work situation; this feedback was used to help participants structure their subjective feelings by providing them with relevant topics for discussion and for their plans to reduce work stress on their ward. They were provided with their ward scores, but not team burnout scores. At the end of the first session, the job stressors that were to be dealt with during the training session were selected. The remaining sessions consisted of an education and an action portion. Subjects included unwanted collective behavior; communication and feedback, building a support network; balancing job-related investments and outcomes; personal experiences; and potential problems with change. During the action component, participants formed problem-solving teams. Outcomes of these sessions were, for example, the introduction of more efficient procedures in regards to reporting about patients and ordering supplies (quantitative demands), the appointment of staff members as "guardian angels" who should watch over team members' well-being (support), and restructuring of the weekly work meetings to enable more participation (voice) of staff members (participation in decision making). Results of multilevel analyses showed that staff in the experimental wards experienced significantly less EE at both Time 2 and Time 3 and less DP at Time 2, compared with the control wards. Moreover, changes in burnout levels were significantly related to changes in the perception of job characteristics over time.

CONCLUSIONS

In conclusion, the stressors and satisfactions in oncology have not changed since the early years of the field but there are new insights into the factors that might contribute to burnout, ways of identifying those at risk of burnout and programs to promote job engagement. As important as workplace interventions are, the responsibility of caregivers to engage in personal wellness programs is essential. Remember the warning when traveling in airplanes and first attach your own oxygen mask.

REFERENCES

1. Vachon MLS, Müeller M. Burnout and Symptoms of Stress. In: Breitbart W Chochinov HM (eds). *Handbook of psychiatry in palliative medicine.* New York: Oxford University Press;2009:559–625.

2. Spickard A Jr. Gabbe SG, Christensen JF. Mid-Career burnout in generalist and specialist physicians. *JAMA.* 2002;288:1447–1450.

3. Maslach C, Leiter MP. Early predictors of job burnout and engagement. *J Appl Psychol.* 2008;93:498–512.

4. Maslach C, Schaufeli WB, Leiter MP. Job burnout. *Annu Rev Psychol.* 2001;52:397–422.

5. Maslach C. Job burnout: new directions in research and intervention. *Curr Dir Psychol Sci.* 2003;12:189–192.

6. Gabbe S, Melville J, Mandel L, Walker E. Burnout in chairs of obstetrics and gynecology. *Am J Obstet Gynecol.* 2002;186:601–612.

7. Warde CE, Moonsinghe K, Allen W, Gelberg L. Marital and parental satisfaction of married physicians with children. *J Gen Int Med.* 1999;14:157–165.

8. Elit L, Trim K, Mand-Bains IH, Sussman J, Grunfeld E, Society of Gynecologic Oncology, Canada. Job satisfaction, stress, burnout among Canadian gynecologic oncologists. *Gynecol Oncol.* 2004;94:134–139.

9. Leiter M, Maslach C. A mediation model of job burnout. In: Antoniou A, Cooper CL (eds). *Research companion to organizational health psychology.* Cheltenham: Edward Elgar Publishing; 2005:544–564.

10. West CP, Huschka MM, Novotny PJ, et al. Association of perceived medical errors with resident distress and empathy: a prospective longitudinal study. *JAMA.* 2006;296:1071–1078.

11. Halbesleben JRB, Rathert C. Linking physician burnout and patient outcomes: exploring the dyadic relationship between physicians and patients. *Health Care Manage.* 2008;33:29–39.

12. Kuerer HM, Eberlein TJ, Pollock RE, et al. Career satisfaction practice patterns and burnout among surgical oncologists: report on the quality of life of members of the Society of Surgical Oncology. *Ann Surg Oncol.* 2007;14:3043–3053.

13. Vachon MLS, Lyall WAL, Freeman SJJ. Measurement and management of stress in health care professionals working with advanced cancer patients. *Death Educ.* 1978;1:365–375.

14. Vachon MLS. *Occupational stress in the care of the critically ill, the dying and the bereaved.* New York: Hemisphere; 1987.

15. Whippen DA, Canellos GP. Burnout syndrome in the practice of oncology: results of a random survey of 1,000 oncologists. *J Clin Oncol.* 1991;9:1916–1920.

16. Ramirez AJ, Graham J, Richards MA, Cull A, Gregory WM, Leaning MS, Snashall DC, Timothy AR. Burnout and psychiatric disorder among cancer clinicians. *Br J Cancer.* 1995;71:1263–1269.

17. Graham J, Ramirez AJ, Cull A, Gregory WM, Finlay I, Hoy A, Richards MA. Job stress and satisfaction among palliative physicians. *Palliat Med.* 1996;10:185–194.

18. Allegra CJ, Hall R, Yothers G. Prevalence of burnout in the US oncology community. *J Oncol Pract.* 2005;1:4:140–147.

19. Asai M, Morita T, Akechi T, et al. Burnout and psychiatric morbidity among physicians engaged in end-of-life care for cancer patients: a cross-sectional nationwide survey in Japan. *Psychooncology.* 2007;16:421–428.

20. Bressi C, Manenti S, Porcellana M, Cevales D, Farina L, et al. Haemato-oncology and burnout: an Italian study. *Br J Cancer.* 2008;98:1046–1052.

21. Cashavelly BJ, Donelan K, Binda KD, Mailhot JR, Clair-Hayes KA, Maramaldi P. The forgotten team member: meeting the needs of oncology support staff. *Oncologist.* 2008;13:530–538.

22. Graham J, Ramirez AJ, Field S, Richards A. Job stress and satisfaction among clinical radiologists. *Clin Radiol.* 2000;55:182–185.

23. Grunfeld E, Whelan TJ, Zitzelsberger L, Willan AR, Montesanto B, Evans WK. Cancer care workers in Ontario: prevalence of burnout, job stress and job satisfaction. *JAMC.* 2000;163:166–169.

24. Grunfeld E, Zitzelsberger LL, Coristine M, Whelan T, Aspelund F, Evans W. Job stress and job satisfaction of cancer care workers. *Psychooncology.* 2005;14:61–69.

25. Escot C, Artero S, Gandubert C, Boulenger JP, Ritchie K. Stress levels in nursing staff working in oncology. *Stress Health.* 2001;17:273–279.

26. Isikhan V, Comez T, Zafer D. Job stress and coping strategies in health care professionals working with cancer patients. *Eur J Onc Nsg.* 2004;8(3):234–244.

27. Kash KM, Holland JC, Breitbart W, Berenson S, Dougherty J, Ouellette-Kobasa S, Lesko L. Stress and burnout in oncology. *Oncology.* 2000;14:1621–1637.

28. Kenny A, Endacott R, Botti M, Watts R. Emotional toil: psychosocial care in rural settings for patients with cancer. *J Adv Nurs.* 2007;60:663–672.

29. Liskopoulou M, Panaretaki I, Papadakis V, et al. Burnout, staff support, and coping in pediatric oncology. *Supp Care Cancer.* 2008;16:143–150.

30. Morita T, Akechi T, Sugawara Y, Chihara S, Uchitomi Y. Practice and attitudes of Japanese oncologists and palliative care physicians concerning terminal sedation: a nationwide survey. *J Clin Oncol.* 2002;20:758–764.

31. Muscatello MRA, Bruno A, Carroccio C, et al. Association between burnout and anger in oncology versus ophthalmology health care professionals. *Psychol Rep.* 2006;99:641–650.

32. Travado L, Grassi L, Gil F, Ventura C, Martins C, Southern European Psycho-Oncology Study (SEPOS) Group. Physician-patient communication among Southern European cancer physicians: the influence of psychosocial orientation and burnout. *Psychooncology.* 2005;14:661–670.

33. Whippen DA, Zuckerman EL, Anderson JW, Kamin DY, Holland JC. Burnout in the practice of oncology: results of a follow-up survey. *J Clin Oncol.* 2004;22:14S:6053.

34. Maslach C, Jackson SE. *The maslach burnout inventory.* Palo Alto, CA: Consulting Psychologists Press; 1981.

35. Shanafelt TD, Novotny P, Johnson ME, et al. The well-being and personal wellness promotion strategies of medical oncologists in the North Central Cancer Treatment Group. *Oncology.* 2005;68:23–32.

36. Ramirez AJ, Graham J, Richards MA, Cull A, Gregory WM. Mental health of hospital consultants: the effect of stress and satisfaction at work. *Lancet.* 1996;16:724–728.

37. Gambles M, Wilkinson S, Dissanayake C. What are you like? A personality profile of cancer and palliative care nurses in the United Kingdom. *Cancer Nurs.* 2003;26:97–104.

38. Taylor C, Graham J, Potts H, Candy J, Richards M, Ramirez A. Impact of hospital consultants' poor mental health on patient care. *Br J Psychiatry.* 2007;190:268–269.

39. Shanafelt T, Chung H, White H, Lyckholm LJ. Shaping your career to maximize personal satisfaction in the practice of oncology. *J Clin Oncol.* 2006;24:4020–4026.

40. Gabbard GO, Menninger RW. The psychology of postponement in the medical marriage. *JAMA.* 1989;261:2378–2381.

41. Kobasa SC. Stressful life events, personality and health: an inquiry into hardiness. *J Pers Soc Psychol.* 1979;37:1–11.

42. Kobasa SC, Maddi SR, Kahn S. Hardiness and health: a prospective inquiry. *J Pers Soc Psychol.* 1982;42:168–177.

43. Kearney M, Mount B. Spiritual care of the dying patient. In: Chochinov HM, Breitbart W (eds). *Handbook of psychiatry in palliative medicine.* New York: Oxford University Press; 2000:357–373.

44. Jackson VA, Mack J, Matsuyama R, et al. A qualitative study of oncologists' approaches to end-of-life care. *J Palliat Med.* 2008;11:893–903.

45. Cohen JS, Erickson JM. Ethical dilemmas and moral distress in oncology nursing practice. *Clin J Onc Nurs.* 2006;10:775–780.

46. Stamm BH. Measuring compassion satisfaction as well as fatigue: developmental history of the compassion satisfaction and fatigue test. In: Figley CF (ed). *Treating compassion fatigue.* New York: Brunner-Routledge; 2002:107–119.

47. Pearlman L, Saakvitne K. *Trauma and the therapist: Countertransference and vicarious traumatization in psychotherapy with incest survivors.* New York: Norton; 1995.

48. Young-Eisendrath P. *The resilient spirit.* Reading MA: Perseus Books; 1996.

49. Hamilton AJ. *The scalpel and the soul.* New York: Jeremy P Tarcher/Putnam.

50. Taylor JB. *My stroke of insight.* New York: Viking; 2006.

51. Katz R. When our personal selves influence our professional work: an introduction to emotions and countertransference in end of life care. In: Katz RS, Johnson TA (eds). *When professionals weep: Emotional and countertransference responses in end-of-life care.* New York: Routledge; 2006:3–12.

52. Institute of Medicine and National Research Council. *From cancer patient to cancer survivor: Lost in transition.* Washington, DC: The National Academies Press; 2006.

53. Haylock PJ, Mitchell SA, Cox T, Temple SV, Curtiss CP. The cancer survivor's Prescription for Living. *Am J Nurs.* 2007;107:58–68.

54. Committee on Psychosocial Services to Cancer Patients/Families in a Community Setting, Institute of Medicine. *Cancer care for the whole patient: Meeting psychosocial health needs.* Washington, DC: The National Academies Press; 2007.

55. Meier DE, Back AL, Morrison RS. The inner life of physicians and care of the seriously ill. *JAMA.* 2001;286:3007–3014.

56. Kearney MK, Weininger RB, Vachon MLS, Mount BM, Harrison R. Self-care of physicians caring for patients at the end of life. 'Being connected...a key to my survival'. *JAMA.* 2009;301:1155–1164.

57. Revisions to Selected Medical Staff Standards. Physician health. Available at: http://www.jcaho.org. Accessed August 14, 2009.

58. Shanafelt T. A career in surgical oncology: finding meaning, balance, and personal satisfaction. *Ann Surg Oncol.* 2008;15:400–406.

59. Marine A, Ruotsalainen J, Serra C, Verbeek J. Preventing occupational stress in healthcare workers. *Cochrane Database of Systematic Reviews.* 4: Art. No. CD002892. DOI 10, 1002/14651858. CD002892. pub.2. 2006.

60. Delvaux N, Razavi D, Marchal S, Brédart A, Farvacques C, Slachmuylder J-L. Effects of a 105 hours psychological training program on attitudes, communication skills and occupational stress in oncology: a randomized study. *Br J Cancer.* 2004;90:106–114.

61. Cohen-Katz JSD, Wiley T, Capuano D, Baker S, Shapiro. The effects of mindfulness-based stress reduction on nurse stress and burnout: a quantitative and qualitative study. *Holist Nurs Pract.* 2004;18:302–308.

62. Fellowes D, Wilkinson S, Moore P. Communication skills training for health care professionals working with cancer patients, their families and/or carers. *Cochrane Library.* 2008;1:1–17. Review.

63. Fallowfield L, Jenkins V, Farewell V, Saul J, Duffy A, Eves R. Efficacy of a Cancer Research UK communication skills training model for oncologists: a randomized controlled trial. *Lancet.* 2002;359:650–656.

64. Fallowfield L, Jenkins V, Farewell V, Solis-Trapala J. Enduring impact of communication skills training: results of a 12-month follow-up. *Br J Cancer.* 2003;89:1445–1449.

65. Razavi D, Delvaux N, Marchal S, Bredart A, Farvacques C, Paesmans M. The effects of a 24-h psychological training program on attitudes, communication skills and occupational stress in oncology: a randomized study. *Eur J Cancer.* 1993;29A:1858–1863.

66. Razavi D, Merckaert I, Marchal S, et al. How to optimize physicians' communication skills in cancer care: results of a randomized study assessing the usefulness of post training consolidation workshops. *J Clin Onc.* 2003;21:3141–3149.

67. Wilkinson S, Perry R, Blanchard K, Linsell L. Effectiveness of a three-day communication skills course in changing nurses' communication skills with cancer/palliative care patients: a randomized controlled trial. *Palliat Med.* 2008;22:365–375.

68. Butow P, Cockburn J, Girgis A, et al. Increasing oncologists skills in eliciting and responding to emotional cues: evaluation of a communication skills training program. *Psychooncology.* 2008;17:209–218.

69. LeBlanc PM, Hox JJ, Schaufeli WB, Taris TW. Take Care!: the evaluation of a team-based burnout intervention program for oncology care providers. *J Appl Psychol.* 2007;92:213–227.

CHAPTER 83

Training Psychiatrists and Psychologists In Psycho-oncology

Andrew J. Roth and Michael A. Hoge

INTRODUCTION

The practice, understanding and art of psycho-oncology have grown over the past 35 years (see Chapter 1). As a multidisciplinary and blended field, contributions and seminal observations have come from oncology, medicine, psychiatry, psychology, nursing, social work, palliative care, ethics, and chaplaincy. The recent report by the Institute of Medicine, "Cancer Care for the Whole Patient" highlighted the psychosocial needs of cancer patients and survivors and the trained workforce necessary to assure they are met.[1] Despite the wide gap between patient's psychosocial needs and available services, there remains a limited number of training opportunities for the disciplines which comprise psycho-oncology.[2]

The care of oncology patients has shifted rapidly to ambulatory care settings over the last 10 years, due to more treatments being delivered at home and an increased emphasis on cost saving. The training of psychologists and psychiatrists in psycho-oncology, primarily conducted on inpatient units in the past, increasingly now focus on the ambulatory setting. This leads to greater training needs in management of treatment side effects, fatigue, pain, anxiety, and depressive symptoms. There is also new attention to survivors' health and well being, as well as patients receiving palliative and end-of-life care. Training must also address the needs of caregivers who give far more medical and psychosocial support today than ever before, while carrying the usual burden of family and work obligations. Considerable challenges exist in the development of optimal ambulatory psychosocial programs which interact with community advocacy organizations.

The economic realities that confront psycho-oncologists in the twenty-first century are formidable, despite the recent passage of the Mental Health Parity Act. Training is strongly hampered by inadequate support and reimbursement for psychosocial services. This chapter describes the present status of training programs for psychiatrists and psychologists, the need for change, and the challenges we face in assembling a trained work force to meet the mandate of the Institute of Medicine Report. The report states that "to give quality cancer care today, the psychosocial must be integrated into routine cancer care."[1]

PSYCHIATRY

Psychiatry is the fourth largest medical specialty in the United States; there are about 45,000 psychiatrists in the United States.[3] They are graduates of medical school and 4 years of general psychiatry residency (the first year as interns). Postresidency fellowship training of one or two additional years is required to attain subspecialty certification. It is economically difficult for many to consider this additional training today.

The psychiatric resident interested in the psychiatric care of the medically ill, including cancer, will be directed to the new subspecialty, Psychosomatic Medicine (PM). Before the subspecialty certification by the Accreditation Council of Graduate Medical Education (ACGME) in 2003, this area of psychiatry was called consultation-liaison psychiatry, addressing the range of complex medical and psychiatric issues that arise in medical and surgical patients. The PM fellowship provides a minimum of 12 months of supervised graduate education, and must be approved by the American Board of Medical Specialties (ABMS), ACGME, and the American Board of Psychiatry and Neurology (ABPN).[4] The subspecialty graduate program must function as an integral part of an accredited psychiatry residency program. There are now 36 accredited programs in PM which provide 50 training slots at present.[5] There are only two programs in the United States that have positions primarily dedicated to Psycho-oncology which train seven psychiatry fellows per year.[1] Many general PM programs offer training in which the fellow can spend time on inpatient oncology services (i.e., bone marrow/stem cell transplant units) or in ambulatory cancer settings (i.e., breast cancer clinics).

The oldest and largest psycho-oncology clinical and research training program in the United States was established in 1979 at Memorial Sloan-Kettering Cancer Center (MSKCC). Over 300 trainees have graduated from the program. This was conceived as a 2-year program that prepared both psychiatrists and psychologists for academic careers and was viewed as a model training program in psycho-oncology. Psychiatrists usually came with strong clinical training, but little or no research; psychologists came with strong research skills and fewer clinical skills. The program addressed this difference and psychologists and psychiatrists were trained clinically together in the same program. With the advent of the ACGME approved PM fellowship program, the training has had to be limited to psychiatrists. The clinical fellowship program at Memorial, one of the largest in PM, is accredited with the Weill Cornell Medical College/New York Presbyterian Hospital (NYPH) psychiatry residency program by the ACGME. The fellows spend 10 months at MSKCC, and 2 months at NYPH where they are assigned to medical and surgical units. The Department of Psychiatry and Behavioral Sciences at MSKCC continues to train psychologists through the research fellowship program, which has been NIH-funded for 25 years. Research fellows participate in clinical activities but there is no formal clinical training program for psychologists at present. However, the Clinical Observer Program invites medical students, social workers, and psychologists for varying periods of time to observe and participate in clinical programs.

GOALS: PSYCHO-ONCOLOGY TRAINING FOR PSYCHIATRISTS

The broad goals of psychiatric training in PM are to develop skills in clinical care, communication, administration, and research. However, psycho-oncology requires development of several additional specific skills.

Necessary skills for the psycho-oncologist

1. perform comprehensive evaluations of cancer patients
2. be able to recognize psychiatric syndromes, cancer-related, and treatment-specific psychiatric problems and understand the psychiatric issues throughout the disease continuum. Knowledge of psychotherapeutic, psychosocial, and psychopharmacological interventions is necessary
3. be able to write clinical and research papers, teach medical staff and give oral presentations
4. be able to evaluate, understand, and conduct research
5. learn organizational and administrative skills needed to manage a psycho-oncology unit or program (see Table 83–1).

Related to these five areas of skills which must be developed, the ability to recognize and diagnose the common psychiatric syndromes and disorders is basic. The fellows must learn those that are common at different sites of cancer and with certain treatments. Often, physiological, medical, or medication problems are masked as psychiatric symptoms.

Table 83–1. Necessary skills for psychiatrists in psycho-oncology

1. Perform comprehensive psychiatric evaluations of cancer patients
   Recognize common psychiatric syndromes, disorders, distress
   Be aware of cancer-, treatment-, and medication-specific psychiatric problems
   Understand the impact of and overlap of psychiatric and cancer issues throughout the cancer continuum
   - Recurrence of disease (Damocles Sword Syndrome)
   - Palliative care: impact of pain, fatigue and nausea on quality of life
   - End-of-life issues
   - Genetic and lifestyle vulnerability
   - Work effectively and supportively in liaison role
2. Appropriately apply interventions for cancer patients, family, and staff
   Choose appropriate psychotherapy for patient situation and medical condition
   Dynamic, supportive, crisis intervention, sexual, bereavement, cognitive behaviorally oriented
   Individual, family, group
   Sychopharmacology: indications for psychotropic medications; drug interactions
   Facilitate understanding of patient and families by oncology staff
3. Communicate psycho-oncology information to others
   Write clinically based or research-oriented scholarly paper
   Teach medical students, house staff including psychiatric residents, nurses and social workers
   Give oral presentations
4. Be able to critically evaluate/understand and/or conduct research in psycho-oncology
5. Learn skills needed to administer a psycho-oncology program

Table 83–2. Six core educational competencies and didactice/ experiential program

Core competencies	Didactic and experiential teaching
Patient care	Introductory ("Core") curriculum
Medical/ psychiatric knowledge	Grand rounds in psycho-oncology in psychiatry/psychology
Professionalism	in oncology/palliative care
System-based practice	rehabilitation/cancer prevention and control Clinically oriented meetings
Practice-based learning and improvement	Case conferences Chairman's rounds Professor's rounds
Interpersonal/ communication skills	Psychotherapy seminars Inpatient rounds Outpatient case conference (referrals to community resources) Mentoring Countertransference rounds Psychosocial care teams Communication skills training Journal club Research seminars Individual supervision, related to patient care, career, and research

It is also essential to be familiar with the medical issues related to specific cancer sites, medications and metabolic and hormonal changes that cause confusion, anxiety, and depression. Management of physical symptoms, which may have a psychological component, particularly fatigue, pain, and nausea, are critical aspects of expertise. Psycho-oncologists must also know in what circumstances to recommend the range of psychosocial interventions: individual, family, group, dynamic, and supportive psychotherapy; crisis intervention; sex therapy; bereavement counseling; and cognitive behaviorally oriented forms of psychotherapy. The overlap of behavioral interventions, such as relaxation and meditation, with complementary therapies means the psycho-oncologist must know the range of interventions to advise patients appropriately.

In terms of psychopharmacology, the trainee must know the indications for specific psychotropic medications, their primary action, and potential drug-drug interactions. Oncologists often rely on the psychiatrist for information in complex situations involving psychotropic drug use and possible side effects.

All psycho-oncologists must be able to work effectively with the multidisciplinary medical team. Assignment to a particular unit permits learning the complex social culture of a single team or unit. Meetings with nursing and social workers, often leads to support activities to address problems on the unit. Learning how to manage a stressful event such as a death of a "special" patient can be highly valuable. At MSKCC, psychiatry fellows attend meetings of the medical team where patient status is reviewed, and often where clinical research is discussed. Psychosocial care teams (PCT's) are comprised of key individuals giving supportive care to a particular patient group. They provide a rich learning experience for the fellow in the range of supportive interventions provided by social workers, art and music therapy, chaplaincy, and complementary therapies. Programs that focus on children and geriatrics also provide settings to learn the problems of children and their parents, and the difficult psychiatric and psychosocial issues around care of the elderly.

Learning about the teaching role is an important part of the training of the fellow who must be able to convey information about the

patient or family to staff who may be frustrated or upset with the patient because of not understanding the psychiatric disorder or psychological problem. Developing good communication skills is a key part of training. At Memorial, the Communication Skills Laboratory has developed a module for PM fellows in which the didactic is coupled with experiential learning by conducting interviews with an actor/patient under supervision.

The psycho-oncology fellow must develop and maintain academic skills by writing scholarly papers with senior faculty, and participating in academic projects, journal clubs and symposia, oral presentations at national and international meetings, and research seminars where methods and statistics are taught. Fellows at MSKCC have two oral presentations per year to the full faculty, presenting a clinical case, a review of a topic, or a research project.

Core educational competencies. Training in Psycho-oncology and PM is based on teaching six core educational competencies:

- Patient care
- Medical and/or psychiatric knowledge
- Professionalism
- System-based practice
- Practice based learning and improvement
- Interpersonal/communication skills

This core of desired skills and knowledge serves as the basis for development of the curriculum and practical experiences for fellows. The Academy of Psychosomatic Medicine (APM) used the concept as the basis of training of psychiatrists in consultation-liaison (CL) psychiatry when the APM served as the oversight professional organization. It has been used by the ACGME in the development of medical and psychiatric residency training. These six core competencies are the basis of receiving certification in PM and psycho-oncology. This concept is valuable because trainees can be evaluated on the basis of these clinical skills. Table 83–2 outlines the six core competencies and the range of didactic and experiential educational activities that address each competency.

Didactic curriculum and training. Psycho-oncology training for psychiatrists requires extensive didactic course work. Table 83–3 outlines the core curriculum which has developed at MSKCC over the past three

Table 83–3. Core curriculum in psycho-oncology

History of psych-oncology
Psychiatric emergencies in oncology setting
Psychopharmacology in the medically ill
Anxiety disorders and adjustment disorders in the oncology setting
Depression and suicide in the medically ill
Delirium in the medically ill
Cancer treatments: neuropsychiatric and other side effects
ABC's of pain
Psychiatric aspects of symptom control: fatigue, nausea, pain
Legal issues/capacity determinations
Palliative care
Ethics and the medically ill
Cognitive-behavioral therapy in psychosomatic medicine
HIV/AIDS
Family interventions in the medical setting
Cancer focused psychotherapy
Pediatric psycho-oncology
Supporting parents with cancer
Alcohol withdrawal
Substance abuse: opioids
Dementia in the medically ill
Countertransference issues
Existential therapy
Neuro-oncology
Women's health
Smoking cessation
Chemotherapy effects on the brain
Bereavement
Psychotherapy with geriatric cancer patients
Cancer survivorship/ psychosocial issues
Psychiatric aspects of specific cancers: prostate, breast, lung and head
    and neck cancers
Psychiatric aspects of bone marrow transplantation
Quality of life research
Gynecological cancer—fertility and sexuality
Fatigue in cancer and AIDS
Couple and family therapy
Men's sexual health
Developed at Memorial Sloan-Kettering as Core Curriculum

ABBREVIATIONS: AIDS, acquired immunodeficiency syndrome; HIV, human
immunovirus.

decades (Table 83–3). The introductory or "core" course is offered early in the year to cover basic areas: management of psychiatric emergencies, depression, suicidal risk, anxiety, delirium, substance abuse and psychotherapy and pharmacology in the medically ill. A pocket handbook of symptom management provides a brief description of the common disorders and their management which reinforces the lectures.[6] Recent textbooks of PM offer fuller descriptions of common problems.[7,8] These didactics reduce anxiety associated with early patient consultations. An ongoing course, "Professor Rounds," throughout the year covers specialty topics.

Another important aspect of the core curriculum is clinically oriented rounds. The format of rounds may be a combination of case conferences, professor rounds, and short specialty conferences that cover a wide range of issues such as pain, bereavement, psychopharmacology, palliative care, cross-cultural psychiatry, pediatric issues, family issues, spirituality, research methods, writing, genetics and prevention, and early detection of cancer and ongoing psychotherapy seminars. At MSKCC, "counter-transference rounds," in which emotional reactions to working with cancer patients are explored, has been a valued seminar for trainees. Finally, trainees should be encouraged to pursue areas of research or review articles of special interest in journal clubs that are jointly facilitated by academic faculty and trainees.

The clinical experience at MSKCC has shown that trainees learn best from the broadest patient exposure coupled with close supervision. Fellows who merely supervise residents, with few patients treated firsthand are at a loss, shortchanged inadvertently. Fellows sometimes report that the amount of supervision in psycho-oncology far surpasses that given in busy residency programs—this is a delicate balance which takes into account the level of greater medical illness of patients under their care versus the need to help the fellow achieve more clinical autonomy. Ideally, good supervision provides close monitoring and support of the trainee early in the process, allowing greater independence later in training.

Faculty. Psycho-oncology faculty members should have extensive experience with the multidisciplinary approach to cancer care. They should have had in-depth clinical experience with patients and their families and have knowledge of the principles related to the medical, psychiatric, and psychological care of the oncology patient. Having faculty with experience in direct patient care is critical to the acceptance of fellows by medical staff.[9] Psychiatry trainees benefit from a broad array of interdisciplinary faculty members, including psychiatrists, psychologists, social workers, and nurses, who have specific experience in dealing with psychosocial service needs. Role-model mentoring by each discipline, including faculty with expertise in insight-oriented psychotherapy, group therapy, psychopharmacology, cognitive-behavioral interventions, and child psychology/psychiatry is valuable.

Mentorship and evaluation. At MSKCC, a training director oversees a fellowship training committee which selects and monitors the progress of trainees, the development of faculty and mentors, and the overall functioning of the program. Every fellow has individual learning objectives developed with a faculty mentor; regular meetings assess progress. Every 6 months supervisors complete written evaluations of fellows. Fellows meet with their supervisor and the Director of Training to discuss their performance and goals for the next 6 months. Fellows also anonymously evaluate their supervisors and the program.

PSYCHOLOGISTS

Psychology is a large and rapidly expanding health profession. It has an increasing role in the provision of psychosocial services in medical centers and a growing, though less formal role, in the provision of mental health services in community settings to individuals with severe and or chronic medical conditions. The size and characteristics of the profession are reviewed below, followed by a discussion of the role of health psychology in this discipline. The development of health psychology has been a major thrust in the field, and offers training most relevant to psycho-oncology. Training programs specific to psycho-oncology occur largely in the context of pre- and postdoctoral internships. A modal internship is briefly presented.

Psychology as a profession. Psychology is the third largest of the traditional mental health disciplines, following social work and counseling. In 2004, there were 85,000 doctoral level psychologists in the United States who were trained to provide clinical care.[10] The discipline has other subgroups, such as experimental and social psychologists, who are not included in this count.

The clinically trained portion of the profession has nearly doubled in size since 1986. In 2004, there were 26,000 students enrolled in accredited doctoral programs.[10] Just over 50% of individuals in the profession are women; however, those from diverse racial and cultural backgrounds comprise only 7% of these professionals.[10] Despite the growth in numbers, there is still a scarcity of psychologists trained to work with children and adolescents, the elderly, individuals with severe mental illness, rural Americans, and individuals with severe or chronic medical illnesses.

GRADUATE TRAINING

The doctoral degree in psychology is the standard educational path for practice as an independent clinical psychologist. Traditionally students obtained a Doctorate in Philosophy (Ph.D.), but many are now pursuing training in more clinically oriented programs that confer a Doctorate of Psychology (Psy.D.). Doctoral programs are typically 5 years in length, of which 1 year is dedicated to a full-time clinical internship. License-eligibility requires an additional year of supervised postdoctoral experience.[11] Postdoctoral internships are not required but are becoming much more common. Individuals with a master's degree in psychology generally cannot practice independently, except for school psychologists and those working in selected rural areas.

The American Psychological Association (APA) accredits three clinically related categories of graduate programs: clinical, counseling, and school psychology. Specialization within these broad categories is possible, but not required. The specialties most relevant to psycho-oncology include clinical health psychology, neuropsychology, rehabilitation psychology, and pediatric psychology.

For all students, basic graduate training in psychology at the doctoral level involves a series of required and elective courses, plus supervised clinical experience gathered through part-time practicum. Depending on the nature of the doctoral program and the degree earned, students may receive minor training or extensive training in research which is combined with experience in conducting independent research.

While accreditation criteria require that all students be taught the biological bases of behavior, the majority of students are not trained to assess or treat the psychosocial impact of acute or chronic medical illnesses. Expertise in this area comes principally from matriculating to a graduate program or internship that offers a training program in health psychology, which has been emerging as a major specialty within applied psychology.

Health psychology as a specialty. Psychology as an organized profession has been engaged over the past decade in an effort to redefine itself. The traditional focus on this discipline as a *mental* health profession is slowly giving way to the broader concept of psychology as a *health* profession. While this language change may appear subtle, the redefined scope promotes a focus on prevention, health promotion, and on nonpsychiatric disorders, including the psychological impact of medical illnesses. The preparation of psychologists to work with cancer patients and their families most often involves specialty training in health psychology, building the core knowledge, principles, and skills that can be applied to any number of medical illnesses, of which cancer is one.

The APA has described the focus of clinical health psychology as the study of interrelationships among behavioral, emotional, cognitive, social, and biological components in health and disease and the application of this knowledge to health promotion and maintenance; medical illness and disability prevention; treatment and rehabilitation; and healthcare system improvement.[12] The specialty is unique in that it draws heavily on both intradiscipline (within psychology) and interdisciplinary foundations. These foundations guide curriculum development and training and have been described by the APA *Commission for the recognition of specialties and proficiencies in professional psychology*:

Biological, cognitive, affective, social, and psychological *bases of health and disease* are bodies of knowledge that, when integrated with knowledge of biological, cognitive affective, social, and psychological *bases of behavior* constitute the distinctive knowledge base of Clinical Health Psychology. This includes broad understanding of biology, pharmacology, anatomy, human physiology and pathophysiology, and psychoneuroimmunology. Clinical Health psychologists also have knowledge of how learning, memory, perception, cognition, and motivation influence health behaviors, are affected by physical illness/injury/disability, and can affect response to illness/injury/disability. Knowledge of the impact of social support, culture, physician–patient relationships, health policy, and the organization of healthcare delivery systems on health and help seeking is also fundamental, as is knowledge of diversity and minority health issues, individual differences in coping, emotional, and behavioral risk factors for disease/injury/disability, human development issues in health and illness, and the impact of psychopathology on disease, injury, disability, and treatment. The specialty also includes special expertise in health research methods and awareness

of the distinctive ethical and legal issues associated with practice in Clinical Health Psychology.[1]

Training in health psychology. From a training and service delivery perspective, the growth of clinical health psychology has been one of the most visible changes in the field. In 1997, the APA recognized this as a professional practice specialty. In 2006, the APA approved 68 doctoral programs that had a training emphasis in health psychology or a medically related area. In 2007, The Association of Psychology Postdoctoral and Internship Centers (APPIC) identified 201 predoctoral internships with a major rotation in health psychology and 381 with minor rotations.[13] It also identified 51 postdoctoral fellowships that offered training related to nonpsychiatric medical illnesses. Data from the APA collected within the past several years suggested that at least 5000 of its members had a "medically related interest area."[14] This is likely an underestimate given that not all psychologists are members of this professional association and many members do not report their interest areas. Graduate training in health psychology involves the core course and experience requirements applicable to any psychology graduate student, plus a set of health psychology courses, both required and elective in nature. Clinical placements focus on medically ill populations and can be diverse in focus, including: chronic pain, asthma, organ transplant, cardiovascular disease, cancer, acquired immune deficiency syndrome, obesity, and hypertension.

The competencies for graduate level health psychology training were initially identified through a 1983 national consensus conference.[14,15] The set of core competencies include

- social, biological, and psychological bases of health and disease;
- health policy, systems, and organizations;
- health assessment, consultation, and intervention;
- health research methods;
- ethical, legal, and professional issues within health psychology;
- interdisciplinary collaboration.

Building off of this core competency set, Belar and colleagues created a tool for self-assessment of knowledge and skills by health psychologists.[16]

There are a variety of problem areas that are frequently at the center of training and practice in health psychology.[17] These include: psychological conditions that are related to disease, injury, and disability; somatic manifestations of psychological problems; psychophysiological disorders (such as migraines); physical problems responsive to behavioral treatments; psychological presentations of organic disease; the psychological and behavioral impact of medical procedures; behavioral risk factors and healthy lifestyles; and behavioral and interpersonal challenges in healthcare delivery. Students receive training in a diversity of intervention techniques on assessment, treatment, and consultation that are tailored to health psychology. Cognitive-behavioral approaches tend to receive considerable emphasis.

Pre- and postdoctoral internships. Disease-specific training is most often obtained through practicum experiences or full-time, full-year pre- and postdoctoral internships. To ascertain the characteristics of internship training focused on cancer care, the *Association of Psychology Postdoctoral and Internship Centers[13]* used its listserv to request information from faculty involved in internships of this nature. This informal survey was conducted on behalf of the Institute of Medicine *Committee on psychosocial services to cancer patients/families in a community setting.[1]*

There were 18 responses in total, most of which contained a brief summary of the training activities in a specific internship. The modal internship described involved clinical experience with cancer patients and families in a hospital setting, supervised by a faculty member who had a specific interest and expertise. As part of the curriculum, many faculty members reported assigning selected readings, while a few internship settings offered a course relevant to cancer care. Most of the training did not appear to be closely linked to an explicit set of competencies. The overall impression is that psychologists are learning to work with cancer patients and their families through an apprenticeship model that involves intensive clinical experience and mentoring by a skilled professional.

The Children's Hospital of Philadelphia has psychology pre- and postdoctoral internships in pediatric psychology that afford specialized training in oncology. This is one of the most highly regarded training programs of this nature.[18] The program combines developmental, ecological/systems, and behavioral approaches as a foundation for training and care delivery. The faculty has adopted an explicit competency model to guide training. There are 55 specific competencies across six domains: psychological assessment; interdisciplinary consultation; prevention and intervention; scientific investigation; diversity and cultural competence; and professional development. Oncology-specific training opportunities are offered in hospital, outpatient, and community settings. The training goals identified by the program are to:

- develop consultation skills as the psychology member of an interdisciplinary team providing care to oncology patients and their families
- gain family-systems and cognitive-behavioral psychotherapy skills for a wide range of issues related to childhood cancer and its treatment, with children, adolescents, and young adults with cancer and their families
- learn to conduct and interpret psychological assessments related to neurotoxic effects of chemotherapy and radiation, with regard to short- and long-term impact on learning and school achievement
- contribute to clinical research as an integral part of clinical care in an academic medical setting.[18]

Financing training. Graduate training in clinical psychology is supported principally by tuition and through government support of state universities. At the postdoctoral level, fellowships are often funded through faculty research grants.

With one major exception, psychology does not receive federal support for training. In contrast, medicine and nursing receive almost $8 billion per year through the graduate medical education (GME) program. The one exception for psychology is the *Graduate Psychology Education (GPE) Program,* established in FY 2002 by the Bureau of Health Professions at $2 million to address the need for "integrated" healthcare services. This included a focus on psychological services for rural and urban underserved populations. The GPE Program added geropsychology as a focus in FY 2003, raising funding levels to $4.5 million. This annual level was maintained through FY 2005 and then reduced again to $2 million in FY 2006.

Reimbursement for psychological services is often viewed as a barrier to the practice of health psychology, which in turn impacts negatively on faculty support and training opportunities for psychologists in this specialty. For example, the carve out of mental health benefits from other healthcare frequently creates confusion or conflict about the identity of the payer responsible for psychological services provided to medically ill individuals. The introduction in 2002 of Medicare Health and Behavior Codes has been viewed as a very positive development, as these cover procedures used by nonphysicians to identify, assess, and intervene with the "…psychological, behavioral, emotional, cognitive, and social factors important to the prevention, treatment, or management of physical health problems."[19] Medicaid coverage for such services remains largely unavailable.

Perhaps the most critical issue regarding training and funding is that it tends to be hospital based. This is certainly an essential element of professional practice with cancer patients and their families. However, the limited nonhospital training options impede development of a workforce that is skilled in caring for persons with cancer in the community, which is the primary context in which care is now delivered.

SUMMARY—PSYCHOLOGISTS AND PSYCHO-ONCOLOGY

Psychologists represent a growing profession, with increasing relevance to cancer care given the expansion of health psychology as a specialty within the discipline. Training at the graduate level tends to focus on developing within young professionals a core knowledge and skill base that is then applied to a broad number of medical problems, of which cancer is one. Skill development related to cancer care happens most often in hospital-based internship programs and primarily from supervised experience rather than formal coursework. Formal competency sets do not appear to play a major role in this apprenticeship model of training. Reimbursement barriers for the psychological services provided to medically ill individuals have a negative effect as they limit support for training faculty and internship positions. The absence of significant federal support for such training further limits the opportunities.

INTERDISCIPLINARY TRAINING

Basic components of a curriculum in psycho-oncology have been reported.[20] However, there is as yet no consensus or standardization of what constitutes a curriculum or clinical training for a psycho-oncologist. The following section discusses the goals, core curriculum and evaluation components of psycho-oncology training for various specialties. The American Psycho-Oncology Society has developed a web-based core curriculum that takes into account different educational needs of various specialties. Topics covered include Symptom Detection and Management: *Delirium; Depression and Suicide; Central Nervous System Effects of Drugs Used in Cancer Treatment; Distress Management in Cancer; Standards and Clinical Practice Guidelines; Cancer-Related Fatigue; Substance Abuse in the Oncology Setting; Anxiety and Adjustment Disorders;* Psychosocial Screening; Psychosocial Interventions: Online Support Groups for Women with Breast Cancer; Counseling Cancer Patients and Their Caregivers; *Cognitive and Behavioral Strategies for Cancer Patients; Psychiatric Emergencies in the Oncology Setting;* Population-Specific Issues; *Cancer Survivorship; Psychosocial Issues and Program Administration; and, Establishing a Psychosocial Program: Challenges and Strategies (http://www.apos-society.org,* 2008).

The International Psycho-Oncology Society (IPOS) also has an international, multilingual online training program in Psycho-Oncology: A Core Curriculum in Psychosocial Aspects of Cancer Care, that includes 1-hour lectures on the following topics: Communication and Interpersonal Skills in Cancer Care ; Anxiety and Adjustment Disorders in Cancer Patients; Distress Management in Cancer; Depression and Depressive Disorders in Cancer Patients and Psychosocial Assessment in Cancer Patients. These core programs are presented in English and the script and slides have been translated to French, German, Hungarian, Italian, and Spanish. In addition, the presentations have been similarly translated into Lithuanian, Polish, Russian, and Japanese. The translations, in each instance, have been modified to be culturally specific. The program is offered on the IPOS web site and on the web site of the European School of Oncology (http://www.ipos-society.org/professionals/meetings-ed/core-curriculum/core-curriculum.htm, 2008).

IPOS/APOS also recently published a pocket handbook for oncologists that focuses on a basic level of knowledge needed to serve the psychosocial needs of cancer patients. This handbook covers basic issues of psychiatric problems encountered in cancer patients and in particular cancer site settings and various treatment modalities including psychopharmacologic and psychotherapeutic interventions: *Quick reference for oncology clinicians: The psychiatric and psychological dimensions of cancer symptom management.*[6] This concise handbook is designed to aid oncology clinicians in addressing the psychological, emotional, and spiritual issues their patients face in coping with their illness. This curriculum adds to the breadth of online education programs offered on the APOS and IPOS web site.[1]

The Wellness Community recently published a manual to help teach psycho-oncologists around the world where resources may be scarce, to teach the basics of psycho-oncology to others. This manual based on international training seminars by a multidisciplinary team, discusses the importance of a seamless delivery of services in the tertiary care cancer center, the community and hospice care. It covers the range of psychotherapeutic and psychopharmacologic interventions from new diagnosis to survivorship and end-of-life issues.[21]

CONCLUSION

Today, organizational structure, departmental philosophies and medical system realities preclude combined training of psychiatrists and psychologists. Though there are separate training programs today, constant "cross pollination" that has resulted from joint responsibilities has led to the mutual enhancement of trainees from all backgrounds. The development of core competencies provides a helpful common ground in which there are great similarities in teaching clinical skills and knowledge. A blurring of boundaries of professional roles was neither a goal nor a result of the training. Rather, individuals from different disciplines have been able to expand their knowledge base about medicine, behavioral medicine, oncology, psychiatry, and psychology, and to learn how combining professional "strengths" and approaches in collaboration can lead to opportunities for novel research and clinical program development.

There will likely be considerable change over the next decade as cancer treatment evolves, as psycho-oncology continues to grow, and as the healthcare system continues to change. A repercussion of changes in the healthcare environment is the mandate issued by third-party payers to reduce costs and demonstrate cost-efficiency of services. This has unfortunately meant that patients often go without psycho-oncology care because they cannot afford it. Psychiatrists and psychologists entering the field of psycho-oncology will require training in basic research methodologies that will allow them to meet the challenge of showing the beneficial outcomes of psycho-oncological care and assure the continuation of psycho-oncology as a discipline.

Those involved in this field will carry the responsibility of furthering the clinical care, research, and development of training programs in psycho-oncology and in guiding other disciplines that are involved in the care of cancer patients and survivors. Educating newcomers to our field and responding to the challenges above with fine-tuning of the training is vital for continued growth and development. Conducting studies to evaluate training programs and curricula will help us surpass basic competence in the most scientific, productive, and caring manner. The preventable cancer agenda has grown as part of the Healthy People 2000 initiative. It will likely continue to grow and the psycho-oncologist of the future should be at the forefront of behavioral science research and application.

Many psycho-oncologists have already begun the process of academic collaboration with hospice physicians and others in the field of palliative medicine. The potential of training psychologists and psychiatrists alongside these other practitioners will enhance psycho-oncologists' abilities in the area of symptom management.

REFERENCES

1. Adler N, Page, A, eds. *Cancer care for the whole patient: Meeting psychosocial health needs.* Institute of Medicine (IOM). 2008.

2. American Psychosocial Oncology Society. 2008; www.apos-society.org.

3. Scully J, Wilk J. Selected characteristics and data of psychiatrists in the United States, 2001–2002. *Acad Psychiatr.* 2003;27:247–251.

4. Academy of Psychosomatic Medicine. 2008; www.apm.org. Accessed August 17, 2009.

5. Accreditation Council for Graduate Medical Education. 2008; www.acgme.org. Accessed August 17, 2009.

6. Holland J, Greenberg D, Hughes M. (eds). *Quick reference for oncology clinicians: The psychiatric and psychological dimensions of cancer symptom management.* APOS; 2006.

7. Levenson J. (ed). *Textbook of psychosomatic medicine.* Washington, DC: American Psychiatric Association; 2005.

8. Strain J, Blumenfeld M. *Psychosomatic medicine.* Philadelphia, PA: Lippincott Williams & Wilkens; 2006.

9. Rainey L, Wellisch D, Fawzy F, Wolcott DL, Pasnau R. Training health professionals in psychosocial aspects of cancer: a continuing education model. *J Psychoso Oncol.* 1983;1(2):41–60.

10. Manderscheid R, Berry J. (eds). *Mental health, united states, 2004.* Rockville, MD: Center for Mental Health Services; 2004.

11. Olvey C, Hogg A. Licensure requirements: have we raised the bar too far? *Prof Psychol: Res Prac.* 2002;33:323–329.

12. American Psychological Association. *Graduate study in psychology.* Washington, DC: APA Books; 2006.

13. APPIC Online Directory. Association of psychology post-doctoral and internship centers. 2007; www.appic.org/directory. Accessed August 17, 2009.

14. Belar C. Issues in training clinical health psychologists. *Psychol Health.* 1990;4:31–37.

15. Stone G. National working conference on education and training in health psychology. *Health Psychol.* 1983;2 (Suppl 5):1–153.

16. Belar C, Brown R, Hersch L, et al. Self-assessment in clinical health psychology: a model for ethical expansion of practice. *Prof Psychol: Res Prac.* 2001;32:135–141.

17. American Psychosocial Association. 2008; www.apa.org. Accessed August 17, 2009.

18. Children's Hospital of Philadelphia. *Psychology Internship Training Program, Training Year 2008–2009.* Philadelphia, PA: Author; 2008.

19. American Medical Association. *CPT 2007.* Chicago: Author; 2006.

20. Die-Trill M, Holland J. A model curriculum for advanced training in psycho-oncology. *Psychooncology.* 1995;4:169–182.

21. Golant M, Roth A, Schachter S. Innovative models of international psychosocial oncology training manual. *Wellness Community.* 2008.

CHAPTER 84

Training Professional Social Workers In Psycho-Oncology

Victoria Kennedy, Kathryn M. Smolinski, and Yvette Colón

INTRODUCTION

The complexity and variability of psychosocial issues associated with cancer has created the demand for highly skilled social work practitioners who are trained to provide screening, assessment, and therapeutic interventions across the cancer continuum— primary prevention, diagnosis, treatment, survivorship, palliative care, end of life and bereavement. Oncology social workers function as dynamic members of the transdisciplinary cancer care team in a wide variety of healthcare settings including academic cancer centers, community hospitals, health systems, community-based agencies, ambulatory clinics, home care, hospice programs, and private practice.

Social workers assist the oncology team in moving beyond the disease process to attend to the practical and emotional matters that may affect the patient's capacity to participate in treatment by serving as a conduit between patient and staff to facilitate optimal responsiveness and communication around treatment goals, disease management, and psychosocial concerns. Issues related to adjustment to illness, treatment decision making, lifestyle changes, discharge planning, and the transition to survivorship become opportunities for the oncology social worker to help patients and families learn and/or strengthen valuable coping and problem-solving skills. In this important role, the social worker becomes a valued team member.

Across cancer care settings, social workers are estimated to provide approximately 75% of the mental health services overall.[1] "Social workers have unique, in-depth knowledge of and expertise in working with ethnic, cultural, and economic diversity; family and support networks; multidimensional symptom management; bereavement; trauma and disaster relief; interdisciplinary practice; interventions across the life cycle; and systems interventions that address the fragmentation, gaps, and insufficiency in health care."[2] In addition, oncology social workers are actively engaged in understanding and promoting teamwork, which includes fostering communication, documenting information, sharing patient and family concerns, problem-solving professional boundaries and ethics, and role modeling self-care.[3]

Emphasis on psychosocial health and well-being is no longer considered ancillary to the medical management of cancer. The 2007 Institute of Medicine (IOM) Report, *Cancer Care for the Whole Patient*, outlines the significance of providing quality psychosocial care to individuals affected by cancer. As the report explains, *Psychological and social problems created or exacerbated by cancer—including depression and other emotional problems; lack of information or skills needed to manage the illness; lack of transportation or other resources; and disruptions in work, school, and family life - cause additional suffering, weaken adherence to prescribed treatments, and threaten patients' return to health ... all patients with cancer and their families should expect and receive cancer care that ensures the provision of appropriate psychosocial health services.*[4]

This chapter describes the roles and skill competencies required of oncology social workers and the multifaceted training and supervision needed to prepare the social worker to work effectively with patients and families. Included are the roles oncology social workers have in training and supervising other social workers, supporting other team members, conducting research, and advocating for systems change.

A VALUED MEMBER OF THE ONCOLOGY TEAM

As a team member in the provision of psychosocial health services, the social work profession has evolved to a central role in the oncology workforce for several reasons. First, when medical social work was established by Ida Cannon, the first hospital social worker at Massachusetts General Hospital in 1919, the role was initiated as it was recognized that

the sources of illness are not exclusively biological; disease onset and recovery and resumption of function are influenced by social forces ... Integration of social work in medical care shifts the emphasis away from an exclusively biologic to a biopsychosocial model in which the patient *is* viewed as an individual with a personal, not only medical, history; with human strengths and frailties and with obligations, responsibilities, and preferences.[5]

Oncology care has been one specialty where medical social workers have practiced in hospitals, outpatient clinics, home care and hospice agencies, community wellness programs, patient advocacy organizations, and other settings. These experiences, and the empirical study of this work, have enabled oncology social workers to accumulate a vast body of knowledge about the interactions of people with cancer in their environments. Oncology social workers also intervene with other oncology professionals who experience significant levels of stress in providing care to this population.[4-8]

Second, oncology social work is founded upon broad exposure in social work training to the variety and breadth of therapeutic interventions that social workers incorporate into their practice. The person-in-environment ecological framework of social work[9] emphasizes both psychological and sociological theories which prepare social workers to design and implement interventions aimed at simultaneously strengthening individual adaptation and environmental responsiveness.[9-11] Therapeutic models introduced in graduate and postgraduate social work education include, but are not limited to, knowledge and skill competencies in systems theory, psychodynamic theories, brief therapies, problem-solving, crisis intervention, cognitive-behavioral approaches, conflict resolution, and supportive-expressive interventions. In addition, graduate academic programs also include training in addressing socio-cultural disparities, social policy, administration, and community organization.

Third, the social worker brings to the oncology team not only a clearly defined set of humanistic values but expert problem-solving skills as well.

Social workers help people solve problems and to make hard decisions, often in the face of great uncertainty. Social workers serve as the connective tissue of the healthcare system by supporting, advocating, informing, educating, sensitizing, counseling, and synergizing all available resources and inherent strengths to the benefit of the patient, family and society.[3]

EDUCATION AND TRAINING

The Council on Social Work Education (CSWE) sets standards for the accreditation of social work degree programs in the United States. A bachelor's degree in social work (BSW) is the minimum education required to become an entry-level social worker in many social service organizations. An undergraduate Bachelor's degree typically requires both general education curricula and social work courses which focus on social work values and ethics, working with diverse populations, social welfare policies, and human growth and development. A Bachelor's degree in social work usually takes 4 years to complete and requires an internship for graduation.

Social workers wishing to further their education and specialize in an area such as healthcare or oncology social work generally must seek an advanced degree. Most oncology social workers have a minimum of a Master's degree in Social Work with state licensure. The Master's of Social Work degree (MSW) requires a bachelor's degree before admission to a MSW program, typically takes 2 years to complete, and requires supervised fieldwork. The MSW is by far the most common degree title used by graduate social work schools; however, some schools may confer an MSSW (Master of Science in Social Work) degree.

The Ph.D. (Doctor of Philosophy in Social Work) and DSW (Doctorate of Social Work) are the final degrees offered in the field of social work. These degrees are available to graduates of Master's degree programs in social work or related fields and typically prepare a social worker for positions in academia, research, program planning, administration, and clinical supervision. The Ph.D. in social work is viewed as a research or academic doctoral degree while the DSW is considered a professional doctoral degree.

All states have licensure requirements for social workers (requirements vary from state to state). States require the completion of a Bachelor's or Master's degree in social work from an accredited school, along with the successful completion of an Association of Social Work Boards (ASWB) examination. The ASWB is the association of boards that regulate social work and develops and maintains social work licensing examinations used in all American states and several Canadian provinces. Continuing education is typically required to maintain licensure, 30 approved hours every 2 years on average.

Continuing education is offered through agency or hospital-based programs such as the oncology social work clinical skills training courses offered in major cancer centers throughout the United States, fellowships in oncology social work provided through the American Cancer Society, professional conferences, online training and programs offered by the Association of Oncology Social Work (AOSW), Association of Pediatric Oncology Social Workers (APOSW), American Psychosocial Oncology Society (APOS), National Association of Social Work (NASW), and other organizations.

Social workers are among the psychosocial care providers whose practice is regulated through professional licensure in every state in the United States, to ensure a high level of professional training and practice. Additionally, an Oncology Social Work Certification (OSW-C) is offered by the Board of Oncology Social Work[12] to individuals who have graduated from a CSWE accredited program and have at least 3 years of postmaster's degree work in oncology social work or a related field. Finally, AOSW has published both the *Oncology social work standards of practice*[13] and *Oncology social work scope of practice*[14] to guide social work professionals in psycho-oncology.

BASIC TENETS OF ONCOLOGY SOCIAL WORK

While providing care and support to patients and families, oncology social workers must be knowledgeable about life stages of development, cancer and its treatments, psychosocial aspects of illness and functioning, cultural and spiritual influences, pain and symptom management, finances, community resources, and innovations in the field of psycho-oncology.[15] The following basic tenets form the core knowledge competencies for the profession.

First, the patient and family are viewed as the focus of care and cancer is viewed as an illness affecting the entire family.[11,16] Social work theory supports a systems focus through its emphasis on working with a person-in-environment approach. This view maintains that all individuals are part of an intricate web whose central ties begin with the family. Training in the biological, psychological, and social theories of development and adaptation, therefore, prepares social workers to assist individuals and their support network. For those individuals with limited social supports, the social worker works to help the

Table 84–1. Basic tenets of oncology social work

1. The patient *and* family are the focus of care
2. Psychosocial concerns can have a significant impact on adjustment to illness, treatment adherence, quality of life and potentially survival itself
3. The diverse and unique needs of patients and families require targeted, evidence-based and culturally-sensitive interventions
4. Patients and families benefit from assistance in removing barriers to accessing the standard of care and valuable community resources

patient develop a new support network. Social work's focus on the larger system of community and society extend the role beyond that of individual counselor or family therapist to ensure that the healthcare system and the larger community are responsive to the needs of individual units.[11,16]

Second, oncology social work promotes the awareness and understanding that there is an interrelationship between the medical condition of the patient and the patient's ever-changing biological, psychological, social, informational, and practical concerns. Social workers promote patient/family independence and self-reliance by using a strengths-based approach focused on skill-building and problem solving. At the very core of this is a belief that people are resilient, have the capacity to adapt, change and maintain hope in the face of uncertainty. Comprehending the need for targeted social work interventions across the psychosocial sequelae is at the core of the oncology social worker's ability to listen to, and understand, the patient's needs within their social and medical context.[3] The social work perspective illuminates the impact various life circumstances and events may have on treatment adherence, quality of life, and potentially survival for the patient and family (Table 84–1).

Third, vast individual differences in the responses to cancer require multimodal approaches for support, problem solving, and rehabilitation. Awareness of diversity is at the heart of social work practice. Social workers understand that patient receptivity to treatment is influenced not only by psychological and social variables but by cultural factors as well. Cultural and developmental factors influence the patient/family's view of the patient role, their reactions to illness and healthcare systems, and the meanings they attach to their illness and its treatment. Social workers are especially attuned and trained to deal with health disparities; focus in training on multiculturalism prepares social workers to address the broad spectrum of people affected by cancer, particularly ethnic, gender, or cultural groups that may not receive as much attention in the training of other professional groups.[17-21]

Fourth, oncology social workers are well versed on navigating complex medical, social, financial, and community systems. The social worker's understanding of the disease, treatment processes, hospital, and community resource systems make the social worker an effective mediator for patients and families who are often overwhelmed by the system and the stressors of the illness. Social workers have frequent contact with patients and families as patients move through the healthcare system and in doing so, often create therapeutic alliances with patients and families that may be at-risk, vulnerable, and most in need of support.[3] Helping patients successfully navigate the healthcare system also benefits the system itself by expediting care and enabling patients to fully realize the possible benefits of treatment with minimal disruptions due to psychosocial complications.[22]

ONCOLOGY SOCIAL WORK: CORE COMPETENCIES

An oncology social worker trains to become expert in understanding the psychological, emotional social, informational, financial, and practical domains of patients and families. This insight leads to a psychosocial formulation of the patient, family, and social system within a context of resiliency and hopefulness that focuses on maximizing internal and external resources in the midst of social change. Within oncology, social workers may further specialize in areas such bone marrow transplant, palliative care, disease-specific clinics, radiation, pediatrics, geriatrics,

Table 84–2. Oncology social work competencies: psychosocial care of the whole patient

Screening, evaluation, and assessment	Conduct psychosocial assessments of patient and family in a brief or comprehensive format while utilizing rapid assessment tools (screening), self-report instruments, online screening programs, and interviews
	Effectively communicate assessment results with patient, family, and heathcare team as appropriate
Counseling for adjustment to illness, treatment, survivorship, and/or end of life	Apply appropriate mental health interventions with individuals, families, and groups including brief therapy, problemsolving, crisis intervention, psychodynamic/psychotherapy, cognitive-behavioral approaches, relaxation and guided imagery, transpersonal, and/or existential psychotherapy, supportive psychotherapy, hypnosis
Pain and symptom management	Perform psychosocial cancer pain assessment and explain how cancer pain differs from and/or co-exists with other kinds of pain
	Describe ways to manage cancer pain across the disease continuum as well as psychosocial factors used to assess cancer pain: family relationships, culture, spirituality, decision making, healthcare beliefs, and co-morbid stressors
	Understand the different pharmacotherapy and nonpharmacotherapy options
	Educate patients and families about the management of cancer pain, including myths, misconceptions and fears of addiction
	Advocate for pain and symptom management throughout the course of the disease continuum, including recurrence, survivorship, and end of life
Discharge and transitional care planning	Conduct assessment of discharge needs in collaboration with team
	Be knowledgeable about insurance, entitlements, and financial resources
	Provide information, patient education, resource linkage, community services, practical assistance, financial aid, environmental interventions as appropriate
Information and referral	Know access and eligibility requirements for institutional, local, and national resources for psychiatric, psychological, social, and spiritual needs
	Share information with staff, patients, and families
	Routinely reevaluate resources for availability and relevance
Advocacy and system navigation	Advocate for patient/family needs, inpatient, outpatient, at home, and in the community with staff, extended family, and caregivers
	Advocate at the administrative and policy level in the local and national arenas
	Provide system navigation support and coordination for seamless delivery of care

and so on.[3,21] The knowledge and skill base of an oncology social worker must therefore be multifaceted and comprehensively framed across the cancer trajectory (Table 84–2).

The National Comprehensive Cancer Network (NCCN) Guidelines for Distress Management (v.1.2008) extensively outlines social work services that are recommended when a cancer patient has a psychosocial or practical problem. These include services such as:

1. screening, evaluation, and assessment;
2. individual, family, and group counseling;
3. pain and symptom management;
4. discharge and transitional care planning;
5. information and referral to valuable resources;
6. advocacy, social change, and patient navigation;
7. administration and clinical supervision;
8. staff intervention and support;
9. training and supervision with volunteers.

Screening, evaluation, and assessment. Oncology social workers utilize a multimodal approach to assessment which has long been a cornerstone of social work practice. Historically, social workers were taught to do lengthy, hand-written assessments using the SOAP format (Subjective, Objective, Assessment, Plan). With the advent of more efficient and effective screening and assessment tools, the social worker can more readily identify the extent and level of urgency of psychosocial need and facilitate the design of appropriate psychosocial interventions. The earliest comprehensive hospital-based screening programs were pioneered by oncology social workers in the early 1990s.[23] Rapid assessment tools such as the distress thermometer and self-report instruments also add informative data to the evaluation process.[23,24] Social workers can use simple standardized tools that can help diagnose or measure pain intensity. For example, a numerical pain intensity scale, measuring pain intensity on a 0–10 Likert-type scale (with 0 = no pain and 10 = worst possible pain) is the most frequently used scale in pain assessment.

Social workers must be competent in the use of various screening and assessment methods, including a working knowledge of the diagnostic categories in the *Diagnostic and statistical manual of mental disorders* (DSM), as well as employing advances that technology.[25] brings into the clinical setting such as touch-screen registration and electronic medical records (EMR). The oncology social worker must also be trained on using the findings from assessment to develop a psychosocial care plan that is focused on early identification of problems, strength-based interventions, and mobilization of practical problem-solving skills that enable the patient and family to identify and link with supportive resources.[2]

Individual, family, and group counseling. Oncology social workers have been instrumental in organizing and facilitating individual, couple and family psychotherapy as well as support groups in hospital and community settings. Through academic coursework and field practicums in MSW graduate programs, theories, and skills of psychotherapy are acquired that allow the social worker to effectively function in the role of psychotherapist or counselor in the oncology setting. Oncology-specific internships and postgraduate training equip the oncology social worker with expertise in the psychosocial issues most relevant to medically ill patients and their families.[5] This training enables the oncology social worker to distinguish, for example, depressive reactions to chemotherapy from endogenous depression and can help the patient and family anticipate and manage commonly experienced effects of treatment.

The counseling role for oncology social workers may at times become over-shadowed by time-sensitive, practical concerns that are necessary to help patients move effectively through the healthcare system. Oncology social workers are adept at integrating brief interventions as well as more structured counseling sessions focused on issues related to adjustment and relationships, anxiety and depression, symptom management, grief, loss, and meaning. With the increasing chronicity of cancer, social workers are also focused on helping families develop lifelong problem solving and coping skills that will sustain the family over the long haul.

Table 84-3. Types of social work referrals

Standard referral	Urgent referral	Emergent referral
Adjustment to illness	Patient and/or family distress related to:	Suicidal ideation
Problem solving	Poor prognosis	Substance abuse
Treatment decision making	Deteriorating condition	Child, spouse, or elder abuse
Support group	Poor test results	Homicidal ideation
Psychoeducational group	Difficult/complex procedures	Signing out AMA
Medical insurance assistance	Diagnostic tests	Treatment refusal
Durable medical equipment	Uncontrolled anxiety and/or depression	
Hospice and homecare services	Pain/symptom management issues	
Transportation options	Nonadherence to treatment	
Housing resources	Social/behavioral issues impacting treatment	
Entitlement programs	Staff distress and/or difficulty coping	
Grief/bereavement support		

Pain and symptom management. Social workers have long provided clinical and educational services in pain clinics and other healthcare settings, which have impacted the patient and family experience of chronic pain. As social workers realized the continuous interplay of physical, emotional, and cognitive factors in the experience of pain, they could more easily identify appropriate practice roles for working with chronic pain patients. Decades ago, social workers were promoting social work involvement in the management of cancer pain, recommending psychosocial and cognitive-behavioral interventions as adjuncts to medical management that included more traditional interventions such as drug therapy and surgery.[26] More recently, the essential role that can be played by social workers in pain and symptom management was outlined, describing the global nature of the psychosocial effects of pain and suggesting that the complex and multidimensional factors that define the experience of pain are a natural fit with a social work profession that incorporates comprehensive assessment of emotional, family, social, practical and environmental issues.[27] While no formal social work core competencies exist for pain and symptom management, NASW addressed the issue in their *Standards for palliative & end of life care.* NASW defines palliative care as

an approach that improves quality of life for patients and their families facing the problems associated with life-limiting illness. This is accomplished through the prevention and relief of suffering by means of early identification and comprehensive assessment and treatment of pain and other physical, psychosocial, and spiritual problems.[2]

Discharge and transitional care planning. Dating back to the days of Ida Cannon at Massachusetts General, medical social workers have been acting as an interface between the hospital and home, hospital and rehabilitation centers, nursing homes and hospice, intervening where necessary to aid in the transition from medical patient to home and community. Often these interventions have been practical in nature, that is, transportation, home medical supplies or equipment, homemaking services, or meals.[28,29] The national expansion of palliative care and hospice programs, complicated insurance reimbursement policies, and shrinking resources requires skilled clinicians to optimally assist cancer patients through these transitions. The National Cancer Institute (NCI) defines this work as "transitional care planning" as it helps create a seamless delivery of care for the patient and family through different phases of the cancer experience. An ability to empathically and assertively advocate for patient communication requires excellent clinical and system negotiation skills. While some functions may be relatively straightforward, because of its complexity, this type of care planning has been and continues to be an important social work role.[30]

Information and referral. Oncology social workers receive and make referrals for psychosocial services. Receiving timely referrals from other members of the healthcare team and/or gaining early access to patients in need enables the oncology social worker to become more quickly engaged to help the patient and family reduce distress and better utilize the healthcare system. Appropriate referrals include requests for help with problem solving, crisis intervention, supportive counseling, psychotherapy, and information and referral to other resources. Once an assessment is completed, the oncology social worker determines a psychosocial care plan, manages the case, and/or makes referrals to services such as nutritional counseling, financial services, support groups, chaplaincy, psychiatry, and community-based and government resources. Patients and families can also self-refer to a social worker. It is important that hospital social work departments and community agencies promote social work services directly to patients and families to facilitate self-referral (Table 84-3).

Advocacy, social change, and patient navigation. Patient and family advocacy is another skill in psychosocial care for which the oncology social worker is uniquely prepared. Coursework and training at the master's level equips social workers with skills that allow them to integrate the specialized needs of patients and families within larger systems. Acting as an advocate with healthcare agencies, government offices, employers, schools, churches, healthcare providers, communities, and others on behalf of the cancer patient and family moves the oncology social worker beyond the psychosocial realm into a humanistic responsibility toward greater societal change. A person-in-environment perspective, therefore, provides many points of intervention and different forms of advocacy efforts.[31] An oncology social worker, no matter the setting, has the skills not only to advocate for patients and families, but to teach those patients and families the skills to communicate and advocate effectively for themselves.

Irrespective of the form of intervention, the resource most needed for advocacy is information. Through research, publication of clinical literature, education and training, oncology social workers are actively engaged in acquiring and sharing information which leads to making communities, and society in general, more responsive to the needs of persons with cancer. The AOSW states in their *Scope of practice* that social workers should provide "advocacy to remove barriers to quality care, to address gaps in service, to help survivors and families secure the protection of existing laws, and to work for any changes needed to policies, programs and legislation."[14]

One form of social work advocacy relates to system navigation. Cancer "patient navigation" is defined as "... individualized assistance offered to patients, families, and caregivers to help overcome health-care system barriers and facilitate timely access to quality medical and psychosocial care from prediagnosis through all phases of the cancer experience."[32] While social workers have been navigating systems for decades, a formalized concept was developed by Harold Freeman, MD in Harlem Hospital in New York City wherein patient navigation was designed to help patients follow through with diagnostic testing, treatment, and follow-up care in an attempt to effect optimal health outcomes. Oncology social workers provide many of these services, sometimes under the title of "Patient Navigator" in their respective setting. It is imperative that oncology social workers champion these programs or collaborate on their design to ensure the highest standards of care for patients and their caregivers.

Social workers, unlike many other psychosocial care providers, are trained in community organization and human rights advocacy which enables them to facilitate collaborative or other efforts on the part of groups, organizations, and communities to effect social action and social change. Several national organizations employ oncology social workers, including executive staff, whom have been instrumental in improving programming, research, funding, and legislation related to cancer. Oncology social workers are consulted as expert advisors to policy makers and bear influence on federal and state healthcare reform initiatives to insure comprehensive psychosocial care of persons affected by cancer. Effecting change at the policy level strengthens the social worker's ability to impact the individual healthcare of patients and is viewed as a necessary role of oncology social work.

Administration and clinical supervision. In addition to serving in the primary role of psychosocial care provider for patients and families with its multiplicity of tasks, oncology social workers are also called upon to serve as administrators, clinical supervisors, and project and/or institutional leaders. As such, administrators and supervisors address the clinical training needs of students and beginning workers, as well as experienced workers through a variety of methods including: the tutorial model of a one-to-one relationship, peer supervision, group supervision, and case consultation. Through these specific educational, administrative, and supportive techniques, oncology social workers at the administrative and supervisory level strive to enhance worker performance, job satisfaction, and social work utilization throughout systems.[6,33]

Stressors for the oncology social worker may include compassion fatigue, cumulated grief and loss, professional boundary discord, and increasing institutional demands amidst diminishing staff resources. Concomitantly, there is a confrontation with and recognition of one's own mortality that is often dealt with by the social worker at an earlier age than is "normal" for the general population. There is the traumatic exposure to mutilation and a constant sense of loss.[10,27] These pressures, and many others, accompany social work practice in oncology, and require a high level of skill and training on behalf of the social worker and supervisor.

Staff intervention and support. The stress of working in an oncology setting is shared by nearly all the members of the oncology team. Stressors often include high patient caseloads, cumulative deaths of critically ill patients, and witnessing patient/family pain, suffering and devastating disability. Increasingly, today's healthcare environment adds to the distress of medical staff who are charged with doing more with less, responding quickly with fewer resources, and seeing cancer patients and their families facing increasing financial and personal distress related to the growing cost of healthcare. While mutual support among the team members may be available, oncology social workers are often called upon to take the lead in supportive interventions with staff. Facilitating staff support groups,[8] providing critical incident stress debriefings (CISD), and meeting one-on-one with individual staff members, both formally and informally, oncology social workers can help to defuse work-related stressors and offer professional psychosocial support at no additional cost to the system.

Training and supervision with volunteers. Recognizing that the effective use of volunteers can significantly enhance patient care, social workers have regularly been involved in volunteer training and supervision. Volunteers provide a range of services from practical assistance to social support including assistance in screening, orientation, diversionary activities, education, fundraising, peer counseling, transportation, and research activities.

As economic considerations deplete the availability of some services, such as transportation, the effective use of volunteer services becomes more significant. Some volunteer tasks, such as providing patients with information about hospital and community programs, may require limited training, but many tasks require in-depth orientation to the psychosocial impact of cancer and the healthcare system for the volunteer

to provide service sensitively and efficiently. Social workers are often instrumental in the training and supervision of volunteers to prepare volunteers to help patients both in the hospital and in the community and provide ongoing supervision and consultation to those volunteers involved in peer support.

ETHICS AND LEGAL ADVOCACY

"Informed consent for treatment and patient participation in decision making implicate social workers because of their role in facilitating communication and mutual understanding between patient and family and professional caregivers."[13,14] Since the advent of the Patient Self-Determination Act of 1990, which requires hospitals and health agencies to develop policies on advance directives, social workers have been leaders in helping patients and families to understand the mandates of the law, in preparing advance directives, and in problem-solving situations when advance directives have not been completed. Schools of social work routinely include ethics in their curriculum, making social workers a valuable resource for patients, families, and the oncology healthcare team in ethical decision making. In fact, social work licensing renewal across the country requires continuing education in ethics training.

PATIENT, STAFF, AND COMMUNITY EDUCATOR

Oncology social workers support and contribute to their own education through the annual national conferences of AOSW and APOS, as well as participation both as attendee and presenter in a vast array of international conferences and workshops. Oncology social workers also play a key role in the education of medical, nursing, and other health professionals regarding the psychosocial impact of cancer.[34,35] Social workers are frequently facilitators of programs such as I Can Cope sponsored by the American Cancer Society and have authored numerous patient-education materials including those published by the NCI, the American Cancer Society, the Leukemia and Lymphoma Society, The Wellness Community, CancerCare, the American Pain Foundation and many other organizations which provide patient and professional education.

PSYCHOSOCIAL ONCOLOGY RESEARCHER

Research is a required component of MSW training as it facilitates the development and teaching of evidence-based knowledge and skills required to practice social work. The Institute for the Advancement of Social Work Research, created in 1992, reflects the profession's recognition of the importance of research in both evaluating practice and furthering knowledge of people and their problems. One of the leading interdisciplinary journals of psychosocial oncology care, the *Journal of Psychosocial Oncology,* which is AOSW's official journal, serves as a forum for sharing research and clinical data. Many of the articles published in this quarterly journal reflect the prevailing practitioner-scholar model, adopted by the oncology social work field, which underscores the need for empirically informed practice.[36–38]

In 1994, AOSW created the Social Work Oncology Research Group (SWORG), which promotes research relevant to oncology social work through multiinstitutional collaboration and function. In 2003, AOSW published *A social work guide to conducting research in psychosocial oncology* to help guide and support AOSW members to engage in evidence-based, empirical research and data collection.[38] Ongoing projects include an exploration of the prevalence of distress across the disease continuum from diagnosis to terminal illness, and an examination of the psychosocial needs of high-distress patients.

TECHNOLOGY AND SOCIAL WORK

As technology rapidly expands into every aspect of medical care, it is critical that oncology social workers be well-informed and trained as to how best integrate technological advances into quality social work practice. NASW and ASWB have developed *Standards for technology in social work practice*[25] which establish a uniform guide for social workers and address critical and pertinent issues related to the integration of technology into evidence-based clinical practice, technical and practice competencies, risk management, and ethical standards. In managing email, electronic referrals and charting, online support groups and educational programs, and other technology-based communication tools, oncology social workers increasingly will be called upon to enhance their skills and understanding of the value, risk, and limitations of using technology in psychosocial cancer care.

CONCLUSION

Oncology social workers are highly trained, skilled clinicians who function as dynamic members of the healthcare team. Social work is dedicated to delivering evidence-based, quality psychosocial care rooted in a value system that empowers individuals, families, communities, and systems toward optimal functioning and quality of life. Oncology social workers require intensive didactic and experiential training beyond the Master's degree which addresses the specific psychosocial issues and social work interventions across the continuum of the cancer experience. To work in oncology, social workers must have compassion, self-awareness, and commitment to teamwork, personal growth, and hope in the face of adversity. The depth of personal and professional satisfaction for the social worker in oncology can be profound and life-changing as one finds a deeper meaning to life and work.

Oncology social workers develop and deliver a wide variety of interventions and programs to facilitate effective coping with cancer, its treatment, survivorship, palliative care, end-of-life, and bereavement services. Empirical studies in psychosocial oncology have documented the efficacy and cost effectiveness of social work interventions. Future social work research and clinical literature will continue to contribute to the understanding of how best to promote psychosocial health and well-being for cancer patients, survivors, and their caregivers by defining and expanding best practices in oncology social work.

REFERENCES

1. Coluzzi PH, Grant M, Doroshow JH, Rhiner M, Ferrell B, Rivera L. Survey of the provision of supportive care services at National Cancer Institute-designated cancer centers. *J Clin Oncl.* 1995;13:756–764.

2. National Association of Social Workers. *NASW standards for palliative and end of life care.* Washington, DC: NASW Press; 2004.

3. Loscalzo MJ. Social workers. The connective tissue of the health care system. In: Emanuel L, Lawrence Librach S, (eds). *Palliative care: Core skills and clinical competencies.* Philadelphia, PA: Saunders; 2007.

4. Institute of Medicine. *Cancer care for the whole patient: Meeting psychosocial health needs.* Washington, DC: National Academies Press; 2007.

5. Lauria M. Oncology social work in *Encyclopedia of social work,* 20th ed. New York, NY: Oxford University Press; 2008;Vol 3:319–322.

6. Supple-Diaz L, Mattison D. Factors affecting survival and satisfaction: navigating a career in oncology social work. *J Psychosoc Oncol.* 1992;10:111–131.

7. Weisman AD. Understanding the cancer patient: the syndrome of caregiver's plight. *Psychiatry.* 1981;44:157–167.

8. McGrath FJ, Dodds-Waugh A. Support group for nurses in an oncology ward. *Aust Soc Work.* 1989;42:29–34.

9. Germain C. An ecological perspective on social work practice in health care. *Soc Work Health Care.* 1977;3:67–76.

10. Black RB. Challenges for social work as a core profession in cancer services. *Soc Work Health Care.* 1989;14:1–13.

11. Berkman B. Knowledge base needs for effective social work practice in health. *J Ed Soc Work.* 1981;17:85–90.

12. Board of Oncology Social Work. 2002 Certification. http://www.oswcert.org/. Accessed January 5, 2009.

13. Association of Oncology Social Work. Standards of practice in oncology social work. 2001. http://www.aosw.org/html/prof-standards.php. Accessed December 20, 2008.

14. Association of Oncology Social Work. Scope of practice in oncology social work. 2001. http://www.aosw.org/html/prof-scope.php. Accessed December 20, 2008.

15. Spiegel, D. Psychosocial interventions with cancer patients. *J Psychosoc Oncol.* 1986;3(4):83–93.

16. Tolley NS. Oncology social work, family systems theory, and workplace consultations. *Health Soc Work.* 1994;19:227–230.

17. LaRosa M. Health care needs of Hispanic Americans and the responsiveness of the health care system. *Soc Work.* 1989;34:104–107.

18. Glajchen M, Blum D, Calder K. Cancer pain management and the role of social work: barriers and interventions. *Health Soc Work.* 1995;20(3):200–206.

19. Sam H, Koopmans J, Mathieson C. The psychosocial impact of a laryngectomy: a comprehensive assessment. *J Psychosoc Oncol.* 1991;9:37–58.

20. Zabora J, Smith E, Baker F, Wingard J, Curbow B. The family: the other side of bone marrow transplantation. *J Psychosoc Oncol.* 1992;10:35–46.

21. Kennedy V. The role of social work in bone marrow transplantation. *J Psychosoc Oncol.* 1993;11(1):103–117.

22. Carlson LE, Bultz BD. Benefits of psychosocial oncology care: Improved quality of life and medical cost offset. *Hlth QoL Outc.* 2003;1(8):1–9.

23. Zabora J, BrintzenhofeSzoc K, Jacobsen P, Curbow B, Piantadosis S, Hooker C. A new psychosocial screening instrument for use with cancer patients. *Psychosom.* 2001;42:241–246.

24. Holland JC, Bultz BD. National Comprehensive Cancer Network (NCCN): the NCCN guideline for distress management. *J Natl Compr Canc Netw.* 2007;5(1):3–7.

25. National Association of Social Workers and Association of Social Work Boards. *NASW and ABSW standards for technology and social work practice.* Washington, DC: Author; 2005.

26. Loscalzo M, Amendola J. Psychosocial and behavioral management of cancer pain. *Adv Pain Res Therapy.* 1990;16:429–442.

27. Altilio T. Pain and symptom management: an essential role for social work. In: Berzoff J, Silverman P, (eds), *Living with dying: A handbook for end-of-life healthcare practitioners.* New York: Columbia University Press; 2004.

28. Bryan J, Greger II, Miller M, et al. An evaluation of the transportation needs of disadvantaged cancer patients. *J Psychosoc Oncol.* 1991;9:23–36.

29. Lurie A, Pinsky S, Tuzman L. Training social workers for discharge planning. *Health Soc Work.* 1981;6:12–18.

30. National Cancer Institute. *Transitional care planning.* Bethesda, MD: National Cancer Institute, 2007. http://www.cancer.gov/cancertopics/pdq/supportivecare/transitionalcare/healthprofessional. Accessed January 28, 2009.

31. Schneider RL, Chester L, Ochieng J. Advocacy. In : Mizrahi T, Davis L, (eds), *Encyclopedia of social work.* 20th ed. New York: Oxford University Press; 2008;1:59–65.

32. C-Change. Defining patient navigation. 2005. http://www.c-hangetogether.org/ pubs/pubs/ CPNDefinition.pdf. Accessed August 15, 2008.

33. Blum D. Clinical supervisory practice in oncology settings. *Clin Supervisor.* 1983;1:17–27.

34. Zayas LH, Dyche LH. Social workers training primary care physicians: essential psychosocial principles. *Soc Work.* 1992;37:247–252.

35. Hunsdon S. The impact of illness on patients and families: social workers teach medical students. *Soc Work Health Care.* 1984;10:41–52.

36. Glajchen M, Magen R. Evaluating process, outcome and satisfaction in community based cancer support groups. *Soc Work Groups.* 1995;18:27–40.

37. Siegel K. Psychosocial oncology research. *Soc Work Health Care.* 1990;15:21–43.

38. Roberts C, BrintzenhofeSzoc K, Zebrack B, Behar L. *A social work guide to conducting research in psychosocial oncology.* Philadelphia, PA: Association of Oncology Social Work ; 2003.

CHAPTER 85

Education of Nurses in Psycho-Oncology

Terry A. Badger, Barb Henry, and Ruth McCorkle

Nurses, the largest of the healthcare professions (approximately 3 million), are commonly on the forefront of patient care in oncology practice. Nurses are responsible for the assessment and referral of psychosocial problems demonstrated by patients and their families, regardless of practice setting.[1] When compared to other professional groups, nurses often experience the most concentrated exposure to intense emotions given the extended time spent with patients and their families. Despite the daily exposure to potent emotions in the practice setting, nurses receive little formal education regarding the psychological aspects of cancer. The purpose of this chapter is to describe the education of nurses, with emphasis as it pertains to psycho-oncology and discuss some ways to address some of the deficiencies that currently exist.

NURSING EDUCATION

Before discussing the specifics of nursing education related to oncology, a general discussion of nursing and nursing education in the United States is warranted. There are three major pathways to becoming a registered nurse (RN): obtaining a 2-year associate's degree in nursing from a community or junior college, a 3-year hospital based diploma, or a 4-year baccalaureate degree from a college or university.[2] All state boards of nursing, except those in North Dakota and New York, accept these three educational paths as appropriate academic preparation for RN licensure.

Nursing curricula are reviewed against specific standards, and there are two organizations that accredit nursing education programs. The National League for Nursing Accrediting Commission (NLNAC) accredits nursing programs across all levels, from practical nursing programs to doctoral programs. The Commission on Collegiate Nursing Education (CCNE), an independent arm of the American Association of Colleges of Nursing (AACN), accredits programs offering baccalaureate, masters, and doctorate of nursing practice degrees in nursing. Although NLNAC does not require institutions to address specific knowledge and skills (e.g., psychosocial), it does require that schools of nursing build their curricula around guidelines for nursing practice selected from those established by a number of recognized nursing organizations. One example is the Pew Health Professions Commission's *21 competencies for the twenty-first century* that recommends a set of core competencies related to psychosocial health services.[3] For example, NLNAC core competencies are that nurses should (1) incorporate the psychosocial-behavioral perspective into a full range of clinical practice competencies, (2) involve patients and their families in decision-making processes, (3) help individuals, families, and communities maintain and promote healthy behavior, and (4) provide counseling for patients in situations where ethical issues arise.

The AACN identifies "nurses practice from a holistic base and incorporating bio-psychosocial and spiritual aspects of health."[4] Content related to psychosocial health services are to be taught throughout the curriculum, and must incorporate the knowledge and skills identified by *The Essentials for baccalaureate education for professional nursing practice*[4] or *The Essentials of master's education for advanced practice nursing.*[5] The current revision of the *Essentials* document[4] lists core knowledge and skills related to psychosocial health services (Table 85–1).

After completion of an accredited nursing program, graduates must pass the National Council Licensure Examination for RNs (NCLEX-RN), administered by the National State Boards of Nursing (NCSBN).

Psychosocial content is a relatively small percentage of questions on the exam, comprising approximately 6%–10%.[6] The scope of nursing practice is determined by the state in which the nurse practices and all practicing nurses must have a current license if working as an RN. All states require nurses to renew their licenses usually annually, with some states requiring evidence of continued education.

Psychosocial oncology content is typically taught in curricula as part of the medical-surgical rotation, and includes a limited number of didactic hours plus clinical experiences with cancer patients. Another typical rotation in which nursing students have experience with cancer patients is during hospice clinical experiences. It would be unusual for the average undergraduate nursing student to not have experiences caring for cancer patients before graduating given the combination of inpatient and community experiences typical of most nursing programs. However, there is limited time in most programs devoted specifically to psychosocial responses to life-threatening illnesses of individuals and their families. Undergraduate nursing students are typically exposed to psychosocial concepts, such as depression and anxiety, as part of their psychiatric-mental health nursing clinical experiences on inpatient psychiatric units or community-based mental health facilities, with little application of these concepts beyond patients with severe mental illnesses.

Although the American Cancer Society (ACS; http://www.cancer.org/) recommended guidelines in the mid-90s regarding the curriculum content they believed was essential for students to learn during their basic education, this psychosocial oncology content is typically not presented adequately.[1] Clinical competencies recommended are that baccalaureate graduates should have the ability to describe the major psychosocial responses of the individual and family to cancer, and to communicate effectively with people with cancer and their families. Although all students need content regarding how depression and anxiety can influence life-threatening illnesses such as cancer, and all graduate nurses need this when practicing in any clinical setting, unfortunately this content is not systematically presented in most basic programs.

There are few programs at the graduate level in which students in oncology nursing have didactic and clinical experiences that focus on psycho-oncology. Nurses receive education in assessment and screening of cancer patients to determine if they need referrals to psychosocial resources.[1] Graduate level education provides advanced knowledge and skills in the theoretical basis of nursing, advanced assessment, diagnosis and treatment, nursing research, trends and issues that influence health care, and concepts such as conflict, change, stress, teaching-learning, and organizational systems and management.

Nurses can also obtain certification from various organizations to recognize their specialized knowledge and skills in a particular practice area. For example, the American Nurses Credentialing Center (ANCC), an arm of the American Nurses Association, certifies nurses in psychiatric-mental health nursing. Nurses who specialize in oncology nursing for either children or adults can be credentialed by the Oncology Nursing Certification Corporation (ONCC). Credentials include Oncology Certified Nurse (OCN), Certified Pediatric Oncology Nurse (CPON), Advanced Oncology Certified Nurse Practitioner (AOCNP), and Advanced Oncology Certified Clinical Nurse Specialist (AOCNS).[7] The oncology exam varies in the percentage of content related to specific areas, but requires that nurses have knowledge and skills in the areas of quality of life, symptom management, psychosocial issues, and psychosocial management. Evidence of continued competency is required when

Table 85–1. Selected core competencies for the essentials of baccalaureate education

Graduates must have the knowledge and skills to

- assist patients to access and interpret the meaning and validity of health information;
- adapt communication methods to patients with special needs, that is, sensory or psychological disabilities;
- use therapeutic communication within the nurse–patient relationship
- provide relevant and sensitive health education information and counseling to patients;
- perform a holistic assessment of the individual across the lifespan, including a health history which includes spiritual, social, cultural, and psychological assessment, as well as a comprehensive physical examination;
- assess physical, cognitive, and social functional ability of the individual in all developmental stages, with particular attention to changes due to aging;
- foster strategies for health promotion, risk reduction, and disease prevention across the life span;
- use information technologies to communicate health promotion/disease prevention information to the patient in a variety of settings;
- evaluate the efficacy of health promotion and education modalities for use in a variety of settings and with diverse populations;
- demonstrate sensitivity to personal and cultural definitions of health;
- assess and manage physical and psychological symptoms related to disease and treatment;
- assess and manage pain;
- demonstrate sensitivity to personal and cultural influences on the individual's reactions to the illness experience and end of life;
- anticipate, plan for, and manage physical, psychological, social, and spiritual needs of the patient and family/caregiver;
- enable individuals and families to make quality-of-life and end-of-life decisions and achieve a peaceful death;
- provide holistic care that addresses the needs of diverse populations across the life span;
- understand the effects of health and social policies on people from diverse backgrounds;
- advocate for healthcare that is sensitive to the needs of patients, with particular emphasis on the needs of vulnerable populations;
- demonstrate knowledge of the importance and meaning of health and illness for the patient in providing nursing care;
- coordinate and manage care to meet the special needs of vulnerable populations, including the frail elderly, to maximize independence and quality of life;
- coordinate the healthcare of individuals across the lifespan utilizing principles and knowledge of interdisciplinary models of care delivery and case management.

SOURCE: Adapted from AACN (2008). *The essentials of baccalaureate education for profession nursing practice.* Accessed at www.aacn.edu.

recertifying to include minimal practice, continuing education, and peer review. Sample competencies for an Oncology Nurse Practitioner are found in Table 85–2.

Currently, the number of certified oncology nurses (OCNs) is small and reflects the national nursing shortage in all areas of practice. Approximately 21 thousand nurses are OCNs with an additional 2600 RNs with advanced preparation and credentials in oncology, (AOCNs). Among RNs with advanced practice preparation and credentials in psychiatry-mental health, there are approximately 20,000. However, the majority of psychiatric-mental health advanced practice nurses (APNs) are working with people with severe mental illnesses not with oncology patients and their families. Clearly, the number of RNs with psycho-oncology education is inadequate for the projected number of cancer survivors and their families.

Table 85–2. Oncology nurse practitioner competencies (ONS, 2007)

Graduates must have the knowledge and skills to

- perform a comprehensive assessment of functional status and the impact on activities of daily living, including but not limited to the following domains:
  - –Psychological
  - –Role
  - –Social
  - –Cognitive
  - –Physical
- assess for the presence of psychological co-morbidities (e.g., anxiety/depression, substance use), past and present coping skills, and the psychosocial impact of the cancer experience
- assess concerns and issues related to sexual function, sexual well-being, and fertility of patients with a past, current, or potential diagnosis of cancer, including the impact on relationships
- assess developmental, ethnic, spiritual, racial socioeconomic, and gender variations in symptom presentation or illness experience of patients with cancer.
- assess the roles, tasks, and stressors of individuals, families, and caregivers and their ability to manage the illness experience (e.g., resources, support services, equipment, transportation, child care, anxiety, depression)
- assess patients' ability to navigate the complex healthcare system and the barriers to continuity, coordination, and communication among multiple care providers
- determine the impact of co-morbidities on the prognosis and treatment of patients with cancer
- diagnose acute and chronic psychological complications (e.g., anxiety, depression, substance abuse) and their influence on the patient's psychological state
- collaborate with the multidisciplinary team, patient, family, and caregivers to formulate a comprehensive plan of care for patients with cancer, including appropriate health education; health promotion; and health maintenance, rehabilitation, and palliative care
- plan therapeutic interventions to restore or maintain an optimal level of functioning
- coordinate care within a context of functional status, cultural considerations, spiritual needs, family or caregiver needs, and ethical principles
- consider co-morbid conditions when implementing cancer treatment
- refer patients and families to appropriate support services
- establish caring relationships with patients, families, and other caregivers to facilitate coping with sensitive issues
- facilitate patient and family decision making regarding complex treatment, symptom management, and end-of-life care
- assist patients with cancer and their families in preparing for and coping with grief and bereavement
- develop interventions with patients and families that are consistent with patients' physiologic and psychological needs and values
- use evidence-based information to help patients with cancer and their families to make informed decisions
- assist patients with cancer and their families and caregivers to negotiate healthcare delivery systems
- refer patients to appropriate local, state, and national patient-support resources.

SOURCE: Adapted from ONCC (2008). ONCC and certification information, 2007.

CURRENT TRENDS TO IMPROVE PSYCHOSOCIAL ONCOLOGY CARE

The recent IOM (2008)[8] report has recommended an intensive focus on five core competencies for health professions to improve workforce performance: (1) patient-centered care; (2) work with interdisciplinary

Table 85–3. Knowledge and skills for providing psycho-oncology care (IOM, 2007)

Communication with patients and families
Screening
Needs assessment
Care planning and coordination
Illness self-management
Collaboration across disciplines/specialties and work in teams
Linking patients to psychosocial services
Outcomes assessment
Informatics

SOURCE: Adapted from IOM (2008), *Cancer care for the whole patient: Meeting the psychosocial health needs.*

teams; (3) employ evidence-based practice; (4) apply quality improvement, and (5) utilize informatics (p. 256). These competencies provide clear direction for the knowledge and skills needed for oncology nurses in the future (Table 85–3).

Most undergraduate and graduate nursing curricula throughout the country include information about patient-centered care, have interprofessional educational opportunities, incorporate evidence-based practice in their didactic and clinical experiences, discuss quality improvement, and have informatics content. Nursing students who are recent graduates have had exposure to the recommended content for workforce improvement.

Nurses who have been in practice for a number of years may be less likely to have these knowledge and skills, depending upon when they graduated. For example, informatics content in curricula has been a fairly recent trend.

The Oncology Nursing Society (ONS), the largest nursing organization dedicated to oncology nursing practice with over 35,000 members, has recognized the need for further nursing education regarding psychosocial oncology care. The ONS Outcomes Resource Area, ons.org/outcomes/measures/summaries.shtml], contains guidelines for high-quality oncology care impacting patient outcomes through evidence-based nursing interventions. *Putting Evidence into Practice* (PEP) cards and web pages are available for nurses to use at the bedside and as online resources. Psychosocial oncology care resources include both measurement and interventions for the following topics: caregiver strain and burden, depression, and anxiety. Resources about many other symptoms such as fatigue, sleep-wake disturbances, nausea, and constipation are also provided. These resources are continuously updated by ONS based on current research and practice. The PEP cards are widely distributed, presented at conferences and the content is also published in *Clinical Journal of Oncology Nursing, Oncology Nursing Forum* and *ONS Connect*. ONS has been a leader in providing continuing education via workshops, congresses, conferences, and web-based offerings.

In the past 10 years, many other organizations have focused on the psychosocial care of care patients and have published guidelines to improve practice. To name just a few of these organizations, American Psychosocial Oncology Society (APOS; http://www.apos-society.org/), ACS, National Comprehensive Cancer Network (NCCN; http://www.nccn.org/), Cancer Care, Lance Armstrong Foundation (LAF; http://www.livestrong.org), National Cancer Institute (NCI; http://www.cancer.gov/), and Wellness Communities (http://www.thewellnesscommunity.org/). Each of these organizations has published guidelines and/or material discussing psychosocial care.[9] Yet, the adoption of these guidelines and standards has been inconsistent. No universal guidelines are recognized.

As evidenced-base care becomes the standard, and required through accreditation organizations, oncology nurses will become more proficient with implementing the current guidelines and standards. Nurses who are involved in cancer care can incorporate routine psychosocial assessment and referral into their comprehensive care, and can take advantage of current educational opportunities to increase their skills.[10] Healthcare institutions can take steps to improve the education of nursing staff by encouraging continued education, certification, and providing supervision for psych-social care. APN's who specialize in psycho-oncology can provide education and supervision to staff nurses to improve psycho-oncology care. Cancer centers that currently do not have these specialized nurses may wish to develop such positions to meet the IOM recommendations, guidelines for obtaining or maintaining designation as a comprehensive cancer center or for Magnet status.[11] In addition, Schwartz Center Rounds (https://www.theschwartzcenter.org) can be used to improve psychosocial care by supporting oncology staff to prevent burnout.

Psychosocial oncology education has improved in the past decade, yet much remains to be done. Organizations must continue to disseminate standards and guidelines for psychosocial care and require that psychosocial care be part of comprehensive cancer care (e.g., APOS, NCI, and ONS[12]). Healthcare institutions should require that all nurses who work in oncology have education in psychosocial care, particularly as this care must be demonstrated as part of accreditation or if seeking Magnet status. Nurses who remain in the forefront of patient care, and who continue to care for patients and their families during intense emotional experiences must rise to the challenge for continuing their own education about guidelines and standards of psychosocial care. Nurses are ideally situated in the healthcare system to assess and refer patients and their families for psychosocial care. Nurses can ensure that patients and their families no longer will report unmet psychosocial needs by working together with other healthcare professions.

REFERENCES

1. McCorkle R, Frank-Stromberg M, Pasacreta JV. Education of nurses in psycho-oncology (Chapter 93). In: J Holland, W Breitbart, PB Jacobson, MS Lederberg (eds), Psycho-Oncology. New York: Oxford University Press; 1998:1069–1073.
2. Institute of Medicine. (IOM). *Improving medical education: Enhancing the behavioral and science content of medical school curriculum.* Washington, DC: The National Academies Press; 2004.
3. National League for Nursing Accrediting Commission. (NLNAC). *NLNAC accreditation manual with interpretive guidelines by program type for post secondary and higher degree programs in nursing.* 2006. http://www/nlnac.org. Accessed January 16, 2008.
4. American Association of Colleges of Nursing. (AACN). *The essentials of baccalaureate education for profession nursing practice.* 2008. www.aacn.edu. Accessed January 15, 2008.
5. American Association of Colleges of Nursing. (AACN) The essentials for master's education for advanced practice nursing. 1996. www.aacn.edu on Accessed January 15, 2008
6. National Council of State Boards of Nursing. (NCSNB). *NCLEX-RN test plan, effective April 2007.* 2006. www.ncsbn.org. Accessed January 16, 2008.
7. Oncology Nursing Certification Corporation. (ONCC). *ONCC and certification information.* 2007. www.ons.org. Accessed January 20, 2008.
8. Institute of Medicine (IOM). *Cancer care for the whole patient: Meeting psychosocial health needs.* Adler NE, Page AE, (eds). Washington, DC: The National Academies Press; 2008.
9. Fulcher CD, Gosselin-Acomb TK. Distress management: practice change through guideline implementation. *Clin J Oncol.* 2007;11(6):817–821.
10. Fieler V, Henry B. *How to give psychological support to patients with cancer.* 2003. Nursing Spectrum CE295. http://www.nurse.com/ce/print.html?CCID=3309. Accessed February, 2008.
11. Aiken LH, Havens D, Sloan D. Magnet nursing services recognition programme. *Nurs Standard.* 2000;14(25):41–46.
12. Oncology Nursing Society. (ONS). ONS homepage plus resources. www.ons.org. Accessed January 20, 2008.

CHAPTER 86

Principles of Communication Skills Training In Cancer Care

Richard F. Brown, Carma L. Bylund, and David W. Kissane

INTRODUCTION

Given the compelling evidence of the importance of doctor–patient communication to patient outcomes, there is a burgeoning interest in developing and evaluating effective ways of improving doctor–patient communication. Communication skills training (CST) research has shown promising results in changing doctors' communication behaviors. Successful CST in cancer has taken a learner-centered approach that is grounded in the assumptions of Adult Learning Theory.[1] Adult learners need to know why they should learn something, prefer to learn the practical as well as the theoretical and are motivated to learn in participatory and active settings. They prefer to take responsibility for their decisions and want to be trusted as capable of self-direction.

In this chapter, we outline evidence for the efficacy of CST in cancer care, provide a core curriculum for CST in oncology, and discuss principles in achieving competence in facilitators. We also consider a range of developmental research agendas, the use of decision aides, and question prompt sheets and finally review training that improves patient communication in the clinical encounter.

A MODEL FOR CST

Several models of physician–patient communication that have served as conceptual frameworks for CST and assessment have been published in the past several years. Our review of these models and the CST literature highlights the need for a model that (1) addressed communication challenges in illness settings that involved continuous and ongoing care; (2) made the skills necessary to meet these challenges explicit and unambiguous; and (3) provided a direct linkage between teaching curriculum and assessment.[2] The Comskil conceptual model addresses these needs by explicitly defining the important components of a consultation.[3]

We propose that communication can be guided by an overarching goal, which is achieved through the use of guidelines or a set of strategies laid out in a clinically relevant sequence. Strategies are achieved through the use of communication skills, defined as a discrete mode by which a physician can further the clinical dialogue. Process tasks, which are sets of dialogues or nonverbal behaviors that create an environment for effective communication, are also critical to achieving strategies. The clinician appraises constantly any cues offered by the patient for information or support, as well as being sensitive to any barriers that impede open communication. Clearly, our definitions of communication goals, strategies, skills, process tasks, and cognitive appraisals are related to one another, as illustrated in the following figure. (See Fig. 86–1)

EFFICACY OF CST

Cegala and Broz[4] reviewed 26 CST projects between 1990 and 2001 and helpfully described methodological challenges. Firstly, they saw little consistency in the use of an overarching theoretical framework to guide CST and encouraged incorporation of the literature on patient–provider communication, communication theory, and educational psychology. Second, they urged the development of more guidance about the optimal timing and sequencing of strategies in the clinical encounter. This concept of time is crucial to the interactive and transactional notion of exchange of both information and meaning. Third, they placed great emphasis on assessment instruments or coding schemas that actually matched the communication skills being taught.

In contrast to the early 1990s, outcomes from training late in the decade revealed improvements in skill counts. These new findings led to the development and validation of coding schemas. Distinctive models of CST emerged in the United Kingdom. Maguire initially recognized several barriers to effective communication and developed a model of recognition and practice through videotaped role play that developed strategies to counter avoidant, blocking behaviors, and fostered a more empathic and patient-oriented approach.[5] Fallowfield preferred to ask clinicians what they found most difficult and then worked with them to resolve at least one of these issues through role play with patient simulators, video review, and group discussion.[6] A third approach by Wilkinson placed greater emphasis on developing assessment skills for nurses, including appraisal of psychological and emotional coping.[7] Each of these styles of approach has proved complementary and worthy of integration into more comprehensive models of CST.

Fallowfield, Lipkin, and Hall compared 1.5 and 3-day training programs in a noncontrolled study of 178 oncologists in the United Kingdom and found a dose effect in self-evaluated improvement in skills.[8] In a further randomized controlled trial of 160 oncologists given a 3-day course of CST, use of open-ended questions and empathic expressions increased significantly.[9] At 12-month follow-up, an enduring effect from asking open-ended questions and making greater use of summaries contrasted with a decline in the use of empathy.[10]

Razavi's group in Belgium has done the most to examine the dose-of-training time needed to sustain improvements in communication skills.[11] Both in training physicians and nurses[12] Razavi and colleagues have shown that consolidation sessions in which learners return for further training after their initial training, significantly increase the retention of skills. Following a basic 2-day program of CST and using a wait-listed design, Razavi exposed subjects to a further 18 hours of consolidation CST after their initial 19 hours of basic training, and found significant increases in open questions, empathic acknowledgments, reality testing utterances, and negotiated agendas.[11] Clearly a dose-of-training effect exists and the more time spent in CST, the greater the likelihood of retention of skills. Moreover, a staggered approach to learning, wherein skills are initially learnt, practiced in the real clinical world for a time, then reinforced with further role play, consolidates the gains as further modules are studied.

Brown and colleagues explored the process of consenting patients to clinical trials given the poor accrual rate seen across oncology units. After training 10 oncologists, the experiences of 90 patients enrolled in phase III trials revealed more shared decision making and greater positive attitude toward trials among patients.[13]

Overall, these studies demonstrate that skills can be taught, and that dose intensity is critical to their maintenance.

CORE CURRICULUM FOR CST IN ONCOLOGY

Communication skills training is initially taught generically in medical schools to guide the opening and closing of clinical interviews, taking a history of the present illness, past medical and social history, guiding discussion of the provisional diagnosis, ordering of investigations, and arranging potential management plans. As doctors enter residency programs, applied CST becomes more discipline specific as clinicians

Table 86–1. Breaking bad news

Strategies	Process tasks	Skills	Examples
1. Establish the consultation framework	Greet patient appropriately Make introductions Ensure patient is clothed Sit at eye-level	Declare your agenda items; Invite patient agenda items; Negotiate agenda	"Today we have the results of your pathology. Before we turn to the results, do you have any issues or concerns that you'd like to put on our agenda?"
2. Tailor the consultation to the patient's needs	Avoid interruptions Invite appropriate third party	Check patient's understanding; Check patient's preference for information	"I'd like to make sure you understand the reasons for the tests." "When I give you the results, guide me with how much information you'd like…an overview, the important facts, or as much detail as possible."
3. Provide information in a way that it will be understood and recalled	Avoid jargon Draw diagrams Write information down Address all questions	Preview information; Categorize Invite patient questions Check patient understanding Summarize	I'm afraid I've got some bad news for you." "The pathology shows that the cancer has spread into nearby lymph glands."
4. Respond empathically to emotion	Maintain eye contact Respect silence Allow time to integrate Offer tissues Provide hope and reassurance	Encourage expression of feelings Acknowledge Normalize Validate	"This is very upsetting news for you. Tears are normal. It's so disappointing, isn't it?"
5. Check readiness to discuss management options	Only proceed if ready Write information down Provide literature Provide web site addresses	Make a "take stock" statement Check patient preference—decision making Preview information	"We have good treatments for your situation. I can tell you about these when you are ready, but patients often like a little time."
6. Close the consultation	Offer to help tell others or respond to their questions Arrange next appointment	Check patient understanding Invite patient questions Summarize Review next steps	"Can you summarize for me what you've learnt so that I can see how much you've been able to take in."

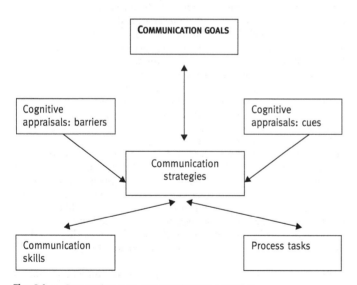

Fig. 86–1. Integrating core communication concepts.

grapple with more sophisticated issues and predicaments. In cancer care, a core curriculum covers the breaking of bad news, how to discuss prognosis, develop shared decision making, how to respond to difficult patients who are grief-stricken or existentially stressed, how to run a family meeting, transition patients to palliative care, and discuss death and dying.

Breaking bad news. Whenever there is a gap between the patient's expectations and the medical reality, the exchange of information will be experienced as "bad news." The diagnosis of cancer, its recurrence, or disease progression, the results of biopsies and multiple tests, outcomes of treatments, surveillance in survivorship, and

end-of-life care—a myriad of opportunities occur across the disease spectrum in which unwelcome news can be delivered. Patients have a right to receive as much information as they desire and its delivery needs to be tailored to suit the individual patient and their family within their own cultural milieu.[14,15] Guidelines for discussing bad news have emerged over recent decades and their common elements are presented in Table 86–1.

Discussing prognosis. Two systematic reviews of over 100 studies conclude that most patients want detailed information about their prognosis, including the extent of their disease, chance of cure, risk of recurrence, and life expectancy, as well as the potential effects of the cancer and its treatments upon their life.[16,17] A small minority prefers not to know, hence the approach to discussing prognosis must be tailored to the needs of each individual and their family. Message framing preferences also differ by individual, their education, and culture so that selection of words, numbers, graphs, bar charts, and 100-person diagrams can also be guided by the patient.[18,19] Use of median survival, interquartile range, best case scenario reflected in the 90th percentile and worse case scenario in the 10th percentile can be considered. A stepwise disclosure is often used across several consultations, with repeated checking of the patient's understanding and need for further information.[20] A guideline for discussing prognosis is presented in Table 86–2. The guideline presented here has been used as the basis of communication skills training for oncology fellows at a large Comprehensive Cancer Center in the United States. The training increased participants' confidence to discuss prognostic information with their patients.[21]

Reaching a shared treatment decision. A set of strategies for reaching shared treatment decisions is presented in Table 86–3. These strategies are based on previous worked by Brown and colleagues and were developed in the context of reaching shared treatment decisions including clinical trial participation.[22,23] These are sensitive to lifestyle and cultural aspects, with evidence of greater satisfaction when these have been recognized.[24] The recent emphasis on patient autonomy does

Table 86-2. Discussing prognosis

Strategies	Process tasks	Skills	Examples
1. Ascertain the patient's need for prognostic information	Check if the patient would like a friend or relative present	Check patient understanding and readiness; Declare your agenda items	"Are you interested in learning about what risks exist for your future?"
2. Negotiate the type and format of prognostic information	Explain limitations and benefits of prognostic formulas (i.e., average statistics) Check type of information preferred: 1. Chances of cure 2. Survival estimates Consider range of formats to present prognosis: 1. Words 2. Numbers 3. Bar charts 4. 100-person diagrams 5. Mixture	Ask open-ended questions Check patient's preference for information Express a willingness to help Invite patient questions Endorse question asking	"Tell me your preferences for the level of detail you like? Some people like statistics, others don't." "It's crucial to understand that statistics are built up around averages, and we cannot expect that you'll conform to the average." "What if we discuss your chances of a cure first and then your chances of getting a recurrence?"
3. Provide information in a manner that is sensitive to the patient's needs and promotes hopefulness	Adhere to the patient's preferences for type and format of information Be culturally sensitive Draw or use diagrams Use mixed framing of prognostic information (i.e., give the chances of cure before the chances of relapse) Avoid jargon Emphasize hope-giving aspects of the information (e.g., extraordinary survivors) Explain source of information (i.e., evidence based medicine)	Preview information Categorize as delivered Invite patient questions Check patient understanding	"In this diagram of 100 people, here is the group that we'd expect to get a recurrence without chemotherapy, and see the change in this group if chemotherapy is given." "The odds of a cure are very high for you…draw hope from this."
4. Respond empathically to emotion	Maintain eye contact Allow time to integrate Offer tissues Provide hope and reassurance Avoid premature reassurance	Encourage expression of feelings Acknowledge Normalize Validate	"Tell me if this situation is what you expected?" "I sense that you are worried by this prognosis? Tell me how you feel."
5. Respond to patient information cues	Review what has not been understood Write information down Address all questions	Clarify and Restate Summarize Invite patient questions Check patient understanding	"Can I clarify for you that it's unwise to consider the average here. Treatment regimens have improved since those statistics were compiled."

not mean that clinicians should be passive and withhold their own recommendation as to the optimal treatment choice.

Responding to difficult emotions. So-called "difficult" encounters tend to be those with intense and highly charged emotions, most easily exemplified by the angry patient,[25] but also including grief which may be difficult for caregivers to manage. A guideline to managing these encounters is offered in Table 86–4.

The goal is to understand the development of the distress, respond empathically to the emotions involved and generate support and problem solving where appropriate.[26] An apology is always helpful if a mistake has been made.

Running a family meeting. In the conduct of a family meeting, co-facilitators need to identify their own leadership roles and agendas before starting the meeting so as to have a coordinated approach to multidisciplinary needs. A typical sequence of strategies, tasks, skills, and exemplary comments are laid out in Table 86–5 and have been published elsewhere.[27]

Here, circular questions involve asking family members for their opinion as to how others in the family are coping, taking turns to collect viewpoints from all present.[28] Reflexive questions explore potential hypotheses and invite family reflection, while strategic questions pose potential solutions, including hypothetically directed, future-oriented questions that may include the possibility of death for the ill family

member.[29] Any family-centered model of care should identify families at risk and in need of continuing care through ongoing therapy.

Transitioning to palliative care and end of life. Understanding each patient's concerns, goals, and values engenders sensitivity when the clinician seeks to transition a patient toward the palliative approach.[30] Bringing the patient's views into consensus building about the goals of care ensures a patient-centered approach.[20,31] Strategies are laid out in Table 86–6, and involve permission being obtained to move toward a discussion of death and dying.[32]

FACILITATOR TRAINING PRINCIPLES

A competent facilitator provides the foundation for successful communication training. The facilitator's goal is to achieve a consistent and reliable experience for learners across role play groups. Role play has been found to be an efficient way of promoting learning at both intellectual and emotional levels, yet the personal style that each facilitator will bring into the process should not alter the basic guidelines for facilitation. The aim is to create a learner-centered experience and this is achieved by prioritizing the learner's agendas and needs.

The basic teaching tasks that facilitators use during group sessions fall into the following categories: (1) start with orientation, creating safety; (2) structure the group's learning with individuals nominating learning goals; (3) run the role play; (4) facilitate the feedback process balancing

Table 86–3. Shared decision making

Strategies	Process tasks	Skills	Examples
1. Establish the consultation framework	Greet patient appropriately; Make introductions of third parties; Ensure patient is clothed; Sit at eye-level	Declare your agenda items; Invite patient's agenda items; Negotiate agenda	"Today we need to develop a treatment plan together." "What issues concern you and should be put on the agenda?"
2. Establish the physician–patient team	Introduce the approach to shared decision making, offering choices to the patient and the goal of reaching a mutual understanding of the choice	Check patient preferences for information and decision-making style; Endorse question asking; Make partnership statements	"Some people like to make the treatment decision on their own, others want to involve their family and doctor. What is your preference?"
3. Develop an accurate, shared understanding of the patient's situation	Begin with patient's understanding of the disease, its prognosis, and any psychosocial needs; Include any third party's understanding when others are present; Correct misunderstandings.	Check patient understanding; Clarify; Invite patient concerns.	"Let's review your understanding of this illness and how it might be treated?"
4. Present established treatment options.	Categorize into chunks; Present treatment benefits, side effects, strength of evidence for each treatment; Avoid jargon; Draw diagrams.	Preview the information; Summarize the information; Check patient understanding; Endorse question asking;	"There are three treatment options you need to consider…surgery, radiation or watchful waiting."
5. Discuss patient's values and lifestyle factors that may impact on the standard treatment decision	Consider the impact of treatment on employment, lifestyle and relationships; Explore patient views and feelings about treatment options; Reinforce value of joint decision making; Avoid interruptions or blocking	Ask open-ended questions; Clarify; Empathically acknowledge, validate, or normalize emotional responses; Make partnership statements	"In considering potential side-effects, it can be helpful to work out which might trouble you the most: incontinence, sexual dysfunction, or rectal bleeding?"
6. Present a clear statement of the recommended treatment option and invite patient choice	It is generally helpful for the clinician to state their treatment recommendation clearly; Work toward consensus and confidence with the treatment choice	Summarize; Ask open-ended questions; Offer decision delay	"While you consider your preferences, I want to make clear my recommendation to you and why I think this would suit you the best."
7. Close the consultation	Arrange for signing of consent forms as needed; Arrange for any additional consultations or referrals; Create plan for next steps	Affirm value of the discussion; Bid goodbye	"Remember that you can take some time to make this decision. Please call me if you have further questions." "Let's arrange for…"

Table 86–4. Responding to difficult emotions

Strategies	Process tasks	Skills	Examples
1. Allow the patient to recount concerns or grievances	Do not act defensively; Avoid interruptions (unless essential for control)	Ask open-ended questions Listen	"Tell me what you thought went wrong, and the events leading up to this."
2. Work toward a shared understanding of the patient's emotional experience	Negotiate the emotion's name proportional to its intensity; Avoid leading questions; Avoid giving premature reassurance	Ask open-ended questions Clarify Restate	"What do you think caused the problem?" "Are you suffering? Can you help me understand what you are feeling and what is making you suffer?"
3. Empathically respond to the emotion/experience	Apologize if appropriate Express understanding	Acknowledge Validate Normalize Praise patient efforts	"I sense this upset you terribly and made you feel quite angry."
4. Explore attitudes and expectations leading to the difficult emotion such as anger	Examine factors contributing to the emotion Direct anger constructively	Ask open-ended questions Restate Clarify Acknowledge	"Have there been prior occasions that have upset you similarly?" "When patients have an appointment, they don't expect to be kept waiting like you were."
5. Facilitate coping and connect to social support	Make referrals; If appropriate, explore problem solving options; Explore patients' networks; Avoid anger causing isolation	Make partnership statements Express a willingness to help	"Let's work together to sort this out with the treatment team." "Let me involve our social worker to see what we can do to help you further."

Table 86–5. Conducting a family meeting

Strategies	Process tasks	Skills	Examples
1. Planning and prior set-up to arrange the family meeting	Consider who should attend and extend invitations; Will the patient be included? Who will co-facilitate? Plan seating, privacy, availability of tissues	Clarify	"I want to invite you to a family meeting to discuss the care of your relative."
2. Welcome and orient the family to the goals of the family meeting	Round of introductions and orientation Include all present at the meeting Normalize anxiety	Declare agenda items and invite family agenda items Negotiate agenda Ask open questions Clarify	"We find it very helpful to meet together to discuss the goals of care, key issues and concerns, and see how care provision is going."
3. Check each family member's understanding of the illness and its prognosis	Clarify name of the illness Clarify seriousness Clarify reasons for admission Clarify everyone's concerns Normalize both concordance and divergence of views Respect culturally sensitive views and urges to protect	Ask open questions Check understanding Acknowledge/ Legitimize distress	"Can you tell me its name and just how serious you understand this illness to be?" "What concerns do you have about this illness?"
4. Check for consensus about the current goals of care	Compare and contrast oncological, nursing, social, psychological, and spiritual goals of care Reality test sensitively where needed Correct misunderstanding	Ask open and circular questions Clarify Summarize	"What are our goals of care in treating this illness?"
5. Identify family concerns about their management of key symptoms or care needs	Consider medication or treatment concerns? Any hygiene issues? Any concerns about walking, moving, transferring? Any concerns about nursing? Any concerns about assessing palliative care resources—extra help? Financial issues? Any need for respite? Any concern about a sense of helplessness? Promote problem solving; Educate as appropriate	Ask open-ended questions Preview information Check understanding Clarify Summarize Make partnership statements	"Are any symptoms proving difficult to control well?" "How might we help you more in your care-giving role?"
6. Clarify the family's view of what the future holds	Are there advanced care directives? Health proxy appointed? Has the place of death been discussed? Consider cultural or religious concerns If at home, who from the family will be providing care? If in the hospital, who will accompany? Help? Support? Educate as appropriate	Ask circular questions Clarify Restate Summarize Make partnership statements	"Can I ask if your affairs are in order?" "Have you appointed a health proxy and an advance directive?" "Who does mum talk to about this illness?" "Who does dad talk to about this illness?"
7. Clarify how family members are coping and feeling emotionally	Review family functioning as a group, asking specifically about their communication, cohesion, and conflict resolution Identify any member considered to be "at risk" or a concern to others Discuss future care needs of family or individuals when concerns exist Avoid premature reassurance	Ask circular questions Acknowledge, legitimize, or normalize any distress as appropriate	"Whom, if anyone, do each of you hold concerns about?" "How effective is your teamwork?" "Do disagreements present any problems?" "What prevents you as a family talking more freely about this illness?"
8. Identify family strengths and affirm their level of commitment and mutual support for each other	Review family traditions, spirituality, accomplishments, mottos, cultural norms	Ask strategic and reflexive questions Praise family efforts Acknowledge, legitimize	"Where do you draw resilience from?" "What traditions guide your decisions?" "Which cultural norms matter to your family?"
9. Close the family meeting by final review of agreed goals of care and future plans	Provide educational resources. Clarify future needs Refer those "at risk" to psychosocial services for further care Consider feedback to patient, if not present	Summarize Make partnership statements Express willingness to help Review next steps	"Let us review the goals of care and family concerns that we've discussed during this meeting." "Going forward, the next steps are…."

Table 86–6. Discussing palliative care and the process of dying

Strategies	Process tasks	Skills	Examples
1. Recognize patient's cue or emergent clinical reality	Ensure setting appropriate for this discussion Consider goals of care	Declare your agenda Invite patient's agenda Negotiate agenda	"The goal of this treatment is to help make you feel better. We will monitor the benefits and side effects of the treatment and talk about the options if the treatment is not helping you."
2. Establish understanding of disease progression, treatment efficacy, and prognosis	Deepen understanding of predicament Correct any misunderstandings Sustain supportive environment and tailor amount of information to patient's need Acknowledge reality	Check patient understanding Invite patient questions Make partnership statements	"Let me check your understanding of where this disease is at?"
3. Discuss patient's values and lifestyle factors that may impact on goals of care; Negotiate appropriate and if need be new goals of care	Introduce palliative approach: a) Contrast cure with care b) Emphasize living in the present c) Emphasize "always something to do to help" d) Commit to continuity of care Establish quality of life goals of importance Acknowledge (anticancer and palliative treatments can be given simultaneously)	Endorse questions Reinforce joint decision making Summarize goals of care Check patient understanding	"I wish that more chemotherapy would help this cancer, but unfortunately at this stage it will only make you sicker. Yet there are many other things we can do to help you deal with your condition." "We want to maintain your quality of life through excellent symptom control."
4. Respond empathetically to emotion	Recognize grief Promote hope Emphasize the living over the dying	Encourage expression of emotions Acknowledge Validate Normalize	"Its' always distressing when you realize this cancer has progressed some more. But we're not giving up on you."
5. Negotiate the shift to discuss the process of dying	Ask permission Describe relevant elements of good symptom control Provide tailored information	Make a "take stock" statement Check patient understanding Check patient's preference for information	"Some people find it helpful to talk through what may lie ahead. Would you like me to do this with you?"
6. Promote understanding of change—illness transitions—and role of courage in accepting one's dying	Explore patient's coping with illness Consider patient's response to family Address specific cultural, spiritual or religious needs Respect any need to "not know" Affirm courage if evident	Validate Summarize Praise patient efforts Express a willingness to help	"What helps you cope with this illness?" "From where do you draw your strength?"
7. Address caregiver's concerns	Examine instrumental care needs Identify value of respite from care position Consider role of community volunteers, health aides	Ask open questions Endorse question asking Make partnership statements	"Families often have questions about how they can help?"
8. Effect referral to palliative care service whenever appropriate	Provide contact details and appointments Write referral letter summarizing goals of care and any needs for parallel, shared care	Make a "take stock" statement Praise patient efforts Express a willingness to help	"We use a lot of parallel care, wherein I'll continue your chemotherapy while one of my colleagues will focus on your pain and symptom control. I'd like to introduce you to one of our palliative care physicians. Is this OK to do?"
9. Close consultation	Remind of availability and commitment to care Affirm progress and focus on continued living Document discussion and inform team members	Summarize Check patient understanding Endorse question asking Review next steps	"Let me summarize before we close. Our goals of care are to . . . . . . We're there to help you as you journey forward. Please don't hesitate to call if you have fresh concerns ahead of our next appointment."

affirmation of strengths with constructive ideas for improvement; (5) rerun the role play to compare varied approaches and use of new skills; and (6) close the session.[33–37] These tasks were developed for use in small-group role play sessions with professional actors,[36] but the principles can be applied to other types of role play sessions as well.

DEVELOPMENTAL AGENDAS IN CST

The future of communication skill training includes the development of many modules focused on optimal framing and communication approaches to specific clinical issues. Examples of these include the discussion of unanticipated adverse events, promotion of treatment adherence, preparation for survivorship, working with interpreters and culturally specific health beliefs, discussing complementary and unproven therapies, and how to respond to queries based on internet information. Research into the incorporation of interactive, web-based decision aides to promote understanding about complex surgical treatments is rapidly enriching the information provided to patients.

DECISION AIDES AND QUESTION PROMPT SHEETS

Decision aides. Decision aides have been developed to help patients make sense of complex information and arrive at a shared decision by clarification of patients' values and treatment preferences. Patients need to understand all treatment options, including respective benefits and limitations. Typical information includes information on the disease/ condition; probabilities of outcomes tailored to personal health risk factors; an explicit values clarification exercise; information on others' opinions; a personalized recommendation on the basis of clinical characteristics and expressed preferences; and guidance or coaching in the steps of decision making and in communicating with others.[38] One illustration is a clinical trial specific decision aide to help patients with trial enrollment.[39]

Question prompt lists. Active patient participation is in part characterized by patients' information seeking behavior. Encouraging patients' questions has been proposed as a means of giving them better control over information flow. Patients who actively participate in consultations by asking questions of the doctor are able to change the focus of the consultation and control the duration and amount of information provided. One method that has demonstrated significant promise in promoting cancer patient participation during their general, surgical, and palliative oncology consultations are Question Prompt Lists (QPLs). QPLs consist of a list of sample written questions separated into content categories, for example, diagnosis and prognosis. Seminal studies by Roter, Butow, and Brown demonstrate the efficacy of QPLs in increasing question asking by patients.

To counter limitations of these studies, (such as limited generalizability and small sample sizes) a randomized trial by Brown et al. evaluated the utility of a QPL, that was actively endorsed by the oncologist, in promoting patient question asking and improving patient outcomes.[40] Patients randomized to receive the QPL asked more questions about prognosis. Additionally, when the value of the QPL was endorsed, patients had less anxiety, better recall, and shorter consultations than other patients. Question topics will undoubtedly vary across oncology contexts. Because of this, researchers developed QPLs with different question sets for the palliative and surgical oncology contexts. The results of pilot testing of these context-specific QPLs have shown them to be acceptable, understandable, and valued by patients. Hence, further rigorous formative research is necessary to develop context-specific QPLs. There is a mounting body of evidence about the communication challenges present in doctor–patient consultations about clinical trials. Brown et al. are developing a QPL that targets patient information needs in this specific context. The goal of this research program is to improve the subsequent quality of informed consent.

Communication and the internet. Between 31% and 60% of patients or caregivers report having used the internet to search for information about cancer.[41–44] The internet has significantly transformed the way patients meet their health-related information needs as it provides patients ready access to information that was previously difficult to obtain. This has also had a leveling effect on the power imbalance in the doctor–patient relationship, specifically in terms of expert power.[45,46]

Alongside this, 44% of oncologists have difficulty handling discussions about internet information.[47] Challenges arise when patients dispute medical information or become confused by too much or conflicting information.[48] Lack of concordance about internet information can prolong consultations and result in conflict.[47,48] Oncologists express concern with the accuracy of cancer-related internet information, with 91% of oncologists in one study suggesting that the internet can harm patients.[48,49]

To help manage these difficult conversations, Bylund and Gueguen[50] suggest six strategies for clinicians: (1) explore the patient's experience with internet information; (2) respond empathically to the patient's experience; (3) acknowledge the patient's efforts; (4) correct any misunderstandings; (5) provide guidance; and (6) reinforce clinician–patient partnership.

Patient Communication Training. Improving clinicians' communication is necessary, but not sufficient to achieve the best possible communication in a clinical encounter. The physician-patient interaction is a dynamic, socially constructed, and reciprocal process[51,52] that relies on at least two participants. Both doctor and patient need to be actively involved and competent communicators. Moreover, patients' communication may, in fact should, influence physicians' responses.[53] Patients face many challenges in clinical consultations, including physicians' ethnic or cultural biases,[52] interruptions,[54] lack of empathic communication,[55] minimal tolerance for patients' desires to talk about internet information,[52] and a lack of physician–patient concordance.[51,56]

The limited literature on comprehensive patient communication training interventions is encouraging about improving patients' active participation and adherence to medical treatments.[57–59] But additional studies are necessary to build a solid evidence base for their effectiveness. Bylund and colleagues propose the following goals for future research: (1) determining the most effective methods of patient communication training, (2) identifying which populations can benefit most from training, and (3) exploring the synergistic nature of physician and patient CST.[60]

CONCLUSION

Effective and compassionate communication is a core component of a medicine that heals illness rather than solely treating disease. CST enhances patient satisfaction, reduces worry, improves understanding, promotes treatment adherence, and reduces litigation. Use of question prompt sheets and decision aides will continue to develop as research explores optimal ways to frame message delivery. Psycho-oncology as a discipline helps the whole treatment team by actively teaching communication skills to healthcare professionals and patients, thus enriching the quality of the care we all deliver as healers.

REFERENCES

1. Knowles MS. *The Adult Learner: A neglected species.* Gulf, Texas: Houston; 1978.

2. Brown RF, Bylund C. Theoretical Models. In: Kissane DW, Bultz B, Butow P (eds). *Handbook of communication in cancer and palliative care.* Oxford: Oxford University Press; 2009.

3. Brown RF, Bylund CL. Communication Skills Training: describing a new conceptual model. *Acad Med.* 2008;83(1):37–44.

4. Cegala DJ, Lenzmeier Broz S. Physician communication skills training: a review of theoretical backgrounds, objectives and skills. *Med Educ.* 2002;36(11):1004–1016.

5. Maguire P, Faulkner A. How to do it: Communicate with cancer patients: Handling bad news and difficult questions. *BMJ.* 1988;297(6653):907–909.

6. Fallowfield L, Jenkins V. Current concepts of communication skills training in oncology. *Recent Results Cancer Res.* 2006;168:105–112.

7. Wilkinson SM, Leliopoulou C, Gambles M, Roberts A. Can intensive three-day programmes improve nurses' communication skills in cancer care? *Psychooncology.* 2003;12(8):747–759.

8. Fallowfield L, Lipkin M, Hall A. Teaching senior oncologists communication skills: results from phase I of a comprehensive longitudinal program in the United Kingdom. *J Clin Oncol.* 1998;16(5):1961–1968.

9. Fallowfield L, Jenkins V, Farewell V, Saul J, Duffy A, Eves R. Efficacy of a Cancer Research UK communication skills training model for oncologists: a randomised controlled trial. *Lancet.* 2002;359(9307):650–656.

10. Fallowfield L, Jenkins V, Farewell V, Solis-Trapala I. Enduring impact of communication skills training: results of a 12-month follow-up. *Br J Cancer.* 2003;89(8):1445–1449.

11. Razavi D, Merckaert I, Marchal S, et al. How to optimize physicians' communication skills in cancer care: results of a randomized study assessing the usefulness of posttraining consolidation workshops. *J Clin Oncol.* 2003;21(16):3141–3149.

12. Razavi D, Delvaux N, Marchal S, et al. Does training increase the use of more emotionally laden words by nurses when talking with cancer patients? A randomised study. *Br J Cancer*. 2002;87(1):1–7.

13. Brown RF, Butow PN, Boyle F, Tattersall MH. Seeking informed consent to cancer clinical trials; evaluating the efficacy of doctor communication skills training. *Psychooncology*. 2007;16(6):507–516.

14. Parker PA, Baile WF, de Moor C, Lenzi R, Kudelka AP, Cohen L. Breaking bad news about cancer: patients' preferences for communication. *J Clin Oncol*. 2001;19(7):2049–2056.

15. Mystakidou K, Parpa E, Tsilila E, Katsouda E, Vlahos L. Cancer information disclosure in different cultural contexts. *Support Care Cancer*. 2004;12(3): 147–154.

16. Hagerty RG, Butow PN, Ellis PM, Dimitry S, Tattersall MH. Communicating prognosis in cancer care: a systematic review of the literature. *Ann Oncol*. 2005; 16(7):1005–1053.

17. Hancock K, Clayton JM, Parker SM, et al. Discrepant perceptions about end-of-life communication: a systematic review. *J Pain Symptom Manage*. 2007;34(2):190–200.

18. Clayton JM, Butow PN, Arnold RM, Tattersall MH. Fostering coping and nurturing hope when discussing the future with terminally ill cancer patients and their caregivers. *Cancer*. 2005;103(9):1965–1975.

19. Hagerty RG, Butow PN, Ellis PM, et al. Communicating with realism and hope: incurable cancer patients' views on the disclosure of prognosis. *J Clin Oncol*. 2005;23(6):1278–1288.

20. Clayton JM, Hancock KM, Butow PN, et al. Clinical practice guidelines for communicating prognosis and end-of-life issues with adults in the advanced stages of a life-limiting illness, and their caregivers. *Med J Aust*. 2007; 186(Suppl 12):S77, S9, S83-S108.

21. Brown R, Brown R, Bylund CL, Eddington J, Gueguen JA, Kissane DW. Discussing prognosis in an oncology setting: Initial evaluation of a communication skills training module. *Psycho-oncology*. 2009;PMID:19441006.

22. Brown RF, Butow PN, Butt DG, Moore AR, Tattersall MHN. Developing ethical strategies to assist oncologists in seeking informed consent to cancer clinical trials. *Soc Sci Med*. 2004;58:379–390.

23. Brown RF, Butow PN, Ellis P, Boyle F, Tattersall MH. Seeking informed consent to cancer clinical trials: Describing current practice. *Soc Sci Med*. 2004;58(12):2445–2457.

24. Charles C, Gafni A, Whelan T, O'Brien MA. Cultural influences on the physician-patient encounter: The case of shared treatment decision-making. *Patient Educ Couns*. 2006;63(3):262–267.

25. Hahn SR, Kroenke K, Spitzer RL, et al. The difficult patient: prevalence, psychopathology, and functional impairment. *J Gen Intern Med*. 1996; 11(1):1–8.

26. Philip J, Gold M, Schwarz M, Komesaroff P. Anger in palliative care: a clinical approach. *Intern Med J*. 2007;37(1):49–55.

27. Gueguen JA, Bylund CL, Brown RF, Levin TT, Kissane DW. Conducting Family Meeting in Palliative Care: Themes, Techniques and Preliminary Evaluation of a Communications Skills Module. *Palliat Support Care*. 2008;7(2): 171–179.

28. Dumont I, Kissane D. Techniques for framing questions in conducting family meetings in palliative care. *Palliat Support Care*. In press.

29. Kissane D, Gueguen J, Bylund C, Brown R, Levin T. Conducting family meetings in palliative care: themes, techniques and preliminary evaluation of a communication skills module. *Palliat Support Care*. In press.

30. Steinhauser KE, Christakis NA, Clipp EC, McNeilly M, McIntyre L, Tulsky JA. Factors considered important at the end of life by patients, family, physicians, and other care providers. *JAMA*. 2000;284(19):2476–2482.

31. Schofield P, Carey M, Love A, Nehill C, Wein S. 'Would you like to talk about your future treatment options'? Discussing the transition from curative cancer treatment to palliative care. *Palliat Med*. 2006;20(4):397–406.

32. Parker SM, Clayton JM, Hancock K, et al. A systematic review of prognostic/end-of-life communication with adults in the advanced stages of a life-limiting illness: patient/caregiver preferences for the content, style, and timing of information. *J Pain Symptom Manage*. 2007;34(1):81–93.

33. Baile WF, Kudelka AP, Beale EA, et al. Communication skills training in oncology. Description and preliminary outcomes of workshops on breaking bad news and managing patient reactions to illness. *Cancer*. 1999;86(5): 887–897.

34. Bylund CL, Brown RF, di Ciccone BL, et al. Training faculty to facilitate communication skills training: development and evaluation of a workshop. *Patient Educ Couns*. 2008;70(3):430–436.

35. Fryer-Edwards KA, Arnold RM, Baile WF, Tulsky JA, Petracca F, Back AL. Reflective teaching practices: An approach to teaching communication skills in a small-group setting. *Acad Med*. 2006;81(7):638–644.

36. Bylund CL, Brown RF, Lubrano di Ciccone B, Diamond C, Eddington J, Kissane DW. Assessing facilitator competence in a comprehensive communication skills training programme. *Med Edu*. 2009;43:342–349.

37. Kurtz S, Silverman J, Draper J. *Teaching and learning communication skills in medicine*. Radcliffe, Abingdon: Medical Press Ltd; 1998.

38. O'Connor AM, Stacey D, Entwistle V, et al. Decision aids for people facing health treatment or screening decisions. *Cochrane Database Syst Rev*. 2003;(2):CD001431.

39. Juraskova I, Butow P, Lopez A, et al. Improving informed consent: pilot of a decision aid for women invited to participate in a breast cancer prevention trial (IBIS -II DCIS). *Health Expect*. 2008;11(3):252–262.

40. Brown RF, Butow PN, Butt DG, Moore AR, Tattersall MHN. Developing ethical strategies to assist oncologists in seeking informed consent to cancer clinical trials. *Soc Sci Med*. 2004;58:379–390.

41. Basch EM, Thaler HT, Shi W, Yakren S, Schrag D. Use of information resources by patients with cancer and their companions. *Cancer*. 2004;100(11); 2476–2483.

42. Metz J, Devine P, DeNittis A, et al. A multi-institutional study of internet utilization by radiation oncology patients. *Int J Radiat Oncol Biol Phys*. 2003;56(4):1201–1205.

45. Monnier J, Laken M, Carter CL. Patient and caregiver interest in internet-based cancer services. *Cancer Pract*. 2002;10(6);305–310.

44. Ranson S, Morrow GR, Dakhil S, et al. *Internet use among 1020 cancer patients assessed in community practice: A URCC CCOP study*. Proc Annu Meet Am Assoc Cancer Res. 2003;22:534.

45. Makoul G. Perpetuating passivity: reliance and reciprocal determinism in physician-patient interaction. *J Health Commun*. 1998;3(3):233–259.

46. Bylund CL, Sabee CM, Imes RS, Sanford AA. Exploration of the construct of reliance among patients who talk with their providers about internet information. *J Health Commun*. 2007;12(1):17–28.

47. Helft PR, Hlubocky F, Daugherty CK. American oncologists' views of Internet use by cancer patients: a mail survey of American Society of Clinical Oncology members. *J Clin Oncol*. 2003;21(5);942–947.

48. Broom A. Medical specialists' accounts of the impact of the internet on the doctor/patient relationship. *Health*. 2005;9(3):319–338.

49. Newnham G, Burns W, Snyder R, et al. Attitudes of oncology health professionals to information from the Internet and other media. *Med J Aust*. 2005;183(4):197–200.

50. Bylund CL, Gueguen J. The effect of internet use on the doctor-cancer patient relationship. In: Kissane D, Butow P, Bultz B, (eds). *Handbook of communication in cancer and palliative care*. Oxford: Oxford University Press; in press.

51. Parker PA, Davison BJ, Tishelman C, Brundage MD. What do we know about facilitating patient communication in the cancer care setting? *Psychooncology*. 2005;14(10):848–858.

52. Street R. Communication in medical encounters: an ecological perspective. In: Thompson T, Dorsey AM, Miller KI, Parrott R, (eds). *Handbook of health communication*. Mahwah, NJ: Lawrence Erlbaum Associates; 2003.

53. Roter DL, Stewart M, Putnam SM, Lipkin MJ, Stiles W, Inui TS. Communication patterns of primary care physicians. *JAMA*. 1997;277(4):350–356.

54. Marvel MK, Epstein RM, Flowers K, Beckman HB. Soliciting the patient's agenda: Have we improved? *JAMA*. 1999;281(3):283–287.

55. Bylund CL, Makoul G. Examining empathy in medical encounters: an observational study using the empathic communication coding system. *Health Commun*. 2005;18(2):123–140.

56. Chewning B, Wiederholt JB. Concordance in cancer medication management. *Patient Educ Couns*. 2003;50(1):75–78.

57. Cegala DJ. Communication skills training for patients: Implications for research into message production in primary care settings. San Francisco: ICA; 1999.

58. Cegala DJ, Marinelli T, Post D. The effects of patient communication skills training on compliance. *Arch Fam Med*. 2000;9(1):57–64.

59. Cegala DJ, McClure L, Marinelli TM, Post DM. The effects of communication skills training on patients' participation during medical interviews. *Patient Educ Couns*. 2000;41(2):209–222.

60. Bylund C, D'Agostino T, Chewning B. Training patients to reach their communication goals: a concordance perspective. In: Kissane D, Bultz B, Butow P, Finlay I, (eds). *Handbook of communication in oncology and palliative care*. Oxford: Oxford University Press; 2009.

CHAPTER 87

Education of Chaplains in Psycho-Oncology

George Fitchett, Stephen D. W. King, and Anne Vandenhoeck

INTRODUCTION

Ministering to the needs of the sick has been a central role of clergy of different faiths for centuries. In the United States, modern healthcare chaplaincy began in 1924 with the appointment of clergyman Anton Boisen as chaplain at a psychiatric hospital in central Massachusetts.[1] The next summer Boisen led a training program for four theological students. In 1930 an organization was formed to promote programs, such as Boisen's, to give theological students experience in supervised care for people in crisis.[2] These training programs came to be called clinical pastoral education (CPE).

In 1939, Russell Dicks, an early hospital chaplain and CPE supervisor, made a presentation on the work of chaplains to the annual meeting of the American Protestant Hospital Association (APHA).[3,4] Dicks' speech moved the APHA to appoint a committee to formulate standards for hospital chaplaincy. The new standards, which the APHA adopted the following year, addressed issues of chaplains' accountability, interdisciplinary collaboration, selection of patients, record keeping, and training. At the APHA meeting in 1946 a group of chaplains active in APHA hospitals formed the Association of Protestant Hospital Chaplains, one of the first organizations of professional healthcare chaplains in the United States.[4,5]

In the rest of this chapter we provide an introduction to healthcare chaplaincy. We begin with a general overview of who healthcare chaplains are, their training, where they work, and what they do. Then we describe healthcare chaplains' work caring for patients with cancer, including their work in hospice and palliative care. These descriptions are largely based on the U.S. context. However, in the following section we describe the training and work of healthcare chaplains in Europe. In the final section we briefly describe future directions for healthcare chaplaincy. A good introduction to professional healthcare chaplaincy can also be found in VandeCreek and Burton.[6]

Before proceeding we need to briefly define two key terms, spirituality and religion. Spirituality is about the ultimate sources of meaning in our lives and our connection with a transcendent dimension of existence. Religion refers to institutions in our culture that play an important role in the development of spirituality for many, but not all, people. For more about these terms see Chapter 59 in this volume and Miller and Thoresen.[7] Because chaplains deal with both religion and spirituality, in this chapter we refer to religion/spirituality (R/S).

WHO ARE PROFESSIONAL HEALTHCARE CHAPLAINS?

The term chaplain is often used in a broad sense to refer to any clergy, or other spiritual counselors, who work in institutional contexts such as hospitals. In the United States, the Joint Commission specifies that patients have a right to care that respects their "spiritual values," and requires a minimal spiritual assessment.[8] Regarding standards for hospital chaplains, Joint Commission guidelines simply state that "clinical chaplains," like other staff should be "qualified...by virtue of...education, training, experience, competence, registration, certification, or applicable licensure, law or regulation."[9] In the absence of more explicit external standards from organizations such as the Joint Commission, hospitals and other healthcare institutions are free to set their own requirements for the chaplains that work there. Consequently, in contrast to other professionals such as physicians or nurses, there can be considerable diversity in the basic training and qualifications of people who are called chaplains.

Some people who are called chaplains are congregational clergy who spend some or all of their time working in the context of a hospital, nursing home or hospice. Often their ministry focuses on people from their own religious tradition. Other people who are called chaplains are clergy who have had additional specialized training in healthcare ministry (e.g., CPE). In recent years the term Board Certified Chaplain (BCC) has emerged to indicate a person who in addition to this specialized training has demonstrated competence in healthcare ministry before a review board.

In North America, six major professional organizations are concerned with specialized ministries of pastoral care, pastoral counseling, and training. Recently these groups formed the Spiritual Care Collaborative (SCC) (The organizations that are part of the Spiritual Care Collaborative [SCC] include the Association of Professional Chaplains [APC], the American Association of Pastoral Counselors [AAPC], the Association for Clinical Pastoral Education, Inc. [ACPE], the National Association of Catholic Chaplains [NACC], the National Association of Jewish Chaplains [NAJC], and the Canadian Association for Pastoral Practice and Education [CAPPE]). In 2004, the groups in the SCC approved a common set of standards for professional chaplains. They also approved Common Standards for pastoral educators/supervisors, those who train healthcare chaplains, and a Common Code of Ethics.

The Common Standards for BCCs begin with endorsement and continued good standing with one's faith tradition. A second basic requirement is completion of both an undergraduate degree and a graduate-level theological degree. The third basic requirement is completion of four units of CPE accredited by one of the SCC groups.

Clinical pastoral education (CPE) is a distinctive form of preparation for professional spiritual care in that it is multifaith; CPE supervisors come from all major faith traditions, as do the students who form the training groups. CPE is also a very experiential form of education. A unit of CPE includes a total of 400 hours of work and 50%–75% of the students' time is usually spent in the supervised practice of spiritual care. In addition to their clinical practice, CPE students participate in didactic seminars and in a peer supervision group where they discuss verbatim or case reports of their clinical practice with their peers and supervisor. Four units of CPE are often completed as a spiritual care residency year. In some cases, students elect to complete a 2-year residency which permits additional training in a specialized area, such as care for patients with cancer and their families.

As noted earlier, chaplains who have faith group endorsement, a graduate theological degree, and at least four units of CPE are eligible to become BCC through one of the certifying groups in the SCC. The process of becoming a BCC includes submitting a written application that includes two reports of one's spiritual care, and an interview with a panel that includes other BCCs. Competencies that must be demonstrated in the application and interview include the ability to formulate a spiritual assessment and plan of care; the ability to provide effective spiritual support to patients and families; the ability to use appropriate religious or spiritual resources in care for patients and families; the ability to provide spiritual care in collaboration with other healthcare professionals; the ability to integrate relevant information from the behavioral sciences into spiritual care; and the ability to reflect on the ethical and theological issues involved in spiritual care.

A key ethical principle, to which BCCs must adhere is to "Demonstrate respect for the cultural and religious values of those they serve and refrain from imposing their own values and beliefs on those served" (Common Ethical Code, Principle 1.3). Casual observers may not be aware of how central this principle of respect for the religious values of others, and prohibition of any attempts to proselytize others, is for modern professional healthcare chaplaincy. Other core ethical principles include promoting the best interests of those served, safeguarding the confidentiality of those served, understanding the limits of one's expertise, and making referrals when appropriate. Part of what is unique about BCCs is the multiple ways in which they are accountable for their work. This begins with accountability to one's faith group which must be documented at the time of certification and every 5 years thereafter. It includes accountability to one's employer. Finally, BCCs must complete 50 hours of annual continuing education and a peer review every 5 years. In the next section we describe what professional healthcare chaplains do.

PROFESSIONAL HEALTHCARE CHAPLAINS—WHAT DO THEY DO?

Healthcare chaplains work in a variety of settings including hospitals, nursing homes, outpatient clinics, hospices, and free standing specialized healthcare settings (e.g., cancer, pediatrics). In most cases these organizations directly employ chaplains. In some cases chaplains work for their own faith group but have hospital privileges to minister to persons from their faith traditions. Infrequently chaplains are volunteers.

Chaplains provide direct R/S care and contribute to the ethos of care in healthcare organizations. Ideally, all healthcare providers provide some R/S care, perhaps by being open to the patient's R/S concerns and inquiring about them in an open, respectful manner. But chaplains usually have greater training and education in R/S care, focus more of their time providing R/S care, and address the more complex depths of a patient's/family member's R/S concerns.[10,11]

Much of a chaplain's work is at the bedside. Establishing a caring relationship with patients/families is primary. For many patients/families, a chaplain may offer empathic listening and faithful presence. Chaplains may represent a caring community or transcendence beyond the identity of the chaplain. Chaplains perform or help establish protocols for R/S screening so that they can better prioritize their ministries. This is important because few healthcare organizations have enough chaplains to see every patient. Chaplains perform R/S assessments that provide insight into the person of the patient, their R/S strengths and concerns, and guiding values that may inform treatment decisions. Chaplains nurture the R/S strengths of those for whom R/S is important, help patients explore R/S concerns, and provide guidance for those seeking to deepen their R/S. Chaplains assess and explore R/S distress that may be manifest or latent.[12–14] Regarding R/S assessment and R/S distress also see Chapter 59 in this book.

Chaplains provide rituals and sacraments. They help process grief regarding losses or potential losses and offer comfort, life review, and care. Chaplains also celebrate good news through words, prayers, or rituals. Chaplains help patients/families in transitions, for example when going home may be scary or when the prognosis is changing for the worse. Chaplains help facilitate communication within families and between patients/families and healthcare providers regarding fears, hopes, realistic prognosis, values, and goals.

One study indicated that chaplains may be even more important to families,[15] especially since families often receive less psychosocial support. Chaplains help patients and family members talk to one another about their common fears, their values regarding end-of-life preferences, the reality of a serious prognosis, and their lives together.[16]

Chaplains often facilitate groups. These might be on-going or term-limited support groups, R/S groups, bereavement groups, and so on. Chaplains also lead worship and meditation services, both on a regular basis and on special occasions.[16,17]

The chaplain may collaborate with representatives of local R/S communities regarding a specific patient or patient group. In some settings, there may be chaplains who primarily minister to patients from the chaplain's faith tradition. More commonly, in nonsectarian healthcare systems, chaplains function as interfaith chaplains, that is, they meet people where they are in their own R/S traditions, addressing broader spiritual issues. When more R/S specific needs are identified, the chaplain will refer to a representative from that tradition (e.g., for a Latter Day Saint blessing).

This raises the question of who really needs a chaplain. Some people are strongly connected to their home R/S community but are now far from home without that strong R/S support. Others have a strong connection with their home R/S community but their clergy may feel uncomfortable in hospital visitation or be overwhelmed with other duties. Many people are spiritual but have no faith community, no one with whom to talk about deeper spiritual issues. All of these persons may benefit from a relationship with a chaplain.

Chaplains function as part of the multidisciplinary team. Within the team, chaplains participate in dialogue about patients and their care, in patient rounds and specific care conferences, in consultation regarding a patient's R/S, and in debriefing and support within the team. Chaplains also chart in the health information/medical record, documenting R/S assessments, care plans, interventions, and outcomes.[6,18–20] But the team also serves the chaplain. Chaplains depend upon other staff for updates about a patient's status or family dynamics as well as for referrals. Enhanced R/S care depends upon staff screening for and engaging patients about R/S needs and appropriately referring to a chaplain.[12,14]

Staff care is another significant ministry for chaplains. This care ranges from informal conversations and relationship building to formal counseling around a personal or professional issue. Conversation topics might include cumulative or disenfranchised grief, the death of a particular patient, vocational discernment, values conflicts at work, work exhaustion and self-care, personal R/S journey, or family issues. Chaplains provide impromptu rituals for staff after the death of a patient, periodic memorial services for staff to remember patients who have died, or memorial services for a colleague who has died. Chaplains may provide rituals of appreciation such as hand blessings or Tea for the Soul.[21,22] Chaplains may provide situation-specific, term-limited staff support groups as well as in-services about various topics, for example, getting in touch with one's own R/S and understandings of death, finding soul at work, grief, self-care, R/S, and cultural diversity, and so on. Many believe that staff who feel appreciated and cared for, a value in its own right, tend to provide better care to their patients, take less sick leave, and stay longer in their jobs.[6,23,24]

Chaplains often contribute to a healthcare organization through participation on committees or other assigned responsibilities. These responsibilities include assisting patients/families with advance directives or in organ donation protocols, participating on ethics committees and consultation teams, providing bereavement care, building relationships with and helping educate local faith communities/clergy regarding S/R and health,[25] and educating about and navigating relationships within multicultural and R/S diversity.[6,26] Chaplains also provide another voice to uphold the ethics and conscience of the organization in the face of competing demands.

Chaplains are involved in ethics decisions formally and informally. Formally, chaplains participate on clinical ethics committees, clinical ethics consultation services, institutional review boards, and research ethics committees. Informally, one dimension of chaplaincy is helping patients/families sort through their values and their implications for healthcare decisions, for example, when to shift from aggressive treatment to comfort care.[6] These values are often rooted in their R/S or cultural tradition.

Chaplains often take the lead in providing care to bereaved families. This care can include follow-up cards or phone calls, providing information about grief and mourning, facilitating a short-term bereavement group, and/or leading memorial services to which families are invited.

CHAPLAINS AND CANCER CARE, PALLIATIVE CARE, HOSPICE

Currently there are no subspecialty certifications in chaplaincy. Either one is or one is not a BCC regardless of context or medical population served. However, some chaplains may have more specialized training in cancer care, palliative care, or hospice care than others. For example, a chaplain who completes a CPE residency in an acute care setting may complete a special project related to oncology chaplaincy. Other chaplains may complete their residency at a major cancer center, or a hospice, or pursue a second year residency/fellowship focusing on oncology, palliative care, and/or hospice.

What we have written above about who chaplains are and what they do also applies to oncology, palliative care, and hospice chaplains. But there are some differences. A diagnosis of cancer may create more fear than other diagnoses, and stimulate questions such as "Will I die from this?" or "How sick will the treatment make me?" or "Will my life ever be the same again?" Indeed, many cancer patients experience their world turned upside down without an adequate map to guide them.[27]

Chaplains in oncology, palliative care, and hospice often develop deep relationships that offer patients/families emotional support and comfort and permit in-depth exploration of important issues. These chaplains are very attentive to theological/existential themes such as hope, forgiveness, healing, finitude, and suffering, what and where is the sacred, the meaning of life, ethical wills (i.e., legacy, what one did and wants to pass on to loved ones), life review, death and how one's life does or does not continue beyond death.[17] Palliative care and hospice chaplains are typically well integrated into multidisciplinary teams, partially because it is mandated by hospice and palliative care standards.

Chaplains must be attentive to developmental issues, especially with children. Developmental stage, as well as culture, impacts personality, understandings of death, locus of safety, and specific concerns (e.g., missing the prom for an adolescent). Pediatric oncology chaplains take different approaches to their patients because of the major developmental differences in the first 18 years of life. Cancer may delay some developments and speed up others (e.g., the child who is "wise beyond her years"). As always, the chaplain must be in the moment; follow the lead of the child; be respectful, genuine, and, sometimes, playful.

With the exception of hospice chaplaincy, which is often home-based, most chaplaincies still occur in the inpatient setting. However, at a few major cancer centers chaplain departments have invested a significant portion of their staff resources to outpatient care. It is in the outpatient setting that patients often learn of a diagnosis or recurrence of disease, of change in prognosis, or of a major complication. The outpatient clinic may be the place where a patient hits the wall, emotionally and physically, after months of treatments, or comes to a place where they want to explore their R/S lives or other important concerns (e.g., relationships, stewardship of one's life, priorities).[28] Furthermore, because treatments are increasingly performed in outpatient settings and can extend over a long period of time, and because cancer in many cases has become a more chronic type of illness, when there is continuity between outpatient and inpatient settings, chaplains can develop long-term relationships that are supportive and often transformative.[29]

While chaplaincy all over the world has many characteristics in common, there are also important national differences in how chaplains are trained, hired, and integrated. We now turn to chaplaincy outside the United States. Since space does not permit us to describe chaplaincy in every part of the world we focus on healthcare chaplaincy in Europe. (For a series of articles about chaplains in countries outside of the United States see the archives of the "Advocacy" column in the chaplaincy e-newsletter, *Plain Views*' [www.plainviews.org], especially Volume 5, 2008. The website of the International Council for Pastoral Care and Counseling [ICPCC] [www.icpcc.net] also has links to chaplaincy networks around the globe. The ICPCC, and other international chaplaincy organizations, reflect a level of shared characteristics among healthcare chaplains across nations.)

CHAPLAINCY IN EUROPE

European chaplains would easily recognize themselves in the preceding description of what chaplains do in general and in the context of cancer and palliative care. Like their North American colleagues, European chaplains work in a variety of settings. The origins of chaplaincy in Europe are similar to those in the United States. Since the rise of Christianity in Europe there has always been some form of attending to the R/S needs of the sick. Countless Christian religious orders founded healthcare institutions where spiritual care was also offered.

As in the United States, changes in healthcare, and developments within theology, led to more professional chaplaincy in the second half of the previous century. In some European countries, like the United Kingdom, chaplains adapted the profession of pastoral counselor. In other countries, like the Netherlands, chaplains adapted the CPE model, but in ways that fit each national context. CPE in Austria, for example, is not part of chaplains' training. Rather, a 3-month unit is required within the first 3 years of employment. Other countries, like Belgium, have never adopted the CPE concept fully and developed their own version of supervision.

This example with CPE illustrates that education, training, and requirements for chaplains in Europe are very diverse. One can simply not talk about the same three basic requirements for European chaplains as exist for BCCs in the United States. Chaplaincy requirements differ by country. Among this great diversity, there are three essential factors that determine the contemporary settings for chaplaincy in each European country: its culture, its healthcare system, and its religious history. Instead of describing those factors for every one of the 27 countries that currently are members of the European Union; we outline the pattern in four major groups of nations.

The first group consists of countries, like Hungary, Bulgaria, or Romania, who struggle to develop professional chaplaincy due to political and economic issues. In these countries, historical, cultural, and healthcare factors are a hindrance in the training, hiring, and integrating of chaplains. Mostly these are European countries who were under a communist regime for a long time. They are still freeing themselves from an ideology that banned all R/S expression. Chaplains in these countries often find that people do not have a language with which to express their R/S needs, hopes, and resources. In these nations, chaplains not only face the lack of language and the gap in religious traditions, but also major financial shortcomings in their healthcare systems. Few chaplains are officially hired by healthcare institutions, and if they are, they can hardly survive.

The second group of countries include those who recently started developing professional chaplaincy and are growing strong. A good example would be Latvia. Latvia was occupied by the Soviet Union until 1990. Some years after the liberation, Lutheran Latvians living and working in the United States started training and funding Latvian Lutherans and Catholics to become chaplains. In 2004 Latvian chaplains participated for the first time in the consultation of the European Network for HealthCare Chaplaincy. In 2005 the Latvian Association for Professionals Chaplains was founded (http://www.lpvaka.lv/lpvaka-eng.html). The Association is a multifaith organization including chaplains from four denominations (the Russian Orthodox Church, the Baptist Church, the Lutheran and Catholic Church). Mostly young women, these Latvian chaplains face the challenge of low wages, low esteem among other healthcare professions, and a lack of supervisors and theological training. Despite their challenges they continue to grow strong as professional chaplains. Other countries in this group would include Estonia, Czech Republic,[30] and Slovakia.[31]

These first two groups were distinguished by where they are in the development of professional chaplaincy. The following two groups are defined by the faith traditions represented in their populations. European countries where one faith group is dominant form the third group. Most chaplains in these countries belong to the dominant faith group. Belgium, Spain, Portugal, Italy, and Austria are examples of countries where the vast majority of hospitals and chaplains are Catholic. The Northern countries like Finland, Denmark, Sweden, and Norway have mostly Protestant chaplains. If one faith group is dominant because the majority of the population belongs to that religious tradition, then multifaith spiritual care services are rare. Chaplains from the majority group generally visit everyone who requests their support or is referred to them. If a patient belongs to another faith group and desires to talk to someone from their tradition, the chaplain will do the necessary work to make that happen. Usually there is a good liaison between chaplains of the majority faith group and chaplains or representatives of minority faith groups. In most Western European countries the proportion of the population who attend church or hold church membership is diminishing. A growing group of people feel they are not affiliated with any religious tradition. This phenomenon does not have a huge impact on the work of Catholic or Protestant chaplains. They visit those people as they always have and try to attend to their spiritual needs, hopes, and resources.

The last group consists of countries who opt for multifaith chaplaincy. The plural society in these countries leads to a need to include chaplains from non-Christian faith groups. The United Kingdom and the Netherlands would be two prime examples. (The Netherlands is also the only European country where representatives from humanism are called spiritual caregivers like their colleagues from religious traditions.) Multifaith chaplaincy in these countries is expressed in mixed teams in each healthcare settings (i.e., each hospital decides which faith groups will be represented). Not all European countries have national chaplaincy associations. In some countries chaplains are organized by denomination or diocese.

Although chaplaincies are organized very differently throughout the nations of Europe, chaplains do come together. The European Network of HealthCare Chaplaincy (ENHCC) gathers representatives of associations and faith groups every 2 years (http://www.eurochaplains.org). This organization was founded about 25 years ago when chaplains from several European countries felt the need to share their experiences. Out of that initiative the European Network was founded in 2000.

The European Network consists of representatives from churches, faith groups, and national associations. It is rooted in Christianity as expressed in European cultures but is open to representatives of other faith groups. During its biannual consultation the network aims to promote high standards for healthcare chaplaincy and to work for the development of professional guidelines required to minister to the spiritual and religious needs of patients, families, and staff. The Network has grown steadily in the number of participating countries and organizations. In recent years the European Network created liaisons with chaplaincy organizations in the United States and with the European Union in Brussels.[32]

During the 2008 consultation, 62 representatives from 23 European countries discussed end-of-life issues. Chaplains in Belgium and the Netherlands have to deal with legalized euthanasia while chaplains in Switzerland and the Netherlands also face legalized physician assisted suicide. Theological, ethical reflection, and case studies were enriching to all and were especially helpful to chaplains in countries facing the process of legalization of euthanasia.

The European Network respects the diversity in the way its members organize chaplaincy. Nevertheless it aims to work on common statements that will inspire and promote chaplaincy. In 2002 the European Network agreed on Standards for healthcare chaplaincy (http://www.eurochaplains.org/turku_standards.htm). The Standards are meant to be a point of reference and a guide for all faiths and denominations. In 2006 the Network agreed on Standards for palliative care (http://www.eurochaplains.org/lisbon06_palliative.doc). The Standards were inspired by the work done in the United Kingdom regarding the value and integration of spiritual care in palliative care (see the work of the Association of Hospice and Palliative Care Chaplains: http://www.ahpcc.org.uk/standards.html). Spiritual care in cancer care and palliative care is a priority to most European chaplains.

FUTURE CHALLENGES

Healthcare chaplaincy has been described as a professionalizing profession, which is a profession that is trying to strengthen its claim for a legitimate place in the healthcare world.[33] The key future challenges faced by healthcare chaplains are related to this process. They include becoming a research-literate and research-informed profession. Chaplains need to be able to read and understand research and learn to integrate insights from relevant research into their professional practice. Chaplains also need research, conducted by themselves or with professional colleagues, that evaluates spiritual care interventions in order both to improve those interventions and to demonstrate the effectiveness of their spiritual care.

Related to the need to become a research-informed profession, healthcare chaplains also need to develop standards for their practice.[34] Healthcare colleagues and the public need to be able to know what they may expect of trained and certified chaplains. For example,

in most healthcare settings chaplains rely heavily on referrals to know where best to focus their limited attention.[35] Having clearer standards for their practice will enable chaplains to provide clearer guidelines to their healthcare colleagues about when they should make a referral to a chaplain. Currently consensus standards of practice for professional chaplains in acute care and long-term care are being developed in the United States.

There are several challenges for healthcare chaplains that are especially relevant for care for cancer patients and their families. One such challenge is expanding the contexts in which chaplains' services are available. With some exceptions, chaplains are not available in the outpatient context where many diagnoses are made and much of cancer treatment occurs.[29,36] In the United States, trained and certified healthcare chaplains are also more likely to be found at larger, urban, teaching hospitals.[37,38] Cancer patients and their families who receive treatment in other contexts are less likely to have access to a chaplain. In light of this, consideration should be given to increasing the number of creative training programs that help clergy and other spiritual counselors become more familiar with and comfortable in addressing the R/S issues faced by cancer patients and their families.[25]

From the time of diagnosis, through difficult treatment, and, in some cases, at the end of life, living with cancer often raises R/S issues for cancer patients and their families. Certified chaplains are members of the healthcare team who have the training and expertise to help cancer patients and their families address these issues and to provide R/S care in this difficult time.

REFERENCES

1. Asquith GH Jr. (ed.) *Vision from a little known country: A Boisen reader.* Decatur, GA: Journal of Pastoral Care Publications, Inc.; 1992.

2. Hall CE. *Head and heart: The story of the clinical pastoral education movement.* Decatur, GA: Journal of Pastoral Care Publications, Inc.;1992.

3. Dicks RL. The work of the chaplain in a general hospital. *Caregiver J.* 1940/1996;12(1):2–5.

4. Peachey K, Phillips CD. The college of chaplains: the first twenty-five years. *Caregiver J.* 1996;12(1):6–17.

5. Montefalcone WR. General hospital chaplaincy. In: R Hunter, (ed). *Dictionary of pastoral care and counseling*, Expanded ed. Nashville, TN: Abingdon Press; 2005:456–457.

6. VandeCreek L, Burton L. Professional chaplaincy: its role and importance in healthcare. *J Pastoral Care.* 2001;55(1):81–97.

7. Miller WR, Thoresen CE. Spirituality, religion, and health: an emerging research field. *Am Psychol.* 2003;58(1):24–35.

8. Joint Commission. Evaluating your spiritual assessment process. *Source.* 2005;3(2):6–7.

9. Joint Commission. *Comprehensive accreditation manual for hospitals: The official handbook.* Oakbrook Terrace, IL: Joint Commission Resources, 2008:GL-20.

10. Gordon T, Mitchell D. A competency model for the assessment and delivery of spiritual care. *Pall Med.* 2004;18:646–651.

11. Koenig HG. *Spirituality in patient care: Why, how, when, and what.* 2nd ed. Philadelphia, PA: Templeton Foundation Press; 2007.

12. Fitchett G. Screening for spiritual risk. *Chaplaincy Today.* 1999a;15(1):2–12.

13. Fitchett G. Selected resources for screening for spiritual risk. *Chaplaincy Today.* 1999b;15(1):13–26.

14. Fitchett G, Risk JL. Screening for spiritual struggle. *J Pastoral Care Counsel.* 2009 Aug;[Online] 63:1,2.

15. VandeCreek L, Lyons M. Ministry of hospital chaplains: patient satisfaction. *J Health Care Chaplain.* 1997;6(2).

16. Goodell E. Cancer and family members. *J Health Care Chaplain.* 1992; 4(1–2):73–85.

17. Handzo G. Where do chaplains fit in the world of cancer care? *J Health Care Chaplain.* 1992;4(1–2):29–44.

18. Ruff RA. "Leaving footprints": The practice and benefits of hospital chaplains documenting pastoral care activity in patients' medical records. *J Pastoral Care.* 1996;50(4):383–391.

19. Sakurai MLD. JCAHO and spiritual care: an invitation for chaplains to educate and advocate. *Vision.* 2000;10(3):6–7.

20. Sakuari M, Tartaglia A, Waff R. JACHO, JCAPS, and pastoral care: significant changes. *Chaplaincy Today.* 1998;14(2):52–56.

21. Brown S. *A blessing of the hands service.* Plain Views. 2008 June 18;5(10). http://www.plainviews.org. Accessed August 17, 2009.

22. Cummings MH. *Random acts of tea*. Plain Views. 2008 April 16;5(6). http://www.plainviews.org. Accessed August 17, 2009.

23. Sharp CG. Use of the chaplaincy in the neonatal intensive care unit. *South Med J*. 1991;84(12):1482–1486.

24. King SD, Jarvis D, Cornwell M. Programmatic staff care in an outpatient setting. *J Pastoral Care Counsel*. 2005;59(3):263–273.

25. Campbell D, Baile W, Galloway A. Advanced training for clergy in psychological oncology: program objectives, curriculum, and evaluation. *CareGiver J*. 1992;9(2–3):71–79.

26. Wilson-Stronks A, Galvez E. *Hospitals, language, and culture: A snapshot of the nation. Exploring cultural and linguistic services in the nation's hospitals. A report of findings*. Oak Brook Terrace, IL: The Joint Commission; 2007.

27. Frank A. *The wounded storyteller: Body, illness, and ethics*. Chicago, CA: The University of Chicago Press; 1995.

28. Samson A, Zerter B. The experience of spirituality in the psycho-social adaptation of cancer survivors. *J Pastoral Care Counsel*. 2003;57(3):329–343.

29. King SD, Jarvis D, Schlosser-Hall A. A model for outpatient care. *J Pastoral Care Counsel*. 2006;60(1–2):95–107.

30. Opatrna M. Why spiritual care in the Czech healthcare system? *Diagnoza v osetrovatelstvi*. 2006;3:105–108.

31. Nadova L, Prasilova M. *Why is it an advantage to have a chaplain in the institution (hospital/hospice)?* Proceedings of the Third International Conference on Hospice and Palliative Care. Trnava: Slovakia; 2005.

32. Vandenhoeck A. *A challenge for the European network of healthcare chaplaincy*. PlainViews. 2005. www.plainviews.org/v2n20/a.html.

33. DeVries R, Berlinger N, Cadge W. Lost in translation: Sociological observations and reflections on the practice of health care chaplaincy. *Hastings Cenr Rep*, 2008:38(6):23–27.

34. Mohrmann ME. Ethical grounding for a professional of hospital chaplaincy. *Hastings Cent Rep*, 2008:38(6):18–23.

35. Galek K, Flannelly KJ, Koenig HG, Fogg SL. Referrals to chaplains: the role of religion and spirituality in healthcare settings. *Ment Health Religion Cult*. 2007;10(4):363–377.

36. Anderson H, Holst LE, Sunderland RH. *Ministry to outpatients: A new challenge in pastoral care*. Minneapolis, MN: Augsburg Press; 1991.

37. Cadge W, Freese J, Christakis NA. The provision of hospital chaplaincy in the United States: a national overview. *South Med J*. 2008;101(6):626–630.

38. Flannelly KJ, Handzo GF, Weaver AJ. Factors affecting healthcare chaplaincy and the provision of pastoral care in the United States. *J Pastoral Care Counsel*. 2004;58(1–2):127–130.

Professional Education in Psychosocial Oncology

Shirley Otis-Green and Betty R. Ferrell

The great aim of education is not knowledge, but action.-Herbert Spencer

THE NEED FOR PROFESSIONAL EDUCATION

Deficits in the delivery of quality oncology care are numerous. Troubling findings continue to emerge regarding disparities in the provision of care, substandard pain and symptom management, poor access to care, high caregiver burden, and communication deficits across the continuum of care.[1-6] Unfortunately, there is an abundance of evidence that these concerns continue to be inadequately addressed.[7-10] The 2009 *National consensus project for quality palliative care: Clinical practice guidelines, Second edition*[11] recognize that psychosocial-spiritual support of patients and their loved ones is essential to maximize opportunities for transformation and growth.

People diagnosed with a serious, potentially life-threatening illness, such as cancer, require competent and compassionate care providers, yet evidence indicates that few healthcare providers are adequately prepared for this critical task.[12-15] The Institute of Medicine Report *Cancer care for the whole patient: Meeting psychosocial health needs*[16] devotes significant attention to the importance of preparing the existing workforce to better address the complex multidimensional needs of patients with cancer. This report explores the educational needs and challenges of physicians, nurses, social workers, and other mental health providers (including psychologists and spiritual care professionals) giving specific recommendations to improve workforce competencies from undergraduate training through continuing education for professionals. This chapter reviews the status of professional education in psychosocial oncology and provides direction for future educational efforts.

The complex interplay of physical, psychological, social, spiritual, existential, medical, financial, and social burdens experienced by cancer patients, make a family perspective and an integrative team approach to care imperative.[16-19] The field of psycho-oncology was developed to address the multiple dimensions of the total cancer experience.[20] Quality oncology care can best be delivered in a collaborative environment that integrates a bio-psychosocial-spiritual model of care and is comprised of skilled medical, nursing, and psycho-oncology professionals.[21-26]

Health professionals must demonstrate compassion and empathy, but without scientific and clinical competence their impact and influence is lessened. To date, most professional education is discipline specific, and few professionals receive specific team building or collaborative-skills training.[27-34] Effective integration of differing disciplines into a cohesive and effective team requires skillful leadership, collaboration, coordination, and communication among all members. Studies indicate that team functioning is best in an environment of trust with an appreciation of the unique perspective each professional contributes to the team.[35-37] Few internship opportunities are available for psychosocial oncology professionals.[38] The challenge is not only to educate future professionals but also, more urgently, to address the training needs of those currently in practice.

Specialization as a psycho-oncology professional requires mastery of several core competencies[39-55] necessary for the delivery of effective care. The *National Comprehensive Cancer Network (NCCN) clinical practice guidelines in oncology* include algorithms for distress management[56] and palliative care[57] which have been adopted in many cancer institutions.

However, the algorithms' success relies upon the necessary institutional infrastructure with teams of skilled personnel in place to implement the recommended interventional strategies.

Although the bio-psychosocial-spiritual dimensions of physical pain are increasingly well-recognized, minimal attention has been given to teaching psychologists, social workers and spiritual care professionals the fundamental skills of pain and symptom management.[58,59] As a result, most psycho-oncology professionals find themselves in the unenviable position of attempting to learn, through trial and error, the necessary skills to address the complex needs for pain and symptom management.[60]

Along with pain and symptom management, oncology professionals should be well-versed in a variety of integrative interventions. For example, knowledge regarding the therapeutic use of heat and cold, exercise and nutrition is helpful. Creative use of music, journaling, poetry, and art can encourage the expression of existential concerns not readily accessed through discussion alone, and assist in the creation of a lasting legacy for loved ones, through an innovative concept called "legacy-building."[61] Although use of the arts can be a powerful and effective interventional tool, few oncology professionals have adequate preparation, training, and skill in this area.[62]

Studies emphasize the importance of developing clear communication skills for use with patients and their families as well as among team members. Collaborative communication-skills training is an essential component of continuing professional education. It is also vital that practitioners involved in the care of oncology patients and families recognize the religious, spiritual, ethnic, and cultural diversities that exist in cancer populations and the particular importance that these variables play throughout the continuum of illness.[63,64] There is tremendous variability regarding communication styles, decision making and use of rituals. Attention to these differences by skillful practitioners is a necessary component of competent healthcare in a diverse society. Yet most healthcare professionals report a lack of confidence in their cultural competence,[65] especially, as related to end-of-life and bereavement care.

Examples of professional education efforts. The authors and their colleagues at the City of Hope (COH) Medical Center Duarte, California, have an extensive record of education, training, and dissemination in areas of pain, quality-of-life (QOL), end-of-life (EOL) care and cancer survivorship. The following is a brief summary of their experiences in conducting national and international education projects related to psychosocial oncology to demonstrate various professional education strategies.

The Department of Nursing Research and Education, under the direction of Dr. Marcia Grant, DNSc, FAAN has a long history of conducting innovative educational programs for cancer professionals.[66] Community-based education began in the late 1980s as the department received multiple requests for education on cancer nursing care from local hospitals where skilled oncology nurses were unavailable. Classes such as Basic Oncology, Chemotherapy, and Vascular Access Devices were developed from materials originally created for COH nurses and included psychosocial aspects of treatment. This record of education has continued over 25 years and in 2006 the Department received the prestigious National Cancer Institute, Cancer Patient Education Network Gold Star Award recognizing more than two decades of excellence in oncology education. In 2007, the Department hosted a total of 18 professional educational ourses (national and international), indicative of the department's continued growth. Following are examples of major training programs.

THE END-OF-LIFE NURSING EDUCATION CONSORTIUM (ELNEC)

ELNEC (http://www.aacn.nche.edu/elnec) is a targeted educational initiative led by Drs. Ferrell and Grant to improve end-of-life care in the United States and abroad. The project provides undergraduate and graduate nursing faculty, continuing education providers, staff development educators, specialty nurses in pediatrics, oncology, critical care and geriatrics, and others with training in end-of-life care so they can teach this essential information to nursing students and practicing nurses. The project, which began in February 2000, was initially funded by a major grant from The Robert Wood Johnson Foundation (RWJF). Additional funding has been received from the National Cancer Institute (NCI), the Aetna Foundation, the Archstone Foundation, and the California HealthCare Foundation. The curriculum is revised regularly on the basis of participant recommendations and new advances in the field and is modified for each distinct audience.

To date, over 10,000 nurses representing all 50 states and over 60 countries have received ELNEC training through these comprehensive courses and are sharing this new expertise in educational and clinical settings. ELNEC trainers are hosting professional development seminars for practicing nurses, incorporating ELNEC content into nursing curriculum, hosting regional training sessions to expand ELNEC's reach into rural and underserved communities, presenting ELNEC at national and international conferences, and improving the quality of nursing care in other innovative ways. Follow-up evaluations have consistently rated the overall course effectiveness as 4.9 on a scale of 0 = low to 5 = high. Numerous papers have been published from the ELNEC project,[66–68] which devotes extensive focus on psychosocial topics including entire modules on Grief, Culture, and Communication.

Dissemination of End-of-Life Education to Cancer Centers (DELEtCC).

DELEtCC was a comprehensive, interdisciplinary project aimed at improving EOL care in cancer centers. Led by Dr. Marcia Grant, the primary objective of this proposal was achieved through four annual workshops for two representatives each from 75 cancer treatment centers. Funded by the NCI R25 mechanism of the National Institutes of Health, which supports the development and implementation of institutional curriculum-dependent programs with core didactic and research requirements, (for more information: http://grants.nih.gov/grants/guide/pa-files/PAR-06–511.html). The first course was held in June, 2002 and the last in April 2005. A total of 405 participants representing 200 institutions attended. Content built on the ELNEC project curricula was expanded to include aspects of change related to institutional commitment, and a framework of continuous quality improvement.[69] Participants were selected from two tiers of staff at cancer centers: Tier 1 consisted of nurses, social workers, administrators, and physicians, and tier 2 consisted of clergy, pharmacists, psychologists, rehabilitation professionals, and unlicensed personnel. An extensive evaluation provided analysis of goals achieved and barriers experienced by participants and formed a basis for the continuing education of healthcare professionals beyond the project period.[70] Examples of institutional change included development of palliative care teams, partnerships with community hospices, and implementing palliative care protocols. The DELEtCC curriculum was also extensively focused on developing psychosocial services in cancer centers. Follow-up evaluation of participants demonstrated excellent progress in areas such as routine screening of psychosocial concerns and strengthening support services.[71]

THE ACE PROJECT: ADVOCATING FOR CLINICAL EXCELLENCE—TRANSDISCIPLINARY PALLIATIVE CARE EDUCATION

The ACE Project (http://www.cityofhope.org/ACEproject) is a 5-year (2006–2011) National Cancer Institute R25 CA 110454 award for development and implementation of a palliative care educational experience for competitively selected psycho-oncology professionals (PI: Otis-Green, Co-I: Ferrell and Grant). The primary aim of this transdisciplinary educational initiative is to improve the delivery of palliative care by competitively selected psychologists, social workers and spiritual care professionals through an intensive advocacy and leadership training program.

This innovative program is conducted by a distinguished faculty of researchers, educators, and leaders in the fields of psycho-oncology and palliative care. The project premise is that more effective team functioning, collaboration, and advocacy are necessary to systemically improve the delivery of palliative care. Although modeled after previously successful COH professional education programs, this project was unique in its transdisciplinary approach to improving the delivery of palliative care, and by its specific focus upon the targeted needs of psycho-oncology professionals. Four annual courses (75 participants/year, for a total N = 300) will be followed by a conference in year 5 that reunites the participants and faculty to reinforce change efforts, share lessons learned, and disseminate findings.

The ACE Project training encourages exploration of role function, improved clinical judgment, advocacy and ethics, professionalism, collaboration, systems thinking, cultural sensitivity, facilitation of learning, accountability, empowerment, and the development of improved interprofessional communication skills. Nine major topic areas are included in the curriculum (Table 88–1).

This course seeks to "change the change agents," by encouraging accountability, growth, and risk taking on behalf of the vulnerable populations that each participant serves. In recognition that working with the dying reminds us of the importance of living an authentic life, opportunities are integrated throughout the course that invite participants to reflect upon their career choices and give consideration to their life purpose and the creation of a personal legacy. Principles of transformational learning theory provide the basis to create an environment that inspires participants to reach personal growth goals. To maximize the effectiveness of course exercises, change concepts taken from the psychology and the business world are applied when appropriate. Course participants receive a binder containing nearly 1000 pages of resources, references, slide content, case studies, and exercises. Extensive evaluations occur immediately postcourse and again at 6 and 12 months following the training. Preliminary findings indicate the success of this format. Expert faculty present didactic information, facilitate small group interactions, and provide mentorship and coaching.[72]

SURVIVORSHIP FOR QUALITY CANCER CARE

The purpose of the NCI R25-funded study—Survivorship for Quality Cancer Care (2005–2010)—is to present and evaluate annual professional interdisciplinary caregiver courses aimed at improving quality care for cancer survivors (PI: Grant; Co-I: Ferrell). Over ten million U.S. cancer survivors are living with late effects of cancer and cancer treatment.[73] Healthcare professionals currently lack the background to identify, design and carry out survivorship activities and do follow-up. The framework of this study is composed of three concepts: institutional change, adult education principles, and the City of Hope Quality of Life Model (COH-QOL) which addresses physical, psychological, social, and spiritual well-being. Four annual courses were designed with precourse and postcourse (6, 12, and 18 month) evaluation data (Table 88–2).

Two-person interdisciplinary teams apply for the course with at least 1 member required to be a nurse, physician, or administrator. One hundred teams applied for the 53 spots available (106 people) in the first course. Participant goals were refined during the course and were evaluated with administrator follow-up evaluations at 6, 12, and 18 months. The overwhelming interest and outstanding faculty resulted in a successful program. Results for the first course revealed attendees rating of quality of content at 4.60 on a scale of 1–5 (5 = best).[70]

PROMOTING EXCELLENCE IN PAIN MANAGEMENT AND PALLIATIVE CARE FOR SOCIAL WORKERS

This two-day national educational program (PI: Otis-Green) was designed to develop the core skills necessary for social work professionals to more effectively address the pain and symptom management

Table 88–1. ACE Project curriculum content

Opening reception

Presentations:

Overview of the course curriculum/key themes/resources
Module 1: Moral imperative
Overview of course participants and project goals
Introduction to faculty with focus on their change efforts

Large group discussion topic:

Integrating the voice of the patient and family (with video)

Day 1: Theme—values-based training

Presentations:

Module 2: Advocacy and change (with video)
Module 3: Personal death awareness
Module 4: Ethical obligations of psycho-oncology professionals in palliative care
Module 5: Transdisciplinary team work and team building
Introduction to goal refinement

Small group discussion topics:

Goal refinement
Ethics case study
Team-building case study (with video)

Activities:

Opening/closing centering practice
Labyrinth (optional)

Day 2: Theme—palliative care knowledge

Presentations:

Module 6: Physical aspects of palliative care (with video)
Module 7: Psychosocial aspects of palliative care (with video)
Module 8: Spiritual aspects of palliative care

Small group discussion topic:

Goal refinement

Large group discussion topic:

Institutional change and participant goals

Activities:

Opening/closing centering practice
Leaf reflection exercise
Labyrinth (optional)

Day 3: Theme—advocacy

Presentations:

Facilitating family conferences
Evolution of "Hands on Harps" program
Module 9: Applying our heart, head and hands: Bringing together passion, knowledge, and action for quality palliative, end of life, and bereavement care

Small group discussion topics:

Goal refinement and completion

Activities:

Opening/closing centering practice
Role play: Family conference
Guided reflection
Labyrinth (optional)

Table 88–2. Key topics in survivorship course

Agenda topics
Introduction to survivorship
Goal refinement
Health education, research, and outcomes for survivors
Models of excellence (Pediatrics, American Cancer Society, Lance Armstrong, Wellness Community, and CancerCare)
State of the science (physical, social, psychological, and spiritual well-being)
National coalition for cancer survivorship and the survivorship movement
Health-related outcomes after pediatric cancer: price of cure
Special survivorship issues for adolescents and young adults
Strategies to partner with diverse communities
Impact of survivorship on QOL
National Cancer Institute and the survivorship research agenda
Partnering with cancer survivors
"A Survivor's Perspective"
Developing a survivorship program
Goal development and institutional change

ABBREVIATION: QOL, quality of life.

these challenges by offering an evidence-based curriculum emphasizing key palliative care competencies. Recognized palliative care leaders are the primary faculty for this course. To date, 4 annual courses have been held with support from community and foundation funding. In 2008 the American Society on Aging recognized the *Promoting excellence* course with their prestigious national Healthcare and Aging Network Award for "innovation and quality in healthcare and aging."

The premise of the program is that more effective social work expertise will increase team functioning and collaboration which is a necessary step to systemically improve the delivery of pain management and palliative care. A QOL model guided the curriculum development. Attention to the family as the primary unit of care and the celebration of diversity were key themes intertwined throughout the course curriculum. Nationally recognized pain management and palliative care leaders were brought together to help create the specific modules within the course curriculum.

Pioneering palliative care and social work leaders were selected as role models for participants and encouraged to offer mentorship and share their expertise with attendees to encourage application of key course concepts within participant settings. Participants in each course were provided with multiple learning opportunities, including lectures, case examples, role play, slides, video clips, and other educational modalities to promote interactive, skill-building and peer-learning time among the attendees.

The course objectives are that participants will:

- Understand the critical role of social workers in pain management and palliative care with special attention to vulnerable populations and the needs of the elderly.
- Identify key aspects of quality pain and symptom management including nontraditional and culturally diverse strategies.
- Link the domains of quality end-of-life care to social work practice.
- Discuss the importance of the social work role in completing a comprehensive bio-psychosocial-spiritual assessment.
- Identify interventions appropriate for social workers to use in the palliative care setting.
- Explore various advocacy strategies to promote excellence in pain management and palliative care within their settings.
- Evaluate the impact of this course on social work practice.

An additional goal of this course is to reach both local and regional social workers across multiple settings such as hospitals, nursing homes, home health, and hospice. An extensive syllabus was modified for each annual course. The syllabus includes copies of all of the PowerPoint

needs of the patients and families that they serve. Social workers, like other healthcare providers, often lack the necessary skills to maximize their interventions in pain and symptom management and to address the complex, yet, critical multidimensional needs facing seriously ill patients and their families. The *Promoting excellence* course addresses slides, exercises, and other handouts to supplement the key teaching concepts in addition to numerous resources for participants to refer to for further information. The curriculum was designed to encourage exploration of the social work role regarding pain management across the continuum of care with a special focus upon the needs of the traditionally underserved.[74]

KEY PRINCIPLES AND LESSONS LEARNED

The above projects illustrate several approaches to improving the psychosocial preparation of professionals in oncology. Across these projects, the investigators have observed some common experiences which may be useful for others in planning educational programs.

Content of education. Creating a course agenda is a challenging task. There is increasing need for content to be evidence based, particularly in psychosocial oncology, where research has been limited and standards of practice are needed. One helpful strategy is to conduct an early needs assessment by surveying professionals in the targeted area. Several of the COH courses have used web-based or e-mailed surveys to determine topics of priority and participant needs. In 2004, the ACE Project investigative team conducted an electronic needs assessment survey of potential participants. A total of 360 psycho-oncology seasoned professionals from across the nation responded. The core competencies (identified from position papers from psychology, social work, and spiritual care) reflected in the needs assessment survey guided module content development, which was further refined by expert consultants representing each of the three disciplines.

Highlights from this survey are reported in Table 88–3. Recipients were asked to complete the tool if they were psycho-oncology professionals (psychologists, social workers, spiritual care professionals) involved in the care of those with advanced, life-limiting illness. The respondents (average age of 49 years) had more than 11 years of work experience with the very ill. Two-thirds of the respondents were female (66%) with the majority employed in hospitals (N = 119) or hospice settings (N = 107). Respondents were asked to rate their formal education on 24 specific core competencies. Respondents reported an average preparedness rating of 2.79 (on a scale of 0 = least prepared to 5 = most prepared) regarding these key skills from their formal professional education. They also identified perceived benefits and barriers to course attendance. Perhaps not surprisingly, course cost and work restrictions were identified as presenting the most significant barriers to attendance.

Developing course content should include peer review by faculty or other experts and requires numerous revisions before an agenda is finalized. Once content is determined, it is also important to determine the appropriate educational strategy, for example, which topics are best presented as lectures, case studies, self-reflection exercises or group discussions. In keeping with adult learning principles, and in recognition of the diversity of participant needs and skill levels represented at each course, we have found it useful to provide learners with a wide variety of reliable resources, texts, tools, and articles to supplement the key content. These references and resources invite participants to apply critical concepts to their individual population and setting.

Targeted audiences. Determining targeted audiences is closely linked to the course objectives. For example, in train-the-trainer courses such as ELNEC, we strive to recruit participants who are in positions to teach others. Courses such as the ACE Project are intended to promote leadership and emphasize advocacy. Many projects are designed with the requirement that participants attend with a partner from their organization so that they have a support system to assist as they return to the busy clinical settings and to enhance the likelihood of successful implementation of their goals. Extensive marketing is done through mailings to past participants, electronic postings on professional listservs and web-site listings, in addition to more conventional marketing efforts. Each course aggressively targets recruitment of minority applicants and applicants from institutions serving minority populations in recognition of the need for culturally diverse voices to be represented in each course.

Table 88–3. ACE Project psycho-oncology needs assessment

How well did your formal education prepare you for[a]	Total N = 360
facilitating support groups?	3.59
facilitating family conferences?	3.54
collaborating with other members of the healthcare team?	3.50
taking a leadership role?	3.47
effectively educating other professionals?	3.26
providing bereavement education, counseling and support?	3.21
addressing cultural and religious diversity concerns at end of life?	3.15
addressing ethical dilemmas at the end of life?	3.12
facilitating decision making at the end of life?	3.07
assessing for indicators of complicated bereavement?	2.92
addressing the multidimensional aspects of suffering?	2.82
advocating for the family's use of culturally relevant rituals in the healthcare setting?	2.79
advocating for change at the institutional level?	2.69
translating research into clinical practice?	2.68
addressing the family as the primary unit of care?	2.54
providing community outreach or education regarding end-of-life concerns?	2.51
managing the personal and professional impact of chronic compassion fatigue?	2.46
providing anticipatory guidance for families regarding what to expect in the final hours of life?	2.45
providing education, support, and guidance regarding advance directives, ethical wills, guardianship concerns, etc?	2.41
using the skills of performance improvement/quality improvement?	2.40
completing a spiritual assessment?	2.32
having competence in basic principles of pain and symptom management?	2.13
completing an integrated psychosocial pain assessment?	2.09
having competence in use of expressive arts?	2.02

[a]Key: Likert-type Scale (0 = least prepared and 5 = most prepared).

Teaching strategies. One of the key "evolutions" in our continuing education projects has been the increasing diversity of teaching strategies. Course lectures that include case studies, small group discussion, videos, journaling, and skill-based sessions on topics such as communication are particularly well received. Adult learners[75] comprehend and retain information best through interactive teaching methods.

For example, we have successfully used various "homework assignments" to encourage reflective learning. These assignments serve the purpose of both "journaling" or given the participants an experience of sharing their experiences and emotions in writing as well as providing valuable qualitative data to the investigators. An example of one homework assignment recently used in an ELNEC Geriatric course is included as Table 88–4. When used during a multiday course, participants are requested to complete the assignment overnight, in preparation for small group discussion on the following day. It is essential to allow sufficient time for group discussion since many participants have vast experiences to share which is of equal importance to planned course content. Interactive learning is essential to enhance knowledge and skills in psycho-oncology.

Reinforcement strategies. Expecting long term outcomes from a short-term experience such as a conference is generally unrealistic. In each of the above projects, the outcomes of participants have been greatly enhanced by postcourse reinforcement efforts. The most effective strategies have been electronic newsletters sent quarterly, as well as

Table 88-4. Sample homework assignment: communication in palliative nursing care

1. Nurses are intimately involved in communication with patients and families facing serious or life-threatening illness. Please describe an important conversation you have had with a patient or family related to this area of nursing that went very well:
2. How difficult are these types of conversations for you?

Rated on a scale of:	0=(not difficult)	–10=(very difficult)
1. Talking with patients once they have received "bad news"		
2. Talking with family members of seriously ill patients		
3. Talking with patients about spiritual/religious concerns		
4. Discussing decisions such as advanced directives, do not resuscitate orders, feeding tubes etc		
5. Remaining silent and listening to difficult feelings from patients or families		
6. Talking with physicians about palliative care issues		
7. Talking with nurse colleagues about palliative care issues		
8. Talking to patients or families about hospice		
9. Talking with patients or families from different cultures		
10. Talking with patients about pain or symptoms		
11. Talking with patients about suffering.		

3. Please share a conversation/communication you have had related to palliative care that *did not* go well:

regularly updated web-based resources. Electronic newsletters are ideal as they are inexpensive, widely accessible, and allow timely sharing of relevant resources and policy updates. We also have used awards programs whereby individuals are honored for successful implementation of their goals in practice. Recognition of these outstanding efforts are promoted through a variety of electronic and print means and have been successful in highlighting excellent work and identifying models for others.

Evaluation strategies. Extensive evaluation of educational projects is needed to demonstrate outcomes and as feedback for continuous quality improvement. Outcome data are also critical to support future funding of psycho-oncology education. Each of the above-mentioned projects uses extensive evaluation methods and designs encompassing precourse, course, and postcourse evaluation. Evaluation begins before the courses through an extensive application process where applicants provide data regarding their own experiences and beliefs as well as the current status of care within their setting or institution. Baseline information is key to demonstrating the impact of the courses.

Precourse assessments also enable participants to come prepared with insight regarding opportunities for the implementation of course content. At each course we collect evaluation data, required for continuing education credit purposes, but also as vital feedback. While the COH investigators have conducted over 100 courses in the past 20 years, we continue to revise each project based on course evaluation data. Course evaluation questions probe areas such as speaker effectiveness and knowledge gained but also aspects such as the application of the content

to clinical practice. Questions that seek to determine what aspects of the course were most meaningful and most professionally useful have offered revealing information regarding the effectiveness of the various course experiences.

Collecting data only at the conclusion of a conference falls short of ideal evaluation. In each of the above projects, follow-up data is collected over multiple time points. The decision as to whether this occurs at 1, 3, 6, 12, 18, or 24 months is influenced by the project design and available resources. Postcourse evaluations strive to determine how course content is applied to practice and serve as a means of reinforcing the efforts of participants. The availability of electronic follow-up surveys has improved the process of collecting evaluation data and increased the percentage of responses received.

FUTURE DIRECTIONS

Growing pressures on health providers ensure the continuing need for efficient and effective professional education. The current workforce requires on-going evidence-based education to meet the needs of the twenty-first century:

- Growing elderly population;
- Increasing uninsured and underinsured populations;
- Limited healthcare resources with increasing disparities in access to quality care;
- Increasingly sophisticated (and resource intensive) technological interventions.

These pressures are magnified when we consider the "graying" of the healthcare workforce. Shortages are expected in upcoming decades in each of the disciplines (physicians, nurses, and social workers). Providing meaningful continuing education is key to retaining a pool of qualified, experienced personnel. Difficult decisions regarding the delivery of care will need to be made as a result of increasing healthcare expenditures, which are considered to be in direct competition with other valued social goods. Politically conscious healthcare providers recognize that choices regarding social justice and the delivery of quality care require an informed cadre of care-providers to meet these challenges. Limited healthcare dollars mean that professional education is necessary to increase competence and to create a sustainable workforce.

The ultimate goal of psychosocial education is to prepare life-long learners who are skilled clinicians committed to offering competent, compassionate, and culturally sensitive care. Leadership is needed across all levels of the healthcare hierarchy to address the disparities in access to quality care that exist at the local, national, and global levels. Today's healthcare professionals are required to be systematic change-agents capable of using data to support recommendations for improvements in the delivery of care throughout the illness trajectory and across settings. Oncology professionals must be capable of applying an evidence base to their selection of interventions to more effectively and efficiently address the psychosocial needs of patients and their families.[16] This multidimensional skill-set includes proficiency as communicators, team collaborators, and patient and family advocates. A multitude of innovative educational initiatives will be necessary to prepare professionals for this challenge.

REFERENCES

1. American Association of Colleges of Nursing. (AACN). *A peaceful death. Report from the Robert Wood Johnson End-of-Life Care Roundtable.* Washington, DC: AACN; 1997.

2. Field, MJ. *Crossing the quality chasm: A new health system for the 21st century.* Washington, DC: Institute of Medicine, National Academy Press; 2001.

3. Last Acts. *Means to a better end: A report on dying in America today.* Washington, DC: Last Acts National Program Office; 2002.

4. The SUPPORT Principal Investigators. A controlled trial to improve care for seriously ill hospitalized patients: the study to understand prognosis and preferences for outcomes and risks of treatment (SUPPORT). *JAMA.* 1995;274:1591–1598.

5. Zabora J, BrintzenhofeSzoc K, Curbow B, Hooker C, Piantadosi S. The prevalence of psychological distress by cancer site. *Psychooncology.* 2001;10:19–28.

6. Foley KM, Gelband H. *Improving palliative care for cancer.* Report of the Institute of Medicine Task Force. Washington, DC: National Academy Press; 2001.

7. Cairns M, Thompson M, Wainwright W, Victoria Hospice Society. *Transitions in dying and bereavement: A psychosocial guide for hospice and palliative care.* Baltimore, MD: Health Professions Press; 2003.

8. Koppelman J. The EOL movement: a historical perspective. *Last Acts Qtrly.* 2004;15:4.

9. Taylor Brown S, Blacker S, Walsh-Burke K, Christ G, Altilio T. *Care at the end of life (best practices series: Innovative practice in social work).* Philadelphia, PA: Society for Social Work Leadership in Health Care; 2001.

10. Werner P, Carmel S, Ziedenberg H. Nurses' and social workers' attitudes and beliefs about and involvement in life-sustaining treatment decisions. *Health Soc Work.* 2004;29(1):27–35.

11. National Consensus Project for Quality Palliative Care. *Clinical practice guidelines for quality palliative care, Second edition.* Brooklyn, NY: National Consensus Project; 2009. http://www.nationalconsensusproject.org

12. Field MJ, Behrman DE. (eds). *When children die: Improving palliative and end-of-life care for children and their families.* Washington, DC: Institute of Medicine, National Academy Press; 2003.

13. Field MJ, Cassel CK. (eds). *Approaching death: Improving care at the end of life.* Washington, DC: Institute of Medicine, National Academy Press; 1997.

14. National Cancer Policy Board. (NCPB), Institute of Medicine. (IOM). Psychosocial services and providers. In: Hewitt M, Herdman R, Simons J, (eds). *Meeting psychosocial needs of women with breast cancer.* Washington, DC: National Academy Press; 1997:70–94.

15. Tuma R. IOM. Psychosocial care in breast cancer improves quality of life, but more attention required. *Oncol Times.* 2004;26(6):8–11.

16. Institute of Medicine (IOM). *Cancer care for the whole patient: Meeting psychosocial health needs.* Washington, DC: The National Academies Press; 2008.

17. Weissman DE. Champions, leaders, and the future of palliative care. *J Pall Med.* 2003;6(5):695–696.

18. Holland JC. Improving the human side of cancer care: psycho-oncology's contribution. *Cancer J.* 2001; 7(6):458–471.

19. Enck RE. Connecting the medical and spiritual models in patients nearing death. *Am J Hosp Palliat Care.* 2003;20(2):88–89.

20. Holland JC. Societal views of cancer and the emergence of psycho-oncology. In: Holland JC, (ed). *Psycho-oncology.* New York: Oxford; 1998:3–15.

21. National Council of Hospice and Palliative Professionals. (NHPCO). Stronger together: reflecting on the hospice interdisciplinary team. *Hosp Pall Care Insights.* 2003;4.

22. Sulmasy DP. A biopsychosocial-spiritual model for the care of patients at the end of life. *Gerontologist.* 2002;42:24–33.

23. McCallin A. Interdisciplinary practice—a matter of teamwork: an integrated literature review. *J Clin Nurs.* 2001;10(4):419–428.

24. Gelfand DE, Baker L, Cooney G. Developing end-of-life interdisciplinary programs in university wide settings. *Am J Hosp Pall Care.* 2003;20(3):201–204.

25. Larson DG. The caring team. In: Larson DG, (ed). *The helper's journey.* Champaign, IL: Research Press; 1993:199–227.

26. Adams D. Movement toward collaboration in clinical palliative care. *amednews.com—The newspaper for America's physicians.* 2001 Aug 20. http://www.ama-assn.org/amednews/2001/08/20/prse0820.htm. Accessed April 29, 2008.

27. Hearn J, Higginson IJ. Do specialist palliative care teams improve outcomes for cancer patients? A systematic literature review. *Pall Med.* 1998;12(5):317–332.

28. Rhiner M, Otis-Green S, Slatkin N. Psychosocial-spiritual responses to cancer and treatment. In: Varricchio C, (ed), American Cancer Society. *A cancer source book for nurses.* 8th ed. Sudbury, MA: Jones and Bartlett Publishers; 2004; 501–511.

29. Arnold, R. The challenges of integrating palliative care into postgraduate training. *J Pall Med.* 2003;6(5):801–807.

30. Reese DJ, Sontag MA. Successful interprofessional collaboration on the hospice team. *Health Soc Work.* 2001;26(3):167–175.

31. Sabur S. Measuring the success of the interdisciplinary team. *Hosp Pall Care Insights.* 2003;4:47–49.

32. DeFord B. Who should lead? Exploring non-medical models of leadership of the hospice team. *Hosp Pall Care Insights.* 2003;4:10–15.

33. Otis-Green S, Sherman R, Perez M, Baird P. An integrated psychosocial-spiritual model for cancer pain management. *Cancer Prac.* 2002;10(Suppl 1):S58-S65.

34. Lynn J, Schuster JL, Kabcenell A, Berwick DM. *Improving care for the end of life: A sourcebook for health care managers and clinicians.* New York: Oxford University Press, Inc.; 2000.

35. Abramson JS, Rosenthal BB. Interdisciplinary and interorganizational collaboration. In: Edwards RL, (ed). in chief. *Encyclopedia of social work.* 19th ed. Washington DC: NASW Press; 1995;2:1479–1489.

36. Bern-Klug M, Gessert C, Forbes S. The need to revise assumptions about the end of life: implications for social work practice. *Health Soc Work.* 2001;26(1):38–47.

37. Cummings I. The interdisciplinary team. In: Doyle D, Hanks GWC, MacDonald N, (eds). *Oxford textbook of palliative medicine.* 2nd ed. New York, NY: Oxford University Press, Inc; 1999:19–30.

38. Fineberg I-C, Wenger NS, Forrow L. Interdisciplinary education: evaluation of palliative care training for pre-professionals. *Acad Med.* 2004;79(8):769–776.

39. National Hospice and Palliative Care Organization. *Competency-based education for social workers.* Arlington, VA: NHPCO; 2001.

40. Gwyther L, Altilio T, Blacker S, et al. Social work competencies in palliative care and end-of-life care. *J Soc Work in End-of-Life Pall Care.* 2005;1(1):87–120

41. Altilio T, Eighmy J, Nahman E. Care of the patient and family. In: Volker B, Watson A, (eds). *Core curriculum for the generalist hospice and palliative nurse.* Dubuque, IA: Kendall Hunt Publishing Company; 2002:155–180.

42. Browning D. Fragments of love: Explorations in the ethnography of suffering and professional caregiving. In: Berzoff J, Silverman P, (eds). *Living with dying: A textbook in end-of-life care for social work.* New York: Columbia University Press; 2004:21–42.

43. Kagawa-Singer M. The cultural context of death rituals and mourning practices. *Oncol Nurs Forum.* 1998;25(10):1752–1756.

44. Hedlund S, Clark E. End-of-life issues. In: Lauria MM, Stearns NM, Hermann JF, (eds). *Social work in oncology: Supporting survivors, families, and caregivers.* Atlanta, GA: American Cancer Society; 2001:299–316.

45. Haley WE, Larson DG, Kasl-Godley J, Neimeyer RA, Kwilosz D. Roles for psychologists in end-of-life care: emerging models of practice. *Prof Psychol: Res Prac.* 2003;34(6):626–633.

46. Fitchett G, Handzo G. Spiritual assessment, screening, and intervention. In: Holland JC, (ed). *Psycho-oncology.* New York: Oxford University Press; 1998: 790–808.

47. Association of Oncology Social Work (AOSW). *Social work and end of life care II: Pain and symptom management.* [AOSW Online Course]. http://www.aosw.org/html/courses.php. Accessed on April 29, 2008.

48. Kramer BJ. Preparing social workers for the inevitable: a preliminary investigation of a course on grief, death, and loss. *J Soc Work Edu.* 1998;34:211–227.

49. Christ G, Sormanti M. Advancing social work practice in end-of-life care. *Soc Work Health Care.* 1999;30(2):81–99.

50. Puchalski C, Kilpatrick SD, McCullough ME, Larson DB. A systematic review of spiritual and religious variables in *Pall Med, Am J Hosp Pall Care, Hosp J, J Pall Care,* and *J Pain Symp Manage. Pall Supp Care.* 2003;1:7–13.

51. American Pain Society Quality of Care Committee. Quality improvement guidelines for the treatment of acute pain and cancer pain. *JAMA.* 1995;274(23): 1874–1880.

52. Holland JC, Chertkov L. Clinical practice guidelines for the management of psychosocial and physical symptoms of cancer. In: Foley KM, Gelband H, (eds). *Improving palliative care for cancer.* Washington DC: National Academy Press; 2001:199–232.

53. National Association of Social Workers. (NASW). NASW standards for social work practice in palliative and end of life care. Washington DC: National Association of Social Workers; 2004.

54. American Psychosocial Oncology Society. *The multidisciplinary curriculum in psycho-oncology.* [Online Education]. http://www.apos-society.org/professionals/meetings-ed/webcasts/webcasts-multidisciplinary.aspx. Accessed on April 29, 2008.

55. Wesley C, Tunney K, Duncan E. Educational needs of hospice social workers: spiritual assessment and interventions with diverse populations. *Am J Hosp Pall Care.* 2004;21(1):40–46.

56. National Comprehensive Cancer Network. *NCCN clinical practice guidelines in oncology: Distress management.* V.1.2008. http://www.nccn.org/professionals/physician_gls/PDF/distress.pdf. Accessed on April 29, 2008.

57. National Comprehensive Cancer Network. *NCCN clinical practice guidelines in oncology: Palliative care.* V.1.2008. http://www.nccn.org/professionals/physician_gls/PDF/palliative.pdf. Accessed on April 29, 2008.

58. Turk DC, Feldman CS. A cognitive-behavioral approach to symptom management in palliative care. In: Chochinov HM, Brietbart W, (eds). *Handbook of psychiatry in palliative medicine.* New York: Oxford University Press; 2000: 223–240.

59. Jarrett N, Payne S, Turner P, Hillier R. 'Someone to talk to' and 'pain control': what people expect from a specialist palliative care team. *Pall Med.* 1999;13(2):139–144.

60. Twillman RK, Cohen BA, Barnett ML. The biopsychosocial model of pain and pain management. In: Lipman AG, (ed). *Pain management for primary care clinicians.* New York: American Society of Health-System Pharmacists; 2004.

61. Bertman S. *Grief and the healing arts creativity as therapy.* Amityville, NY: Baywood Publishing Company Inc; 1999.

62. Otis-Green S. Legacy building. *Smith Coll Stud Soc Work.* 2003;73(3): 395–404.

63. Williams BR. Dying young, dying poor: a sociological examination of existential suffering among low-socioeconomic status patients. *J Pall Med.* 2004; 7(1):27–37.

64. Smedley BD, Stith AY, Nelson AR, (eds). *Unequal treatment: Confronting racial and ethnic disparities in health care.* Washington DC: National Academy Press; 2003.

65. Doorenbos AZ, Schim SM. Cultural competence in hospice. *Am J Hosp Pall Care.* 2004;21(1):28–32.

66. Ferrell BR, Virani R, Grant M, et al. Evaluation of the end-of-life nursing education consortium undergraduate faculty training program. *J Pall Med.* 2005;8(1):107–114.

67. Paice JA, Ferrell BR, Virani R, Grant M, Malloy P, Rhome A. Graduate nursing education regarding end-of-life care. *Nurs Outlook.* 2006;54(1):46–52.

68. Malloy P, Ferrell BR, Virani R, et al. Evaluation of end-of-life nursing education for continuing education and clinical staff development educators. *J Nurs Staff Develop.* 2006;22(1):31–36.

69. MacDonald DJ, Sand S, Kass FC, et al. The power of partnership: Extending comprehensive cancer center expertise in clinical cancer genetics to breast care in community centers. *Semin Breast Dis.* 2006;9:39–47.

70. Grant M, Hanson J, Mullan P, Spolum M, Ferrell B. Disseminating end-of-life education to cancer centers: overview of program and of evaluation. *J Cancer Edu.* 2007;22(3):140–148.

71. Grant M, Economou D, Ferrell B, Bhatia S. Preparing professional staff to care for cancer survivors. *J Cancer Surviv: Res Prac.* 2007;1(1):98–106.

72. Otis-Green S, Ferrell B, Spolum M, et al. An overview of the ACE Project - advocating for clinical excellence: transdisciplinary palliative care education. *J Cancer Edu.*2009;24(2):120–126.

73. Hewitt M, Greenfield S, Stovall E. *From cancer patient to cancer survivor: Lost in transition.* Washington DC: The National Academy Press; 2005.

74. Otis-Green S, Lucas S, Spolum M, Ferrell B, Grant M. Promoting excellence in pain management and palliative care for social workers. *J Soc Work End-of-Life Pall Care.* 2008;4(2):120–134.

75. Knowles MS. *The adult learner: A neglected species.* Houston, TX: Gulf Publishing; 1973.

PART XIV

Ethical Issues

Marguerite S. Lederberg, ED

CHAPTER 89

Care Ethics: An Approach to the Ethical Dilemmas of Psycho-Oncology Practice

Antonella Surbone

SUMMARY

In a 1990 editorial in the *New England Journal of Medicine* about ethical imperialism in medical, the Editor, Dr. Marcia Angell, wrote that *"Knowledge, although important, may be less important to a respectable society than the way it is obtained."*[1] Clinical practice is based on medical knowledge, which should always be taught in compliance with the ethical standards that have developed over time in response to the medical abuses that have been perpetrated throughout history. Furthermore, clinical activities involve a complex and emotionally laden relationship between two or more human beings who are deeply, but asymmetrically, engaged. Hence, clinical practice must constantly be held to high ethical standards in all areas: the physical, intellectual, psychological, and moral dimensions that coexist in human relationships.

Learning the basics of bioethics and the complexities of bedside ethical dilemmas must become a standard part of the expertise of psycho-oncologists. The aim of this chapter is, first, to offer a balanced and comprehensive review of the theoretical basis of bioethics, with special reference to care ethics, and to provide insight into the application of such principles in negotiating and solving the most common ethical dilemmas encountered in oncology practice. Second, the chapter analyses the role of cross-cultural differences in many bedside ethical problems. As cultural differences in disclosure of information to cancer patients are common, an in-depth discussion of truth telling serves to illustrate the influence of culture on ethical norms. Throughout the chapter, I reference clinical cases encountered in my own practice as a medical oncologist in the United States and in Italy to illustrate common difficulties in ethical deliberation. Some information has been modified to protect patients' confidentiality.

INTRODUCTION

The word "ethics" derives from ancient Greek, which could mean either "custom" or "character," and was used to refer to the appropriate norms of conduct in all aspects of life.[2] Ethics has always had a relevant role in medicine. The Hippocratic Oath of 420 BC, considered to be the first document of medical ethics in western cultures was based on the paternalistic role of physicians, who held center stage in the patient–doctor relationship, and swore not to harm their patients and to provide them beneficent care, according to their best judgement.[3] The next authoritative western document on medical ethics was the *Code of medical ethics* written by Sir Thomas Percival in 1803, which also considered professional conduct in hospitals.[4] The American Medical Association published its first *Code of ethics* in 1847, subsequently revised it, and updates it regularly to meet the new challenges posed by rapid developments in modern medicine.[5]

In contrast with the Hippocratic tradition, modern western medicine has moved from a paternalistic to a participatory model, where patients and physicians share rights and responsibilities within the therapeutic relationship. Doctors must always strive to respect the patient's autonomy while they face the many ethical issues that may arise throughout the course of the patient's illness. The word "bioethics," from the Greek bios = life and ethos = ethics, was coined by the U.S. oncologist Potter in 1971, who applied it in a descriptive, naturalistic way to all ethical issues related to medicine and biotechnologies.[6] Bioethics has since rapidly grown into a well-defined scholarly field, with many different theories and schools of thoughts. Bioethics is now integrated in most medical curricula, and it is taught in dedicated courses for health professionals at all major medical schools worldwide.

New medical interventions have positively changed the fate of humankind through the rise of new biotechnologies and the expansion of diagnostic and therapeutic possibilities. However, they bring a greater moral responsibility regarding health-related matters, since biomedical interventions can also be inappropriate or create new problems at the ethical and social levels. Consider the example of genetic testing for cancer predisposition: on the one hand, it may enable members of high-risk families to find out whether they carry genetic mutations allowing them to engage, if they choose, in measures of prevention or early diagnosis. On the other hand, experts, patients, and the public have expressed concern about the value of cancer genetic testing, because of the potential for negative repercussions at the psychosocial and ethical levels.[7] Mutation carriers, for example, may be subject to different forms of discrimination. *A BRCA positive patient told me she was equally worried about passing onto her daughters the risk of cancer, and of their being exposed to discrimination because of her diagnosis. "With good laws, she said, my daughters may find great jobs, but they may still not be seen as ideal spouses or mothers."* Until recently, many at-risk individuals have foregone genetic testing for cancer susceptibility to avoid potential discrimination. Most medical societies, including the American Society of Clinical Oncology, have therefore cautioned physicians and strongly advised them to inform all patients of the potentially negative psychological, social, and ethical implications of genetic testing, including the risk of genetic discrimination.[7] In many countries, such as in the United States, where the Genetic Information Nondiscrimination Act (GINA) was approved by Congress on May 1st 2008, legislators have relied on the contributions of bioethicists to address the ethical issues raised by the new developments in genetics.[8]

Bioethics is, in fact, related to both medicine and the law, in its four main functions and scopes. First, in its analytic function, bioethics evaluates relevant innovations in medicine and biotechnologies with regard to the range of morally acceptable actions and of the possible constraints to such actions. Second, bioethics provides methodological and procedural guidelines to healthcare professionals: not necessarily offering predetermined solutions, but rather teaching ways to tackle different ethical issues in clinical practice. Third, in its pragmatic function, bioethics looks for practical solutions to bedside ethical dilemmas, taking into account the different perspectives of the involved parties. Fourth and finally, bioethics has an anticipatory function with regard to the directions that medicine may take: it explores and debates the potential moral and social consequences of new and developing medical interventions and technologies.

BIOETHICS AND THE PATIENT–DOCTOR RELATIONSHIP

In 1988, Drs. Pellegrino and Thomasma in their pivotal textbook of bioethics entitled *"For the patient's good: The restoration of Trust in Medicine"* assert that the philosophical foundations of bioethics are rooted in the nature of the patient–doctor relationship.[9] The relationship is based on the fiduciary act that arises when a person in need—the patient—seeks the help of a fellow human being—the physician—who has specific medical knowledge and expertise. Patients and physicians establish a therapeutic alliance based on reciprocal obligations in view of a common therapeutic goal. Within their alliance, they trust each others as fellow human beings, with both reason and emotions, who are committed to the same healing purpose.

In opposition to the old paternalistic model, today we increasingly see the patient–doctor relationship in terms of a partnership based on patient's autonomy and right to share in decision making.[9,10] The nature of this relationship, however, is not to be interpreted as a usual contract among peers, but rather a covenant—historically, a special form of contract that entails a moral obligation bound by reciprocal trust, despite the differing roles of those involved.[9] The patient–doctor relationship is an asymmetric relationship of help. Asymmetry between patient and doctor has three main dimensions: the existential one, related to the different positions that patient and doctor have with respect to illness; the epistemic one, related to their different degrees of knowledge and expertise with regard to the patient's illness; and the social one, related to their respective roles within the relationship and with respect to society.[11] A power imbalance results from the asymmetry in the patient–doctor relationship, and reciprocity is born out of a special connection between nonequal partners.[12]

ETHICAL DELIBERATION IN CLINICAL MEDICINE AND THE ROLE OF PRINCIPLES

Ethical deliberation in clinical medicine is a complex process that requires knowledge, principles, and virtues. Illness enhances vulnerability and dependence, making care and trust indispensable, particularly as ethical issues and dilemmas arise.[13,14] These deliberations require open discussion and honest mediation[15] and it must always be kept in mind that patients and doctors do not necessarily share similar values or norms. When cross-cultural differences give rise to bedside misunderstandings or even conflicts, it has been said that *"the patient and the physician must negotiate their different views of illness and of health, as well as their different perceptions of the patient-doctor relationship, to achieve their common therapeutic goal."*[16]

Ethical deliberation in clinical contexts often makes use of the so called *prima facie* principles of *nonmaleficence, beneficence, autonomy,* and *justice*. These four principles were first applied to bioethics by Beauchamp and Childress in their textbook entitled *"Principles of Biomedical Ethics."*[10] They are called *prima facie* principles, because they are essential, basic ethical principles that may come into conflict; one principle can render the others inoperative. The high degree of universality and practicality of these four principles provides a basic framework for the resolution of ethical dilemmas within existing pluralism, although they may conflict with each other. For example, a cancer patient or his or her family may demand additional chemotherapy at an advanced stage of cancer, while the physician believes that continued treatment would not be beneficial to the patient, and potentially even harmful. In this instance, the principles of autonomy and beneficence come into conflict.

Moreover, the same *prima facie* principle could be invoked to justify opposing ethical choices at the bedside.[17] In truth telling to cancer patients, either disclosure or nondisclosure can be justified in the name of autonomy or beneficence, when applied to different individual and cultural contexts. In certain cultures outside the Anglo-American world, withholding information is considered an act of beneficence to protect cancer patients from painful truths and their possible negative psychological consequences. By contrast, in most industrialized countries, informing patients is considered the physicians' duty, because it respects patient autonomy.[18] The principles of autonomy and beneficence, in this and many other cases, are in fact interrelated, rather than conflicting.[19] Full disclosure to the patient is simultaneously an act of autonomy and beneficence, as it gives the patient information enabling him to make the best choices according to his own values.[17] Thus, while the principles of bioethics can be a very useful tool for a preliminary reading of clinical ethical dilemmas, ethics of virtue and care are necessary to account for the complexity of ethical deliberation in clinical medicine.

ETHICS OF CARE AND RELATIONAL AUTONOMY

Care ethics, born out of the major contributions of women philosophers to contemporary moral debate, is based on the recognition that not all the relationships that we establish in our life are symmetrical.[12,14,20,21] Throughout the course of our lives, we also engage in relationships

---

Textbox 89–1. Relational autonomy means that:

We define and exercise our *autonomy* within the context of our *connectedness* to others.
Autonomy is more than a matter of individual *rights and choices*.
Autonomy refers to the capacity *to make choices* and the *possibility of enacting them*.
Both *internal factors* and *external resources* contribute to one's autonomy.

---

where our vulnerability is at stake and we need to establish trust in other people from whom we receive help and assistance. Care ethics, which has been successfully applied to clinical practice and the patient–doctor relationship, starts with the recognition of the asymmetry of knowledge and power between patients and health professionals. The patient–doctor relationship is a concrete relationship between "particular others," each with a body, mind, and soul.[13,21] Patients do not consult a doctor to acquire general medical knowledge, but to find specific answers and gain an understanding of their particular illness. Physicians respond to patients in view of their knowledge and personal expertise on a certain illness or treatment.[22] Equality in the patient–doctor relationship is different than equality among peers, and it rather arises from the relationship itself.

Care ethics in clinical medicine also takes into account the relational nature of patient autonomy.[18,23–25] Autonomy has traditionally been understood in terms of an individual's right to make his or her own choices. The act of choosing is meaningless without action, as an individual's choices influence, and result from, many internal, external, and contextual variables: Choice does not occur in a vacuum. As a result, understanding autonomy in a relational way entails not only recognizing the importance of the responsibilities that arise from our connections to others, but also acknowledging the internal and external factors that shape our choices, while respecting varying cultural, socio-economic, and contextual aspects of decision making (Textbox 89–1).

For example, a woman who has discovered that she carries a *BRCA* mutation predisposing her to a very high chance of developing breast or ovarian cancer, will not only make decisions about the best prevention and management of her own health, but will also be faced with the question of whether to inform her children and relatives, who may also carry the same genetic mutation and future cancer risks.[7] A lung cancer patient living in a rural area may be offered the chance to participate in a clinical trial run at a distant cancer center. The patient may wish to enroll in the trial, yet he is living alone and is limited by financial and transportation issues, which ultimately prevent him from participation. For many female cancer patients who are mothers with multiple responsibilities, participation in clinical trials may depend on external factors such as the availability or affordability of child care. *I once offered palliative care to one of my long-time patients with extensive metastatic breast cancer, who had been through multiple unsuccessful chemotherapy and radiation treatments over the course of several years. She told me that she agreed with me about the futility of trying to a different chemotherapy, except for the fact that she was the only caregiver to her two handicapped sons, both in their twenties. To her, even one extra day of life was worth.*

Care ethics in clinical medicine is based upon *attention, responsibility, responsiveness, integrity,* and *trust.* Patients should be able to trust their physicians and healthcare professionals, institutions, and healthcare structures, but also science itself. Care ethics is not always sufficient to cover all domains of bioethics, but can be extremely helpful in providing guidance in bedside dilemmas. Care ethics utilizes the guiding moral principles of bioethics, with the principle of justice serving as the unifying element in ethical dilemmas that arise due to the relational aspects of care ethics.[25]

ETHICAL DILEMMAS IN ONCOLOGY PRACTICE

Ethical dilemmas in medicine are extremely complex and are often magnified in oncology by several factors: the severity of the illness and the negative metaphoric implications that a cancer diagnosis may carry within a patient's cultural context; the physical and psychological suffering of the patient, which can become extreme during difficult treatments or at end of life; the medical, psychological, and social ramifications of living with cancer, including social stigmatization and discrimination; the uncertainty related to cancer prognosis and treatment, standard or experimental; the use of multimodal therapies that result in fragmentation of care and subsequent involvement with many oncology professionals; and finally, the patient's difficulty in attempting to balance her desire to be involved in her own care with the desire to be guided by oncologist while still feeling respected and supported in the psychological and spiritual journey through and with cancer.[18]

Many of the ethical dilemmas that oncology professionals encounter in clinical practice relate to different aspects of communication and information with cancer patients. These can arise from a wide range of issues, such as: diagnosis and prognosis; decision making in different phases of cancer, especially regarding end-of-life care, experimental treatments, and integrative therapies; and counseling about genetic risks and testing (Textbox 89–2).

Dilemmas may also arise from cultural differences between patients and members of their treating oncology teams.[16,26,27] For example, giving bad news to an uninformed cancer patient whose family has requested the physician not to do so, is an example of cultural insensitivity often encountered in multicultural oncology practices. *In my clinical practice, I find myself presenting the information to cancer patients and their families differently, depending on whether I am practicing in Italy or in the United States, where the cultural expectations are still divergent. In the United States I am often expected to convey statistical information on risks and prognosis during the initial chemotherapy consultation, while in Italy this would generally be inappropriate, as patients may feel overwhelmed and confused by such information, rather than helped.* High ethical standards in communication require that oncologists avoid being blunt and, rather, convey information in a sensitive timely manner. The notion of "offering the truth" to cancer patients, based on allowing individual patients to choose their own paths, has been proposed as an effective way to respect patients' autonomy in light of their own cultural norms.[28] But a closer understanding of care ethics would lead one the patient context and culture carefully before following any predetermined route in a straight line.

CROSS-CULTURAL DIFFERENCES IN ONCOLOGY AND THE IMPORTANCE OF CULTURAL COMPETENCE

Cross-cultural encounters in the clinic are increasingly frequent and they are reported as a common source of bedside ethical dilemmas. Cultural differences between patients and health care professionals may give rise to conflicts with respect to truth telling, end-of-life choices, prevention and screening, and involvement in clinical trials (Textbox 89–3).[16,29] The acquisition of knowledge and skills in delivering culturally sensitive care has, therefore, become a requirement in medical training in many increasingly multiethnic societies, such as the United States. The American Academy of Family Physicians *Guidelines on end of life care* states that *"Health professionals should recognize, assess, and address the psychological, social, spiritual and religious issues, and cultural taboos realizing that different cultures may require significantly different approaches."*[30]

Culture has profound implications in all aspects of society, and is present at many levels. For example, medicine, oncology, and psycho-oncology are all individual cultures: they each have their own language and status within. Depending on the extent to which the patient and the physician are engaged in their relationship, every clinical encounter is an exercise in cultural competence, as each person carries his own personal and cultural identity.[11] Cultural differences influence the interpretation of ethical principles and norms, especially with regard to the meaning and role of patient autonomy.[18,31]

Culture, described in complex ways in the anthropological and sociological literatures, can be defined as the sum of the integrated patterns of knowledge, beliefs and behaviors of a given community.[32] Culture influences our attitudes toward truth telling; the focus and style of decision making and end-of-life decisions; our views of the therapeutic relationship; and the trust we have in physicians, nurses, and institutions.[29] Cultural differences also play a significant role in the existing disparities in access to cancer care and research.[33]

The acquisition of cultural competence in oncology is a multilayered task that presupposes awareness *of one's own culture, beliefs, and values.* One cannot understand cultural differences without being aware of the culture of medicine. Cultural competence also requires the *acquisition of specific knowledge, skills, and attitudes*, and in individual caregivers, qualities *of humility, empathy, curiosity, respect, sensitivity, and awareness.* It needs awareness of the risks of stereotyping, *racism, classism, sexism, ageism, and many culture-specific prejudices* which, often contribute to a distorted view of culture.[29]

It has been shown that cultural competence improves appreciation of differences in healthcare values among people belonging to different cultures, furthers communication between patients and physicians, and facilitates the solution of ethical dilemmas in the clinic, which, in turn, leads to improved therapeutic outcomes and decreased disparities in medical care (Textbox 89–4).[33,34] These goals are better achieved if the caregivers are practicing in a culturally competent healthcare system, flexible enough to meet the needs of different patients or groups of patients.[33] Teaching cultural competence requires providing caregivers with relevant information about different cultures with respect to many health issues, including the role of patient autonomy, the involvement of families, and the meaning of suffering and dying. Patients themselves are the best teachers of their own beliefs and preferences.[29,34,35]

ETHICS OF TRUTH TELLING AND WORLDWIDE EVOLUTION OF ATTITUDES AND PRACTICES OF DISCLOSURE

Truth telling is at the core of bioethics. It relates to both the role of patient autonomy and to the influence of culture on the modulation and expression of ethical norms.[22] Bioethics originated within the Anglo-American context and its long standing tradition of respect for individual rights, including the right to self-governance, privacy, and personal liberties. Patients must be fully informed about their diagnosis, treatment options, risks, and prognosis, to be able to exercise their autonomy. Information leads to better patient participation in decision making and increases patient compliance and satisfaction.[36]

While the doctrine of informed consent was born in 1947 as a result of the Nuremberg Trial, a milestone study of truth-telling practices in the United States published in *JAMA* in 1961, showed that 10% of surveyed physicians would never reveal a cancer diagnosis.[37] Over the following two decades, physicians' truth-telling practices in the United States changed dramatically and in the late 1970s 98% of surveyed U.S. physicians revealed a cancer diagnosis to their patients.[38]

In nonwestern cultures, including some ethnic minorities within the United States, truth-telling attitudes and practices were rarely discussed until the late 1980s.[39] During the 1990s, numerous reports suggested major cross-cultural differences in truth telling.[40–42] In cultures centered on family and community values, the word "autonomy" was often perceived more as synonymous with "isolation" than of "freedom," and a protective role with respect to the ill person was attributed to families and physicians.[40] Basic information and bad news were often withheld from patients, or strongly censored, to avoid taking away hope or causing them severe distress, while physicians tended to tell the full truth only to one or two close relatives. In this "conspiracy of silence," doctors and relatives were often caught in the web of half-truths, and patients were left to suffer alone, deprived of the chance to ask questions and receive answers, put in order their affairs, or say good-bye to their loved ones.[40] Some patients responded heroically by becoming the protectors of those who are trying to protect them.

In my first years of oncology training patients were treated with state-of-art oncology therapies, yet I met several young women with bone metastases from breast cancer. Those patients had agreed to be treated for severe arthritis by doctors and family members who wanted to protect them from knowledge of their dire prognosis. Yet, a few of these women were clearly aware that their cancer had metastasized, but feigned ignorance because they wanted to protect their families and especially their small children. A 17-year-old boy with advanced lymphoma asked me not to disclose to his family the failure of his last treatment, something he had obviously perceived from the continuous growth of his lymph nodes and his increasing systemic symptoms. He asked to see me one night when I was on call and explained that his mother had already lost two small infants and she should be able to talk to him about his dead sisters until his last day. A middle-aged engineer with metastatic gastrointestinal (GI) cancer asked me to make a house call because of respiratory distress. When I arrived at his home, he was sitting quietly at his desk, and told me he needed to know the truth about his prognosis, because he had to make important work decision that would have affected his large family. He reassured me, though, that he would have never let them understand that we had spoken and that he knew the truth.

A dramatic shift in truth-telling attitudes and practices has occurred worldwide in the past two decades, especially in European, Middle Eastern, and Asian countries.[43] A 1999 study of western and nonwestern American Society of Clinical Oncology (ASCO) members attending the annual meeting showed no difference in disclosure rates of cancer diagnosis.[44] The reasons for the evolution of truth-telling attitudes and practices worldwide appear remarkably similar to those that determined the shift in the United States between the early 1960s and the late 1970s.[27] Among the main contributing factors are therapeutic advances in the field of oncology, growing public knowledge of the nature and treatment of cancer, adequate training of physicians in palliative and end-of-life care, increasingly strict legal requirements for information and informed consent, and patient and public activism.

The international literature now suggests that cancer patients across cultures share similar communication needs and preferences and that content, style, and setting are all essential aspects of communication. However, cross-cultural differences in truth-telling still persist, and literature reviews suggest that only a relative minority of cancer patients in nonwestern countries expect truthfulness about their illness or wish to participate in the decision making, as compared to an overwhelming majority in western countries.[45] Patients' awareness of the severity and curability of their cancer is reported as still poor in many countries. In addition, the actual rate of disclosure remains low even among physicians who believe in patients' right to information, as documented in a 2000 survey of 675 Northern Italian physicians conducted by Dr. Grassi and colleagues.[46] A 2008 study of Italian oncologists in southern and northern Italy, however, shows that most of them now inform their patients.[47]

Variability in truth-telling rates worldwide can be attributed to several factors: age and gender, urban versus rural residence, type of treating institution, and family involvement.[48] The extent and modalities of family involvement varies, and sometimes in some countries, families make decisions in place of the uninformed relative. In many countries, especially in Asia, the family is always consulted before revealing a cancer diagnosis to the patient, and many nonwestern families still oppose truth-telling to cancer patients.[15,49] A survey of the relatives of 150 Turkish cancer patients showed that 66% requested that the truth be withheld from the patient.[50] As families take part in the care of their sick relatives in every culture, they cannot be excluded from the process of information and communication unless it is the expressed wish of the patient.[51] A common ethical dilemma arises when a family requests the hospital staff not to disclose the truth to the cancer patient in a country, such as the United States, with strict requirements for informed consent.[26,27]

In my oncology clinic, I have met elderly cancer patients from nonwestern countries who wish to be informed of their treatment options, including ongoing clinical trials, despite their family's strong opposition. An Islamic patient, affected by metastatic breast cancer, who always came for her visits accompanied by several family members, once left me a note written in broken English that she knew exactly how widely spread was her cancer and that she didn't want any life support measures. In the note, she had also asked me not to tell her family about what she knew.

A recent study of a multicultural patient population being treated at a large cancer center, suggests that information should be tailored to individual, family, and community values, especially when dealing with specific requests to withhold or to downplay the truth.[26] However, oncology professionals must adhere to the ethical norms and legal requirements of their own country. If those norms see withholding the truth as an infringement on the patient's autonomy, they should explain to family members that they have a duty to inform the patient, but that they will do so gradually and with extreme sensitivity.[26,27] In most cases, it is advisable to ask cancer patients how much they wish to be informed, and it is important to repeat such question at different times during the course of the illness and treatment. Furthermore, in the course of a chronic illness such as cancer, which often entails frequent visits to specialists and periods of hospitalization, almost all patients will inevitably be told or will overhear the truth at some point. As a result, they may lose trust in the treating physicians and team members who have withheld information from them.[26,27]

CARE ETHICS AND THE ROLE OF CANCER PATIENTS' FAMILIES

Cancer affects not only sick individuals, but also their families. As Drs. Baider, Cooper, and Kaplan De-Nour discuss in their textbook *"Cancer and the Family,"* a successful healing process requires that physicians interact effectively with patients' families and loved ones.[52] Cancer alters the internal dynamics of the family, whose members, mostly women, take on increased care giving responsibilities, especially at the end of the cancer patient's life. It is therefore necessary to address the psychosocial and ethical needs not only of cancer patients, but also of their families and communities. Primary caregivers always deserve special attention.

In many cultures, patients' relatives are the first, and sometimes the only people, to receive adequate information, and may be the locus of decision making. Studies of sources of support for breast cancer survivors of differing ethnicities show differences in their perceptions of their own role within their families and of the importance of their families in helping them make important medical decisions.[53,54]

Each family has distinct informational needs, and requires guidance and support when faced with ethical dilemmas.[55,56] While the intervention of relatives may add a layer of complexity to the patient–doctor relationship, oncologist and psycho-oncologists now learn how to address the concerns of family members, while respecting patients' information and decision-making needs.[56]

CONCLUSION

Pluralism is an enriching reality in modern societies, but it has also become the source of major ethical quandaries in the practice of clinical oncology. In caring for cancer patients, oncologist and psycho-oncologists must learn to respect cultural differences without falling into cultural determinism or ethical relativism. As the basic principles of human dignity apply to all individuals in every social and cultural context, sensitivity to individual and cultural differences should not prevent oncology professionals from respecting and fostering their patients' rights to self-determination. They can do this by investing the time and energy to know their patients and understand their wishes, before ethical dilemmas arise. The adequate practice of care ethics is an ongoing process.

An ethics of principles, virtues, and care must also acknowledge the limitations of medicine and physician. Because the care ethics model values the role played by people outside the medical team in most healing processes, it always includes families, friends, and communities in ethical analysis and deliberation. The ethical role of families as the ultimate caregivers for our cancer patients can never be underestimated. Miscommunication and conflicts, however, can occur between cancer patients and family members. Improving understanding and concordance among patients, family caregivers, and physicians is part of the ethical responsibilities of oncology professionals. Psycho-oncologists have special professional qualifications and ethical duties to assess and clarify the underlying tensions that could lead to future ethical dilemmas, and to find shared solutions to ethical dilemmas on the basis of respect and trust.

REFERENCES

1. Angell M. "Ethical Imperialism?: Ethics In International Collaborative Clinical Research." *New Engl J Med.* 1988;319:1081–1083.

2. Aristotles. *Nichomachean ethics.* Ross D, trans. Oxford and New York: Oxford University Press; 1925.

3. Hippocrates. *Oath of Hippocrates.* In: WHS Jones, (eds). *Hippocrates.* Cambridge: University Press; Harvard 1868.

4. Percival T. *Medical ethics: A code of institutes and precepts, adapted to the professional conduct of physicians and surgeons.* Manchester: S. Russel; 1803.

5. American Medical Association. *History. Council on ethical and judicial affairs. Code of medical ethics. Current opinions with annotations.* American Medical Association; 1997:v–vi.

6. Potter VR. *Bioethics: Bridge to the future.* Englewood Cliffs, NJ: Prentice Hall; 1971.

7. American Society of Clinical Oncology. "Statement of the American Society of Clinical Oncology: Genetic Testing for Cancer Susceptibility." *J Clinic Oncol.* 1996;(14):1730–1736.

8. Hudson KL, Holohan MK, Collins FS. Keeping peace with the times—The Genetic Information Nondiscrimination Act of 2008. *N Engl J Med.* 2008;358:2661–2663.

9. Pellegrino ED, Thomasma DC. *For the patient's good: The restoration of beneficence in health care.* New York and London: Oxford University Press; 1988.

10. Beauchamp T, Childress JF. *Principles of biomedical ethics.* 4th ed. New York: Oxford University Press; 1994.

11. Surbone A, Lowenstein J. Asymmetry in the patient-doctor relationship. *J Clinic Ethics.* 2003;14:183–188.

12. Held V. "Feminism and Moral Theory." In: Kittay EF, Meyer D, (eds). *Women and moral theory.* Savage, MD: Rowman & Littlefield; 1987:111–128.

13. Pellegrino ED. Altruism, self interest, and medical ethics. *JAMA.* 1987;(258):1939–1940.

14. Baier A. Moral prejudices. Essays on ethics. Cambridge, Massachusetts & London, UK: Harvard University Press; 1994.

15. Edgar A. A discourse ethics approach to quality of life measurements. In: Surbone A, Zwitter M, (eds). *Communication with the cancer patient. Information and truth.* Annals of the New York Academy of Sciences; 1997:30–39.

16. Kagawa-Singer M, Blackhall LJ. Negotiating cross-cultural issues at the end of life. *JAMA.* 2001;286:2993–3001.

17. Tuckett AG. Truth-telling in clinical practice and the arguments for and against: a review of the literature. *Nurs Ethics.* 2004;11:500–513.

18. Surbone A. Telling truth to patients with cancer: what is the truth? *Lancet Oncol.* 2006;7:944–950.

19. Pellegrino ED. Is truth-telling to patients a cultural artifact? (Editorial) *JAMA.* 1992;268:1734–1735.

20. Noddings N. *Caring: A feminine approach to ethics and moral education.* Berkley: University of California Press; 1984:91–94.

21. Kittay EF. *Love's labor. Essays on women, equality and dependency.* New York and London: Routledge; 1999.

22. Surbone A. Truth telling. In: Cohen-Almagor R, (ed). *Medical ethics at the dawn of the 21st century.* New York: New York Academy of Sciences; 2000; 52–62.

23. Sherwin S. A relational approach to autonomy in health care. In: S Sherwin, Coordinator, The feminist health Care Ethics Research Network, *The politics of women's health: Exploring agency and autonomy.* Philadelphia: Temple University Press; 1988:19–44.

24. Donchin A. Understanding autonomy relationally: toward a reconfiguration of bioethical principles. *J Med Phil.* 2001;26:365–386.

25. Mahowald MB. *Genes, women, equality.* New York, Oxford: Oxford University Press, 2000.

26. Anderlik MR, Pentz RD, Hess KR. Revisiting the truth telling debate: a study of disclosure practices at a major cancer center. *J Clin Ethics.* 2000;11:251–259.

27. Surbone A. Cultural aspects of communication in cancer care. In: Stiefel F, (ed). *Communication in cancer care. Recent results in cancer research.* Heidelberg: Springer Verlag; 2006(168):91–104.

28. Freeman B. Offering truth. One ethical approach to the uninformed cancer patient. *Arch Intern Med.* 1993;153:572–576.

29. Kagawa-Singer M. A strategy to reduce cross-cultural miscommunication and increase the likelihood of improving health outcomes. *Acad Med.* 2003;78:577–587.

30. Russell Searight H, Gafford J. Cultural diversity at the end of life: issues and guidelines for family physicians. *Am Fam Physician.* 2005;71:515–522.

31. Blackhall LJ, Murphy ST, Frank G, Michel V, Azen S. Ethnicity and attitudes toward patient autonomy. *JAMA.* 1995;274:820–825.

32. Olweny C. The ethics and conduct of cross-cultural research in developing countries. *Psychooncology.* 1994;3:11–20.

33. Surbone A. Cultural competence: why? *Ann Oncol.* 2004;15:697–699.

34. Betancourt JR, Green AR, Carrillo JE, Ananeh-Firempong II O. Defining cultural competence: a practical framework for addressing racial/ethnical disparities in health and health care. *Public Health Rep.* 2003;188:293–302.

35. Betancourt JR. Cultural competence and medical education: many names, many perspectives, one goal. *Acad Med.* 2006;81:499–501.

36. Fallowfield LJ, Jenkins VA, Beveridge HA. Truth can hurt but deceit hurts more: communication in palliative care. *Palliat Med.* 2002;16:297–303.

37. Oken D. What to tell cancer patients. *JAMA.* 1961;175:1120–1128.

38. Novack DB, Plumer S, Smith Rl, Ochitill H, Morrow GR, Bennett JM. Changes in physicians' attitudes toward telling the cancer patient. *JAMA.* 1979;241:897–900.

39. Holland JC, Geary N, Marchini A, Tross S. An international survey of physician attitudes and practices in regard to revealing the diagnosis of cancer. *Cancer Invest.* 1987;5:151–154.

40. Surbone A. "Truth Telling To The Patient." *JAMA.* 1992;268:1661–1662.

41. Carrese J, Rhodes L. Western bioethics on the Navajo reservation: benefit or harm? *JAMA.* 1995;274:826–829.

42. Authors Various. In: Surbone A, Zwitter M, (eds). *Communication with the cancer patient: Information and truth.* 2nd ed. Baltimore: Johns Hopkins University Press; 2000.

43. Mystadikou K, Parpa E, Tsilila E, Katsouda E, Vlahos L. Cancer information disclosure in different cultural contexts. *Support Care Cancer.* 2004;12:147–154.

44. Baile WF, Lenzi R, Parker PA, Buckman R, Cohen L. Oncologists' attitudes toward and practices in giving bad news: an exploratory study. *J Clin Oncol.* 2002;20:2189–2196.

45. Surbone A. Persisting differences in truth-telling throughout the world. (Editorial) *Supp Care Cancer.* 2004;12:143–146.

46. Grassi L, Giraldi T, Messina EG, Magnani K, Valle E, Cartei G. Physicians' attitudes to and problems with truth-telling to cancer patients. *Supp Care Cancer.* 2000;8:40–45.

47. Bracci R, Zanon E, Cellerino R, et al. Information to cancer patients: a questionnaire survey in three different geographic areas in Italy. *Supp Care Cancer.* 2008;16:866–877.

48. Seo M, Tamura K, Shijo H, Morioka E, Ikegame C, Hirasako K. Telling the diagnosis to cancer patients in Japan: attitude and perceptions of patients, physicians and nurses. *Palliat Med.* 2000;14:105–110.

49. Ozdogan M, Samur M, Bozcuk HS, et al. "Do not tell": what factors affect relative' attitudes to honest disclosure of diagnosis to cancer patients? *Supp Care Cancer.* 2004;12:497–502.

50. Farber SJ, Egnew TR, Herman-Bertsch JL, Taylor TR, Guldin GE. Issues in end-of-life care: patient, caregiver and clinical perceptions. *J Palliat Medicine.* 2003;6:19–31.

51. Baider L, Cooper CL, De-Nour K. (eds). *Cancer and the family*. 2nd ed. Sussex, England: Wiley & Sons, Ltd; 2000.

52. Kagawa-Singer M, Nguyen TU. A cross-cultural comparison of social support among Asian-American and Euro-American women following breast cancer. In: Baider L, Cooper CL, De-Nour K, (eds). *Cancer and the family*. 2nd ed. Sussex, England: Wiley & Sons, Ltd; 2000.

53. Phipps E, Ture G, Harris D, et al. Approaching end of life: attitudes, preferences, and behaviors of African-American and White patients and their family care-givers. *J Clin Oncol*. 2003;21:549–554.

54. Surbone A. The role of the family in the ethical dilemmas of oncology. In: Baider L, Cooper CL, De-Nour K, (eds). *Cancer and the family*. 2nd ed. Sussex, England: Wiley & Sons, Ltd; 2000:513–534.

55. Clayton JM, Butow PN, Tattersall MHN. The needs of terminally ill patients versus those of caregivers for information regarding prognosis and end of life issues. *Cancer*. 2005;103:1957–1964.

56. Holland J, Johansen C, Surbone A, Baider L. Care giving in context. *Am Soc Clinic Oncol Educational Book*. 2006;27:151–163.

Negotiating the Interface of Psycho-Oncology and Ethics

Marguerite S. Lederberg

INTRODUCTION

The name psycho-oncology defines the interface between the challenges of cancer and cancer treatment, and the human stresses it engenders. It ranges from relatively calm periods, through the whole gamut of human experience with illness, sometime cure, but sometimes the slide into death. This still young discipline has grown in response to those stresses, endured by patients, their families, and in a different way, the medical caregivers.

The runaway success of medical science in improving care and survival of cancer is cause for celebration. But it continues to bring, at an accelerating rate, situations which cannot be foreseen. Not only unknown, many of them are unimaginable until their dramatic appearance into clinical situations. Novel situations generate novel problems. We must never forget that the most difficult ones are unrelated to science per se. But they are deeply connected to humanity's inadequacy in managing the socio-cultural, psychological, and ethical correlates of scientific advances.

In the clinical setting, these inadequacies translate into new ethical questions. This chapter will review the special features of the psycho-oncology hospital and clinic settings and will outline a method that helps the consultant who is called into an intense, complicated situation where physical, psychological, and moral issues are all in play and the participants are highly invested and emotionally involved.

BOUNDARIES IN THE IN-PATIENT SETTING

Characteristics of a hospital stay. During a patient's hospital admission, the patient, family, and staff are thrown together for days at a time during which severe physical and emotional suffering is endured and life-changing decisions are required. Privacy vanishes, as patients become dependent, regressed, and in pain. They are deeply frightened, sometimes repelled by their body, confused about their condition, their future, and what difficult treatments await them. Yet they are often asked to make major decisions from this tenuous platform.

Families linger anxiously, some angry, some exhausted by grief, offering various ratios of support to intrusiveness. The demand of their caregiving role often cause major disruptions in family life. They will have long-lasting consequences. When the patient no longer has capacity, the decisional role some of them must assume often leaves them with a sense of guilt and responsibility that the years will not extinguish.

Lastly the staff become more intimately involved with all the participants.[1] They become witness to intimate moments and painful conflicts that are normally private, and are sometimes even drawn into family dramas. The poignancy and intensity of what they share may resonate with their own life experiences, leading to an emotional involvement that is deeper than they realize. Such involvement, conscious or not, often has an impact on case management.

This is the milieu in which psycho-oncologists are called to function. They must be able to involve themselves deeply enough to understand all the dynamics, yet keep themselves apart enough to remain objective. It becomes easier over time, but self-awareness should always be part of their evaluation and training.

About boundaries. The way young psychotherapists learn to maintain their objectivity begins with understanding and respecting boundaries.

Much has been written about them and many ethical codes created to clarify them. Some writers are concerned about too much looseness, citing the "slippery slope" problem, while others worry that too much rigidity is an obstacle to treatment.[2] Boundary events have been broken down into two categories, boundary violations versus boundary crossings.[3] The first includes blatantly inappropriate acts like sexual contact that demand a corrective response when they are exposed, no matter what their context.

On the other hand, a boundary crossing is "a deviation from classical therapeutic activity that is harmless, nonexploitative and possibly supportive of the therapy itself."[4] The harm, if there is any, will derive not from the action itself, but from the patient's subjective experience of it. Therefore context is all important.[3,4] When the therapist is fully aware of himself and is keeping the patient's welfare at the forefront of his thinking, boundary crossings should not disturb the therapeutic frame, and may actually help the therapy. Even when an action is misjudged, if the therapist takes responsibility and immediately opens a dialogue to clarify and rectify the situation, it does not automatically qualify as a boundary violation. It demands careful self-examination and possibly consultation for the therapist.[5] The therapist must remain responsible for maintaining the proper setting.[4]

A psychiatry resident or psychotherapy trainee's first exposure to boundaries is the protocol of the interview. She is taught a physical, verbal, mental, and emotional discipline that prevents distractions and keeps the focus firmly on the patient's therapeutic needs. It is awkward at first, but its benefits become clear over time and each therapist develops her personal way of honoring them.

Boundaries with in-patients. However, hospital settings make a mockery of the usual guidelines. Boundaries are often nearly dissolved and must be renegotiated repeatedly because of forced intimacy. The therapist comes upon a patient who may be lying in pain and poorly covered because she cannot change positions, preoccupied with catheters and drains, and intent upon getting the attention of the nursing staff. Helping with sheets and pillows to ease pain and protect privacy, alerting the nursing staff to problems, and delaying the interview if needed is an appropriate prologue to the requested interview.

The patient's body has become her constant preoccupation. She needs to talk about it and may even occasionally expose a part of it. If the therapist is not comfortable in managing the situation, the patient will feel embarrassed and humiliated. But keep in mind that even a well-covered patient is vulnerable to feeling the same way, given the powerlessness of the patient position. Recognizing this, the therapist must demonstrate genuine comfort with the patient's physical situation, without any undue familiarity. It is humane, but also establishes rapport with the patient. After all, the therapist will ask the patient to discuss very intimate things with only a curtain to provide a semblance of privacy. An interviewer who displays a comfortable level of interest and supportiveness for the patient's gritty physical reality will inspire trust and develop a deeper understanding of the patient.

Boundaries crossings are inevitable in psychosomatic medicine and the therapist must deal with them in a way that make them benign or better yet, therapeutic. If he feels confident about his goals, he may institute boundary crossings himself. But the psychiatrist cannot forget that some aspects of showing respect for the patient in this setting would be considered a violation in another. The patient's welfare must remain uppermost and the therapist should always be clear about what he is doing and why he is doing it. Making the switch from office to medical hospital setting, and back again, does not always come naturally. Some elaboration is needed to make the shift a more conscious and comfortable one for all therapists.

Boundaries between the psycho-oncologist and medical staff. The first lesson a medical student learns in the hospital is the importance of accurate chart notes to good patient care. Once she becomes a psychiatry resident, that same student is told about the absolute duty to honor patient confidentiality. It is an ethical obligation for the whole medical profession which is firmly buttressed by law and cultural expectation. But it has special significance for psychiatrists who deal with the thoughts and feelings that patients do not share with anyone else. Thus, having gracefully navigated the intrusion on the patient's physical privacy, the psycho-oncologist must now negotiate the sharing of his emotional privacy.

The psychiatric consultant owes a duty to the physician who called for him. Yet he also owes a duty to the patient. If he foresees a conflict between the two, as when he must disclose something the patient is doing that could impact negatively on his care, he must inform the patient about what he must do. The problem of dual agency must be recognized and managed with careful attention. Cancer patients who are sick enough to be hospitalized usually cooperate when given clear explanations as to why the disclosure is in their best interest.

With less controversial aspects of the history, it is clear that all facts necessary to optimize medical care must be shared. There must be enough documentation to support the diagnosis and recommendations, but the level of personal detail can be minimal. A history of substance abuse must be documented, but particular incidents can be left out if they do not add something definitely useful. A difficult relationship should be noted if it clarifies aspects of case management. Care must be taken to protect the privacy of individuals who figure in the patient's narrative, whether family member or friend. Other people's names should not appear in the chart unless needed as contacts.

Some therapists write generic notes with the minimum personal information. But it can be useful to add certain positive highlights that will humanize the patient and elicit a warmer, more individualized response from the staff, while enhancing the patient's connection to his healthy self. It is good for the patient if a nurse or house officer walks in saying: "I hear you used to be a tennis champion. That's terrific!" On the other hand, if the patient is currently famous, write-ups must be circumspect and discussions among the staff who are becoming close to VIP, must be dampened to avoid accidental breaches of confidence in the nursing station.

Boundaries between medical staff and patient/family. During a hospital stay, the medical caregivers assume enormous importance to the patient and family for whom the interactions are highly emotionally loaded. Some families argue, criticize, and reject, others attach themselves and try to extract more of an emotional response from the staff members. The latter's own reactions range from the most common comfort zone of friendly neutrality to much deeper personal feelings that can be problematic, whether they are positive or negative. Decision making can be impaired and intrastaff conflicts may develop around the favorite patient as readily as around the difficult patient. It is the overinvolvement that matters, not its valence! The psycho-oncologist may be in a position to recognize some of the latent issues and can help the team reach a consensus, trying to focus on events rather than individuals.

Therapist boundaries with families. The boundaries faced by therapists in dealing with families are multidimensional, variable, and sometimes conflicting. Family members sleep in the room; some haunt the corridors for many hours. How many individuals are involved? How do they relate to each other—to the patient?—to the staff? What is the patient's understanding of his separateness or closeness to his family as a group and as individuals? What does he want whom to know? How does the therapist evaluate the dynamics when answering anxious questions? How does he deal with conflicted families? Even when families are in

harmony, misunderstandings may occur, so he must consciously direct his communications toward bringing members closer to each other, not accidentally driven apart in confusion.

This requires spending time with them in the room or the hallway together and/or individually. There is no escaping family members. Nor should they be escaped. Some are devoted allies, others intrude with their own needs or inject family stressors into the hospital room. How far does the psycho-oncologist go to protect the patient? Especially a weak and conflicted patient? How deeply should the psycho-oncologist be involved in supporting needy family members? He should play a role in dealing with any family member who interferes with patient care or is disruptive to the ward milieu, working closely with the staff, social work, and security as necessary. But his responsibility extends to inquiring about care for the disturbed person, encouraging it, offering a referral and answering other family member's questions. He continues to explore the situation and give support to patient and family at the bedside and outside the room, if the ward does not have a dedicated space. If he prescribes medication, he should realize that he now has an ethical and fiduciary responsibility for his patient. It is not wise to do it casually, and many, though not all hospitals have rules against it, unless the family member formally registers as a patient. Even then, one should be very selective. There are situations where it might be the best thing to do, such as for a family member who is far from home, without any resource of her own, and anxious to the point of interference with her own well-being and her supportive role for the patient. She can register, and when she returns home, she would be given a local referral. Therapists in private practice or working in a small clinic may not have any choice. Judgements are always required despite the lack of obvious guidelines.

The patient's wishes must be determined, in as much detail as necessary. Respecting them is both a moral duty and a legal requirement. When family relations are close and the patient able to communicate, it can be easy. Everyone is on the same team. But families are not always harmonious. In many Western cultures, there is a primary duty to honor the patient's desires, and a secondary duty to minimize the distress of the family members as much as possible. In other cultures, individuals are raised to defer to the good of a unit greater than themselves and honoring an alternate good is culturally acceptable or even expected. Modern mores require that medical caregivers be culturally competent, hence able to work within the patient's cultural framework.

When the patient loses decisional capacity about his medical care, or manifests a rapidly shifting mental state, constant efforts must be made to improve patient capacity, but decisions cannot always wait and the need for a designated health proxy is obvious. Lacking one, a good surrogate may present himself. But when none appears, the therapist must use his skills to elicit the optimal solution among the available family members and other sources of support.

In some venues, a generic list of succession dictates who should be the next in line to be proxy is. But medical caregivers who have worked with indifferent, unprepared, unwilling, or personally incapable proxies know that patients deserve better than this, and they will make every effort to negotiate a better compromise.

BOUNDARIES IN THE OUT-PATIENT SETTING

Boundaries between doctor and patient. In the clinic with patients who are currently well enough to come for appointments, there is much less exposure and less intensity. Hence, boundaries can function as they do in standard psychotherapy. But wheelchair patients are common, as are some who are too fatigued or in too much pain to concentrate on anything else. The therapist should be solicitous of any ill patient who has made the effort to attend an out-patient session, making him as comfortable as possible and gearing the interview to his level of tolerance. Checking in with a frail patient about his comfort during the session is perfectly appropriate. In fact, cancellations due to ill health are accepted unless they are being clearly abused and phone consults are more readily arranged, although they are seldom as useful as face to face sessions.

Therapy proceeds with the standard ground rules, except that doctor and patient share an intense interest in the cancer experience which both may pursue actively. The therapist is more likely to remain in close touch with the oncologist and be openly directive to insure that the patient sees the appropriate physicians. The dual agency problem remains unchanged and the rules of confidentiality should be followed with the same care as on the ward. But patients may see their psychotherapist more often than their other doctors, a fact which may facilitate a more timely referral.

Termination. Since cancer is a chronic disease, even patients who live far away will reappear, so continuity is an issue.

Many patients have a positive transference with the therapist and want to begin dealing with preexisting psychological issues. Whether to proceed or not depends on the therapist and the demands of his particular position. If possible, he should continue to treat the patients who is actively ill or has a poor prognosis. But he may transfer the patient who can realistically hope for a cure or a significant remission and will do as well as dealing with life issues near home.

With patients who have been coming for some time and are getting sicker without acknowledging it, the therapist must neither violate nor collude with their denial. She must remain alert for any hints or openings and be able to tolerate expressions of profound grief and fear. When they appear, being securely present is one of the most meaningful things a therapist can offer at this time, followed as it often is, by more openness and a certain sense of relief. However, unlike standard outpatient therapy, it is highly desirable to bring family members into this process.

Boundaries involving family members. Boundaries with family members are quite different from standard psychotherapy since the relatives are much more present and intimately involved. The patient may insist on their presence during the interview. Some of them insist on coming with the patient who usually agrees. The patient may need them, knowing that they are the only ones who can provide much of the information. Often the patient and selected relatives are interviewed separately. Maintaining each one's confidence may be difficult, and must be negotiated. Discussing the issue ahead of time, or asking permission to discuss some topics and explaining the reasons why, may be sufficient.

It is difficult when patients refuse to involve relatives who are essential to their care, yet are not legally incompetent. If the patient is unable to care for himself and the situation severe enough, their denial can be over ridden with or without any legal input depending on the country or culture involved. The psycho-oncologist will usually be involved and needs to be culturally sensitive and clear about all the laws and local regulations that bear on these issues.

But most patients are eager for support and the therapist is always well advised to inquire about, and meet the most involved family members, alone or in any combination deemed productive. Their information is critical to the management, and they are owed support as well, by reason of their need, even if it is not a legal requirement.

Family sessions are useful in all cases anyway, since good communication is such a fundamental feature of family and patient adjustment while silence or miscommunications are so common. Communication is the most efficient way to bring everyone to the same page while giving the therapist a much better insight into family dynamics, strengths, and weaknesses.

With very ill patients, all members of the family should receive attention because they are all living through an experience which will mark them for life. They may not all accept it, but some always do and the others may come onboard later. This includes all generations. Children in particular are often shunted aside "for their protection," a common self-protective maneuver from parents who are overwhelmed and cannot deal with their children. If the therapist is not comfortable with children or young adolescents, he should get access to someone who is. He can either refer the children or obtain supervision until he becomes more proficient. Frail grandparents or great-grandparents are also protected. If they are very ill themselves, and perhaps marginally competent, it is a family judgment call whether to expose them to such pain. But "protecting them" should not be an excuse. If they are healthier and will live long enough to find out anyway or even suspect something, or feel left out, they too should be included in a thoughtful, supportive way.

The emotional and ethical burden of end-of-life decision making on surrogate, proxies and family members is underestimated. Psychoeducation and support are essential to minimize their frequent guilt and exaggerated sense of responsibility for the outcome, feelings which remain vivid for decades like other kinds of traumatic learning.

Transitions between sites. Ideally, the same psycho-oncologist should follow the patient in both in and out-patient settings whenever possible. It becomes impossible when scattered sites are involved. The out-patient therapist must facilitate the transfer by alerting her in-patient colleagues and they, in turn, will refer the patient back to her upon discharge. When patients have moved to a new location for treatment, they will return periodically, so it is important for the same therapist to make herself available, while also helping them locate help in their home town. Both treatments should be coordinated and the therapist should play an active role to make it happen if the patient is not well enough to be proactive on his own behalf. When a therapist has followed a patient to the end of the road, it is often therapeutic to be very active in helping the patient accomplish end-of-life goals that he can no longer do alone. This is often described as "lending the patient your ego," something uniquely valuable at this time.

MAKING A SITUATIONAL DIAGNOSIS

Reactions to stress. Other than boundary issues which are inherent to the milieu, most of the ethical questions that arise in psycho-oncology are intimately embedded in the story of a given case, magnified by the high stress settings and the painful realities to be confronted by exhausted individuals thrown together in unnatural proximity.

In such conditions, ethical dilemmas generate dysfunctional psychological reactions strong enough to obscure the original ethical problem, generating a pseudo-psychiatry consultation. On the other hand, preexisting psychological dysfunction in patient and family may lead to ethical conflicts because of poor judgment and distorted communication, generating a pseudo-ethics consultation. The interactions are so fluid and bidirectional (see Fig. 90–1) that it may be difficult to accurately access the chain of events.[6] But in fact, many cases are complex and include both ethical and psychiatric elements.

There may be a large cast of characters, many with strongly held opinions. The level of involvement may be such that the patient is a silent figure in the eye of the emotional storm that involves not only family members, but also staff members whose neutrality has been moderately eroded by the intensity of the situation. Interference with care, visible emotional abuse, or neglect will generate strong responses in the staff, as will the iconic "difficult" patient. Staff involvement is usually responsive to clarification, while the family and patient may cling to powerful, predetermined emotional responses. The psychiatric consultant faced with such confusion does well to have a systematic way of establishing the chain of cause and effect. Otherwise, he is at risk for his own reactions to be co-opted by the most persuasive participant.

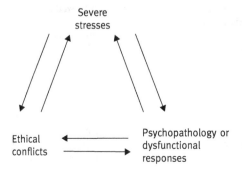

Fig. 90–1. Constant state of bidirectional flux between components of a complex clinical situation.[7]

Table 90–1. The situational diagnosis

Components of the situational diagnosis	Related interventions
I. Patient/ family issues: 1. Is there a psychological problem or treatable psychiatric disorder affecting the patient or any relevant family member? 2. Psychologically, what issues are driving the situation? 3. Whom do they involve?	**I. Patient/ family issues** • Establish patient's decisional capacity • If absent, treat and optimize it • Treat or refer acute psychiatric disorders in family members • If not, minimize and/or neutralize them • Answer questions and educate • Promote communication and mutual support • Address family conflicts as required
II. Staff issues: 4. Is there disagreement about medical management? 5. Is some other interstaff conflict being played out?	**II. Staff issues:** • Involve relevant caregivers • Discuss conflicts, focusing on issues, not individuals • Circumvent intrastaff/systemic issues unless discussion is required for patient care
III. Joint issues: 6. What is the nature of the relationship between the staff and the patient and family? 7. What is the understanding and explicit labeling of the issues by different participants?	**III. Joint issues:** • Explain patient/family issues to staff in ways that promote accurate empathy • Address overinvolvement and rejection, dealing with observable events rather than individuals • Recognize and minimize cultural/religious incongruences. Call in bridging cultural/religious figures • Allow everyone to ventilate
IV. Legal issues: 8. Are there laws or regulations, federal, state or local that impinge upon the case? 9. Are there institutional constraints that impinge upon the case? 10. Are there advances directives/proxy issues that need attention? 11. Could any of these create a potential conflict? What is the nature of that conflict?	**IV. Legal/institutional issues:** • Ensure that participants know and understand any of these constraints • Discuss their impact on the particular case • Clarify the advance directives situation • If needed and possible, complete them • Discuss the existing conflicts and resolve the ones that have a clear solution

Components and related interventions for the first four components of the situational diagnosis.

Table 90–2. Components of the ethical issues and related interventions

Ethical analysis	Related actions
Are there remaining conflicts that have not been addressed?	Identify the remaining issues
Do they involve moral values? What are they?	Identify the hierarchy of values, if needed.
If there is more than one moral conflict, which one should take priority?	Identify the major protagonist and the secondary ones
Who are the major protagonists?	If psychological issues are primary, explain the situation to all concerned
Who are secondary protagonists?	Then see if you can loosen the ethical stalemate
Is this issue leading to psychological problems or are they driving the moral conflict?	
If it is a moral conflict:	
What is the range of possible scenarios to respond to the primary conflict?	**If not, describe the range of scenarios to all participants in a narrative fashion that is easy to follow, along with their moral consequences. Facilitate constructive discussion**
What are the moral consequences of each one?	**Use legal or ethical consultation if stalemated**
How can all these options be most usefully described in a narrative fashion that will be followed by all participants?	
Address the second rank of moral conflicts unless they fade, once the major one is addressed	

The situational diagnosis is an organizational tool that can be used after the initial information has been collected to verify that nothing has been overlooked, to identify the psychological and ethical issues and to make an informed judgment about the chain of cause and effect. An accurate understanding of this sequence enable the psycho-oncologist to make better sense of the whole situation and to point his interventions more judiciously.

Using the situational diagnosis. The situational diagnosis has five components: (1) Patients and family issues (2) Staff issues (3) Joint issues (4) Legal/institutional issues and lastly (5) Ethical issues.[7] Table 90–1 outlines the first four in more detail and matches them with corresponding interventions. An educational component is always needed in all of them, that must match the needs and understanding of the parties involved. It is not included in the table because it is so individual to each

Table 90–3. Therapeutic approaches

Dealing with patient and family:
The family needs a nonjudgmental therapeutic approach, establishing what they understand and building on it
Involve religious or cultural bridging figures as needed (Keep a roster of different ones)
Dealing with staff:
Use this as a learning opportunity in staff meeting
Encourage an open lively discussion of the moral issues
Normalize variations if appropriate
Work to enable the staff to deal more effectively with the patient and family, and perhaps each other

Table 90–4. Basic principles guiding ethical analysis in the clinical setting

RESPECT FOR PERSONS: accepting the right of a person to decide what is done to his body
NONMALEFICENCE: the injunction against inflicting harm
BENEFICENCE: the duty to always act in the best interests of the patient
JUSTICE: the duty to treat all patients with the same dedication

case. Provision of information is critical to the emotional well-being of patients and families, and the earlier the better, before dysfunctional patterns become solidified.[7]

Working through the list of issues outlined in Table 90–1, identifies many problems. They may not be all resolved, but addressing them and thinking about them clarifies what needs to be done. Examples include

1. Establishing the need to get a family member into therapy
2. Seeing the need to defuse intrastaff issues at least sufficiently to allow more rational attitudes in this particular case
3. Humanizing the patient so the staff can become accurately empathic
4. Cutting through the confusion and floating affect to focus on legal requirement or firm institutional guidelines that are creating controversy.

After this analysis is completed, unaddressed issues will stand out clearly and these will be ethical dilemmas which are addressed in Part 5 of the situational diagnosis. See Table 90–2. Even when the conflicts emerge, they still deserve careful examination following the questions outlined in the table. One possible solution is mentioned in the right column which is that sometimes a careful discussion of the entire situation as it has been analyzed may be enough to loosen the ethical stalemate. This can occur because participants can alter their attitudes as their understanding of the dynamics of the situation improves. Otherwise, it may be necessary to use further legal or ethical consultation.

Each consultant will have his own personal style, however Table 90–3 describes guidelines that differentiate the therapeutic approach in dealing with patients and family versus the different methods that are effective with medical staff.

Ethical analysis. With the wide distribution of the first (1977) edition of Beauchamp's Principles of Biomedical Ethics, the principles of autonomy, nonmaleficence, beneficence, and justice, defined in Table 90–4, became widely adopted as guides to ethical analysis in most hospitals

and training programs.[8] Over time, some limitations became clearer and other theories were also expounded, leading to a more pluralistic approach. Autonomy is now called "respect for persons," a significant change because it narrows the definition to "an individual's freedom to decide what can be done to his body," which is not as overinclusive as autonomy had become over time. It no longer implies that the individual is a totally self-determining agent and leaves room for others such as family or community to have some standing. This has been promulgated in what is referred to as "care ethics" and its relevance is poignantly obvious in psycho-oncology.[9]

It should be noted that the basic principles are not derived from a comprehensive ethical theory. In particular, beneficence may be orthogonal to respect for persons. But when applied to a given situation, they have been found sufficiently comprehensive to insure that most issues are addressed, although they are geared to Western cultures. Ethics of care or a communitarian ethics may present other issues.[8] Any analysis must optimize them for the protagonists through a close examination of the situation that allows the consultant to answer the questions and carry out the tasks outlined in Table 90–2. Table 90–3 describes the different stances that distinguish transactions with the staff from those with patients families.

CONCLUSION

Consultation-liaison (C-L) psychiatry, as the clinical arm of psychosomatic medicine has been known, has always required an ability to move comfortably into different settings, relate to different medical teams, and deal with patients suffering from a multiplicity of acute diseases, injuries, fears, and losses. Psycho-oncologists are becoming increasingly integrated in medical, pediatric, and surgical oncology services, and are called more frequently for the very ill patients than the ones doing well. The relational, social, and intellectual demands of the work are added to the emotional impact of the human tragedies that engage them, tragedies that strike so ubiquitously that they are bound to hit home occasionally, even with the sturdiest practitioner. The fluidity of boundaries typical of this work, and the ever-present problem of dual agency make additional demands. Finally, the likelihood of having to make sense of stressful situations where one cannot always tell where psychological and ethical problems begin and stop, makes the task daunting indeed. This chapter has attempted to give some clarification about boundary issues and to provide tools to bring order to chaotic situations,[6,7] but self-monitoring and consultation, informal or otherwise, remain essential.

REFERENCES

1. Peteet J, Ross DM, Medeiros C, Walsh-Burke K, Rieker P. Relationships with patients in oncology: can a clinician be a friend? *Psychiatry.* 1992;55:223–229.
2. Glass L. The gray areas of boundary crosings and violations. *Am J Psychother.* 2003;57(4):429–444.
3. Gutheil T, Gabbard GO. Misuses and misunderstandings of boundary theory in clinical and regulatory settings. *Am J Psychiatry.* 1998;155(3):409–414.
4. Gutheil T, Simon RI. Non-sexual boundary crossings and boundary violations: the ethical dimension. *Psychiatr Clin N Am.* 2002;25:585–592.
5. Gutheil T, Gabbard GO. The concept of boundaries in clinical practice: theoretical and risk-management dimensions. *Am J Psychiatry.* 1993;150(2):188–196.
6. Lederberg M. Making a situational diagnosis: psychiatrists at the interface of psychiatry and ethics in the consultation-liaison setting. *Psychosomatics.* 1997;38(4):327–338.
7. Lederberg M. Disentangling ethical and psychological issues: a guide for oncologists. *Acta Oncologica.* 1999;38(6):771–779.
8. Beauchamp T. *Principles of biomedical ethics.* 1st ed. USA: Oxford University Press; 1977.
9. Winzelberg G, Hanson LC, Tulsky JA. Beyond autonomy: diversifying end-of-life decision-making approaches to serve patients and families. *JAGS.* 2005;53:1046–1050.

Research Ethics in Psycho-Oncology

Donald L. Rosenstein and Franklin G. Miller

INTRODUCTION

Clinical research is deeply integrated into the practice of oncology. Since President Nixon's 1971 declaration of a "war on cancer," the Federal government's funding of research into the causes and treatment of cancer, primarily through the National Cancer Institute (NCI), has grown to nearly five billion dollars a year.[1] There are now more than sixty NCI-designated Cancer Centers in the United States charged with conducting research, which typically operate in the same medical settings where standard (nonresearch) cancer care is provided.[2] In the case of pediatric oncology, over half of American children with cancer who are younger than 14 receive their treatment in clinical trials within a research network.[3] Over the past two to three decades, this tightly coordinated effort to standardize and improve cancer treatment for children and adolescents has contributed to a dramatic reduction in pediatric cancer mortality.[4] During this same timeframe, industry and foundation-sponsored funding of oncology research has grown in parallel with Federal funding and has fueled an expansion of cancer trials beyond academic medical centers to community-based oncology settings.

Despite the great complexity of cancer biology, research-driven advances in basic and translational science have led to major advances in cancer treatment. Furthermore, for some cancer patients, there might even be a "trial effect" such that participants in a research study have a better clinical outcome than nonparticipants.[5] Nonetheless, the nature of clinical research in oncology (i.e., how it is conducted, by whom and under what clinical and contextual circumstances) raises several ethical issues that are important to the practice of psycho-oncology. For example, psycho-oncologists (i.e., psychiatrists, psychologists, nurses, social workers, and other healthcare providers who work with cancer patients) are often asked to evaluate potential research subjects for their ability to provide informed consent for a research study or to render an opinion about whether emergent mood, cognitive or behavioral symptoms are attributable to an experimental cancer treatment. Today, clinically oriented psycho-oncologists are more likely than ever before to provide supportive care to cancer patients who are enrolled in a research study. In addition, there has been substantial recent growth in research protocols specifically focused on psychosocial aspects of cancer care. Consequently, the psycho-oncologist, either in her role as a clinician or an investigator, should have a meaningful appreciation of clinical research ethics and how these issues stem from the related but different goals of medicine and science.

Our aim in this chapter is to describe ethical issues in clinical research that are relevant to the psycho-oncologist and provide a general framework for the analysis of these issues. The premise underlying our approach is that the oncology setting is particularly conducive to a conflation of the ethics of medical care with the ethics of clinical research, based on a failure to appreciate the ethically significant differences between clinical research and medical care. In routine medical care, physicians are obligated to offer personalized therapy to particular patients consistent with the professional standard of care. Risks of diagnostic and treatment interventions are justified exclusively by the prospect of medical benefits to the patient. In contrast, clinical trials differ from medical care in their purpose, characteristic methods, and justification of risks. A clinical trial is an experiment designed to answer a scientific question, not a form of personal therapy. Clinical trials aim at developing knowledge that can lead to improving the medical care of future patients, not at promoting the best medical interests of enrolled patient-subjects. Unlike routine medical care, randomized clinical trials assign patient-subjects treatment (or placebo) by a random method; they are often conducted under double-blind conditions; and they typically restrict the dosing of experimental and control treatments and the use of concomitant treatments in accordance with the study protocol. In addition, clinical trials include procedures, such as blood draws, biopsies, lumbar punctures, and imaging procedures, designed to measure trial outcomes (rather than to guide clinical management), which carry some degree of risk of harm or discomfort to participants without compensating benefits to them. These risks of clinical research are justified by the value of knowledge to be generated. In sum, clinical research routinely incorporates features of study design that are not justifiable within the ethical framework of medical care but can be justified within a research ethics analysis.

Several factors contribute to this confusion between clinical research and medical care: cancer research subjects are often quite ill and motivated to enroll in a study hoping for remission or cure; many cancer clinical trials test experimental approaches that are similar to or minor modifications of currently available treatments; oncology clinical trials take place in hospitals, clinics, and doctors' offices and employ the same types of procedures and interactions as would occur with routine treatment; and the studies are typically carried out by the same physicians and nurses who would otherwise provide nonstudy related care. Together, these contextual realities of oncology research contribute to a therapeutic orientation to clinical trials that can obscure important ethical distinctions between standard oncology care and clinical research.[6] The consequences of this blurring of care and research can include flawed study design, compromised informed consent, and problems in the development of a concept of professional integrity that is appropriate to clinical research. It is our contention that an increased awareness of and formal education in these distinctions is the best approach to ensure the ethical conduct of human subjects research.[7,8]

KEY ETHICAL ISSUES IN THE ONCOLOGY RESEARCH SETTING

Ethical considerations enter into every phase of the clinical research enterprise from study design choices through the conduct, analysis, and reporting of trial results. For example, should a promising novel cancer treatment be tested in an "add-on" fashion or head-to-head against the "standard of care"? Are there circumstances under which the use of placebos can be employed in oncology trials?[9] The answer to these questions will depend on factors such as the severity and natural course of the malignancy under study, the effectiveness and toxicity of available treatments, and the hypothesized "effect size" of the experimental agent. Investigators often complicate the risk:benefit assessment for a clinical trial by adding research diagnostic procedures that do not offer therapeutic benefit but carry with them risks of discomfort or harm (e.g., research biopsies or invasive imaging). A related design issue is the selection of the study endpoint. Is the primary outcome measure toxicity

The opinions expressed are those of the authors and do not necessarily reflect the position or policy of the National Institutes of Health, the Public Health Service, or the Department of Health and Human Services.

(as in Phase I trials), a narrowly defined measure of tumor regression, time-limited disease-free survival or mortality? The potential for miscommunication or mismatched expectations between investigators and subjects about this critical issue is considerable.

Eligibility criteria and subjects' capacity to provide informed consent reflect study choices that also have an impact on the ethical analysis of the research. Some studies require subjects to have failed multiple prior treatments and carry a dire prognosis to meet eligibility criteria and thus raise concerns about vulnerability and voluntariness. Who will be responsible for determining the ability of potential subjects to provide informed consent? Should the designation of a holder of a durable power of attorney (DPA) be required for certain cancer patients at high risk of diminished decision-making capacity (e.g., those with central nervous system [CNS] lesions or paraneoplastic syndromes) or protocols which administer neurotoxic agents (e.g., corticosteroids or interleukin-2)? Will decisionally impaired subjects be eligible? If so, what are the procedures for ensuring adequate surrogate research authorization?[10] Given the growing body of evidence that research subjects, surrogate decision makers, and even investigators are often confused about important details of the study under consideration or subject to the "therapeutic misconception,"[11-15] what additional protections are written into the protocol to prevent the exploitation of medically ill and potentially vulnerable subjects?

Once a given study is underway, the ongoing monitoring of subjects for safety and emergent adverse events presents multiple decision points regarding possible dose adjustments or study discontinuation. Protocol definitions of adverse events and how they will be managed have direct and tangible effects on the experience of research subjects. For example, subjects may be removed from a cancer trial for toxicity, tumor progression, or reasons unrelated, or tangentially related, to their cancer (e.g., nonadherence, substance abuse, suicidal thinking, behavioral problems). Tensions may arise between the desire of investigators to continue gathering critical research data and the wish on the part of subjects and their families to stop study participation so as to minimize toxicity and transition to palliative care. Each of these decisions translates into real consequences for investigators, research subjects, and the clinicians who manage their care during the study.

In reporting research results in the professional literature, authors and journal editors have an obligation to fully disclose details about the ethical conduct of the study. Manuscripts should specify that the study was approved by an Institutional Review Board (IRB) (or exempted from review) and that informed consent was obtained from research subjects or their legally authorized representatives (unless the requirement for informed consent was waived by the IRB). One revealing example of the confusion between the ethics of research and the ethics of medical care is reflected in the Methods section of published articles. Often, manuscripts are silent about IRB review and informed consent. In other cases, authors have taken the position that IRB review and informed consent was not necessary because the study procedures were very similar to standard clinical practice. To some extent, this practice is a carryover from an earlier time when reporting case series and clinical observations were viewed as direct extensions of academic medical practice. However, whenever systematic procedures are employed for purposes of research and personally identified data are collected from subjects, IRB approval and research authorization are necessary unless these requirements are explicitly waived under appropriate research regulations.

Finally, a central ethical issue relevant to all clinical research concerns the professional integrity of investigators and clinicians who support patients enrolled in research. The challenges to professional integrity may be more acute for oncology researchers than other investigators. In contrast to other fields of medical research in which the use of certain research designs reveal sharp distinctions between medical care and clinical research (e.g., placebo-controlled trials; washout studies, symptom-provoking, or "challenge" studies), in oncology, the clinical trial comparing two or more treatments is the overwhelmingly predominant research paradigm. This fact, coupled with the poor prognosis of many cancer research subjects, challenges the professional integrity of oncology researchers who have dual obligations to the well-being of their patients and the fidelity of their research findings.[16]

MULTIPLE ROLES OF THE PSYCHO-ONCOLOGIST IN THE CANCER RESEARCH SETTING

The specific ethical challenges facing psycho-oncologists depend critically on their role in the research setting. Psycho-oncologists have traditionally supported research efforts through the provision of clinical care to study subjects. However, growing numbers of academically oriented psycho-oncologists are principal or associate investigators who conduct psychosocial research with cancer patients. Many also serve as members of a hospital ethics consultation service, ethics committee, IRB or Data and Safety Monitoring Board (DSMB).[17-21] In addition, psycho-oncologists function in other supportive roles such as a study coordinator, research nurse, consultant, or patient educator. Although many professionals are simultaneously engaged in both clinical and research activities, the following analysis considers the clinically oriented psycho-oncologist who is a member of a multidisciplinary research team separately from the psycho-oncologist acting as an investigator conducting her own research with cancer patients.

Most psycho-oncologists bring to their work an exclusively or predominantly clinical orientation and are guided by a deep professional socialization process that emphasizes the patient's best interests above all else. In importance, all cancer patients, whether they are enrolled in research or not, require team-oriented clinical care. However, even when a psycho-oncologist is engaged in a "purely" clinical role with a research subject, she may be asked to make judgments about a subject's protocol eligibility or risk of enrollment (e.g., Will a patient's history of bipolar disorder prevent their successful completion of a study?). Similarly, she may be engaged in trying to increase the subject's chances of successfully completing the research by helping the subject maintain sobriety or adhere to concurrent mental health treatment. Other common requests of clinical psycho-oncologists are to assess capacity to provide informed consent for research, monitor and evaluate CNS toxicity, or render judgments that influence study endpoints and trial discontinuation. Disagreements can arise around each of these issues and their resolution may depend on the psycho-oncologist's standing within the primary research team. Role tensions related to "dual-agency," inescapable for the physician–researcher, have also been described for nurses, social workers and other clinicians working at the interface of clinical care and research.[22-24]

Managing the tensions between promoting research and providing appropriate clinical care for patient-subjects posed by these, and related, examples requires that psycho-oncologists are clear about what they are doing and why. Specifically, they need to be clear about when they are addressing the medical needs of patient-subjects and when they are helping to facilitate continued participation in research. While these functions may overlap and be mutually achievable, in other cases they may conflict. Careful assessment of morally relevant considerations and clinical judgment are indispensable to managing potentially competing role responsibilities.

The following examples are drawn from clinical experience in a research hospital and illustrate some of the ethical issues facing clinically oriented psycho-oncologists. How should a social worker respond to evidence of impaired reasoning and judgment in a research participant with a brain tumor who has just been enrolled in a phase I clinical trial by an enthusiastic investigator and the encouragement of a desperate and hopeful spouse? In another case, a psychiatrist was asked to consult on a depressed subject who was demonstrating only modest tumor regression during a phase II trial of a promising new chemotherapy. During the psychiatric evaluation, the research subject revealed active suicidal ideation, which was listed in the protocol as a grade IV toxicity and mandated trial discontinuation. Should there have been a different outcome if the actively suicidal subject had demonstrated a robust tumor response?

A different set of ethical challenges face the psycho-oncologist researcher as compared to the psycho-oncologist clinician. Two central issues for psycho-oncology investigators are related to the risks of psychosocial research and ancillary-care obligations of researchers. A frequent concern expressed by psychosocial investigators is that there is a double standard with respect to what are considered acceptable research risks in studies of cancer patients. Some investigators have charged that bio-medically oriented IRBs have substantially greater tolerance for physical research risks associated with chemotherapy, surgery, or radiation than they do for the anticipated risks of emotional distress that might accompany questions about coping, sexuality, depression, suicide, and death.[25,26] To be sure, investigators and IRBs should be thoughtful about the potential cumulative distress burden on sick cancer research subjects asked to volunteer for studies involving lengthy interviews, psychological testing, or brain imaging. However, there is no compelling empirical evidence to suggest that cancer patients find psychosocial research distressing, and they may well find it personally beneficial.[27]

What are the clinical obligations of a psychologist conducting research on the coping strategies of patients with recurrent breast cancer? It would be expected that some study subjects would express clinically meaningful levels of anxiety, depression, and even thoughts of suicide. Is it sufficient for the investigator to make a referral for further evaluation and care or should the psychologist-investigator also treat that study subject/cancer patient?[28] We contend that the ancillary-care obligations for the psychosocial investigator are no different from any clinical investigator and should be guided by a framework that is based on important distinctions between the ethics of medical care and the ethics of clinical research.

ETHICAL FRAMEWORK

A standard approach to thinking about the ethics of clinical research is to invoke the four principles of biomedical ethics-respect for autonomy, beneficence, nonmaleficence, and justice.[29] In our view, this approach is not a helpful way to articulate a workable and satisfactory ethical framework for clinical research. The four principles are highly abstract, such that they apply to both clinical practice and clinical research, despite fundamental ethical differences between these two activities. Thus, by themselves, they provide no determinate guidance for research ethics.

Moreover, two of the four principles, which are more familiar and better understood in the context of medical care, are apt to be applied to clinical research in a way that fundamentally distorts the ethics of this activity. With respect to medical care, beneficence and nonmaleficence are understood as having a distinctly therapeutic meaning. Beneficence entails the obligation of the healthcare professional to do what is best medically for particular patients. Nonmaleficence entails the obligation to avoid exposing patients to harms or risks of harm that are not compensated by the prospect of medical benefits to them. By way of contrast, in clinical research, beneficence must be understood primarily as directing investigators to promote social value by means of generating scientific knowledge; and nonmaleficence as requiring that risks are minimized and justified by the potential value of the knowledge to be gained by the research. In other words, the exclusively patient-centered, therapeutic meaning of beneficence and nonmaleficence in medical care do not properly apply to the design and conduct of clinical research, owing to the fundamentally different purpose of the latter and the ethically different way in which risks to subjects are justified as compared to that of patients in medical care.

For these reasons, we avoid appeal to the general principles of biomedical ethics in developing an ethical framework for clinical research; what is required instead is an ethical framework tailored to clinical research. Emanuel and colleagues have proposed such a framework, which draws on codes of ethics, commission reports, research regulations, and the bioethics literature[30] and consists of seven requirements: (1) social value, (2) scientific validity, (3) fair subject selection, (4) favorable risk-benefit ratio, (5) independent review, (6) informed consent, and (7) respect for enrolled subjects. We briefly describe each of these requirements.

Social value. Clinical research is designed to answer socially valuable scientific questions concerning the understanding, treatment, or prevention of disease. Clinical research is not worth undertaking unless it is directed to answering a valuable question with the potential to contribute to improving medical care or promoting health. In addition, the risks to research subjects in studies lacking such value cannot be justified, making them unethical. As the risks increase, the value of the science should be proportionately more compelling. However, the fact that a study has great potential social value does not imply that grave risks are justifiable. The most basic ethical challenge is to balance the moral value in developing knowledge aimed at improving health with the moral imperative to protect the rights and well-being of subjects.

Scientific validity. To achieve the potential value of clinical research, studies must be designed with sufficient methodological rigor to provide a scientifically valid test of their hypotheses or to contribute to generalizable knowledge. If the study design lacks such rigor, if it cannot produce interpretable results or valid data, then it is not worth conducting. In the case of poorly designed research, risks to participants cannot be justified.

Fair subject selection. Fairness in subject selection typically concerns groups of human subjects regarded as "vulnerable" because their characteristics or situation render them less than fully capable of making voluntary, informed decisions about research participation. This is often relevant to oncology research either because of the poor health of subjects or their altered ability to provide initial and ongoing informed consent. As a general rule, subjects who lack or have grossly impaired decision-making capacity should not be enrolled in research as long as the research question can be answered with people who are capable of giving informed consent or unless the prospect of direct medical benefit through study participation is compelling. Likewise, children should not be enrolled in studies if the research question can be examined by recruiting competent adults. However, based on the disorder under investigation or the nature of the research question, it may be necessary to involve subjects incapable of giving informed consent, in which case special protections, including authorization by surrogate decision makers, are required.

Favorable risk-benefit ratio. Risk-benefit assessment is ethically required to judge whether the risks to which participants are exposed are justified by the potential benefits, either to them or to future patients and society. Three dimensions of risk are relevant: probability, magnitude, and duration of harm. Accordingly, three questions must be addressed. First, what is the chance that research interventions will produce various harms to the health or well-being of participants? Second, how serious is the potential harm? Third, how long is the potential harm expected to last?

Achieving a favorable risk-benefit ratio requires that risks are minimized to the extent possible. This does not mean that risks must be eliminated, for that would make almost all clinical research impossible to conduct. Study designs should be evaluated to determine if they can be modified to pose less risk without compromising the validity of data generated.

Multiple dimensions of the design and conduct of clinical research are relevant to the requirement of minimizing risks. Exclusion criteria for eligible participants should rule out those who can be predicted to be at increased risk from experimental interventions. Procedures posing higher risks or serious discomfort need to be carefully scrutinized to judge whether they are necessary to produce valuable data. Alternative, less risky ways to test hypotheses should be explored. Finally, to minimize risks, careful procedures must be in place to monitor the condition of participants and end their participation if their safety is endangered.

Should there be limits to the level of risk that can be justified in clinical research regardless of the value of the knowledge to be gained? This is an unsettled issue of research ethics. U.S. Federal regulations provide no guidance for limits on acceptable risk for competent adults.[31] The Nuremberg Code, developed in the wake of the Nazi concentration camp experiments, states that "No experiment should be conducted where there is an *a priori* reason to believe that death or disabling injury will occur; except, perhaps, in those experiments where the experimental physicians also serve as subjects."[32] The qualification of an *a priori* reason is critical. Because a subject dies or is seriously injured as a result of an experiment, it does not follow that the research was unethical. The ethical justification of risk must be evaluated prospectively, based on knowledge available at the time a study is reviewed and approved.

How can it be determined whether the potential value of knowledge to be gained from a given study can justify the risks posed to subjects? There are no formulas available. The assessment calls for carefully considered and deliberated judgments by research sponsors, investigators, and research ethics committees.

Independent review. Prospective independent review of research protocols by research ethics committees, known as IRBs, was mandated by the U.S. Federal Government in response to revelations in the 1960s of abuses of research subjects.[33] Self-regulation by investigators was no longer considered to be ethically adequate. Independent review is a key safeguard for protecting participants from the inherent potential of research to compromise their rights or welfare. Independent review also serves the value of public accountability, since clinical research exposes participants to risks for the good of society. The task of the research ethics committee is to apply the other six ethical requirements in the review, modification, approval, and oversight of scientific protocols.

When appropriate, typically in multicentered randomized trials, independent DSMBs are used, with the primary role of deciding whether it is ethically necessary to stop a trial early owing to unexpected adverse events, a determination that the primary research question has been answered, or a judgment that it is futile to continue the trial because there is little likelihood that further accrual of subjects would contribute to answering the question.[34]

Informed consent. Investigators have no right to conduct an experiment without the consent of subjects or their authorized representatives. The point of informed consent in the case of competent adults is to assure that participation reflects their free choice and self-determination. As the term "informed consent" implies, this requirement includes two basic components. First, prospective subjects must be adequately informed about what research participation involves: especially, the nature of the study, the procedures administered, the risks and potential benefits (if any), alternatives to participation (including receiving standard treatment in clinical practice), and the right to decline or withdraw without penalty. Second, participants must voluntarily agree to participate.

It is important to recognize, however, that the informed consent of subjects is not necessary for research to be ethical. Research enrolling children and incompetent adults can be ethical, provided that adequate safeguards are employed, including informed authorization by parents or surrogate decision makers. Although controversial, research evaluating treatments in emergency settings may be ethically justified, despite the inability of subjects to consent and the lack at the time of enrollment of surrogate authorization.

Respect for enrolled subjects. Clinical research must be conducted with adequate safeguards to protect the welfare and rights of participants during the course of the study. These include procedures to protect privacy and confidentiality, monitoring the condition of subjects to assure their safety, terminating participation in the case of adverse events, and informing subjects about risks discovered in the course of research or new information about risks reported in the medical literature. IRBs should review and approve written plans to monitor the condition of participants. In the case of higher risk research, it may be desirable to institute independent safety monitors to determine when it is appropriate to withdraw participants for reasons of safety. Adverse event reports must be prepared by investigators and submitted to IRBs in timely fashion so that determinations can be made about whether to modify the study design, change informed consent documents, and notify subjects about new risks, or to stop the research. In addition, respect for subjects includes debriefing at the conclusion of their participation to discuss any medical implications and communicate individual results.

CONCLUSION

Biomedical and psychosocial research in the oncology setting promise important improvements in cancer care. Nonetheless, the nature of conducting research with patients suffering from cancer raises ethical questions and professional integrity challenges for the psycho-oncologist, whether in her role as a clinician or investigator. We have argued that contextual aspects of the oncology research setting foster an ethically problematic therapeutic orientation to cancer clinical trials and that tensions between promoting clinical research and patient care are inevitable and call for thoughtful management. In addition, we have described an ethical framework that is well-suited to guide psycho-oncologists in their interface with clinical research.

REFERENCES

1. National. *National Institutes of Health FY 2008 enacted appropriation.* National Institutes of Health; 2008. Available at http://officeofbudget.od.nih.gov/ui/2008/FY%202008%20IC%20Distribution%20and%20PriorYrs.pdf. Accessed October 20, 2008.

2. National Cancer Institute. *Cancer centers program.* National Cancer Institute; 2008. Available at http://cancercenters.cancer.gov/cancer_centers/index.html. Accessed October 16, 2008.

3. National Cancer Institute. *Care for children and adolescents with cancer: Questions and answers.* National Cancer Institute; 2008. Available at http://www.cancer.gov/cancertopics/factsheet/NCI/children-adolescents. Accessed October 16, 2008.

4. Ries LAG, Melbert D, Krapcho M, et al. *SEER cancer statistics review, 1975–2005.* National Cancer Institute; 2008. Available at http://seer.cancer.gov/csr/1975_2005/index.html. Accessed October 16, 2008.

5. Peppercorn JM, Weeks JC, Cook EF, Joffe S. Comparison of outcomes in cancer patients treated within and outside clinical trials: conceptual framework and structured review. *Lancet.* 2004;363:263–270.

6. Miller FG, Rosenstein DL. The therapeutic orientation to clinical trials. *N Engl J Med.* 2003;348:1383–1386.

7. Preisman RC, Steinberg MD, Rummans TA, et al. An annotated bibliography for ethics training in consultation-liaison psychiatry. *Psychosomatics.* 1999;40:369–379.

8. Rosenstein DL, Miller FG, Rubinow DR. A curriculum for teaching psychiatric research bioethics. *Biol Psychiatry.* 2001;50:802–808.

9. Daugherty CK, Ratain MJ, Emanuel EJ, Farrell AT, Schilsky RL. Ethical, scientific, and regulatory perspectives regarding the use of placebos in cancer clinical trials. *J Clin Oncol.* 2008;26:1371–1378.

10. Rosenstein DL, Miller FG. Research involving those at risk for impaired decisionmaking capacity. In: Emanuel EJ, Grady C, Crouch RA, Lie R, Miller F, Wendler D (eds). *The Oxford textbook of clinical research ethics.* New York: Oxford University Press; 2008:437–445.

11. Joffe S, Cook EF, Cleary PD, Clark JW, Weeks JC. Quality of informed consent in cancer clinical trials: a cross-sectional survey. *Lancet.* 2001;358:1772–1777.

12. Appelbaum PS, Lidz CW, Grisso T. Therapeutic misconception in clinical research: frequency and risk factors. *IRB.* 2004;26:1–8.

13. Kodish E, Eder M, Noll RB, et al. Communication of randomization in childhood leukemia trials. *JAMA.* 2004;291:470–475.

14. Joffe S, Weeks JC. Views of American oncologists about the purposes of clinical trials. *J Natl Cancer Inst.* 2002;94:1847–1853.

15. Ellis PM, Dowsett SM, Butow PN, Tattersall MHN. Attitudes to randomized clinical trials amongst out-patients attending a medical oncology clinic. *Health Expect.* 1999;2:33–43.

16. Miller FG, Rosenstein DL, DeRenzo EG. Professional integrity in clinical research. *JAMA.* 1998;280:1449–1454.

17. Youngner SJ. Consultation-liaison psychiatry and clinical ethics: historical parallels and diversions. *Psychosomatics.* 1997;38:309–312.

18. Bourgeois JA, Cohen MA, Geppert CMA. The role of psychosomatic-medicine psychiatrists in bioethics: a survey study of members of the Academy of Psychosomatic Medicine. *Psychosomatics.* 2006;47:520–526.

19. Geppert CMA, Cohen MA. Consultation-liaison psychiatrists on bioethics committees: opportunities for academic leadership. *Acad Psychiatry.* 2006;30:416–421.

20. Leeman CP. Psychiatric consultations and ethics consultations: similarities and differences. *Gen Hosp Psychiatry.* 2000;22:270–275.

21. Lederberg MS. Understanding the interface between psychiatry and ethics. In: Holland JC, (ed). *Psycho-oncology.* New York: Oxford Press; 1998:1123–1131.

22. Cox K. Setting the context for research: exploring the philosophy and environment of a cancer clinical trails unit. *J Adv Nurs.* 2000;32:1058–1065.

23. Martin W, Grey M, Webber T, et al. Balancing dual roles in end-of-life research. *Can Oncol Nurs J.* 2007;17:141–147.

24. Brody H, Miller FG. The clinician-investigator: unavoidable but manageable tension. *Kennedy Inst Ethics J.* 2003;13:329–346.

25. Luebbert R, Tait RC, Chibnall JT, Deshields TL. IRB member judgments of decisional capacity, coercion, and risk in medical and psychiatric studies. *JERHRE.* 2008;3:15–24.

26. Oakes JM. Risks and wrongs in social science research. An evaluator's guide to the IRB. *Eval Rev.* 2002;26:443–479.

27. Pessin H, Galietta M, Nelson CJ, Brescia R, Rosenfield B, Breitbart W. Burden and benefit of psychosocial research at the end of life. *J Palliat Med.* 2008;11:627–632.

28. Richardson HS, Belsky L. The ancillary-care responsibilities of medical researchers: an ethical framework for thinking about the clinical care that researchers owe their subjects. *Hastings Cent Rep.* 2004;34:25–33.

29. Beauchamp TL, Childress JF. *Principles of biomedical ethics, fifth edition.* New York: Oxford University Press; 2001.

30. Emanuel EJ, Wendler D, Grady C. What makes clinical research ethical? *JAMA.* 2000;283:2701–2711.

31. Department of Health and Human Services. *Protection of human subjects. Code of federal regulations, title 45, public welfare: Part 46;* 1991.

32. The. *The Nazi doctors and the Nuremberg code: Human rights in human experimentation.* New York: Oxford University Press; 1992.

33. Faden RR, Beauchamp TL, King NMP. *A history and theory of informed consent.* New York: Oxford University Press; 1986.

34. Slutsky AS, Lavery JV. Data safety and monitoring boards. *N Engl J Med.* 2004;350:1143–1147.

PART XV

The Future of Psycho-Oncology Research

Paul B. Jacobsen, ED

CHAPTER 92

Basic and Translational Psycho-Oncology Research

Michael Stefanek

"There is not pure science and applied science but only science and the applications of science"-Louis Pasteur
"A science, such as physics or chemistry or mathematics, is not the sum of two discrete parts, one pure and the other applied. It is an organic whole, with complex interrelationships through-out."
-Vannevar Bush

Basic research aims to increase *understanding*. Its essential quality is the contribution it seeks to make to the general knowledge of a field of science. Applied research pertains to use or *function,* that is, research *directed toward* some individual need or use. Thus, for some time, basic and applied research was believed to represent conflicting goals and this view promoted a consistent tension between basic and applied research. A common simplistic linear paradigm was often displayed when describing this basic-applied relationship (Fig. 92–1).

What is striking about this simplistic notion is that as you move toward one pole, you move away from the other—clearly not the paradigm needed to move psycho-oncology research forward. This view oversimplifies the complicated process of give and take between basic and applied research. Rather, consider a sports analogy: compare the simple view of a relay race, with one runner passing the baton to the next, with the more engaging analogy of the basic-applied relationship as a rugby game, during which the ball gets passed, dribbled, and kicked back and forth, with the direction of the ball not always known very far in advance, and with many passes not being terribly accurate. However, after much work, a few dirty uniforms, cuts, and scrapes, a goal is scored-and research is advanced. In this framework, the teams score with the ball moving both up and down the field (basic → applied, applied → basic). I would argue that this is the appropriate paradigm for our vision of basic and applied research. Breakthroughs (goals) achieved by applied research can lead to further basic research, just as breakthroughs in basic research might lead to further applied work.

There is a now maturing recognition that to maximize our ability to improve human health, basic behavioral research must be translated into practical applications. Such basic research might provide new assessment tools or provide guidance into the decision-making processes of individuals which may inform clinical approaches and interventions. Moving from applied to basic, clinical researchers and practitioners must provide necessary information to those engaged in basic research about the key issues facing cancer patients and survivors, so that such potential applications can be considered in areas of basic research such as decision making, risk perception, motivation to change behavior, and communication processes.

Such translational research in both biomedical and behavioral research is driving the clinical research engine. As translational research becomes more the norm, and the value of basic behavioral research in psychosocial care of cancer patients and caregivers is increasingly valued, more and more of the artificial barriers separating each research arena will dissolve, and patients and caregivers will benefit greatly.

BASIC BEHAVIORAL RESEARCH

Behavioral research has played a role in the health of our nation for quite some time. Indeed, while its value is often underappreciated in this role, it is recognized as an important component, along with biomedical research, of the mission of the National Institutes of Health.[1] A separate office exists within the National Institutes of Health, the Office of Behavioral and Social Sciences Research (OBSSR) (http://obssr.od.nih.gov/content) to foster behavioral research. This office, established in 1995, has as one of its primary goals to integrate biobehavioral interdisciplinary perspectives into all NIH research areas. Defined by this office, basic behavioral and social research is divided into three categories:

1. Research on behavioral and social processes;
2. Biopsychosocial research;
3. Research on the development of procedures for measurement, analysis, and classification.

Basic research thus helps us to understand *basic behavioral and social phenomena* in and of themselves, aids in the understanding of the mechanisms that link behavioral factors to health outcomes, and helps us to understand how such mechanisms interrelate with biomedical factors in disease and health.

Many of us consider basic behavioral research as focused only on the individual or even intraindividual phenomena only (motivation, consciousness, expectancy, etc). However, a broader view of basic behavioral research embraced by the OBSSR includes not only the level of the individual (animal or human) but also the basic research examining small groups, institution, organization, community, or even population level analyses. Research also includes the study of the interactions within and between these levels,[2,3] such as the study of environmental or community variables on individual behavior (e.g., the role of segregation or socio-economic status on availability of neighborhood resources and subsequent impact on health behaviors such as physical activity, smoking, or nutritional intake).

Biopsychosocial (or biobehavioral) research includes work done examining the interactions of biological factors with behavioral or social variables. This body of work includes behavioral genetics, psychoneuroimmunology, and cognitive neuroscience, for example. The role of gene–environment interactions in health and health behavior and the identification of biopsychosocial stress markers are included here.

Finally, basic behavioral research includes work involving *measuring and analyzing behavior, psychological functioning, or the social environment*. Such work might include domains of statistical techniques (multilevel modeling), memory assessment, or new assessment techniques ("real time" data collection strategies such as ecological momentary assessment). In sum, this area focuses on the development of research tools that might be utilized across behavioral or even biomedical research (e.g., pain assessment).

BASIC BEHAVIORAL RESEARCH: LEVELS OF ANALYSIS

Anderson[2] was one of the first to illustrate the value of considering and categorizing the various levels of analysis in basic behavioral research. Although initially applied to the larger domain of health research, these

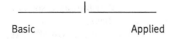

Basic   Applied

Fig. 92–1. The traditional basic-applied research paradigm.

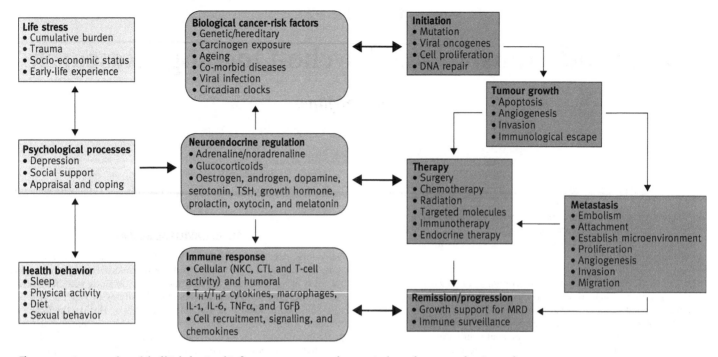

Fig. 92–2. Integrated model of biobehavioral influences on cancer pathogenesis through neuroendocrine pathways.
SOURCE: Reprinted by permission from Macmillan Publishers Ltd: [Nature Reviews Cancer] (Antoni MH, Lutgendorf SK, Cole SW, et al. The influence of bio-behavioural factors on tumour biology: pathways and mechanisms. *Nat Rev Cancer.* 2006;6(3):240–248), Copyright (2006).

levels include the molecular, cellular, organ systems, behavioral/psychological, and social/environmental. This framework fits nicely with the view promoted in this chapter of basic behavioral research ranging from "cells to society," not restrained by the traditional view of such research restricted to the individual level.

Basic work both within and across these levels can again not only be informative as producers of knowledge about basic behavioral or social phenomena, but also can inform next steps in the research process which may lead to interventions impacting health and health behavior.

The range of research spanning the "basic" realm that might apply to behavioral and psychosocial oncology includes work investigating the influence of biobehavioral factors on tumor biology[4] to the role of social networks and the "spread" of obesity over time.[5] A model of biobehavioral research is shown below in Fig. 92–2 and displays the importance of basic research across this model.

There are virtually limitless areas of research within each box in the model that will provide additional information about phenomena (e.g., sleep, cytokines, neuroendocrine regulation and the proposed pathways). Basic research in each of these will help us test proposed models, and consider applied research and clinical applications, contingent upon how well the model holds as we gather additional information about factors within each "box." Basic research related to stress, chronic depression, and other psychosocial factors will lead to understanding of both the biological and clinical significance of such factors on cancer incidence, tumor growth, and metastasis. Historically, this is a research domain that has suffered as we have not appreciated the need for basic research to inform more applied work. As one example, over the past 2 decades, psychosocial research has made far too premature a leap with intervention trials to determine the role of support groups on survival among cancer patients.[6] Clearly needed was a firm foundation in basic behavioral (and biomedical) research examining the multiple factors involved in Fig. 92–2 to determine the merit of more applied intervention trials with survival as an endpoint. While hindsight is 20:20, much more value would have accrued if the time, cost, and intellectual energy needed for the host of clinical trials testing the psychosocial support-survival link had been spent investigating the role of mechanisms involving biobehavioral factors, the hypothalamic pituitary axis (HPA) and autonomic nervous system (ANS) and their effects

on the immune and neuroendocrine processes possibly involved in cancer development and progression.

While the biobehavioral work above is work most clearly identified as "basic," research extending beyond the biology of the individual can be just as cleanly in the basic research realm. While research in network analysis at a cellular level has exploded in the last decade, leading to new insights into disease processes and gene activity, it is only very recently that "social" networks have been explored. While clearly our social networks impact health in the sense that we spread pathogens to our friends and contacts in a variety of forms (and vice versa), Christakis et al.[3,7] have expanded this idea of "network medicine" to include outcomes linked to health behaviors in a way that reminds us that networks may impact us in ways not previously explored. More specifically, it appears that network phenomena are linked to obesity and tobacco use-that both may well be "spread" through network ties. This is clearly relevant to behavioral and psycho-oncology, given the clear tobacco-cancer link and the growing and clear connection between obesity and cancer development, along with its role in cancer survival across a number of cancer sites.[8]

In an example of basic research at a social level involving obesity, Christakis[5] used a densely interconnected sample of participants from the Framingham Heart study (n = 12,067) with body mass index (BMI) data available for subjects. Longitudinal statistical models examined whether weight gain in one person was associated with weight gain among friends, siblings, spouses, and neighbors. A person's chance of becoming obese (BMI >30) increased by 57% (95%; CI, 6%–123%) if he or she had an obese friend, sibling (40%; 95% CI, 21%–60%) or spouse (37%; CI, 7%–73%). These findings support the hypothesis that obesity (and other health behaviors) spread in social networks in quantifiable ways that depend in part on the nature of the social ties.

This example of basic behavioral research, while informing us of the impact of social networks and behavior, also has clinical applications, as we understand how "bad" and "good" behaviors may transfer socially. It may be that interventions that modify a social network may indeed impact behavior, leading, perhaps, to medical, behavioral, and public health interventions that may be more cost effective, given this expanding knowledge that change in one individuals behavior may spread to others.

There are a number of findings in basic behavioral research that may have clinical applications. For instance, Parent, Ward, and Mann[9] investigated how health information is processed under one of two systems: the "hot" system (focusing on emotions) and the "cool" system (more cognitively based, emotionally neutral). In their study among college undergraduates, messages were presented that focused on each of these systems (the "cool" system message emphasizing facts and statistics; the "hot" system involving side effects described as somatic sensations). Why might this matter? As one potential application, perhaps such work may inform health educators how best to fashion a message that grabs the attention of listeners and motivates them to engage in healthy behaviors, such as increasing activity or adhering to treatment regimens. Such an application may have an impact in cancer prevention, early detection, or survivorship. One advantage to such work with an undergraduate sample in a laboratory setting is that a variety of hypotheses can be explored quickly, such as use of "hot" and "cold" messages, where placement might occur in the message, and pairing of messages, to assess intent to engage in health behaviors. Such work allows promising hypotheses with the potential for application in cancer control to be further explored.

Another research area with potential application to behavioral and psycho-oncology is the domain of health disparities. In the United States, consistent differences exist in treatment patterns among people of different race and ethnicity who have the same disease. Kaufman[10] has noted that some hypothesize that individual choices (related to smoking, diet, and screening) may be partially or primarily related to such disparities, or inherent differences between groups, such that culture or genetics may contribute significantly to such disparities. Thus, if racial or ethnic groups value health states differently and as a result make different choices related to health and healthcare, the disparities are simply a function of these free choices. Gaskin and Frick[11] examined this issue by reviewing data from 21,362 adult respondents to the Medical Expenditure Panel Survey (MEPS) and their answer to items assessing how health states were valued. The finding that race and ethnicity were not associated with differences in valuation of health states (although health status, age, poverty were indeed predictors of health valuations), leads back to the importance of healthcare and provider-related factors.

This issue of basic research in health disparities, cultural issues and even aging is a critical one. As Whitfield[12] has noted, current projections suggest that by the year 2050 the total number of non-Hispanic whites aged 65 and older will double, the number of blacks aged 65 and older will more than triple and the number of Hispanics is expected to increase 11-fold. Do we have theory-driven explanatory models for health behavior and decision making that incorporate basic research in gerontology and cultural issues?

There are a host of other promising areas of basic behavioral research that may well provide knowledge informing more applied work across the cancer continuum:

1. Affective Forecasting—how individuals accurately (or not) evaluate the pleasure, satisfaction, or reward to be derived as a result of different decisions;
2. Cross-cultural understanding of others emotions—while not clear, some data support the hypothesis that accuracy is lower when attempting to read the emotional expressions of individuals in cultures different than our own;
3. The role of emotion in attentional processes and decision making with aging—how emotion influences both attention and memory and how such influence changes over the life span;
4. Affective and deliberative risky decision making in children, adolescents, and adults—it may be that affective/emotional processes and experiential learning are more critical factors among adolescents than deliberative processes;
5. Ambiguity Aversion and decision making—people often face ambiguous information about their risks and risk-reducing behavior that may present a conflicting view of costs and benefits (e.g., prostate screening tests). How do people cope with such information and how are decisions made?

In sum, much of our applied work in psycho-oncology, from determining how best to develop a decision aid or discuss health behavior change with patients or caregivers to developing psychosocial interventions with components most likely to have lasting emotional and behavioral impact is potentially informed by the knowledge resulting from basic behavioral research. Utilizing the extensive accomplishments of many of our professional colleagues outside of oncology and psycho-oncology research in the areas of decision making, motivation, beliefs and attitudes and psychoneuroimmunology promises to advance work in cancer control from prevention to end-of-life care of cancer patients.

TRANSLATIONAL BEHAVIORAL RESEARCH

The traditional Basic (Bench)→Applied (Bedside) view of translational research has appropriately expanded to one more consonant with advancing use of research findings into the community (Fig. 92–3).

The boxes are purposefully the same size to indicate that none of the boxes is more critical than any other, and that all three are needed to maximize the impact of "evidence-based" psycho-oncology research into the cancer community. The bidirectional arrows extending from Basic↔Dissemination indicate that the impact of basic research does not simply reach the applied stage of research, but also necessarily impacts the effectiveness of the intervention, once the intervention is moved to the "trenches." In addition, once in the application phase, engrained in community practice, there may still be findings from basic research that find their way to the community implementation, or evaluation of accepted community interventions may raise questions best addressed back in the basic behavioral laboratory.

It may be helpful to utilize nomenclature that clearly distinguishes basic→ applied translational work from applied→ dissemination. One option is to simply refer to the first link as *T1* (moving research from bench to bedside) and *T2* (the translation of results from clinical studies into everyday clinical practice), with T2 including what might be considered "knowledge translation" plus widespread promotion.[13] This chapter focuses on *T1* while the accompanying chapter by Jacobsen in this text addresses many issues related to *T2*.

In one of the seminal papers examining the evolution of cancer control research, Best et al.[14] noted the importance of "…a continuing (and nonlinear) examination of the underlying knowledge base" for cancer control science, along with "fundamental and applied scientists working together…," a clear call not only for transdisciplinary approaches but also for continuing focus on *T1* research to eventually inform *T2*.

Anderson[2] nicely formulated the importance of basic research in his description of convergent and reciprocal causation. In such a model the interaction of levels of analyses ranging from **molecular→ cellular→ organ systems→ behavioral/psychological→ social/environmental** result in health outcomes or pathogenic processes. In one example, the initiation of smoking (behavioral level) may be strongly tied in adolescents to peer influences and advertising (social and environmental level). Smoking may then become addictive which contributes to continued smoking behavior. Basic research at each level of analysis (when does smoking become habitual? What are the decisional processes involved in starting or stopping smoking? What is it about advertising that pulls in adolescents? How do social networks "spread" smoking? What brain and other physiological changes "mark" addiction?) has informed or continues to inform our knowledge of tobacco addiction and cessation. Such work clearly links to applied research by informing intervention development and potentially tailoring interventions to subgroups to maximize the efficacy of a given intervention.

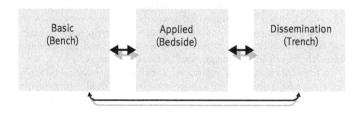

Fig. 92–3. Translational research: the new paradigm.

Translational research *(T1)* involves moving findings from basic research, at times conducted without a specific health problem in mind, or indeed, without addressing health at all, to applied research in the health domain, utilizing these findings in an intervention trial. At other times, basic research may be conducted knowing full well that it applies to an unresolved issue in an applied health field. Indeed, this is part of the bidirectional communication in translational research. That is, it is critical for applied researchers to inform basic researchers on key needs in the "trenches" just as it is critical for basic researchers to teach applied researchers what relevance their work may have in cancer control. Two such examples of basic research being guided directly from needs in the "trenches" comes from work currently being conducted by the Centers of Excellence in Cancer Communication Research (CECCR) (http://dccps.nci.nih.gov/hcirb/ceccr/), a major funded initiative from the National Cancer Institutes Division of Cancer Control and Population Sciences.

Hinyard and Kreuter[15] assessed the impact of breast cancer information presented in personal experience narratives from African-American breast cancer survivors among low-income African-American women. Outcomes included ratings of the viewers' engagement in the videos, judgments of trust, expertise and liking of the survivors, and how such ratings impacted positive reactions to the videos. The goal of the study was to *understand* the predictors of positive reactions to the videos and to develop a randomized trial to test the effects of narrative versus didactic videos on African-American women's use of mammography.

A second study clearly linking basic research to planned applied research involved a biobehavioral evaluation of antitobacco public service announcements (PSA's).[16] This project was interested in determining whether argument quality and message sensation value influence smokers' psychophysiological, cognitive, and behavioral responses when viewing antitobacco PSA's and to assess the relationship between physiological responses and persuasiveness of the PSA's. The goal again was to *understand* the biological basis of the persuasiveness of antismoking PSA's and to develop and evaluate counter-marketing strategies based on such understanding. Such developed and evaluated strategies may thus make the transition from the bench to the bedside to the trenches *(T1 to T2)*.

(T1) TRANSLATIONAL RESEARCH: MAKING IT HAPPEN

I hope the importance of *T1* translational research is clear from the rationale and examples provided in this chapter. However, for those who have not systematically engaged in "reaching back" to basic behavioral research to inform applied work in psycho-oncology, it may be challenging to begin this process. One first step is to become familiar with organizations and sponsored conferences that support such work. While all of us may regularly attend meetings that center upon applied work in psycho-oncology (American Psycho-Oncology Society (APOS); International Psycho-Oncology Society (IPOS), the Society of Behavioral Medicine (SBM) and a host of others in our respective disciplines (psychiatry, psychology, social work, nursing, etc.), other meetings hold promise for informing us of more basic research relevant to our work. A far from exhaustive list might include the Association for Psychological Science (APS), the Society for Judgment and Decision Making (SJDM), and the Psychoneuroimmunolgy Research Society (PNIRS). Each of these organizations sponsors its own journal which may provide links to work of interest and potential collaborators from the basic behavioral science arena. In the area of cancer prevention, including cancer survivors and second primaries, the American Association for Cancer Research (AACR) sponsors an annual Frontiers in Cancer Prevention meeting, with a growing presence of behavioral science and integration of behavioral and biomedical research. As noted previously, the National Science Foundation (NSF) supports basic behavioral research, and within the National Cancer Institute, the Basic and Biobehavioral Research Branch (BBRB) promotes *T1* translational work.

In terms of establishing partnerships with basic behavioral researchers, successful collaborations can be complex and challenging, involving close and active relationships with investigators that are typically a step away from applied research in psycho-oncology and the *T2* phase. Clearly, movement toward a "shared" project involves the formulation of

a sound hypothesis supported by compelling "preclinical" data.[17] Such a hypothesis may help drive the design of the more applied work-sample, outcome variables, or even timing of the outcome measurements. Such "preclinical" data may also function to test hypotheses about moderators and mediators of behaviors and behavior change as part of the continuum from theory to research to practice. As noted by Glanz, Rimer, and Viswanath[18] and Anderson[2] it is critical to consider all levels of behavioral influence to determine the optimal partners for collaboration: intrapersonal, interpersonal, institutional or organizational, community, and public policy. As noted previously, basic behavioral research extends from "cells to society" and the selection of basic behavioral research partners is determined in part by the level(s) of intervention of most interest.

Critically important to applied and basic researchers alike is finding a partner(s) who is committed to extending his/her work to a more translational paradigm, and one who shares your enthusiasm about partnering, so that jointly you may investigate a specific applied problem in your research area. There needs to be tight integration between the "bench" and the "bedside" investigators, and involvement in smaller, pilot projects to determine if the right chemistry exists between potential partners.

Finally, in terms of academia and promotions, it is often the case that promotion and/or recognition within a department hinge on first or senior author publications. This has clearly played a role as a barrier to interdisciplinary and "big science," and it also may pose a barrier connecting with colleagues who may not initially serve as a Principal Investigator on a first collaborative effort. In addition to developing plans to alternate first or senior authorships over time depending upon the focus of a given study, many journals now encourage noting the contributions of each author. Such visibly noted significant contributions to a manuscript can help when the time comes for promotions or tenure decisions. It is also important to note that, with such collaboration, the impact of the work (and possibly the impact factor of the journal) will likely be superior to work done without such informed collaboration. In addition, many institutions are becoming more sensitive to the push for translational work, interdisciplinary work, multidisciplinary work, and "big science" involvement of investigators, now more common across both biomedical and behavioral disciplines. Thus, many are in the evolving process of reconsidering standard promotional criteria with the evolution of such a major shift in how research is done. Such changes include movement toward a more inclusive framework, rewarding those who engage in translational work including multiauthored papers.

As Jain[17] notes, some institutions are now providing awards (e.g., "Team Science Awards") for collaborative successes, and the same could easily be done for *T1* or *T2* translational science projects.

THE FUTURE

In the next chapter, Jacobsen addresses the issue of *T2* translational research. As the fields of cancer control and psychosocial oncology move forward, *T2* research will clearly receive ongoing emphasis, given the need to move behavioral science research out of the journal pages into hospital and community settings. The growing presence of community-based participatory research (CBPR) is evidence of the recognition to apply research in ways that move it from "efficacious" to "effective," and a ray of hope in our ability to do so. Actively engaging with community partners is one way of ensuring the relevance of the work to the community setting and very likely increases the chances for a successful intervention. Both work involving the diffusion and dissemination of research evidence is needed, and research on the diffusion and dissemination process. While researchers often believe that translation and dissemination of their work is not their responsibility, practitioners often feel that such dissemination is the work of researchers. Sharing of this responsibility of dissemination and implementation must be accomplished for behavioral science findings to have maximum impact.

Basic behavioral and T1 translational science has suffered from far too little "cross-talk" between basic and applied behavioral scientists. Many applied researchers have not recognized the value of basic behavioral science to their work, and many basic scientists have not considered the application of their findings. It is clear that basic research in risk perception, mood, emotion, decision making, motivation, communication, and a host of other areas are indeed intimately tied to the care of cancer patients. Likewise, the issues facing cancer patients and healthcare providers provide a rich resource of research questions for basic scientists that can lead to further research questions relevant to morbidity, survival, and quality of life of cancer patients. The degree to which both groups work to close this historic gap is the degree to which they will ultimately contribute to the quality of the care we provide to cancer patients and their loved ones.

REFERENCES

1. Stefanek M, Hess S, Nelson W. Behavioral and social science research at the National Institutes of Health: is the mission being fulfilled? *APS Observer.* 2005;18:1.

2. Anderson NB, Scott PA. Making the case for psychophysiology during the era of molecular biology. *Psychophysiology.* 1999;36:1–13.

3. Abrams DB. Applying transdisciplinary research strategies to understanding and eliminating health disparities. *Health Educ Behav.* 2006;33(4):515–531.

4. Antoni MH, Lutgendorf SK, Cole SW, et al. The influence of bio-behavioural factors on tumour biology: pathways and mechanisms. *Nat Rev Cancer.* 2006;6(3):240–248.

5. Christakis NA, Fowler JH. The spread of obesity in a large social network over 32 years. *N Engl J Med.* 2007 July 26;357(4):370–379.

6. Coyne JC, Stefanek M, Palmer SC. Psychotherapy and survival in cancer: the conflict between hope and evidence. *Psychol Bull.* 2007;133(3):367–94.

7. Christakis NA, Fowler JH. The collective dynamics of smoking in a large social network. *N Engl J Med.* May 22, 2008;358(21):2249–58.

8. American Cancer Society. *Cancer facts & figures 2008.* Atlanta: American Cancer Society; 2008.

9. Parent SJ, Ward A, Mann T. Health information processed under limited attention: is it better to be "hot" or "cool"? *Health Psychol.* 2007;26(2):159–164.

10. Kaufman JS. Dissecting disparities. *Med Decis Making.* 2008;28(1):9–11.

11. Gaskin DJ, Frick KD. Race and ethnic disparities in valuing health. *Med Decis Making.* 2008;28(1):12–20.

12. Whitfield KE. Studying biobehavioral aspects of health disparities among older adult minorities. *J Urban Health.* 2005;82(2):103–110.

13. Graham ID, Tetroe J. Nomenclature in translational research. *JAMA.* 2008 May 14;299(18):2149–2150.

14. Best A, Hiatt RA, Cameron R, Rimer BK, Abrams DB. The evolution of cancer control research: an international perspective from Canada and The United States. *Cancer Epidemiol Biomarkers Prevent.* 2003;12:705–712.

15. Hinyard LJ, Kreuter MW. Using narrative communication as a tool for health behavior change: a conceptual, theoretical, and empirical overview. *Health Educ Behav.* 2007;34(5):777–792.

16. Strasser A, Capella J, Jepson C, et al. Experimental evaluation of anti-tobacco PSAs: effects of message content and format on physiological and behavioral outcomes. *Nicotine Tob Res.* 2009 Mar;11(3):293–302. Epub 2009 Feb 26.

17. Jain RK. Lessons from multidisciplinary translational trials on anti-angiogenic therapy of cancer. *Nat Rev Cancer.* 2008;8(4):309–316.

18. Glanz K, Rimer B, Viswanath V. (eds). *Health behavior and health education: Theory, research and practice.* 4th ed. San Francisco, CA. Jossey-Bass Inc; August 2008.

CHAPTER 93

Translating Psychosocial Oncology Research to Clinical Practice

Paul B. Jacobsen

In the previous chapter of this volume, Dr. Michael Stefanek described how scientific progress often moves through three phases: basic research followed by applied research followed by dissemination. In this schema, basic science discoveries are determined to have clinical applications that are then evaluated through applied research which, in turn, yield positive findings that should be disseminated and guide everyday clinical practice. In colloquial terms, these phases have been described as moving from the bench (basic research) to the trench (dissemination) via the bedside (applied research). The emphasis in the previous chapter was on the movement of research from the bench to the bedside. This chapter focuses on the movement of research from beside to the trench or, in other words, the translation of clinical research findings into everyday clinical practice.

EFFORTS TO LINK CLINICAL RESEARCH WITH CLINICAL PRACTICE

A considerable body of work suggests there are major challenges in the moving from the bedside (clinical research) to the trench (everyday clinical practice). Numerous reports and publications have documented that many patients fail to receive the care shown in clinical research to be effective for their disease or condition.[1-4] One example is a widely cited study which found that medical patients typically received only 55% of the care that would be recommended for them based on their history and health status.[4] Within oncology, recognized problems with the quality of care include the underuse of certain screening tests (e.g., mammography) as well as several forms of therapy (e.g., adjuvant chemotherapy for breast cancer) known to be effective based on clinical research.[1]

The field of evidence-based medicine arose, in part, to address problems such as these.[5,6] Like many frequently used terms, evidence-based medicine has been defined in numerous different ways. According to its major proponents, the practice of evidence-based medicine involves integrating individual clinical experience with the best available external clinical evidence from systematic research.[7] The practice of medicine based only on clinical experience is viewed as running the risk of becoming rapidly out of date to the detriment of patients.[7] On the other hand, without the benefit of clinical experience, the practice of medicine is viewed as running the risk becoming tyrannized by evidence that is inapplicable to or inappropriate for an individual patient.[7] As noted by the same proponents,[7] the evidence that should be used to practice evidence-based medicine is not limited to randomized controlled trials (RCTs) or meta-analyses of the research literature, even though these are recognized as the "gold standard" of clinical research evidence. In many instances, no randomized trial or meta-analysis has been conducted that is directly relevant to a particular clinical decision. Under these circumstances, the recommendation is that practice should be guided by the next best available external evidence.[7]

Efforts to translate research findings into clinical practice are conceived as occurring through three distinct processes: diffusion, dissemination, and implementation (see Fig. 93-1).[8]

Diffusion is defined as a passive process in which information with relevance to clinical practice is simply made available to potentially interested readers, typically in the form of articles in peer-reviewed journals.[8] This form of communication is seen as effecting change only when the information provided carries with it clear and unambiguous implications for clinical practice.[8] Even then, the impact will most likely be limited to individuals sufficiently motivated to seek out the information. Dissemination is defined as a more active process in which information relevant to clinical practice may be targeted or tailored for the intended audience.[8] Examples of such forms of communication include systematic reviews and meta-analyses as well as practice guidelines and consensus statements issued by professional organizations or government bodies. These secondary sources of information are considered to be more likely to reach their intended audience and raise awareness than primary sources such as published results of individual studies.[8] Implementation is defined as an even more active process that seeks to address barriers and identify strategies that enable healthcare providers to deliver care in a manner consistent with published findings.[8] Work in this area focuses on examining and changing the underlying organizational issues that influence how care is delivered. Similar to the use of evidence to guide the content of care, efforts to implement changes in clinical practice (i.e., processes of care) should also be evidence-based. With regard to implementation, relevant research can be found in the areas of social and behavioral science, human factors engineering, and health services.[9]

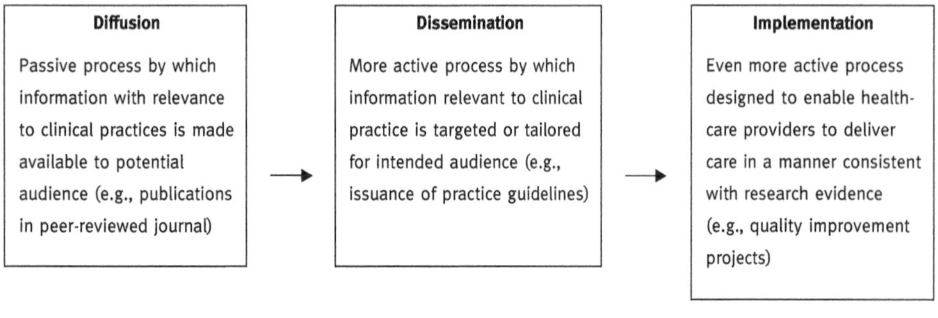

Diffusion	Dissemination	Implementation
Passive process by which information with relevance to clinical practices is made available to potential audience (e.g., publications in peer-reviewed journal)	More active process by which information relevant to clinical practice is targeted or tailored for intended audience (e.g., issuance of practice guidelines)	Even more active process designed to enable health-care providers to deliver care in a manner consistent with research evidence (e.g., quality improvement projects)

Fig. 93-1. Diffusion, dissemination, and implementation continuum.
SOURCE: Adapted from http://cancer-control.cancer.gov/d4d/definitions.html. Accessed July 14, 2008.

RECOMMENDATIONS FOR PSYCHOSOCIAL CARE OF CANCER PATIENTS

To illustrate the issues and challenges inherent in attempting to use clinical research to inform everyday clinical practice, the current chapter focuses on the status of efforts to provide evidence-based psychosocial care to cancer patients. This topic is a timely one as reflected by a 2007 report of the U.S. Institute of Medicine titled, "Cancer Care for the Whole Patient: Meeting Psychosocial Health Needs."[10] One of the report's major conclusions is that, despite good evidence for the effectiveness of services in meeting patients' psychosocial health needs, cancer care often fails to address these needs.[10] The reasons for this failure are many and include the tendency of oncology care providers to underestimate distress in patients[11] and to not link patients to appropriate services when needs are identified.[12] To address these problems, the report recommends that provision of appropriate psychosocial services should be adopted as a standard of quality cancer care.[10] The report also identifies a model for the effective delivery of psychosocial services that specifies the implementation of processes for (1) facilitating effective communication between patients and care providers; (2) identifying patients' psychosocial needs; (3) designing and implementing a plan that links patients with needed psychosocial services, coordinates their biomedical and psychosocial care, and engages and supports them; and (4) systematically following-up on, reevaluating, and adjusting the plan.[10]

These recommendations are similar to those embodied in Clinical Practice Guidelines for the Management of Distress first issued by the National Comprehensive Cancer Network (NCCN) in 1999.[13] The NCCN guidelines were developed based on the recognized need for better management of distress and with the intent of promoting best practices for the psychosocial care of cancer patients. Although too detailed to be fully summarized here, the NCCN guidelines are presented in the form of clinical pathways that describe recommended procedures for evaluating patients and recommended uses of psychological, psychiatric, social work, and pastoral care services to treat a wide range of problems. Similar to the Institute of Medicine report,[10] the NCCN guidelines recommend that all patients be routinely screened to identify the level and source of their distress. The specific services and resources subsequently recommended are designed to be appropriate to the nature and severity of the problems identified through screening and further evaluation.[13]

By specifying standards of care and identifying clinical pathways, the Institute of Medicine report and the NCCN guidelines have the potential to improve the quality of psychosocial care received by cancer patients. Among their notable limitations, however, is the limited use made of the existing evidence base in psychosocial oncology of RCTs. Most of the recommendations offered in the NCCN guidelines are identified as being based on lower level evidence that includes clinical experience.[13] This situation is true even though higher level evidence could be cited in several instances. For example, the NCCN guidelines recommend that psychotherapy be considered in the management of anxiety and depression.[13] Although several psychosocial interventions have been found to be effective against anxiety and depression in RCTs with cancer patients,[14] these research-supported interventions are not identified in the guidelines. With regard to the Institute of Medicine report, it is noteworthy that there is no explicit statement in the standards of care that the psychosocial care provided to care patients should be evidence-based.[10]

USE OF EVIDENCE TO GUIDE CLINICAL PRACTICE IN PSYCHOSOCIAL ONCOLOGY

The examples cited above illustrate how much needs to be accomplished to promote translation of research findings from psychosocial oncology into everyday clinical practice. Part of the problem reflects limitations in the existing evidence base in psychosocial oncology and part of the problem reflects the way in which this evidence base has been used. Consider, for example, evidence on the efficacy of psychosocial interventions against anxiety and depression in cancer patients. Over 60 RCTs have been conducted in which the effects of psychosocial interventions

on anxiety or depression in adult cancer patients have been evaluated and several systematic reviews and meta-analyses have been conducted summarizing the results of these studies.[14–18]

A recent summary of these reviews and meta-analyses identified three major weaknesses in this evidence base.[19] First, the research is characterized by inconsistent findings One systematic review examined whether at least 75% of the trials evaluating a specific strategy yielded statistically significant positive results.[15] Only one strategy was found to have met this criterion for anxiety and none met it for depression.[15] This lack of consistency can be attributed, in part, to differences across studies evaluating the same intervention strategy in the demographic, disease, and treatment characteristics of the samples recruited, the number and timing of the outcome assessments performed, and the outcome measures used. In addition, there appears to be considerable variation across studies in the number and content of sessions for interventions that share the same name (e.g., relaxation training).

The quality of the studies is the second major weakness. Inadequate reporting of study methodology appears to be a major problem. One review of this literature found that only 3% of trials provided sufficient information to permit evaluation of 10 indicators of study quality.[15] However, problems are also evident when study methodology is adequately described. For example, the majority of studies conducted in the 1990s failed to account for patients lost to follow-up in the outcome analyses that were performed.[15]

The general lack of research on patients experiencing clinically significant levels of anxiety and depression is the third major weakness. One review found that only 5% of studies limited eligibility to patients experiencing some degree of anxiety, depression, or psychological distress.[14] On the basis of the reported prevalence of anxiety and depression in oncology settings,[20,21] the average patient in most intervention studies was likely to be experiencing low levels of anxiety and depression at the time they were recruited. In addition to limiting the statistical power to detect intervention effects, the lack of eligibility criteria based on current anxiety or depression raises questions about whether the findings are generalizable to patients experiencing clinically significant symptomatology. This issue is important since clinical practice guidelines, such as those developed by NCCN,[13] recommend the use of psychosocial interventions specifically for patients experiencing heightened distress. This recommendation is also consistent with everyday clinical practice, where resources for psychosocial care are usually scarce and are provided primarily to patients experiencing heightened distress.

As noted previously, part of the problem in promoting the translation of research findings from psychosocial oncology into everyday clinical practice reflects the way in which the evidence base is used. Systematic reviews and meta-analyses of the research literature often focus only on providing an overall conclusion regarding the efficacy of psychosocial interventions for cancer patients. Depending on how the evidence is weighed, the conclusions arrived at may be quite different. For example, two recent reviews of many of the same publications reached very different conclusions about the overall effectiveness of psychosocial interventions for cancer patients. While one review[22] concluded that, "the preponderance of evidence furnished by these systematic reviews, particularly that gleaned from meta-analyses, suggests that psychological interventions are effective in managing distress," the other review[23] concluded that, "our review of reviews, particularly the more systematic reviews, provides no compelling evidence of broadly effective psychological interventions for reducing a wide range of distress outcomes in cancer patients."

Rather than attempt to reach an overall conclusion about the efficacy of psychosocial interventions, it may be more useful for efforts to translate research into practice to use research findings to derive specific evidence-based recommendations for the psychosocial care of cancer patients. One such approach developed by the author and others is to summarize the literature in terms of the number of RCTs that have positive results for a particular endpoint based on intervention type and patient disease or treatment status.[19] Table 93–1 illustrates how this approach was used to generate evidence-based recommendations for the use of psychosocial interventions to manage anxiety and depression.

Specifically, Table 93–1 lists RCTs published between 1980 and 2003 (the period covered by the systematic review) for which significant ($p < 0.05$) effects were obtained for an intervention relative to a control

Table 93–1. Evidence-based recommendations for use of psychosocial interventions according to intervention type and disease or treatment status

Relaxation techniques, alone or with education/skills training, are effective in preventing or relieving:
anxiety[24,25] and depression[24–26] in newly diagnosed patients
anxiety[27] and depression[27] in patients in the terminal phase of illness
anxiety[28–33] and depression[28–32] in patients undergoing chemotherapy
anxiety[34,35] and depression[34–36] in patients undergoing radiotherapy
anxiety[37,38] and depression[38,39] in patients undergoing surgery
anxiety[40] and depression[41] following completion of active treatment

Psycho-education is effective in preventing or relieving:
anxiety[42,43] and depression[42] in newly diagnosed patients
anxiety[44] and depression[45] in patients undergoing surgery
anxiety[46] in patients undergoing chemotherapy
depression[47] in patients undergoing chemotherapy

Supportive and supportive-expressive therapies are effective in preventing or relieving:
anxiety[48,49] and depression[48,50] in patients with metastatic disease
anxiety[32] and depression[32] in patients undergoing chemotherapy
anxiety[35] and depression[35] in patients undergoing radiotherapy
depression[51] in patients undergoing surgery

Couples counseling is effective in preventing or relieving:
depression[52] in patients undergoing surgery

Cognitive-behavioral therapy is effective in preventing or relieving:
depression[50] in patients with metastatic disease
anxiety[53] in patients undergoing surgery

Cognitive therapy is effective in preventing or relieving:
depression[54] in patients undergoing chemotherapy

SOURCE: Adapted from Jacobsen PB, Jim HS. Psychosocial interventions for anxiety and depression in cancer patients: Achievements and challenges. *CA - Cancer J Clin.* 2008;58:214–230.

condition. Providing this information to practitioners can serve several useful purposes. First, practitioners can readily determine when in the disease course or at what point in the treatment process a specific intervention strategy has been shown to be effective in preventing or relieving anxiety or depression. Second, the number of unique citations next to each listing identifies the strength of evidence for the specific use of that intervention strategy. Finally, the citations themselves identify publications that provide information about the content and delivery of the intervention strategy and the methodology used to evaluate it.

A variant of this approach was used by the National Breast Cancer Centre and the National Cancer Control Initiative in Australia to develop their "Clinical Practice Guidelines for the Psychosocial Care of Adults with Cancer."[55] These guidelines are presented in the form of a series of recommendations, accompanied by identification of the levels and sources of research support. An assumption underlying these guidelines is that evidence collected from other populations is generalizable to cancer patients. That is, some of the evidence cited to support recommendations comes from systematic reviews and randomized trials conducted on populations other than cancer patients.

DIFFUSION, DISSEMINATION, AND IMPLEMENTATION OF EVIDENCE-SUPPORTED PSYCHOSOCIAL INTERVENTIONS

Current efforts to translate psychosocial oncology research into clinical practice consist mostly of the diffusion of information via publication of research studies and the dissemination of information via publication of systematic reviews and meta-analyses. As described

earlier in this chapter, there have also been limited efforts by individuals and organizations to disseminate information via evidence-based recommendations.[19,55]

A project recently initiated by the U.S. National Cancer Institute and several other governmental bodies represents an important step forward in efforts to disseminate and promote implementation of evidence-supported interventions for psychosocial care of cancer patients. The project, Cancer Control P.L.A.N.E.T. (Plan, Link, Act, Network with Evidence-Based Tools), consists of a website (http://cancercontrolplanet.cancer.gov) that provides a link to a list of interventions relevant to the prevention, detection, and control of cancer. To be listed, an intervention must meet several criteria including having been developed with funding from a peer-reviewed research grant and having been evaluated in a study published in a peer-reviewed journal. In addition to describing an intervention, the web site provides ratings by peer reviewers of its dissemination capability, the strength of the research evidence supporting its efficacy, and its gender, cultural, and age appropriateness. There are also links that provide information about how to obtain the training manuals and other materials that may be necessary to deliver the intervention. Beyond this, the web site offers a web-based course designed to promote implementation by providing instruction in how to adapt a research-tested intervention program to a local community context.

Although Cancer Control P.L.A.N.E.T. and similar resources can facilitate the dissemination and implementation of existing research-tested intervention, several impediments to implementation remain in place. One major impediment to efforts to promote greater implementation of evidence-based psychosocial care of distress in cancer patients is the general lack of research on integrated models of care delivery. As noted previously, the NCCN guidelines describe a model of care that features screening to identify patients' level and source of distress, selection, and use of appropriate intervention strategies that may include psychotherapy and pharmacotherapy, and follow-up evaluations of patients' status.[13] Contrast this approach with most RCTs of interventions for anxiety and depression in cancer patients. These trials have generally accepted participants regardless of their level of distress and have generally focused on psychosocial rather than pharmacological or combined modality interventions.[14] Consequently, most of the evidence base in psychosocial oncology has little bearing on the NCCN model of care, a model that probably reflects how psychosocial care is being delivered in many oncology settings.

Investigators in psychosocial oncology seeking examples of research on integrated models of care delivery may wish to consider studies evaluating collaborative care for depression in primary care settings. Although the specific elements vary from study to study, most collaborative care interventions share certain basic elements: depression screening to identify cases; use of evidenced-based protocols for treatment of depression; structure collaborations between primary care providers and mental health specialists; and active monitoring of adherence to treatment and outcomes.[56] A recent meta-analysis identified 37 randomized studies that have evaluated collaborative care for depression among patients seen in primary care settings.[57] Overall, findings indicated that collaborative care yielded significantly ($p < 0.05$) better outcomes on standardized measures of depression at 6 months, with significant effects still present at 5 years in those studies that included a long-term follow-up assessment. The evidence for the efficacy of this intervention is considered to be sufficiently strong as to raise questions about whether further trials of collaborative care in the primary care setting are necessary.[56,57]

Although this model of care is of considerable relevance to psychosocial oncology, it has received limited research attention to date. A search of the literature identified only two studies in which the collaborative care model for depression has been studied with cancer patients. In the first study, described as a pilot project, 55 low-income Latina patients with breast or cervical cancer found to have comorbid depression through screening in an oncology clinic, were randomly assigned to usual care or a collaborative care intervention.[58] The intervention included initial and follow-up sessions with a master's level social worker trained to provide problem-solving therapy, support for antidepressant medication adherence, and assistance with systems navigation. Findings showed significantly ($p < 0.03$) better outcomes for the collaborative care group. Specifically, 37% of women in the collaborative care condition and only 12% of women in the control condition displayed a clinically significant reduction in depressive symptomatology by the 4-month follow-up assessment.

In the other study, 200 cancer patients being treated at a regional center who were found to have major depressive disorder through screening, were randomly assigned to usual care or usual care plus a collaborative care intervention.[59] The intervention consisted of up to ten sessions with a cancer nurse that included education about depression and its treatment (including antidepressant medication) and problem-solving therapy to overcome feelings of helplessness. In addition, the nurse communicated with each patient's oncologist and primary care doctor about management of major depressive disorder. Findings showed significantly ($p < 0.05$) better scores on a measure of depressive symptomatology 3 months after randomization for patients who received the collaborative care intervention. These differences are reflected in the percentages of usual care patients (45%) versus collaborative care patients (68%) whose major depressive disorder had remitted in the 3-month period. The beneficial effects of collaborative care observed at 3 months were still evident at 6-month and 12-month follow-up assessments.

These two studies provide strong evidence that an integrated model of care delivery, which includes routine screening and care delivered according to a standardized protocol, can improve the management of depression in cancer patients beyond usual care. It is noteworthy both interventions incorporated a form of psychotherapy (i.e., problem-solving therapy) found previously to be effective against depressive symptomatology in a RCT with cancer patients.[60] Thus, both studies provide excellent examples of how a research-tested intervention can be incorporated into a broader intervention strategy designed for dissemination into clinical practice. The next phase in the development of this collaborative care model would be to identify strategies to facilitate its dissemination to professionals working with cancer patients and to promote its implementation in oncology settings.

FINAL THOUGHTS ON TRANSLATING RESEARCH INTO CLINICAL PRACTICE

The rationale for promoting the translation of psychosocial oncology research into clinical practice is straightforward. With a growing body of research demonstrating the efficacy of psychosocial interventions in improving the prevention, detection, and control of cancer, clinicians have an obligation to deliver care in a manner consistent with this evidence. Although the rationale may be straightforward, there are major challenges to achieving the goal of translating psychosocial research into clinical practice.

One challenge involves the nature of the evidence. Many intervention strategies, although shown to be effective, have little potential for dissemination because of the time, expense, and resources required to implement them. This challenge is not insurmountable and can be addressed by designing new interventions with dissemination in mind or redesigning existing interventions to make them more disseminable.

Making practitioners aware of evidence that is relevant to their clinical practice is another challenge. Passive diffusion of evidence, such as the publication of studies in peer-reviewed journals, generally has limited impact on practice given the volume of findings published and the complexities of implementing many psychosocial interventions. Targeted dissemination of information, such as the issuance of evidence-based guidelines, has greater potential to influence clinical practice, especially if the recommendations are based on evidence from multiple studies. A valuable resource for identifying and reviewing evidence-based guidelines relevant to psychosocial oncology is the National Guideline Clearinghouse maintained by the U.S. Agency for Health Care Research and Quality (accessible at www.guideline.gov). There, for example, one can find evidence-based guidelines for smoking cessation, genetic cancer risk assessment and counseling, and long-term follow-up of survivors of childhood, adolescent, and young adult cancers.

Getting practitioners to implement evidence-based interventions is perhaps the most difficult challenge. Evidence from psychosocial oncology suggests that awareness of clinical guidelines does not translate into adherence to clinical practice guidelines.[61] As noted previously, this last challenge requires active efforts to address barriers and identify strategies that enable practitioners to deliver care in a manner that is evidence-based. One useful conceptual framework for understanding and addressing this challenge is the push-pull infrastructure model (see Fig. 93–2).[62]

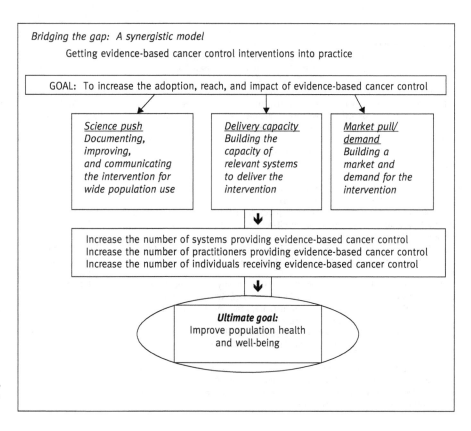

Fig. 93–2. Push-pull infrastructure model.
SOURCE: Adapted from Bindemann S, Soukop M, Kaye SB. Randomised controlled study of relaxation training. *Eur J Cancer.* 1991;27(2):170–174.

The model stipulates that efforts to "push" knowledge from science into practice must be accompanied by increased demand (i.e., "pull") for evidence-based approaches by patients and providers and an increase in the capacity of the infrastructure to deliver evidence-based interventions. According to the model, when all three factors work in concert, the number of individuals providing and receiving evidence-based interventions should increase, thereby leading to improved outcomes.[62] To date, efforts to promote evidence-based psychosocial care have focused mostly on the push part of the model. For greater progress to be achieved, the model suggests that more attention needs to be devoted to fostering greater demand for evidence-based psychosocial care among providers and the public and increasing capacity to deliver such care.

REFERENCES

1. Institute of Medicine. *Ensuring quality cancer care*. Washington: National Academy Press; 1999.

2. Institute of Medicine. *Crossing the quality chasm: A new health system for the 21st century*. Washington: National Academy Press; 2001.

3. Jencks SM, Cuerdon T, Burwen DR, et al. Quality of medical care delivered to Medicare beneficiaries: a profile at state and national levels. *JAMA*. 2000;284(13):1670–1676.

4. McGlynn EA, Asch SM, Adams J, et al. The quality of health care delivered to adults in the United States. *New Engl J Med*. 2003;348(26):2635–2645.

5. Berwick DM. Disseminating innovations in health care. *JAMA*. 2003;289(15):535–542.

6. Lenfant C. Clinical research to clinical practice-Lost in translation? *New Engl J Med*. 2003;349(9):868–874.

7. Sackett DL, Rosenberg WM, Gray JA, Haynes RB, Richardson WS. Evidence based medicine: What it is and what it isn't. *Brit Med J*. 1996;312:71–72.

8. Lomas J. Diffusion, dissemination, and implementation: who should do what? *Ann NY Acad Sci*. 1993;703:226–235.

9. Shortell SM, Rundall TG, Hsu J. Improving patient care by linking evidence-based medicine and evidence-based management. *JAMA*. 2007;298(6):673–676.

10. Institute of Medicine. *Cancer care for the whole patient: Meeting psychosocial health needs*. Washington: The National Academies Press; 2007.

11. Fallowfield L, Ratcliffe D, Jenkins V, Saul J. Psychiatric morbidity and its recognition by doctors in patients with cancer. *Brit J Cancer*. 2001;84:1011–1015.

12. Institute of Medicine. *Implementing cancer surivorship care planning*. Washington: The National Academies Press; 2007.

13. Anonymous. NCCN practice guidelines for the management of psychosocial distress. *Oncology (Huntington)*. 1999;13:113–147.

14. Jacobsen PB, Donovan KA, Swaine ZN, Watson IS. Management of anxiety and depression in adult cancer patients: Toward an evidence-based approach. In: Chang AE, Ganz PA, Hayes DF, Kinsella TJ, et al. (eds). *Oncology: An evidence-based approach*. New York: Springer-Verlag; 2006:1552–1579.

15. Newell SA, Sanson-Fisher RW, Savolainen NJ. Systematic review of psychological therapies for cancer patients: overview and recommendations for future research. *J Natl Cancer Inst*. 2002;94(8):558–584.

16. Rodin G, Lloyd N, Katz M, Green E, Mackay JA, Wong RK. The treatment of depression in cancer patients: a systematic review. *Support Care Cancer*. 2007;15(2):123–136.

17. Sellick SM, Crooks DL. Depression and cancer: an appraisal of the literature for prevalence, detection, and practice guideline development for psychological interventions. *Psychooncology*. 1999;8(4):315–333.

18. Sheard T, Maguire P. The effect of psychological interventions on anxiety and depression in cancer patients: results of two meta-analyses. *Br J Cancer*. 1999;80(11):1770–1780.

19. Jacobsen PB, Jim HS. Psychosocial interventions for anxiety and depression in cancer patients: achievements and challenges. *CA—Cancer J Clin*. 2008;58:214–230.

20. Kerrihard T, Breitbart W, Dent R, Strout D. Anxiety in patients with cancer and immunodeficiency virus. *Semin Clin Neuropsych*. 1999;4(2):114–132.

21. Pirl W. Evidence report on the occurrence, assessment, and treatment of depression in cancer patients. *J Natl Cancer I Mono*. 2004;(32):32–39.

22. Andrykowski MA, Manne SL. Are psychological interventions effective and accepted by cancer patients? I. Standards and levels of evidence. *Ann Beh Med*. 2006;32(2):93–97.

23. Lepore SL, Coyne JC. Psychological interventions for distress in cancer patients: a review of reviews. *Ann Beh Med*. 2006;32(2):85–92.

24. Arakawa S. Relaxation to reduce nausea, vomiting, and anxiety induced by chemotherapy in Japanese patients. *Cancer Nurs*. 1997;20(5):342–349.

25. Bindemann S, Soukop M, Kaye SB. Randomised controlled study of relaxation training. *Eur J Cancer*. 1991;27(2):170–174.

26. Edgar L, Rosberger Z, Collet JP. Lessons learned: outcomes and methodology of a coping skills intervention trial comparing individual and group formats for patients with cancer. *Int J Psychiatry Med*. 2001;31(3):289–304.

27. Liossi C, White P. Efficacy of clinical hypnosis in the enhancement of quality of life of terminally ill cancer patients. *Cont Hypn*. 2001;18(3):145–160.

28. Burish TG, Lyles JN. Effectiveness of relaxation training in reducing adverse reactions to cancer chemotherapy. *J Behav Med*. 1981;4(1):65–78.

29. Burish TG, Carey MP, Krozely MG, Greco FA. Conditioned side effects induced by cancer chemotherapy: prevention through behavioral treatment. *J Consult Clin Psychol*. 1987;55(1):42–48.

30. Carey MP, Burish TG. Providing relaxation training to cancer chemotherapy patients: a comparison of three delivery techniques. *J Consult Clin Psychol*. 1987;55(5):732–737.

31. Jacobsen PB, Meade CD, Stein KD, Chirikos TN, Small BJ, Ruckdeschel JC. Efficacy and costs of two forms of stress management training for cancer patients undergoing chemotherapy. *J Clin Oncol*. 2002;20(12):2851–2862.

32. Mantovani G, Astara G, Lampis B, et al. Evaluation by multidimensional instruments of health-related quality of life of elderly cancer patients undergoing three different "psychosocial" treatment approaches. A randomized clinical trial. *Support Care Cancer*. 1996;4(2):129–140.

33. Morrow GR. Effect of the cognitive hierarchy in the systematic desensitization treatment of anticipatory nausea in cancer patients: a component comparison with relaxation only, counseling, and no treatment. *Cog Ther Res*. 1986;10(4):421–446.

34. Decker TW, Cline-Elsen J, Gallagher M. Relaxation therapy as an adjunct in radiation oncology. *J Clin Psychol*. 1992;48(3):388–393.

35. Evans RL, Connis RT. Comparison of brief group therapies for depressed cancer patients receiving radiation treatment. *Public Health Rep*. 1995;110(3):306–311.

36. Pruitt BT, Waligora-Serafin B, McMahon T, et al. An educational intervention for newly-diagnosed cancer patients undergoing radiotherapy. *Psychooncology*. 1993;2(1):55–62.

37. Cheung YL, Molassiotis A, Chang AM. The effect of progressive muscle relaxation training on anxiety and quality of life after stoma surgery in colorectal cancer patients. *Psychooncology*. 2003;12(3):254–266.

38. Petersen RW, Quinlivan JA. Preventing anxiety and depression in gynaecological cancer: a randomised controlled trial. *BJOG*. 2002;109(4):386–394.

39. Fawzy FI, Cousins N, Fawzy NW, Kemeny ME, Elashoff R, Morton D. A structured psychiatric intervention for cancer patients. I. Changes over time in methods of coping and affective disturbance. *Arch Gen Psychiatry*. 1990;47(8):720–725.

40. Elsesser K, van Berkel M, Sartory G. The effects of anxiety management training on psychological variables and immune parameters in cancer patients: a pilot study. *Beh Cog Psychoth*. 1994;22:13–23.

41. Simpson JS, Carlson LE, Trew ME. Effect of group therapy for breast cancer on healthcare utilization. *Cancer Pract*. 2001;9(1):19–26.

42. McQuellon RP, Wells M, Hoffman S, et al. Reducing distress in cancer patients with an orientation program. *Psychooncology*. 1998;7(3):207–217.

43. Wells ME, McQuellon RP, Hinkle JS, Cruz JM. Reducing anxiety in newly diagnosed cancer patients: a pilot program. *Cancer Pract*. 1995;3(2):100–104.

44. Ali NS, Khalil HZ. Effect of psychoeducational intervention on anxiety among Egyptian bladder cancer patients. *Cancer Nurs*. 1989;12(4):236–242.

45. McArdle JM, George WD, McArdle CS, et al. Psychological support for patients undergoing breast cancer surgery: a randomised study. *BMJ*. 1996;312(7034):813–816.

46. Jacobs C, Ross RD, Walker IM, Stockdale FE. Behavior of cancer patients: a randomized study of the effects of education and peer support groups. *Am J Clin Oncol*. 1983;6(3):347–353.

47. Rawl SM, Given BA, Given CW, et al. Intervention to improve psychological functioning for newly diagnosed patients with cancer. *Oncol Nurs Forum*. 2002;29(6):967–975.

48. Goodwin PJ, Leszcz M, Ennis M, et al. The effect of group psychosocial support on survival in metastatic breast cancer. *N Engl J Med*. 2001;345(24):1719–1726.

49. Spiegel D, Bloom JR, Yalom I. Group support for patients with metastatic cancer. A randomized outcome study. *Arch Gen Psychiatry*. 1981;38(5):527–533.

50. Edelman S, Bell DR, Kidman AD. A group cognitive behaviour therapy programme with metastatic breast cancer patients. *Psychooncology*. 1999;8(4):295–305.

51. Watson M, Denton S, Baum M, Greer S. Counselling breast cancer patients: a specialist nurse service. *Counsel Psychol Quart*. 1988;1(1):25–34.

52. Christensen DN. Postmastectomy couple counseling: an outcome study of a structured treatment protocol. *J Sex Marital Ther*. 1983;9(4):266–275.

53. Moynihan C, Bliss JM, Davidson J, Burchell L, Horwich A. Evaluation of adjuvant psychological therapy in patients with testicular cancer: randomised controlled trial. *BMJ*. 1998;316(7129):429–435.

54. Marchioro G, Azzarello G, Checchin F, et al. The impact of a psychological intervention on quality of life in non-metastatic breast cancer. *Eur J Cancer*. 1996;32(9):1612–1615.

55. National Breast Cancer Centre and National Cancer Control Initiative. *Clinical practice guidelines for the psychosocial care of adults with cancer*. Camperdown: National Breast Cancer Centre; 2003.

56. Simon G. Collaborative care for depression. *Brit Med J*. 2006;332: 249–250.

57. Gilbody S, Bower P, Fletcher J, Richards D, Sutton AJ. Collaborative care for depression: a cumulative meta-analysis and review of longer-term outcomes. *Arch Int Med*. 2006;166(21):2314–2321.

58. Dwight-Johnson M, Ell K, Lee PJ. Can collaborative care address the needs of low-income Latinas with comorbid depression and cancer? Results from a randomized pilot study. *Psychosomatics*. 2005;46:224–232.

59. Strong V, Waters R, Hibberd C, et al. Management of depression in people with cancer (SMaRT oncology 1): a randomised trial. *Lancet*. 2008;372(9632): 40–48.

60. Nezu AM, Nezu CM, Felgoise SH, McClure KS, Houts PS. Project Genesis: assessing the efficacy of problem-solving therapy for distressed adult cancer patients. *J Consult Clin Psychol*. 2003;71(6):1036–1048.

61. Jacobsen PB, Ransom S. Implementation of NCCN distress management guidelines by member institutions. *J Natl Comp Cancer Net*. 2007;5(1):99–103.

62. Kerner JF, Guirguis-Blake J, et al. Translating research into improved outcomes in comprehensive cancer control. *Cancer Cause Control*. 2005;16(Suppl 1): 27–40.

CHAPTER 94

How to Design and Analyze Screening Studies

Alex J. Mitchell

WHAT IS SCREENING?

When epidemiologists talk of screening they are referring to the application of a test to individuals who are currently asymptomatic. In cancer settings this is usually a population strategy whereby large numbers of people in the community are screened for cervical, colon, breast, or prostate cancer. The aim of screening is establish those who probably have the disorder, ideally at an early stage and at the same time rule-out (reassure) those who are healthy. Once an individual comes to medical attention the attempt to establish a disorder is often called case-finding. In this chapter I will focus on psychological screening, such as methods to identify depression and distress (Textbox 52–1).

In both screening and case finding the aim is to make an accurate diagnosis and thereby offer help where help is wanted. The main difference is that screening is typically applied when prevalence is low thus screening tests must be efficient, highly acceptable and usually emphasize the ability to rule-out noncases with minimal false negatives. A lower rule-in accuracy (positive predictive value, PPV) may be acceptable in population screening because a second stage assessment is recommended in those who screen positive as a possible case. These multistep strategies which begin simply and progress to a more complex but more accurate second step are also known as algorithm approaches. Just as with the introduction of a new drug, a new screening test cannot be assumed to be efficacious without testing. In fact, like a new drug, a screening test may have unforeseen adverse consequences or it may simply be ignored by health professionals. To be effective a screening method must have not only accuracy and acceptability but adequate uptake and linked methods to improve quality of care.

DESIGNING STUDIES TO TEST NEW SCREENING METHODS

Screening study design. Despite the huge promise of better screening methods for psychological disorders the evidence that any particular method improves patient outcomes is still lacking. The problem lies with a poverty of studies that have examined implementation of screening as opposed to testing just the accuracy (or more correctly diagnostic validity) of a given tool. The evaluation of screening methods should be viewed in a wider context of tool development (Table 94–1). In the preclinical phase the tool itself is developed, often by borrowing items from existing scales and usually by consensus rather than by scientific testing. No matter how plausible the new tool, it is essentially untested at this stage. In phases I and II preliminary testing occurs, ideally in a clinically representative sample with several competing comparison groups. For example, the ability of a tool to detect major or minor depression in cancer compared to those with no symptoms of depression and those with subsyndromal symptoms alone. This "diagnostic validity" testing is an important step which shows the maximum potential of a scale. However, it does not show the real-world ability of the test. By analogy, a phase II drug trial may demonstrate potential efficacy of a drug but the effectiveness in clinical practice is unknown to this stage.

The next steps are probably the most important, but most often overlooked. In phase III of screening tool development a randomized control trial (RCT) is conducted to directly compare the results of clinicians using the new tool with those using either an older established method or an unassisted "diagnosis as-usual" (or ideally both). This is akin to the drug RCT and the outcome of interest is the number of additional cases correctly diagnosed or ruled out compared with assessment as usual. In the final step, phase IV, the success or otherwise of the new method is monitored in the field. In short, the question here is how much does the tool influence the outcome of patients once implemented and also how well is the tool accepted by clinicians (uptake). Ultimately the value of a tool must be proven in the clinical environment by comparison against either an established tool or clinical skills alone. The acceptability, availability, and cost of the tool will ultimately influence its uptake as much as its theoretical accuracy.

Refinement of existing scales and tools. Given that there are a large number of imperfect, but widely used instruments, it follows many could be refined by adding or removing items or changing the weighting of scoring or possibly the diagnostic algorithm. There have been recent attempts to improve efficacy of screening instruments using modern psychometrics, most notably using Rasch models. The models are part of a family of measurement models developed for educational psychology, increasingly employed in test development and refinement in medicine. Frequently it is found that conventional instruments may be shortened in length without significantly reducing screening efficacy. Occasionally the abbreviation of the original is dramatic, but there is may be a limit to the reducibility. Further, the ability of these adapted instruments to identify a key outcome variable such as distress warranting an intervention usually remains less than perfect. Combining items drawn from a number of instruments into an item bank may improve screening efficacy, whilst at the same time minimizing the number of questions patients are required to answer and consequently reducing patient burden. Item banks, such as these and computer-adaptive tests, which tailor the questions presented to patients' responses have already been successfully developed for assessing emotional distress in a psychiatric population.[1,2]

ANALYZING THE RESULTS OF A SCREENING STUDY

Basic measures of accuracy. Attempts to separate those with a condition from those without on the basis of a test or clinical method are best represented by the 2 × 2 table which generates sensitivity (Se), specificity (Sp), positive predictive value (PPV) and negative predictive value (NPV) (Fig. 94–1).[3] It is important to understand the difference between looking vertically across cells and looking horizontally. Vertically, the denominator is the number of cases with or without the condition, a number which is unknown to the clinician. Horizontally, the dominator is the number of positive or negative screens, a number that is known and hence the reason why PPV and NPV are often more important than Se and Sp. Performance of most tests varies with the baseline prevalence of the condition. Put easy it is simple to detect cases when nothing but cases exist (prevalence = 100%) but conversely it is hard for to detect cases when such cases are very rare.[4] Rule in and rule out accuracy should be considered independent variables although a test may perform well in both directions. Rule-in accuracy is best measured by the PPV but a very high Sp also implies few false positives and hence any positive screen will suggest a true case.[5] Rule-out accuracy is best measured by the NPV where the denominator is all who test negative but again if the Se is very high there will be few false negatives and hence any negative implies a true noncase (Textbox 94–1).[5]

Table 94–1. Stages in the evaluation of the screening tool or diagnostic test

Stage	Type	Purpose	Description
Preclinical	Development	Development of the proposed tool or test	Here the aim is to develop a screening method that is likely to help in the detection of the underlying disorder, either in a specific setting or in all setting Issues of acceptability of the tool to both patients and staff must be considered in order for implementation to be successful
Phase I_screen	Diagnostic validity	Early diagnostic validity testing in a selected sample and refinement of tool	The aim is to evaluate the early design of the screening method against a known (ideally accurate) standard known as the criterion reference In early testing the tool may be refined, selecting most useful aspects and deleting redundant aspects to make the tool as efficient (brief) as possible whilst retaining its value
Phase II_screen	Diagnostic validity	Diagnostic validity in a representative sample	The aim is to assess the refined tool against a criterion (gold standard) in a real-world sample where the comparator subjects may comprise several competing condition which may otherwise cause difficulty regarding differential diagnosis
Phase III_screen	Implementation	Screening RCT; clinicians using vs not using a screening tool	This is an important step in which the tool is evaluated clinically in one group with access to the new method compared to a second group (ideally selected in a randomized fashion) who make assessments without the tool
Phase IV_screen	Implementation	Screening implementation studies using real-world outcomes	In this last step the screening tool/method is introduced clinically but monitored to discover the effect on important patient outcomes such as new identifications, new cases treated, and new cases entering remission

	Gold standard disorder	Gold standard no disorder	
Test +ve	A	B	A / A + B **PPV**
Test -ve	C	D	D / C + D **NPV**
Total	A / A + C **Se**	D / B + D **Sp**	

Fig. 94–1. Generic 2 × 2 table.

Textbox 94–1. Basic measures of diagnostic accuracy

Sensitivity (Se) a/(a + c)
A measure of accuracy defined the proportion of patients with disease in whom the test result is positive: a/(a + c)

Specificity (Sp) d/(b + d)
A measure of accuracy defined as the proportion of patients without disease in whom the test result is negative

Positive Predictive Value a/(a+b)
A measure of rule-in accuracy defined as the proportion of true positives in those that screen positive

Negative Predictive Value c/(c+d)
A measure of rule-out accuracy defined as the proportion of true negatives in those that screen negative

Composite (summary) measures of diagnostic accuracy. Optimal accuracy is often achieved by choosing one test for ruling-in (case-finding) and another for ruling-out (screening) but not uncommonly where resources are limited only a single test can be applied and this single test must perform as well as possible in both directions. Here summary statistics are used to test accuracy. These use a combination of either Se and Sp or PPV and NPV. Reciprocal measures are also becoming more common and offer a "number needed" estimate. All such methods work well when the optimum cutoff is known or in binary (yes/no) tests, but where performance varies according to the cutoff threshold then sensitivity versus specificity for each cutoff generates a receiver operating characteristic (ROC) curve and the area under the curve gives a measure of the overall performance. More advanced methods are needed when multiple tests need to be compared (each with different Se and Sp values). For example, results can be combined in a summary receiver operator curve (sROC),[6] or even a hierarchical sROC that combines all results meta-analytically.

Youden's J index. Youden's J is based on the characteristics of sensitivity and specificity as follows: $J = sensitivity + specificity -1$.[7] If a test has no diagnostic value J = −1 and if perfect then $J = +1$. Youden's index is probably most useful where sensitivity and specificity are equally important and where prevalence is close to 0.5. A qualitative rating is >0.90 = excellent; >0.80 = good; > 0.70 = modest performance.

The reciprocal of Youden's *J* was originally suggested as a method to calculate the number of patients that need to be examined to correctly detect one person with the disease. This has been called the *number needed to diagnose* (NND). Thus NND = 1/(Sensitivity − [1 − Specificity]). However, the NND statistic is distorted as the Youden score approaches 0 and is no longer recommended.

The predictive summary index. Unlike sensitivity and specificity, PPV and NPV are measures of discrimination (or gain) that are strongly influence by prevalence. A measure of gain in the certainty that a condition is present is the difference between the posttest probability (the PPV) and the prior probability (the prevalence) when the test is positive. The gain in certainty that there is no disease is the difference between NPV and the probability of no disease (1−prevalence). This is best illustrated in a Bayesian plot of conditional probabilities (Fig. 94–2). In the Bayesian plot shown in Figure 94–2 the pretest probability is plotted (black line) and the posttest probability the dotted line. The overall benefit of a test from positive to negative is a summation of (PPV − Prevalence) + (NPV − [1 − Prevalence]) = PPV+NPV − 1. This is the predictive summary index (PSI). A qualitative rating is >0.90 = excellent; >0.80 = good; > 0.70 = modest performance.

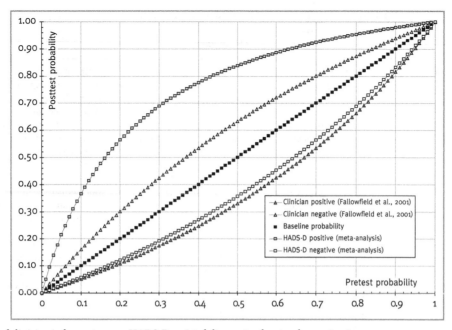

Fig. 94–2. Bayesian plot of clinician judgment versus HADS-D assisted diagnosis of major depression in cancer.
SOURCE: Clinician Data from Fallowfield L, Ratcliffe D, Jenkins V, Saul J. Psychiatric morbidity and its recognition by doctors in patients with cancer. Br J Cancer. 2001;84:1011-1015; HADS-D data from unpublished meta-analysis Mitchell AJ.

An improvement upon the NND is to take the reciprocal of the PSI. This was proposed by Linn and Grunau (2006) and called the number needed to predict (NNP) which is the reciprocal of the predictive summary index.

Overall accuracy (fraction correct). A third approach to calculating accuracy is to measure the overall fraction correct. The overall fraction correct is given by A+D/A+B+C+D (Fig. 94–1). 1 minus the fraction correct (1-FC) is the fraction incorrect. The fraction correct can be useful because it reveals the real number of correct versus incorrect identifications. The fraction correct minus the fraction incorrect can serve as a useful "identification index" which can be converted into a number needed to screen.

The number needed to screen = 1 / FC – (fraction incorrect) or 1/ Identification index. Unlike the Youden score or NND, the clinical interpretation of the NNS is clinically meaningful. It is the actual number of cases that need to be screened to yield one additional correct identification (case or noncases) beyond those misidentified.

Take a hypothetical example of a new screening test for depression tested in 100 with the condition and 1000 without which yields a Se of 0.90 and a Sp of 0.50. The Youden score is thus 0.4 and the NND 2.5 suggesting 2.5 individuals are needed to diagnose one person with depression. In fact, out of every 100 applications of the test there would be nine people with depression (prevalence × 100) of whom 90% would be true positives (=8.2), and 81 without depression (1 – prevalence × 100) of whom 50% would be negatives (=45.5). In this example there would be 53.6 true cases per 100 screened (fraction correct per 100 cases) but at the expense of 46.4 errors (fraction incorrect) per 100 screened; a net gain of 7.3 identified cases per 100 screened. Thus, the number to screen (NNS) would be 13.75 applications of the test to yield one true cases *without error*.

Meta-analytic measures of diagnostic accuracy. A meta-analysis attempts to combine data from individual studies, placing more emphasis on those with larger samples. The main problem is accounting for heterogeneity as studies usually vary by setting and prevalence. It is therefore recommended to pool data for sensitivity and specificity as these are relatively independent of prevalence and then calculate PPV and NPV according to local prevalence rates. Many statistical

programs can perform such a meta-analysis but recently Reitsma and colleagues developed the command "metandi" for Stata 10 as a bivariate diagnostic meta-analysis that purports to separate interdependence of sensitivity and specificity.[8] This method was originally developed as a mixed effects regression model for meta-analysis of trials and modified more recently for studies of diagnostic accuracy. Pooled results can be plotted in a summary Bayesian plot of conditional probabilities (Fig. 94–2). Area under the Bayesian curve allows statistical comparison of accuracy across all possible prevalence values and can be calculated simply using Microsoft Excel. Case-finding (rule-in) success is therefore the area under the positive curve (AUC+) and screening (rule-out) success given by the area above the negative curve (AUC-).

CLINICAL INTERPRETATION OF DIAGNOSTIC ACCURACY

Clinical utility index (occurrence and discrimination combined). We have considered the strengths and limitations of various measures of diagnostic accuracy. Se and Sp are essentially measures of occurrence. If 8 out of 10 with anxiety score positive on the distress thermometer then the sensitivity of the distress thermometer for anxiety is 80%. Contrastingly PPV and NPV are essentially measures of discrimination. If nine of those with anxiety to every one without anxiety scores positive on the distress thermometer then the PPV will equal 90%. These two attributes, occurrence and discrimination should both be high for an ideal test. Consider the example of a new "Depression Thermometer" test which if positive has a 90% PPV but is only positive in half of depressed individuals (Se 50%). Clinically relevant rule in accuracy would be product of the PPV and Se. This called the +ve utility index (UI+ = Se × PPV). Similarly clinically relevant rule out accuracy would be product of the NPV and Sp. This called the –ve utility index (UI– = Sp × NPV). The utility index is a measure of the clinical value of a diagnostic test when applied in a specific setting and can be graded using the following scale: <0.5 poor, ≥0.5 <0.64 fair, ≥0.64 <0.81 good and ≥0.81 ≤1 excellent (Textbox 94–2).

Clinical feasibility. Even a test with high performance measures cannot be assumed to be beneficial. A number of factors determine whether a screening tool can be usefully translated into a screening program. Guidelines from the U.K. National Screening Committee are helpful here. Feasibility asks whether a tool is practical both in

Textbox 94–2. UK National Screening Committee Guidelines

The condition should:

- Be an important health issue
- Have a well-understood history, with a detectable risk factor or disease marker
- Have cost-effective primary preventions implemented.

The screening tool should:

- Be a valid tool with known cutoff
- Be acceptable to the public
- Have agreed diagnostic procedures.

The treatment should:

- Be effective, with evidence of benefits of early intervention
- Have adequate resources
- Have appropriate policies as to who should be treated.

The screening program should:

- Show evidence that benefits of screening outweighing risks
- Be acceptable to public and professionals
- Be cost effective (and have ongoing evaluation)
- Have quality-assurance strategies in place.

Adapted from: *UK National Screening Committee Criteria for appraising the viability, effectiveness and appropriateness of a screening programme* http://www.nsc.nhs.uk/pdfs/criteria.pdf

screening program those who receive a worthwhile screening should have 1. a high satisfaction with care 2. improved interaction with clinical staff 3. a higher likelihood of appropriate treatment 4. a better chance of remission 5. improved health related quality of life.

CONCLUSIONS

Decades of intensive research in psycho-oncology have yielded instruments that offer a diagnostic performance close to that generated by longer psychiatric interviews. Yet there is a paucity of research examining whether these methods actually improve quality of care and almost no direct comparison with clinicians unassisted (routine) diagnoses. The development and evaluation of diagnostic (screening) tests should be approached using the same high standard that is afforded to the evaluation of new drugs. For example, a screening RCT would involve evaluation of diagnoses in one group of patients assessed with the new tool compared to a second group randomized to assessment using conventional methods. Existing tools can often be refined, simplified, or combined to optimize efficiency. The aim is to preserve accuracy in the briefest, most efficient package. Many statistical techniques are available to test accuracy including the newly developed utility index and bivariate diagnostic meta-analysis. However the rate limiting step in the effectiveness of any screen is its acceptability (for discussion see Mitchell and Coyne, 2008).[10] Acceptability to health professionals influences clinicians' willingness to apply a screening test and acceptability to patients influences a persons willingness to attend for screening.

application and scoring to gain acceptance by health professionals and patients. This has been poorly studied in relation to depression severity scales. However, in one example Bermejo et al. (2005) looked at attitudes to the Patient Health Questionnaire (PHQ9) in primary care in Germany.[9] In this study 1034 patients from 17 GPs were enrolled and both patients and health professionals asked about acceptability. Patients found the instrument highly acceptably but 62.5% of the GPs felt that the questionnaire as too long and 37.5% too time-consuming, even though it typically took 1–2 minutes. 50% of the GPs rated the PHQ as an impediment to daily practice and 75% thought it was impractical compared with only 25% of patients. One proxy for feasibility is willingness of clinicians to use the test. Any screening roll out will be compromised if front line staff find the tool too difficult to administer or score.

Feasibility and uptake can be measured, as can satisfaction of patients and health professionals. Together with improvements in patient outcomes, these are important components of demonstrating the clinical value of screening tests.

Clinical Benefit. Ultimately a screening test should bring tangible patient benefits. These should go beyond increased detection per se. A screening tool linked with an intervention, staff training and patient monitoring is called a screening program. In a trial of a hypothetical

REFERENCES

1. Fliege H, Becker J, Walter OB, Bjorner JB, Klapp BF, Rose M. Development of a computer-adaptive test for depression (D-CAT). *Qual Life Res.* 2005;14:2277–2291.

2. Walter OB, Becker J, Bjorner JB, Fliege H, Klapp BF, Rose M. Development and evaluation of a computer adaptive test for 'Anxiety' (Anxiety-CAT). *Qual Life Res.* 2007;16:S143-S155.

3. Yerushalmy J. Statistical problems in assessing methods of medical diagnosis, with special reference to X-ray techniques. *Pub Health Rep.* 1947;62:1432–49.

4. Whiting P, Rutjes AWS, Dinnes J, Reitsma JB, Bossuyt PMM, Kleijnen J. *Development and validation of methods for assessing the quality of diagnostic accuracy studies.* Health Technology Assessment; 2004:Vol 8: number 25.

5. Sackett DL, RB Haynes. The architecture of diagnostic research. This is the second in a series of five articles. *BMJ.* 2002;324:539–541.

6. Macaskill P, Empirical Bayes estimates generated in a hierarchical summary ROC analysis agreed closely with those of a full Bayesian analysis. *J Clin Epidemiol.* 2004;57:925–932.

7. Youden WJ. Index for rating diagnostic tests. *Cancer.* 1950;3:32–35.

8. Reitsma JB, Glas AS, Rutjes AWS, Scholten RJPM, Bossuyt PM, Zwinderman AH. Bivariate analysis of sensitivity and specificity produces informative summary measures in diagnostic reviews. *J Clinl Epidemiol.* 2005;58:982–990.

9. Bermejo I, Niebling W, Mathias B, Harter M. Patients' and physicians' evaluation of the PHQ-D for depression screening. *Prim Care Commun Psychiatr.* 2005;10(4):125–131.

10. Mitchell AJ, Coyne J. Screening for postnatal depression: barriers to success. *Br J Obst Gyn.* 2008; online first.

PART XVI

International Psycho-Oncology

Jimmie C. Holland, ED

CHAPTER 95

International Psycho-Oncology: Present and Future

Christoffer Johansen and Luigi Grassi

INTRODUCTION

The overall principle behind all psychological and social treatment of cancer is that it is a bio-psycho-existential-social disease, which afflicts all aspects of life. The psychosocial aspects of cancer are treated by a range of clinical approaches, which vary according to the socioeconomic status of the region or country in which such treatment is given. Thus, an oncology nurse in a country with scarce resources and a low gross national product will concentrate on palliation or treating the immediate side effects of cancer that arise from insufficient capacity to manage cancer in general and its complications. Cultural and general belief systems affect the interpretation of cancer as an illness, influence the expectations of patients and relatives and alter the treatment approach. Access to basic treatment options, such as specialists, X-ray equipment, chemotherapy, and opioids, is an important determinant of psychosocial reactions to cancer. The availability of sickness leave, the social security system in the country, access to treatment with or without a health insurance, the prices of the drugs required, access to outpatient follow-up clinics and to psychologists and other persons who can address the psychological problems of cancer patients also affect treatment. Most psychosocial support systems, clinical research, guidelines, and training of specialists in psychosocial oncology are found in affluent countries, reflecting not advances in the discipline but the global distribution of wealth.

The international spread of psychological and social treatment of cancer is discussed below in the framework of scientific benchmarks and by reviewing advances in clinical practice and access to psychosocial support. This chapter starts with a brief history of psychosocial support in cancer treatment; then, we highlight some of the major scientific achievements and examine the growth in international collaboration. In a further section, examples are given of guidelines for providing psychosocial care in overall cancer treatment. In the last section, international organization and future aspects of international collaboration are described to support our vision of psychosocial clinical care and research.

HISTORY OF PSYCHOSOCIAL ONCOLOGY

The history of psychosocial oncology is both brief and extremely long.[1] Thus, it has a brief history as a specialty in the area of oncology but a long history as part of the relationship between the healthcare professional and the cancer patient. Its history also reflects different cultural and scientific environments. In Europe, there is a long tradition of socioeconomic health research, based mainly on continuing advances in public health systems which aim to secure equal access to all health services. This tradition has been reflected in European scientific and clinical psychosocial interventions for centuries.

In developing countries, belief systems, and limited access to economic resources are the main reasons for clinical and scientific focus on psychosocial treatment of cancers at more advanced stages. Psychosocial oncology in Asia (mainly Japan) and the United States grew out of a medical tradition of focusing on the psychiatric effects of cancer and its treatment. In all regions, countries, and clinics, however, cancer patients experience more than a biological event. Psychosocial oncology thus relies on an understanding of the illness as a biological, psychological, and social event, and this is the driving force behind the clinical interventions offered to cancer patients. The psychological and social

aspects of illness have not always been considered equal to the biological aspects; however, and the treatment of cancer has focused mainly on the latter. This position is often defended by arguing that patients must survive before side effects can be treated. Nevertheless, the psychosocial aspects of every illness, including cancer, must be treated, even for patients with a poor prognosis.

Modern psychosocial oncology began in the United States, with several prospective studies on the effect of illness on psychological and social outcomes. In some remarkable and still informative studies conducted during the decade 1951–1961, A.M. Sutherland and colleagues investigated several key issues in psychosocial oncology, such as adaptation to a colostomy,[2] depressive reactions after surgery and psychological barriers to rehabilitation,[3] how mothers of children with cancer cope with the loss of a child,[4,5] reactions to mastectomy for breast cancer or to a hysterectomy after uterine cancer,[6,7] adaptation by the spouses of rectal cancer patients with a colostomy,[8] communication between cancer patients and doctors.[9] These studies cover almost all the subjects addressed during the past six decades, and these seminal papers, in which Sutherland and his colleagues described the obvious physical changes after treatment, were a first step in unifying the work of clinicians, psychologists, social workers, nurses, and psychiatrists in what became the discipline of psychosocial oncology.

Communication between doctors and patients and how doctors announce a diagnosis, possible side effects of treatment and the prognosis became important issues. The 1968 student revolt gave rise to social demands for democratic transparency and human rights, including the right to be told the truth about a diagnosis of disease. A book by Kubler-Ross (1969)[10] addressed this demand and drew medical attention to the need for continuous dialogue with cancer patients about their disease. In the United States, the beginning of the 1970s saw the start of training in psycho-oncology for clinicians, who began to record the psychological and social effects of cancer, in addition to their daily work. The first intervention groups, consisting of cancer survivors and led by psychiatrists, were also set up in the United States, and soon such groups were formed by national cancer societies in other countries. These societies were nongovernmental organizations, which focused more and more on the psychosocial aspects of cancer, reflecting the worldwide sociopolitical changes.

The next step was the acceptance of psychology as a discipline that would benefit cancer patients, spouses, and relatives as well as professionals working in oncology. In the larger European countries, such as France, Germany, Italy, and the United Kingdom, the establishment of national societies formalized the activity. These organizations encouraged integration of the psychosocial aspects of cancer treatment at a level of equal importance with biological treatment. Other European countries soon followed this trend, and scientific research in the field increased rapidly. In contrast to practice in the United States, psychologists formed the basic staff assigned to the psychosocial care of cancer patients. In a survey of psychosocial care for cancer patients in 38 countries, psychosocial screening instruments were found to be used in about one-third; however, only half of the countries reported the existence of guidelines for psychosocial interventions. Most of the countries from which information was reported were industrialized ones.[11]

Training of personnel for psychosocial services for cancer patients in developing countries differs substantially from that in Australia,

Europe, Japan, and the United States. In India, lack of proper treatment facilities at most cancer treatment centers, poor infrastructure, and illiteracy often result in poor survival rates, and the focus of cancer treatment has thus been on the quantity rather than the quality of life.[12] Furthermore, quality of life is considered to be related to financial status, distance from the treating hospital, educational level, and marital status, rather than the psychological aspects of the disease.[13] In South America, studies published in English of psychosocial effects in cancer patients involved few patients or were based on qualitative methods, making it difficult to determine which psychosocial problems are of particular importance for cancer patients in that part of the world. Studies on the health behavior of cancer patients in sub-Saharan Africa show that most come to a clinic when their disease is in a late stage, and most have not heard about the symptoms of cancer.[14] Likewise, women with breast cancer in a study in Nigeria were unaware of important aspects of the disease and its early detection. In addition, it was shown that public health workers were not the main source of information and that most patients heard about the disease from their elders, neighbors, and friends.[15] A study of 1600 cancer patients in Morocco illustrated the interaction of cultural beliefs and religious practice among Muslim patients with cancer. Most patients changed their behavior, and almost 95% of patients who were characterized as not religious before diagnosis initiated some religious activity.[16] These examples illustrate the wide variety of issues that are of relevance in developing countries and point to the need for better access to treatment of cancer. They also show that psychological, social, religious, and existential problems are important all over the world.

MAJOR ACHIEVEMENTS IN INTERNATIONAL PSYCHOSOCIAL ONCOLOGY

The most important achievement is recognition of the fact that the psychological and social needs of patients require intervention by health professionals. This is the result of thousands of publications published in the peer-reviewed literature since the papers by Sutherland's group.

The next important benchmark is the design and testing of psychometric measures and quality-of-life scales, which can be used to detect a need for some form of intervention other than physical treatment of cancer. Aaronson[17] in Europe and Cella et al.[18] in the United States concurrently reported quality-of-life measures, consisting of core modules and cancer site-specific modules that can be applied to almost all cancers. This was the beginning of a series of scales to measure the life situation of cancer patients. At the same time, the first reports of severe depression were published;[19] later, it was shown that the risk of cancer patients for suicide is higher than that of the general population.[20] These findings pointed to the need for interventions for patients who, in the aftermath of cancer treatment, react with depressive symptoms. The 1980s saw the first reports of the benefits of psychological interventions, not only in terms of lower prevalences of depression and anxiety but also better survival.[21,22]

Acquiring evidence for an association between interventions and survival depends on a number of methodological considerations. Most research on psychosocial intervention and survival has been characterized by studies with few patients, poorly validated measures of psychological function, retrospective and cross-sectional designs, no information on the biology of the tumor or treatment and *a priori* theory of an association. It is possible that the earlier findings of improved survival can be explained by methodological problems inherent in the design of the studies. The most solid criticism of the studies by the groups of Spiegel and Fawzy, for instance, is that the control groups differed from the intervention groups.

The results of the latest replication studies indicate that the hypothesis that psychotherapy alone or therapy for specific states of mind (e.g., depression, hopelessness or helplessness, poor quality of life, life crisis, existential problems) improves survival should be abandoned. The evidence shows rather that investigations should address the interactions between the psychological, social and health behavior components of intervention programs. It also indicates the need for targeted treatment of late effects in cancer patients, as these effects might be the main

reason for inability to change behavior, such as increasing the amount of physical activity. The finding of a social gradient in cancer survival, even in countries with free, tax-paid health systems, indicates the need for targeted intervention programs among socially disadvantaged populations of cancer survivors.[23]

Patients with cancer need support in several aspects of their lives. Treatment can comprise a combination of surgery, radiation, chemotherapy, and endocrine therapy, and these treatments, in combination with the biology of the disease, give rise to late effects, which require as much attention as the disease itself. Psychological and social problems must also be addressed, and interventions are needed with regard to the lifestyle of the patient. The last issue has been highlighted in a number of studies, which show that physical training,[24] changes in alcohol consumption, quitting smoking, and change of diet in particular can improve the overall quality of life, improve physical functioning, change the severity of side effects and perhaps improve survival. These outcomes are being confirmed, as few controlled studies have been carried out in this area of behavioral intervention, and this area of study has a promising future.

A further achievement is elucidation of the concept that mind causes cancer. This is a prevalent hypothesis in populations at risk and has been investigated in several large studies. In a review of studies of psychological factors and cancer, it was concluded, however, that the studies published so far give no indication that these factors play a major role in cancer causation when the roles of bias, confounding, and chance have been taken into account. Insufficient sample size and length of follow-up and large numbers of analyses make it hard to rule out the possibility that chance played a role in the results of many of the studies in this area. Furthermore, loss to follow-up and inadequate ascertainment of cancer cases limit the interpretation, especially of those studies that showed the strongest effects[25] (see Chapter 7). In principle, therefore, mind does not cause cancer.

INTERNATIONAL GUIDELINES

In 1997, the National Comprehensive Cancer Network in the United States was established, consisting of a multidisciplinary team to determine how to integrate psychosocial care into routine cancer care. The team chose the word "distress" to describe the psychological, social and spiritual aspects, and experiences of cancer. The term can be considered to cover everything from normal fears, worry, and sadness to disabling problems such as a clinical depression, generalized anxiety, or an existential crisis.[26] In 2003, the Distress Management Panel of the Network published revised standards for the psychosocial care of cancer patients, which for the first time established measures for managing distress.[27] The guidelines cover: recognition and monitoring of distress, screening of patients regularly and when their disease status changes, identification of the level and nature of distress and assessment and management of distress according to clinical practice guidelines. This work is a cornerstone of the worldwide effort to integrate measures of distress or outcomes close to distress in clinical work with cancer patients.

Up until now, healthcare providers have focused on physical vital signs, that is, temperature, respiration, heart rate, blood pressure, and pain. These vital signs are indicators of the patient's physical state and are used as navigation points to help the healthcare provider establish the appropriate treatment to achieve wellness and survival. During the trajectory of a cancer, 25%–70% of patients in various countries and regions of the world experience emotional distress, and it has been demonstrated that health systems see clear benefits in terms medical costs when psychosocial services are provided. In 2005 in Canada, the strategy for cancer control was amended by the addition of emotional distress as the sixth vital sign, implying that monitoring of emotional distress is a vital indicator of a patient's state of being, needs and progress through the disease.[28]

In 2005, the United States Congress established a working group under the auspices of the Institute of Medicine to study the capacity for addressing the psychosocial needs of cancer patients review the available training programs and identify barriers to access to cancer-related mental health services. The main conclusion of the group's report[29] was that there is enough evidence for the inclusion of psychosocial health services in cancer care. The standard of care should ensure appropriate psychosocial health services by facilitating communication between patients and healthcare providers, identifying the needs of each patient, contain a plan to link patients with the psychosocial services they need and systematic follow-up, reevaluation and adjustment of the plan. The report shows growing understanding that communication is a *sine qua non* and is the platform for other activities; it also highlights the need for training of healthcare providers in all aspects of communication. It points to the need for psychosocial screening, as not all cancer patients need such services. The idea of designing a plan for psychosocial care which undergoes continuous review is important, given the change in the treatment paradigm to cancer therapy tailored to the individual, which might not follow a standard protocol.

The European Council has adopted a policy that clearly acknowledges the importance of psychosocial aspects of cancer care.[30,31] The *Council conclusions on reducing the burden of cancer* state that "to attain optimal results, a patient-centered comprehensive interdisciplinary approach and optimal psycho-social care should be implemented in routine cancer care, rehabilitation and posttreatment follow-up for all cancer." Furthermore, they emphasize that "cancer treatment and care is multidisciplinary, involving the cooperation of oncological surgery, medical oncology, radiotherapy, chemotherapy as well as psycho-social support and rehabilitation and, when cancer is not treatable, palliative care. Services providing care to the individual patient and support to the patient's family must be effectively coordinated." Lastly, they invite Member States "to take into account the psycho-social needs of patients and improve the quality of life for cancer patients through support, rehabilitation and palliative care."

Comprehensive clinical guidelines have also been prepared in Australia (www.nhmrc.gov.au), and a manual entitled "Psychosocial clinical practice guidelines: providing information support and counseling for women with breast cancer" was published in 2000 by the National Breast Cancer Centre. On the basis of that experience, a multidisciplinary steering group subsequently prepared "Clinical practice guidelines for the psycho-social care of adults with cancer," which were published by the National Breast Cancer Centre and the National Cancer Control Initiative and were approved by the National Health and Medical Research Council in 2003. The guidelines will be reviewed in 2008. In the United Kingdom, the National Institute for Clinical Excellence (http://www.nice.org.uk/), an independent organization responsible for providing national guidance on promoting good health and preventing and treating ill health, prepared a series of guidelines for various areas of public health and clinical practice, including oncology. In 2004, within the cancer service guidance, it published guidelines on "Improving supportive and palliative care for adults with cancer," with the objective of ensuring that cancer patients, their families and carers are well informed, cared for, and supported. Specifically, they recommend that people with cancer be involved in cancer services; that there be good communication, and that people with cancer be involved in decision making; that information be available free of charge; that people with cancer be offered a range of physical, emotional, spiritual, and social support; that services be available to help people living with the after-effects of cancer to manage the effects themselves; that people with advanced cancer have access to a range of services to improve their quality of life; that there be support for people dying from cancer; that the needs of families and other carers of people with cancer be met; and that there be a trained workforce to provide these services.

INTERNATIONAL COLLABORATION

There is some international collaboration in the field of psychosocial oncology. Most is in training and education, as illustrated by the numerous scholarships and exchange options available from large international cancer foundations. There is also a need to meet and exchange ideas and viewpoints and to present data from clinical practice and from scientific studies. As mentioned above, national societies of clinicians and

scientists dedicated to psychosocial aspects of cancer were formed in the 1970s in a number of countries and regions. In 1984, these societies unified their forces into the International Psycho-Oncology Society (IPOS), which has become a truly international organization, today consisting of more than 5000 members in 75 countries; it holds an annual meeting, and a scientific journal, *Psycho-oncology*, is published monthly (www.ipos-society.org).

At the annual world congress and through its web site, IPOS inspires professionals in diverse fields to discuss ways of improving cancer care at an international level and to devise strategies to ensure that psychosocial support is integrated in all aspects of cancer control. IPOS is collaborating increasingly with the World Health Organization (WHO) and is preparing an application for recognition as a nongovernmental organization in official relations with WHO. For the first time, the global cancer control programs supported by WHO will incorporate the social, psychological, and behavioral aspects of prevention, diagnosis, treatment, and palliative care, with IPOS members providing the expertise. According to WHO,[32] the global burden of cancer will increase from 10 to 15 million new cases each year by 2020, and 60% of the new cases will occur in developing countries. Experts estimate that one-third of cancer cases are preventable, and one-third of cases are curable if they are found early enough and standard treatment is available and accessible. Tragically, cancer remains undiagnosed at curable stages in most of the developing world. WHO has assisted countries in preparing national cancer control program guidelines covering five basic areas of cancer control: prevention, early diagnosis, screening, therapy, and palliative care. Although psychological, social, and behavioral forces play a major role in each of these areas and the outcome of control programs depends in many ways on successful treatment of psychological, social, and behavioral factors, little attention is paid to them. Representatives of the IPOS contributed to the latest edition of the WHO cancer control program (www.who.int/cancer).

IPOS collaborated with the European School of Oncology in preparing a core curriculum for psychosocial oncology in English, French, German, Hungarian, Italian, and Spanish. The curriculum has also been translated into Japanese and in Portuguese. It is available in webcast format to all health professionals who care for cancer patients and their families (www.ipos-society.org or www.eso.net). It can also be used for training students in health professions, such as medicine, nursing, and rehabilitation. Preliminary results from 4239 evaluations rated the ability of the webcast to meet the stated objectives as excellent (19%), very good (49%), and good (19%); in comparison with other e-learning systems, the IPOS core curriculum was rated as much better (21%), better (46%), or of the same quality (31%). The tool was found to be useful by 97% of respondents.[33]

FEDERATION OF PSYCHO-ONCOLOGY SOCIETIES AND FUTURE PERSPECTIVES

International collaboration among professionals in the field of psycho-oncology is also ensured by single research and training groups in different countries, which have conducted many cross-cultural and cooperative studies. Establishing dialogue in a more formal network of societies of psycho-oncology throughout the world is the main objective of the IPOS, which favors exchanges of opinions, projects, and proposals at every meeting. In a survey conducted by IPOS in 2006 to determine which countries had established a psycho-oncology association, formal national societies were reported in about 20 countries, while other working groups and associations existed in others. This survey also showed that at least 5000 professionals are active in the field.

When the findings of the survey were presented at the IPOS world congress in Venice in 2006 (www.ipos2006.it), participants concluded that help in establishing psycho-oncology organizations should be given to countries that do not have the resources to establish a society. In view of the important potential role of psycho-oncology societies, a proposal was made for an international federation of national societies, within IPOS, to create a powerful force for advocacy, education, and training and research. At a meeting held in London in 2007 (www.ipos-society. org/ipos2007/), a firm commitment was made to establish a mechanism by which the international psycho-oncology movement would be represented by one powerful voice, to facilitate action, progress, and collaboration. It was recognized that IPOS was the most effective organ for promoting psycho-oncology globally, as it reaches and serves the thousands of members of existing national psycho-oncology societies and supports the setting up of national societies where they do not exist. It was therefore decided to create an IPOS federation of national and regional psycho-oncology societies, to be called the IPOS Federation. The Federation was established at the annual congress in Madrid in 2008 (www.ipos-society.org/ipos2008/) and the board of the Federation was established at the annual congress in Vienna (www.ipos-society.org/ ipos2009/) with the involvement of 21 national psycho-oncology societies in 20 countries (Australia, Austria, Brazil, Canada, China, Colombia, France, Greece, Hungary, India, Ireland, Israel, Italy, Lithuania, the Netherlands, Portugal, Serbia, Spain, Turkey, and the United States). Other countries can join the Federation simply by application.

The main objective of the Federation is to represent psycho-oncology worldwide, communicating a compelling, unified message that all cancer patients and their families, throughout the world, should receive optimal psychosocial care at all stages of the disease and survival. As the Federation represents all members of all national psycho-oncology societies, activities to influence the cancer treatment policies of WHO, the European Union, and other major regional organizations can be initiated. The Federation also supports national psycho-oncology organizations in integrating psycho-oncology into their national healthcare structures and in establishing standards of care and training. It facilitates collaboration on issues of advocacy, education, training, and research in order to strengthen psycho-oncology globally, regionally, and within countries.

As psycho-oncology is a multidisciplinary field, it is faced with many projects and challenges. Some of the most important are training and research and close networking with other societies active in oncology and palliative care, from the point of view of both health professionals and patients. Interactions with world cancer associations, such as the International Union against Cancer, the American Society of Clinical Oncology, and the European Society of Medical Oncology, should be strengthened to formulate common programs for training, education and research. IPOS and the IPOS Federation should ensure that cancer societies consider psychological aspects of cancer as having the same importance as pain and other problems that affect cancer patients. Influential documents, such as the *World cancer declaration* of the International Union against Cancer, should include the psychosocial consequences of cancer.

Cooperation between the International Association for Hospice and Palliative Care and IPOS, in response to a request from the Cancer Control Programme of WHO, is already influencing the updating of the list of essential medicines for palliative care, including psychotropic drugs. Cooperation with the European Association of Palliative Care may improve the assessment and treatment of depression, which is being addressed by the European Palliative Care Research Collaborative.

Cooperation with the World Psychiatric Association and its Section on Psycho-Oncology and Palliative Care (www.wpanet.org/) could help to sensitize mental health professionals about psycho-oncology. The concept that there is no health without mental health[34] could broaden the view of psychiatrists concerning the needs not only of the general population but also of physically ill patients, and specifically cancer patients.

A further area for development is the relation between psycho-oncology as a discipline and advocacy and cancer patient movements. The Wellness Community in North America and some movements elsewhere, such as in India, Ireland, and the United Kingdom, provide free support, education, and hope to people with cancer and their families. The emotional aspects of cancer and the role of psycho-oncological treatment are part of their programs. In Europe, the goal of the European Cancer Patient Coalition (www.ecpc-online. org/), with 250 national members, is to represent the views of cancer patients in the European healthcare debate and to give them a forum for exchanging information and sharing experiences of best practice. Both the discipline of psycho-oncology and advocacy movements should be considered in psycho-oncology projects, so that the quality of care of cancer patients and their families around the globe can really be improved.

REFERENCES

1. Holland JC. History of psycho-oncology: overcoming attitudinal and conceptual barriers. *Psychosom Med.* 2002;64:206–221.

2. Sutherland AM, Orbach CE, Dyk RB, Bard M. The psychological impact of cancer and cancer surgery. I. Adaptation to the dry colostomy; preliminary report and summary of findings. *Cancer.* 1952;5:857–872.

3. Sutherland AM, Orbach CE. Psychological impact of cancer and cancer surgery. II. Depressive reactions associated with surgery for cancer. *Cancer.* 1953;6:958–962.

4. Bozeman MF, Orbach CE, Sutherland AM. Psychological impact of cancer and its treatment. III. The adaptation of mothers to the threatened loss of their children through leukemia. *Cancer.* 1955;8:1–19.

5. Sutherland AM. Psychological barriers to rehabilitation of cancer patients. *Postgrad Med.* 1955;17:523–526.

6. Bard M, Sutherland AM. Psychological impact of cancer and its treatment. IV. Adaptation to radical mastectomy. *Cancer.*, 1955;8:656–672.

7. Bieber I, Drellich MG, Sutherland AM. The psychological impact of cancer and cancer surgery. VI. Adaptation to hysterectomy. *Cancer.* 1956;9: 1120–1126.

8. Dyk RB, Sutherland AM. Adaptation of the spouse and other family members to the colostomy patient. *Cancer.* 1956;9:123–138.

9. Sutherland AM. Communication between the doctor and the cancer patient. *CA Cancer J Clin.* 1958;8:119–121.

10. Kubler-Ross E. *On death and dying.* New York, Macmillian; 1969.

11. Mehnert A, Koch U. Psychosocial care of cancer patients—international differences in definition, healthcare structures, and therapeutic approaches. *Support Care Cancer.* 2005;13:579–588.

12. Pandey M. Quality of life of patients with cancer in India: challenges and hurdles in putting theory into practice. *Psychooncology.* 2004;13:429–433.

13. Pandey M, Thomas BC, Ramdas K, Nandamohan V. Factors influencing distress in Indian cancer patients. *Psychooncology.* 2006;15:547–550.

14. Kazaura MR, Kombe D, Yuma S, Mtiro H, Mlawa G. Health seeking behavior among cancer patients attending Ocean Road Cancer Institute, Tanzania. *East Afr J Public Health.* 2007;4:19–22.

15. Oluwatosin OA, Oladepo O. Knowledge of breast cancer and its early detection measures among rural women in Akinyele Local Government Area, Ibadan, Nigeria. *BMC Cancer.* 2006;6:271–274.

16. Errihani H, Mrabti H, Boutayeb S, et al. Impact of cancer on Moslem patients in Morocco. *PsychoOncology.* 2008;17:98–100.

17. Aaronson NK. Methodologic issues in assessing the quality of life of cancer patients. *Cancer.* 1991;67:844–850.

18. Cella D, Tulsky D, Gray G, et al. The functional assessment of cancer therapy (FACT) scale: development and validation of the general version. *J Clin Oncol.* 1993;11:570–579.

19. Dalton SO, Johansen C. Risk for depression in cancer patients. *J Clin Oncol.* 2009;27:1440–1445.

20. Yousaf U, Christensen M-LM, Engholm G, Storm HH. Suicides among Danish cancer patients 1971–1999. *Br J Cancer.* 2005;92:995–1000.

21. Spiegel D, Bloom JR, Kraemer HC, Gottheil E. Effect of psychosocial treatment on survival of patients with metastatic breast cancer. *Lancet.* 1989;ii: 888–891.

22. Fawzy FI, Fawzy NW, Hyun CS, et al. Malignant melanoma. Effects of an early structured psychiatric intervention, coping, and affective state on recurrence and survival 6 years later. *Arch Gen Psychiatry.* 1993;50:681–689.

23. Boesen EH, Johansen C. Impact of psychotherapy on cancer survival: Time to move on ? *Curr Opin Oncol.*, 2008;20:372–377.

24. Holick CN, Newcomb PA, Trentham-Dietz A, et al. Physical activity and survival after diagnosis of invasive breast cancer. *Cancer Epidemiol Biomarkers Prevent.* 2008;17:379–386.

25. Dalton SO, Boesen EH, Ross L, Schapiro I, Johansen C. Mind and cancer—do psychological factors cause cancer? *Eur J Cancer.* 2002;38:1313–1323.

26. National Comprehensive Cancer Network. NCCN practice guidelines for the management of psychosocial distress. *Oncology (Williston Park).* 1999;13: 113–147.

27. Holland JC, Andersen B, Breitbart WS, et al. Distress management clinical practice guidelines in oncology. *J Natl Compr Canc Netw.* 2003;1:344–374.

28. Bultz BD, Carlson LE. Emotional distress: the sixth vital sign—future directions in cancer care. *Psychooncology.* 2006;15:93–95.

29. Institute of Medicine. *Cancer care for the whole patient. Meeting psychosocial health needs.* Washington, DC: National Academies Press; 2008.

30. Council of the European Union. *Council conclusions on reducing the burden of cancer.* Luxembourg; 2008. Available at www.eu2008.si/en/News_and_Documents/Council_Conclusions/June/0609_EPSCO_cancer.

31. Grassi L, Travado L. The role of psycho-social oncology in cancer care. In: Coleman MP, Alexe DM, Albreht T, McKee M (eds). *Responding to the challenge of cancer in Europe.* Ljubljana, Slovenian Institute of Public Health; 2008:211–231.

32. WHO. The 58th World Health Assembly approved resolution on cancer prevention and control, May 2005. www.who.int/cancer. Accessed August 17, 2009.

33. Grassi L, Johansen C. E-learning: the on-line IPOS/ESO multilingual core curriculum on psychosocial aspects of cancer care. *Psychooncology.* 2006;15:S9-S10.

34. Prince M, Patel V, Saxena S, et al. No health without mental health. *Lancet.* 2007;370:859–877.

PART XVII

Policy Issues

Jimmie C. Holland, ED

CHAPTER 96

Branding Distress—as the 6th Vital Sign; Policy Implications

Barry D. Bultz and Neil J. Berman

The focus of cancer care continues to be based on traditional biomedical perspectives despite evidence that 35%–45%[1-4] of cancer patients and their families experience significant clinical distress as defined by the National Comprehensive Cancer Network (NCCN).[5] This seemingly all or none focus of cancer care on life extension is rational, but imposes significant avoidable/preventable costs on patients, healthcare providers, and healthcare systems and may, in fact, not encompass the best interests of all concerned.

After being diagnosed with breast cancer, 45-year-old author (Susan Sontag) wrote *Illness as a metaphor*[6] stating that cancer as an illness is synonymous with death, pain, and suffering. Nowadays, despite significant advances in oncology treatments' extension of life, societies continue to provide billions of dollars for laboratory bioscience, clinical trials, and complementary/alternative medicine in attempts to extend life. Although a plethora of evidence exists to show that enhancing quality of life and survivorship lets patients achieve the best outcomes of their cancer journey, this research and care area remains impoverished. A likely cause is the view of many hospital directors and fundraisers that psychosocial oncology is a "difficult sell" or "not sexy enough" to garner investment of resources. Given these barriers, psycho-oncology has been blocked from attaining seats at heath policy tables where decisions about budget, space, and recruitment issues are addressed.

THE ARGUMENTS

Prior to pioneering work on terminal illness and the publication of *On death and dying* (Elizabeth Kubler-Ross, 1969[7]), the healthcare sector had little to offer patients when options to extend life had been exhausted. Following this work, it was realized that reductions in suffering were achievable and patients' quality of life enhanceable. These realizations encouraged a change in healthcare to incorporate the role of palliative care near the end of life. Subsequently, a new language and social movement—developed in the healthcare system—mobilized to improve quality of life for patients facing terminal illness. This was the impetus for inclusion of palliative care into core service offerings of hospitals, cancer centres,[8-11] medical schools and was deemed an essential component of care by accreditation bodies.[12] This dramatic shift towards enhancing patient experience at the end of life also served to extend focus of attention on patient experience from the time of cancer diagnosis onwards. Despite the emergence of research proving psychosocial intervention benefits on depression, anxiety, sleep, antiemetic use, and broadly speaking quality of life, psychosocial oncology received only token acknowledgement.[13,14]

Given the impetus from Kubler-Ross's palliative care concepts, cancer centers capitalized on the lessons learned around the developments of the "Death and Dying movement" and began directing financial support to enhance cancer patients' experience by creating psychosocial oncology departments and programs.

One of the catalysts for increased attention to the benefits of psychosocial oncology was spawned by Spiegel's[15] claim that group psychotherapy (Supportive-Expressive Therapy), in the treatment arm of a randomized group of advanced breast cancer patients, extended

life by up to 18 months compared to the standard care control group. Despite later criticism[16,17] and failure to replicate Spiegel's findings,[18] his work continued to impact the cancer community, patients, and care-givers, through the belief that therapeutic benefits of psychosocial oncology impacted not only patients' quality of life but also the holy grail of extension of life. However, despite the plethora of research, to date only limited changes in practice and policy have been implemented.

THE FOCUS ON DISTRESS

With good scientific evidence and growing understanding that distress has a key impact on patient experience, several distress prevalence studies began to emerge.[1,2,19-24] Prevalence rates of clinically significant distress in these studies were consistently discovered in cancer patients: 35%–45% range for outpatients and higher for inpatients. The two largest patient samples came from the United States[1] and Canada.[2] A convenience cross-sectional sample of 3000 patients attending the Tom Baker Cancer Centre (TBCC) was screened over 1 month; the 37.5% clinically significant prevalence rate was similar to those discovered by the Johns Hopkins study. In addition to high prevalence rates, studies highlighted the types of problems rated by patients as having a major negative impact on quality of life: fatigue, sleeplessness, pain, anxiety, depression, and distress about the financial burden associated with cancer and its treatments.

Despite the existence of NCCN's standards and guidelines[25] and the revealed high prevalence rates of distress, studies consistently demonstrated that clinicians were not assessing patients' psychosocial status. In a large British study,[26] 143 physicians in 34 cancer centers were asked to assess the psychological status of their patients: of nearly 2300 patients assessed, 35% (800) were found to be misclassified. A subsequent study[27] presented alarming data showing that while 70% of palliative care providers screened for distress, only 58% of oncologists did so and 14% never tried. Perhaps of most concern, 64% of oncologists relied solely on clinical acumen and less than 10% routinely used standardized questionnaires (i.e., screening tools). Furthermore, a 2007 survey[28] of 18 NCCN affiliated institutions revealed that only three cancer centers conducted routine screening for distress.

Such findings raised queries of why cancer care professionals do not routinely screen all their patients for distress? Schofield et al.,[29] postulated that cancer specialists are biomedically focused, have limited expertise and time, and are more likely to rely on concerns raised by patients. While not surprising, these reasons should be of concern to all healthcare providers and their care systems/communities.

USING AND MARKETING RESEARCH TO GENERATE POLICY CHANGE

In many developed countries worldwide, national cancer control strategies are being used to reform/generate national directions, priorities, and policies. In Canada, the federal government and the cancer sector developed the Canadian Strategy for Cancer Control (CSCC; 1999–2005) to explore and implement pragmatic ways to guide, enhance, and standardize cancer care services across the country. Recognizing significant disparities in resources and outcomes across Canada, "Working Groups" were established within the CSCC to develop recommendations through multiple aspects of cancer control including standards, guidelines, human resources, and patient-based experience (Rebalance Focus Working Group-which focused on psychosocial oncology, palliative care, survivorship, rehabilitation, and supportive care). In 2006, the Canadian government established a nonprofit corporation—Canadian Partnership Against Cancer (CPAC)—to implement and expand on the CSCC recommendations, via federal funding and collaborative partnerships with cancer control-related institutions/jurisdictions/entities across the country.[30]

The CSCC Cancer Screening Working Group addressed population-based screening for breast, colorectal, and gynaecological cancers, focussing on increased screening programs to elevate early detection and thereby provide a subsequent reduction in morbidity and mortality for the diagnosed population. On the basis of the discussions about population-based screening impacts it seemed surprising that psychosocial oncology was not looked at to have standardized distress screening implemented as part of routine cancer practice policies. Communication on this issue required translations into healthcare providers' language and policy approaches to patient care, in a more comprehensive and integrative way. Given that four "Vital Signs" (body temperature, pulse rate, blood pressure, respiratory rate) are standard screening in medical settings; and given that the Joint Commission on the Accreditation of Healthcare Organizations in the US assigned pain as the 5th Vital Sign (1999),[12] it made sense to add to this initiative by recommending that Distress be deemed the 6th Vital Sign in Cancer Care. With submissions on this rationale, in June 2004 the 6th Vital Sign—Emotional Distress—was endorsed by the CSCC as a key policy aspect for the delivery of comprehensive cancer care.[31]

Cancer agencies/institutions in Canada rapidly endorsed naming emotional distress as a standardized vital sign. Building on this momentum and using the branding of distress as the 6th Vital Sign to reinforce the process of change in healthcare practice and policy, psychosocial oncology leaders have published papers[32-36] and presented at conferences and hospital seminars to advocate for the implementation of distress as the 6th Vital Sign in cancer care. Change of medical practice to incorporate distress screening and the psychosocial aspects of cancer must be seen as a critical aspect of a fully integrated comprehensive cancer care system. Psychosocial care not only facilitates adjustment to a very difficult disease, but also relieves the associated emotional burden, can reduce the financial cost to the healthcare system and the strain on the already overburdened healthcare system and its practitioners.[37,38] In recognition of these discussions, The Canadian Council of Health Services Accreditation (CCHSA)—the sole national accreditation body—has just acknowledged the importance *of assessment to evaluate and monitor the client's emotional distress...as the sixth vital sign* and has included this standard as part of the accreditation review process.[39] With success building on success, and with increased attention to the branding of distress as a "vital sign," CPAC deemed screening as a priority direction with the intention of working to see screening initiated and implemented in cancer care programs across Canada (CPAC 2008—Annual Report[40]). Without question, moving from the patient experience, to research, to policy, and subsequent change of practice is a long process. Partnerships, collaborations, and good evidence are the tools to implement change of policy. Support from multiple agencies assures policy makers that the decisions they are endorsing are sound, worthy, and implementable. As a part of a cancer care community it is essential to build on each others' successes to attain a common goal of what is best for both the patient and healthcare systems. Branding Distress as the 6th Vital Sign generates an understandable and marketable message into the complicated language of healthcare. It also enables health policy officials, healthcare administrators and providers to collaboratively hook a desired evidence-based intervention discovery (i.e., improved fiscal, biopsychosocial outcomes) into an existing policy bucket ("Vital signs") used across healthcare systems. Additional drivers for policy makers are similar policy changes and implementations by their peers in comparable institutions/countries and jurisdictions, particularly those with similar healthcare systems.

FUTURE STEPS

To expand the number of decision makers (responsible for "point of care" service systems policies) that incorporate this "branded" distress monitoring package into standards of cancer care, the 6th Vital Sign requires incorporation into policy changes at the global sector. Hence national/international leaders, organizations, and jurisdictions (e.g., national psychosocial societies, IPOS, UICC, WHO, hospital and cancer program accreditation bodies, etc.) need to be motivated to incorporate such policy changes into their expert/evidence-based standards for enhancing cancer control outcomes at national, regional, local, and global levels.

SUMMARY

Care services for any illnesses, including cancer, focus primarily on life extension; however, given the growth of evidence proving the significant prevalence of clinical distress in cancer patients, care services require incorporation of a focus on patients' quality of life into official cancer care policies. The existence of substantial and long-term scientific evidence of interventions that are proven to produce beneficial changes to patient care is not fully sufficient to motivate comprehensive incorporation of such interventions into institutional and health systems' official policies. Human interactions within multiple jurisdictions, sectors, levels, and in particular by international leaders with their peers and respected experts, are the practical effective activities that enable research outcomes to impact the evolution of health systems policies. Use of language/branding like the "6th Vital Sign" enables healthcare practitioners to rapidly understand that patients' experience with cancer is as vital as the extension of their lives, and hence is a key indicator of health status. Incorporating the "6th Vital Sign" into the *common health language* helps healthcare settings match their psychosocial care capacity to patients' needs via official changes in practice and policy.

ACKNOWLEDGMENTS

Thanks to Joshua Lounsberry for assistance with editing and Bejoy Thomas for referencing.

REFERENCES

1. Zabora J, BrintzenhofeSzoc K, Curbow B, Hooker C, Piantadosi S. The prevalence of psychological distress by cancer site. *Psychooncology*. 2001 01;10(1):19–28.

2. Carlson LE, Angen M, Cullum J, et al. High levels of untreated distress and fatigue in cancer patients. *Br J Cancer*. 2004 06/14;90(12):2297–2304.

3. Cella DF, Jacobsen PB, Orav EJ, Holland JC, Silberfarb PM, Rafla S. A brief POMS measure of distress for cancer patients. *J Chronic Dis*. 1987;40(10):939–942.

4. Walker MS, Zona DM, Fisher EB. Depressive symptoms after lung cancer surgery: their relation to coping style and social support. *Psychooncology*. 2006 Aug;15(8):684–693.

5. National Comprehensive Cancer Network. NCCN practice guidelines for the management of psychosocial distress. *Oncology (Williston Park)*. 1999;13:113–147.

6. Sontag S. *Illness as metaphor*. New York: Farrar, Straus and Giroux; 1978.

7. Kubler-Ross E. *On death and dying*. New York: Macmillian; 1969.

8. Porzsolt F, Tannock I. Goals of palliative cancer therapy. *J Clin Oncol*. 1993 Feb;11(2):378–381.

9. Hearn J, Higginson IJ. Do specialist palliative care teams improve outcomes for cancer patients? A systematic literature review. *Palliat Med*. 1998 Sep;12(5):317–332.

10. Dobkin PL, Morrow GR. Biopsychosocial assessment of cancer patients: methods and suggestions. *Hosp J*. 1986;2(3):37–59.

11. Syrjala KL, Chapko ME. Evidence for a biopsychosocial model of cancer treatment-related pain. *Pain*. 1995 Apr;61(1):69–79.

12. National Pharmaceutical Council. Pain: current understanding of assessment, management and treatments. 2001(29).

13. Greer S, Moorey S, Baruch JD, Watson M, Robertson BM, Mason A, et al. Adjuvant psychological therapy for patients with cancer: a prospective randomised trial. *BMJ*. 1992 Mar 14;304(6828):675–680.

14. Bosanquet N, Sikora K. The economics of cancer care in the UK. *Lancet Oncol.* 2004 Sep;5(9):568–574.

15. Spiegel D, Bloom JR, Kraemer HC, Gottheil E. Effect of psychosocial treatment on survival of patients with metastatic breast cancer. *Lancet.* 1989 Oct 14;2(8668):888–891.

16. Fox BH. Rejoinder to Spiegel et al. *Psychooncology.* 1998 Nov-Dec;7(6):518–519.

17. Fox BH. A hypothesis about Spiegel et al.'s 1989 paper on Psychosocial intervention and breast cancer survival. *Psychooncology.* 1998 Sep-Oct;7(5):361–370.

18. Goodwin PJ, Leszcz M, Ennis M, et al. The effect of group psychosocial support on survival in metastatic breast cancer. *N Engl J Med.* 2001 Dec 13;345(24):1719–1726.

19. Thomas BC, Carlson LE, Bultz BD. Cancer patient ethnicity and associations with emotional distress—the 6th vital sign: a new look at defining patient ethnicity in a multicultural context. *J Immigr Minor Health.* 2009 Aug;11(4):237–248.

20. Thomas BC, Pandey M, Ramdas K, et al. Identifying and predicting behaviour outcomes in cancer patients undergoing curative treatment. *Psychooncology.* 2004 Jul;13(7):490–493.

21. Pang SM, Chan KS, Chung BP, et al. Assessing quality of life of patients with advanced chronic obstructive pulmonary disease in the end of life. *J Palliat Care.* 2005 Autumn;21(3):180–187.

22. Awadalla AW, Ohaeri JU, Gholoum A, Khalid AO, Hamad HM, Jacob A. Factors associated with quality of life of outpatients with breast cancer and gynecologic cancers and their family caregivers: a controlled study. *BMC Cancer.* 2007 Jun 19;7:102.

23. Khatib J, Salhi R, Awad G. Distress in cancer inpatients in King Hussein Cancer Centre (KHCC): a study using the Arabic-modified version of the distress thermometer. *Psychooncology.* 2004;12(1):S42.

24. Eapen V, Revesz T. Psychosocial correlates of paediatric cancer in the United Arab Emirates. *Support Care Cancer.* 2003 Mar;11(3):185–189.

25. National Comprehensive Cancer Network, Inc. Clinical practice guidelines in oncology: distress management. V.1.2008.

26. Fallowfield L, Ratcliffe D, Jenkins V, Saul J. Psychiatric morbidity and its recognition by doctors in patients with cancer. *Br J Cancer.* 2001 Apr 20;84(8):1011–1015.

27. Mitchell AJ, Kaar S, Coggan C, Herdman J. Acceptability of common screening methods used to detect distress and related mood disorders-preferences of cancer specialists and non-specialists. *Psychooncology.* 2008 Mar;17(3):226–236.

28. Jacobsen PB, Ransom S. Implementation of NCCN distress management guidelines by member institutions. *J Natl Compr Canc Netw.* 2007 Jan;5(1):99–103.

29. Schofield P, Carey M, Bonevski B, Sanson-Fisher R. Barriers to the provision of evidence-based psychosocial care in oncology. *Psychooncology.* 2006 Oct;15(10):863–872.

30. Harper S. *Prime minister announces Canadian partnership against cancer.* 2007; Available at: http://www.pm.gc.ca/eng/media.asp?id=1417. Accessed July 18, 2008.

31. Rebalance Focus Action Group. A position paper: screening key indicators in cancer patients-pain as a 5th vital sign and emotional distress as a 6th vital sign. *Can Strategy Cancer Control Bull.* 2005;(Suppl 7):4.

32. Holland JC, Bultz BD, National comprehensive Cancer Network. (NCCN). The NCCN guideline for distress management: a case for making distress the sixth vital sign. *J Natl Compr Canc Netw.* 2007 Jan;5(1):3–7.

33. Bultz BD, Carlson LE. Emotional distress: the sixth vital sign—future directions in cancer care. *Psychooncology.* 2006 Feb;15(2):93–95.

34. Bultz BD, Holland JC. Emotional distress in patients with cancer: the sixth vital sign. *Commun Oncol.* 2006;3(5):311–314.

35. Bultz BD, Carlson LE. Emotional distress: the sixth vital sign in cancer care. *J Clin Oncol.* 2005 Sep 10;23(26):6440–6441.

36. Bultz BD, Thomas BC, Stewart DA, Carlson LE. Distress—the sixth vital sign in cancer care: Implications for treating older adults undergoing chemotherapy. *Geriatrics Aging.* 2007;10(10):647–653.

37. Carlson LE, Bultz BD. Efficacy and medical cost offset of psychosocial interventions in cancer care: making the case for economic analyses. *Psychooncology.* 2004 Dec;13(12):837–849.

38. Chiles JA, Lambert MJ, Hatch AL. The impact of psychological interventions on medical cost offset: a meta-analytic review. *Clin Psychol: Sci Prac.* 1999;6:204–220.

39. Accreditation Canada. Qmentum Program 2009 Standards: Cancer Care and Oncology Services. 2008;Ver 2.

40. Canadian Partnership Against Cancer. *Annual report 2007–2008.* 2008. Toronto, ON: Canada.

CHAPTER 97

The New Standard of Quality Cancer Care in the US: *The Institute of Medicine (IOM) Report, Cancer Care for the Whole Patient: Meeting Psychosocial Needs*

Jimmie C. Holland and Talia R. Weiss

"To ignore these factors while we pour billions of dollars into new technologies is like spending all of one's money on the latest model car and then not have the money left to buy gas to run the car."
-Nancy Adler, PhD

Chair, IOM Committee in Psychosocial Care[1]

INTRODUCTION

The Institute of Medicine (IOM) has undertaken a series of reports which have had a profound effect on the quality of US healthcare. *Crossing the quality chasm: A new health system for the 21st century* was the first of a series of reports which have addressed improving care of both physical and mental disorders.[2] In 2007, the IOM published a report which examined the psychological, behavioral, and social problems that occur with serious illness. While the report focuses on cancer, the recommendations from the report *Cancer care for the whole patient: Meeting psychosocial needs* are relevant to the care of patients with other serious and complex medical conditions[1] (Figs. 97–1 and 97–2). The conclusions and the recommendations made by the committee are important for clinicians, health policy makers, and organizations responsible for quality standards. In fact, the multidisciplinary committee noted that while cancer treatment in the United States is among the most advanced in the world, the psychological and social aspects of patient care have lagged far behind. A review of research found that there is a strong evidence base for psychosocial and behavioral interventions to reduce distress,

enhance patients' ability to adhere to treatment which improves outcomes, and positively effect behaviors affecting health.

The report concludes that to fail to address psychosocial needs of patients being treated for cancer today is to give less than quality care. The report states that a new standard of quality care now exists which requires psychosocial care be integrated into routine cancer care and treatment. The committee concluded that

Attending to psychosocial needs should be an integral part of quality cancer care. All components of the health care system that are involved in cancer care should explicitly incorporate attention to psychosocial needs in their policies, practices and standards addressing clinical health care. These policies, practices and standards should be aimed at ensuring the provision of psychosocial health services to all patients who need them.[1]

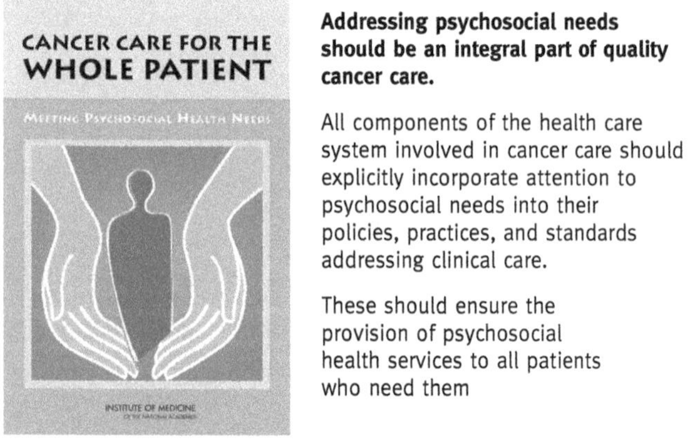

BACKGROUND OF IOM REPORT

The IOM Report came about because there was a growing awareness from patients with cancer that their psychological and social problems were not being addressed. They reported that oncologists did not consider psychological care as part of cancer treatment. Furthermore, the physicians did not identify or understand their psychosocial needs, and did not know when or to whom to refer to when problems were found.[3] Through the continuum of care beginning with diagnosis, patients report dissatisfaction with the amount and type of information given to them; and, frequent absence of effective communication which they could use to make decisions and manage their illness.[4] Oncologists tend to underestimate the psychological distress patients are experiencing.[5,6] Significant levels of anxiety and depression were reported in 35% of 5000 new patients treated for cancer at Johns Hopkins; it is often unrecognized and untreated.[7] In addition, patients increasingly complain of the cost of health insurance and medications, which many cannot afford. They lack financial means to pay for transportation and care. This amounted to 12 million people (1 in 5) in 2007 whose family had trouble paying medical bills.[8] Many delayed or decided against treatment because of costs. Five percent of the 1.5 million American families who filed for bankruptcy noted cancer contributed.[9]

Given the existential meaning to most people of a cancer diagnosis, and the rigorous treatment and life-threatening potential, one must ask why this neglect has been so far reaching. Particularly, this question continues in the context that unmet psychosocial needs negatively impact treatment outcome. Social isolation is comparable to smoking and cholesterol as risk factors for chronic disease.[1] In women with breast cancer, women who reported being isolated had a 66% greater chance

Addressing psychosocial needs should be an integral part of quality cancer care.

All components of the health care system involved in cancer care should explicitly incorporate attention to psychosocial needs into their policies, practices, and standards addressing clinical care.

These should ensure the provision of psychosocial health services to all patients who need them

Fig. 97–1. Cancer care for the whole patient.

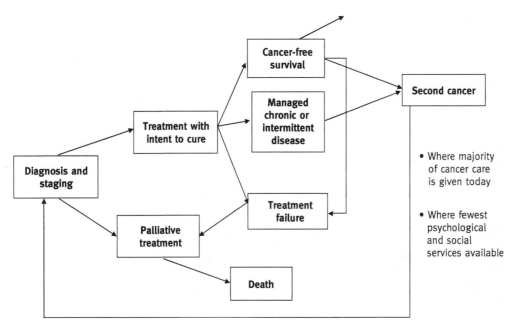

Fig. 97–2. Community oncology offices.

of mortality by 6 years.[10] Several factors contributed to the continued neglect of this aspect of care:

1. Most cancer care today occurs in overworked busy ambulatory care settings, as compared to earlier times when most cancer care was given in the hospital. When care shifted to being primarily outpatient based care, there was no shift of support personnel (especially social work and psychology) to the clinic. In small community oncology offices of only a few oncologists, there is often no social support staff.

2. Reimbursement for ambulatory psychological and social services is so low through private and public health insurances, that small oncology practices cannot sustain the cost of social workers and psychologists. Fig. 97–1 notes where most cancer treatment is given in the ambulatory setting and ironically, where least psychological and social services are available.

3. Often routine office practices are not designed to direct attention to psychosocial needs—oncologists have little time to explore issues not directly bearing on treatment decisions.

4. Patients want to be perceived as "good" and hesitate to complain of psychological problems of anxiety, depression, or sexual problems since there is a continuing fear of being labeled as having a "psychiatric" problem or being perceived by the doctors as "morally weak."

5. Families bear a far greater burden of care today as patients remain at home and much of their informal care must be given, often at great personal cost, by family or friends. This burden leads to significant distress in family members, neglect of young children in the home, and the caregivers' inattention to their own health leading at times to premature death.[11]

6. Patients who are at highest risk of psychological problems are likely to go unrecognized in routine care: elderly who are isolated; patients with preexisting mental disorders; those with language or cultural barriers; and those with poor economic resources.

COMMITTEE CHARGE

It was because of these prescient reasons that 1 million dollars was allocated by Congress in 2005 to the National Institute of Health (NIH) to study the barriers to access to psychosocial services in ambulatory oncology settings, with particular emphasis on community practices. The charge included the mandate to study how services are developed and delivered, current capacity of mental health and cancer treatment teams to meet the challenge and needed additional training and resources as well as an action plan to reduce the barriers and improve psychosocial care. Susan Solomon, Ph.D., at the NIH was the initial Project Officer

Table 97–1. IOM committee

NANCY E. ADLER (*Chair*), University of California—San Francisco
RHONDA J. ROBINSON BEALE, United Behavioral Health
DIANE BLUM, CancerCare Inc.
PATRICIA GANZ, UCLA Schools of Medicine and Public Health and Jonsson Comprehensive Cancer Center
SHERRY GLIED, Mailman School of Public Health, Columbia University
JESSIE GRUMAN, Center for the Advancement of Health
MICHAEL HOGE, Yale University School of Medicine
JIMMIE HOLLAND, Memorial Sloan-Kettering Cancer Center
MELISSA HUDSON, St. Jude Children's Research Hospital
SHERRIE KAPLAN, University of California at Irvine School of Medicine
ALICIA MATTHEWS, University of Illinois,
RUTH MCCORKLE, Yale University School of Nursing
HAROLD ALAN PINCUS, New York-Presbyterian Hospital
LEE SCHWARTZBERG, The West Clinic
EDWARD WAGNER, Group Health Cooperative and W.A. McColl Institute
TERRIE WETLE, Brown Medical School

and Julia Rowland, Ph.D., Director, Office of Cancer Survivorship, National Cancer Institute followed her. The grant was given to the IOM which appointed a Project Director, Ann Page, and a 16-member multidisciplinary Committee on Psychosocial Services to Cancer Patients/Families in a Community Setting. The Committee included members from medicine, oncology, nursing, social work, mental health, economics, and policy (Table 97–1 lists members and their affiliations).

DEFINITION OF PSYCHOSOCIAL HEALTH

Since the charge to the Committee was broad, the first requirement was to determine the parameters to be considered as part of psychosocial care. Psychosocial Health services were defined by the Committee as the following:

Psychosocial health services are psychological and social services and interventions that enable patients and their families, and health care providers to optimize biomedical health care and to manage the psychological/behavioral and social aspects of illness and its consequences so as to promote better health.[1]

This definition was determined to include assessing patients' psychosocial needs and developing a treatment plan which coordinated with medical care and referred to a proper psychosocial resource.

PSYCHOSOCIAL NEEDS AND SERVICES: LITERATURE SEARCH

The committee sought to determine first: what are the essential psychosocial needs? Table 97–2 (IOM Summary) outlines seven areas: obtaining information; help in coping; help in managing illness; changing behaviors that impact illness; material resources; help with work, family; and financial advice. The existing services which address each psychosocial need were identified. A extensive literature search was then undertaken to determine if there was evidence of efficacy in relation to one or more of several outcomes: survival, functional status, quality of life, symptom reduction (pain, fatigue), reduced psychiatric co-morbidity; improved care coordination, and patient management; and improved family function. In deliberations over 1 year, the Committee analyzed the literature with particular attention to randomized trials and meta analyses. They also consulted with a wide range of organizations and individuals, both from cancer and from other chronic diseases particularly heart disease and diabetes where a greater amount of psychosocial research has been done. A strong evidence base was found for the benefits of services in these areas:

- Communication between patient and provider
- Psychotherapy and counseling
- Psychopharmacologic interventions
- Self-management (from diabetes, cardiovascular) literature
- Behaviors (e.g., smoking, diet)
- Support for the family caregiver

The Committee concluded that there is sufficient evidence from the literature to support a new standard of care which mandates that psychosocial care be integrated into routine cancer treatment. Clinical practice guidelines and organizations setting standards must take this into account (Table 97–3).

A UNIFYING MODEL FOR DELIVERY OF PSYCHOSOCIAL HEALTH SERVICES

The Committee reviewed the range of existing models for delivery of psychosocial services. They varied in type and resources required.

However, the Committee sought to recommend a single model plan that could be implemented in any treatment setting, irrespective of level of resources (Fig. 97–3).

Fig. 97–3 shows the four components of the model which begins with the basic assumption (with a strong evidence base) that psychosocial care (as well as medical care overall) depends on effective communication between patient and providers. "Effective communication" is defined by the NCI Report by Epstein and Street (2007) as "fostering healing relationships, exchanging information, responding to emotions, managing uncertainty, making decisions and enabling self management."[4] The model notes that communication must include the patients' family and the providers' medical team members.

The second part of the model notes the necessity to identify psychosocial needs. Patients often do not volunteer information and both nurses and physicians frequently fail to recognize depression (in cancer and primary care).[5,6]

The routine screening for psychosocial needs is recommended for all patients at the initial or an early visit. There are now "ultra-short" instruments suitable for use in the waiting room of oncologists' offices that give a broad stroke "first phase" approach which indicates that the patient may be at risk for psychosocial problems. If the first phase is positive then a "second phase" is needed with more in depth-questioning by the oncologist, nurse or social worker of those who score at a vulnerable level.[12,13] (The range of valid instruments are listed in Chapter 4.) The National Cancer Center Networks (NCCN) Clinical Practice Guidelines for Management of Distress outlines this approach and recommends use of the Distress Thermometer and Problem List as a brief "first phase" screening tool)[14] www.nccn.org.

Increasing use of touch screen technology as compared to pencil and paper self report suggests that screening can be even more rapidly done with this method.

Identifying psychosocial needs must be followed by development of a psychosocial treatment plan that (1) coordinates with the medical care; (2) supports the patient with needed information, identifies needs, provides emotional support and helps the patient manage illness and treatment; (3) and links the patient to appropriate psychosocial services. The ideal situation is to have a social worker, psychologist or mental health professional on site in the clinic or nearby so that the patient experiences a seamless referral to a psychosocial resource. Navigators and case managers help in many places to assist patients who are more vulnerable by virtue of language or culture. If there is no on site source, then the oncology office team must keep a list of available resources in the

---

Table 97–2. IOM summary

IOM Report Recommendations For Action

1. The standard of psychosocial care
   Facilitate effective communication between patients and care providers;
   - Identify each patient's psychosocial health needs;
   - Design and implement a plan that
     - links the patient with needed psychosocial services,
     - coordinates biomedical and psychosocial care,
     - engages and supports patients in managing their illness and health; and
   - Systematically follows up on, reevaluate, and adjust plans.
2. Health care providers' Responsibility
   To ensure that every cancer patient within their practice receives care that meets the standard for psychosocial health care.
3. Patient & Family education and advocacy organizations' Responsibility
   To educate patients with cancer and their family caregivers to expect, and request when necessary, care that meets the standard for psychosocial care.
   To continue to work on strengthening the patient side of the patient–provider partnership by enabling patients to participate actively in their care by providing tools and training in how to:
   - obtain information,
   - make decisions,
   - solve problems, and
   - communicate more effectively with their health care providers.

4. Support for dissemination and uptake

The NCI, CMS, and the AHRQ should conduct a large-scale evaluation of various approaches to the efficient provision of psychosocial health care in accordance with the standard of care. This program should demonstrate how the standard can be implemented in different settings, with different populations, and with varying personnel and organizational arrangements.

5. Support from payers

Group purchasers of health care coverage & health plans should fully support the evidence based interventions necessary to deliver effective psychosocial health services. Group purchasers should:

- Ensure coverage and reimbursement of mechanisms for identifying the psychosocial needs of cancer patients & linking them with appropriate providers who can meet those needs, and coordinating psychosocial services with patients' biomedical care.
- Review cost-sharing provisions that affect mental health services and revise those that impede cancer patients' access to such services.
- Ensure that their coverage policies do not impede cancer patients' access to providers with expertise in the treatment of mental health conditions in individuals undergoing complex medical regimens such as those used to treat cancer.
- Include incentives for the effective delivery of psychosocial care in payment reform programs—such as pay-for-performance and pay-for-reporting initiatives—in which they participate.

6. Quality oversight

The NCI, CMS, and AHRQ should fund research focused on the development of performance measures for psychosocial cancer care. Organizations setting standards for cancer care and other standards-setting organizations should:

- Create oversight mechanisms that can be used to measure and report on the quality of ambulatory oncology care (including psychosocial health care).
- Incorporate requirements for identifying and responding to psychosocial health care needs into their protocols, policies, and standards.
- Develop and use performance measures for psychosocial health care in their quality oversight activities.

7. Workforce competencies

a. Educational accrediting organizations, licensing bodies, and professional societies should develop their standards for licensing and certification criteria as fully as possible in accordance with a model that integrates biomedical and psychosocial health care.

b. Congress and federal agencies should support and fund the establishment of a Workforce Development Collaborative on Psychosocial Care during Chronic Medical Illness. This cross-specialty, multidisciplinary group should comprise educators, consumer and family advocates, and providers of psychosocial and biomedical health services and be charged with

- identifying, refining, and broadly disseminating to health care educators information about workforce competencies, models, and preservice curricula relevant to providing psychosocial services to persons with chronic medical illnesses and their families;
- adapting curricula for continuing education of the existing workforce using efficient workplace-based learning approaches;
- drafting and implementing a plan for developing the skills of faculty and other trainers in teaching psychosocial health care using evidence-based teaching strategies; and
- strengthening the emphasis on psychosocial health care in educational accreditation standards and professional licensing and certification exams by recommending revisions to the relevant oversight organizations.

c. Organizations providing research funding should support assessment of the implementation in education, training, and clinical practice of the workforce competencies necessary to provide psychosocial care and their impact on achieving the standard for such care.

8. Standardized nomenclature

To facilitate research on and quality measurement of psychosocial interventions, the NIH and AHRQ should create and lead an initiative to develop a standardized, transdisciplinary taxonomy and nomenclature for psychosocial health services. This initiative should aim to incorporate this taxonomy and nomenclature into such databases as the National Library of Medicine's Medical Subject Headings (MeSH), PsycINFO, CINAHL and EMBASE.

9. Research priorities

Organizations sponsoring research in oncology care should include the following areas among their funding priorities:

- Further development of reliable, valid, and efficient tools and strategies for use by clinical practices to ensure that all patients with cancer receive care that meets the standard of psychosocial care. These tools and strategies should include:
  - approaches for improving patient–provider communication and providing decision support to cancer patients;
  - screening instruments that can be used to identify individuals with any of a comprehensive array of psychosocial health problems;
  - needs assessment instruments to assist in planning psychosocial services;
  - illness and wellness management interventions; and
  - approaches for effectively linking patients with services and coordinating care.
- Identification of more effective psychosocial services to treat mental health problems and to assist patients in adopting and maintaining healthy behaviors, such as smoking cessation, exercise, and dietary change. This effort should include:
  - identifying populations for whom specific psychosocial services are most effective, and psychosocial services most effective for specific populations; and
  - development of standard outcome measures for assessing the effectiveness of these services.
- Creation and testing of reimbursement arrangements that will promote psychosocial care and reward its best performance.

10. Promoting uptake and monitoring progress

The NCI/NIH should monitor progress and report its findings on at least a biannual basis to:

oncology providers,

consumer organizations,

group purchasers and health plans,

quality oversight organizations, and

other stakeholders.

These findings could be used to inform an evaluation of the impact of the report and each of its recommendations. Monitoring activities should make maximal use of existing data collection tools and activities.

Table 97-3. Psychosocial needs and formal ways to address them (1/2)

Psychosocial need	Health services
Information about illness, treatments, health, services	Provision of info; e.g., on illness, treatments, effects on health, and psychosocial services, and helping patients/families understand and use this info
Help coping with emotions	Assistance changing behaviors to minimize impact of disease
Help managing illness	Material and logistical resources, e.g., transportation
	Help managing disruptions in work, school, and family life
	Financial advice/assistance
Assistance changing behaviors to minimize impact of disease	Behavioral/health promotion interventions; e.g.,
	Provider assessment/monitoring of health behaviors (e.g., smoking, exercise)
	Brief counseling
	Patient education
Material and logistical resources, e.g., transportation	Provision of resources
Help managing disruptions in work, school, and family life	Family/caregiver education
	Assistance with ADLs, chores
	Legal protections / services, legal protection services
	Cognitive testing/educational assistance
Financial advice / assistance	Financial planning/counseling/daily managementInsurance (e.g., health, disability) counselingEligibility assessment/counseling for benefits; e.g., Supplemental financial grants

ABBREVIATION: ADL, activities of daily living.

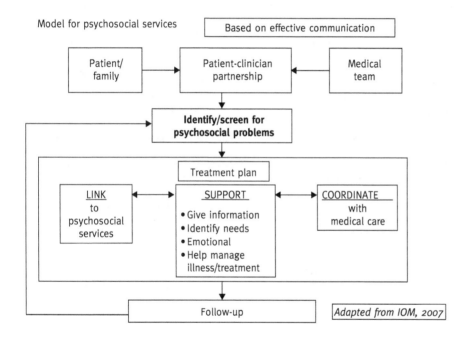

Fig. 97-3. Model for psychosocial services. Adapted from IOM, 2007.

community (e.g., advocacy organizations and individuals in private practice who have experiences with cancer). In absence of professional services in the community, the many resources available by telephone and online should be identified and recommended. Patients should be given the 800 numbers and web sites to ease there ability to access these *free* services. However, it is clear that many physicians are not aware of the psychosocial services in their community or those that are provided by telephone or online by the over 40 site-specific advocacy organizations that exist. (Chapter 5 gives the national organizations, their missions, telephone numbers and e-mail addresses.) Helplines are increasingly available 24/7 for a range of advice about cancer, including financial needs. Notable are the NCI, American Cancer Society, and Cancer Care. The American Psychosocial Oncology Society (APOS) has a Helpline to assist patients and families to find a counselor in their own community (1-866-APOS4HELP/ 1-866-276-7443).

The last part of the model requires that a follow up be done and the patient reevaluated as clinically appropriate (e.g., transitions in treatment or status) and the psychosocial treatment plan modified to fit the current situation.

RECOMMENDATIONS FOR ACTION

The Committee outlined 10 recommendations to overcome the barriers identified and ensure that psychological issues become an integral part of routine cancer care.[1]

Recommendation 1: the standard of care. All parties establishing or using standards for the quality of cancer care should adopt the following as a standard:

All cancer care should ensure the provision of appropriate psychosocial health services by

- facilitating effective communication between patients and care providers.[4]

- identifying each patient's psychosocial health needs.
- designing and implementing a plan that:
  - links the patient with needed psychosocial services.
  - coordinates biomedical and psychosocial care.
  - engages and supports patients in managing their illness and health.
- systematically following up, reevaluating, and adjusting the plan as needs change, including into survivorship.

Recommendation 2: healthcare providers. All cancer care providers should ensure that every cancer patient within their practice receives care that meets the new standard for psychosocial healthcare. The National Cancer Institute should help cancer care providers implement the standard of care by maintaining an up-to-date directory of free psychosocial services available through national advocacy organizations.

The committee believes that *all* providers can and should implement the recommendation, despite the fact that individual clinical practices vary by patient population, community setting, and available resources. Because of this, *how* individual healthcare practices implement the standard of care and the level at which it is done may vary. Nevertheless, as this report describes, the committee believes that it is possible for all providers to meet this standard in some way. The committee believes that the inability to solve all psychosocial problems permanently should not preclude attempts to remedy as many as possible—a stance akin to oncologists' commitment to treating cancer even when the successful outcome of every treatment is not assured.

Recommendation 3: patient and family education. Patient education and advocacy organizations should educate patients with cancer and their family caregivers to expect, and request when necessary, cancer care that meets the standard for psychosocial care. These organizations should also continue their work on strengthening the patient side of the patient–provider partnership. The goals should be to empower patients to participate actively in their care by providing educational tools and training in how to better obtain information, make decisions, solve problems, and communicate more effectively with their healthcare providers.

Recommendation 4: support for dissemination and uptake. The National Cancer Institute, the Centers for Medicare and Medicaid Services (CMMS), and the Agency for Healthcare Research and Quality (AHRQ) should, individually or collectively, conduct a *large-scale demonstration* and evaluation of various approaches to the efficient provision of psychosocial health care in accordance with the new standard of care. This program should demonstrate how the standard can be implemented in different settings, with different populations, and with varying personnel and organizational arrangements.

Because policies set by public and private purchasers, oversight bodies, and other healthcare leaders shape how healthcare is accessed, what services are delivered, and the manner in which they are delivered, group purchasers of healthcare coverage and health plans should take a number of actions to support the interventions necessary to deliver effective psychosocial health services. The National Cancer Institute, CMMS, and AHRQ also should spearhead the development and use of performance measures to improve the delivery of these services.

Recommendation 5: support from payers. Group purchasers, both public and private, of healthcare coverage and health plans should fully support the evidence-based interventions necessary to deliver effective psychosocial health services:

- Group purchasers should include provisions in their contracts with health plans that ensure coverage and reimbursement of mechanisms for identifying the psychosocial needs of cancer patients, linking patients with appropriate providers who can meet those needs, and coordinating psychosocial services with patients' biomedical care.
- Group purchasers should review cost-sharing provisions that affect mental health services and revise those that impede cancer patients' access to such services.

- Group purchasers and health plans should ensure that their coverage policies do not impede cancer patients' access to providers with expertise in the treatment of mental health conditions in individuals undergoing complex medical regimens such as those used to treat cancer. Health plans whose networks lack this expertise should reimburse for mental health services provided by out-of-network practitioners with this expertise who meet the plan's quality and other standards (at rates paid to similar providers within the plan's network).
- Group purchasers and health plans should include incentives for the effective delivery of psychosocial care in payment reform programs—such as pay-for-performance, and pay-for-reporting initiatives —in which they participate.

Mental healthcare providers "with expertise in the treatment of mental health conditions in individuals undergoing complex medical regimens such as those used to treat cancer" include mental health providers who possess this expertise through formal education (such as specialists in psychosomatic medicine) as well as mental health care providers who have gained expertise though their clinical experiences, for example, mental health clinicians (from nursing, social work, psychology, psychiatry) who are a part of an interdisciplinary oncology practice.

Recommendation 6: quality oversight. The National Cancer Institute, Center for Medicare and Medicaid Services, and AHRQ should fund research focused on the development of performance measures for psychosocial cancer care. Jacobsen and his colleagues have spearheaded an initiative in Florida which has developed performance measures of two components: identifying the distressed patient and linking to appropriate resources (www.cas.usf.edu/~jacobsen).[15] He also leads a group exploring this further in the APOS. Organizations setting standards for cancer care (e.g., NCCN, American Society of Clinical Oncology, American College of Surgeons' Commission on Cancer, Oncology Nursing Society, APOS) and other standards-setting organizations (e.g., National Quality Forum, National Committee for Quality Assurance, URAC, JACHO, Joint Commission) should

- Create oversight mechanisms that can be used to measure and report on the quality of ambulatory oncology care (including psychosocial healthcare).
- Incorporate requirements for identifying and responding to psychosocial health care needs into their protocols, policies, and standards.
- Develop and use performance measures for psychosocial health care in their quality oversight activities.

Recommendation 7: workforce competencies. There are inadequate numbers of professionals who are selecting the health professions as their careers, and this is particularly true in the field of oncology. There is a need to explore ways to encourage young investigators and clinicians into this area by grants for postgraduate work and early career support.

Educational accrediting organizations, licensing bodies, and professional societies should examine their standards, licensing, and certification criteria to identify competencies of its members in delivering psychosocial healthcare and developing them as fully as possible in accordance with a model that integrates biomedical and psychosocial care.

Congress and federal agencies should support and fund the establishment of a Workforce Development Collaborative on Psychosocial Care during Chronic Medical Illness. This cross-specialty, multidisciplinary group should comprise educators, consumer and family advocates, and providers of psychosocial and biomedical health services and be charged with

- Identifying, refining, and broadly disseminating to healthcare educators information about workforce competencies, models, and preservice curricula relevant to providing psychosocial services to persons with chronic medical illnesses and their families.
- Adapting curricula for continuing education of the existing workforce using efficient workplace-based learning approaches.

- Drafting and implementing a plan for developing the skills of faculty and other trainers in teaching psychosocial healthcare using evidence-based teaching strategies.
- Strengthening the emphasis on psychosocial health care in educational accreditation standards and professional licensing and certification examinations by recommending revisions to the relevant oversight organizations in keeping with the new standard of care.

Organizations providing research funding should support assessment of the implementation in education, training, and clinical practice of the workforce competencies necessary to provide psychosocial care and their impact on achieving the standard for such care set forth in Recommendation 1.

Recommendation 8: standardized nomenclature. To facilitate research on and quality measurement of psychosocial interventions, the National Institutes of Health (NIH) and AHRQ should create and lead an initiative to develop a standardized, transdisciplinary taxonomy and nomenclature for psychosocial health services. This initiative should aim to incorporate this taxonomy and nomenclature into databases, particularly the National Library of Medicine's Medical Subject Headings (MeSH), PsycINFO, CINAHL (Cumulative Index to Nursing and Allied Health Literature), and EMBASE. Clarifying and standardizing the often unclear and inconsistent language used to refer to psychosocial services will be facilitated.

In addition, improving the delivery of psychosocial health services requires targeted research. This research should aim to clarify the efficacy and effectiveness of new and existing services and to identify ways of improving the delivery of these services to various populations in different geographic locations and with varying levels of resources.

Recommendation 9: research priorities. Organizations sponsoring research in oncology care should include the following areas among their funding priorities:

- Further development of reliable, valid, and efficient tools and strategies for use by clinical practices to ensure that all patients with cancer receive care that meets the standard of psychosocial care set forth in Recommendation 1. These tools and strategies should include
  - approaches for improving patient-provider communication and providing decision support to cancer patients.
  - screening instruments that can be used to identify individuals with any type of psychosocial health problems.
  - needs assessment instruments to assist in planning psychosocial services.
  - illness and wellness management interventions.
- Approaches for effectively linking patients with services and coordinating healthcare to assist patients in adopting and maintaining healthy behaviors, such as smoking cessation, exercise, and dietary change. This effort should include
- Identifying populations for whom specific psychosocial services are most effective, and psychosocial services most effective for specific populations.
  - Development of standard outcome measures for assessing the effectiveness of these services.
  - Creation and testing of reimbursement arrangements that will promote psychosocial care and reward its best performance. Research on the use of these tools, strategies, and services should also focus on how best to ensure delivery of appropriate psychosocial services to vulnerable populations, such as those with low literacy, older adults, the socially isolated, and members of cultural minorities.

Recommendation 10. promoting uptake and monitoring progress. The National Cancer Institute/NIH should monitor progress toward improved delivery of psychosocial services in cancer care and report its findings on at least a biannual basis to oncology providers, consumer organizations, group purchasers and health plans, quality oversight organizations, and other stakeholders. These findings could be used to inform an evaluation of the impact of this report and each of its recommendations. Monitoring activities should make maximal use of existing data collection tools and activities.

Implementation of recommendations. The impact of the Report's recommendations on improving psychosocial care will depend on national efforts to disseminate the information to key professional and advocacy organizations in cancer. The APOS focused its annual meeting on the IOM Report in 2008, hosting a session of approximately 30 individuals representing major patient advocacy organizations (The Wellness Community, Gilda's Club, and others) and the key professional groups (American Cancer Society, ASCO, AOSW, ONS, and others). An Alliance of Organizations to disseminate and implement the IOM Report recommendations has been established. An Executive Committee has a monthly conference call to execute the mission. The major effort will be two-pronged: to enlist patient and families through the advocacy organizations to educate patients to request that the new standard be respected in oncology offices from which they secure services, and to advocate at a national level for needed policy changes, particularly adequate reimbursement for supportive services. The second prong will be directed toward the professional oncology organizations to improve training in psychosocial care, to include these issues in accreditations and standards, as well as clinical practice guidelines. The Alliance will serve as the infrastructure from which the breadth of activities ensure change will be directed.

SUMMARY

The 2007 IOM Report has provided a landmark document that gives psychosocial aspects of cancer care credibility from a major independent national organization that influences public and private policy. The NIH utilizes their findings in determining research and policy decisions. The IOM Committee, after a yearlong analysis of the literature, determined that the evidence base suggests that a new standard has been established for quality cancer care: it must integrate the psychosocial domain into routine cancer care. Clinical practice guidelines developed by professional organizations will be expected to include this dimension in their recommendations. Performance measures for psychosocial care have been developed; it will soon be possible for accrediting bodies to assess the level of psychosocial care in an office or clinic's report card on quality of psychosocial care using validated performance measures. No longer can this area be viewed as "soft science" which can be disregarded as part of the research agenda in cancer and in clinical care. The science from the "bench" now supports application of this information to "bedside" care. A new benchmark for psychosocial care has been established.

To obtain the IOM report: 800-624-6242 or on the web at: www. nap.edu.

REFERENCES

1. IOM. *Cancer care for the whole patient.* Washington, DC: The National Academies Press; 2007.

2. IOM. *Crossing the quality chasm: A new health system for the 21st century.* Washington, DC: The National Academies Press; 2003.

3. President's Cancer Panel. *Living beyond cancer: Finding a new balance. President's Cancer Panel 2003-2004 annual report.* Bethesda, MD: National Cancer Institute, National Institutes of Health, Department of Health and Human Services; 2004.

4. Epstein RM, Street RL. *Patient-centered communication in cancer care: Promoting healing and reducing suffering.* Bethesda, MD: National Cancer Institute; 2007.

5. Fallowfield R, Jenkins S. Psychiatric morbidity and its recognition by doctors in patients with cancer. *Br J Cancer.* 2001;84:1011–1015.

6. Keller, Sommerfeldt, Fischer, et al. Recognition of distress and psychiatric morbidity in cancer patients: a multi-method approach. *Eur Soc Med Oncol.* 2004;15:1243–1249.

7. Zabora J BrintzenhofeSzoc K, Curbow B, et al. The prevalence of psychological distress by cancer site. *Psychooncology.* 2001;10:9–28.

8. May JH, Cunningham PJ. *Tough trade-offs: Medical bills, family finances and access to care.* Washington, DC: Center for Studying Health System Change; 2004.

9. Himmelstein DU, Warren E, Thorne D, Woolhandler S. Market watch: illness and injury as contributors to bankruptcy. *Health Affairs.* 2005;w5:63–73.

10. Kroenke CH, Kubzansky LD, Schernhammer ES, Holmes MD, Kawachi I. Social networks, social support, and survival after breast cancer diagnosis. *J Clin Oncol.* 2006;24:1105–1111.

11. Kurtz ME, Kurtz JC, Given CW, Given BA. Depression and physical health among family caregivers of geriatric patients with cancer—a longitudinal view. *Med Sci Monitor.* 2004;10:CR447–CR56.

12. Mitchell AJ, Coyne JC. Do ultra-short screening instruments accurately detect depression in primary care? *Br J Gen Prac.* 2007;57(535):144–151.

13. Mitchell AJ. Are one or two simple questions sufficient to detect depression in cancer and palliative care? A Bayesian meta-analysis. *Br J Cancer.* 2008;98: 1934–1943.

14. Holland J, Andersen B. The NCCN distress management clinical practice guidelines in oncology. *J NCCN.* 2007;5:66–98.

15. Jacobsen PB, Jim HS. Psychosocial interventions for anxiety and depression in adult cancer patients: achievements and challenges. *CA Cancer J Clin.* 2008;58:214–230.

INDEX